D1090931

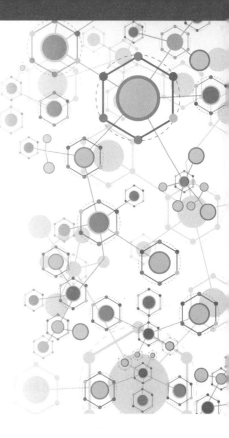

Health Information Management

Concepts, Principles, and Practice

Fifth Edition

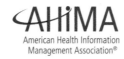

American Health Information
Management Association®

Copyright ©2016 by the American Health Information Management Association. All rights reserved. Except as permitted under the Copyright Act of 1976, no part of this publication may be reproduced, stored in a retrieval system, or transmitted, in any form or by any means, electronic, photocopying, recording, or otherwise, without the prior written permission of the AHIMA, 233 North Michigan Avenue, 21st Floor, Chicago, Illinois, 60601-5809 (https://secure.ahima.org/publications/reprint/index.aspx).

ISBN: 978-1-58426-514-6
AHIMA Product No.: AB103315

AHIMA Staff:
Caitlin Wilson, Assistant Editor
Ashley Latta, Production Development Editor
Pamela Woolf, Director of Publications

Limit of Liability/Disclaimer of Warranty: This book is sold, as is, without warranty of any kind, either express or implied. While every precaution has been taken in the preparation of this book, the publisher and author assume no responsibility for errors or omissions. Neither is any liability assumed for damages resulting from the use of the information or instructions contained herein. It is further stated that the publisher and author are not responsible for any damage or loss to your data or your equipment that results directly or indirectly from your use of this book.

The websites listed in this book were current and valid as of the date of publication. However, webpage addresses and the information on them may change at any time. The user is encouraged to perform his or her own general web searches to locate any site addresses listed here that are no longer valid.

CPT® is a registered trademark of the American Medical Association. All other copyrights and trademarks mentioned in this book are the possession of their respective owners. AHIMA makes no claim of ownership by mentioning products that contain such marks.

For more information, including updates, about AHIMA Press publications, visit http://www.ahima.org/publications/updates.aspx

American Health Information Management Association
233 North Michigan Avenue, 21st Floor
Chicago, Illinois 60601-5809
ahima.org

Health Information Management

Concepts, Principles, and Practice

Fifth Edition

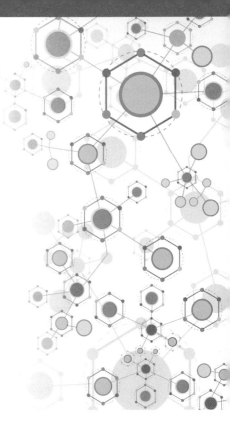

Volume Editors

Pamela Oachs, MA, RHIA, CHDA, FAHIMA

Amy Watters, EdD, RHIA, FAHIMA

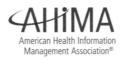

AHIMA
American Health Information
Management Association®

Brief Table of Contents

Online Appendices

Detailed Table of Contents

Online Appendices

About the Volume Editors

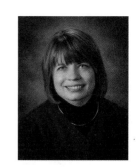

Pamela K. Oachs, MA, RHIA, CHDA, FAHIMA is an assistant professor and director of the health information management undergraduate program in the College of St. Scholastica's health informatics and information management department. She teaches courses related to health information technology, workflow redesign, healthcare management, and data analytics. She has more than 15 years of healthcare experience. Her career has included a variety of positions, both managerial and professional, in the areas of utilization management, quality improvement, medical staff credentialing, Joint Commission coordination, information technology, project management, and patient access. She has been involved in system implementations, both small and large, in a variety of healthcare settings. She has served on the board of directors of the Minnesota Health Information Management Association and the Northeastern Minnesota Health Information Management Association, has served as a commissioner on the Commission on Certification for Health Informatics and Information Management, and is on the editorial board for Perspectives in Health Information Management.

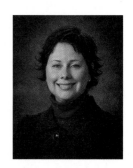

Amy L. Watters, EdD, RHIA, FAHIMA, is an associate professor and director of the health information management graduate program at the College of St. Scholastica. She teaches courses related to health information technology, best practices in HIM, and applied research and writing. She has more than 15 years of HIM experience in a variety of areas, such as release of information, HIM and admitting management in acute-care settings, product management at a software and consulting firm, and HIPAA security at a multispecialty physician group. In addition to serving as coeditor of this textbook, Dr. Watters has coauthored chapters related to privacy and security in two textbooks, and published work in various peer reviewed publications. She has served on the board of directors of the Minnesota Health Information Management Association and the Minnesota Healthcare Information and Management Systems Society, has been President of the Northeastern Minnesota Health Information Management Association, and was appointed to the CAHIIM HIM Accreditation Council. She is also on the editorial review board for Perspectives in Health Information Management. In addition to both a bachelor's and master's degree in HIM, she has a doctoral degree in education, focusing her research on community and its impact on online learning.

About the Authors

Margret K. Amatayakul, MBA, RHIA, CHPS, FHIMSS, is president of Margret\ A Consulting, LLC, in Schaumburg, Illinois, a consulting firm specializing in electronic health records, HIPAA and HITECH, and associated HIM standards and regulations. She has more than 40 years of experience in national and international HIM. A leading authority on electronic health record (EHR) strategies for healthcare organizations, she has extensive experience in EHR selection and project management, and she formed and served as executive director of the Computer-based Patient Record Institute (CPRI). Other positions held include adjunct faculty at the College of St. Scholastica, associate executive director of AHIMA, associate professor at the University of Illinois, and director of medical record services at the Illinois Eye and Ear Infirmary. She is a much-sought-after speaker, has published extensively, and has earned several professional service awards.

Danika E. Brinda, PhD, RHIA, CHPS, HCISPP is an assistant professor in the health information and informatics department at the College of St. Scholastica. She is also the owner of TriPoint Healthcare Solutions, which focuses on advising, educating, and operationalizing privacy and security requirements. Dr. Brinda has over 10 years of experience in healthcare privacy and security practices. She received her certified in healthcare privacy and security (CHPS) designation from the American Heath Information Management Association (AHIMA) and her healthcare information security and privacy practitioner (HCISPP) from (ISC)². She also holds AHIMA's registered health information administrator (RHIA) credential. Dr. Brinda is a local and national speaker regarding a wide variety of topics in healthcare privacy and security. Her expertise includes HIPAA risk assessment, HIPAA risk mitigation, privacy and

security policy creation and management, privacy and security education, creation of privacy and security audits, Meaningful Use requirements, and evaluating best practices in privacy and security. Dr. Brinda has worked closely with both covered entities and business associates regarding HIPAA compliance. Dr. Brinda received her bachelor's degree in health information management and computer science/information systems from the College of St. Scholastica. She also received her master's degree from the College of St. Scholastica in health informatics and information management. She completed her PhD in information technology with a focus in information governance and security in 2015.

Cindy Glewwe Edgerton, MHA, MEd, RHIA is the HIM program director at Charter Oak State College. Her professional background includes 20 years of experience as an educator and program director in health information management degree programs, having developed one of the first online HIM associate degree programs. Currently, Cindy has created and designed curriculum for countless residential and online courses. This experience has been instrumental in many successful accreditations of HIM programs. She has been very involved in the American Health Information Management Association at both the national level and the state level (Minnesota Health Information Management Association). She has been an elected board member for MHIMA and was an appointed member of the AHIMA Council for Excellence in Education. She has presented at the national AHIMA Assembly on Education conference for several years and was a presenter for the Train-the-Trainer Personal Health Record initiative. Cindy graduated with a bachelor's degree in health information administration with a minor in management from the College of St. Scholastica. In 2007, she obtained her master of education degree with a specialization in leadership in higher education from Capella University. She earned a second master's degree, in healthcare administration, from Kaplan University in 2015. She has been a registered health information administrator since 1987.

Elizabeth Forrestal, PhD, RHIA, CCS, FAHIMA, is a professor emerita in the department of health services and information management at East Carolina University. She previously worked at Hennepin County Medical Center and the University of Minnesota Hospitals, both in Minneapolis, from 1974 through 1990. Dr. Forrestal worked in several departments, such as third-party reimbursement, credit and collections, account auditing, outpatient registration, inpatient admissions, research studies, and quality management. In 1990, Dr. Forrestal joined the faculty of the Medical College of Georgia in Augusta. While on the faculty, she also consulted for the physicians' practice group. Dr. Forrestal successfully sat for the first CCS examination in 1992. In 2001, she was awarded the designation of fellow of the American Health Information Management Association, one of the first two individuals in the country to receive this award. She is the coauthor of *Principles of Healthcare Reimbursement*, published by AHIMA in 2006 and currently in its fifth edition, for which she and her coauthor were recipients of AHIMA's Legacy Award in 2007. She contributed chapters to the fourth edition of *Health Information Management: Concepts, Principles, and Practice* and coauthored *Health Informatics Research Methods: Principles and Practice*, both AHIMA publications. She was the first editor of *Perspectives in Health Information Management* and has delivered presentations at numerous AHIMA events. She earned her baccalaureate degree from the University of Minnesota. While working, she earned her associate's degree in medical record technology. She completed St. Scholastica's progression program to earn her postbaccalaureate certificate in health information administration. She earned her master's degree in organizational leadership from the College of St. Catherine's and her doctorate in higher education from Georgia State University.

Sandra R. Fuller, MA, RHIA, FAHIMA, is senior vice president and executive consultant at eCatalyst Healthcare Solutions. Her practice includes information governance, strategic health information management consulting, and revenue cycle project management. Prior to joining eCatalyst, she was the executive vice president and chief operating officer at AHIMA, where she led the professional and membership facing services of the association. Sandra was the director of patient data services at the University of Washington Medical Center. Her volunteer activities included serving on the board of directors of AHIMA and acting as president of the Washington State Health Information Management Association. She was awarded the WSHIMA Professional Achievement Award in 1996. She authored the book *Secure and Access Guidelines for Managing Patient Information*, published in 1997 by AHIMA.

Leslie L. Gordon, MS, RHIA, FAHIMA, is an associate professor and the HIM program director at the University of Alaska Southeast. She earned her MS from the College of St. Scholastica and has been teaching at UAS since 2003. Before teaching she worked as a reimbursement manager and data analyst at a hospital in Sitka, Alaska for many years. She is an active member of the Alaska CSA and has served in many positions on the AKHIMA Board. She is a fellow of AHIMA and currently serves on the CAHIIM board of commissioners.

Morley L. Gordon, RHIT, is an HIM analyst for Home Health and Hospice at Evergreen Hospital in Washington State. Prior to this she was the director of health information management at a long-term care facility in central Washington. She graduated from the University of Alaska's HIT program and is continuing her education at Western Governors College. Morley credits her mom in getting her into the field of HIM and is grateful for the opportunities that have opened up because of it.

Anita C. Hazelwood, MLS, RHIA, FAHIMA, is a professor in the HIM department at the University of Louisiana at Lafayette and serves as the program director. She has been a credentialed registered health information administrator (RHIA) for more than 39 years. Anita has actively consulted in hospitals, nursing homes, physician's offices, clinics, facilities for the developmentally challenged, and other educational institutions. She acts as the health information management consultant to the Louisiana Mental Health Advocacy Service. She has conducted numerous ICD-10-CM/PCS, ICD-9-CM, and CPT coding workshops throughout the state for hospitals and physicians' offices and has written numerous articles and coauthored chapters in several HIM textbooks. Anita has coauthored and edited several AHIMA publications including *ICD-9-CM and ICD-10-CM Coding and Reimbursement for Physician Services, Certified Coding Specialist—Physician-Based Exam Preparation, Clinical Coding Workout: Practice Exercises for Skill Development*, and *ICD-10-CM Preview*, for which she won AHIMA's Legacy Award in 2003. She has coauthored a chapter in AHIMA's *Effective Management of Coding Services*. Anita has been an AHIMA member for over 39 years and has served on various committees and boards. She is a member of the Louisiana Health Information Management Association (LHIMA) and was selected as its 1997 Distinguished Member. She has served throughout the years as president, president-elect, treasurer, strategy manager, and board member and has directed numerous committees and projects.

T.J. Hunt, PhD, RHIA, FAHIMA, is an associate dean and associate professor of health information management at Davenport University. His HIM experience prior to transitioning to the education field includes leadership roles with Sparrow Health System, ProMedica Health System, and Mercy Health Partners. He earned an associate's degree from Mercy College of Ohio, a bachelor's degree from Cleary University, a master's degree from Davenport University, and a doctorate degree at Indiana Institute of Technology. He is a registered health information administrator and fellow of the American Health Information Management Association. He is a past president of the Michigan Health Information Management Association. T.J. has presented at state, national, and international conferences including the International Federation of Health Information Management Associations (IFHIMA) Congress and General Assembly, AHIMA Convention and Exhibit, and AHIMA Assembly on Education.

Merida Johns, PhD, RHIA, has more than 40 years health information management experience on national and international levels and is a noted author and presenter in the field. She has over 50 published articles and has authored several books and chapters in health information management and healthcare informatics. Dr. Johns holds BA and BS degrees from Seattle University; a master's in community services administration from Alfred University, New York; and PhD from The Ohio State University. She began her career in 1973 and has held positions of director of quality assurance, assistant and director of medical record departments. Dr. Johns held tenured positions at The Ohio State University and the University of Alabama at Birmingham where in 1991 she was the founding director of the nation's first master's program in health informatics for the training of healthcare CIOs. Dr. Johns has held numerous elected and appointed professional positions with AHIMA, AMIA, CAHIIM, HIMSS, and professional state associations and nonprofit community groups. She served as AHIMA's president in 1997 and has received three AHIMA national honors including Professional Achievement, Champion, and Distinguished Member awards. Most recently in 2013 she received the Illinois Health Information Management Association's Professional Achievement Award. Currently Dr. Johns heads The Monarch Center for Women's Leadership Development, a company she founded that provides leadership coaching and workshops to help women help themselves fulfill their leadership and economic potential and break the glass ceiling.

Madonna M. LeBlanc, MA, RHIA, FAHIMA is an assistant professor in the health informatics and information management program (HIIM) in the School of Health Science (SHS) at the College of St. Scholastica (CSS) and is a graduate of CSS's master's in HIM program. Prior to her teaching role, she managed health information services at St. Mary's/Duluth Clinic Health System in

Superior, Wisconsin. Her responsibilities included a broad spectrum of acute-care HIM functions, from physician education to Joint Commission survey coordination. LeBlanc's field experience also includes cancer registry and physician peer review. She was co-faculty for six years in the SHS interdisciplinary health science leadership course designed to provide transdisciplinary collaboration and problem solving in the healthcare setting. Madonna served six years on Minnesota Health Information Management Association's (MHIMA) board of directors as delegate director and president. She was the CSA community education coordinator for the American Health Information Management Association's (AHIMA) myPHR campaign, volunteered on the AHIMA Council for Excellence in Education (CEE) Community workgroup, and volunteered on the AHIMA Scholarship Committee.

Charisse Madlock-Brown, PhD, MLS, is an assistant professor in the department of health informatics and information management at the University of Tennessee Health Science Center, joining the faculty in 2015. She recently graduated with a PhD in health informatics from the University of Iowa, and has a background in library and information science. Her research area is scientometrics with a focus on biomedicine. Scientometrics is the study of scientific communication and communities. It has been used by funding agencies and institutions to evaluate research activities, and monitor changes. Her research goals are to ground research policy and planning into a concrete framework for evaluation and assessment. Her dissertation project offers a framework for emerging topic detection in medical literature. Policy makers, funding agencies, and researchers could all benefit from a robust emerging topic detection application. Dr. Madlock-Brown is currently working on developing an online system that can be used in real-time. She also conducts "team science" research, and has presented several times at the national Science of Team Science conference. Her research within that community includes the assessment of the impact of publication subject diversity on research performance for individuals, understanding the relationship

between gender disparities and collaborative behavior, and assessing the impact of the Clinical and Translational Science Awards (CTSA) on collaborative research patterns. Her work will soon become part of the CTSASearch system, a federated search engine published by members of the CTSA Consortium. In summer 2015, she presented her work on CTSA institutions at the international Advances in Social Network Analysis and Mining conference. Other recent projects include large scale analysis of biomedical literature for purposes of article retraction trend analysis, using data mining algorithms to find interesting groupings of gene-related data, and developing personal information management tools.

David T. Marc, PhD, CHDA is an assistant professor and the graduate program director for health informatics at the College of St. Scholastica in the department of health informatics and information management. Dr. Marc is an accomplished speaker and researcher with a breadth of experience around health data analytics. Previously, he was employed at a biotech company where he developed predictive data models for the diagnosis of neurological and immunological diseases. Dr. Marc has a master's degree in biological sciences and a PhD in Health Informatics from the University of Minnesota.

Phillip G. McCann, MSC, MS, RHIA, CISSP is the information systems and project leader for security and awareness training at Northwestern Memorial Healthcare and is also an adjunct instructor in the HIM department at Herzing University. In the capacity of project leader, he is responsible for information security policy development and maintenance; design of security policy education, training and awareness activities; monitoring compliance within the health system to internal policy, and applicable local, state and federal laws. Phillip also serves as the DIRECT messaging expert and the HIPAA compliance and risk management coordinator for the health information exchange. Phillip was previously a program manager of operations for the Metro-Chicago Health Information Exchange (MCHIE), a division of the Illinois Health and Hospital Association (IHA). Prior to

MCHIE, Phillip served at the Illinois Health Information Technology Regional Extension Center at Northern Illinois University as a multipurpose expert for a range of projects encompassing research, communications and training for Meaningful Use, telemedicine, Medicare and Medicaid policy, and health information exchange across Illinois. Before moving into healthcare Phillip worked as a consultant in strategic internal business communications for Fortune 500 corporations in the hospitality, manufacturing, healthcare training, and foodservice industries. As a consultant he developed programs, training modules, and events focused on innovation, total quality management, and operational excellence. Phillip holds a MS in health information management from the College of St. Scholastica, a graduate certificate in adult education from DePaul University, and a MSC in communication systems strategy and management from Northwestern University.

Susan E. McClernon, PhD, FACHE, currently serves as the CEO and president of Innovative Healthcare Leadership, a healthcare consulting firm based in Duluth, Minnesota. She also serves as adjunct faculty for the College of St. Scholastica and serves as faculty director for the UMN College of Continuing Education (CCE) program in health services management and applied business. Sue previously served as a chief operating officer and administrator for large tertiary hospitals including St. Mary's Medical Center in Duluth, Minnesota, and Brackenridge Hospital in Austin, Texas. Brackenridge Hospital was named a top 100 hospital in 2001, 2002, and 2003 by Modern Healthcare's Solucient Benchmarking process during Sue's tenure as administrator. She is an active fellow in the American College of Healthcare Executives and was named Hospital Administrator of the Year in 2007 by HCAAM and MHA. She received her bachelor's degree in healthcare management from the College of St. Scholastica and her master's degree in healthcare administration from the University of Minnesota. She completed her doctorate in health research, policy, and administration through the University of Minnesota's School of Public Health in 2013. Sue has also been active in the American Hospital Association and Catholic Healthcare Association.

Colleen Malmgren, MS, RHIA, is the corporate director of charge capture, charge master and pricing for Fairview Health Services in Minneapolis, Minnesota. Previously, she served as director of HIM for Fairview Lakes Hospital in Wyoming, Minnesota, and was the HIM and quality management director at a California-based healthcare facility. She is has been an adjunct professor for the College of St. Scholastica, teaching online courses in healthcare revenue cycle improvement and an adjunct professor for St. Catherine University, teaching courses in coding. She is an alumnus of the College of St. Scholastica's health information management program and earned her master's in healthcare administration at Central Michigan University. She has served in several board positions for the Minnesota Health Information Management Association and presented at the local and state levels on revenue cycle improvement efforts.

Rosann M. O'Dell, DHSc, MS, RHIA, CDIP is a clinical assistant professor and academic progression manager in the department of health information management at the University of Kansas Medical Center (KUMC). In her role at KUMC, she teaches introduction to healthcare management, healthcare reimbursement and financing, and information governance in healthcare in a bachelor of science in health information management (BS in HIM) program. Her duties also include student advising and program management in the department's online RHIT to RHIA degree completion, healthcare management minor, and BS in HIM/ Master of Health Services Administration Bridge programs. Rosann is actively engaged in volunteerism and professional service at the state and national level. She is currently an elected commissioner of the Commission on Certification for Health Informatics and Information Management. Previously she served on various AHIMA committees such as the AHIMA Consumer Engagement Practice Council, Clinical Terminology and Classification Practice Council, as well as the AHIMA Foundation's Research and Periodicals Workgroup and working groups for the Global Health Workforce Council. She has also served on the Kansas Health Information Management Association's Nominating Committee, Communications Committee, and Information Governance Committee. Prior to her career in academia, Rosann had diverse experiences managing personnel, operations, and information systems in areas such as cancer registry, clinical classification, clinical documentation support, and release of information. Her career experiences additionally include program management in continuing medical education and regulatory aspects of clinical research. She has served on institutional committees including HIPAA Privacy, HIPAA Security, oncology services, and clinical ethics. She earned a BS in HIM from the University of Kansas, an MS in management from Friends University, followed by a graduate certificate in clinical healthcare ethics from Saint Louis University. Her doctorate in health sciences with a concentration in global health is from A.T. Still University. Additionally, she is an AHIMA-approved ICD-10-CM/PCS Trainer.

Brandon D. Olson, PhD, PMP is the chair of the computer information systems department at the College of St. Scholastica. Dr. Olson holds a PhD in information technology with a specialization in project management and a master's degree in computer information resource management. His research interests include project management, knowledge management, and IT strategy. Prior to entering academia, Dr. Olson worked as a project manager in the pharmaceutical, healthcare, and business services industries. He also directs outreach programs for the Minnesota chapter of the Project Management Institute.

Brooke Palkie, EdD, RHIA, is an associate professor at the College of St. Scholastica in the health informatics and information management department. She teaches courses related to clinical quality, compliance, and clinical classifications, vocabularies, terminologies and data standards. She recently led a collaborative and interdisciplinary grant assisting an independent behavioral health organization transition to DSM-5 and ICD-10 for

documentation, billing, and reporting purposes. Her healthcare experience includes management and professional positions in health information management, quality, corporate compliance, and consulting. She is a frequent presenter at both state and national meetings and conferences and has authored several articles, white papers, and textbook chapters related to health informatics and information management. She has also served in several capacities at the state, regional, and national levels of the Minnesota and American Health Information Management Associations.

Karen R. Patena, MBA, RHIA, FAHIMA, is a clinical associate professor and director of HIM programs, department of biomedical and health information sciences, College of Applied Health Sciences, at the University of Illinois at Chicago (UIC). She earned an MBA from DePaul University and is an alumnus of the University of Illinois health information management program. Previously, Karen was director of the independent study division of AHIMA and a faculty member at Indiana University and Prairie State College. She also has extensive experience in hospital medical record department management, including computer systems planning and implementation. Her areas of expertise include management, quality improvement and TQM, the use of computers in healthcare and systems analysis, and online curriculum development; and has presented tutorials at local, state, and national levels. She has served in numerous volunteer roles at AHIMA, and currently is a member of the panel of accreditation surveyors for the Commission on Accreditation for Health Informatics and Information Management Education (CAHIIM) and sits on the Virtual Lab Strategic Advisory Board and the PPE workgroup of the Council for Excellence in Education.

Rick Revoir, EdD, MBA, CPA, is an associate professor and chair of accounting, finance, and economics at the College of St. Scholastica, where he teaches healthcare finance, business ethics, and accounting courses. He has 11 years of healthcare finance experience in a variety of positions including director of financial analysis, senior financial analyst, and cost accountant. He serves as commissioner and treasurer of the Duluth Seaway Port Authority. He is a member of the Healthcare Financial Management Association and the American Institute of Certified Public Accountants.

Rebecca B. Reynolds, EdD, RHIA, is a professor and department chair in health informatics and information management. She is past-president of the Tennessee Health Information Management Association and has served on the AHIMA Nominating Committee. She is a recipient of the Tennessee Health Information Management Association's Distinguished Member Award and the Outstanding New Professional Award. Rebecca was a 2006 recipient of AHIMA's Faculty Development Stipend Award and is a member of the inaugural class of AHIMA's HIM Research Training Institute. She received a master's degree in healthcare administration and her EdD in higher education leadership from the University of Memphis. She is currently on the Editorial Review Board for Perspectives in Health Information Management and most recently coedited and coauthored *Fundamentals of Law for Health Informatics and Information Management*, published by AHIMA and whose editors received the 2010 AHIMA Legacy Award for the textbook.

Laurie A. Rinehart-Thompson, JD, RHIA, CHP, FAHIMA is the interim director and an associate professor of clinical health and rehabilitation sciences in the health information management and systems program at The Ohio State University in Columbus. She earned her BS in medical record administration and her law degree from The Ohio State University. In addition to education, her professional experiences include behavioral health, home health, and acute care. She has served as an expert witness in civil litigation testifying as to the privacy and confidentiality of health information. She has served and continues to serve on AHIMA committees and is on the board of directors of the Ohio Health Information Management Association. A frequent speaker on the HIPAA Privacy Rule, she is a coeditor of *Fundamentals of Law for Health*

Informatics and Information Management (AHIMA) and a contributing author to numerous other textbook publications. She has also published in *Perspectives in Health Information Management.*

Ryan H. Sandefer, MA, CPHIT, is chair and assistant professor in the health informatics and information management department at the College of St. Scholastica. He teaches research methods, program evaluation, technology applications, and consumer informatics. He has coedited the textbook *Data Analytics in Healthcare Research: Tools and Strategies*. He is currently engaged in multiple research projects, including projects related to electronic clinical quality measure reporting in rural hospitals, usability of mobile technologies, and consumer personal health information management. Ryan regularly presents at national and local meetings of HIM and HIT professionals and has published articles in the areas of health policy, health workforce, and health informatics. He is a member of the American Health Information Management Association, American Medical Informatics Association, and Health Information Management Systems Society. He is currently pursuing a PhD in health informatics from the University of Minnesota–Twin Cities. He received both his undergraduate and graduate degrees in political science from the University of Wyoming.

Marcia Y. Sharp, EdD, MBA, RHIA, is an associate professor and graduate program director in the department of health informatics and information management at the University of Tennessee Health Sciences Center. She has had an outstanding career in health information management and in human resource management. She is an active member of the Memphis Health Information Management Association, serving as former treasurer, and the Tennessee Health Information Management Association, serving as Tennessee delegate to the AHIMA House of Delegates and former member of the Tennessee Nominating Committee. She received a master's degree in business administration and holds an EdD in higher education leadership. She is currently a member of the Council for Excellence in Education and the Editorial Review Board for

Perspectives on Health Information Management (PHIM). She has written articles and contributed chapters to several AHIMA publications including *Health Information Management Technology: An Applied Approach* and *Fundamentals of Law for Health Informatics and Information Management.*

C. Jeanne Solberg, MA, RHIA, is a director at Prism Healthcare Partners LTD, a healthcare consulting firm focusing on helping hospitals, health systems, and academic medical centers improve their financial, operational, and clinical performance. Her work experience includes roles as president/CEO of a health information management consulting firm; director of business processes at a large healthcare insurer; EHR manager of patient access at a multihospital and clinic organization; senior implementation consultant for a large publicly traded healthcare services company; manager of decision support services and clinical decision support at large tertiary care hospitals in the East and Midwest; and director of HIM, quality assessment, and utilization management in acute-care hospitals with large ambulatory care practices. She is a past director on the American Health Information Management Association (AHIMA) Board; served as chair of the Commission on Accreditation of Health Informatics and Information Management Education (CAHIIM), and chaired AHIMA's Program Committee. Jeanne has a strong interest in health information and data governance, revenue cycle management, clinical and financial decision support, and business management and leadership development.

David X. Swenson, PhD, is a professor of management in the School of Business and Technology at the College of St. Scholastica, where he teaches strategic management, organization development, leadership, marketing, and thesis research. He is also the program director of a new online MBA program for rural health professionals. He has a part-time consulting practice in organization development and forensic psychology, also holding a post-doctoral diplomate in the latter field. David has worked in the field of psychology for more than 40 years and has served as director of

student development at the College of St. Scholastica and director of clinical services at the Human Resource Center of Douglas County, Wisconsin. He has authored more than 100 publications, including *Stress Management for Law Enforcement.* A doctoral graduate of the University of Missouri at Columbia in counseling and personnel services, David also has master's degrees in management, school counseling, educational media and technology, and information technology leadership.

Carol A. Venable, MPH, RHIA, FAHIMA, is a retired professor and department head of HIM at the University of Louisiana at Lafayette and has been an HIM professional for over 35 years. She is still involved with AHIMA's Board of Accreditation Surveyors and several other committees as well as the Louisiana Health Information Management Association, where she has held many leadership positions and was selected as Distinguished Member in 1991. She has served throughout the years as president, president-elect, treasurer, strategy manager, and board member and has also directed numerous projects and committees. Previously, she was director of medical records at Lafayette General Medical Center, has consulted in a variety of healthcare facilities and educational institutions, and conducts coding workshops for hospitals and physician offices. Venable has written, coauthored, and edited numerous publications, including AHIMA's *ICD-10-CM and ICD-9-CM Diagnostic Coding and Reimbursement for Physician Services, Certified Coding Specialist—Physician-Based (CCS-P) Exam Preparation, Clinical Coding Workout,* and *ICD-10-CM and ICD-10-PCS Preview,* for which she was awarded AHIMA's Legacy Award in 2003. She frequently serves as a reviewer for publishers of HIM-related textbooks, certification exams, and electronic materials.

Valerie J.M. Watzlaf, PhD, RHIA, FAHIMA, is an associate professor within the department of health information management in the School of Health and Rehabilitation Sciences at the University of Pittsburgh. She also holds a secondary appointment in the Graduate School of Public Health. In those capacities, she teaches and performs research in the areas of HIM and epidemiology. She has worked and consulted in several healthcare organizations in health information management, long-term care, and epidemiology. She is very active in professional and scientific societies having served on several AHIMA committees, as a board member of AHIMA and the AHIMA Foundation, and as the chair of the Council for Excellence in Education of the AHIMA Foundation. She is currently serving on the IG Task Force of the CEE. She is also on the Editorial Advisory Board for the Journal of AHIMA and for Perspectives in Health Information Management. Dr. Watzlaf has published extensively in the field of HIM and is the recipient of numerous awards and professional accolades including AHIMA's Research Award and PHIMA's Distinguished Member Award. She is currently working as a partner with IOD/Healthport as part of the CareInnoLab conducting research in HIM applications.

Susan E. White, PhD, RHIA, CHDA, is the administrator of analytics at the James Cancer Hospital at The Ohio State University Wexner Medical Center and an associate professor—clinical in the health information management and systems division at The Ohio State University. She teaches statistics, healthcare finance, and database design and development courses. Prior to that appointment, she was the vice president of research and development for Cleverley + Associates and vice president of data operations for CHIPS/Ingenix. Dr. White has written numerous books and articles regarding the benchmarking of healthcare facilities, healthcare financial management, and the application of statistical techniques in analyzing healthcare data. She is the author of AHIMA's *A Practical Approach to Analyzing Healthcare Data* and *Principles of Finance for Health Information and Informatics Professionals* texts. Dr. White received her PhD in statistics from The Ohio State University. She is a member of AHIMA, the American Statistical Association, and the Healthcare Financial Management Association. She has presented to both national and local meetings of healthcare executives and HIM professionals.

Foreword

"The Times They Are A-Changin'" is a song written by Bob Dylan and released as the title track of his 1964 album of the same name (Dylan 1964). It was an everlasting message of change and the lyrics are as appropriate now as they were more than five decades ago. And yet, despite all of the changes we are facing in healthcare, it is an amazing time to become part of the health information management (HIM) profession.

Hospitals and Health Networks published an article by Laura Jacobs called "Looking Ahead in 2016: Top Trends in Health Care" (Jacobs 2016). Of the ten trends cited, including consolidation, value-based payment, reaching across the care continuum, information technology and data governance, all will require healthcare leaders to use information to support decision making. It is now more important than ever that the HIM professional understand the world of information so that they can provide data and information that leaders can then turn into knowledge. This knowledge will subsequently support the changes needed for healthcare providers to remain viable in the market while reducing costs, improving quality and taking care of the populations and communities being served. Only through *trusted* information can decision makers take appropriate action and accelerate innovation and value.

The volume of information HIM professionals manage will continue to grow. Howard Solomon says in the article, "The Amount of Data We're Creating is Out of This World," that "the sheer volume of the world's digital data would fill a stack of iPad air tablets extending two-thirds distance to the moon. By 2020, this stack would extend from the earth to the moon 6.6 times due to the rate of data growth." (Solomon 2014). Someone will need to manage the exponentially increasing amounts of information and that person is the HIM professional.

In our roles, we must be knowledgeable of all the topics in this edition of *Health Information Management: Concepts, Principles, and Practice* including the delivery system; legal issues in health information management; data governance and information governance; health record content and documentation; clinical classifications, vocabularies, terminologies and standards; data management; reimbursement methodologies; revenue cycle management; compliance and risk; data privacy, confidentiality and security; technology; systems strategic planning; consumer health informatics; health information exchange; statistics; data analytics; data visualization; research methods; biomedical and research support; clinical quality management; managing and leading during organizational change; human resource management; employee training and development; work design and process improvement; financial management; project management; ethical issues in health information management; and strategic thinking and management.

It may seem overwhelming that all of these topics need to be understood in order to be an effective HIM professional in today's world. However, with this rich background you will be able to pursue a myriad of opportunities as you enter your career. AHIMA's current Career Map outlines over 60 different job types across 120 different settings. The fact that there is so much opportunity and a diversity of choices in our profession is what makes HIM such an exciting field of study. It is also rewarding to know that with information there is power to improve decision making and healthcare overall. This text will provide you with the background you need to succeed.

Yes, the "Times They Are A-Changin'" but we as HIM professionals will lead the healthcare transformation with information that can be trusted and has integrity. We will help change our healthcare world for the better.

Lynne Thomas Gordon, MBA, RHIA, FACHE
Chief Executive Officer
American Health Information Management Association

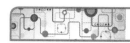 References

Dylan, B. *The Times They Are A-Changin.* Album. Columbia Records. January 13, 1964.

Jacobs, L. "Looking Ahead in 2016: Top 10 Trends in Healthcare," *Hospitals and Health Networks.* January 5, 2016.

Soloman, H. "The Amount of Data We're Creating is Out of This World," *IT World Canada.* April 15, 2014.

Acknowledgments

The editors and publications staff would like to express appreciation to the many authors who contributed chapters to this textbook. They willingly shared their expertise, met tight deadlines, accepted feedback, and contributed to building the body of knowledge related to health information management. Writing a chapter is a time-consuming and demanding task, and we are grateful for the authors' contributions.

We would also like to thank authors who contributed to previous editions of this textbook:

- Rita K. Bowen, MA, RHIA, CHPS
- Elizabeth D. Bowman, RHIA, FAHIMA
- Bonnie S. Cassidy, MPA, RHIA, FHIMSS, FAHIMA
- Nadinia Davis, MBA, CIA, CPA, RHIA, FAHIMA
- Chris R. Elliott, MS, RHIA
- Mehnaz Farishta, MS
- Susan H. Fenton, MBA, RHIA
- Margaret M. (Maggie) Foley, PhD, RHIA, CCS
- Kathy Giannangelo, RHIA, CCS, CPHIMS, FAHIMA
- Michelle A. Green, MPS, RHIA, CMA
- Matthew J. Greene, RHIA, CSS
- J. Michael Hardin, PhD
- Laurinda B. Harman, PhD, RHIA, FAHIMA
- Loretta A. Horton, MEd, RHIA
- Diana Lynn Johnson, PhD
- Linda L. Kloss, MA, RHIA, FAHIMA
- Deborah Kohn, MPH, RHIA, CPHIMS, FHIMSS
- Mary Cole McCain, MPA, RHIA
- Carol E. Osborn, PhD, RHIA

- Susan L. Parker, MEd, RHIA
- Carol Ann Quinsey, MS, RHIA, CHPS
- Uzma Raja, PhD
- Lynda A. Russell, EdD, JD, RHIA, CHP
- Rita Scichilone, MHSA, RHIA, CCS, CCS-P, CHC-F
- Patricia B. Seidl, RHIA
- Kam Shams, MA
- Carol Marie Spielman, MA, RHIA
- Cheryl Stephens, MBA, PhD
- Karen Wager, DBA
- Janelle A. Wapola, RHIA, MA
- Andrea Weatherby White, PhD, RHIA
- Frances Wickham Lee, DBA, RHIA
- Vicki Zeman, MA, RHIA

We also would like to thank the following reviewers who lent a critical eye to this endeavor. *Current edition reviewers:*

- Karen Bakuzonis, PhD, MS, RHIA
- Hertencia V. Bowe, EdD, RHIA, MHSA
- Karen Clancy, MBA
- Dilhari R. DeAlmeida, PhD, RHIA
- Lois Hitchcock, MHA, RHIA, CPHQ
- Deborah J. Honstad, MA, RHIA

Previous edition reviewers also include

- Janie L. Batres, RHIT, CCS
- Donna Bowers, JD, RHIA, CHP
- June E. Bronnert, RHIA, CCS, CCS-P
- Jill Burrington-Brown, MS, RHIA
- Christopher G. Chute, MD, DrPH
- Jill S. Clark, MBA, RHIA
- Kathryn DeVault, RHIA, CCS, CCS-P
- Julie A. Dooling, RHIT

- Claire Dixon-Lee, PhD, RHIA, FAHIMA
- Michelle L. Dougherty, RHIA, CHP
- Melanie A. Endicott, MBA/HCM, RHIA, CCS, CCS-P
- Susan H. Fenton, MBA, RHIA
- Leslie A. Fox, MA, RHIA, FAHIMA
- Jennifer Garvin, PhD, RHIA, CPHQ, CCS, FAHIMA
- Kathy Giannangelo, RHIA, CCS
- Barry S. Herrin, Esq.
- Beth Hjort, RHIA, CHPS
- Susan Hull, MPH, RHIA, CCS, CCS-P
- Lolita M. Jones, RHIA, CCS
- Karen Kostick, RHIT, CCS, CCS-P
- Donald T. Mon, PhD, FHIMSS
- Carol Ann Quinsey, RHIA, CHPS
- Harry Rhodes, MBA, RHIA, CHPS

- Theresa Rihanek, MHA, RHIA, CCS
- Dan Rode, MBA, FHFMA
- Angela Dinh Rose, MHA, RHIA, CHPS
- Rita A. Scichilone, MHSA, RHIA, CCS, CCS-P, CHC
- Stephen A. Sivo, PhD
- Mary H. Stanfill, RHIA, CCS, CCS-P
- Diana M. Warner, MS, RHIA, CHPS, FAHIMA
- Valerie J.M. Watzlaf, PhD, RHIA, FAHIMA
- Lou Ann Wiedemann, MS, RHIA, CPEHR, FAHIMA
- Maggie Williams, MA
- Ann Zeisset, RHIT, CCS-P, CCS

Finally the editors wish to acknowledge Ashley Latta, production development editor, for her guidance throughout this project.

Introduction

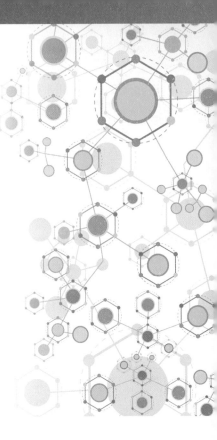

Pamela K. Oachs, MA, RHIA, CHDA, FAHIMA
and Amy Watters, EdD, RHIA, FAHIMA

As the healthcare industry recognized the importance of clinical recordkeeping and its impact on patient care and delivery, the health information management (HIM) profession emerged. Originally referred to as medical record science, the field of HIM has been a recognized profession for over 90 years. Today, health information management is described as the practice of acquiring, analyzing, and protecting digital and traditional medical information vital to providing quality patient care (AHIMA n.d.).

Once known as medical record librarians, the role of the HIM professional has changed significantly with the times. Changes in healthcare reimbursement systems, new healthcare delivery models, and advancements in medicine and technology have all contributed to the array of skills that HIM professionals possess, and the diversity of jobs and settings in which they work. These professionals affect the quality of patient information and patient care at every point in the healthcare delivery cycle and serve as a bridge to connect the clinical, operational, and administrative functions (AHIMA n.d.).

Although the core of the HIM profession has always been to collect and maintain high-quality health data, the methods to do so have changed as healthcare has become more technology driven.

The HIM professional's knowledge and skills have transitioned from paper-based records and manual systems, to a focus on managing electronic content. This makes for an information-rich environment requiring a unique mix of clinical, management, and information technology competencies (LaTour et al. 2013).

AHIMA's Core Model identifies the roles in which HIM professionals participate and their impact across the healthcare industry. See figure 0.1. The center of the model encompasses the HIM professional's varied interactions with health information, which is at the heart of health information governance and stewardship. Through these activities HIM professionals impact policy, standards, education, and research (AHIMA 2011), all of which are critical to meeting the Triple Aim of healthcare.

The Triple Aim refers to the simultaneous pursuit of three dimensions of healthcare: improving the patient experience of care, improving the health of populations, and reducing the per capita cost of healthcare (Institute for Healthcare Improvement n.d.). Many healthcare organizations, including federal agencies like the Centers for Medicare and Medicaid Services (CMS), are using the Triple Aim

Figure 0.1.   AHIMA core model

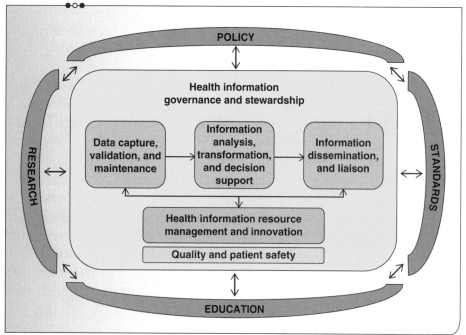

Source: AHIMA 2011.

as a framework to achieve their goals and improve healthcare. Although there are currently many healthcare-related government and industry initiatives in existence with varying goals, each initiative relates to the Triple Aim in some way; and with their clinical, technical, and management expertise, HIM professionals are poised to lead the way.

Proper management of health information is critical for the success of these challenging initiatives, requiring HIM professionals to continue to develop, utilize, and market their skills. AHIMA's Council for Excellence in Education (CEE) is the leading force in education strategy for the HIM profession, guiding the academic community and workforce through improvements to education, coursework, and curricula (AHIMA Foundation n.d.). The curriculum, designed to prepare the HIM student, includes the following domains for all levels of HIM education:

- Data content, structure, and standards
- Information protection: access, disclosure, archival, privacy and security
- Informatics, analytics, and data use
- Revenue management

- Compliance
- Leadership (AHIMA Foundation 2013)

In addition, supporting foundational knowledge in the areas of pathophysiology, pharmacology, anatomy and physiology, medical terminology, computer concepts and applications, and statistics provides HIM professionals with a combination of skills and competencies that differentiate them from other healthcare professionals. Interwoven through all areas of the academic content are critical thinking and personal branding where the ability to work independently, use judgment skills effectively, be innovative, take personal accountability, and be reliable and self-sufficient are key (AHIMA Foundation 2013).

Content expertise is undeniably critical to success as a HIM professional, however the academic community and healthcare industry also recognize the importance of soft skills when developing a leader in the field. Development around communication skills, professionalism, and the concept of understanding organizational culture are critical for new and current HIM professionals alike (see figure 0.2).

Communication skills include not only being able to write and speak clearly, but also to listen

Figure 0.2. Components of HIM leadership

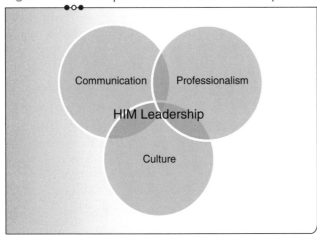

The ability to respectfully achieve results, meet goals, build relationships and network with others, adapt to change, be open to new ideas, and offer creative solutions are all characteristics of a strong leader. One can be a leader in their role or area of expertise by being confident in their knowledge, being honest and thoughtful, dependable, and collaborative. Being professional in all situations instills confidence and trust from others, which is essential for HIM professionals who serve as a bridge among people, systems, and concepts.

Understanding the workplace culture, and what impacts it, is another critical proficiency for the HIM leader. Thoughtful and effective communication skills along with consistent professional behavior create a culture of creativity, respect, and openness in the workplace. An environment where individuals are encouraged to share ideas, gain new skills, experience opportunities outside of their usual routine, and feel comfortable stating their opinions supports the development of strong leaders in HIM who can effect change (Mancilla et al. 2015). It is the efforts of these leaders who will impact the success of the Triple Aim and make lasting contributions to the transformation of the healthcare industry.

carefully. At its most basic level, communication is the exchange of information, which is central to health information management; effective communication is the foundation for quality care, efficient processes, strong relationships, collaboration, and a positive work environment. Communication skills are a key component of professional behavior as well as an organizational culture based on respect.

Professionalism is as integral to gaining respect in a chosen field as technical or content expertise.

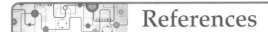

References

American Health Information Management Association. n.d. Health Information 101: What is Health Information? http://www.ahima.org/careers/healthinfohttp://www.ahima.org/careers/healthinfo

http://www.ahimafoundation.org/education/cee.aspx

American Health Information Management Association. 2011. A New View of HIM: Introducing the Core Model. Retrieved from http://library.ahima.org/xpedio/groups/public/documents/ahima/bok1_049283.pdfhttp://library.ahima.org/xpedio/groups/public/documents/ahima/bok1_049283.pdf

http://www.ihi.org/engage/initiatives/tripleaim/Pages/default.aspx

AHIMA Foundation. n.d. Council for Excellence in Education. http://www.ahimafoundation.org/education/cee.aspx

http://www.ahimafoundation.org/education/cee.aspx

AHIMA Foundation. 2013. Academic Competencies. http://www.ahimafoundation.org/downloads/pdfs/2014%20Side-by-Side_Curriculum_Map.pdf

Institute for Healthcare Improvement. n.d. The IHI triple aim. http://www.ihi.org/engage/initiatives/tripleaim/Pages/default.aspxhttp://www.ihi.org/engage/initiatives/tripleaim/Pages/default.aspx

LaTour, K.M., S. Eichenwald Maki, P.K. Oachs. 2013. *Health Information Management: Concepts, Principles and Practice,* 4th ed. Chicago: AHIMA.

Mancilla, D., C. Guyton-Ringbloom, and M. Dougherty. 2015 (June). Ten skills that make a great leader. *Journal of AHIMA* 86(6):38–41.

PART I
Data Content, Standards, and Governance

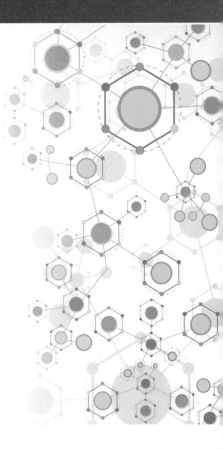

1

The US Healthcare Delivery System

Sandra R. Fuller, MA, RHIA, FAHIMA

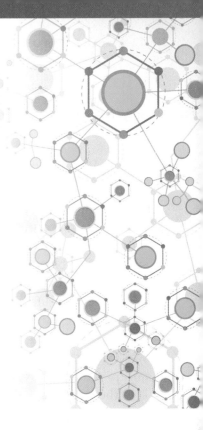

Learning Objectives

- Construct a timeline of the history of the healthcare delivery system from ancient times to the present
- Identify the basic organization of the various types of hospitals and healthcare organizations
- Describe the impact of external forces on the healthcare industry
- Identify the various functional components of an integrated delivery system
- Describe the systems used for reimbursement of healthcare services
- Articulate the role of government in healthcare services
- Discuss the impact of regulatory change on the healthcare delivery system

Key Terms

Accountable care organization (ACO)
Accreditation
Acute care
Allied health professional
Ambulatory care
Biotechnology
Centers for Medicare and Medicaid Services (CMS)
Certification
Chief executive officer (CEO)
Clinical privileges
Continuum of care
Deemed status
For-profit

Health maintenance organization (HMO)
Health savings account (HSA)
Home healthcare
Hospice care
Hospital
Hospital outpatient
Inpatient
Integrated delivery system (IDS)
Investor-owned hospital chain
Licensure
Long-term care
Managed care
Managed care organization (MCO)
Medicaid

Medical device
Medical staff bylaws
Medical staff classification
Medicare
Mission
Multihospital system
Network
Not-for-profit
Organized healthcare delivery
Patient-focused care
Peer review
Point of service (POS) plan
Post-acute care
Preferred provider organization (PPO)

Retail clinics

Skilled nursing facility (SNF)

Surgeon general

Telehealth

TRICARE

Values

Value-based purchasing

Vision

Workers' compensation

A broad array of healthcare services are available in the United States today, ranging from simple preventive measures such as vaccinations to complex lifesaving procedures such as heart transplants. An individual's contact with the healthcare delivery system often begins with family planning and prenatal care before he or she is born and continues through end-of-life planning and hospice care.

Healthcare services are provided by physicians, nurses, and other clinical providers who work in ambulatory care, acute care, rehabilitative and psychiatric care, and long-term care facilities. Healthcare services also are provided in the homes of hospice and home care patients. Assisted living centers, industrial medical clinics, and public health department clinics also provide services to many Americans.

While most healthcare is experienced locally and individually, healthcare is the single largest part of the US economy, consuming 18.3 percent of the gross domestic product (GDP) in 2014 (Wilson 2014). It is delivered by an ever-expanding variety of providers from large multi-institutional integrated delivery networks (IDNs) to nurse practitioners within the neighborhood drug store. Although the growth in healthcare spending has been slowing since 2003, it continues to outpace the overall growth in the US economy; and US healthcare spending rose to $2.8 trillion in 2014 (Wilson 2014).

In 2013, there were 5,686 registered hospitals in the United States according to the American Hospital Association (AHA 2014). Almost 5,000 of those were community hospitals, which include nonfederal, short-term general hospitals and other specialty hospitals. They also include academic medical centers and teaching hospitals not owned by the federal government. About 20 percent of the community hospitals were for-profit and investor-owned, and over 3,000 were part of a system (AHA 2015). **Multihospital systems** include two or more hospitals owned, leased, sponsored, or contract managed by a central organization. Hospitals can also be part of a **network**, which is a group of hospitals, physicians, and other providers and payers that collaborate to coordinate and deliver services to their community.

In addition to hospital systems and networks there are other forms of organized healthcare delivery. **Organized healthcare delivery** can be defined as "that care providers have established relationships and mechanisms for communicating and working to coordinate patient care across health conditions, services, and care settings over time" (Kovner et al. 2011, 206). A multispecialty physician group practice that includes a health insurer is another example of organized care. Recent healthcare reform legislation, economic pressure, and the opportunity to provide better care through coordination and improved access to information continue to move healthcare away from the traditional freestanding solo practice of the past.

This chapter discusses the origin and history of the healthcare industry in the United States. Included in this history is the impact of external forces that have shaped the healthcare system of today.

History of Western Medicine

Modern Western medicine can be traced to the ancient Greeks who developed surgical procedures, documented clinical cases, and created medical books. Before modern times, European, African, and Native American cultures all had traditions of folk medicine based on spiritual healing and herbal cures. The first hospitals were created by religious orders in medieval Europe to provide care and respite to religious pilgrims traveling back and forth from the Holy Land. However, it was not until the late 1800s that medicine became a scientific discipline. More progress and change occurred during the 20th century than over the preceding 2,000 years. The past few decades have seen dramatic developments in the way diseases are diagnosed and treated as well as the way healthcare is delivered.

The medical knowledge that had been gained by ancient Greek scholars such as Hippocrates was lost during the Middle Ages. The European Renaissance, a historical period beginning in the 14th century, revived interest in the classical arts, literature, and philosophy as well as in the scientific study of nature. This period also was characterized by economic growth and concern for the welfare of workers at all levels of society. With this concept came a growing awareness that a healthy population promoted economic growth.

North America's First Hospitals

Early settlers in the British colonies of North America appointed commissions to care for the sick, to provide for orphans, and to bury the dead. It was also recognized that a place was needed to isolate new immigrants who may have contracted a communicable disease.

In Philadelphia, Benjamin Franklin and other colonists persuaded the legislature to develop a hospital for the community. It was the first hospital in the British colonies of North America. The Pennsylvania Hospital was established in Philadelphia in 1752 and served as a model for the organization of hospitals in other communities. The New York Hospital opened in 1771 and started its first register of patients in 1791. Boston's Massachusetts General Hospital opened in 1821.

Standardization of Medical Practice

Medical practice began evolving in ancient civilizations even before the ancient Greeks invented the construct of a medical diagnosis and prognosis and introduced ethics into medicine. In the 12th century universities in Italy began training doctors. The discovery of germ theory in the 19th century eventually lead to more effective treatments for many diseases. However, there was very little standardization in the training or practice of medicine.

An individual's early medical education consisted of serving as an apprentice to an established practitioner. In the late 1700s it was recognized that medical results varied between practitioners and leaders and that standardization or regulation could improve overall results. The first attempts at regulation took the form of licensure. The first licenses to practice medicine were issued in New York in 1760. As the population of the United States grew and settlers moved westward, the demand for medical practitioners far exceeded the supply. To staff new hospitals and serve a growing population, many private medical schools appeared almost overnight. However, these schools did not follow an established course of study, and some graduated students with as little as six months of training. The result was an oversupply of poorly trained physicians. The American Medical Association (AMA) was established in 1847 to represent the interests of physicians across the United States (AMA 2015). In 1876, the Association of American Medical Colleges (AAMC) was established (AAMC 2015). AAMC's mission was to standardize the curriculum for medical schools in the United States and to increase the public's awareness of the need to license physicians.

Early in the 20th century the need for curriculum reform in medical schools and licensure of physicians was recognized. In 1906, Abraham Flexner initiated a four-year study of medical colleges, visiting every medical college and carefully documenting his observations (Flexner 1910). In 1910, he presented his findings of the poor quality of medical training to the Carnegie Foundation, the AMA, and the AAMC. Based on his report and recommendations by the AMA's Committee on Medical Education, several reforms were adopted. These reforms included that medical school applicants hold a college degree, that medical training be founded on science and that medical students receive practical hospital-based training. These reforms had two consequences across the following decade, about half of the medical schools closed while the others adopted the change so that by 1920 most of the medical colleges in the United States met the standards of the AAMC (Cooke et al. 2006).

Today, medical school graduates must pass a test administered by state medical boards before they can obtain a license to practice medicine. Many states now use a standardized licensure test developed in 1968 by the Federation of State Medical Boards of the United States. However, passing scores for the test vary by state. Most physicians also complete several years of residency training in addition to medical school.

Specialty physicians also complete extensive postgraduate medical education. Board certification for the various specialties requires the completion of postgraduate training as well as a passing score on a standardized examination. Common medical specialties include:

- Internal medicine
- Pediatrics
- Family practice
- Cardiology
- Psychiatry
- Neurology
- Oncology
- Radiology

Common surgical specialties include:

- Anesthesiology
- Cardiovascular surgery
- Obstetrics and gynecology
- Orthopedics
- Urology
- Ophthalmology
- Otorhinolaryngology
- Plastic and reconstructive surgery
- Neurosurgery

Some medical and surgical specialists undergo further graduate training to qualify to practice subspecialties. For example, the subspecialties of internal medicine include endocrinology, pulmonary medicine, rheumatology, geriatrics, and hematology. Physicians also may limit their practices to the treatment of specific illnesses such as an endocrinologist limiting his or her practice to the treatment of diabetes. Surgeons can work as general surgeons or as specialists or subspecialists. For example, an orthopedic surgeon may limit his practice to surgery of the hand, knee, ankle, or spine.

Some physicians and healthcare organizations employ physician assistants (PAs) and surgeon assistants (SAs) to help them carry out their clinical responsibilities. Such assistants may perform routine clinical assessments, provide patient education and counseling, and perform simple therapeutic procedures. Most PAs work in primary care settings and most SAs work in hospitals and ambulatory surgery clinics. PAs and SAs always work under the supervision of licensed physicians and surgeons.

Standardization of Hospital Care

In 1910, Dr. Franklin H. Martin, who became the first editor of the *Journal of the American College of Surgeons*, suggested surgical care needed to pay better attention to patient outcomes (ACS 2015). Martin learned these concepts from Dr. Ernest Codman, a British physician who thought that patient outcomes should be tracked over time to determine what treatment delivered the best results (Hazelwood et al. 2005).

At that time, Martin and other American physicians were concerned about the conditions in US hospitals. It was thought that the lack of an organized medical staff and lax professional standards contributed to the problems. In the early 20th century hospitals were used mainly for performing surgery. Most nonsurgical medical care was still provided in the home. It was natural, then, for the force behind improved hospital care to come from surgeons.

The push for hospital reforms eventually led to the formation of the American College of Surgeons in 1913. The organization faced a difficult task. In 1917, the leaders of the college asked the Carnegie Foundation for funding to plan and develop a hospital standardization program. The college then formed a committee to develop a set of minimum standards for hospital care and published the formal standards under the title of the Minimum Standards.

Adoption of the Minimum Standards was the basis of the Hospital Standardization Program and marked the beginning of the modern accreditation process for healthcare organizations. To this day, accreditation standards are developed to reflect reasonable quality standards, and the performance of each participating organization is evaluated annually against the standards. The accreditation process is voluntary. Healthcare organizations choose to participate in order to improve the care they provide to their patients.

The American College of Surgeons continued to sponsor the hospital accreditation program until the early 1950s. In 1952 a new organization called the Joint Commission on Accreditation of Hospitals was formed by the American College of Physicians, the AMA, the American Hospital Association (AHA) and the Canadian Medical Association. The Joint Commission began performing accreditation surveys in 1953 (Carter and Shaw 2000).

The Joint Commission continues to survey several types of healthcare organizations today, including:

- Acute-care hospitals
- Long-term care facilities
- Ambulatory care facilities
- Psychiatric facilities
- Home health agencies

Several other organizations also perform accreditation of healthcare organizations. These include the American Osteopathic Association (AOA), the Commission on Accreditation of Rehabilitation Facilities (CARF), and the Accreditation Association for Ambulatory Health Care (AAAHC).

Professionalism of the Allied Health Professions

After World War I, many of the roles previously played by nurses and nonclinical personnel began to change. With the advent of modern diagnostic and therapeutic technology in the middle of the 20th century, the complex skills needed by ancillary medical personnel fostered the growth of specialized training programs and professional accreditation and licensure.

Allied health professionals work with physicians and nurses and have received specialized training. "Allied health professionals are the segment of the workforce that delivers services involving the identification, evaluation, and prevention of diseases and disorders; dietary and nutrition services; and rehabilitation and health systems management"(ASAHP 2015). Allied health professionals comprise nearly 60 percent of the healthcare workforce and include careers such as dental hygienists, diagnostic medical sonographers, dietitians, medical technologists, occupational therapists, physical therapists, radiographers, and speech language therapists (ASAHP 2015). All 50 states require licensure for some allied health professions (physical therapy, for example). Practitioners in other allied health professions (occupational therapy, for example) may be licensed in some states, but not in others.

Check Your Understanding 1.1

Instructions: **On a separate piece of paper, write down the word or term that correctly completes each of the sentences.**

1. The ancient _____ developed surgical procedures, documented clinical cases, and created medical books.
   A. Chinese
   B. Greeks
   C. Phoenicians
   D. Egyptians

2. The _____ was established in 1847 to represent the interests of physicians across the United States.
   A. American Association of Medical Colleges
   B. American College of Surgeons
   C. Committee on Medical Education
   D. American Medical Association

3. Today, medical school students must pass a test before they can obtain a _____ to practice medicine.
   A. degree
   B. residency
   C. specialty
   D. license

4. The Flexner Report recommended that medical schools should
   A. require applicants to hold a college degree.
   B. include hospital-based training.
   C. include training in the basic sciences.
   D. All of the above

5. In 1910, Dr. Franklin H. Martin suggested that the surgical area of medical practice needed to become more concerned with _____.
   A. patient care
   B. professional standards
   C. patient outcomes
   D. nonsurgical medical care

6. Adoption of the Minimum Standards marked the beginning of the modern _____ process for healthcare organizations.
   A. accreditation
   B. licensing
   C. reform
   D. educational

7. Physical therapists and occupational therapists are part of what segment of the healthcare workforce?
   A. Home health
   B. Nursing care
   C. Ambulatory care
   D. Allied health

Modern Healthcare Delivery in the United States

The 20th century was a period of tremendous change in American society. Advances in medical science promised better outcomes and increased the demand for healthcare services. But medical care has never been free. Even in the best economic times, many Americans have been unable to take full advantage of what medicine has to offer because they cannot afford it.

Concern over access to healthcare was especially evident during the Great Depression of the 1930s. During the Depression, America's leaders were forced to consider how the poor and disadvantaged could receive the care they needed. Before the Depression, medical care for the poor and elderly had been handled as a function of social welfare agencies. During the 1930s, however, few people were able to pay for medical care. The problem of how to pay for the healthcare needs of millions of Americans became a public and governmental concern. Working Americans turned to prepaid health plans to help them pay for healthcare, but the unemployed and the unemployable needed help from a different source.

Effects of the Great Depression

The concept of prepaid healthcare, or health insurance, began with the financial problems of one hospital—Baylor University Hospital in Dallas, Texas (AHA 1999, 14). In 1929, the administrator of the hospital arranged to provide hospital services to Dallas's schoolteachers for 50 cents per person per month. Before that time, a few large employers had set up company clinics and hired company physicians to care for their workers, but the idea of a prepaid health plan that could be purchased by individuals had never been tried before.

The idea of public funding for healthcare services also dates back to the Great Depression. The decline in family income during the 1930s curtailed the use of medical services by the poor. In 10 working-class communities studied between 1929 and 1933, the proportion of families with incomes under $150 per capita had increased from 10 to 43 percent. A 1938 Gallup poll asked people whether they had put off seeing a physician because of the cost and the results showed that 68 percent of lower-income respondents had put off medical care, compared with 24 percent of respondents in upper-income brackets (Starr 1982, 271).

The decreased use of medical services and the inability of many patients to pay meant lower incomes for physicians. Hospitals were in similar trouble. Beds were empty, bills went unpaid, and contributions to hospital fundraising efforts tumbled. As a result, private physicians and charities could no longer meet the demand for free services. For the first time, physicians and hospitals asked state welfare departments to pay for the treatment of people on relief.

The push for government-sponsored health insurance continued in the late 1930s during the administration of President Franklin D. Roosevelt. However, compulsory health insurance (required by law) stood on the margins of national politics throughout the New Deal era. It was not made part of the new Social Security program and it was never fully supported by President Roosevelt.

Postwar Efforts Toward Improving Healthcare Access

After World War II, the issue of healthcare access finally moved to the center of national politics. In the late 1940s, President Harry Truman expressed unreserved support for a national health insurance program. However, the issue of compulsory health insurance became entangled with America's fear of communism. Opponents of Truman's healthcare program labeled it "socialized medicine," and the program failed to win legislative support.

The idea of national health insurance did not resurface until the administration of Lyndon Johnson and the Great Society legislation of the 1960s. The Medicare and Medicaid programs were legislated in 1965 to pay the cost of providing healthcare services to the elderly and the poor, respectively. The issues of healthcare reform and national health insurance were again given priority during the first four years of President Bill Clinton's administration in the 1990s. However, the complexity of American healthcare issues at the end of the 20th century doomed reform efforts. Healthcare continues to be a major political issue—significant healthcare reform legislation was proposed by President Barack Obama and passed in 2010. The Patient Protection and Affordable Care Act (ACA) addresses healthcare costs, coverage, and quality, but it remains highly controversial and is scheduled to take years to be fully enacted.

Influence of Federal Legislation

During the 20th century, Congress passed many pieces of legislation that had a significant impact on the delivery of healthcare services in the United States. Many of these legislative efforts are described in table 1.1.

Table 1.1. Federal healthcare legislation

Title	Date of enactment	Key provisions	Impact
Biologics Control Act	1902	Regulated the vaccines and serums sold via interstate commerce	Launched the research laboratories that later became the National Institutes of Health (NIH)
Social Security Act	1935	Provided states matching funds for maternal and infant care, rehabilitation of crippled children, general public health work, and aid for dependent children	Extended the federal government's role in public health.
Hospital Survey and Construction Act (also known as the Hill-Burton Act)	1946	Authorized grants for states to construct new hospitals	Created a boom in hospital construction; hospitals grew from 6,000 in 1946 to a high of 7,200
Public Law 89-97	1965	Amendments to Social Security that created Medicare and Medicaid	Medicare provides healthcare benefits to citizens over the age of 65 Medicaid supports medical and hospital care for the medically indigent
Public Law 92-603	1972	Expanded initial Medicare and Medicaid requirements for utilization review to include concurrent review; established the professional standards review organization (PSRO) program	Efforts to curtail the rising costs of the Medicare and Medicaid programs by evaluating patient care services for necessity, quality, and cost-effectiveness
Health Planning and Resources Development Act	1974	Created a system of local organizations called health systems agencies to make service and technology decisions	Along with other legislation of this type, it was unsuccessful in slowing cost increases and was repealed in 1986
Utilization Review Act	1977	Required hospitals to conduct continued stay reviews to determine medical necessity of hospitalization, also included fraud and abuse regulations	An additional effort to control growing healthcare costs
Peer Review Improvement Act	1982	Redesigned the PSRO program	Hospitals began to review medical necessity and appropriateness of hospitalizations prior to admission; in 2002, they were given a new name of Quality Improvement Organizations (QIOs)
Tax Equity and Fiscal Responsibility Act (TEFRA)	1982	Introduced the prospective payment system for Medicare reimbursement to control the rising cost of providing healthcare services to Medicare beneficiaries	Changed Medicare reimbursement from a fee-for-service model to a predetermined level of reimbursement
Prospective Payment Act/Public Law 98-21	1982/1983	Defined the prospective payment system and the use of diagnosis related groups (DRGs) as the methodology for inpatient care	Prospective payment was successful at slowing the rate of growth of healthcare spending so it was expanded to other service modalities like outpatient services in 2000
Consolidated Omnibus Budget Reconciliation Act (COBRA)	1985	Allowed the federal government to deny reimbursement for substandard services provided to Medicare and Medicaid beneficiaries	Began establishing a link between quality and reimbursement for services in the Medicare and Medicaid programs
Healthcare Quality Improvement Act	1986	Established the National Practitioner Data Bank (NPDB)	Provides a clearinghouse for medical practitioners who have a history of malpractice suits and other quality problems
Omnibus Budget Reconciliation Act	1989	Instituted the Agency for Healthcare Policy and Research now known as the Agency for Healthcare Research and Quality (AHRQ)	The mission of AHRQ is to develop outcome measures to evaluate the quality of healthcare services

Table 1.1. Continued.

Title	Date of enactment	Key provisions	Impact
Health Insurance Portability and Accountability Act (HIPAA)	1996	Addressed issues related to the portability of health insurance after leaving employment and administrative simplification of healthcare	Reduced the barriers to changing employers due to existing health conditions and created a federal floor for healthcare privacy
Mental Health Parity Act	1996	If mental health benefits are provided by an employer, it sets the annual and life-time benefits equal to those for medical and surgical benefits provided	Began the discussion of equating mental health benefits with other health benefits; provided increased coverage for those with severe, disabling brain disorders
American Recovery and Reinvestment Act and the Health Information Technology for Economic and Clinical Health (HITECH)	2009	Accelerated the adoption of and use of information technology in healthcare through economic incentives and planned future financial penalties. Expanded HIPAA privacy protections and established regional extension centers	In 2013, 59% of hospitals and 48% of physicians had at least a basic electronic health record (EHR), respective increases of 47 percentage points and 26 percentage points since 2009 (ONC 2014)
Patient Protection and Affordable Care Act (ACA)	2010	Requires most US citizens to have healthcare coverage through increased access to health insurance, tax credits to employers offering health insurance, expansion of the Medicaid programs, and tax penalties for those who choose not to purchase coverage. Expands Medicaid to all non-Medicare eligible people under age 65 with incomes up to 133% of the federal poverty level. This provision was made optional by a Supreme Court ruling (Kaiser Family Foundation 2013)	At the end of the second enrollment period in February, 2015, 11.6 million people signed up for coverage through the healthcare marketplace created under the ACA; 10.8 million people gained Medicaid coverage compared to a baseline period from July through September of 2013; and growth in Medicaid increased by 27% in states that expanded Medicaid compared to 7% in states that did not adopt Medicaid expansion (Kaiser Family Foundation 2015)

Future Federal Planning

Legislation and federal policy have a significant impact on healthcare. As the largest payer of healthcare services, the US government has a dual role of protecting the health of the population and ensuring that federal money is well spent. Beyond the legislative activities outlined previously, the Department of Health and Human Services (HHS) is responsible for almost one-quarter of all federal spending, and its mission is to enhance the health and well-being of Americans by providing for effective health and human services and by fostering sound, sustained advances in the sciences underlying medicine, public health, and social services (HHS 2010). Updated every four years, HHS's strategic plan for the years from 2014 to 2018 contains four goals (HHS 2015):

- Strengthen healthcare.
- Advance scientific knowledge and innovation.
- Advance the health, safety, and well-being of the American people.
- Increase efficiency, transparency, accountability, and effectiveness of HHS programs.

In setting these goals HHS advances their mission and establishes strategic direction for programs over the time period. These priorities are demonstrated in research and policy initiatives.

Biomedical and Technological Advances in Medicine

Rapid progress in medical science and technology during the late 19th and 20th centuries revolutionized the way healthcare was provided. One of the most important scientific advancements was the discovery of bacteria as the cause of infectious disease. An important technological development was the use of anesthesia for surgical procedures. These 19th-century advances formed the basis for the development of antibiotics and other pharmaceuticals and the application of sophisticated surgical procedures in the 20th century. Figure 1.1 offers a timeline of key biological and technological advances at a glance.

These scientific advances continue today through research and development in the diverse discipline of biotechnology. **Biotechnology** is "the field devoted to applying the techniques of biochemistry, cellular biology, biophysics, and molecular biology to addressing practical issues related to human beings, agriculture, and the environment" (Stedman's Medical Dictionary 2000). Two examples of the types of companies in the field of biotechnology are pharma (a pharmaceutical or drug company) and medical device companies. These companies conduct research on, develop, market, and distribute drugs for the healthcare industry.

A **medical device** company produces devices such as instruments, machines, or an implement or apparatus intended for use in the diagnosis of disease or for monitoring or treatment of a condition. A medical device is used by a physician for a patient who has a condition whereby a body part does not achieve any of its primary intended purposes such as a heart valve. Medical devices can be used for life support, such as anesthesia ventilators; as well as for monitoring of patients, such as fetal monitors; and other uses, such as incubators (WHO 2015).

Figure 1.1. Key biological and technological advances in medicine

Time	Event
1842	First recorded use of ether as an anesthetic
1860s	Louis Pasteur laid the foundation for modern bacteriology
1865	Joseph Lister was the first to apply Pasteur's research to the treatment of infected wounds
1880s–1890s	Steam first used in physical sterilization
1895	Wilhelm Roentgen made observations that led to the development of x-ray technology
1898	Introduction of rubber surgical gloves, sterilization, and antisepsis
1940	Studies of prothrombin time first made available
1941–1946	Studies of electrolytes; development of major pharmaceuticals
1957	Studies of blood gas
1961	Studies of creatine phosphokinase
1970s	Surgical advances in cardiac bypass surgery, surgery for joint replacements, and organ transplantation
1971	Computed tomography first used in England
1974	Introduction of whole-body scanners
1980s	Introduction of magnetic resonance imaging
1990s	Further technological advances in pharmaceuticals and genetics; Human Genome Project
2000s	NIH creates roadmap to accelerate biomedical advances, creates effective prevention strategies and new treatments, and bridges knowledge gaps in the 21st century

Check Your Understanding 1.2

Instructions: **On a separate piece of paper, match the descriptions with the appropriate legislation.**

1. _____ Hospital Survey and Construction (Hill-Burton) Act

2. _____ Tax Equity and Fiscal Responsibility Act

3. _____ Public Law 89-97 of 1965

4. _____ Utilization Review Act

5. _____ Omnibus Budget Reconciliation Act of 1989

6. _____ Public Law 92-603 of 1972

7. _____ Healthcare Quality Improvement Act of 1986

8. _____ Biologics Control Act

9. _____ Patient Protection and Affordable Care Act of 2010

A. Amendments to the Social Security Act that brought Medicare and Medicaid into existence

B. Authorized grants for states to construct new hospitals

C. Required concurrent review for Medicare and Medicaid patients

D. Launched laboratories that became the NIH

E. Required hospitals to conduct continued-stay reviews for Medicare and Medicaid patients

F. Established the National Practitioner Data Bank

G. Requires most US citizens to have healthcare coverage

H. Required extensive changes in the Medicare program to control the rising cost of providing healthcare services to Medicare beneficiaries (PPS general implementation)

I. Instituted the Agency for Health Care Policy and Research (now the Agency for Healthcare Research and Quality)

Healthcare Providers and Settings

According to the US Department of Labor, a healthcare provider or health professional is an organization or a person who delivers proper healthcare in a systematic way professionally to any individual in need of healthcare services (29 CFR 825.118). Healthcare delivery is more than hospital-related care. It can be viewed as a continuum of services that cuts across services delivered in ambulatory, acute, sub-acute, long-term, residential, and other care environments. This section describes several of the alternatives for healthcare delivery along this continuum.

Organization and Operation of Modern Hospitals

The term **hospital** can be applied to any healthcare facility that has the following four characteristics:

- An organized medical staff,
- Permanent inpatient beds,
- Around-the-clock nursing services, and
- Diagnostic and therapeutic services.

Most hospitals provide acute-care services to inpatients. **Acute care** is the short-term care provided to diagnose and treat an illness or injury. The individuals who receive acute-care services in hospitals are considered inpatients.

An **inpatient** is a person who is provided with room, board, and continuous general nursing services in an area of an acute-care facility where patients generally stay at least overnight (AHIMA 2014a). "The physician or other practitioner responsible for a patient's care at the hospital is also responsible for deciding whether the patient should be admitted as an inpatient. The decision to admit a patient is a complex medical judgment that can be made only after the physician has considered a number of factors, including the patient's medical history and current medical needs, the types of facilities available to inpatients and to outpatients, the hospital's bylaws and admissions policies, and the relative appropriateness of treatment in each setting. Factors to be considered when making the decision to admit include such things as:

- The severity of the signs and symptoms exhibited by the patient;
- The medical predictability of something adverse happening to the patient;
- The need for diagnostic studies that appropriately are outpatient services (that is, their performance does not ordinarily require the patient to remain at the hospital for 24 hours or more) to assist in assessing whether the patient should be admitted; and
- The availability of diagnostic procedures at the time when and at the location where the patient presents" (CMS 2015a).

The average length of stay (ALOS) in an acute-care hospital is 30 days or less. Hospitals that have ALOSs longer than 30 days are considered long-term care facilities. (Long-term care is discussed in detail later in this chapter.) With ongoing advances in surgical technology, anesthesia, and pharmacology, the ALOS in an acute-care hospital is currently 4.8 days (CDC 2015). In addition, many diagnostic and therapeutic procedures that once required inpatient care can now be performed on an outpatient basis.

For example, before the development of laparoscopic surgical techniques, a patient might be hospitalized for 10 days after a routine appendectomy (surgical removal of the appendix). Today, a patient undergoing a laparoscopic appendectomy might spend only a few hours in the hospital's outpatient surgery department and go home the same day. The influence of managed care and the emphasis on cost control in the Medicare and Medicaid programs also have resulted in shorter hospital stays.

In large acute-care hospitals, hundreds of clinicians, administrators, managers, and support staff must work closely together to provide effective and efficient diagnostic and therapeutic services. Most hospitals provide services to both inpatients and outpatients. A **hospital outpatient** is a patient who receives hospital services without being admitted for inpatient (overnight) clinical care. Outpatient care is considered a kind of ambulatory care. (Ambulatory care is discussed later in this chapter.)

Types of Hospitals

Modern hospitals are complex organizations. Much of the clinical training for physicians, nurses, and allied health professionals is conducted in hospitals. Medical research is another activity carried out in hospitals. Hospitals can be classified in many different ways according to the following items:

- Number of beds
- Type of services provided
- Type of patients served
- For-profit or not-for-profit status
- Type of ownership

The following sections describe each of these criteria in detail.

Number of Beds

A hospital's number of beds is based on the number of beds that it has equipped and staffed for patient care. The term *bed capacity* is sometimes used to reflect the maximum number of inpatients for which the hospital can care. Hospitals with fewer than 100 beds are usually considered small. Most of the hospitals in the United States fall into this category, but some large, urban hospitals have more than 500 beds. The number of beds is usually broken down by adult beds and pediatric beds; the number of maternity beds and other special categories may be listed separately. Hospitals also can be categorized on the basis of the number of outpatient visits per year. The number of hospital beds declined dramatically in the late 1900s with shorter length of stays and more procedures being done on an outpatient basis.

Type of Services Provided

Some hospitals specialize in certain types of service and treat specific illnesses. For example:

- *Rehabilitation hospitals* provide long-term care services to patients recuperating from debilitating or chronic illnesses and injuries such as strokes, head and spine injuries, and gunshot wounds. Patients often stay in rehabilitation hospitals for several months.

- *Psychiatric hospitals* provide inpatient care for patients with mental and developmental disorders. In the past, the ALOS for psychiatric inpatients was longer than it is today. Rather than months or years, most patients now spend only a few days or weeks per stay. However, many patients require repeated hospitalization for chronic psychiatric illnesses. (Behavioral healthcare is discussed in detail later in this chapter.)

- *General acute-care hospitals* provide a wide range of medical and surgical services to diagnose and treat most illnesses and injuries.

- *Specialty hospitals* provide diagnostic and therapeutic services for a limited range of conditions (for example, burns, cancer, tuberculosis, obstetrics and gynecology).

Type of Patients Served

Some hospitals specialize in serving specific types of patients. For example, children's hospitals provide specialized pediatric services in a number of medical specialties. Cancer centers offer integrated treatment regimens for cancer diagnosis and therapies. There are also hospitals that specialize in surgical cases and even further specialization for cardiac or orthopedic surgeries.

For-Profit or Not-for-Profit Status

Hospitals also can be classified on the basis of their ownership and profitability status. **Not-for-profit** healthcare organizations use excess funds to improve their services and to finance educational programs and community services. **For-profit** healthcare organizations are privately owned. Excess funds are paid back to the managers, owners, and investors in the form of bonuses and dividends.

Type of Ownership

The most common ownership types for hospitals and other kinds of healthcare organizations in the United States include the following:

- *Government-owned hospitals* are operated by a specific branch of federal, state, or local government as not-for-profit organizations. Government-owned hospitals are sometimes called public hospitals. They are supported, at least in part, by tax dollars. Examples of federally owned and operated hospitals include those operated by the Department of Veterans Affairs to serve retired military personnel. The Department of Defense operates facilities for active military personnel and their dependents. Many states own and operate psychiatric hospitals. County and city governments often operate public hospitals to serve the healthcare needs of their communities, especially those residents who are unable to pay for their care.

- *Proprietary hospitals* may be owned by private foundations, partnerships, or investor-owned corporations. Large corporations may own a number of for-profit hospitals, and the stock of several large US hospital chains is publicly traded.

- *Voluntary hospitals* are not-for-profit hospitals owned by universities, churches, charities, religious orders, unions, and other not-for-profit entities. They often provide free care to patients who otherwise would not have access to healthcare services.

Organization of Hospital Services

The organizational structure of every hospital is designed to meet its specific needs. For example, most acute-care hospitals are made up of a board of directors, a professional medical staff, an executive administrative staff, medical and surgical services, patient care (nursing) services, diagnostic and laboratory services, and support services (for example, nutritional services, environmental safety, health information management services).

Board of Directors

The board of directors has primary responsibility for setting the overall direction of the hospital. In some hospitals, the board of directors is called the governing board or board of trustees. The board works with the chief executive officer (CEO) and the leaders of the organization's medical staff to develop the hospital's strategic direction as well as its mission, vision, and values:

- *Mission:* A statement of the organization's purpose and the customers it serves
- *Vision:* A description of the organization's ideal future
- *Values:* A descriptive list of the organization's fundamental principles or beliefs

Other specific responsibilities of the board of directors include the following:

- Establishing bylaws in accordance with the organization's legal and licensing requirements
- Selecting qualified administrators
- Approving the organization and makeup of the clinical staff
- Monitoring the quality of care

The board's members are elected for specific terms of service (for example, five years). Most boards also elect officers, commonly a chair, vice chair, president, secretary, and treasurer. The size of governing boards varies considerably. Individual board members are called directors, board members, or trustees. Individuals serve on one or more standing committees such as the executive committee, joint conference committee, finance committee, strategic planning committee, and building committee.

The makeup of the board depends on the type of hospital and the form of ownership. For example, the board of a community hospital is likely to include local business leaders, representatives of community organizations, and other people interested in the welfare of the community. The board of a teaching hospital, on the other hand, is likely to include medical school alumni and university administrators, among others.

Boards of directors face strict accountability in terms of cost containment, performance management, and integration of services to maintain fiscal stability and to ensure the delivery of high-quality patient care.

Medical Staff

The medical staff consists of physicians who have received extensive training in various medical disciplines (for example, internal medicine, pediatrics, cardiology, obstetrics and gynecology, orthopedics, surgery). The medical staff's primary objective is to provide high-quality care to the patients who come to the hospital. The physicians on the hospital's medical staff diagnose illnesses and develop patient-centered treatment regimens. Moreover, physicians on the medical staff may serve on the hospital's governing board, where they provide critical insight relevant to strategic and operational planning and policy making.

The medical staff is the aggregate of physicians who have been granted permission to provide clinical services in the hospital. This permission is called **clinical privileges**. An individual physician's privileges are limited to a specific scope of practice. For example, an internal medicine physician would be permitted to diagnose and treat a patient with pneumonia but not to perform a surgical procedure. Most members of the medical staff are not employees of the hospital. However, there are exceptions as many hospitals employ radiologists, anesthesiologists, and hospitalists. Additionally, hospitals may contract with companies to provide physicians for specific services like emergency room physicians or radiologists.

Medical staff classification refers to the organization of physicians according to clinical assignment. Typical medical staff classifications include active, provisional, honorary, consulting, courtesy, and medical resident assignments. Depending on the size of the hospital and on the credentials and clinical privileges of its physicians, the medical staff may be separated into departments such as medicine, surgery, obstetrics, pediatrics, and other specialty services.

Officers of the medical staff usually include a president or chief of staff, a vice president or chief of staff elect, and a secretary. These offices are authorized by vote of the entire active medical staff. The president presides at all regular meetings of the medical staff and is an ex officio member of all medical staff committees. The secretary ensures that accurate and complete minutes of medical staff meetings are maintained and that correspondence is handled appropriately.

The medical staff operates according to a predetermined set of policies. These policies are called the **medical staff bylaws**. The bylaws spell out the specific qualifications that physicians must demonstrate before they can practice medicine in the hospital. The bylaws are considered legally binding. Any changes to the bylaws must be approved by a vote of the medical staff and the hospital's governing body.

Administrative Staff

The leader of the administrative staff is the **chief executive officer (CEO)**. The CEO is responsible for implementing the policies and strategic direction set by the hospital's board of directors. He or she also is responsible for building an effective executive management team and coordinating the hospital's services. Today's healthcare organizations commonly designate a chief financial officer (CFO), a chief operating officer (COO), and a chief information officer (CIO) as members of the executive management team.

The executive management team is responsible for managing the hospital's finances and ensuring that the hospital complies with the federal, state, and local regulations, standards, and laws that govern the delivery of healthcare services. Depending on the size of the hospital, the CEO's staff may include healthcare administrators with job titles such as vice president, associate administrator, department director or manager, or administrative assistant. Department-level administrators manage and coordinate the activities of the highly specialized and multidisciplinary units that perform clinical, administrative, and support services in the hospital.

Healthcare administrators may hold advanced degrees in healthcare administration, nursing, public health, or business management. A growing number of hospitals are hiring physician executives to lead their executive management teams. Many healthcare administrators are fellows of the American College of Healthcare Executives.

Patient Care Services

Most of the direct patient care delivered in hospitals is provided by professional nurses. Modern nursing requires a diverse skill set, advanced clinical competencies, and postgraduate education. In almost every hospital, patient care services constitute the largest clinical department in terms of staffing, budget, specialized services offered, and clinical expertise required.

Nurses are responsible for providing continuous, around-the-clock treatment and support for hospital inpatients. The quantity and quality of nursing care available to patients are influenced by a number of factors, including the nursing staff's educational preparation and specialization, experience, and skill level. The level of patient care staffing is also a critical component of quality.

Traditionally, physicians alone determined the type of treatment each patient received. However, today's nurses are playing a wider role in treatment planning and case management. They identify timely and effective interventions in response to a wide range of problems related to the patients' treatment, comfort, and safety. Their responsibilities include performing patient assessments, creating care plans, evaluating the appropriateness of treatment, and evaluating the effectiveness of care. At the same time that they provide technical care, effective nursing professionals also offer personal caring that recognizes the patients' concerns and the emotional needs of patients and their families.

Diagnostic and Therapeutic Services

The services provided to patients in hospitals go beyond the clinical services provided directly by the medical and nursing staff. Many diagnostic and therapeutic services involve the work of allied health professionals. Allied health professionals receive specialized education and training, and their qualifications are registered or certified by a number of specialty organizations.

Diagnostic and therapeutic services are critical to the success of every patient care delivery system. Diagnostic services include clinical laboratory, radiology, and nuclear medicine. Therapeutic services include radiation therapy, occupational therapy, and physical therapy.

Clinical Laboratory Services The clinical laboratory is divided into two sections: anatomic pathology and clinical pathology. Anatomic pathology deals with human tissues and provides surgical pathology, autopsy, and cytology services. Clinical pathology deals mainly with the analysis of body fluids, principally blood, but also urine, gastric contents, and cerebrospinal fluid.

Physicians who specialize in performing and interpreting the results of pathology tests are called pathologists. Laboratory technicians are allied health professionals trained to operate laboratory equipment and perform laboratory tests under the supervision of a pathologist.

Radiology Radiology involves the use of radioactive isotopes, fluoroscopic and radiographic equipment, and CT and MRI equipment to diagnose disease. Physicians who specialize in radiology are called radiologists. They are experts in the medical use of radiant energy, radioactive isotopes, radium, cesium, and cobalt as well as x-rays and radioactive materials. They also are experts in interpreting x-ray, MRI, and CT diagnostic images. Radiology technicians are allied health professionals trained to operate radiological equipment and perform radiological tests under the supervision of a radiologist.

Nuclear Medicine and Radiation Therapy Radiologists also may specialize in nuclear medicine and radiation therapy. Nuclear medicine involves the use of ionizing radiation and small amounts of short-lived radioactive tracers to treat disease, specifically neoplastic disease (that is, nonmalignant tumors and malignant cancers). Because of the mathematics and physics of tracer methodology, nuclear medicine is widely applied in clinical medicine. However, most authorities agree that medical science has only scratched the surface in terms of nuclear medicine's potential capabilities.

Radiation therapy uses high-energy x-rays, cobalt, electrons, and other sources of radiation to treat human disease. In current practice, radiation therapy is used alone or in combination with surgery or chemotherapy (drugs) to treat many types of cancer. In addition to external beam therapy, radioactive implants and therapy performed with heat (hyperthermia) are available.

Occupational Therapy Occupational therapy is the medically directed use of work and play activities to improve patients' independent functioning, enhance their development, and prevent or decrease their level of disability. The individuals who perform occupational therapy are credentialed allied health professionals called occupational therapists. They work under the direction of physicians. Occupational therapy is made available in acute-care hospitals, clinics, and rehabilitation centers.

Providing occupational therapy services begins with an evaluation of the patient and the selection of therapeutic goals. Occupational therapy activities may involve the adaptation of tasks or the environment to achieve maximum independence and to enhance the patient's quality of life. An occupational therapist may treat decreased functionality related to developmental deficits, birth defects, learning disabilities, traumatic injuries, burns, neurological conditions, orthopedic conditions, mental deficiencies, and psychiatric disorders. Within the healthcare system, occupational therapy plays various roles. These roles include promoting health, preventing disability, developing or restoring functional capacity, guiding adaptation within physical and mental parameters, and teaching creative problem solving to increase independent function.

Physical Therapy and Rehabilitation Physical therapy and rehabilitation services have expanded into many medical specialties—especially in neurology, neurosurgery, orthopedics, geriatrics, rheumatology, internal medicine, cardiovascular medicine, cardiopulmonary medicine, psychiatry, sports medicine, burn and wound care, and chronic pain management. It also plays a role in community health education. Credentialed allied health professionals administer physical therapy under the direction of physicians.

Medical rehabilitation services involve the entire healthcare team: physicians, nurses, social workers, occupational therapists, physical therapists, and other healthcare personnel. The objective is to either eliminate the patients' disability or alleviate it as fully as possible. Physical therapy can be used to improve the cognitive, social, and physical abilities of patients impaired by chronic disease or injury.

The primary purpose of physical therapy in rehabilitation is to promote optimal health and function by applying scientific principles. Treatment modalities include therapeutic exercise, therapeutic massage, biofeedback, and applications of heat, low-energy lasers, cold, water, electricity, and ultrasound.

Respiratory Therapy Respiratory therapy involves the treatment of patients who have acute or chronic lung disorders. Respiratory therapists work under the direction of qualified physicians and surgeons. The therapists provide such services as emergency care for stroke, heart failure, and shock patients. They also treat patients with chronic respiratory diseases such as emphysema and asthma.

Respiratory treatments include the administration of oxygen and inhalants such as bronchodilators. Respiratory therapists set up and monitor ventilator equipment and provide physiotherapy to improve breathing.

Ancillary Support Services

The ancillary units of the hospital provide vital clinical and administrative support services to patients, medical staff, visitors, and employees.

Clinical Support Services The clinical support units provide the following services:

- Pharmaceutical services
- Food and nutrition services
- Health information management (health record) services
- Social work and social services
- Patient advocacy services
- Environmental (housekeeping) services
- Purchasing, central supply, and materials management services
- Engineering and plant operations

Health information management (HIM) services are managed by credentialed health information management professionals—RHIAs and RHITs. The pharmacy is staffed by registered pharmacists and pharmacy technologists. Food and nutrition services are managed by registered dietitians (RDs), who develop general menus, special-diet menus, and nutritional plans for individual patients. Social work services are provided by licensed social workers and licensed clinical social workers. Patient advocacy services may be provided by several types of healthcare professionals, most commonly, registered nurses and licensed social workers.

Administrative Support Services In addition to clinical support services, hospitals need administrative support services to operate effectively. Administrative support services provide business management and clerical services in several key areas, including

- Admissions and central registration
- Claims and billing (business office)
- Accounting
- Information services
- Human resources
- Public relations
- Fund development
- Marketing

✓ Check Your Understanding **1.3**

Instructions: **On a separate piece of paper, write the best terms to complete the following sentences.**

1. _____ is short-term care provided to inpatients.
   A. Outpatient care
   B. Ambulatory care
   C. Acute care
   D. Long-term care

2. Hospitals can be classified according to which of the following?
   A. Number of beds
   B. State in which they reside
   C. Medical staff
   D. Age

3. _____ hospitals may be owned by private foundations, partnerships, or investor-owned corporations.
   A. Government-owned
   B. Voluntary
   C. State-owned
   D. Proprietary

4. Selecting qualified administrators is the responsibility of:
   A. The board of directors
   B. Hospital administration
   C. The medical staff
   D. The nursing staff

5. _____ is the medically directed use of work and play activities to improve patient's functioning.
   A. Physical therapy
   B. Occupational therapy
   C. Social services
   D. Nursing

6. Rehabilitation services include which of the following?
   A. Nursing
   B. Health information
   C. Medical staff
   D. Physical therapy

7. The _____ is responsible for implementing the policies and strategic direction of the hospital.
   A. Chief financial officer
   B. Chief executive officer
   C. Chief nursing officer
   D. Chief information officer

8. _____ is divided into two sections, anatomic and clinical pathology.
   A. Radiology
   B. Nursing
   C. Health information
   D. Clinical laboratory services

Organization of Ambulatory Care

Ambulatory care is the provision of preventative or corrective healthcare services on a nonresident basis in a provider's office, clinic setting, or hospital outpatient setting (AHIMA 2014a). Ambulatory care encompasses all the health services provided to individual patients who are not residents in a healthcare facility. Such services include the educational services provided by community health clinics and public health departments. Primary care, emergency care, and ambulatory specialty care (including ambulatory surgery) can all be considered ambulatory care. Ambulatory care services are provided in a variety of settings including urgent care centers, school-based clinics, public health clinics, and neighborhood and community health centers.

Current medical practice emphasizes performing healthcare services in the least costly setting possible. This change in thinking has led to decreased utilization of emergency services, increased utilization of nonemergency ambulatory facilities, decreased hospital admissions, and shorter hospital stays. The need to reduce the cost of healthcare also has led primary care physicians to treat conditions they once would have referred to specialists.

Physicians who provide ambulatory care services fall into two major categories: physicians working in private practice and physicians working for ambulatory care organizations. Physicians in private practice are self-employed. They work in solo, partnership, and group practices set up as for-profit organizations. Alternatively, physicians who work for ambulatory care organizations are employees of those organizations. Ambulatory care organizations include the following:

- health maintenance organizations
- hospital-based ambulatory clinics
- walk-in and emergency clinics
- hospital-owned group practices and health promotion centers
- freestanding surgery centers
- freestanding urgent care centers
- freestanding emergency care centers
- health department clinics
- neighborhood clinics
- home care agencies
- community mental health centers
- school and workplace health service agencies
- prison health services agencies

Ambulatory care organizations also employ other healthcare providers including nurses, laboratory technicians, podiatrists, chiropractors, physical therapists, radiology technicians, psychologists, and social workers.

Private Medical Practice

Private medical practices are physician-owned entities that provide primary care or medical and surgical specialty care services in a freestanding office setting. The physicians have medical privileges at local hospitals and surgical centers but are not employees of those healthcare entities.

Hospital-Based Ambulatory Care Services

In addition to providing inpatient services, many acute-care hospitals provide various ambulatory care services.

Emergency Services and Trauma Care

Hospital-based emergency departments provide specialized care for victims of traumatic accidents and life-threatening illnesses. In urban areas, many also provide walk-in services for patients with minor illnesses and injuries who do not have access to regular primary care physicians.

Many physicians on the hospital staff also use the emergency care department as a setting to assess patients with problems that may either lead to an inpatient admission or require equipment or diagnostic imaging facilities not available in a private office or nursing home. Emergency services function as a major source of unscheduled admissions to the hospital.

Outpatient Surgical Services

Ambulatory surgery refers to any surgical procedure that does not require an overnight stay in a hospital. It can be performed in the outpatient surgery department of a hospital or in a freestanding ambulatory surgery center. Over the past decade the number of visits to freestanding ambulatory surgery centers increased dramatically while the rate of visits to hospital-based surgical centers remained about the same (CDC 2009). The increased number of procedures performed in an ambulatory setting can be attributed to improvements in surgical technology and anesthesia and the utilization management demands of third-party payers.

Outpatient Diagnostic and Therapeutic Services

Outpatient diagnostic and therapeutic services are provided in a hospital or one of its satellite facilities. Diagnostic services are those services performed by a physician to identify the disease or condition from which the patient is suffering. Therapeutic services are those services performed by a physician to treat the disease or condition that has been identified.

Hospital outpatients fall into different classifications according to the type of service they receive and the location of the service. For example, emergency outpatients are treated in the hospital's emergency or trauma care department for conditions that require immediate care. Clinic outpatients are treated in one of the hospital's clinical departments on an ambulatory basis. And referral outpatients receive special diagnostic or therapeutic services in the hospital on an ambulatory basis, but responsibility for their care remains with the referring physician.

Community-Based Ambulatory Care Services

Community-based ambulatory care services refer to those services provided in freestanding facilities that are not owned by or affiliated with a hos-

pital. Such facilities can range in size from a small medical practice with a single physician to a large clinic with an organized medical staff (Masters and Nester 2001). Among the organizations that provide ambulatory care services are specialized treatment facilities. Examples of these facilities include birthing centers, cancer treatment centers, renal dialysis centers, and rehabilitation centers.

Freestanding Ambulatory Care Centers

Freestanding ambulatory care centers (ACCs) provide emergency services and urgent care for walk-in patients. Urgent care centers (sometimes called emergicenters or immediate care centers) provide diagnostic and therapeutic care for patients with minor illnesses and injuries. They do not serve seriously ill patients and most do not accept ambulance cases.

Two groups of patients find these centers attractive. The first group consists of patients seeking the convenience and access of emergency services without the delays and other forms of negative feedback associated with using hospital services for nonurgent problems. The second group consists of patients whose insurance treats urgent care centers preferentially compared with physicians' offices.

As they have increased in number and become familiar to more patients, many of these centers now offer a combination of walk-in and appointment services. In 2000, the first retail clinics opened and their number increased rapidly. From 2006 to 2014, retail clinics grew from 200 to 1,800 and the number of visits grew from 1.5 million to 10.5 million in 2012 (Rand Health 2015). These **retail clinics** treat non–life-threatening acute illnesses and offer routine wellness services such as flu shots, sports physicals, and prescription refills. These visits are covered by most insurers including Medicare.

Freestanding Ambulatory Surgery Centers

Generally, freestanding ambulatory surgery centers provide surgical procedures that take anywhere from 5 to 90 minutes to perform and that require less than a four-hour recovery period. Patients must schedule their surgeries in advance and be prepared to return home on the same day. Patients who experience surgical complications are sent to an inpatient facility for care.

Most ambulatory surgery centers are for-profit entities. They may be owned by individual physicians, managed care organizations, or entrepreneurs. Generally, ambulatory care centers can provide surgical services at lower cost than hospitals can because their overhead expenses are lower.

Public Health Services

Although the states have constitutional authority to implement public health, a wide variety of federal programs and laws assist them. HHS is the principal federal agency for ensuring health and providing essential human services. All its agencies have some responsibility for prevention. Through its 10 regional offices, HHS coordinates closely with state and local government agencies, and many HHS-funded services are provided by these agencies as well as by private-sector and nonprofit organizations.

The Office of the Secretary of HHS has two units important to public health: the Office of the Surgeon General of the United States and the Office of Disease Prevention and Health Promotion (ODPHP). ODPHP has an analysis and leadership role for health promotion and disease prevention.

The **surgeon general** is appointed by the president of the United States and provides leadership and authoritative, science-based recommendations about the public's health. The surgeon general has responsibility for the public health service (PHS) workforce (HHS 2012).

Home Care Services

Home healthcare is a wide range of healthcare services that can be delivered in the home and it is the fastest-growing sector to offer services for Medicare recipients (Medicare.gov 2015a). The primary reason for this is increased economic pressure from third-party payers. In other words, third-party payers want patients released from the hospital more quickly than they were in the past to reduce cost. Moreover, patients generally prefer to be cared for in their own homes. In fact, most patients prefer home care, no matter how complex their medical problems. Research indicates that the medical outcomes of home care patients are similar to those of patients treated (Medicare.gov 2015b) in skilled nursing facilities (SNFs) for similar conditions.

In 1989, Medicare rules for home care services were clarified to make it easier for Medicare beneficiaries to receive such services. Patients are eligible to receive home health services from a qualified Medicare provider when they are homebound; when they are under the care of a specified physician who will establish a home health plan; and when they need physical or occupational therapy, speech therapy, or intermittent skilled nursing care.

Skilled nursing care is defined as both technical procedures, such as tube feedings and catheter care, and skilled nursing observations that are required on an intermittent basis and can be delivered at home (Medicare.gov 2015b). Intermittent is defined as up to 28 hours per week for nursing care and 35 hours per week for home health aide care (Medicare.gov 2015b). Many hospitals have formed their own home healthcare agencies to increase revenues and at the same time allow them to discharge patients from the hospital earlier.

Voluntary Agencies

Voluntary agencies provide healthcare and healthcare planning services, usually at the local level and to low-income patients. Their services range from giving free immunizations to offering family planning counseling. Funds to operate such agencies come from a variety of sources, including local or state health departments, private grants, and different federal bureaus.

One common example of a voluntary agency is the community health center. Sometimes called neighborhood health centers, community health centers offer comprehensive, primary healthcare services to patients who otherwise would not have access to them. Often patients pay for these services on a sliding scale based on income or according to a flat rate, discounted fee schedule supplemented by public funding.

Some voluntary agencies offer specialized services such as counseling for battered and abused women. Typically, these are set up within local communities. An example of a voluntary agency that offers services on a much larger scale is the Red Cross.

Check Your Understanding 1.4

Instructions: **On a separate piece of paper, indicate whether the following statements are true or false (T or F).**

1. _____ Current medical practice emphasizes performing healthcare services in the least costly setting possible.

2. _____ Emergency services are not a major source of unscheduled admissions to a hospital.

3. _____ Improvements in surgical technology and anesthesia have increased the number of surgical procedures performed in an ambulatory setting.

4. _____ Community-based ambulatory care services are provided in a freestanding facility not owned or affiliated with a hospital.

5. _____ Retail clinics treat life-threatening acute illnesses.

6. _____ CMS is the principal federal agency for ensuring health and providing essential human services.

7. _____ One common example of a voluntary agency is the community health center.

8. _____ Voluntary agencies do not offer specialized services.

9. _____ Patients in post-acute care do not require ongoing medical management or therapeutic, rehabilitative, or nursing services.

10. _____ Living environments that are more homelike and less institutional are known as residential care facilities.

Telehealth

Telehealth uses communication technology between the patient and the provider or the provider and a specialist to deliver healthcare services. This could be monitoring blood sugar or vital signs and providing that information to a clinician or video-conferencing to deliver consultations or surgical support. Ideally, the clinical content will provide two-way communication of not just physiological information (namely vital signs) but education and compliance information as well. Rich clinical content provides diagnosis-specific information, including programs for comorbidity diagnoses that takes patient responses into account when determining the next question. For instance, if a congestive heart failure patient does not demonstrate an understanding of the significance of shortness of breath or the importance of taking medications each day, the system uses branching logic to transmit appropriate educational information. This individualizes each encounter the patient has with the telehealth system.

Daily documentation of patient information using telehealth technology allows the care provider to track health patterns over time and detect deviations in patient data that may indicate a decline in health before it becomes acute. A telehealth system can provide alerts that are activated when patient-specific baselines exceed a given parameter—weight, for instance.

Long-Term Care

Long-term care is the healthcare rendered in a non–acute-care facility to patients who require inpatient nursing and related services for more than 30 consecutive days. Skilled nursing facilities, nursing homes, long-term care facilities, and rehabilitation hospitals are the principal facilities that provide long-term care. Rehabilitation hospitals provide recuperative services for patients who have suffered strokes and traumatic injuries as well as other serious illnesses. Specialized long-term care facilities serve patients with chronic respiratory disease, permanent cognitive impairment, and other incapacitating conditions.

Long-term care encompasses a range of health, personal care, social, and housing services provided to people of all ages with health conditions that limit their ability to carry out normal daily activities without assistance. People who need long-term care often have multiple physical and mental disabilities. Moreover, their need for the mix and intensity of long-term care services can change over time.

Long-term care is mainly rehabilitative and supportive rather than curative. Moreover, healthcare workers other than physicians can provide long-term care in the home or in residential or institutional settings. For the most part, long-term care requires little or no technology, however, there is growing adoption of electronic health records in long-term care facilities (AHIMA 2014b).

Long-Term Care and the Continuum of Care

The availability and cost of long-term care is one of the most important health issues in the United States today. In the United States in 2010, 13 percent of the population was over the age of 65 and by 2030 that number is expected to jump to 19 percent. In this population, the number of individuals experiencing two or more functional limitations will increase to 21 million in 2040 (Robert Wood Johnson Foundation 2014).

As discussed earlier, healthcare is now viewed as a **continuum of care**. That is, patients are provided care by different caregivers at several different levels of the healthcare system. In the case of long-term care, the patient's continuum of care may have begun with a primary provider in a hospital and then continued with home care and eventually care in an SNF. That patient's care is coordinated from one care setting to the next.

Moreover, the roles of the different care providers along the patient's continuum of care are continuing to evolve. Health information managers play a key part in providing consultation services to long-term care facilities with regard to developing systems to manage information from a diverse number of healthcare providers.

Post-Acute Care

Post-acute care supports patients who require ongoing medical management or therapeutic, rehabilitative, or skilled nursing care (AHA 2010b). Patients require frequent physician oversight and advanced nursing care but no longer require the acute interventions and diagnostic services of acute-care settings. It is delivered in a variety of environments, including long-term acute-care hospitals, skilled nursing facilities, rehabilitation centers, and at home-by-home health services (AHA 2010a). In 2015, there were 428 long-term acute-care hospitals (LTACHs) in the United States (LTPAC HIT 2015). Covered by Medicare, LTACHs provide intensive long-term services for patients with complex medical problems (AHA 2015). To qualify as an LTACH for Medicare payment, a facility must meet Medicare's conditions of participation for acute-care hospitals and have an average inpatient length of stay greater than 25 days.

Delivery of Long-Term Care Services

Long-term care services are delivered in a variety of settings. Among these settings are SNFs or nursing homes, residential care facilities, hospice programs, and adult day care programs.

Skilled Nursing Facilities or Nursing Homes

The most important providers of formal, long-term care services are nursing homes. **Skilled nursing facilities (SNFs)**, or nursing homes, provide medical, nursing, and, in some cases, rehabilitative care around the clock. The majority of SNF residents are over age 65 and quite often are classified as the frail elderly.

Many nursing homes are owned by for-profit organizations. However, SNFs also may be owned by not-for-profit groups as well as local, state, and federal governments. Nursing homes are no longer the only option for patients needing long-term care. Various factors play a role in determining which type of long-term care facility is best for a particular patient, including cost, access to services, and individual needs.

Residential Care Facilities

New living environments that are more homelike and less institutional are the focus of much attention in the current long-term care market (assisted living and memory care centers, for example). Residential care facilities now play a growing role in the continuum of long-term care services. Having affordable and appropriate housing available for elderly and disabled people can reduce the level of need for institutional long-term care services in the community. Institutionalization can be postponed or prevented when the elderly and disabled live in safe and accessible settings where assistance with daily activities is available.

Hospice Programs

Hospice care is provided mainly in the home to the terminally ill and their families. Hospice is based on a philosophy of care imported from England and Canada that holds that during the course of terminal illness, the patient should be able to live life as fully and as comfortably as possible but without artificial or mechanical efforts to prolong life.

In the hospice approach, the family is the unit of treatment. An interdisciplinary team provides medical, nursing, psychological, therapeutic, pharmacological, and spiritual support during the final stages of illness, at the time of death, and during bereavement. The main goals are to control pain, maintain independence, and minimize the stress and trauma of death.

Hospice services have gained acceptance as an alternative to hospital care for the terminally ill. The number of hospices is likely to continue to grow because this philosophy of care for people at the end of life has become a model for the nation.

Adult Day Care Programs

Adult day care programs offer a wide range of health and social services to elderly persons during the daytime hours. Adult day care services are usually targeted to elderly members of families in which the regular caregivers work during the day.

Many elderly people who live alone also benefit from leaving their homes every day to participate in programs designed to keep them active. The goals of adult day care programs are to delay the need for institutionalization and to provide respite for the caregivers. They are also known as day health centers.

Behavioral Health Services

From the mid-19th century to the mid-20th century, psychiatric services in the United States were based primarily in long-stay institutions supported by state governments and patterns of practice were relatively stable. Over the past 50 years, however, remarkable changes have occurred. These changes include a reversal of the balance between institutional and community care, inpatient and outpatient services, and individual and group practice.

The shift to community-based settings began in the public sector, and community settings remain dominant. The private sector's bed capacity increased in the 1970s and 1980s, including psychiatric units in nonfederal general hospitals, private psychiatric hospitals, and residential treatment centers for children. Substance abuse centers and child and adolescent inpatient psychiatric units grew particularly quickly in the 1980s, as investors recognized their profitability. In the 1990s, the growth of inpatient private mental health facilities leveled off and the number of outpatient and partial treatment settings increased sharply. The number of mental health organizations providing 24-hour services (hospital inpatient and residential treatment) increased significantly over the 32-year period from 1970 to 2002 (Foley et al. 2004). Because of deinstitutionalization and the closure of public psychiatric hospitals, community hospitals are the primary source of inpatient psychiatric care delivered in either designated psychiatric units or in scatter beds throughout the medical units (Mark et al. 2010). In 2010, the AHA reported only 406 dedicated nonfederal psychiatric hospitals (AHA 2014).

Residential treatment centers for emotionally or behaviorally disturbed children provide inpatient services to children under 18 years of age.

The programs and physical facilities of residential treatment centers are designed to meet patients' daily living, schooling, recreational, socialization, and routine medical care needs.

Day hospital or day treatment programs occupy one niche in the spectrum of behavioral healthcare settings. Although some provide services seven days a week, many programs provide services only during business hours. Day treatment patients spend most of the day at the treatment facility in a program of structured therapeutic activities and then return to their homes until the next day. Day treatment services include psychotherapy, pharmacology, occupational therapy, and other types of rehabilitation services. These programs provide alternatives to inpatient care or serve as transitions from inpatient to outpatient care or discharge. They also may provide respite for family caregivers and a place for rehabilitating or maintaining chronically ill patients. The number of day treatment programs has increased in response to pressures to decrease the length of hospital stays.

Insurance coverage for behavioral healthcare has always lagged behind coverage for other medical care. Although treatments and treatment settings have changed, rising healthcare costs, the absence of strong consumer demand for behavioral health coverage, and insurers' continuing fear of the potential cost of this coverage have maintained the differences between medical and behavioral healthcare benefits. Although the majority of individuals who are covered by health insurance have some outpatient psychiatric coverage, the coverage is often quite restricted. Typical restrictions include limits on the number of outpatient visits, higher copayment charges, and higher deductibles.

Behavioral healthcare has changed significantly over the past 40 years, as psychopharmacologic treatment has made possible the shift away from long-term custodial treatment. Psychosocial treatments continue the process of care and rehabilitation in community settings. There are fewer large state hospitals; they have been replaced by psychiatric units in general hospitals, new outpatient clinics, community mental health centers, day treatment centers, and halfway houses. Treatment has become more effective and specific, based on our growing understanding of the brain and behavior (Kovner et al. 2011).

Integrated Delivery Systems

Many hospitals have responded to financial pressures by rapidly merging, acquiring, and entering into affiliations and various risk-sharing reimbursement agreements with other acute and nonacute providers, hospital-based healthcare systems, physicians and physician group practices, and managed care organizations. Transactions have included mergers of nonprofit organizations into either investor-owned or other nonprofit entities.

The goal of integrated delivery systems (IDSs) is to organize the entire continuum of care, from health promotion and disease prevention to primary and secondary acute care, tertiary care, long-term care, and hospice care, to maximize its effectiveness across episodes of illness and pathways of wellness.

Managed care and healthcare organization integration have placed enormous pressure on information systems. The need for cost data, as well as the integration of data from the various components of integrated systems, has placed many demands on systems technology and personnel. A healthcare provider that cannot completely analyze the cost of delivery when dealing with an insurer is at a distinct disadvantage. Similarly, an inability to integrate patient data across a system can produce increased costs, inefficiencies, and even medical errors.

An **integrated delivery system (IDS)** combines the financial and clinical aspects of healthcare and uses a group of healthcare providers, selected on the basis of quality and cost management criteria, to furnish comprehensive health services across the continuum of care (AHIMA 2014a). An IDN may also be called integrated health system, integrated delivery system (network), integrated care system (network), organized delivery system, community care network, integrated healthcare organization, integrated service network, or population-based integrated delivery system. These are all referring to the same thing.

The Affordable Care Act created a new model of integrated delivery system called the **accountable care organization (ACO)**. An ACO is a group of service providers that work together to manage and coordinate care to Medicare fee-for-service beneficiaries. Guidelines for the establishment of an ACO are under the purview of the secretary of HHS, but they may include quality reporting, e-prescribing, and the use of electronic health records.

Check Your Understanding 1.5

Instructions: On a separate piece of paper, indicate whether the following statements are true or false (T or F).

1. _____ Ambulatory care is the short-term care provided to diagnose and treat an illness or injury.

2. _____ The influence of managed care and the emphasis on cost control in the Medicare and Medicaid programs have resulted in shorter hospital stays.

3. _____ Hospitals can be classified on the basis of their type of ownership.

4. _____ Government hospitals are operated by a specific branch of federal, state, or local government as for-profit organizations.

5. _____ The board of directors has primary responsibility for setting the overall direction of the hospital.

6. _____ Medical staff classification refers to the organization of physicians according to clinical assignment.

7. _____ A registered nurse qualified by advanced education and clinical and management experience usually administers patient care services.

8. _____ Physicians who specialize in radiology are called radiology technicians.

9. _____ Occupational therapy is made available in acute-care hospitals, clinics, and rehabilitation centers.

10. _____ The ancillary units of the hospital provide vital clinical and administrative support services to patients, medical staff, visitors, and employees.

Forces Affecting Hospitals

A number of developments in healthcare delivery have had far-reaching effects on the operation of hospitals in the United States.

Development of Peer Review and Quality Improvement Programs

The goal of high-quality patient care is to "promote, preserve, and restore health. High-quality care is delivered in an appropriate setting in a manner that is satisfying to patients. It is achieved when the patient's health status is improved as much as possible. Quality has several components, including the following:

- Appropriateness (the right care is provided at the right time)

- Technical excellence (the right care is provided in the right manner)

- Accessibility (the right care can be obtained when it is needed)
- Acceptability (the patients are satisfied)" (Stokes 2004)

Peer Review

In **peer review**, a member of a profession assesses the work of colleagues within that same profession. Peer review has traditionally been at the center of quality assessment and assurance efforts. The medical profession's peer review efforts have emphasized the scientific aspects of quality. Appropriate use of pharmaceuticals, postoperative infection rates, and accuracy of diagnosis are among the measures of quality that have been used. Peer review is a requirement of both CMS and the Joint Commission.

Quality Improvement

Quality improvement (QI) programs have been in place in hospitals for years and have been required by the Medicare and Medicaid programs and accreditation standards. QI programs have covered medical staff as well as nursing and other departments or processes.

Efforts to encourage the delivery of high-quality care take place at the local and national levels. Such efforts are geared toward assessing the efforts of both individuals and institutions. Currently, professional associations, healthcare organizations, government agencies, private external quality review associations, consumer groups, managed care organizations, and group purchasers of care all play a role in trying to promote high-quality care. (Refer to chapter 21 for more detail on clinical quality improvement).

Meaningful Use of Electronic Health Records The ARRA legislation passed in 2009 provides for economic incentives for hospitals and eligible providers who can demonstrate meaningful use of certified electronic health records. The incentive program started in October 2010 and if hospitals have not met the criteria by 2015 they are subject to payment penalties (CMS 2015c). Hospitals must first ensure that they possess a certified EHR. This may be done by acquiring a new system that is certified through an accredited certification body or by having current systems certified by that

body. Then hospitals must meet a set of required performance objectives and choose from a list of elective measures that they must attest are being used in their organization. Some of the core objectives include the following:

- Maintain active medical allergy list
- Record standardized patient demographics
- Record vital signs and chart changes
- Maintain an active medication list
- Implement systems to protect patient privacy and security of patient data in the EHR
- Maintain a current problem list
- Engage patients through electronic access to their information and the ability to email providers

Finally, the EHR must be able to directly report quality measures to CMS. In 2015, over 4,800 hospitals and almost 531,000 medical professionals had taken part in this program (CMS 2015c). This has dramatically changed the landscape for health information management practice as an unprecedented investment in technology is underway and resulted in systems that are implemented and used to manage care. Because meaningful use impacts many aspects of healthcare delivery, it is discussed in a number of chapters in this book. The primary source for locating information about the Meaningful Use Incentive Payment Program can be found on the CMS website (CMS 2015c).

Malpractice

The federal government became involved in the quality-of-care and malpractice issues through the establishment of the NPDB under the Healthcare Quality Improvement Act of 1986. Congress enacted this legislation to

- moderate the incidence of malpractice,
- allow the medical community to demonstrate new willingness to weed out incompetence, and
- improve the base of timely and accurate information on medical malpractice.

The act required hospitals to request information from the data bank whenever they hire, grant privileges, or conduct periodic reviews of a practitioner. (See chapter 2 for additional discussion of malpractice and other legal issues affecting HIM.)

Growth of Managed Care

Managed care is a generic term for a healthcare reimbursement system that manages cost, quality, and access to services. Most managed care plans do not provide healthcare directly. Instead, they enter into service contracts with the physicians, hospitals, and other healthcare providers who provide medical services to enrollees in the plans.

Managed care systems control costs primarily by presetting payment amounts and restricting patient access to healthcare services through precertification and utilization review (UR) processes. (Managed care is discussed in more detail in chapter 7.) Managed care delivery systems also attempt to manage cost and quality by:

- Implementing various forms of financial incentives for providers
- Promoting healthy lifestyles
- Identifying risk factors and illnesses early in the disease process
- Providing patient education

Restructured initiatives and increased use of technology have streamlined operations and improved operational efficiencies over recent years for the managed care industry. There are three types of managed care plans—health maintenance organizations, preferred provider organizations, and point of service plans. The more flexible a plan, the higher the cost. **Health maintenance organizations (HMOs)** usually only pay for care within their own network and the primary care doctor coordinates care. A **preferred provider organization (PPO)** usually will pay for care delivered outside the network, but it may cost the individual more. A **point of service (POS) plan** lets the beneficiary choose between the HMO or PPO model each time care is accessed.

Efforts at Healthcare Reengineering

During the 1980s and 1990s, healthcare organizations attempted to adopt continuous quality improvement (CQI) processes. Lessons learned from other areas of business were applied to healthcare settings. Reengineering came in many varieties, such as focused process improvement, major business process improvement, and business process innovation; total quality management (TQM); and CQI. Regardless of the approach, healthcare organizations attempted to look inside and think "process" as opposed to traditional "department" thinking. Healthcare organizations formed cross-functional teams that collaborated to solve organizational problems. At the same time, the Joint Commission reengineered the accreditation process to increase its focus on process and systems analysis. Gone were the days of thinking in a "silo." All of those silos were turned over and healthcare teams learned from each other. The drivers of reengineering included cost reduction, staff shortages, patient satisfaction, and implementation of technology.

Value-Based Purchasing

Medicare launched the **value-based purchasing** program in fiscal year 2013 as required by the ACA. The intent is to pay for care that rewards better value, patient outcomes, and innovation rather than just the volume of care provided. The Hospital Inpatient Quality Reporting measure infrastructure is used to identify quality care. Hospitals are evaluated and assigned points based on their performance compared to peer groups and their own performance improvement over time. Clinical process and patient experience criteria are both included in the evaluation. Because the funding for the incentive increase is taken out of the overall pool of prospective payment funds, hospitals that do not qualify for payment increases may experience reduction in payment. Certainly data collection, management, and reporting will be an important part of successful compliance.

Emphasis on Patient-Focused Care

Patient-focused care is a concept developed to contain hospital inpatient costs and improve quality by restructuring services so that more of them take place in the nursing units (patient floors) and not in specialized units in dispersed hospital locations. The emphasis is on cross-training staff in the nursing units to perform a variety of functions for a small group of patients rather than one set of functions for a large number of patients. Some organizations have achieved patient-focused care by assigning multiskilled workers to serve food, clean patients' rooms, and assist in nursing care. However, some organizations have experienced low patient satisfaction with this type of worker because the patients are confused and do not know who to ask to do what.

Hospital staff spend most of their time performing activities in the following nine categories:

- Medical, technical, and clinical procedures
- Hotel and patient services
- Medical documentation
- Institutional documentation
- Scheduling and coordination
- Patient transportation
- Staff transportation
- Management and supervision
- Preparation activities

Hospitals have had difficulty in fully and rapidly implementing patient-focused care for the following reasons: the high cost of conversion; the extensive physical renovations required; resistance from functional departments; and other priorities for management, such as mergers and considering potential mergers.

Licensure, Certification, and Accreditation of Healthcare Facilities

Under the 10th Amendment of the US Constitution, states have the primary responsibility for public health, which includes disease and injury prevention, sanitation, water and air pollution, vaccination, isolation and quarantine, inspection of commercial and residential premises, food and drinking water standards, extermination of vermin, fluoridation of municipal water supplies, and licensure of physicians and other healthcare professionals. Each state has a division or an agency that is dedicated to promoting high-quality patient care and safety in healthcare facilities and outpatient services by conducting regular on-site surveys. State and federal licensing and certification programs require that high-performance standards be met in the provision of medical care and in the construction and maintenance of the healthcare facility.

State Licensure

Licensure gives legal approval for a facility to operate or for a person to practice within his or her profession. States require that hospitals, sanatoria, nursing homes, and pharmacies be licensed to operate; although the requirements and standards for licensure may differ from state to state. State licensure is mandatory. Federal facilities such as those of the Department of Veterans Affairs (VA) do not require licensure.

Although licensure requirements vary, healthcare facilities must meet certain basic criteria that are determined by state regulatory agencies. These standards address such concerns as adequacy of staffing, personnel employed to provide services, physical aspects of the facility (equipment, buildings), and services provided, including health records. Licensure typically is performed annually, and facilities must usually meet the minimum acceptable standards for operation.

Certification for Medicare Participation

In 1965, the Social Security Act established both Medicare and Medicaid. Medicare was the responsibility of the Social Security Administration (SSA), but federal assistance to the state Medicaid programs was administered by the Social and Rehabilitation Service (SRS). SSA and SRS were agencies in the Department of Health, Education, and Welfare (HEW). In 1977, the Health Care Finance Administration (HCFA) was created under HEW to effectively coordinate Medicare and Medicaid. In 1980, HEW was divided into the Department of Education and the Department of Health and Human Services. In 2001, HCFA was renamed the **Centers for Medicare and Medicaid Services (CMS)**, an agency of HHS.

CMS maintains oversight of the survey and certification of nursing homes and continuing care providers (including hospitals, nursing homes, home health agencies, end-stage renal disease facilities, hospices, and other facilities serving Medicare and

Medicaid beneficiaries) and makes information about these activities available to beneficiaries, providers and suppliers, researchers, and state surveyors. In November 2002, CMS began the national Nursing Home Quality Initiative (NHQI). The goals of the initiative are essentially twofold: (1) to give consumers an additional source of information about the quality of nursing home care by providing a set of Minimum Data Set (MDS)-based quality measures on Medicare's Nursing Home Compare website, and (2) to help providers improve the quality of care for their residents by giving them access to clinical resources, quality improvement materials, and assistance from the QIOs in every state (CMS 2015b). From the beginning of the NHQI, CMS has insisted that the quality measures be dynamic and continue to be refined as part of CMS's ongoing commitment to quality.

To be eligible for Medicare and Medicaid reimbursement, providers must become Medicare-certified by demonstrating compliance with the conditions of participation. **Certification** is the process by which government and nongovernment organizations evaluate educational programs, healthcare facilities, and individuals as having met predetermined standards. The certification of healthcare facilities is the responsibility of the states. However, Section 1865(a)(1) of the Social Security Act specifies that facilities accredited by the Joint Commission and the American Osteopathic Association must be deemed in compliance with the Medicare conditions of participation for hospitals; those accredited are said to have deemed status (CMS 2015d).

Voluntary Accreditation

Accreditation agencies create standards for medical care, construct measurements of quality, and determine which organizations meet their standards. Provider organizations seek **accreditation** in order to prove that they meet the standards of legitimate and appropriate medical practice.

The Joint Commission operates voluntary accreditation programs for hospitals and other healthcare services. It certifies hospitals as having met the conditions of participation required for reimbursement under the federal Medicare pro-

gram. The definition of federal **deemed status** is as follows:

> In order for healthcare organizations to participate in and receive payment from the Medicare and Medicaid programs, [they] must be certified as complying with the conditions of participation, or standards, set forth in federal regulations. (Joint Commission 2014)

A majority of state governments also recognize the Joint Commission accreditation as a condition of licensure and receiving Medicaid reimbursement. Inspections are typically triannual with accreditation and survey findings made publicly available. The standards are based on the premise that healthcare organizations exist to maximize the health of the people they serve while using resources efficiently. When an organization is found to be in substantial compliance with the Joint Commission standards, accreditation may be awarded for up to three years. Hospitals must undergo a full survey at least every three years.

The Joint Commission publishes accreditation manuals with standards for hospitals, non–hospital-based psychiatric and substance abuse organizations, long-term care organizations, home care organizations, ambulatory care organizations, and organization-based pathology and clinical laboratory services.

Much like the Joint Commission, the American Osteopathic Association (AOA) Hospital Accreditation Program is a voluntary program that accredits osteopathic hospitals. Those hospitals that are accredited are recognized by HHS as having deemed status and thus are eligible to receive Medicare funds (AOA 2015).

The AOA has been accrediting healthcare facilities for more than 30 years under Medicare. It is one of only two voluntary accreditation programs in the United States authorized by CMS to survey hospitals under Medicare. In addition, the program is a cost-effective, user-friendly means to validate the quality of care provided by a facility.

The AOA accreditation program was developed in 1943 and 1944 and implemented in 1945. Under this program hospitals were surveyed each year. In this manner, the AOA was able to ensure that osteopathic students received their training through rotating internships and residencies in facilities that provided high-quality patient care. In 1995, the AOA applied for and received deeming authority to accredit laboratories within AOA-accredited hospitals under the Clinical Laboratory Improvement Amendments of 1988. The AOA also has developed accreditation requirements for ambulatory care and surgery, mental health, substance abuse, and physical rehabilitation medicine facilities (AOA 2015).

Check Your Understanding 1.6

Instructions: **On a separate piece of paper, write the best terms to complete the following sentences.**

1. Quality has several components including appropriateness, technical excellence, _____, and acceptability.
   A. accuracy of diagnosis
   B. continuous improvement
   C. connectivity
   D. accessibility

2. _____ programs have been in place in hospitals for years and have been required by the Medicare and Medicaid programs and accreditation standards.
   A. Quality assurance
   B. Peer review
   C. Managed care
   D. Quality improvement

3. Today, _____ refers to the level of skilled care needed by patients with complex medical conditions, typically Medicare patients who have multiple medical problems.
   A. acute care
   B. ambulatory care
   C. post-acute care
   D. high-quality care

4. _____ is a generic term for a healthcare reimbursement system that manages cost, quality, and access to services.
   A. Quality improvement
   B. Subacute care
   C. Managed care
   D. Patient-focused care

5. _____ attempts to contain hospital inpatient costs and improve quality by restructuring services.
   A. Continuous quality improvement
   B. Patient-focused care
   C. Managed care
   D. Acute care

6. Managed care and healthcare organization integration have placed enormous pressure on _____.
   A. integrated delivery systems
   B. acute-care facilities
   C. rehabilitation facilities
   D. information systems

7. Healthcare organizations seek _____ in order to prove they meet the standards of legitimate and appropriate medical practice.
   A. insurance contracts
   B. accreditation
   C. licensure
   D. medical staff

Reimbursement of Healthcare Expenditures

In the United States healthcare is paid for by the government, employers, and individuals. As healthcare technology and treatments have advanced and become more expensive, the payment systems have evolved. Originally dominated by fee-for-service payment systems now, Medicare and Medicaid programs and the managed care insurance industry have virtually eliminated fee-for-service reimbursement arrangements.

Evolution of Third-Party Reimbursement

The evolution of third-party reimbursement systems for healthcare services began in the 1940s. The evolution created a need for systematic and accurate communications between healthcare providers and third-party payers. Commercial health insurance companies (for example, Aetna) offer medical plans similar to Blue Cross/Blue Shield plans. Traditionally, Blue Cross organizations covered hospital services and Blue Shield covered inpatient physician services and a limited amount of office-based care. Today, Blue Cross plans and commercial insurance providers cover a full range of healthcare services, including ambulatory care services and drug benefits. (Healthcare reimbursement systems are discussed in more detail in chapter 7.)

Most commercial health insurance is provided in the form of group policies offered by employers as part of their fringe benefit packages for employees. Unions also negotiate health insurance coverage during contract negotiations. In most cases, employees pay a share of the cost and employers pay a share. Individual health insurance plans can be purchased through the health insurance marketplace created through the ACA. Individuals with preexisting medical conditions cannot be denied coverage. Individuals who are not covered by any of these options are required to pay a healthcare tax.

Commercial insurers also sell major medical and cash payment policies. Major medical plans are directed primarily at catastrophic illness and cover all or part of treatment costs beyond those covered by basic plans. Major medical plans are sold as both group and individual policies. Cash payment plans provide monetary benefits and are not based on actual charges from healthcare providers. For example, a cash payment plan might pay the beneficiary $150 for every day he or she is hospitalized or $500 for every ambulatory surgical procedure. Cash payment plans are often offered as a benefit of membership in large associations such as AARP.

Government-Sponsored Reimbursement Systems

Until 1965, most of the poor and many of the elderly in the United States could not afford private healthcare services. As a result of public pressure calling for attention to this growing problem, Congress passed Public Law 89-97 as an amendment to the Social Security Act. The amendment created Medicare (Title XVIII) and Medicaid (Title XIX). Medicare and Medicaid are not issuers of health insurance. They are public health plans through which individuals obtain health coverage.

Medicare

Medicare was first offered to retired Americans in July 1966. Today, retired and disabled Americans who are eligible for Social Security benefits automatically qualify for Medicare coverage without regard to income. Coverage is offered under two coordinated programs: hospital insurance (Medicare Part A) and medical insurance (Medicare Part B).

Medicare Part A is financed through payroll taxes. Initially, coverage applied only to hospitalization and home healthcare. Subsequently, coverage for extended care in nursing homes was added. Coverage for individuals eligible for Social Security disability payments for over two years and those who need kidney transplantation or dialysis for end-stage renal disease also was added.

Medical insurance under Medicare Part B is optional. It is financed through monthly premiums paid by eligible beneficiaries to supplement federal funding. Part B helps pay for physicians' services, outpatient hospital care, medical services and supplies, and certain other medical costs not covered by Part A. At the present time, Medicare Part B does not provide coverage of prescription drugs. (Medicare Parts A and B are discussed in greater detail in chapter 7.) In January 2006, Medicare Part D was implemented to provide prescription drug coverage for Medicare beneficiaries who select this option. Commercially offered Medicare plans, called Medicare Advantage plans, are sometimes referred to as Medicare Part C. They offer Medicare Parts A and B coverage and often include vision, dental, and hearing benefits (Medicare.gov 2015c).

Medicaid

Medicaid is a medical assistance program for low-income Americans. The program is funded partially by the federal government and partially by state and local governments. The federal government requires that certain services be provided and sets specific eligibility requirements. Medicaid covers the following benefits:

- Inpatient hospital care
- Outpatient hospital care
- Laboratory and x-ray services
- SNF and home health services for persons over 21 years old
- Physicians' services
- Family planning services
- Rural health clinic services
- Early and periodic screening, diagnosis, and treatment services

Individual states sometimes cover services in addition to those required by the federal government.

Services Provided by Government Agencies

Federal health insurance programs cover health services for several additional specified populations including active and retired military and their families and Native Americans. In partnership with state governments additional insurance coverage is provided to children whose families cannot afford medical coverage although they do not qualify for Medicaid (Medicaid.gov 2015).

TRICARE, which was originally referred to as the Civilian Health and Medical Program for the Uniformed Services (CHAMPUS), pays for care delivered by civilian health providers to retired members of the military and the dependents of active and retired members of the seven uniformed services. The Department of Defense administers the TRICARE program. The program also provides medical services to active members of the military.

The Veteran's Health Administration (VA) provides healthcare services to eligible veterans of military service. The VA hospital system was established in 1930 to provide hospital, nursing home, residential, and outpatient medical and dental care to veterans of World War I. Today, the VA operates more than 1,700 sites of care including hospital, clinics, counseling centers and other medical facilities throughout the United States (US Department of Veteran Affairs 2015).

Through the Indian Health Service, HHS also finances the healthcare services provided to Native Americans who are enrolled members of a federally recognized tribe. Healthcare services are provided either at an Indian Health Services facility or through contracted services. Indian Health Services, like other federally funded healthcare programs, must submit an annual report to Congress on the quality of care provided (Indian Health Services 2015).

State governments often operate healthcare facilities to serve citizens with special needs, such as the developmentally disabled and mentally ill. Some states also offer health insurance programs to those who cannot qualify for private healthcare insurance. Many county and local governments also operate public hospitals to fulfill the medical needs of their communities. Public hospitals provide services without regard to the patient's ability to pay.

Workers' Compensation

Workers' compensation is an insurance system operated by the individual states. Each state has its own law and program to provide covered workers with some protection against the costs of medical care and the loss of income resulting from work-related injuries and, in some cases, illnesses. The first workers' compensation law was enacted in New York in 1910; and by 1948, every state had enacted such laws. The theory underlying workers' compensation is that all accidents that occur at work, regardless of fault, must be regarded as risks of industry and that employer and employee should share the burden of loss (Kovner et al. 2011, 55).

Insurance

Healthcare insurance was created to spread risk over a large pool of people and to protect assets in the event of a catastrophic illness or injury. Health insurance guards against financial devastation in the face of serious health problems. In 2013, 86.6 percent of Americans had health insurance (Smith and Medalia 2014).

Managed Care

Managed care encompasses several types of prepaid health insurance plans. There are three major types of managed care plans, health maintenance organizations (HMOs), preferred provider organizations (PPOs), and point-of-service (POS) plans.

The development of managed care was an indirect result of the federal government's enactment of the Medicare and Medicaid amendments in 1965. Medicare and Medicaid legislation stimulated the growth of university medical centers and prompted the development of **investor-owned hospital chains**, publicly traded for-profit groups of hospitals.

The new healthcare programs for the elderly and poor laid the groundwork for increased corporate control of medical care delivery by third-party payers. This was done through the government-mandated regulation of fee-for-service and indemnity payments for healthcare services. After years of unchecked healthcare inflation, the government authorized corporate cost controls on hospitals, physicians, patients, prospective payment systems, and the resource-based relative value scale.

Further federal support for the corporate practice of medicine resulted from passage of the HMO Act of 1973. Amendments to the act enabled managed care plans to increase in numbers and expand enrollments through healthcare programs financed by grants, contracts, and loans.

Impact of Managed Care Organizations

With more and more Americans receiving their health insurance through **managed care organizations (MCOs)**, where healthcare organizations assume the financial risk as well as provide healthcare services for a defined population of patients. The responsibilities of primary care providers have changed. In the fee-for-service model, the primary care provider is responsible only for the patients actually seen in his or her office, and a practice is viewed as being made up of individual patients. In a fully capitated managed care setting, however, particularly when the provider is paid through a capitation system rather than by a modified fee-for-service system, he or she is responsible for providing care to a defined population of patients assigned by the MCO. The MCO may audit the provider's practice to determine whether standards of care are being met. In the capitated MCO setting, providers are often held responsible for each patient on their panels, whether or not the patient ever comes to the office to be seen (Kovner et al. 2011).

The advent of managed care appeared to tame healthcare cost inflation during the early and mid-1990s, but costs are once again rising rapidly. In particular, the total cost of pharmaceuticals is skyrocketing. The managed care industry faces continued financial challenges. At the same time, it remains under intense public scrutiny and is facing continued attempts at increased government legislation and regulation. In addition, for many years costs increased faster than premiums could rise to cover them. Thus, escalating costs have forced employers to ask workers to pay for a larger share of healthcare. Political and market forces and the weakness of any stabilizing influences are eroding the ability of managed care firms to control underlying healthcare costs.

Although managed care deserves much of the credit for taming the rampant, double-digit healthcare inflation of the 1980s and early 1990s, the relief from rising medical bills that Americans enjoyed for several years is over, and increases in premiums have both HMOs and employers, especially smaller ones, scrambling for countermeasures.

Consumer-Driven Healthcare

An emerging issue in the private insurance market is that of consumer-driven healthcare. This strategy seems to be gaining momentum in an effort to both allow employees more choice in their healthcare decisions and to stabilize healthcare costs. The design of consumer-driven plans varies, but, essentially, it focuses on making consumers more price conscious by setting a large deductible before individuals receive insurance benefits. It is very different than managed care in that people have more choice but face sizeable personal financial risk (Kovner et al. 2011, 58). See figure 1.2 for an overview breakdown of the 2011 health insurance premiums for US covered workers.

Health Savings Accounts

Health savings accounts (HSAs), also called medical savings accounts, offer participants the opportunity to control how their healthcare dollars are spent. HSAs were created by the Medicare bill signed by President George W. Bush in December 2003 and are designed to help individuals save for future qualified medical and retiree health expenses on a tax-free basis.

The benefit of an HSA is that the member pays for the deductible with pretax dollars, which allows a member to save the money that ordinarily would have gone to pay taxes. When members pay off the deductible, the insurance company begins to pay. The money in the HSA earns interest and is owned by the member who holds the account. In 2013, 13.5 million Americans had a health savings account (AHIP 2014).

Figure 1.2. Average annual firm and worker premium contributions and total premiums for covered workers for single and family coverage, by plan type, 2014

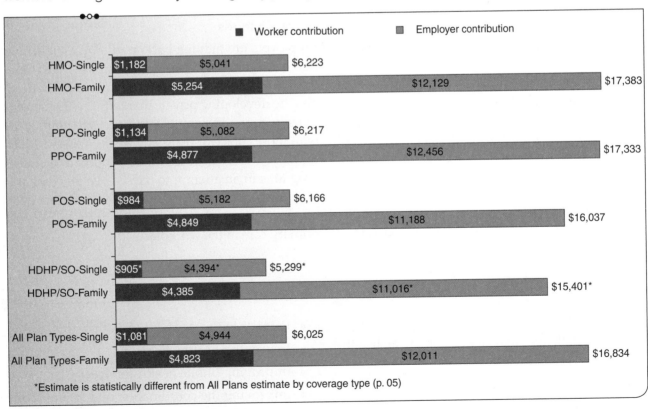

*Estimate is statistically different from All Plans estimate by coverage type (p. 05)

Reprinted with permission from the Kaiser Family Foundation.

Figure 1.3. Average health insurance costs as a share of payroll for employees with access to coverage, by establishment size, 1999 and 2010

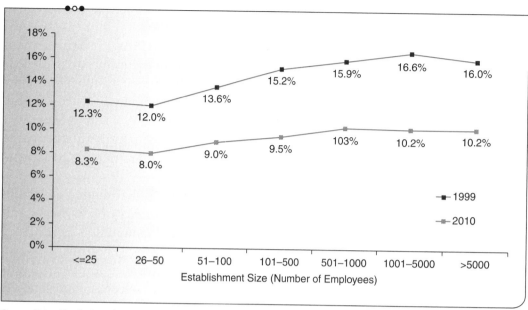

Source: Kaiser Family Foundation calculations based on data from the National Compensation Survey, 1999 and 2010, conducted by the Bureau of Labor Statistics. Reprinted with permission from the Kaiser Family Foundation.

Continued Rise in Healthcare Costs

The rising cost of healthcare has moderated since the recession however it continues to exceed the increase in wages. Average insurance premiums increased 34 percent between 2004 and 2009 (Kaiser 2014), however wages only grew 15.7 percent in that same period (SSA 2013). In the next five years, between 2009 and 2014, premiums grew 26 percent (Kaiser 2014), 8 percent less than the previous period, however wages only grew 12 percent (SSA 2013). See figure 1.3. Employees and employers are getting squeezed by the price of healthcare. The struggle to control health costs is viewed as crucial to improving wages and living standards.

The catalysts for employers' annual cost for healthcare coverage increases include the cost of prescription drugs, medical innovation, and a growing acceptance of higher-premium health plans that offer greater flexibility in choice of providers.

Payer Changes

Employers are fighting back, partly by establishing new benefit methods that can accomplish much more than simply raising workers' copayments. Companies are developing private marketplaces that incentivize insurers to compete and provide employees with more choice of plans and costs (Abelson 2014). Employers have increased their support of wellness programs in an attempt to reduce overall costs and improve productivity and some employers are even hiring in-house physicians and nurses to provide primary care in the workplace.

Future of American Healthcare

Six major challenges that face the American healthcare system today include:

- Improving quality and safety
- Improving access and coverage
- Reining in the growth of healthcare costs
- Improving healthy behavior
- Improving public health services
- Improving the coordination and accountability of healthcare services

Although other challenges like health disparity and workforce issues exist, addressing these six would dramatically improve the system (Kovner et al. 2011).

As other industries like banking and retail have been transformed by technology, healthcare now has the opportunity to dramatically change how care is delivered. Digital technology has the promise to increase communication between care-givers and to increase communication between clinicians and patients. Technology will also allow patients to perform basic diagnostic testing and to better manage chronic disease with the use of applications (PWC 2014). These advances will place the emphasis on maintaining health instead of treating disease.

Check Your Understanding 1.7

Instructions: On a separate piece of paper, indicate whether the following statements are true or false (T or F).

1. _____ Most commercial health insurance is provided in the form of group policies offered by employers as part of their fringe benefit packages for employees.

2. _____ Today, retired and disabled Americans who are eligible for Social Security benefits automatically qualify for Medicare coverage.

3. _____ Medicaid is a medical assistance program for upper-income Americans.

4. _____ Blue Cross plans and commercial insurance providers cover a full range of healthcare services.

5. _____ The Department of Defense administers the TRICARE program.

6. _____ Employers provide employees with a personal care account in consumer-driven healthcare.

7. _____ The development of managed care was an indirect result of the federal government's enactment of the Medicare and Medicaid amendments in 1965.

8. _____ The federal government became involved in the quality-of-care and malpractice issues through the establishment of the National Practitioner Data Bank under the Healthcare Quality Improvement Act of 1986.

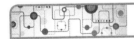

References

Abelson, R. 2014 (March 16). Companies Test Plans to Cut Their Health Costs. *New York Times.* http://www.nytimes.com/2014/03/07/business/companies-turn-to-private-exchanges-to-control-health-care-costs.html?_r=0

American College of Surgeons. 2015 (May 26). Franklin H. Martin, First JACS Editor. https://www.facs.org/publications/jacs/history/martin

American Health Information Management Association. 2014a. *Pocket Glossary of Health Information Management and Technology,* 4th ed. Chicago: AHIMA.

American Health Information Management Association. 2014b. Electronic health record adoption in long-term care. *Journal of AHIMA* 85:11: expanded web version.

American Health Insurance Plans. 2014 (May 30). Health Savings Account Growth Reaches 13.5 Million. https://www.ahip.org/News/Press-Room/2012/Health-Savings-Account-Enrollment-Reaches-13-5-Million.aspx

American Hospital Association. 2015. (May 28). Long-term Care Hospitals. http://www.aha.org/advocacy-issues/postacute/ltach/index.shtml

American Hospital Association. 2014. (June 1) Fast Facts on US Hospitals. http://www.aha.org/research/rc/stat-studies/fast-facts.shtml

American Hospital Association. 2010a (June). Accountable Care Organizations—AHA Research Synthesis Report. http://www.aha.org/research/cor/content/ACO-Synthesis-Report.pdf

American Hospital Association. 2010a. Maximizing the Value of Post-Acute Care. http://www.aha.org/research/reports/tw/10nov-tw-postacute.pdf

American Hospital Association. 2010b (November). Maximizing the Value of Post-acute Care, Trendwatch, p. 1–14.

American Hospital Association. 1999. *100 Faces of Healthcare*. Chicago: Health Forum.

American Medical Association. 2015. Our History. http://www.ama-assn.org/ama/pub/about-ama/our-history.page?

American Osteopathic Association. 2015 (May 30). Healthcare Facilities Accreditation Program. http://www.hfap.org/about/overview.aspx

Association of American Medical Colleges. 2015. About the AAMC. https://www.aamc.org/about/

Association of Schools of Allied Health Professionals. 2015 (May 25). Allied Health Professionals. http://www.asahp.org/wp-content/uploads/2014/08/Health-Professions-Facts.pdf

Carter, D. and P. Shaw. 2000. *Quality and Performance Improvement in Healthcare: Theory, Practice, and Management*. Chicago: AHIMA.

Centers for Disease Control and Prevention. 2015 (May 26). Hospital Utilization. http://www.cdc.gov/nchs/fastats/hospital.htm

Centers for Disease Control and Prevention. 2009. Health care in America: Trends in utilization. http://cdc.gov/nchs/datawh/nchsdefs/postacutecare.htm

Centers for Medicare and Medicaid Services. 2015a (May 26). Medicare Benefit Policy Manual. https://www.cms.gov/Regulations-and-Guidance/Guidance/Manuals/downloads/bp102c01.pdf

Centers for Medicare and Medicaid Services. 2015b (May 26). Nursing Home Quality Initiative. http://www.cms.gov/Medicare/Quality-Initiatives-Patient-Assessment-Instruments/NursingHomeQualityInits/index.html?redirect=/NursingHomeQualityInits/45_NHQIMDS30TrainingMaterials.asp

Centers for Medicare and Medicaid Services. 2015c. (May 30). EHR Incentive Program. http://www.cms.gov/Regulations-and-Guidance/Legislation/EHRIncentivePrograms/Downloads/March2015_SummaryReport.pdf

Centers for Medicare and Medicaid Services. 2015d (Oct 24). Accreditation. https://www.cms.gov/Medicare/Provider-Enrollment-and-Certification/SurveyCertificationGenInfo/Accreditation.html

Cooke, M., D. Irby, W. Sullivan, and K.M. Ludmerer. 2006. American medical education 100 years after the Flexner report. *New England Journal of Medicine* 355:1339–1344.

Department of Health and Human Services. 2015. (May 26). HHS Strategic Plan. http://www.hhs.gov/about/strategic-plan/index.html

Department of Health and Human Services. 2012. Office of the Surgeon General. http://www.surgeongeneral.gov/about/index.html

Department of Health and Human Services. 2010. Strategic Plan and Priorities. http://www.hhs.gov/secretary/about/priorities/priorities.html

Flexner, A. 1910. Medical Education in the United States and Canada Bulletin Number Four. The Carnegie Foundation for the Advancement of Teaching. http://archive.carnegiefoundation.org/publications/medical-education-united-states-and-canada-bulletin-number-four-flexner-report-0

Foley, D.J., R.W. Manderscheid, J.E. Atay, J. Maedke, J. Sussman, and S. Cribbs. 2004. Chapter 19: Highlights of Organized Mental Health Services in 2002 and Major National and State Trends. In *Mental Health, United States, 2004*. HHS Publication No. (SMA) 06-4195. http://mentalhealth.samhsa.gov/publications/allpubs/sma06-4195/chapter19.asp.Harris-

Hazelwood, A., E. Cook, and S. Hazelwood. 2005. The Joint Commission on Healthcare Organization's Sentinel Events Policy. *Academy of Healthcare Management Journal*. Annual.

Indian Health Services. 2015 (Nov 9). Frequently Asked Questions. https://www.ihs.gov/forpatients/index.cfm/faq/

Joint Commission. 2014 (May 30). Facts About Federal Deemed Status and State Recognition. http://www.jointcommission.org/facts_about_federal_deemed_status_and_state_recognition/default.aspx

Kaiser Family Foundation. 2015 (May 25). ACA 101: What You Need to Know. http://kff.org/health-reform/event/aca-101-what-you-need-to-know-2015/

Kaiser Family Foundation. 2014 (June 1). 2014 Employer Health Benefits Survey. http://kff.org/report-section/ehbs-2014-summary-of-findings/

Kaiser Family Foundation. 2013 (May 25). Summary of the Affordable Care Act. http://kff.org/health-reform/fact-sheet/summary-of-the-affordable-care-act/

Kovner, A., J. Knickman, and V. Weisfeld. 2011 (May 25). *Health Care Delivery in the United States*, 10th ed. New York: Springer Publishing Company. Kindle Edition.

Long Term and Post Acute Care Health Information Technology (LTPAC HIT). 2015 (Oct 24). About Long

Term and Post Acute Care. http://www.ltpachealthit.org/content/about-long-term-and-post-acute-care

Mark, T., E. Stranges, and K. Levit. 2010 (September 7). Using Healthcare Cost and Utilization Project State Inpatient Database and Medicare Cost Reports Data to Determine the Number of Psychiatric Discharges from Psychiatric Units of Community Hospitals. Agency for Healthcare Research and Quality (AHRQ). http://www.hcup-us.ahrq.gov/reports.jsp

Masters, P.A. and C. Nester. 2001 (Jan.). A study of primary care teaching comparing academic and community-based settings. *Journal of General Internal Medicine* 16(1): 9–13.

Medicaid.gov. 2015 (Oct. 24). Benefits. http://www.medicaid.gov/chip/benefits/chip-benefits.html

Medicare.gov. 2015a (Oct. 24). What's Home Healthcare and What Should I Expect? http://www.medicare.gov/what-medicare-covers/home-health-care/home-health-care-what-is-it-what-to-expect.html

Medicare.gov. 2015b (Oct 24). Medicare and Home Health Care. https://www.medicare.gov/Pubs/pdf/10969.pdf

Medicare.gov. 2015c (Oct 24). Medicare Part C, Medicare Advantage. https://medicare.com/medicare-advantage/medicare-part-c/

Office of the National Coordinator for Health Information Technology. 2014 (June 1). Update on the Adoption of Health Information Technology and Related Efforts to Facilitate the Electronic use and Exchange of Health Information. http://healthit.gov/

PricewaterhouseCoopers. 2014 (May 31). Healthcare Delivery of the Future: How Digital Technology Can Bridge Time and Distance Between Clinicians and Consumers. http://www.pwc.com/en_US/us/health-industries/top-health-industry-issues/assets/pwc-healthcare-delivery-of-the-future.pdf

Rand Health. 2015 (Oct. 21). Organizing Health: In Depth. http://www.rand.org/health/key-topics/organizing-care/in-depth.html

Robert Wood Johnson Foundation. 2014 (Oct 24). Long Term Care: What Are the Issues? http://www.rwjf.org/content/dam/farm/reports/issue_briefs/2014/rwjf410654

Smith, J. and C. Medalia. 2014. U.S. Census Bureau, Current Population Reports, P60-250, Health Insurance Coverage in the United States: 2013. Washington, DC: U.S. Government Printing Office.

Social Security Association. 2013 (June 1). Measures of Central Tendency for Wage Data. http://www.ssa.gov/OACT/COLA/central.html

Starr, P. 1982. *The Social Transformation of American Medicine.* New York: Basic Books.

Stedman's Medical Dictionary. Biotechnology. 2000. http://www.stedmans.com.

Stokes, M. D. 2004. (January 26). The Impact of Obesity on Healthcare Delivery. *For the Record* 16 (2): 34.

US Department of Veteran Affairs. 2015. (Oct 24). Veterans Health Administration. http://www.va.gov/health/

World Health Organization. 2015 (October 20). Medical Devices. http://www.who.int/medical_devices/definitions/en/

Wilson, K. 2014 (May 28). Healthcare Costs 101. California Healthcare Foundation. http://www.chcf.org/~/media/MEDIA%20LIBRARY%20Files/PDF/H/PDF%20HealthCareCosts14.pdf

29 CFR 825.118: What is a health care provider? 1995.

2

Legal Issues in Health Information Management

Laurie A. Rinehart-Thompson, JD, RHIA, CHP, FAHIMA

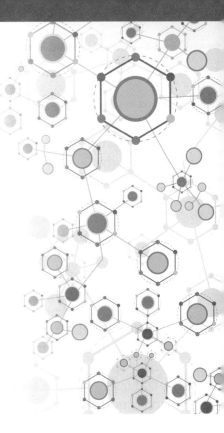

Learning Objectives

- Identify the three related subsystems of government
- Identify the sources of law
- Diagram the state and federal court systems
- Differentiate public law and private law
- Differentiate civil law and criminal law
- Apply the process for civil litigation
- Apply the process for criminal proceedings
- Examine healthcare causes of action as they relate to tort liability
- Examine healthcare causes of action as they relate to breach of contract
- Verify the external forces that impact the form and content of the health record
- Identify the purpose of and challenges associated with defining the legal health record

- Examine liabilities associated with the electronic health record
- Verify the internal and external forces that impact health record retention
- Apply legal principles in determining health record ownership and access
- Demonstrate how the health record can be used as evidence in legal proceedings, including e-discovery
- Examine release of information principles for proper disclosure of health information, including highly sensitive information
- Identify types and consequences of medical identity theft
- Identify types of quality improvement activities and examine the risk of documents associated with these activities being deemed discoverable

Key Terms

Acceptance
Accreditation
Acquittal
Adhesion contract
Administrative law
Administrative system

Advance directive
Answer
Apology statute
Appellate court
Arbitration
Arm's length transaction

Arraign
Assault
Assumption of risk
Authentication
Authenticity
Battery

Breach of warranty
Burden of proof
Charitable immunity
Circuit
Circuit court
Civil law
Common law
Comparative negligence
Complaint
Consent
Consideration
Contract
Contract law
Contributory negligence
Corporate negligence
Counterclaims
Criminal law
Criminal negligence
Cross-claim
Defamation of character
Default judgment
Defendant
Deposition
Designated record set
   (DRS)
District court
Diversity jurisdiction
Do-Not-Resuscitate Order
   (DNR)
Durable Power of Attorney for
   Healthcare Decisions
e-discovery
Electronic health record (EHR)
Evidence
Express warranty
False imprisonment
Federal Register
Felony
Fraud
Freedom of Information Act
   (FOIA)

General consent
General jurisdiction
Good Samaritan Statutes
Governmental immunity
Grand jury
Gross negligence
Health Insurance Portability
   and Accountability Act
   (HIPAA)
Hung jury
Implied warranty
Incident
Incident report
Indictment
Infliction of emotional distress
Informed consent
Intent
Interrogatories
Invasion of privacy
Joinder
Judicial system
Jurisdiction
Legal health record (LHR)
Legal hold
Legal system
Legislative system
Libel
Licensure
Limited jurisdiction
Litigation
Living will
Malfeasance
Mediation
Medical identity theft
Metadata
Misdemeanor
Misfeasance
Motion for summary judgment
Negligence
Nonfeasance
Offer

Ordinary negligence
Original jurisdiction
Patient Self-Determination Act
Persuasive authority
Petition for writ of certiorari
Physician-patient privilege
Plaintiff
Potentially compensable
   event
Precedent
Preemption
Privacy Act of 1974
Private law
Privilege
Prosecutor
Protected health information
   (PHI)
Public law
Punitive damages
Regulations
Request for production
Respondeat superior
Restitution
Right to privacy
Settlement
Slander
Spoliation
Standard of care
Stare decisis
Statute of limitations
Statutes
Statutory (legislative) law
Strict liability
Subject matter jurisdiction
Subpoena
Summons
Supreme Court
Tort
Trial court
Trier of fact
Writs

To understand the health information management (HIM) professional's role in protecting confidential health information, one must first understand basic legal concepts and the principles of appropriate access and disclosure. Because health records are often central to litigation, which is the sum of the proceedings in a legal case, the HIM professional should be very comfortable with the legal process. The following sections present basic and crucial information about the American legal system, including healthcare causes of action and legal considerations that must accompany the management of health information.

Organization of Government

The legal system in the United States consists of three related subsystems: a judicial system, a legislative system, and an administrative system.

The judicial system, which is the court system, provides an avenue to enforce both rights and obligations. Through the courts, a person or entity has the opportunity to bring a civil action against another person or entity believed to have caused harm. A wide variety of civil actions can be brought against an alleged wrongdoer, while a defense can be prepared at the same time. The judicial system also provides a mechanism for a government to charge a person or entity with a crime. At the same time, the system allows the charged person or entity the opportunity to defend against the charge or charges.

The legislative system, which enacts laws, controls many activities related to industry, including the healthcare industry. These controls exist as statutes. Statutes are laws created by legislative bodies and often set forth what action is required.

The administrative system, which controls governmental administrative operations, operates through federal and state administrative agencies that enact regulations. Regulations are rules derived from or brought forward by administrative agencies subsequent to the passage of statutes. They set forth how statutory actions are to be carried out. Regulations have the same force of law, or level of authority, that statutory laws do.

Understanding the American judicial, legislative, and administrative systems within a governmental organization at any level (federal, state, or local) gives an HIM professional an appreciation for the health record as a legal document and its role in each of these systems.

Sources of Law

The laws that rule all Americans' lives come from many sources, resulting in a rather complex legal system. Overall, there is a federal legal system, 50 individual state legal systems, and myriad of local legal systems. Regardless of the source, the legal system is a process through which members of society settle disputes. These disputes may be between private individuals and organizations or between either of these entities and the government, whether state, federal, local, or a combination.

Constitutional Law

Much of the law governing society is set out in the state and federal constitutions. The Constitution of the United States is the highest law in the land. It takes precedence over constitutions and laws in the individual states and local jurisdictions (Rinehart-Thompson 2012a). The US Constitution defines the federal government's general organization and grants powers to it. It also places limits on what federal and state governments may do. State constitutions have the same effect within the borders of each state. Some state constitutions are very elaborate and govern everything from state lotteries to retirement plans for state workers.

Common Law

English common law is the primary source of many legal rules and principles and was based initially on tradition and custom. Common law (also known as judicial law, judge-made law, or case law), is regularly referred to as unwritten law originating from court decisions where no applicable statute exists. As the English legal system developed, it included juries that heard complaints from the king's subjects. Since there were few written laws at the time, principles that evolved from these court decisions became known as "common law" (Pozgar and Santucci 2016).

Subsequent to the American Revolution, most states adopted all or part of English common-law principles (Pozgar and Santucci 2016). States continue to add to the body of common law through court decisions (also referred to as a court's holding) when existing statutes do not apply to the issue before the court. Because each state adds to the common law within its boundaries, there is no body of national common law. Thus, a common-law principle established in one state has no effect in another state unless the second state also adopts the principle. Even then, it may be applied differently. After a court establishes a new common-law principle, that principle becomes a precedent or binding force for future cases addressing the same issues in that state. The body of common law in a given state is continually evolving by being modified, overturned, repealed, or created by court decisions. Although a precedent in one state does not bind courts in other states, states may use each other's precedents as persuasive authority, or guidance, in analyzing a specific legal problem (Rinehart-Thompson 2012a). Lower courts must look to higher courts in the same court system for precedent; however, the higher courts are not bound by the decisions held in the lower courts in the same court system. Courts on the same level within the same court system are not obligated to follow the decisions of one another (Rinehart-Thompson 2012a).

Another legal principle of note is *stare decisis*, which means "let the decision stand" (Rinehart-Thompson 2012a). This principle states that in cases in a lower court involving a fact pattern similar to that in a higher court within the court system, the lower court is bound to apply the decision of the higher court (Rinehart-Thompson 2012a).

Statutory Law

Statutory (legislative) law is written law established by federal and state legislatures. It may be amended, repealed, or expanded by the legislature. Statutory law also may be upheld or found by a court to violate or conflict with the state or federal constitution. Further, it may be found to conflict with a different state law or a federal law.

Courts also interpret laws in terms of how they apply to a given situation. Thus, statutory law may be "revised" by a court ruling in terms of its constitutionality and applicability. However, if the legislature disagrees with the court's interpretation, it can revise the statute. The legislative revision then becomes the law instead of the court's revision based on its interpretation.

Administrative Law

Federal and state legislatures often delegate their legislative authority to regulate in technical or complex areas to appropriate federal and state administrative agencies, respectively. These agencies are empowered to enact regulations that have the same force of law as statutory law and can often impose criminal penalties for noncompliance. Accordingly, administrative law is the branch of law that controls the government's agency, or administrative, operations. Administrative agencies include licensing bodies, Medicare, Medicaid, and other federal and state government programs. Additionally, regulatory agencies can at times function in a legislative, adjudicative, and enforcement role regarding their own regulations (Pozgar and Santucci 2016).

Federal administrative agencies function under the Administrative Procedure Act, which sets forth the following parameters:

- The procedures under which administrative agencies must operate
- The procedural responsibilities and authority of administrative agencies
- The legal remedies for individuals or entities harmed by agency actions (Pozgar and Santucci 2016)

The act also requires administrative agencies to make agency rules, opinions, orders, records, and proceedings available to the public (Administrative Procedure Act §552). The publication used to accomplish this is the *Federal Register*, which is issued by the US Government Printing Office every business day.

Agencies must publish proposed administrative rules and revisions to existing rules for which they have responsibility and authority. They are published in the *Federal Register* for a comment period and the public is invited to make comments on the applicability and impact of the proposed rules. After the comment period, the applicable administrative agency may or may not finalize the rules. If the rules are finalized, the notice and the final rule are published in the *Federal Register*. The final rule is also codified and published in the appropriate code section. The Medicare Conditions of Participation regulations and HIPAA's Administrative Simplification rules are examples of healthcare regulations published in the *Federal Register*. Courts can review regulations and administrative decisions if there is a question as to whether an agency has overstepped its bounds or misinterpreted a law. Most states have similar administrative procedure acts, but they are generally less elaborate than that of the federal government.

The Court System

The American court system is composed of state court systems and the federal court system. The nature of the issue determines which court has **jurisdiction**—the right to hear and decide the controversy in a given case—over an issue. Matters in the following three categories belong only to federal courts: **subject matter jurisdiction**, which includes federal crimes, such as racketeering and bank robbery, and constitutional issues, which deal with interpretations of the US Constitution; and **diversity jurisdiction**, where the parties do not live in the same state. Other civil and criminal cases are heard in the state court systems.

State Court Systems

Typically, each state court system has several levels. In most states, the lowest level consists of specialty courts or local courts that hear cases involving traffic and small claims issues. State civil and criminal cases are initiated in the lower-level **trial courts**, which have the authority to first hear a case on a given matter, referred to as **original jurisdiction**. Some trial courts at this level have **limited jurisdiction** and may only hear certain types of cases, and include probate, family, juvenile, surrogate, and criminal courts. Other trial courts at this same level have **general jurisdiction** and may hear cases of all types. Decisions made in a court at this level may be appealed to the intermediate courts, usually known as the **appellate court** (or court of appeals). State appellate courts have general jurisdiction.

State legal systems also include a court at the highest level, usually referred to as the **supreme court** of that state. Supreme courts also have general jurisdiction over all cases heard in the state's trial and appellate courts. Decisions coming from the highest state court hearing a case become the law of that state unless a state legislative process enacts a statute to override the court's decision, or unless it is overturned by another case.

Federal Court System

The 94 trial-level federal courts are referred to as the US **district courts** (Rinehart-Thompson 2012a). Specialized federal courts have exclusive jurisdiction over certain matters such as bankruptcy, customs, and claims against the federal government. These cases cannot be filed in a state court.

The federal appellate level is composed of the US courts of appeals, each court covering a geographic area known as a **circuit**. There are 13 of these appellate courts, also known as **circuit courts**, in the United States (Rinehart-Thompson 2012a). These appellate courts have several purposes:

- Reviewing cases heard in federal district courts within the court's circuit
- Reviewing orders issued by certain administrative agencies
- Issuing original **writs**, or written commands, in cases as appropriate (Pozgar and Santucci 2016)

The US Supreme Court is the highest court in the US legal system and hears appeals from the federal appellate courts and the highest state courts. It most frequently considers cases that have risen through the federal court system. The US Supreme Court has considerable discretion in determining which cases it will and will not hear. A request for the US Supreme Court to consider a case is a **petition for writ of certiorari**. The Court will either grant certiorari (that is, will hear the case) or denies certiorari (that is, declines to hear the case). The majority of requests are denied certiorari.

The Legal Process

The HIM professional can better serve patient interests if he or she has an understanding of the legal process. This includes understanding the distinction between public law and private law, as well as civil and criminal law, because healthcare organizations can be affected by cases in any of these areas.

Public Law vs. Private Law

Public law involves the relationship between the government at any level with individuals and organizations. The purposes of public law are defining, regulating, and enforcing rights where the government is a party. Criminal law, discussed later, is public law because it is the government that brings a criminal action (prosecution) against an individual or entity. Public law also encompasses statutory and administrative law because it involves the carrying out of statutes and regulations created by a governmental body. Public statutory and administrative law can be civil or criminal, depending on how the statute or regulation is written. **Private law** involves the relationship between private entities or individuals; the government is not a party. Private law often includes torts, contracts, and property issues. Because torts are civil (noncriminal) wrongs that result in injury, they are the basis for medical and other professional malpractice cases.

Civil Law

Civil law involves relations between individuals, corporations, government entities, and other organizations. Most actions encountered in the healthcare industry are based on civil law. Typically, the remedy for a civil wrong is monetary, but it may also include carrying out or stopping some action.

The party bringing the action or complaint in a civil case is the **plaintiff**. The plaintiff or an attorney on the plaintiff's behalf begins the process by filing a **complaint**, a legal document that sets forth the facts and claims, in the appropriate court and serving a **summons** (or notice) and the complaint to the **defendant**, the one who is accused of

committing the wrong. The defendant or an attorney on the defendant's behalf prepares an **answer** (or response) and files it in the same court where the original complaint was filed. The plaintiff has the burden of proving that a wrong occurred, that the defendant committed the wrong, that the wrong harmed the plaintiff, defining what the harm was, and naming the expected **restitution** or compensation. The plaintiff presents **evidence**, which is supporting information, before a judge or a jury that is compelling enough to meet the **burden of proof**—the required degree of belief as presented by the evidence. There are different burdens of proof and they vary based on the type of case; for example, the burden of proof is higher in a criminal case than in a civil case because the stakes—jail or prison—are higher than monetary damages, which is the potential consequence in a civil case (Brodnik and Sharp 2012).

Other actions may be taken before a case is resolved. The defendant may bring a claim against the plaintiff (**counterclaim**), one party may bring a claim against another party who is on the same side of the litigation (**cross-claim**), or the defendant may bring a claim against an outsider as a co-defendant (**joinder**) (Rinehart-Thompson 2012a).

A case may be resolved in one of five ways:

- A judge can dismiss the plaintiff's case for procedural reasons. The plaintiff's complaint may not set forth a claim recognized by law, the summons and complaint may not have been properly served on the defendant, or the court may not have jurisdiction. Depending on the reason, the judge may permit the plaintiff to correct the error and refile the case.

- If the defendant fails to file a timely answer, the court will find in favor of the plaintiff and enter a **default judgment** against the defendant.

- A case may be settled out of court before it goes to trial or at any time during trial before the **trier of fact** (judge or jury) announces the decision. In addition to **settlements**, or official agreements, cases may be submitted to

arbitration, where a decision is made by an impartial third-party, or **mediation**, where a case is heard by a mediator but the parties reach a mutual agreement.

- Presuming the case does not settle or is not dismissed or no default judgment is entered, the case will proceed with pretrial activities by both plaintiff and defendant. Such activities, known as pretrial discovery, include but are not limited to the taking of witnesses' **depositions**, or sworn statements; the serving of **interrogatories**, or formal questions; **requests for production**, legal requests for documents from the opposing party; and the issuing of **subpoenas**, directives to attend or respond to legal proceedings, as necessary. The court (the judge assigned to the case) will set dates according to the law by which pretrial discovery must be completed. At the conclusion of this stage, in most cases one or both parties present **motions for summary judgment**, in which they argue that there are (or are not) any facts remaining in dispute and that one or the other is (or is not) entitled to a judgment being entered without the intervention of the trier of fact. If the judge grants such a motion, the case is over and has the same effect as if the case had proceeded to trial.

- If a motion for summary judgment is not successful or is not made, the case will proceed to trial before the trier of fact. In most civil cases, the plaintiff must prove his or her case by the burden of proof known as a "preponderance of the evidence." In simple terms, this means that there is enough evidence to tip the scales, even slightly, in favor of the plaintiff's case. This is a substantially lower burden of proof than a criminal case, in which the government must prevail "beyond a reasonable doubt." Upon conclusion of the trial, a verdict is given. In civil cases, a verdict is more commonly referred to as being *liable* or *not liable*. If a party is found to be liable, a judgment is rendered against the party determined to be wholly or partially liable for the harm. Either party may appeal the judgment to an appellate court and possibly even to the highest court in that state.

Criminal Law

Criminal law addresses crimes, which are wrongful acts against public health, safety, and welfare. Criminal laws also include punishment for those persons violating the law. Criminal cases involve matters between individuals or groups of people and the government. Crimes are either a felony or a misdemeanor as defined by state or federal law. A **felony** is the more serious type of crime and includes, among others, murder, thefts of items or cash in excess of a certain value set by statute, assault, and rape. A **misdemeanor** is a lesser offense and includes wrongs such as disorderly conduct and thefts of small amounts of property. Information theft crimes (such as hacking, computer destruction, spamming, and the like) can be either misdemeanors or felonies. The criminal provisions of the HIPAA Privacy Rule, described in chapter 11, include only felony crimes.

An investigation is begun when law enforcement learns that a crime has or may have been committed. The government initiates a criminal action against those individuals or groups of people it believes have committed the crime based on the law enforcement investigation. When the **prosecutor** (prosecuting attorney), also known as the district or state attorney (depending on the state) or the US attorney (in the federal system), determines sufficient evidence is present, he or she files charges against the defendant on behalf of the government. In some states, a **grand jury** must return an **indictment**, or formal charge, for a felony crime to be prosecuted. The grand jury has the authority to issue subpoenas for its investigative process and all evidence considered by the grand jury remains confidential unless an indictment is returned. The court **arraigns**, or calls before the court, the charged person on the prosecutor's charge and the prosecutor brings those charges against the defendant. The prosecutor has the burden of proving the charges against the defendant. In virtually all criminal cases, the government must prove the defendant's guilt beyond a reasonable doubt.

The accused defendant may plead guilty and be sentenced to probation or imprisonment and/or pay a fine. He or she may instead plead not guilty, which results in a trial. Upon conclusion of the trial, a verdict of either guilty or not guilty is rendered. When a defendant is found not guilty, the charges are dismissed. To be found guilty or not guilty, all of the triers of fact (for example, all the members of a jury) must agree on the defendant's guilt or lack of proven guilt (**acquittal**). If all individuals cannot agree, this results in a **hung jury**. A defendant found to be guilty is sentenced to probation or imprisonment and/or to pay a fine. In most jurisdictions, only a defendant who is found guilty at trial can proceed through the appellate process.

Check Your Understanding 2.1

Instructions: **Answer the following questions on a separate piece of paper.**

1. What are the three related subsystems of government?
2. What are the four sources of laws in the United States?
3. What are the two types of jurisdictions that determine whether a case will be brought in federal court?
4. What are the three tiers in the federal and state court systems?
5. What is the court of last resort in the United States legal system?
6. What is the difference between public law and private law?
7. What is the difference between civil law and criminal law?
8. What are the parties and processes in civil litigation?
9. What are the parties and processes in a criminal case?
10. In civil and criminal cases, who has the burden of proof?

Healthcare Causes of Action

The healthcare industry is involved most often in civil cases and less often in criminal cases. However, because government is increasing its investigations into and prosecutions for healthcare fraud, health information privacy violations, and refusal to treat patients based on financial status, the healthcare industry will be faced with more criminal cases. However, this chapter focuses on civil actions. The types of civil legal actions that most typically affect the healthcare industry are torts and contracts. The vast majority of claims founded in tort and contract law are resolved without appearing in court, many before a lawsuit is filed.

Torts

A **tort** is an action brought when one party believes that another party caused harm through wrongful conduct and the party bringing the action seeks compensation for that harm. In addition to compensation, a second reason for bringing a tort action is to discourage the wrongdoer from committing further wrongful acts. Three categories of tort liability exist: negligence, intentional torts, and strict and products liability. Most healthcare incidents arise in the negligent tort category.

Negligent Torts

Negligence results when a person does not act the way a reasonably prudent person would act under the same circumstances. A negligent tort occurs when a person acts or fails to act as a reasonably prudent person in a particular situation. Negligence also may occur in cases where an individual has evaluated the alternatives and the consequences of those alternatives and has not exercised his or her best possible judgment. A person can also be found negligent when he or she has failed to guard against a risk that he or she knew could happen. Furthermore, negligence can occur in circumstances where it is known, or should have been known, that a particular behavior would place others in unreasonable danger. If an individual's behavior is categorized as reckless disregard or deliberate indifference, he or she may be found liable for **criminal negligence**.

Typically, negligence is conduct that is outside the generally accepted standard of care. **Standard of care** is defined as what an individual is expected to do or not do in a given situation. Standards of care are established in a variety of ways: by professional associations or accrediting bodies, by statute or regulation, or by practice. Such standards are considered to represent expected behavior unless a court finds differently. Therefore, standards also are established by case law. Standards not established by a governmental body do not by themselves have the force of law. In healthcare, the standard of care is the exercise of reasonable care by healthcare professionals having similar training and experience in the same or similar communities. The law relies on industry or national standards instead of community standards because courts hold that the standard of care should not vary by geographic area. This is particularly true in an era when patients can be referred to providers where more sophisticated technology exists or consultations can occur via telemedicine.

The standard of care does not apply only to direct patient care. It also applies to the physical safety of the premises for patients, staff, visitors, vendors, and members of the general public who come onto the premises. Physical safety means being free from physical defects in buildings and grounds and from being harmed by patients, nonstaff members, or staff members. In addition, healthcare organizations must address staff safety as it relates to treatment of violent or uncontrolled patients (for example, a patient under the influence of drugs or alcohol while being treated in the emergency department).

Negligence can further be categorized in various ways. For example, negligent torts can be categorized as one of the following:

- **Malfeasance:** The execution of an unlawful or improper act
- **Misfeasance:** The improper performance of an act resulting in injury to another
- **Nonfeasance:** The failure to act when there is a duty to act as a reasonably prudent person would act in similar circumstances (Pozgar and Santucci 2016)

Further, negligence can be categorized by the degree of wrongdoing. **Ordinary negligence** is failure to do what a reasonably prudent person would do, or doing something that a reasonably prudent person would not do, in the same or a similar situation. **Gross negligence** is an extreme departure from the ordinary standard of care and it represents reckless disregard (Proels 2012).

To recover damages caused by negligence, the plaintiff must show that all four elements of negligence are present (Pozgar and Santucci 2016):

- There must be a *duty of care*. For this element to be present in a medical malpractice case, a physician–patient, nurse–patient, therapist–patient, or other caregiver–patient relationship must exist at the time of the alleged wrongful act (there must be an obligation to meet a standard of care).
- There must have been a *breach of the duty of care*. The plaintiff must present evidence that the defendant acted unreasonably under the circumstances (either a failure to follow a standard of care or a deviation from the standard of care).

- The plaintiff must have *suffered an injury* as a result of the defendant's negligent act or failure to act. Injury includes not only physical harm but also mental suffering, pain, loss of income or reputation, and the invasion of a patient's rights and privacy.

- The plaintiff must show that the defendant's conduct *caused* the plaintiff's harm. As an example, varying from a recognized procedure is insufficient to justify the plaintiff's recovery of damages. The plaintiff must show that the variance was unreasonable and that it caused the harm. The plaintiff must show not only that the defendant's conduct actually caused the harm, but that the breach was also the proximate (foreseeable) cause of the injury.

When no statute exists to define what is reasonable, the trier of fact determines what a reasonably prudent person would have done. This is a "nonexistent, hypothetical person who is put forward as the community ideal of what would be considered reasonable behavior" (Pozgar and Santucci 2016). The trier of fact considers defendant characteristics such as age, sex, training, education, mental capacity, physical condition, and knowledge in defining the reasonably prudent person. After the behavior of a reasonably prudent person is defined for the given circumstances, the trier of fact compares the defendant's behavior against that definition. If the defendant's behavior meets or exceeds the definition, no negligence has occurred. On the other hand, if the defendant's behavior does not meet the reasonably prudent person standard and injury or damages result, negligence has occurred. In such a case, the trier of fact must determine whether the harm that would result from the failure to meet the reasonably prudent person standard could have been foreseen and negligent act caused harm to the plaintiff (Pozgar and Santucci 2016).

Intentional Torts

Although most torts experienced in healthcare are based on negligence, an occasional intentional tort

is committed. The element of intent is the difference between an intentional tort and negligent tort. **Intent** means the person committed an act purposely or knowing that harm would likely occur.

This section of the chapter provides a review of several intentional torts and an idea of how they may occur in a healthcare setting. These intentional torts include assault, battery, false imprisonment, defamation of character (slander or libel), fraud, invasion of privacy, and infliction of emotional distress.

Assault Assault is a deliberate threat, along with apparent ability, to cause contact with another person that can either be offensive or cause physical harm. For example, a large male nurse in the emergency department tells a frail elderly woman that he will break her arm if she does not do what he tells her to do. His comment is a deliberate threat and his size gives him the apparent ability to harm the woman. In this example, the woman does not need to suffer actual damage or even come in contact with the nurse. The apprehension that the threat creates is sufficient to constitute assault.

Battery Battery is the intentional and nonconsensual touching of another person's body (Proels 2012). In healthcare, laws regarding battery are especially important because of the requirement for consent for medical and surgical procedures. The patient does not need to be aware that battery has occurred. For example, battery occurs to the patient who is sedated and has surgery performed on him or her without either implied or express consent. Thus the hospital and the treating healthcare professionals may be held liable for harm caused by the lack of a proper patient consent. Further, even if the outcome of the procedure benefits the patient, touching the patient without proper consent may make the healthcare professional liable for battery.

False Imprisonment False imprisonment is another intentional tort. A healthcare provider's efforts to prevent a patient from leaving a hospital may result in false imprisonment. Although physical force is not required for one to be held liable for false imprisonment, when excessive force is used to restrain a patient the healthcare provider may be held liable for both false imprisonment and battery. It is not false imprisonment when a patient with a contagious disease or a mentally ill patient who is likely to cause harm to others is required to remain in the hospital. In general, restriction on a person's right to move about must be legally justifiable. A patient's insistence on leaving the facility should be documented in his or her health record, and the patient should be asked to sign a discharge against medical advice form that releases the facility from responsibility.

Defamation of Character

Defamation of character is a false communication about someone to a person other than the subject that may injure that person's reputation. The communication may be either oral or written—**libel** is the written form of defamation, and **slander** is the spoken form. To recover damages in an action for defamation, the plaintiff must prove that

- The defendant made a false and defamatory statement about the plaintiff
- The statement was not a "privileged" publication and was made to a third person
- At least negligence occurred
- Actual or presumed damages occurred

There are four situations where the plaintiff is not required to show proof of actual harm to his or her reputation when the defendant allegedly performs one of the following acts, because harm is presumed:

- Accuses the plaintiff of a crime
- Accuses the plaintiff of having a loathsome disease
- Uses words that affect the plaintiff's profession or business
- Calls a woman unchaste

However, healthcare professionals are protected against libel claims for reporting communicable diseases that the patient may consider loathsome, if such reporting is required by law (Proels 2012).

The defendant has two principal defenses available to a defamation action:

- Truth: There is no defamation liability if the statement was true
- Privilege: There is no defamation liability if the communication was made in good faith, on the proper occasion, in the proper manner, and to persons who have a legitimate reason to receive the information (Proels 2012).

The defense of privilege is relevant when the person making the communication has an obligation to report such information. For example, a director of nursing wrote a letter to a nurse's professional registry stating that the hospital wanted to discontinue a particular registry nurse's services because narcotics were disappearing whenever the nurse was on duty (*Judge v. Rockford Memorial Hospital* 1958). The court upheld the defense of privilege because the director of nurses had a legal duty to make the communication in the interests of society (Pozgar and Santucci 2016). Thus, the court denied the nurse's claim for damages. Two additional defenses—authorization of the disclosure by the plaintiff and lack of publication—are also viable (Proels 2012).

Fraud

Fraud is a prevalent concern in today's healthcare environment. Fraud is intentional misrepresentation that can harm another. For example, physicians can be held liable for fraud if they claim that a particular procedure will cure a patient's ailment when they know it will not; or if they charge a third-party payer for a medical procedure they did not actually perform. To prove fraud, the plaintiff must show

- An untrue statement known to be untrue by the party making the statement and made with an intent to deceive
- The victim's justifiable reliance on the truth of the statement
- Damages resulting from that reliance (Pozgar and Santucci 2016)

Invasion of privacy Invasion of privacy, the intrusion upon one's solitude, is another major concern in healthcare. A person's right to privacy is the right "to be let alone" (Warren and Brandeis 1890). This includes the rights of individuals to be free from surveillance and interference, as well as the right to keep one's information from being disclosed (Rinehart-Thompson and Harman 2006). The United States Constitution does not specifically grant a right to privacy; however, courts have interpreted the Constitution to give privacy rights in various subject matters (Rinehart-Thompson 2012a). Although a constitutional right to privacy with respect to health information does not exist, privacy of such information has been established through various court decisions, state laws, and federal laws, specifically the HIPAA Privacy Rule (45 CFR 160 and 164) (Rinehart-Thompson 2012a). Causes of action exist to protect patients when healthcare providers disregard a patient's right of privacy. One major actionable offense of concern in healthcare involving invasion of privacy is the unlawful disclosure of a patient's health information.

Infliction of emotional distress The intentional or reckless infliction of emotional distress for which a person can be held liable includes mental suffering resulting from such things as despair, shame, grief, and public humiliation (Pozgar and Santucci 2016). If the plaintiff shows that the defendant (the one inflicting the distress) intended to cause mental distress and knew or should have known that his or her actions would do so, the plaintiff can recover damages (Pozgar and Santucci 2016). Although this section focuses on the intentional infliction of emotional distress, a plaintiff may have a cause of action for negligent infliction of emotional distress as well, or as an alternative.

The distinction between negligence torts and intentional torts is far from academic. In most state legal systems, punitive damages—those damages awarded to punish or deter wrongful conduct over and above compensation for injury—are limited in negligence cases and may, in fact, be capped in medical malpractice cases. However, most states permit punitive damages as a matter of right in cases of intentional torts and these damages usually fall outside the scope of state laws capping jury awards or damages. Consequently, it is possible for a battery case involving a failure to obtain surgical consent (an intentional tort) to have more economic value than a medical malpractice case (a negligence tort) due to the presence or absence of punitive damages.

Products Liability

Products liability is the legal doctrine under which a manufacturer, seller, or supplier of a product may be liable to a buyer or other third party for injuries caused by a defective product (Pozgar and Santucci 2016). The injured person may bring an action based in negligence; breach of warranty, either implied or express; or strict liability.

To prevail in a products liability case based on *negligence,* the plaintiff must show all four elements of a negligence case: there was a duty; the duty was breached; injury resulted; and the breach was found to cause the injury. The manufacturer will not be held liable for injuries if they resulted from the user's negligent use of the product. However, manufacturers will be held liable for injuries resulting from a bad product design; thus manufacturers often provide instructions on the proper use of their product or otherwise face potential negligence liability (Pozgar and Santucci 2016). Defective packaging and a failure to warn of dangers associated with normal, proper use of the product can also result in the manufacturer being held liable in negligence (Pozgar and Santucci 2016).

Second, to recover under the theory of breach of warranty, or a broken promise, the plaintiff must show there was an express or implied warranty. Through an express warranty, the seller makes specific promises to the buyer, whereas an implied warranty exists when the law implies such a warranty exists "as a matter of public policy" to protect the public from harm (Pozgar and Santucci 2016).

The third basis on which a plaintiff may base a product's liability claim is strict liability, which occurs when a person or entity is held for acts or omissions regardless of whether there was fault (Proels 2012). To prevail, the plaintiff only must show an injury resulted while using the product in the proper manner. The plaintiff does not need to show negligence by the manufacturer. The elements for a strict liability case are the following:

- The defendant manufactured the product
- The product was defective when it left the hands of the manufacturer or seller; defects typically consist of
  - Manufacturing defects
  - Design defects
  - Absent or inadequate warnings for product use
  - The specific product must have injured the plaintiff
  - The defective product must have been the proximate, or immediate, cause of the injury (Pozgar and Santucci 2016)

Under strict liability, the manufacturer also may be held liable pursuant to *res ipsa loquitur* (the thing speaks for itself). To recover under this concept, the plaintiff must show that

- The product did not perform in the way intended
- Neither the buyer nor a third person had tampered with the product
- The defect in the product existed when it left the manufacturer (Pozgar and Santucci 2016)

Defenses

A healthcare provider may raise a number of defenses in response to a lawsuit. These include the following:

- **Statute of limitations** exceeded: A statutorily set time frame within which a lawsuit must be brought or the court must dismiss the case.
- **Contributory negligence:** The plaintiff's conduct contributed in part to the injury the plaintiff suffered and, if found to be sufficient, can preclude the plaintiff's recovery for the injury.
- **Comparative negligence:** The plaintiff's conduct contributed in part to the injury the plaintiff suffered, but the plaintiff's recovery

is reduced by some amount based on his or her percentage of negligence.

- **Assumption of risk:** The plaintiff who voluntarily places himself or herself at risk to a known or appreciated danger may not recover damages for injury resulting from the risk (McWay 2010).
- **Consent:** The plaintiff agreed to the act that is now alleged to have been wrongful
- **Good Samaritan statutes:** Statutes that protect physicians and other rescuers from liability for their acts or omissions in providing emergency care in a nontraditional setting such as at an automobile accident site when no charge for services is made and standard medical equipment is generally not available.
- **Charitable immunity:** Charitable institutions such as charity hospitals often were protected from liability for torts occurring on its property or by its employees.
- **Governmental immunity:** Precludes anyone from bringing a lawsuit against a governmental entity unless that entity consents to the lawsuit (McWay 2010).

The charitable immunity and governmental immunity defenses have been either significantly limited or abolished as defenses by state and federal laws (McWay 2010). Further, the assumption of risk defense is not frequently used in healthcare cases because voluntariness is generally lacking in a patient seeking medical care (Proels 2012).

A common fear by healthcare providers is that apologies made to a patient or patient's family members will be considered an admission of liability and will be used against providers who are named as defendants in lawsuits. Many states have created **apology statutes** ("I'm Sorry" laws) that protect a healthcare provider's apology from being admitted into evidence during a court proceeding as an admission of liability (Klaver 2012a).

Defenses specific to products liability cases include assumption of risk, intervening cause, contributory negligence, comparative fault, and disclaimers (Pozgar and Santucci 2016).

Contract

Lawsuits under contracts are the other type of civil claim arising in the healthcare industry. A **contract** is a written or oral agreement that, in most cases, is enforceable through the legal system. Contracts must not violate state or federal policy or state or federal statute, rule, or regulation. **Contract law**, which addresses the creation of contracts and the resolution of contract disputes, is based on common law. However, some states have replaced common law with statutory law or administrative agency regulations. In those states, the statutes or administrative regulations control. One example of how contractual issues affect healthcare is a contract for services between the hospital and a contracting physician or a physician group, such as pathologists, radiologists, anesthesiologists, and emergency medicine physicians. The parties to a contract must have the capacity to enter into the agreement, such as being competent adults, being of the age of majority, not being incapacitated by medication or alcohol, and not being mentally incapacitated. The provider-patient relationship is also based on a contractual agreement.

The elements of a contract must be stated clearly and specifically. A contract cannot exist unless all the following elements exist: there must be an *agreement* between two or more persons or entities, and the agreement must include a valid offer, an exchange of consideration, and acceptance.

In an **offer**, one party promises to either do something or not do something if the other party agrees to either do something or not do something (Klaver 2012b). The party making the offer must communicate it to the other party so that it can be accepted or rejected.

A contract must be supported by legal and bargained-for **consideration**, which is what the parties will receive from each other in exchange for performing the obligations of the contract (Klaver 2012b). There also must be **acceptance**, which requires a meeting of the minds between the parties about terms that are sufficiently definite and complete (Klaver 2012b).

A contract action arises when one party claims that the other party has failed to meet an obligation set forth in a valid contract. In other words, the other party has breached the contract. The resolution available is either compensation (monetary damages) or performance of the obligation. To succeed in a breach of contract action, the plaintiff must show that

- Parties entered into a valid contract
- Plaintiff performed as specified
- Defendant did not perform as specified
- Plaintiff suffered an economic loss as a result of the defendant's failure to perform (Pozgar and Santucci 2016)

The defendant can raise a variety of defenses to a breach of contract action including fraud (the nonperforming party was misled on a material contract term); mistake of fact (both parties relied on a mistake); duress (unlawful threat or pressure was used to execute the contract); impossibility (contract was impossible to perform); or illegality (contract was for illegal purposes or against public policy). A contract provision that places a healthcare provider in a significant position of power over a patient who relies on the provider's services may be against public policy and is called an **adhesion contract**.

Check Your Understanding 2.2

Instructions: **Answer the following questions on a separate piece of paper.**

1. What are the two most common types of civil healthcare causes of action?

2. What tort causes of action exist that relate to healthcare?

3. What are the three categories of negligence, and what are the four elements of negligence?

4. What are the types of intentional torts that were discussed in the text?

5. How might defamation of character be committed by a healthcare organization?

6. What defenses are available to an individual or organization defending against a tort action?

7. What is a contract and what elements must be present for a contract to exist?

8. What types of healthcare situations relate to a breach of contract?

9. What must occur for a contract action to arise?

10. When might a healthcare contract be against public policy and deemed an adhesion contract?

Legal Aspects of Health Information Management

The patient's health record is a legal document that serves as evidence of a patient's treatment and continuity of care. It is important for all HIM professionals to understand the statutes and regulations that affect access to and creation, maintenance, and retention of the health record.

Form and Content of the Health Record

The health record is a complete, accurate, and current report of the medical history, condition, and treatment that a particular patient receives during an encounter with a healthcare provider. (See a discussion of a legal health record later in this chapter.) An encounter may be either inpatient or outpatient, and it may reflect one episode of treatment or an accumulation of all episodes of treatment (a longitudinal record).

The health record is composed of demographic information and clinical information. Most of the demographic information is collected at the time of admission or registration for treatment. It includes, among other items, the patient's name, sex, age, insurance information, and the person to contact in case of emergency. The clinical information consists of the patient's complaint, history of present illness, medical history, family history, social history, continuing documentation of ongoing medical care, report of diagnostic tests, x-ray reports, surgery and other procedure reports, consultant reports, nursing documentation, various graphs, and the final diagnoses.

The content of health records maintained by a healthcare provider may be determined based on multiple requirements. Content is often determined by state law via statutes and regulations, which may be prescriptive or broad in scope. For example, some laws detail what a proper health record must contain and the information to be retained; others specify broad categories of information required; and still others simply require that the health record be accurate, adequate, and complete. Medicare providers must also follow the Medicare Conditions of Participation, which include minimum requirements for health record content. Third-party payers also dictate how health records for their insured must be maintained and kept. Accrediting bodies also determine a provider's health record content. Joint Commission and the American Osteopathic Association (AOA), as well as others, also have health record content requirements. The HIM professional must be aware of the most prescriptive definition of the health record content that his or her organization must follow. The following sections outline external forces that impact, to varying degrees, the forms and content of the health record maintained by healthcare providers: licensing agencies, accrediting bodies, and statutory and regulatory law.

Licensing Agencies

Typically, state legislatures grant authority to designated state administrative agencies to

- Develop standards that hospitals and other healthcare providers must meet
- Issue licenses to those hospitals and other healthcare providers that meet the standards
- Monitor continuing compliance with the standards
- Penalize hospitals and other healthcare providers that violate the standards

Licensure is government regulation that is mandatory for hospitals and other healthcare organizations, depending on state law. Licensure is issued to organizations as a whole. It addresses policies and procedures, staffing, and hospital building integrity among many other facets of the organization. Some states require additional licenses for specific services. For example, laboratory, pharmacy, radiology, renal dialysis, medical equipment, and substance abuse services in a hospital may require separate licenses in addition to the organization's license. Hospitals cannot operate without a license or equivalent type of approval. Those that violate licensure standards may lose their licenses or be penalized in other ways, such as fines.

Accrediting Bodies

Accreditation is offered through nongovernmental organizations. Accreditation is considered voluntary and is not legally mandated, but it is very important to healthcare organizations because it provides an organization with a designation as a high-quality healthcare provider. One of the most prominent accrediting bodies for acute-care hospitals is Joint Commission, but it also accredits organizations in other types of settings (for example, behavioral health, ambulatory services, and home health). Other accrediting bodies, such as the Commission on Accreditation of Rehabilitation Facilities (CARF), occupy a larger space in care settings outside the acute-care hospital, such as long-term care.

Joint Commission develops standards that organizations must meet to be accredited. An organization first applies to Joint Commission, pays an accreditation fee, and submits to an extensive survey to ensure compliance with Joint Commission's published standards. Joint Commission addresses record content, privacy, information security, confidentiality, ethical behavior, patient rights training, and whether the organization complies with applicable laws, regulations, and standards. Similarly, the American Osteopathic Association accredits osteopathic hospitals through its Healthcare Facilities Accreditation Program (HFAP) and functions in much the same way as Joint Commission. Some states accept Joint Commission or AOA accreditation as a basis for partial or full licensure with a limited or no additional survey by a state agency. This "deeming" authority gives Joint Commission and AOA a significant amount of power they would not otherwise have. In addition to Joint Commission and AOA surveys that focus on an entire organization, there are also accrediting processes that focus on specific services such as laboratory and radiology. These surveys can be offered by Joint Commission, AOA, or other accrediting bodies.

Statutory and Regulatory Law

An organization must consult its applicable state and federal statutes and regulations to determine which ones apply. The federal Medicare regulations apply to any provider that participates in the Medicare program, and the majority of providers fit within this definition. In order to be reimbursed by Medicare, providers must comply with the requirements in the Medicare Conditions of Participation. The Medicare program also recognizes organizations that have Joint Commission or AOA accreditation as meeting most of the Conditions of Participation, and it grants them deemed status. An organization would typically undergo an additional survey only if a special Medicare inspection finds noncompliance.

Privacy There are many sources of law mandating the privacy of health information. The federal Health Insurance Portability and Accountability Act of 1996 (HIPAA) Privacy Rule occupies a large space in this area. However, HIM professionals must also consult their individual state statutes and regulations for specific applications that provide privacy protections in addition to those provided by HIPAA.

Although the US Constitution does not specifically grant a right to privacy, in 1965 the US Supreme Court recognized an implicit constitutional right of privacy in *Griswold v. Connecticut (1965)*. In this case, the court limited government authority over contraception (Showalter 2012). Some states, such as California, Arizona, and Florida, also have recognized the right to privacy in their state constitutions (California Constitution, Article 1, Declaration of Rights, Section 1; Arizona Constitution, Section 8, Right to privacy; Florida Constitution, Article I, Section 23, Right of privacy).

The **Privacy Act of 1974** was an early piece of federal legislation that addressed the right to privacy. This act was written to give individuals some control over the large amounts of information collected about them by the federal government and its contractors (Rinehart-Thompson 2012b). It does not apply to records maintained by institutions in the private sector (McWay 2010). Under the Privacy Act of 1974, people have the right to learn what information has been collected about them; view and obtain a copy of that information; and maintain limited control over the disclosure of that information to other persons or entities (Hughes 2002). Because the act only applies to federal agencies and contractors, its applicability in healthcare is limited to federal healthcare organizations such as the Veterans Health Administration (VHA), the Indian Health Service, and their contractors (Hughes 2002).

The **Freedom of Information Act (FOIA)** of 1967 is a federal law through which individuals can seek access to information without authorization of the person to whom the information applies. The underlying premise of FOIA is government accountability and transparency; however, access exceptions exist for medical records to protect their privacy in most situations. This act, like the Privacy Act, also applies only to federal agencies so its applicability to healthcare organizations is generally limited to those owned and operated by the Veterans Health Administration and Defense Department.

The Medicare Conditions of Participation requires that healthcare organizations have procedures in place to protect the confidentiality of patient records (Rinehart-Thompson 2012b). This includes the protection of records against unauthorized access and alteration. Further, original records may be removed from the facility only in accordance with federal and state laws (Hughes 2002). However, the Conditions of Participation regulate only providers who receive funds from Medicare and Medicaid (Rinehart-Thompson 2012b).

The **Health Insurance Portability and Accountability Act (HIPAA)** was enacted by Congress on August 21, 1996. This legislation initially focused on making it easier for employees to retain health coverage when they changed jobs or their family status changed. The HIPAA legislation addressed waste, fraud, and abuse in the healthcare system. It also focused on simplifying the administration of health insurance. To address simplification, Congress added the Administrative Simplification provisions, which created a single federal standard electronic claims format for electronic data interchange. With these provisions, the legislature intended to improve the efficiency and effectiveness of the healthcare system. However, Congress continued to express concerns about privacy and security of patient information in an electronic environment. Consequently, HIPAA required the Department of Health and Human Services (HHS) to develop and implement electronic transaction standards and to develop regulations to protect the privacy and security of individually identifiable health information (HIPAA 1996).

As a result, HHS issued three sets of standards: Transactions and Code Sets (45 CFR 160 and 162), Privacy, and Security (45 CFR 160 and 164). All rules for these three sets of standards have been promulgated and issued. Covered entities as defined in HIPAA were required to be in compliance with the Privacy Rule by April 14, 2003, with the Transactions and Code Sets Rule by October 16, 2003, and with the Security Rule by April 20, 2005. The compliance dates for small health plans were extended by one year for each set of rules.

In February 2009, President Barack Obama signed the American Recovery and Reinvestment Act (ARRA) of 2009, which included the Health Information Technology for Economic and Clinical Health (HITECH) Act provisions. HITECH strengthened the requirements included in the HIPAA Privacy and Security Rules. ARRA is discussed in other chapters throughout this book.

The Legal Health Record

In 2006, the AHIMA House of Delegates passed a resolution stating that "AHIMA advocates that organizations define one set of health information that meets the legal and business needs of the organization and complies with state and federal laws and regulations" (AHIMA 2007b). This resolution set the stage for the legal health record (LHR), but did not define its parameters. The **legal health record (LHR)**—as defined by a specific organization—includes those documents and data that the organization determines it will disclose pursuant to a legal request, and whether that information meets the rules of evidence requirements and health record content, maintenance, and retention requirements. As the LHR transforms from a paper-based record to an **electronic health record (EHR)**, laws and regulations continually change to reflect technological changes. Adding to the complexity of defining the LHR is the existence of health records in many different formats (paper, imaged, electronic, hybrid) and rapid movement toward the EHR, where information is created and retrieved at the point of care and data fields can be managed.

Defining the Legal Health Record

Factors the HIM professional should consider in defining or assessing whether the current record is a LHR, regardless of format, include:

- Purpose of the health record
- State and federal laws, regulations, and standards defining health record content
- Internal documents
- Risks the organization faces if its health record does not meet business record or legal health record requirements or the rules of evidence, especially if it is an EHR

Pursuant to the Federal Rules of Evidence (FRE) for business records, the health record qualifies as a business record. It is created and kept in the normal course of business, made at or near the time of the matter recorded, and made by a person within the business with knowledge of the events recorded (FRE 803(6)). The business is providing healthcare. As a business record, the health record contains documentation of patient care, which can be used for continuity of care and for billing. Further, it serves as a communication tool for caregivers. The organization uses the health record for operational activities such as evaluating quality of care and as a resource for medical research and education.

The health record as a business record can also serve as "testimony" in legal proceedings (AHIMA 2007c). The legal standards that control whether a record is admissible in court apply regardless of whether the health record is paper or electronic (AHIMA 2007a). Such standards include the presumption that information recorded in conjunction with business practices is trustworthy and has potential evidentiary value. Thus, based on its status as a business record and a generally admissible document, the health record is the organization's "legal health record" (Rinehart-Thompson et al. 2012).

Once that determination is made, however, organizations must consider what documentation is included in and excluded from the legal health record. State and federal statutes, regulations, licensure requirements; accrediting body standards; and internal documents such as medical staff bylaws provide guidance by defining health record content, maintenance, and documentation requirements; however, these vary widely by practice setting (McLendon 2012; Rinehart-Thompson et al. 2012). Thus, there is no boilerplate definition of the LHR. Rather, it is as each organization defines it.

The LHR definition was much simpler to attain when only paper-based records were used, but in today's electronic health record environment it is more difficult to define the LHR. Not only is EHR technology impacting the definition, but so too is the evolving content of the health record (AHIMA 2011). Health records now consist of a "facility's record, outpatient diagnostic test results or therapies, pharmacy records, physician records, other care providers' records, and the patient's own personal health record" (AHIMA 2011). The health record may also have administrative, financial, and clinical data intermingled. However, the organization can apply the same criteria it used to define the paper legal health record to define its legal heath record in today's environment:

- What information can be stored long term?
- What information is clinically useful for the long term?
- What are the storage costs?
- How can the EHR be effectively and succinctly assembled for long-term use? (AHIMA 2011)

The healthcare organization may define its LHR in terms of the data set to be released in response to a legal request such as a subpoena by cataloging and using policies and procedures to state what will be divulged pursuant to a legal request (McLendon 2007). Because most healthcare organizations have moved to some level of electronic health record, the LHR definition may include information in both paper and electronic format, typically referred to as a hybrid health record (McLendon 2012). The organization must broaden its assessment of what makes up the LHR by considering data such as "electronic-structured documents, images, audio files, video files, and paper documents" (Rinehart-Thompson et al. 2012). In EHRs, the HIM professional must account for source EHR systems that feed into what the organization has defined as its legal EHR (McLendon 2007). Organizations should develop and maintain a source system matrix (McLendon 2012). Therefore, regardless of format, defining the LHR is a multidisciplinary responsibility. To define the legal EHR, in addition to writing new policies as needed, HIM professionals utilize a list of documents that defines the paper-based LHR. An organization's legal counsel should participate in policy and procedure development (McLendon 2012).

Record Authenticity

Those who use information in the health record rely on it as being correct, accurate, and complete. It must not have been changed either intentionally or accidentally (Rinehart-Thompson et al. 2012). Reliability and integrity of the health record are critical to meeting the standards of evidence in a court of law and thus being classified as the organization's LHR (Rinehart-Thompson et al. 2012).

Inextricably linked to reliability and integrity is **authenticity**, which means that the record is genuine and "is what it purports to be" (Rinehart-Thompson et al. 2012; FRE 901(a)). Authenticity relates both to the reliability of the system on which information is created and stored, and to the information itself. System reliability includes such features as user access controls, system security, access tracking and auditing capabilities, and operational stability (dependability and availability). These features are particularly important because of the concern that electronically stored information can easily be changed (Rinehart-Thompson et al. 2012). In both paper and EHR environments, information authenticity includes both the content and the authors of health record entries. **Authentication** establishes information authenticity. In paper records, authentication is accomplished by a handwritten signature or initials, both in ink. Electronic or digital signatures and computer keys are examples of authentication methods in EHRs (Rinehart-Thompson et al. 2012). Whatever approach is decided upon, it must comply with applicable laws and regulations as well as accrediting body requirements (Olenik 2008). Additional authentication considerations are counter-signatures (which may be required when one professional practices under the direct supervision of another) and documents such as assessments that require authentication by all staff members involved

Other issues that need to be considered when defining the LHR and maintaining a legally defensible health record include the appropriate uses of abbreviations; legibility; changes such as revisions, additions, deletions, and version management; timeliness and completeness; and control over printing so that paper printouts do not contain more current information than the electronic record (McLendon 2012; Rinehart-Thompson et al. 2012).

As concerns about inappropriate abbreviations and legibility have lessened with the electronic health record, another problem has replaced it.

This is the "cut and paste" function enabled in some systems. Risks include:

- Copying information to the wrong patient
- Copying information to the wrong encounter for the correct patient
- Inadequate identification of the original author and date of the entry, thus creating authorship issues
- Determinations that such conduct is unethical or illegal in circumstances such as clinical trials (Olenik 2008)

Other factors that affect the integrity of the legal electronic health record include granting appropriate access to the various portions of the record by staff based on their roles in the organization (role-based access); designating the custodian(s) of the record, which is an information governance issue; determining procedures for retention, destruction, and permanent archiving; system and network security; and disaster recovery and data backup (McLendon 2007, 2012).

The Legal Health Record vs. Designated Record Set

One last point that must be made regarding the LHR is its distinction from the HIPAA-defined **designated record set (DRS)**. HIPAA defines the DRS as those medical records and billing records about an individual that a HIPAA-covered entity maintains or that the covered entity uses to make decisions about individuals (45 CFR 164.501). Because the DRS may include documents from other providers and electronic communications (for example, e-mails) between providers and between provider and patient, the DRS encompasses more information than what has historically been included in an organization's paper-based LHR (Rinehart-Thompson et al. 2012). The DRS is described in greater detail in chapter 11.

The Electronic Health Record

The move toward a fully electronic health record (EHR) brings special liability issues with it. In particular, liability issues can be classified in two categories:

- Those in which the information in the EHR serves as proof in a lawsuit of the quality of patient care provided
- Those that arise from unauthorized access to, or the careless handling of, patient information in a computerized environment (McWay 2010)

The first issue focuses on whether information in the EHR can be admitted as evidence. This raises the hearsay rule, which excludes certain out-of-court statements as inherently unreliable, and how it can be overcome for electronically stored medical records. Although admissibility of such records has been tested on a limited basis, federal courts have allowed a computer printout into evidence where the foundation, trustworthiness, and accuracy requirements were shown to have been met (McWay 2010).

The second issue focuses on legal requirements to keep EHRs safe and secure. The EHR must be subject to all three components of the HIPAA Security Rule: administrative safeguards (policies, procedures, risk assessment [45 CFR 164.308]); physical safeguards (facility access control [45 CFR 164.310]); and technical safeguards (access control [45 CFR 164.312]). Further, ARRA charges healthcare providers to follow security and privacy regulations issued by HHS (McWay 2010, 289).

Retention of the Health Record

The health record serves several purposes and must be retained to meet those purposes. These purposes include patient treatment, communication among providers, and continuity of care; proof of services provided to justify reimbursement; evidence in legal proceedings; evaluation of quality and efficiency of care; source of information for statistics, research and education; and facilitation of an organization's operations management (Rinehart-Thompson et al. 2012). These varied purposes influence how long health records must be kept (that is, their retention period). Equally as important as defining retention periods is ensuring that information is private and secure during the time it is retained.

Federal and state statutes and regulations often determine retention periods. For example, the

Medicare Conditions of Participation require a five-year retention period for hospital records (42 CFR 482.24(b)(1)). For those periods determined by state law, the state defines what the minimum retention period will be. Some states are more specific than others and may set specific retention requirements for particular parts of the health record (for example, x-rays or mammography studies) or for particular patient types (for example, minors, mentally ill, deceased) (Gaffey and Groves 2011). Additionally, organizations must take into consideration the applicable statutes of limitations for bringing a legal action (for example, for medical malpractice or breach of contract actions), so the record will still exist if needed for legal proceedings. This consideration is particularly important for retaining the records of minors (should they file lawsuits on their own behalf once they reach the age or majority) or incompetent individuals (should their mental incompetence be lifted by the court system) (Rinehart-Thompson et al. 2012). The HIM professional must be aware of all applicable retention laws and statutes of limitations in his or her state.

In addition to legal sources, other factors affect retention decisions. Organizations such as professional associations (for example, AHIMA) offer guidance, as do accrediting bodies. The Joint Commission does not mandate specific retention periods, but defers to an organization's applicable statutes, regulations, and patient care and operational needs (Rinehart-Thompson et al. 2012). Organizations' retention periods, although bound by the period required by applicable laws, may vary otherwise among each other. Some organizations will opt for longer retention periods than others based on factors such as cost and operational needs including availability of information for statistics, research, and education.

Finally, technology continues to affect retention. The EHR allows many organizations to retain records for longer periods of time, but retention decisions associated with EHRs are also impacted by federal and state e-discovery rules. Organizations must know how long information is stored, in what form(s) it exists, and when it will be destroyed. They must also know where informa-

tion is stored including hidden locations such as document drafts, shadow records, and electronic backup systems. Retention schedules must also be developed for metadata (for example, logs showing when electronic documents are created, accessed, and changed) (Klaver 2012a).

Ownership and Access to the Health Record

Patients often believe they own their health record. While it is true that the information in the record is that of the individual and he or she has the right to access it, the organization that created and maintains the physical record is responsible for its integrity and security, and thus is the legal custodian. The HIM professional must be able to advise the patient regarding the actual ownership and control of the physical health record and the patient's rights to the information contained in it.

The emergence of the electronic health record has clouded the ownership question because the accepted ownership rule has been based on "original hard copy documents" (Jergesen 2011). Historically, the physical health record was considered the property of the healthcare provider that maintained it because it was the healthcare provider's business record and there was only one original copy to control. However, regardless of whether the medical record format is paper or electronic, the organization responsible for its creation and maintenance continues to be legally obligated to "to maintain its basic integrity, and particularly to protect it from loss, destruction, or improper alteration" (Jergesen 2011). This principle is reinforced by the HIPAA privacy and security rules as well as by some state laws and accrediting bodies such as Joint Commission (Jergesen 2011). In effect, then, the organization that is responsible for the record "owns" it even though it is electronically stored.

HIPAA grants individuals the right to access their **protected health information (PHI)**, which is information specifically protected by HIPAA. This right will be described in more detail in chapter 11; however, it is important for HIM professionals to understand that although the organization owns the record patients have the right to access the record with exceptions noted in HIPAA. Also, many state laws give individuals the right of access to their own health information. However, if state law does not provide individuals with the same degree of access that HIPAA allows, the state law will be superseded by HIPAA through the principle of **preemption**, which gives federal law precedence over state law. The right of access is continuously becoming more ubiquitous as individuals are not only able to access their information via patient portals, but are encouraged to do so per Stage 2 Meaningful Use requirements.

Check Your Understanding 2.3

Instructions: Answer the following questions on a separate piece of paper.

1. What are the two types of information collected in the health record? Discuss what information constitutes each type.

2. What is the primary difference between licensure and accreditation of healthcare organizations?

3. What external factors must be taken into consideration when a healthcare organization makes decisions about the form and content of its health records?

4. What was the holding regarding privacy issued by the court in *Griswold v. Connecticut*?

5. In addition to HIPAA, what pieces of legislation are discussed that address privacy?

6. Why is the Privacy Act of 1974 of limited use to individuals with respect to their health information?

7. What steps should an organization take to define its legal health record? What special considerations should be taken into account for defining a legal *electronic* health record?

8. What types of liabilities does the electronic health record present?

9. Legally, what factors *must* be taken into consideration when developing health record retention schedules? What factors *should* be taken into consideration? Which of these are internal factors and which are external factors?

10. Who owns the information contained in the health record, whether paper or computer based?

The Health Record as Evidence

The health record is key evidence in many types of legal proceedings. It serves as documentation of care provided in civil cases such as medical malpractice (for example, a patient alleges wrongdoing against healthcare providers) or other personal injury (for example, vehicle accidents) and in criminal cases (for example, rape, homicide, and healthcare fraud).

Admissibility of the Health Record

The health record may be valuable evidence in a legal proceeding. To be admissible, the court must be confident that the record

- Is complete, accurate, and timely (recorded at the time the event occurred),
- Was documented in the normal course of business, and
- Was made by healthcare providers who have knowledge of the "acts, events, conditions, opinions, or diagnoses appearing in it" (AHIMA e-HIM Work Group on Maintaining the Legal EHR 2005).

The court must accept that the information was recorded as the result of treatment, not in anticipation of a legal proceeding. Furthermore, to be admissible, the health record must be relevant and proper. The health record is considered hearsay because the healthcare providers made the entries in the record and not in court under oath (McWay 2010). However, the business records exception to the prohibition against using hearsay as evidence will often permit it to be admitted (Klaver 2012a).

For an electronic health record to be admissible, the court must be confident that the system from which the record was produced is accurate and trustworthy. Characteristics used to support a system's accuracy and trustworthiness are:

- The type of computer used and that computer's acceptance as standard and efficient equipment
- The record's method of operation
- The method and circumstances of preparation of the record (AHIMA e-HIM Work Group on Maintaining the Legal EHR 2005)

Medical witnesses may refer to the health record to refresh their recollection. The custodian of records, typically the health information manager, may be called as a witness to identify the record as the one subpoenaed. He or she also may be called to testify as to policies and procedures relevant to the following:

- Creation of the record including the system or process used
- Maintenance of the record to prevent it from being altered
- Maintenance of the record to prevent it from being accessed without proper authorization

The actual admissibility as evidence depends on the facts and circumstances of the case and the applicable state and federal rules of evidence.

Consent and Advance Directives

Consents and advance directives play an important evidentiary role in health information management. It is vital to know an individual's wishes regarding the receipt of healthcare and for those wishes to be documented. Consent is one's agreement to receive medical treatment. Consent can either be written (preferred because it offers greater proof) or spoken; express (communicated through words) or implied (communicated through conduct or a mechanism other than words, such as an unconscious person who is brought to the emergency room). Healthcare organizations obtain a **general consent**, which permits healthcare providers to perform overall medical care, from a patient for routine treatment. Failure to obtain general consent can result in a legal action, generally for battery. When a treatment or procedure becomes more risky or invasive, it is important that the **informed consent** process be completed to ensure the patient has a basic understanding of diagnosis, the nature of the treatment or procedure, along with the risks, benefits, alternatives (to include opting out of treatment), and individuals who will perform the treatment or procedure. It is the responsibility of the provider who will be rendering the treatment or performing the procedure to obtain the patient's informed consent and answer the patient's questions. Failure to obtain informed consent can result in legal action generally based on negligence (Klaver 2012c).

An **advance directive** is a special type of consent that communicates an individual's wishes to be treated or not to be treated should the individual become unable to communicate on his or her own behalf. Through a **durable power of attorney for healthcare decisions**, an individual—while competent—designates another person (proxy) to make healthcare decisions consistent with the individual's wishes on the individual's behalf. The term *durable* indicates that the document is in effect when the individual is no longer competent. A **living will** is executed by a competent adult, expressing the individual's wishes to limit treatment should the individual become afflicted with certain conditions (for example, a persistent vegetative state or a terminal condition) and can longer communicate on his or her own behalf. Living wills often address extraordinary lifesaving measures such as ventilator support and either the continuation or removal of nutrition and hydration. The lack of advance directives, where controversy erupted regarding the undocumented wishes of individuals, has sparked such high-profile end-of-life cases as

Karen Ann Quinlan, Nancy Cruzan, and Terri Schiavo (Klaver 2012c).

A third type of document, which always specifies an individual's wish not to receive treatment (specifically, cardiopulmonary resuscitation or CPR) is the **do-not-resuscitate (DNR) order**. Most often used by individuals who are elderly or in chronically ill health, it directs healthcare providers to refrain from performing the otherwise standing order of CPR should the individual experience cardiac or respiratory arrest. Prior to executing a DNR, the patient and physician should have a discussion, a consent form should be signed by the patient, and the physician is to write an order in the patient's medical record. State law provides the framework for completing DNR orders and forms. Joint Commission-accredited organizations are required to implement policies regarding advance directives and DNR orders (Klaver 2012c). Table 2.1 differentiates between these three types of advance directive documents.

In 1990, Congress passed the **Patient Self-Determination Act**, which requires healthcare institutions that are Medicare or Medicaid providers to provide adult patients with information about advance directives; document in the health record whether patients have an advance directive or not; and treat patients equally despite the presence or absence of an advance directive (Klaver 2012c).

e-Discovery

Responsibility for responding to requests for health records involved in litigation, either for depositions or in the courtroom, has long rested with HIM professionals. However, this process is changing rapidly as health records transition to hybrid or completely electronic formats. What HIM professionals are experiencing is known as **e-discovery**, which is a pretrial process through which parties obtain and review electronically stored data. With the increased prevalence of electronically stored data and the ease of searching these data, the legal discovery process in civil and criminal cases is focusing more on e-discovery (McLendon 2012). The e-discovery amendments to the Federal Rules of Civil Procedure (FRCP) became effective December 1, 2006 (Klaver 2012a). Although the FRCP applies only to cases in federal district courts, states have implemented similar e-discovery rules that apply to state civil and criminal cases.

Issues associated with e-discovery that need to be addressed include identifying what needs to be preserved, the format that it will be presented in, the locations of all electronically stored information (ESI), legal holds, record retention and destruction policies, disaster recovery, and business continuity (Klaver 2012a). In the past, HIM professionals were involved in the pretrial discovery phase through a subpoena for records or by testifying at a deposition. With e-Discovery, the HIM professional's involvement begins much earlier in litigation with pretrial conferences. During pretrial conferences, attorneys for the parties meet to reach agreement on matters related to document discovery and to discuss whether documents are even available. The involvement of information technology (IT) personnel in the early stages of litigation becomes very important. Although the

Table 2.1. Comparison of advance directives

Durable power of attorney for healthcare decisions	Executed by a competent adult on his or her own behalf.
	Designates another person (proxy) to make healthcare decisions consistent with the individual's wishes on the individual's behalf.
Living will	Executed by a competent adult on his or her own behalf.
	Expresses one's wishes to limit treatment if a medical condition renders the individual unable to communicate on his or her own behalf.
	May be limited to certain medical conditions (for example, vegetative state), depending on state law.
Do-not-resuscitate order	Most often used elderly or in chronically ill health.
	Directs healthcare providers to refrain from CPR if the individual experiences cardiac or respiratory arrest.

entity producing the ESI can object, it must produce the information in "the form in which it is ordinarily maintained or a reasonably usable form" (DeLoss 2008).

Defining what constitutes the legal health record for disclosure purposes becomes particularly important in e-discovery (McLendon 2007). With EHR technology, vast volumes of information can be created and stored. Therefore, much more extensive information is subject to discovery than in the paper record environment. Any data stored electronically can serve as evidence (for example, e-mails, voicemails, texts, instant messages, drafts of documents, information on personal mobile devices, calendar files, websites) (AHIMA e-Discovery Task Force 2008; Olenik et al. 2012). The concept of "any and all records" has taken on a new meaning with e-discovery.

HIM professionals must now be familiar with documents stored in what is natural or "native file format," including **metadata**—electronic data about data that include information not previously available in paper documents such as time stamps that show when and by whom a document or entry was created, accessed, or changed (Klaver 2012a). It is important to establish policies and procedures that define how to produce "the designated business record, including the native file format and metadata" (McLendon 2012).

The concepts of a legal hold and spoliation continue under the e-discovery rule. A **legal hold** is typically issued by a court to lock or disengage any editing capabilities to a health record, whether paper or electronic, when there is concern that information relevant to a legal proceeding or an audit could be destroyed. This hold would suspend any normal disposition activities including destruction. The following events can prompt the HIM professional to place a health record under a legal hold:

- Complaints
- Civil investigative demands
- Subpoenas
- Demand letters
- Prelitigation discussions with opposing counsel

- Preservation letters
- Written notices from opposing counsel
- Government investigations or inquiries (DeLoss 2008)

Spoliation is "intentional destruction, mutilation, alteration, or concealment of evidence" (Klaver 2012a). A trier of fact may reasonably infer that destruction of evidence related to a legal proceeding was done so with a consciousness of guilt or nefarious motive; however, courts will generally allow the spoliator to rebut the inference and show that there was no bad faith (Klaver 2012a). HIM professionals should review the organization's information management plan in order to know how it defines its records, including the business record, legal health record, and designated record set. They should also know the various locations (for example, source systems and databases) where information is stored, as well as the types of information stored (Dimick 2007). The HIM professional knows which departments feed clinical information into the legal health record whether in the paper or electronic format; they must now also become familiar with what systems are used by these different departments. The locations in which information can be electronically stored both at home and at work include:

- Laptops and desktops
- Servers and shared drives
- Handheld devices such as PDAs and cell phones
- Removable storage devices such as flash drives, thumbnails, CDs (compact discs)
- Websites
- Databases (DeLoss 2008)

The location of ESI must also be addressed from the perspective of ancillary services, clinical services, remote access, personal equipment, and e-mail. With regard to ancillary services, the HIM professional must know or determine whether the information is integrated into the EHR or maintained separately. One should ask if external providers are networked and if data resides on equipment such as an MRI, digital x-ray, IV medication pumps, dictation systems, robotics, equipment for emergency or "crash" situations, or personal health records (PHRs) (DeLoss 2008).

Complying with an e-discovery request or subpoena most likely involves many systems. This is complex because the standards for what will be discoverable and what electronic information needs to be part of the health record are still being developed. HIM professionals should store only what is vital because if it is stored, it is likely subject to e-discovery (Dimick 2007). Having good policies, procedures, standards, and information management plans are an important start.

The organization must also develop a litigation response plan and healthcare organizations should take five key steps to develop and implement such a plan:

- Evaluate applicable rules—federal-, state-, and local-level e-discovery rules

- Form a litigation response team—an interdisciplinary group to implement and conduct ongoing review of the e-discovery process

- Analyze issues, risks, and challenges that may arise from e-discovery—this analysis is the basis for policy and procedure development

- Develop or revise organizational policies and procedures to incorporate e-discovery

- Develop and implement an ongoing monitoring and evaluation process to ensure continued compliance with policies and procedures (AHIMA e-Discovery Task Force 2008)

So what is the role of the HIM professional in e-discovery? As the volume of discoverable information increases as electronic health record systems advance, there must be people who are knowledgeable about how to store, manage, and access the information (Dimick 2007).

Privileges

Professional relationships between the patient and specific groups of caregivers further affect use of the record and its contents as evidence. These relationships are referred to as **privileges**. The information exchanged between patient and caregiver pursuant to a privilege is a confidential communication that the patient anticipates will be held confidential. One such widely recognized privilege is the **physician–patient privilege**. This privilege provides that the physician is not permitted to testify as a witness about certain information gained as a result of this relationship without the patient's consent.

The information included in the physician–patient privilege is insulated from the discovery process when there is no patient authorization, waiver, or overriding law or public policy (Gaffey and Groves 2011). State laws address the scope of privilege (for example, whether a court can order an examination that is not protected by the privilege and whether or not the privilege survives if a third party was present during a physician–patient communication) (Klaver 2012a). Depending on the state, similar privileges exist between psychotherapist and patient, sexual assault victim and counselor, and domestic violence victim and counselor. In states where these professional relationships are recognized, they apply when the caregiver is being compelled to testify as a witness concerning information obtained as a result of the relationship. However, these privileges do not preclude the caregiver from making reports as required by law.

The patient may release the caregiver from the privileges discussed through words or actions. This release is known as a waiver of the privilege. For example, a patient who placed his or her treatment at issue in a trial could not continue to claim a privilege to protect the information. The caregiver then could be compelled to testify regarding the information previously considered confidential.

Government's Right of Access to Health Records

The government, whether federal or state, has the right to access health information with or without patient authorization in certain circumstances, such as Medicare or Medicaid. Medicare is a federal program that provides insurance for medical care for the elderly and disabled (Showalter 2012). Medicaid is a joint federal and state program to provide insurance for medical care to individuals unable to pay for care. As the payers, both programs may request information from the health record to support the healthcare provider's bill submitted for payment. By signing up with Medicare or Medicaid, the patient gives permission for the healthcare provider to disclose confidential health information to the appropriate agency without further authorization.

The government also may require access to health information for other investigative purposes such as pursuant to the federal fraud and abuse statutes that require information-sharing arrangements to be undertaken in an arm's length transaction and pursuant to a written agreement (Kadzielski 2011). An **arm's length transaction** is a transaction in which "parties are dealing from equal bargaining positions, neither party is subject to the other's control or dominant influence, and the transaction is treated with fairness, integrity, and legality" (Trautmann 2003).

Another important federal statute for which the government may need access to health information as part of an investigation is the Emergency Medical Treatment and Labor Act (EMTALA) (Cohen 2011). This statute protects any patient seeking emergency care in a Medicare-participating hospital, but its efforts to prevent "patient dumping" evolved because of hospitals that transferred, discharged, or refused to treat patients who were unable to pay (Klaver 2012d).

Check Your Understanding 2.4

Instructions: **Answer the following questions on a separate piece of paper.**

1. What may a custodian of health information be called as a witness to testify about regarding the health record?

2. Per the Federal Rules of Evidence, what factors qualify the health record as a business record?

3. What are three types of advance directives and how do they differ from one another?

4. What is e-discovery and why does it present challenges for health information professionals?

5. Why might the health record be valuable as evidence in legal proceedings including e-discovery?

6. What are metadata? Give examples of metadata and explain why they are important to e-discovery.

7. What does the physician–patient privilege protect? When does it not provide protection?

8. Give two examples of government access to health information with or without patient authorization.

9. Is there a difference between ownership of and access to the health record?

10. What laws give individuals access to their health records?

Release of Information

Managing the release of information (ROI) requires the HIM professional to be fully aware of federal and state statutes and regulations affecting the use and disclosure of PHI, as well as accrediting body standards. In organizations where the ROI function is decentralized and carried out by multiple areas, all departments in the organization that perform the ROI function must follow standardized policies and procedures that adhere to external requirements. ROI staff must also be familiar with the HIPAA authorization requirement, disclosing information pursuant to an authorization at all times that one is required, being aware of authorization exceptions, and understanding when organizational policy mirrors HIPAA's permissiveness (where authorization is not required) or places more stringent authorization requirements on such disclosures. Any alleged HIPAA violations by ROI staff in the disclosure process must be investigated as potential breaches. Breaches are discussed in more detail in chapter 11.

Handling Highly Sensitive Information

Certain types of health information, because of the stigma and sensitivity associated with them, require special protections. Although they are not categorically addressed separately by HIPAA nor subject to a different set of requirements under HIPAA, other laws come into play in order to protect them. Highly sensitive information includes behavioral health, substance abuse, HIV/AIDS, genetic testing, and adoption records.

Behavioral health information is highly safeguarded because of its sensitive nature and the stigma associated with it. HIM professionals should consult their relevant state laws in order to know of any additional safeguards afforded to behavioral health information. Further, best practice dictates that authorizations for the disclosure of behavioral health information provide a designated area for individuals to authorize the disclosure of that information specifically.

The Confidentiality of Alcohol and Drug Abuse Patient Records federal regulation (42 CFR 2 Part 2) was issued in 1987 to particularly describe the situations when substance abuse information could be disclosed either with or without the patient's authorization. It applies to information created for patients treated in a federally assisted drug or alcohol abuse program that holds itself out as providing alcohol or drug abuse diagnosis, treatment, or referral for treatment. The program may be a standalone, a unit within a general medical facility, or personnel within in a general medical facility (Brodnik and Sharp 2012). This rule specifically protects the identity, diagnosis, prognosis, or treatment of these patients. The rule also specifies the circumstances under which information can be released without patient authorization and requires that language

generally prohibiting redisclosure be attached to all released information concerning drug or alcohol treatment. Redisclosure of health information related to this treatment is prohibited except as needed in a medical emergency or when authorized by an appropriate court order (AHIMA 2013).

HIV/AIDS information is also highly safeguarded because of its sensitive and stigmatic nature. Because it is protected specifically by state law, HIM professionals should be familiar with relevant state laws in order to become aware of special safeguards afforded to this type of information. Best practice dictates that authorizations for the disclosure of HIV/AIDS information provide a designated area for individuals to authorize the disclosure of that information specifically.

With the availability of genetic testing and information that pertains to one's propensity for developing a certain disease or condition, laws have been created at both the federal and state levels to safeguard genetic information. The federal Genetic Information Non-Discrimination Act of 2008 (GINA) serves to protect individuals from being discriminated against by health insurers and employers based on genetic information. There are state laws in place that provide similar protections. Best practice provides that individuals specifically authorize the disclosure of their genetic information.

Adoption records have historically been sensitive because of the many closed adoptions that took place. Where closed adoptions still exist, this information must receive special protection. Adoption information is protected by individual state laws. Unless court order mandates it, the health record is not the usual location for the identity of a birth parent or birth child to be identified. Requests for such information should be referred to the appropriate agency, such as a state department of health or vital statistics, or the adoption agency that was involved in the adoption being asked about (Brodnik and Sharp 2012).

Wrongful Disclosure

Individuals are personally liable for their own acts of unauthorized disclosure of confidential health information. The individual's liability is based on fault because he or she did something wrong or failed to do something he or she should have done. Employers also may be held liable for any job-related acts of their employees or agents per the doctrine of *respondeat superior* ("let the master answer") (Proels 2012). Healthcare organizations are less likely to be found liable for a breach of confidentiality by the members of its medical staff if they are not deemed to be employees or agents of the organization. However, the organization may be liable for the consequences of any unauthorized disclosure under the doctrine of **corporate negligence**, whether by employees,

agents, or medical staff members, because of the breach of its duty to maintain information confidential. The injured person benefits from these concepts of fault because he or she can sue the employer, the employee, or both.

Unauthorized disclosure by various healthcare professionals also may be addressed in professional licensing and certifying laws or regulations. These provisions subject the professional to potential discipline by the licensing or certifying agency for breach of confidentiality because it is considered unprofessional conduct.

Medical Identity Theft

A significant legal challenge facing healthcare organizations today, and the HIM profession in particular, is **medical identity theft**. It is the inappropriate or unauthorized misrepresentation of another's identity to do one of two things: obtain medical services or goods or falsify claims for medical services in an attempt to obtain money (Dixon 2006). In both types of medical identity theft, the individual's health information is either created under the wrong name or altered, leading to potentially deadly consequences.

There are two types of medical identity theft. External medical identity theft is committed by individuals from outside an organization. Although much attention has been paid to this type because it includes the use of the victim's insurance information so the perpetrator can obtain medical services in the victim's name, the second type—internal medical identity theft—is more common (Olenik et al. 2012). Individuals inside an organization, with access to vast amounts of patient information,

commit internal medical identity theft. These individuals may act alone or may be part of a larger crime ring that has intentionally infested the organization to gain access to information (Olenik et al. 2012).

What makes medical identity theft unique as compared to other types of identity theft is that it affects both the victim's financial information and medical information. When incorrect information is entered into a victim's health record, improper medical treatment could result. Although laws in the financial industry provide significant protections for victims of financial identity theft, much is left to be done to protect people from medical identity theft. Many states have breach notification laws, but they are not tailored to medical information. The HIPAA breach notification requirement, created by ARRA/HITECH and discussed in detail in chapter 11 provides the greatest outlet by which victims can become aware that their health information has been breached by inappropriate use or disclosure (Olenik et al. 2012).

Confidentiality of Quality Improvement Activities

Quality improvement (QI) is the process of evaluating and improving medical care and potentially

decreasing healthcare costs. (This process is discussed more fully in chapter 21.)

QI activities can be carried out on a concurrent review basis (as care is being given) or on a retrospective basis (after an encounter has ended). The healthcare organization is responsible for reviews that take the form of a focused study based on a pattern of questionable care. Questionable care that is deemed to be due to professional practice which is not at the expected level of care may result in educational intervention. If warranted, more stringent steps, such as suspension or termination of a physician's medical staff privileges, or termination of a provider's employment, may be taken.

These review activities involve collecting outcomes and performance data on how a healthcare provider performed. Physician reviews may affect continued medical staff membership. Understandably, the contents of these reviews are potentially of great interest to individuals contemplating or involved in litigation related to medical malpractice or wrongful termination actions. These records will be sought for discovery purposes, with attempts to admit them into evidence. Many states have statutes that specifically protect the confidentiality of records of this type (Carroll 2011). For example, California Evidence Code Section 1157 protects from discovery the proceedings and records of organized peer review committees responsible for the evaluation and improvement of the quality of care. Without such specific statutory protection, however, these types of records are often deemed discoverable.

Incident Reports

An occurrence that is inconsistent with the standard of care is generally defined as an **incident**. Standards of care are not related only to direct patient care. Therefore, incidents do not relate only to patient care either. Anyone witnessing or involved in an incident should complete an incident report as soon as possible after the incident as a way to capture the details of what happened. The **incident report** is one tool staff can use to report unusual incidents to administration. Data should be collected from the incident reports and analyzed to determine whether trends are developing.

Because incident reports contain facts, hospitals strive to protect their confidentiality. In some states, incident reports are protected under statutes protecting QI studies and activities (Carroll 2011). They also may be protected under attorney–client

privilege (Carroll 2011; McWay 2010, 264). Protection under this doctrine may be based on whether the primary purpose of the incident report is to provide information to the hospital's attorney or liability insurer (Carroll 2011; McWay 2010).

Incident reports themselves are not a part of the clinical record and are considered confidential and privileged in many states (Gaffey and Groves 2011; McWay 2010). Even though the facts regarding the incident and the resolution should be documented, there should be no reference to completion of an incident report nor to risk management involvement in the clinical record (Bunting and Benton 2011; Gaffey and Groves 2011). Such a reference to the incident report in the clinical record would likely render the incident report discoverable because it is mentioned in a document that is discoverable in legal proceedings. To further ensure incident report confidentiality, no copies should be made or disseminated (Carroll 2011).

To encourage staff to complete and submit incident reports, staff must be assured that there will be no punishment or retribution for reporting according to organizational policy (Carroll 2011; Woodfin 2011). Incident reports showing a repeated error such as medication errors that lead to patient injury by a single practitioner might involve some form of discipline with a focus on the acts that contributed to the error (Carroll 2011).

When dealing with incident reports or other potentially compensable events for which documentation has been created or received, the health information manager and the risk manager should work as a team. The risk manager depends on the health information manager to alert him or her to **potentially compensable events**. These are events that could result in a settlement or judgment against the organization, further resulting in a payout of funds whether through insurance or from an organization's internal funds. Such events can be identified through coding and abstracting and various health information review activities conducted by HIM department staff. The health information manager also can advise the risk manager when an attorney requests a copy of a health record. The risk manager then can review records identified by any of these methods to determine whether further action is necessary from a risk management standpoint.

Check Your Understanding 2.5

Instructions: **Answer the following questions on a separate piece of paper.**

1. What are five types of highly sensitive information that require special disclosure protections?

2. What are two legal theories under which employers may be held liable for wrongful disclosure of health information by their employees?

3. What is medical identity theft and what type of harm can it cause its victims?

4. What are the types of medical identity theft?

5. Distinguish between concurrent and retrospective quality review activities.

6. Why do healthcare organizations strive to maintain the confidentiality of QI records, including incident reports?

7. Define an incident as it relates to the healthcare environment and identify one doctrine under which incident reports may be protected.

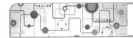 # References

Administrative Procedure Act, 5 U.C.S. §500-576 (Law. Co-op. 1989).

AHIMA e-Discovery Task Force. 2008. Litigation response planning and policies for e-Discovery. *Journal of AHIMA* 79(2):69–75. http://www.ahima.org/e-him.

AHIMA e-HIM Work Group on Maintaining the Legal EHR. 2005. Update: Maintaining a legally sound health record—Paper and electronic. *Journal of AHIMA* 76(10):64A–L. http://www.ahima.org/e-him.

American Health Information Management Association. 2013. Redisclosure of patient health information (updated). *Journal of AHIMA* 84(11): expanded web version. http://ww.ahima.org.

American Health Information Management Association. 2011. Fundamentals of the legal health record and designated record set. *Journal of AHIMA* 82(2): expanded online version. http://www.library.ahima.org.

American Health Information Management Association. 2007a. Is your electronic record a legal record? *Journal of AHIMA* 78(1):54.

American Health Information Management Association. 2007b. Resolution on the legal health record. *Journal of AHIMA* 78(1):53.

American Health Information Management Association. 2007c. The legal EHR: Trials and errors. *AHIMA Advantage* 11:4. http://www.ahima.org.

Arizona Constitution, Article 2, Section 8, Right to privacy. http://azleg.state.az.us/const/2/8.htm.

ARRA/HITECH. American Recovery and Reinvestment Act of 2009. Public Law 111-5.

Brodnik, M.S. and M. Sharp. 2012. Access, Use, and Disclosure/Release of Health Information. Chapter 12 in *Fundamentals of Law for Health Informatics and Information Management*. Edited by M.S. Brodnik, L.A. Rinehart-Thompson, and R.B. Reynolds. Chicago: AHIMA.

Bunting, R.F., Jr. and J.H. Benton. 2011. Managing Risk in the Ambulatory Environment. Chapter 15 in *Risk Management Handbook for Healthcare Organizations. Volume 2 Clinical Risk Management*, 6th ed. Series edited by R. Carroll. Volume edited by S.M. Brown. San Francisco: Jossey-Bass.

California Constitution, Article 1, Declaration of rights, Section 1. http://leginfo.ca.gov/.const/.article_1.

Carroll, R. 2011. Early Warning Systems for the Identification of Organizational Risks. Chapter 6 in *Risk Management Handbook for Healthcare Organizations. Volume 1 The Essentials*, 6th ed. Series edited by R. Carroll. Volume edited by P.L. Nakamura and R. Carroll. San Francisco: Jossey-Bass.

Cohen, M. 2011. Statutes, Standards, and Regulations. Chapter 1 in *Risk Management Handbook for Healthcare Organizations. Volume 3 Business Risk: Legal, Regulatory, and Technology Issues*, 6th ed. Series edited by R.

Carroll. Volume edited by G.T. Troyer. San Francisco: Jossey-Bass.

DeLoss, G.E. 2008. Electronic health records: An overview of legal liability, discovery and donation issues. California Health Information Management Association 2008 State Convention and Exhibit. San Jose, CA: CHIA.

Dimick, C. 2007. E-Discovery: Preparing for the coming rise in electronic discovery requests. *Journal of AHIMA* 78(5):24–29.

Dixon, P. 2006. Medical identity theft: the information crime that can kill you. World Privacy Forum. http://www.worldprivacyforum.org.

Emergency Medical Treatment and Labor Act (EMTALA). Social Security Act 1867, codified as 42 USC. §1395dd; 42 CFR 489 and others. (Term *active* removed from title in 1989.)

Federal Rules of Evidence (FRE) 803(6): Hearsay Exceptions: Availability of Declarant Immaterial (2000).

Federal Rules of Evidence (FRE) 901: Requirement of Authentication or Identification (1975).

Florida Constitution, Article I, Section 23, Right of privacy. http://www.leg.state.fl.us.

Gaffey, A. and S. Groves. 2011. The Clinical Record. Chapter 13 in *Risk Management Handbook for Healthcare Organizations. Volume 1 The Essentials*, 6th ed. Series edited by R. Carroll. Volume edited by P.L. Nakamura and R. Carroll. San Francisco: Jossey-Bass.

Griswold v. Connecticut, 381 U.S. 479 (1965).

Health Insurance Portability and Accountability Act of 1996. Public Law 104-191.

Hughes, G. 2002. Practice brief: Laws and regulations governing the disclosure of health information (updated). http://library.ahima.org.

Jergesen, A.D. 2011. Who owns the medical record? *CHIA Journal* 63(5):1, 12.

Judge v. Rockford Memorial Hospital, 17 Ill. App. 2d 365, 150 N.E. 2d 202 (1958).

Kadzielski, M.A. 2011. Physician and Allied Health Professional Credentialing. Chapter 14 in *Risk Management Handbook for Healthcare Organizations. Volume 1 The Essentials*, 6th ed. Series edited by R. Carroll. Volume edited by P.L. Nakamura and R. Carroll. San Francisco: Jossey-Bass.

Klaver, J.C. 2012a. Evidence. Chapter 4 in *Fundamentals of Law for Health Informatics and Information Management*. Edited by M.S. Brodnik, L.A. Rinehart-Thompson, and R.B. Reynolds. Chicago: AHIMA.

Klaver, J.C. 2012b. Corporations, Contracts, and Antitrust Legal Issues. Chapter 6 in *Fundamentals of Law for Health Informatics and Information Management*. Edited by M.S. Brodnik, L.A. Rinehart-Thompson, and R.B. Reynolds. Chicago: AHIMA.

Klaver, J.C. 2012c. Consent to Treatment. Chapter 7 in *Fundamentals of Law for Health Informatics and Information Management*. Edited by M.S. Brodnik, L.A. Rinehart-Thompson, and R.B. Reynolds. Chicago: AHIMA.

Klaver, J.C. 2012d. Risk Management and Quality Improvement. Chapter 14 in *Fundamentals of Law for Health Informatics and Information Management*. Edited by M.S. Brodnik, L.A. Rinehart-Thompson, and R.B. Reynolds. Chicago: AHIMA.

McLendon, W.K. 2012. *The Legal Health Record Regulations, Policies and Guidelines*. Chicago: AHIMA.

McLendon, K. 2007 (Feb). Record disclosure and the EHR: Defining and managing the subset of data disclosed upon request. *Journal of AHIMA* 78(2): 58–59.

McWay, D.C. 2010. *Legal and Ethical Aspects of Health Information Management*. Clifton, NY: Delmar.

Olenik, K. 2008. How to create your legal EHR policy. California Health Information Management Association 2008 State Convention and Exhibit. San Jose, CA: CHIA.

Olenik, K., M.S. Brodnik, R.B. Reynolds, and L. Rinehart-Thompson. 2012. Security Threats and Controls. Chapter 11 in *Fundamentals of Law for Health Informatics and Information Management*. Edited by M.S. Brodnik, L.A. Rinehart-Thompson, and R.B. Reynolds. Chicago: AHIMA.

Pozgar, G.D. and N. Santucci. 2016. *Legal Aspects of Health Care Administration*. Sudbury, MA: Jones and Bartlett.

Proels, S.E. 2012. Tort Law. Chapter 5 in *Fundamentals of Law for Health Informatics and Information Management*. Edited by M.S. Brodnik, L.A. Rinehart-Thompson, and R.B. Reynolds. Chicago: AHIMA.

Rinehart-Thompson, L.A. 2012a. The Legal System in the United States. Chapter 2 in *Fundamentals of Law for Health Informatics and Information Management*. Edited by M.S. Brodnik, L.A. Rinehart-Thompson, and R.B. Reynolds. Chicago: AHIMA.

Rinehart-Thompson, L.A. 2012b. The HIPAA Privacy Rule. Chapter 9 in *Fundamentals of Law for Health Informatics and Information Management*. Edited by M.S. Brodnik, L.A. Rinehart-Thompson, and R.B. Reynolds. Chicago: AHIMA.

Rinehart-Thompson, L.A., R.B. Reynolds, and K. Olenik, 2012. The Legal Health Record: Maintenance, Content, Documentation, and Disposition. Chapter 8 in *Fundamentals of Law for Health Informatics and Information Management.* Edited by M.S. Brodnik, L.A. Rinehart-Thompson, and R.B. Reynolds. Chicago: AHIMA.

Rinehart-Thompson, L.A. and L. B. Harman, 2006. Ethical Challenges in the Management of Health Information. Chapter 3 in *Privacy and Confidentiality.* Edited by L.B. Harman. Sudbury, MA: Jones and Bartlett Publishers.

Showalter, J.S. 2012. *The Law of Healthcare Administration.* Chicago and Washington, D.C.: Health Administration Press and AUPHA Press.

Trautmann, C.O. 2003. Dictionary of Small Business. http://www.small-business-dictionary.org/default.asp

Warren, S.D., and Brandeis, L.D. 1890. The right to privacy. *Harvard Law Review.*

Woodfin, K. 2011. Risk Management Considerations in Home Healthcare. Chapter 16 in *Risk Management Handbook for Healthcare Organizations. Volume 2 Clinical Risk Management,* 6th ed. Series edited by R. Carroll. Volume edited by S.M. Brown. San Francisco: Jossey-Bass.

42 CFR 2 Part 2: Confidentiality of Alcohol and Drug Abuse Patient Records. 1987.

42 CFR 482.24(b)(1): Condition of participation: Medical record services. 2012.

45 CFR 160 and 162: General Administrative Requirements; Administrative Requirements. 2003.

45 CFR 160 and 164: General Administrative Requirements; Security and Privacy. 2003.

45 CFR 164.308: Administrative safeguards. 2003.

45 CFR 164.310: Physical safeguards. 2003.

45 CFR 164.312: Technical safeguards. 2003.

45 CFR 164.501: Definitions. 2003.

3

Data Governance and Stewardship

Merida Johns, PhD, RHIA

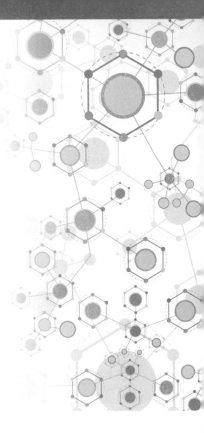

Learning Objectives

- Explain data governance concepts
- Provide a definition of data governance
- Discuss the functions of data governance
- Explain the benefits of a data governance program
- Discuss the importance of a business case for a data governance program
- Compare and contrast the data management domains

- Describe a typical data governance organizational structure
- Distinguish between data and information governance
- Given a case study, determine and suggest a successful data governance program development roadmap

Key Terms

Accountability
Artifacts
Business case
Business intelligence (BI)
Content management
Controls
Cross-functional
Data architecture
Data governance
Data governance steering committee
Data governance office (DGO)
Data life cycle
Data quality management

Data security
Data security management
Data stakeholders
Data steward
Data, information, knowledge, and wisdom (DIKW) hierarchy
Decision rights
Enterprise health information management
Executive data governance council
Framework
Goal
Information governance

Iterative process
Key performance indicators
Master data management
Metadata
Mission statement
Planning
Process
Rules of engagement
Stakeholder analysis
Strategic IM plan
Structured data
Terminology and classification management
Unstructured data

While the phrase *data governance* appears to define itself, there are many definitions of data governance (DG). Over the past decade, DG has received a lot of attention in popular business magazines and blogs and is a key topic at information management meetings and conventions. As healthcare struggles with the bombardment of digital data and regulatory reporting requirements, DG has also received a good deal of hype. Service companies, consultants, and vendors have latched onto the term, but the divergence of thought on DG sometimes makes the concept and its implementation tough to pin down (Johns 2015). In many cases the definition of DG is subjective and difficult for organizations to implement. Fortunately, several professional organizations and academic researchers are treating DG with the respect it deserves and are helping to create a roadmap for developing sound principles and practices for DG in healthcare. The focus of this chapter is to help clarify the concept of DG, provide approaches for applying DG, and suggest best practices for establishing a DG effort in a healthcare environment.

Distinction between Data and Information Governance

Data governance (DG) and **information governance** (IG) are sometimes used interchangeably in popular literature and by vendors and consultants. However, they are not the same (Dimick 2013). DG is concerned with governing the input (data), whereas IG is concerned with governing the output (information) of an information system.

The distinction between DG and IG begins with examining the difference between the assets that are being governed, namely data and information. The differences are best illustrated through the **data, information, knowledge, and wisdom (DIKW) hierarchy** that is an essential principle of computer information and library sciences (figure 3.1). In the DIKW hierarchy, data are facts. For example, blood pressure readings of 140/90, 150/95, 138/95 have no particular meaning other than they are recorded as fact. When a fact is related to some other fact (data), the relationship produces a piece of information. For instance, if the blood pressure readings are associated with a specific patient, such as Mrs. Smith, the data that compose the relationship become information. Interpreting Mrs. Smith's blood pressure over time and recognizing a pattern suggestive of a

Figure 3.1. DIKW pyramid

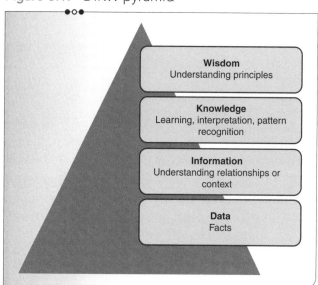

©Merida L. Johns

prehypertensive stage transforms information to knowledge.

Each level in the DIKW hierarchy is dependent on the previous levels. For instance, there can be no information without data. Likewise, there is no knowledge without information. While a relationship exists between data and information, it is apparent that they are not the same thing. Therefore, the way data and information are governed would be expected to be different (Kooper et al.

Figure 3.2. Comparison of DG and IG functions

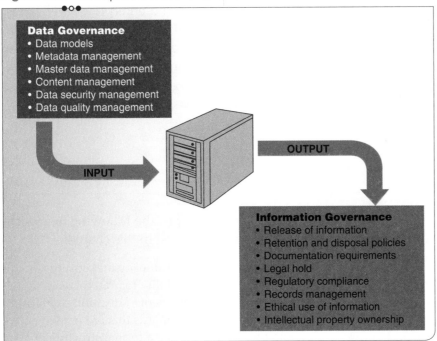

©Merida L. Johns

2011). In DG, the input (data) into an information system is the governed asset. The form of data may include text, video, and images. DG encompasses oversight functions that establish policies and standards for data quality and how data are defined, captured, structured, stored, and retrieved (Johns 2015). These usually include functions associated with data life cycle management, data modeling, metadata management, master data management, and data security, among others.

IG is concerned with governing the output (information) of an information system (Johns 2015). IG focuses on the control and use of the actual documents, reports, and records created from data (Smallwood 2013). Consequently IG establishes policies and standards for governing how information is used, shared, and analyzed. These may include policies and standards that apply to information confidentiality, ethical use of information, record retention and disposal, and regulatory or legal compliance (Johns 2015). Figure 3.2 illustrates some of these distinctions between DG and IG functions. For example, policies about the maintenance of data models, development and maintenance of metadata schema, requirements for master and reference data, and processes for assessing and measuring data quality would fall under DG while policies on legal holds for records, amendments and deletion of clinical notes, ethical use of statistical data, and release of information would fall under IG.

Governance

Governance is defined as "the establishment of policies and the continual monitoring of their proper implementation for managing organization assets to enhance the prosperity and viability of the organization" (BusinessDictionary 2015). Governance is an enterprise activity that exercises authority across the entire organization and includes an enforcement component (Ladley 2012). The top organization authority exercises governance by applying a framework of policies, standards, rules, and decision rights and implementing these through formal structure of assigned roles, responsibilities, and accountabilities. The purpose of governance is to influence the behaviors of the organization's employees and other stakeholders in support of organizational goals (Foss and Klein 2008). Governance at the enterprise level is visible in every aspect of an organization. Examples where enterprise governance is typically applied include accounting and audit management, human resources management, financial reporting, record keeping and risk management.

Data Governance Definition and Concepts

As noted previously, there are many definitions of DG. The following is a sampling of these definitions:

- DG is the organization and implementation of policies, procedures, structures, roles, and responsibilities that outline and enforce rules of engagement, decision rights, and accountabilities for the effective management of information assets (Ladley 2012, 115).

- DG is the exercise of authority and control (planning, monitoring, and enforcement) over the management of data assets (DAMA 2010, 37).

- DG is a system of decision rights and accountabilities for information-related processes, executed according to agreed-upon models that describe who can take what actions with what information, when and under what circumstances, and using what methods (Data Governance Institute 2013).

While the definitions vary, there are several core concepts. These include:

- Enterprise-level authority and accountability for effective data asset management

- Establishing and monitoring data policies, standards, practices, decision rights, and accountabilities for managing, using, improving, and protecting organizational information corporate data

- Execution of policies, standards, and practices through formal structures, roles, and responsibilities (Johns 2015, 81)

Based on these concepts, the following is a working definition of DG used in this chapter:

> DG is the enterprise authority that ensures control and accountability for enterprise data through the establishment of decision rights and data policies and standards that are implemented and monitored through a formal structure of assigned roles, responsibilities, and accountabilities (Johns 2015, 81).

The purpose of DG is to influence the behaviors of organization stakeholders toward the effective and efficient use of data to support the organization's strategy and meet its goals.

The term *data governance* emerged in the 1990s when the value of data was recognized beyond its use in operational transactions and extended to decision support functions (Chen 2010). During this period, technology had advanced to a point where data from different functional areas could be consolidated in data warehouses for strategic and tactical decision support. While the technology could consolidate data, it could not guarantee data quality. As data were consolidated from across the organization, data quality issues such as inconsistent data types, invalid values, missing values, and duplicate data materialized. Because of these and other data quality issues, organizations recognized that policies and standards were needed to govern data that would ensure data across the organization were consistently defined, structured, accurate, and current before being loaded into the data warehouse. At first the concept of data governance applied to only structured data commonly stored in databases. However, over the past two

Figure 3.3. EHIM model of HIM practice

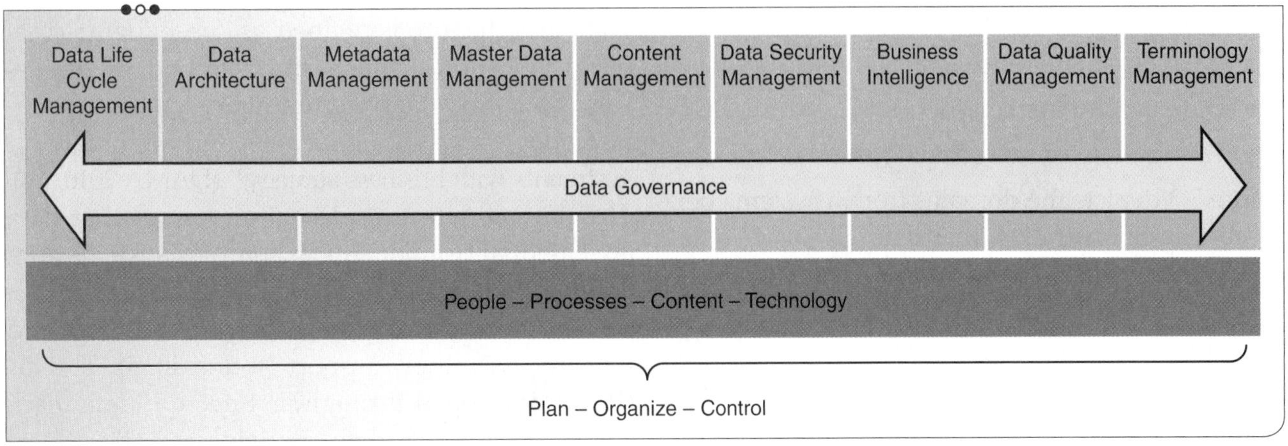

©Merida L. Johns

decades, data governance has broadened from the oversight of structured data for data warehousing purposes to include the governance of all enterprise data in any format (DAMA 2010).

Today DG is accomplished through a formal organizational structure and applied to several data management domains such as data architecture management, master data management, metadata management, content management, and data security (figure 3.3). A principal purpose of DG is to coordinate and synchronize all of the data management domains and the scope of the DG effort varies among organizations. For example, some organizations may take a focused approach and apply the DG effort to one or two data management domains, such as master data management

and data security. Others may take a broad scope and apply the DG effort to several or all data management domains depicted in figure 3.3.

The organizational structure, discussed later in the chapter, depends on organization culture, size, and scope of the DG program. Typically DG is a collaborative effort with responsibility for authorization of the program vested in a high-ranking steering committee composed of executive level organization officials. A DG council, authorized by the DG steering committee, is usually responsible for establishing DG policy and standards and monitoring their implementation. DG policies and standards are coordinated and implemented in a variety of ways, such as through data steward committees or councils.

Data Management Domains

A model for describing how data governance is applied requires understanding the typical data management domains (figure 3.3), though their definitions vary. For example, the Data Management Association (DAMA) framework identifies 11 data management domains (DAMA 2010). Others, like the Data Governance Institute (DGI) consolidate these into fewer domains or include variations of these domains. Taken together these domains are frequently referred to as enterprise

information management (EIM) (Johns 2015). For the purposes of this chapter, the following are considered the data management domains for **enterprise health information management** (EHIM) and are closely aligned with those included in the DAMA framework:

- Data life cycle management
- Data architecture management
- Metadata management
- Master data management

- Content management
- Data security management
- Business intelligence management
- Data quality management
- Terminology management (Johns 2015)

Figure 3.3 depicts the domains from a systems perspective; demonstrating that data governance applies to the set of all data management domains. The policies, standards, and accountabilities that govern the planning, organizing, and controlling of data in each domain are developed by the data governance process. The descriptions of each of the data management domains are provided (Johns 2015).

Data Life Cycle Management

Data management is based on the assumption that all data have a life cycle. A life cycle is made up of a series of successive stages and has beginning and end points. Plants, animals, and businesses all have life cycles. They have beginning, developmental, maturation, declining, and ending stages. Each stage in the life cycle has a function and must be managed appropriately to fulfill its purpose. From a systems perspective, a life cycle is a component of a larger system. In addition to the functions performed within each life cycle stage, inputs from and outputs to a larger system are accommodated.

There are many models of the data life cycle and while each portrays a slightly different view of life cycle stages, there are striking similarities among them (Chung 2010). A typical **data life cycle** includes the following stages: data planning, data inventory and evaluation, data capture, data transformation and processing, data access and distribution, data maintenance, data archival, and data destruction (Johns 2015). Typical data life cycle functions requiring data governance include:

- Establishing what data are to be collected and how they are to be captured
- Setting standards for data retention and storage
- Determining processes for data access and distribution
- Establishing standards for data archival and destruction (Johns 2015)

Data Architecture Management

Data architecture is defined as "an integrated set of specification artifacts (models and diagrams) used to define data requirements, guide integration and control of data assets, and align data investments with business strategy," (DAMA 2010, 63). The data architecture domain assumes that data are essential components in complex systems and, as such, require abstractions and models to describe data and the relationships among data and the processes they support (Johns 2015). The **artifacts** developed through architecture data management—such as data models, use cases, data flow diagrams, and data dictionaries—are as important to data management as the blueprints prepared by an architect are to a building design and maintenance. Data architecture provides the underpinning of an organization's information system. Typical functions of data architecture management requiring data governance include:

- Establishing standards, policies, and procedures for the collection, storage, and integration of enterprise data and design of information systems
- Identifying and documenting data requirements that meet the needs and support the processes of the organization
- Developing and maintaining enterprise and conceptual data and process models that represent the organization's business rules (Johns 2015)

Metadata Management

Metadata are often referred to as "data about data." Metadata are structured information used to increase the effective use of data. By describing data, metadata makes it easier to locate, retrieve, use, and manage (NISO 2004, 1). There are several types of metadata. For example, some metadata describe data for the purposes of locating data; search engines use this type of metadata. Other metadata describe when data were created or changed; this kind of metadata is used in computer audit trails. Another type of metadata describes who has access rights to create, review, update, and delete data. This metadata is used for access control and security purposes. One of the most familiar types of metadata is used to describe data in databases. Data element name, data type, and field length are examples of this kind of metadata. There are numerous metadata standards, many of which are industry sector-specific.

Metadata play an important role in achieving interoperability among different computer systems and providing search and navigation capabilities. Metadata are used for discovery purposes to maintain, update, and retain data to meet regulatory and legal obligations and may be embedded with the data they describe or may be maintained in large metadata repositories. Usual metadata management functions requiring data governance include:

- Managing data dictionaries
- Establishing enterprise metadata strategy
- Developing policies, goals, and objectives for metadata management and use
- Adopting metadata standards
- Establishing and implementing metadata metrics
- Monitoring procedures to ensure metadata policy implementation (Johns 2015)

Master Data Management

Master data management refers to master data that an enterprise maintains about key business entities such as customers, employees, or patients, and to reference data that is used to classify other data or identify allowable values for data such as codes for state abbreviations or products. A good healthcare example of master data is the master patient index that includes master data on the key entity—the patient—and usually includes patient medical record number; patient last, middle, and first names; birthdate; gender; and address. Since master and reference data are used across the organization, it is critical that they be consistent. Data quality issues are often attributable to poor management of one or both of these types of data. Inconsistencies or redundancies among either can have profound, negative effects on data quality and make it impossible to share data across

computer applications both internal and external to the organization. Typical functions associated with master data management include:

- Identifying reference data sources (such as databases and files)
- Maintaining authoritative reference data values lists and associated metadata
- Implementing change management processes for reference data
- Establishing organizational master data sets
- Defining and maintaining match rules for master data
- Identifying duplicate master data and reconciling to provide the "system of record" or "single source of truth"
- Establishing policies and procedures for applying data quality and matching rules, and incorporating data quality checks for master data
- Implementing change management processes for master data (Johns 2015)

Content Management

Content management encompasses managing both **structured data** (for example, data stored in databases) and **unstructured data** (such as data contained in text documents). Structured data commonly refer to data that are organized and easily retrievable and interpreted by traditional databases and data models. Unstructured data are data that do not have a predefined data model or are not stored in a traditional database structure. Unstructured data are typically found in documents, e-mails, and images. To manage data in both forms, policies and standards must be established for the creation, storage, and retrieval of documents and records as well as the cataloguing and the categorizing of information within these. Typically, content management functions requiring data governance include:

- Developing and implementing policies and procedures for the organization and categorization of unstructured data (content) in electronic, paper, image, and audio files for its delivery, use, reuse, and preservation.

- Developing and adopting taxonomic systems for the indexing, cataloging, and categorizing of data for purposes of information searching and retrieval.

- Developing and maintaining an information architecture and metadata schema that identify links and relationships among documents and define the content within a document (Johns 2015).

Data Security Management

Data security includes protection measures and tools for safeguarding data and information. **Data security management** includes policies and procedures that address confidentiality and security concerns of organizational stakeholders (for example, patients, providers, and employees), protecting organizational proprietary interests, and compliance with government and regulatory requirements while accommodating legitimate access needs. The typical functions of data security management that require data governance include:

- Data security planning and organization

- Developing, implementing, and enforcing data security policies and procedures

- Establishing a data security risk management program

- Developing a business continuity plan

- Monitoring audit trails to identify potential and actual security violations

- Managing employee, contractor, and business partner security and confidentiality agreements

- Implementing employee security awareness training (Johns 2015)

Information Intelligence and Big Data

Business intelligence (BI) is defined as "a broad category of applications and technologies for gathering, storing, analyzing, and providing access to data to help enterprise users make better business decisions," (Brannon 2010, 2). BI systems use structured data extracted from organizational transactional databases that are stored in data warehouses. Since unstructured data such as those found in word processed documents and e-mails, make up for a large percentage of an organization's data, more attention is being given to using techniques to analyze this type of data. However, unstructured data are difficult to define and categorize. Therefore, special text analysis tools are used to process, extract, and create clusters of text that are subsequently arranged in a data model and can be analyzed. Usual functions associated with enterprise information intelligence that require data governance include:

- Identifying enterprise intelligence needs

- Assessing current intelligence resources and use

- Determining scope and defining requirements and architecture for enterprise intelligence

- Developing and implementing policies and procedures for enterprise information intelligence

- Identifying, assessing, and resolving data quality issues

- Implementing data warehouses and data marts that store massive amounts of data

- Identifying and implementing appropriate business intelligence tools and interfaces (Johns 2015)

Data Quality Management

All enterprise operations depend upon accurate data. The purpose of data quality management is to ensure that data meet quality characteristics such as accuracy, completeness, accessibility, precision, relevance, and timeliness. **Data quality management** is characterized as "a continuous process for defining the parameters for specifying acceptable levels of data quality to meet business needs, and for ensuring that data quality meets these levels." (DAMA 2010, 291). Typical functions of a data quality management program that require data governance include:

- Identifying data quality requirements and establishing data quality metrics

- Identifying and implementing data quality projects

- Profiling data and measuring conformance to established quality metrics and business rules
- Identifying data quality problems and assessing their root cause
- Managing data quality issues
- Implementing data quality improvement measures
- Providing training for ensuring data quality (Johns 2015)

Terminology and Classification Management

Terminology and classification management consists of the processes for managing the breadth of healthcare terminologies, vocabularies, classification systems, and data sets that an organization may use and also serves as a terminology authority for the enterprise. Typical functions assumed by this domain that require data governance include:

- Ensuring appropriate adoption, maintenance, dissemination, and accessibility of vocabularies, terminologies, classification systems, and code sets for semantic interoperability and data integrity
- Developing algorithmic translations, concept representations, and mapping among clinical nomenclatures
- Providing oversight for clinical and diagnostic coding to ensure compliance with established standards (Johns 2015)

Check Your Understanding 3.1

Instructions: **Choose the best answer.**

1. Which of the following best describes DG?
   A. Enterprise authority that ensures control and accountability for enterprise data
   B. A set of policies, procedures, and standards that manage data
   C. Decision rights and accountabilities for data
   D. A network of data stewards that function collaboratively across the organization

2. Which of the following data management domains would be responsible for establishing standards for data retention and storage?
   A. Data architecture management
   B. Metadata management
   C. Data life cycle management
   D. Master data management

3. Which of the following is often referred to as "data about data"?
   A. Master data
   B. Metadata
   C. Structured data
   D. Unstructured data

4. Which of the following synchronizes and coordinates all of the data management domains?
   A. Data architecture management
   B. Data life cycle management
   C. Data governance
   D. Data security management

5. Which of the following would not be considered a DG function?
   A. Developing policies for identifying master data management
   B. Enforcing data security policies
   C. Assessing the ethical use of statistical data
   D. Establishing policies for data model maintenance

Data Governance Program Plan

Development of a DG program plan should be incorporated with the organization's strategic information management (IM) planning efforts. A **strategic IM plan** is developed so that all information management efforts are aligned with the organization's strategic plan and ensure that information management goals and strategies support the organization's high-level initiatives. An IM plan usually includes a description of the business needs for information management. Business needs are identified from the organization's strategic plan and by conducting an external and internal environmental analysis of the current status and future projection of needs. An IM plan typically states the IM vision, mission, values, and high-level goals. The IM plan includes the key objectives, activities, and timeline for reaching each goal as well as establishing the metrics for evaluating the plan's success. To illustrate the connection between these planning processes consider the process depicted in figure 3.4. An organization's strategic plan includes a goal of having in place an IM infrastructure that advances quality patient care, efficient operations, competitive advantage and decision making, and also ensures compliance with data regulations and mandates. To support the organization's strategic objective, the IM plan includes a goal for enabling enterprise data management. The IM plan identifies the development of a DG plan as one of the key activities for meeting the strategic objective.

Development of a DG program includes the typical management processes of planning, organizing, directing, and controlling. The Data Governance Institute (DGI), a vendor-neutral organization founded in 2003, incorporates these processes for developing a DG program, called a roadmap, and consists of the following steps:

1. Develop a value statement
2. Prepare a program roadmap
3. Plan and fund the program
4. Design the program
5. Deploy the program
6. Govern the data
7. Monitor the program, measure program effectiveness, report results (Thomas 2014)

Figure 3.4. Relationship among organizational planning efforts

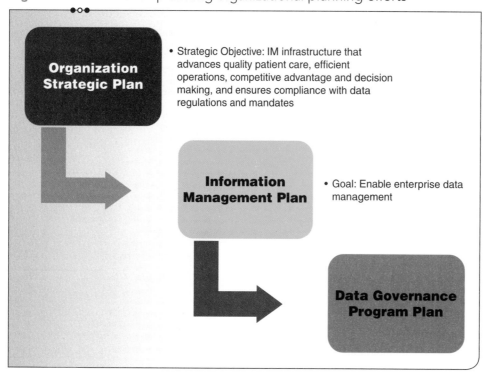

In launching any organizational effort, determining what must be done and why it should be accomplished is called **planning**. In developing a DG program, identifying the purpose and value of the program should be the first step. Sometimes this is referred to as the **business case** or value proposal. The business case lays out the benefits and value for the organization that implementation of the DG program can obtain by anticipating a positive change from the current status. For instance, the current status may be framed by stating: Business efficiency and effectiveness rests on timely access to accurate data. Inaccurate data leads to rework and reduces efficiency; incomplete data leads to wasted time and inefficiencies; late data leads to idle resources and increases costs. Based on this example, the business case or outcome of a DG program might be stated in the following way:

- If we reduce duplicate records in our master patient index, then clinical and administrative errors will be reduced, which should lead to better patient care.

- If we improve the integration of our data, then we will increase our efficiency, which should lead to lower costs and faster efficiency.

- If we establish an organization-wide data dictionary, then we will have better interoperability among different information systems, which should lead to better and quicker clinical and administrative decision making (Johns 2015, 88).

After a business case is established, executive support for the program is solicited, usually in the form of an executive sponsor. At this stage, a data governance executive council (described later) is formed and the planning process commences. Development of a DG mission statement, identification of program scope and priorities, and establishment of an organizational structure are the usual outcomes of the initial planning process.

Tackling all of the data management domains requiring data governance can be an overwhelming effort. Therefore, organizations usually start a DG program by focusing on a specific area or activity, such as master data management, content management, business intelligence, or customer relationship management. It is best to start the DG program by completing small steps that bring immediate value to the organization.

After the mission, scope, and focus of the program is established, identifying and organizing resources for the program is typically the next step. This includes identifying which individuals and organizational bodies will be included or created, establishing lines of authority and responsibility, and determining how funding will be obtained. A data governance office and DG steering committee (explained in the next section) may be established to begin the initial DG work. Once the appropriate organizational bodies and people are in place, DG goals are usually refined, tasks and timelines are developed, and controlling processes are put in place.

Data Governance Implementation and Stewardship

Data governance is the glue that synchronizes the management of all of the data management domains. It is the overarching authority that ensures policies, standards, and accountabilities are in place and enforced for data management. Data governance is implemented through a formal organizational structure with both authority and responsibility for managing an organization's data assets. The governance structure varies among organizations, but is normally headed by a high-level data governance committee (sometimes called a data governance council or similar name) that is sponsored by the highest levels of organizational authority and supported by a network of data stewards. Typical data governance functions include:

- Advocating for the data asset
- Establishing data strategy
- Establishing data policies
- Approving data procedures and standards
- Communicating, monitoring, and enforcing data policy and standards
- Ensuring regulatory compliance
- Resolving data issues
- Approving data management projects
- Coordinating data management organization (Johns 2015)

Data Governance Frameworks

There are many frameworks available for implementing DG. A **framework** is a conceptual structure for classifying, organizing, and showing interrelationships among activities used as a guide for taking action to achieve a goal. In the case of DG, a framework assists an organization in determining what constitutes the DG mission and scope, and DG responsibilities, authority, organizational structure, and governance processes. Examples of DG frameworks include the Method for an Integrated Knowledge Environment (MIKE2.0), Data Governance Institute Framework, Data Management Association Framework, and Contingency Approach to Data Governance. While all frameworks differ in varying degrees, they all assume the following:

- DG views data as a corporate asset requiring the same priority for management as other high stake organizational assets.
- DG is an enterprise-wide program, linked to organizational strategy, and supported by a business case. The portfolio of DG initiatives is determined by organizational strategy.
- DG is an **iterative process**. It initially prioritizes initiatives and focuses on small select business imperatives that quickly deliver value and expand as the program matures.

- DG is a collaborative effort requiring participation from all organizational levels and stakeholders.
- DG specifies who has the authority and accountability for data decisions and who is responsible for carrying out the activities associated with these decisions. This requires identification and codification in written documents of the priorities, goals, main activities, roles, and responsibilities that are undertaken.
- The DG program includes an executive sponsor, a high-level and strategic oversight committee, and supporting committees or task forces composed of data stewards.
- The DG program is usually supported by a DG office, headed by the chief data steward, chief data officer (CDO), or other senior data management professional.

Data Governance Institute and Data Management Association Frameworks

There is no one right way to structure the DG program. The structure and reporting lines of the DG program will vary among organizations and are usually based on the mission and scope of the DG program and the customary way the organization operates.

The DGI and DAMA frameworks encompass many of the key characteristics of other DG frameworks and are closely associated with organizational management concepts, so they are exemplary of how a DG program can be implemented.

The DGI framework consists of three overarching parts each consisting of several components (table 3.1). The three major parts of the framework are: rules and rules of engagement, people and organizational bodies, and DG processes (Data Governance Institute n.d.). Each of these and their components are explained in the following sections.

Rules and Rules of Engagement   Operation of a DG program depends upon having rules in place for program operation. Rules are a set of principles and regulations; examples include policies, standards, controls, and accountabilities. **Rules of engagement** specify the way that policy makers,

Table 3.1. Data governance operation

Rules and rules of engagement	People and organizational bodies	Data governance processes
• Creating a mission statement	• Data stakeholders	• Establishing rules and processes for governing data
• Developing DG goals	• Data governance council	• Establishing rules and process for coordinating the DG program
• Establishing DG metrics	• Data stewards	
• Determining funding strategies	• Data steward program committee	
• Developing data rules and definitions	• Data governance office	
• Assigning decision rights		
• Assigning accountabilities		
• Establishing controls		

data owners, data stewards, and other stakeholders interact with each other. The following are considered essential rules of engagement in the DGI framework.

Creating a Mission Statement A mission statement identifies the fundamental purpose, scope, and high-level goals of the DG program so that all stakeholders understand and agree on what is to be accomplished. A good mission statement helps to unify and motivate stakeholders, keeps the DG program on track, and holds the organization accountable for achieving the stated goals. The mission of a DG program will vary among organizations and depends upon overall organizational strategy as well as the scope of the program. One example mission statement may be: To improve data search and retrieval and integration of transactional data for executive decision making. In this case the DG program scope may be narrowly focused on metadata management and developing a business intelligence infrastructure. For another organization the DG mission statement may be: To increase data integrity to improve operational performance. In this case the DG program scope may be focused on data architecture and master data management. In some cases the DG mission statement may be very broad such as: To increase data integrity, best practices in data management, reporting standards, and information consistency. Here the DG scope would likely include governance of all of the data management domains.

Developing DG Program Goals A goal is a desired end result expressed in measurable terms. Goals should be SMART: specific, measurable, attainable, realistic, and time-related. The goals of a DG program depend on the program's mission and scope and vary among organizations. For example, the initial goals of a DG program with a mission and scope to ensure master data quality may include the following:

• Develop a master data model for master patient data within 12 months

• Develop a master data model for provider data within 12 months

• Map source data to the master patient data model within 18 months

• Map source data to the master provider data model within 18 months

Another organization with a DG mission to provide a sound data architecture may have the following goals:

• Develop and implement data modeling standards within 6 months

• Develop enterprise data dictionary within 18 months

• Develop enterprise data model within 12 months

As the DG program matures and initial goals are achieved, new goals are developed. Take the goal to develop and implement data modeling standards within 6 months, for example—once data modeling standards are established and implemented, the goal might change to "all database projects will comply with data modeling standards," or "data dictionary naming conventions are used 100 percent of the time."

Establishing DG Metrics and Success Measures

Success measures, often called **key performance indicators** (KPIs), are developed to assess the effectiveness of a DG program. Without the use of agreed upon KPIs, it is impossible to determine the value of a DG program. KPIs depend upon the DG program mission and goals and vary among organizations. Examples of KPIs of a DG program may include the following:

- Degree of compliance with data governance security policies
- Degree of master data accuracy over time
- Degree of compliance with data model development standards
- Length of time in which data issues are remediated

Determining DG Funding Strategies   All DG programs require funding and resources to support them. Funding is provided through budget allocations that support, among other items, DG program staff salaries, technology and infrastructure investments and maintenance, and DG projects. Funding of a DG program depends upon the organization's structure and the DG program scope, mission, and goals. Strategies for funding can range from budget support for a standalone unit, inclusion as a line item in project budgets, and charge-back to business units, to being included in departmental IT budgets (Johns 2015). The DGI outlines four specific DG funding needs:

- The initial design and implementation of the data governance program
- Ongoing data governance/stewardship/ compliance/access management efforts
- Ongoing data stewardship/data quality efforts
- Recommended projects and efforts that come from governance-led issue analysis (**Data Governance Institute** 2015).

Developing Data Rules and Definitions

At its basic level, DG entails policy development, implementation, and enforcement. Typically, a DG program will include:

- Policies on data availability, access accountability, and ownership that clarify who is accountable for the quality and security of critical data
- Specific roles and responsibilities of data committees, data stewards, and data custodians
- Established data capture and validation standards and reference data rules
- Data access and usage rules
- Standards security, privacy rules, and master data, metadata, data definition, and data model standards (Johns 2015)

Assigning Decision Rights   Assignment of **decision rights** is defined as appointing authority to specific individuals or categories of individuals to make data-related decisions and designating when and how those decisions are made. Assigning decision rights specifies commitments and is a precursor for establishing accountability for data decisions and is a critical component of the rules of engagement. Decision rights must be clearly defined to avoid conflict and inconsistencies. For example: Who has the decision rights for establishing data policies and standards for the master data model? Who has the decision rights for developing data security policies and standards? Who has the decision rights for establishing standards for data element naming conventions, determining the length of a data field, or determining data access?

Assigning Accountability   DG involves more than establishing policies and standards. A critical part of DG includes assigning accountability for policy and standards implementation and monitoring. Specific questions considered with each policy and standard include who does what, when, how, and why. For example, when a security breach occurs the following accountabilities should be established: who is responsible for the

response, what must they do, when must they do it, and why must it be done. Or, when data access rights are granted the following accountabilities should be established: who should grant data access, when they should grant access, how they should grant access, and what access should they grant.

Establishing Controls   Controls are measures and functionality established for the purpose of preventing and mitigating risks (Johns 2015). Data are at risk for corruption, improper use, breach, and destruction at every point of the data life cycle. During the data capture life cycle stage, data are at risk for being incomplete or incorrect. To mitigate this risk, data capture controls might include forced field completion, use of drop-down lists of predefined terms, and automatic data type and format edit checks. When data are updated in a database, data concurrency controls are used to ensure data integrity. A DG program will assign accountabilities to individuals and groups of individuals for establishing, implementing, and monitoring a variety of controls that mitigate data risk.

People and Organizational Bodies   The second part of the DGI framework specifies those responsible for the operation of the DG program. This includes identifying data stakeholders and those responsible for DG policy development and DG decisions, enforcement, implementation, and operation. As noted earlier, implementation of DG requires establishing a formal organizational structure that is given the authority and responsibility by the highest executive level to carry out DG functions. While the governance structure varies among organizations, the structure in figure 3.5 is typical of many of these.

Data Stakeholders   Data stakeholders are those who have an interest or stake in organizational data (Johns 2015). Stakeholders can include customers, frontline workers, business units, managers, executives, and even external groups such as state and federal agencies, accreditation bodies, and others. Among internal stakeholders are executive and senior management, business units, service units, and information technology groups. Among external stakeholders are patients, public health

Figure 3.5.   Example DG program organization

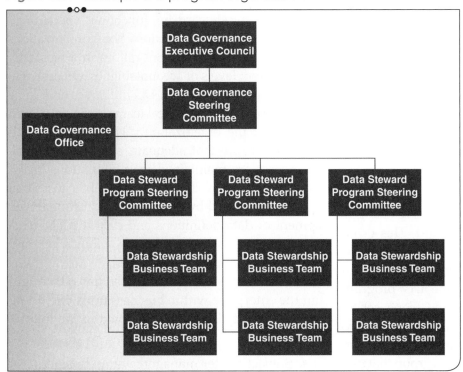

© Merida L. Johns

and state and federal governmental agencies, other healthcare providers, and vendors (Johns 2015).

Because an important DG purpose is to serve stakeholder interests, understanding stakeholder needs is pivotal to DG program success. For example, a top data priority of a senior executive may be to retrieve timely and aggregated operational data for strategic decision making whereas the human resource unit may need timely personnel and staffing data for daily staffing decisions. These are very different needs and may require different approaches for DG. Determining stakeholder needs can be assessed by conducting a stakeholder analysis with key stakeholders. A **stakeholder analysis** is a process that identifies and analyzes the attitudes or opinions of stakeholders. How the analysis is designed depends on the mission, scope, and specific projects undertaken by the DG program. For example, the analysis may take the form of a focus group or survey that targets determining the type of data needed for the most critical organization operations and decisions or the most frequent uses of data for operational, tactical, and strategic decision making. The analysis should evaluate the stakeholder's level of influence such as decision maker, policy maker, auditor, or user; stakeholder role in data creation, transformation, and use; data used and processes supported; and interactions with other stakeholder groups (Sharpe et al. 1999). A representative of each key stakeholder group falling within the scope of the DG program should be identified as a liaison between the group and the DG program. Frequently, these individuals will serve as part of the DG data steward council or on a DG project team (Johns 2015).

Executive Data Governance (DG) Council

Typically the DG program is led by a high-level committee, frequently referred to as the **executive data governance council**, committee, or board. This group of executives and senior level managers are responsible to make the business case for the DG program, provide the authorization for the DG program, establish the program's mission and scope, set the program's strategic direction, secure funding and resources for the program, and evaluate and measure the overall program success. It is this group that usually has the final responsibility and authority for approving enterprise-wide DG policies and standards

and resolving data-related issues that cannot be decided at lower levels of the DG program.

Data Governance (DG) Steering Committee

The **DG steering committee** is usually composed of representatives from various business or functional organizational units. This group serves as the coordinating body for the DG program. It develops the goals of the DG program, identifies and sequences project and task priorities, coordinates the data steward committees, monitors DG program outcomes, recommends policy and standards, and reports the status of the DG program to the executive data governance council.

Data Stewards and Data Steward Program Committees

There are many definitions of a **data steward**, but the central concept includes an individual appointed with responsibility and accountability for data, usually in a specific domain. **Accountability** is the duty of an individual, group, or organization to be answerable for specific activities. Data stewardship is therefore a formalization of accountability for data across its life cycle. It involves a range of stewardship responsibilities from data capture through data disposition and is carried out by a network of data stewards.

The way the stewardship function is operationalized varies among organizations. Some organizations arrange stewardship responsibilities in a hierarchy with different levels of accountabilities. Others organize the function based on DG initiatives and some may have designated tactical teams by business unit throughout the organization. "The data steward's role is to ensure that adequate, agreed-upon quality metrics are maintained on a continuous basis" (Berson and Dubov 2011, 116). Some of the tasks that may be performed by data stewards include development of data definitions and data models, resolution of data issues, data quality monitoring, and testing of data security procedures.

Data stewards are typically designated throughout the enterprise within business units, including IT. Data stewards may be classified in the following way:

- Subject matter managers within business areas who have a high level of accountability for the management of the data, but not necessarily the day-to-day hands-on responsibilities.

- Data definition stewards who function in a business, as opposed to a technical role; major responsibilities include identifying the specific data needed to operate business processes, recording business definitions and metadata, identifying and enforcing quality standards, communicating data issue concerns, and communicating new or changed business requirements.

- Data production stewards who can be either in a business or technical role and are responsible for inserting, updating, and deleting business and technical data in IT systems; validating data that enters and exits business processes; coding and editing data quality standards such as format and content; and communicating data issue concerns and new or changed business requirements.

- Data usage stewards who are data users who access and use data for its intended purpose; access information about the data (metadata); ensure the quality, completeness, and accuracy of data usage; and communicate data issue concerns and new or changed business requirements (Seiner 2005).

Data stewards may be organized in program teams focused on specific initiatives that support the organization's DG mission and scope. Usually these teams are cross-functional, meaning they are composed of individuals that represent different business units, including IT. For example, an organization whose DG focus is on master data management may have a cross-functional stewardship team composed of representatives from health information management, human resources, finance and business, registration and admissions, medical staff services, procurement, compliance, and information technology. All of these units have a vested interest in ensuring the quality of master data, such as master person data, master vendor data, and master provider data. A sample of the tasks this team may perform include identifying deficiencies in the organization's master data and determining resolutions for these, developing a master

data model, ensuring data from source systems are mapped to the master data model, recommending data quality metrics for monitoring master data quality, and drafting policies and standards for the management of master data and recommending these to the DG steering committee.

Data Governance Office   A DG program should have an assigned staff that administratively supports efforts of the various DG committees, maintains DG documentation, and provides communication among all DG parties. Most DG efforts are supported by a **data governance office** (DGO) that is led by an individual with the title of chief data officer (CDO) or data governance program director. Among the responsibilities of the office are:

- Providing centralized communication and archive for DG initiatives
- Working with stakeholders
- Coordinating DG initiatives
- Facilitating and coordinating data steward committees, task forces, and meetings
- Supporting the data governance council
- Collecting and analyzing DG metrics (Johns 2015)

The number of staff required for the DG program depends upon the size of the organization and scope and structure of the DG program.

Data Governance Processes   Processes are specific steps or actions that are taken to achieve a goal or outcome. DG processes are the steps required for governing data and ensuring compliance with DG policies and standards. The following 12 processes are considered DG best practices that should be incorporated into any DG program.

- Aligning policies, requirements, and controls
- Establishing decision rights
- Establishing accountability
- Performing stewardship
- Managing change
- Defining data
- Resolving data issues
- Specifying data quality requirements

- Building governance into technology
- Providing stakeholder care
- Communications and program reporting
- Measuring and reporting value (Data Governance Institute 2013, 16)

Processes can be proactive, reactive, or ongoing. Proactive processes are those that anticipate events and are associated with initiating change. Reactive processes, on the other hand, are those that are initiated as a response to an immediate and specific incident and usually do not continue beyond the event. Ongoing processes are those that maintain a steady state and stability within a system. Ideally, DG processes should be both proactive and ongoing, like those listed here.

Check Your Understanding 3.2

Instructions: **Choose the best answer.**

1. Which of the following best describes the definition of a business case?
   A. Best return on investment
   B. Positive revenues
   C. Proposal for executing a new idea
   D. Desired outcome of implementing a business change

2. Which of the following describes a real or conceptual structure that organizes a system or concept?
   A. Maturity model
   B. Framework
   C. Mission statement
   D. Vision statement

3. Normally, which of the following is the highest decision-making authority in a DG program?
   A. DG officer
   B. Data steward committee
   C. DG council
   D. Data steward

4. Which of the following is the best definition of decision rights?
   A. Granting authority to specific individuals to make data-related decisions
   B. Granting permission to specific individuals to access data
   C. Granting responsibility for making policy decisions
   D. Granting individuals security clearance

5. Which of the following is an individual appointed with responsibility and accountability for data, usually in a specific domain?
   A. Data stakeholder
   B. Data owner
   C. Data steward
   D. Data officer

6. Which of the following identifies the fundamental purpose, scope, and high-level goals of the DG program?
   A. Program charter
   B. Mission statement
   C. Vision statement
   D. Business case

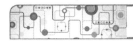

References

Berson, A. and L. Dubov. 2011. *Master Data Management and Data Governance.* New York: McGraw Hill.

Brannon, N. 2010. Business intelligence and e-discovery. *Intellectual Property & Technology Law Journal* 22(7):1–5. http://search.proquest.com/docview/504044279?accountid=10224

Businessdictionary.com. 2015. Governance. http//:www.businessdictionary.com

Chen, W. 2010. A Brief History of Data Governance. http://blog.kalido.com/a-brief-history-of-data-governance/

Chung, C. 2010. Data Life Cycle. https://blogs.princeton.edu/onpopdata/2012/03/12/data-life-cycle/.

Data Administration Management Association. 2010. *The DAMA Guide to the Data Management Body of Knowledge.* Bradley Beach: Technics Publications LLC.

Data Governance Institute. (n.d.). The DGI Data Governance Framework. http://www.datagovernance.com/the-dgi-framework/

Data Governance Institute. 2015. Funding Models: Funding Data Governance. http://www.datagovernance.com/funding-models-funding-data-governance/

Data Governance Institute. 2013. Definitions of Data Governance. http://www.datagovernance.com/adg_data_governance_definition/

Dimick, C. 2013 (Nov-Dec). Governance apples and oranges: Differences exist between information governance, data governance, and IT governance. *Journal of the AHIMA* 84(11):60–62.

Foss, N. and P. Klein. 2008. Organizational Governance. Prepared for R. Wittek, T. Snijders, and V. Nee, eds. *The Handbook of Rational Choice Social Research.* New York: Russell Sage Foundation. http://web.missouri.edu/~kleinp/papers/08061.pdf

Johns, M. 2015. *Enterprise Health Information Management and Data Governance.* Chicago: AHIMA.

Kooper, M.N. R. Maes, and R. Lindgreen. 2011. On the governance of information: Introducing a new concept of governance to support the management of information. *International Journal of Information Management* 31:195–200.

Ladley, J. 2012. *Data Governance: How to Design, Deploy and Sustain and Effective Data Governance Pro*gram. Waltham, MA: Elsevier.

National Information Standards Organization. 2004. Understanding Metadata. Bethesda: NISO Press. http://www.niso.org/publications/press/UnderstandingMetadata.pdf

Sharpe, H, A. Finkelstein, and Galan, G. 1999. Stakeholder Identification in the Requirements Analysis Process. http://eprints.ucl.ac.uk/744/1/1.7_stake.pdf

Smallwood, R. 2013. *Managing Electronic Records Methods, Best Practices and Technologies.* Hoboken: John Wiley & Sons.

Seiner, R. 2005 (Oct). Data steward roles and responsibilities. *Real-World Decision Support Journal* 1(29). http://www.ewsolutions.com/resource-center/rwds_folder/rwds-archives/issue.2005-10-06.9442499950/document.2005-10-06.1879501317

Thomas, G. 2014. The Data Governance Framework. Data Governance Institute. http://www.datagovernance.com/category/guidance-by-gwen/focus-areas-of-data-governance/

4

Health Record Content and Documentation

Rebecca B. Reynolds, EdD, RHIA, FAHIMA and Marcia Sharp, EdD, RHIA

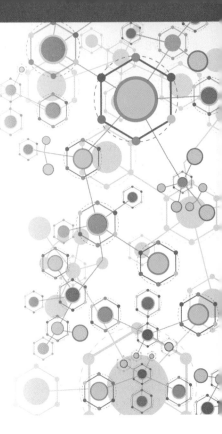

Learning Objectives

- Identify the factors that determine the content of the health record
- Identify the organizations and standards for the content of the health record
- Compare the major content areas of the health record, including administrative and demographic data, clinical data, and specialized content
- Examine the flow of health record information from initial encounter to final format
- Identify examples of general requirements for the primary documentation required in most health records, including the history and physical examination, progress notes, orders, and discharge summary
- Examine forms and documentation requirements specific to facilities other than acute care hospitals, including ambulatory care, home care, hospice care, rehabilitation care, and long-term care facilities
- Differentiate between the personal health record and patient portals
- Differentiate between quantitative and qualitative record analysis
- Identify the purposes of the following processes: concurrent analysis and discharge analysis, open-record review, record review, point-of-care review, and continuous record review
- Define an incomplete health record and a delinquent health record
- Examine the role of the health information management (HIM) professional in the design and control of forms
- Evaluate how new developments such as voice recognition technology will change the role of the medical transcriptionist
- Compare and contrast the unit and serial-unit systems of record numbering and filing and the appropriate use of each, including methods of number assignment
- Examine the basic rules of terminal digit filing and the advantages of using terminal digit filing concepts for productivity
- Assess policies and procedures on health record storage, retention, and destruction
- Identify the functions of the master patient index
- Examine issues related to identity management

Key Terms

Advance directive	Durable power of attorney	Overlap
Authentication	Electronic signature	Overlay
Bylaws	Emergency Medical Treatment	Patient/member web portal
Care path	and Active Labor Act	Personal health record (PHR)
Case manager	(EMTALA)	Problem-oriented medical
Charting by exception	History	record
Closed record	Hybrid record	Progress notes
Closed-record review	Informed consent	Qualitative analysis
Computerized provider order	Integrated health record	Quantitative analysis
entry (CPOE) system	Joint Commission	Retention
Concurrent analysis	Longitudinal health record	Scanning
Consent	Master patient index (MPI)	Serial-unit numbering system
Consultation	Medicare	Source-oriented health record
Delinquent health record	Medication administration	Straight numeric filing system
Digital dictation	record (MAR)	Terminal-digit filing system
Discharge summary	Notice of Privacy Practices	Unique identifier
Disposition	Open-record review	Unit numbering system
Do not resuscitate (DNR) order	Optical imaging technology	Voice recognition technology

The patient health record takes many forms in healthcare organizations, from paper-based to an electronic format. Indeed, most healthcare facilities currently maintain their health records using a combination of the two formats (sometimes referred to as a hybrid health record system) in order to accommodate the many different ways in which patient information is gathered and stored. Today's health records include digital images as well as handwritten notes. Data arrive via electronic transfer from computerized laboratory or radiological testing or examination, through direct voice entry into documentation systems, and from provider wireless devices. However, the paper-based health record continues to be utilized in today's healthcare system. The momentum to move away from paper is increasing dramatically, but a fully operational electronic health record (EHR) for all types of healthcare providers and facilities remains a future goal for the healthcare system.

This chapter traces the evolution of the health record and describes the different kinds of information it contains and the different formats in which it is kept. The chapter also focuses on the health information management (HIM) professional's role in managing patient information through the record life cycle, from the creation and storage of information to its long-term retention and eventual destruction, and in ensuring its accuracy, completeness, and security. Finally, this chapter describes the functions of the master or enterprise patient index, which is critical for proper patient identification and record linkage.

Evolution of the Health Record

The patient health record has evolved as medicine and medical technology have evolved. Once simply the notation of the patient's name and a brief description of his or her illness or injury, today's health record has evolved into a detailed collection of handwritten entries, transcribed reports, electronic data, and digital images reflecting the contributions of numerous healthcare providers.

Historical Overview

Health records have existed as long as there has been a need to communicate information about patient treatment. Archeological evidence indicates that maintaining information on patient care and treatment techniques is an ancient art.

Health records are maintained by all organizations that deliver healthcare services including physician and provider offices, long-term care facilities, emergency clinics, rehabilitation facilities, home health agencies, behavioral health facilities, correctional institutions, and numerous types of delivery systems and organizations. Health records are also generated by patients with the increasing use of personal heath monitoring devices and the ability of individuals to record and transmit data to providers. Records vary depending on the type of facility. Healthcare records in acute-care hospitals, for example, require rapid documentation by many providers. Patients are often in the hospital for life-threatening injuries or conditions, and various healthcare practitioners access and record information in the patients' health records. Records in nonacute-care hospital settings have much of the same content found in the acute-care settings. The records also contain specialized content to meet requirements related to those settings. Although format and content of the health record may differ among healthcare settings, all providers of care must maintain information to meet patient care needs and to comply with relevant laws, standards, and regulations.

Today's health information management professional is responsible for records that still contain paper and are maintained in a variety of formats other than paper. There is an increasing demand to share information among providers on a regional basis to improve continuity of care. The multiple formats of today's records are a challenge to the goal of uniform sharing of information. The skills of the HIM professionals are in great demand to ensure the quality and integrity of shared health information.

Factors Influencing the Content of the Health Record

A variety of factors influence what is included in the health record and how it is formatted. In the physician office, for example, provider preference may influence what and how much data are collected about the patient. The process of providing healthcare is another factor. The healthcare provider must gather enough information to determine a diagnosis and to direct treatment. That data must then be structured in a way that is useful for all users of the record. For many settings, such as acute care, long-term care, and home health, data sets have been developed that indicate what data elements should be found in records for that type of facility. Finally, there are accrediting and certifying bodies' external standards and regulations and state licensure standards, in addition to internal standards such as medical staff bylaws that outline requirements for content of the health record. Meaningful Use incentives also drive the content and format of the health record as providers are required to collect and transmit certain data elements electronically.

Documentation and Maintenance Standards for the Health Record

Health records provide proof of what has been done for the patient. As the complexity of care has evolved, so has the need for improved documentation. Standards for record documentation and maintenance have been established and are refined and revised constantly. These standards and regulations have a major impact on what is documented in the health record. The following includes an overview of the common sources of documentation and maintenance standards for the health record.

The American College of Surgeons and the Joint Commission

The American College of Surgeons (ACS) provided the impetus for standardizing health records when it developed minimum standards for hospitals early in the 20th century. It was evident to the ACS that standards were needed because candidates for membership were unable to produce proof of their experience with various types of surgical cases. Records were either nonexistent or of poor quality. The ACS Minimum Standard of 1917 included specific requirements for maintaining patient health records.

The **Joint Commission** is the successor organization to the ACS in the area of standardization. It assumed responsibility for the accreditation process in 1952 as a joint effort of the ACS, American College of Physicians, American Medical Association, and the American Hospital Association. Initially responsible for the accreditation of hospitals, the Joint Commission has since expanded its accreditation process to home health, long-term care, and other types of healthcare facilities.

The major source of information about the hospital or any healthcare facility is the health record. Joint Commission surveyors routinely review the health records of current patients to obtain knowledge about the facility's performance and process of care.

Medicare Conditions of Participation

In 1965, the federal government passed legislation creating the **Medicare** program, which provides healthcare insurance coverage to Americans age 65 or older. Since then, the legislation has been expanded to cover persons disabled for two years as well as persons with chronic kidney disease. The Centers for Medicare and Medicaid Services (CMS) is the division of the federal Department of Health and Human Services responsible for developing and enforcing regulations regarding the participation of healthcare providers in the Medicare program.

The regulations for health record content and documentation were originally established in the Conditions of Participation—guidelines and regulations under which facilities are allowed to participate in Medicare and Medicaid programs. As health record documentation became increasingly important, CMS began to focus on reviewing it for medical necessity and compliance with the decision-making rules established by the federal government. In addition, CMS published guidelines for documenting histories and physical examinations and medical decision making that affect physician reimbursement.

State Licensure

Every state has licensure regulations that healthcare facilities must meet in order to operate. Licensure regulations may include very specific requirements for the content, format, retention, and use of patient records. These regulations are established by state governments, usually under the direction of state departments of health.

Internal Standards

Bylaws, rules, and regulations are developed by the medical staff and approved by the board of trustees or governing body in healthcare facilities. In addition to describing the organization's manner of operation, **bylaws** outline the content of patient health records, identify the exact personnel who can enter information in health records, and may restate applicable Joint Commission and CMS requirements. In addition, bylaws describe the time limits for completing patient health records. External surveyors review the bylaws to ensure that healthcare facilities abide by their own established rules and regulations and that the bylaws are in agreement with current standards and regulations. All medical staff personnel are required to abide by the approved bylaws. The HIM professional must be able to work effectively with the medical staff to ensure that they follow the medical staff bylaws and regulations and adhere to the many laws and regulations that specify the need for proper documentation.

Of great importance to the HIM professional is the adherence of individual medical staff members to bylaws related to completion of medical records and compliance with documentation guidelines and requirements. The HIM professional supports the patient care process by ensuring quality and timely documentation in the patient record. This also supports the patient safety and quality efforts of the facility. The typical medical staff bylaws contain provisions for timely and proper completion of medical records, including the requirements to write legibly or utilize the hospital information system to record patient notes; for communicating and coordinating the care of the patient with other members of the staff; and for dictating reports of history and physical examinations, operative notes, and other required documents based on best practices and facility policies. Failure to comply with any of the provisions of medical record documentation may result in progressive discipline up to and including suspension of medical staff membership. One common process is suspending admission privileges until the delinquent health records are completed. Suspension limits the ability of the practitioner to schedule time in the operating room or admit patients. Hospitals typically have procedures to notify the admissions department, surgical care department, and other key hospital departments when a practitioner's privileges are suspended. Sometimes a suspended practitioner may ask his or her partners to admit patients for him or her. This can create patient care and safety issues for the patients and requires the HIM professional to become an active participant in the patient care team. This is a common situation that involves the HIM professional to provide access to the patient records and generate reports to look at the admission pattern changes to ensure that suspended practitioners are following the suspension regulations set forth in the bylaws.

There is generally a medical staff committee responsible for health information management and patient record issues including electronic health records. Information about incomplete and delinquent medical records is typically reported by the director of the health information management department during committee meetings. Because of this, it is important that the HIM professional know the medical staff bylaws, Joint Commission standards, the CMS Conditions of Participation, any state statutes, and other facility licensure requirements regarding the timely completion of medical records.

Today's Health Record

Today's health record includes the contributions of numerous healthcare providers. In addition, it includes information provided by the patient or a person acting on his or her behalf describing the reasons for the patient's visit to the healthcare provider and other pertinent background facts. The modern health record is patient centered, meaning that the patient is the focus of all documentation of the activities that revolve around him or her while under the provider's care.

The patient health record is the foundation for most of the decisions made in any healthcare facility. Decisions relative to patient care and financial reimbursement depend on the quality of documentation in the health record. The health record is the communication tool among the members of the patient's healthcare team. It is evidence of what was done for the patient, and the information it contains is used to evaluate the quality of care and to provide important information for research and public health needs. The information in the healthcare record protects the legal interests of both the patient and the facility. The traditional saying in healthcare, "if it wasn't documented, it wasn't done," is a reminder of how important the record is for the patient, the facility, and the numerous other users of the record and the information it contains.

Definition of the Health Record

The health record must outline and justify the patient's treatment, support diagnosis of the patient's condition, describe the patient's progress and response to medications and services, and explain the outcomes of the care provided. The health record promotes continuity of care among all the providers who treat the patient by documenting all of the activities that revolve around the patient.

Functions of Health Records and Health Information

To providers, the health record is valuable as the principal source of information in determining care for the patient. To the healthcare facility, it is valuable as a primary source of information in determining the reimbursement for care. In addition, new payment models that emphasize value-based purchasing strengthen the need for health records to be accessible and provide timely, accurate, and a complete picture of the patient care.

The primary functions of the health record are as follows:

- Facilitate the ongoing care and treatment of individual patients
- Support clinical decision making and communication among clinicians

- Document the services provided to patients in support of reimbursement
- Provide information for the evaluation of the quality and efficacy of the care provided
- Provide information in support of medical research and education
- Help facilitate the operational management of the facility
- Provide information as required by local and national laws and regulations

Ongoing Care and Treatment of Individual Patients   The most important use of the health record is patient care, and the person to whom the record is of most value is the patient. When physicians were the only caregivers, they knew the patient and family and decided how detailed the patient's records needed to be. Often a small card or a ledger listing the patient's problem at a particular time was all the recordkeeping physicians needed. As healthcare has come to depend on technology and the skilled personnel to use it, health records have become more complex. Patients often have multiple caregivers. Providers cannot remember all the information provided by the available technology to a large number of patients, and fast access to past information about the patient's care is vital to the continuity of care.

Clinical Decision Making and Communication   Health information serves the vital function of allowing all the patient's providers to enter and analyze information and to make decisions. Each member of the healthcare team must have access to the information to review what others are doing and communicate with them through the record. Thus, the health record is the healthcare team's primary reference and communication tool. This is extending outside of the healthcare organization as the amount of data sharing and reporting increases with meaningful use reporting and health information exchange efforts.

Reimbursement Including Meaningful Use   Information in the health record is used to document the services provided to the patient so that coding and payment for the care provided can be made by those responsible for creating the bill. Insurance companies, managed care organizations, and CMS require that specific information be submitted to support the services billed to the patient and to demonstrate that the care provided was medically necessary and effective. The role of the patient record in reimbursement is becoming more complex with the CMS present on admission criteria and Meaningful Use requirements, which both rely on documentation in the health record and can impact reimbursement.

Evaluation of the Quality and Efficacy of Care   The health record is used as a legal document to assess the quality of care rendered by the healthcare provider and serves as the legal business record of the organization. The documentation in the record provides information for accrediting and licensing activities. The content of the health record also provides evidence of compliance with evidence-based medicine guidelines.

Medical Research and Education   Data from many health records can be aggregated and analyzed for research studies and can provide statistical information on medical conditions and treatment modalities. As an example, public health agencies need data on certain diseases and conditions to develop prevention and control procedures as well as to monitor disease trends. Moreover, the information in health records serves to provide continuing education for students in a variety of health professions.

Operational Management   Information gathered from health records helps facilities plan for the future based on the types of patients and diagnoses treated. Aggregate statistical information provides data on the use of services, provider patterns, and other important issues. Management often uses the information to make comparisons with other facilities. Finally, the quality of information in the health record aids managerial decision making in terms of improving the quality of patient care.

Legal Purposes The health record serves the legal interests of the patient, the provider, and the facility. It serves as evidence in legal cases addressing the treatment received by the patient or the extent of injuries. It serves to prove the patient's allegations in a malpractice case and also is used by the clinical provider and the facility to defend the care they provided the patient. The record is admissible as evidence in court under the business records provision because the documentation occurs routinely as part of the healthcare facility's daily operation. This is one of the roles of the HIM professional as the custodian of the health record. More information about the role of the record custodian and the admissibility of health records in legal proceedings is found in chapter 2.

The health record itself is the property of the healthcare facility. However, the patient has the right to be informed about the use of his or her protected health information (PHI). Federal Health Insurance Portability and Accountability Act (HIPAA) regulations require that the patient be notified of the uses of PHI through the Notice of Privacy Practices. See chapter 11 for more information related to HIPAA and patient privacy.

The Longitudinal Health Record

The **longitudinal health record** is a record compiled about an individual that contains health records from various encounters and from numerous healthcare delivery settings. This is not a new concept but is commonly being accomplished via health information exchange (HIE) projects in the United States. It is valuable because all the information about a patient is maintained and accessible. It serves as a reference of past history and helps the provider avoid repetition of details and duplication of testing for the same conditions. Moreover, the longitudinal health record helps to prevent medical errors because information on allergies, drug interactions, surgeries, and past medical problems can be made available before treatment decisions are made. The practitioner can review the details of a patient's care and retrieve information needed at a later date. Refer to chapter 15 for more detail on health information exchange.

Responsibility for Quality Documentation

Ensuring data accuracy of health record content is one of the primary responsibilities of the HIM professional. HIM professionals must lead the effort in healthcare organizations to ensure that availability of quality health information. Integrity of health information is one of the biggest challenges to health record quality.

One issue to address is copy paste functionality, which is also called cloning or copy forward. This occurs when a provider copies a note from a previous patient encounter either into the same health record or the health record of another patient. Organizational policies should be established addressing copy past functionality in the health record. The prevalence of copy and paste in the health record creates many issues beyond the accuracy of clinical information. For the HIM professional, there is concern about how to certify the health record as a legal record when the original source of entries in the health record is difficult to establish. There is also concern when a copied patient note may be disclosed to an individual as part of the patient record that is not the patient's information and creates a breach of PHI.

Making corrections and amendments to the health record has occurred in paper and electronic formats and is not a new issue in health records; however, EHRs complicate the process of making corrections in the health record. The HIM professional must ensure that the original entry in the health record is preserved when changes are made to the health record. Many systems allow various mechanisms for correction of entries in the health record and the HIM professional must be involved in the process of how these functions are enabled and monitored.

Legacy systems and standalone source systems in ancillary areas like radiology and other diagnostic areas can create issues for the HIM professional in records management. Before these systems are discontinued, it must be determined whether or not the data have been interfaced into the current system or if there is a need for the data. This requires the consideration of the record retention policies to know what data need to be maintained.

Patient identity management is a huge issue in today's connected environment. Ensuring that the right patient is connected with the right information relies on accurate patient identity management. The master patient index (MPI) is discussed later in this chapter.

The provider of care is responsible for ensuring that entries made in the record are of high quality.

Although the facility's medical staff bylaws establish the rules and regulations for record content, the individual care providers are ultimately responsible for the quality of entries they make and authenticate. Figure 4.1 presents general documentation guidelines that every practitioner who writes or enters information in the patient health record should follow.

Figure 4.1. Guidelines for documenting and maintaining the patient health record

These guidelines are considered standard or typical health information practices. Individual facilities develop their own policies based on institutional needs and laws and regulations.

1. All entries in the health record must be authenticated to identify the author (name and professional status) and dated.
2. All entries in the paper health record should be in ink. Photocopying or scanning should be considered when colored ink or colored forms are used because some colors do not reproduce well.
3. No erasures or deletions should be made in the health record. This applies to paper and electronic records.
4. If a correction must be made in a paper health record, one line should be neatly drawn through the error, leaving the incorrect material legible. The error then should be initialed and dated so that it is obvious that it is a corrected mistake. If a correction must be made in an electronic health record, the original entry should be noted and hidden but the incorrect entry should still be part of the health record.
5. The original report should always be maintained in the health record. Cumulative laboratory reports or computerized nursing notes may be replaced with the latest cumulative report. Faxed copies of admission orders and histories and physicals may be used as originals in the record. The usual signature requirements should be followed.
6. Blank spaces should not be left in progress and nursing notes. If blanks are left, they should be marked out with an X so that additional information cannot be inserted on the paper out of proper date sequence.
7. All blanks on forms should be completed, especially on consent forms.
8. When health records are filed incomplete (as directed by medical staff or health record committee policy), a statement should be attached to indicate that this is the case. The statement should be signed by the chief of staff or chair of the health record committee as specified in the policy.
9. Chart folder labeling, dotting, or other methods of identifying at a glance a particular type of patient, such as one with a drug or alcohol diagnosis or HIV-positive status, should be discouraged to prevent inadvertent breaches of patient confidentiality.

Check Your Understanding 4.1

Instructions: **Answer the following questions on a separate sheet of paper.**

1. What is the primary purpose of patient health information?
2. What are six other purposes or uses of patient health information?
3. What factors influence the content of the health record?
4. What is the role of each of the following in the development of standards for health information: Joint Commission, Centers for Medicare and Medicaid Services, state licensure, and medical staff bylaws?
5. Why is a longitudinal health record valuable, and why is a longitudinal health record in a hybrid system difficult to achieve?
6. Who is responsible for ensuring the quality of health record documentation?

Content of the Health Record

All health records contain information that can be classified into two broad categories: (1) administrative and demographic data or (2) clinical data. All health record entries must be legible, complete, dated, and authenticated according to the healthcare organization's policies. Health records may be paper based, electronic, or hybrid (a combination of formats). As health records evolve from paper to electronic and digital formats, the term **hybrid record** is used to describe the record information format that includes both paper-based and electronic health information. Because the hospital record is the most complex in content, it will be used in describing the content of the record.

Administrative and Demographic Information

Administrative and demographic information is generally found on the front page or face sheet of the paper health record and on the login screen or dashboard in an EHR. The information entered provides data that identify the patient and data related to payment and reimbursement and other operational needs of the healthcare facility. This information is entered into the system by administrative staff when the patient presents for care or may be entered electronically by the patient or staff from a physician's office. Facility patient portals may allow for patients to enter this information prior to an elective admission or edit after discharge from the facility.

Demographic Data

Demographic data represent one type of administrative information.

Demographic information includes facts such as:

- Patient's name
- Patient's address
- Patient's telephone number
- Patient's date of birth
- Patient's next of kin
- Other identifying information specific to the patient

A **unique identifier** number is assigned to each health record, which is often called the medical record number. More information about medical record number assignment is covered later in this chapter. Facilities use the unique identifier to ensure that all information about the patient is entered in the correct record and that the correct record is accessed when a query is entered into the computer system. Demographic information helps to specifically identify the patient and can be aggregated from many patients to provide statistical information that is vital for planning, research, statistics, and other needs.

Consent to Treatment

Through the **consent** process, the patient agrees to undergo the treatments and procedures to be performed by practitioners. A general consent is often part of the admission or intake process into the healthcare facility and allows the facility to provide routine care. However, this general consent does not replace the individual consent forms the patient must complete and sign for each operation or special procedure to indicate that he or she is fully informed about the care to be provided. Written consents signed by the patient for experimental drugs and treatment and for participation in research also must be included in the health record. Refusal of treatment or procedures likewise must be written to ensure that the consequences of the decision to refuse treatment have been explained and the patient is aware of them.

Consent to Use or Disclose Protected Health Record Information

Under HIPAA, at the time of admission to the facility or prior to treatment by the provider, patients must be informed about the use of individually identifiable health information. This **Notice of Privacy Practices** must explain and give examples of the uses of the patient's health information for treatment, payment, and healthcare operations, as well as other disclosures for purposes established in the regulations. If a particular use of information is not covered in the Notice of Privacy Practices, the patient must sign an authorization form specific to the additional disclosure before his or her information can be released. (See figure B.21 in appendix B.) HIPAA and the Privacy Rule are discussed in chapter 11.

Consent to Special Procedures

In cases where the patient is coming to the facility for a specific procedure, an informed consent spelling out the exact details of the treatment must be signed by the patient or his or her legally authorized representative. This consent must show that the patient, or the person authorized to act for the patient, understands exactly what the procedure, test, or operation is going to be, including any possible risks, alternative methods, and outcomes.

Advance Directives

An advance directive is a written document, such as a living will, that states the patient's preferences for care in the event that the patient's condition prevents him or her from making care decisions. It also can be in the form of a durable power of attorney for healthcare in which the patient names another person to make medical decisions on his or her behalf in the event he or she is incapacitated. A durable power of attorney for healthcare is a document that names someone to make decisions for the patient if the patient is unable to make these decisions. This person is often called a proxy or a healthcare agent and may be a provider, a family member, or a friend of the patient. The advance directive goes into effect when the physician determines the patient is no longer able to communicate about healthcare decisions.

When the patient has a written advance directive, its existence must be noted in the health record. Patients or family members may bring the document to the facility to show the patient's wishes in case of terminal disease, traumatic injury, or cardiac arrest. The advance directive can be included as a part of the health record, although its inclusion may not be required. Rather than a formal written document, there may be documentation by the physician outlining the discussion with the patient or the family about the patient's wishes. Patients must be informed that they have the right to have an advance directive. Further, they must be notified of the provider's policies regarding its refusal to comply with advance directives. Caring Connections is a program of the National Hospice and Palliative Care Organization and provides links to information about advance directives in each state. This information is helpful for HIM professionals since legal processes and procedures are primarily dictated by state law.

Acknowledgment of Receipt of Patient's Rights Statement

CMS requires that Medicare patients be informed of their rights, including the right to know who is treating them, the right to confidentiality, the right to determine what visitors the patient wants to have, and the right to be informed about treatment. The patient's rights statement also must explain the patient's right to refuse treatment, to participate in care planning, and to be safe from abuse. The patient must sign a statement that these rights have been explained, and the signed statement must be made part of the health record. States often have laws and regulations regarding which rights must be explained to patients, such as the right to privacy in treatment, to refuse treatment, and to refuse experimental treatments and drugs.

Property and Valuables List

Although facilities encourage patients to leave jewelry and other valuables at home, patients often will have clothing, dentures, eyeglasses, hearing aids, and other personal articles. Patients may be asked to list these items and sign a release of responsibility form to absolve the facility of responsibility for loss or damage to their personal property. This form then becomes part of the patient health record.

Clinical Data

Clinical data include information related to the patient's condition, course of treatment, and progress. The patient health record includes mainly clinical data.

Medical History

The history is a summary of the patient's illness from his or her point of view. Its purpose is to allow the patient or his or her authorized representative to give the practitioner as much background information about the patient's illness as possible.

Documentation guidelines for histories and physical examinations and medical decision making published by CMS affect physician reimbursement and are discussed further in chapter 7.

Components of the Medical History

The medical history has several components, including the following:

- *Chief complaint (CC):* Told in the patient's own words (or those of the patient's representative), the chief complaint is the principal reason the patient is seeking care.
- *Present illness or history of present illness (HPI):* This component addresses what the patient feels the problem is and includes a brief description of the duration, location, and circumstances of the complaint.
- *Past medical history:* This section consists of questions designed to gather information about past surgeries and other illnesses that might have a bearing on the patient's current illness. The practitioner asks about childhood and adult illnesses, operations, injuries, drug sensitivities, allergies, and other health problems.
- *Social and personal history:* The social history uncovers information about habits and living conditions that might have a bearing on the patient's illness, such as marital status, occupation, environment, and such. Consumption of alcohol or tobacco products also may affect a patient's health, and information about these habits is included in the social history. This section also should address the patient's psychosocial needs.
- *Family medical history:* The questions in this component allow the physician to learn whether the patient's family members have conditions that might be considered genetic. Common questions concern cardiovascular

diseases or conditions, renal diseases, history of cancer or diabetes, allergies, health of immediate relatives, and ages of relatives at death and causes of their deaths.

- *Review of systems (ROS):* This component consists of questions designed to cue the patient to reveal symptoms he or she may have forgotten, did not think were important, or neglected to mention when providing the historical information.

It is important that the person recording the history document whether the information was given by the patient or by another person in cases where the patient is unable to communicate. Table 4.1 lists the information usually included in a complete medical history

Physical Examination

The physical examination is the actual comprehensive assessment of the patient's physical condition through examination and inspection of the patient's body by the practitioner. The practitioner usually tailors the physical examination to symptoms described in the patient's history and begins an assessment. The end of the physical examination should include the impression, which is a list of the patient's problems based on the information obtained. Thus, the history and physical (H&P) provides a base on which the practitioner can develop an initial plan of care. Appropriate treatment can then begin.

Components of the Physical Examination

The physical examination is conducted by observing the patient, palpating or touching the patient, tapping the thoracic and abdominal cavities, listening to breath and heart sounds, and taking the blood pressure. In a comprehensive physical examination, each body system of the patient is examined thoroughly. If the patient is admitted for a particular procedure, a more focused physical examination may take place.

Time Frame of the History and Physical Examination

The facility must have a policy that establishes a time frame for completing the history and physical. Most facilities set the time frame as within the

Table 4.1.   Information usually included in a complete medical history

Components of the history	Complaints and symptoms
Chief complaint	Nature and duration of the symptoms that caused the patient to seek medical attention as stated in his or her own words
Present illness	Detailed chronological description of the development of the patient's illness, from the appearance of the first symptom to the present situation
Past medical history	Summary of childhood and adult illnesses and conditions, such as infectious diseases, pregnancies, allergies and drug sensitivities, accidents, operations, hospitalizations, and current medications
Social and personal history	Marital status; dietary, sleep, and exercise patterns; use of coffee, tobacco, alcohol, and other drugs; occupation; home environment; daily routine; and so on
Family medical history	Diseases among relatives in which heredity or contact might play a role, such as allergies, cancer, and infectious, psychiatric, metabolic, endocrine, cardiovascular, and renal diseases; health status or cause of and age at death for immediate relatives
Review of systems	Systemic inventory designed to uncover current or past subjective symptoms that includes the following types of data: • *General:* Usual weight, recent weight changes, fever, weakness, fatigue • *Skin:* Rashes, eruptions, dryness, cyanosis, jaundice; changes in skin, hair, or nails • *Head:* Headache (duration, severity, character, location) • *Eyes:* Glasses or contact lenses, last eye examination, glaucoma, cataracts, eyestrain, pain, diplopia, redness, lacrimation, inflammation, blurring • *Ears:* Hearing, discharge, tinnitus, dizziness, pain • *Nose:* Head colds, epistaxis, discharges, obstruction, postnasal drip, sinus pain • *Mouth and throat:* Condition of teeth and gums, last dental examination, soreness, redness, hoarseness, difficulty in swallowing • *Respiratory system:* Chest pain, wheezing, cough, dyspnea, sputum (color and quantity), hemoptysis, asthma, bronchitis, emphysema, pneumonia, tuberculosis, pleurisy, last chest x-ray • *Neurological system:* Fainting, blackouts, seizures, paralysis, tingling, tremors, memory loss • *Musculoskeletal system:* Joint pain or stiffness, arthritis, gout, backache, muscle pain, cramps, swelling, redness, limitation in motor activity • *Cardiovascular system:* Chest pain, rheumatic fever, tachycardia, palpitation, high blood pressure, edema, vertigo, faintness, varicose veins, thrombophlebitis • *Gastrointestinal system:* Appetite, thirst, nausea, vomiting, hematemesis, rectal bleeding, change in bowel habits, diarrhea, constipation, indigestion, food intolerance, flatus, hemorrhoids, jaundice • *Urinary system:* Frequent or painful urination, nocturia, pyuria, hematuria, incontinence, urinary infections • *Genitoreproductive system:* Male—venereal disease, sores, discharge from penis, hernias, testicular pain, or masses; Female—age at menarche, frequency and duration of menstruation, dysmenorrhea, menorrhagia, symptoms of menopause, contraception, pregnancies, deliveries, abortions, last Pap smear • *Endocrine system:* Thyroid disease; heat or cold intolerance; excessive sweating, thirst, hunger, or urination • *Hematologic system:* Anemia, easy bruising or bleeding, past transfusions • *Psychiatric disorders:* Insomnia, headache, nightmares, personality disorders, anxiety disorders, mood disorders

first 24 hours following admission and require that the history and physical be completed by the practitioner who is admitting the patient. CMS Conditions of Participation requires that the history and physical examination be completed no more than 30 days before or 24 hours after admission and the report must be placed in the record within 24 hours after admission (42 CFR 482.24(4)(i)(A)). If the history and physical have been completed within the 30 days prior to admission, there must be an updated entry in the medical record that documents an examination for any changes in the patient's condition since the original history and physical examination, and this entry must be included in the record within the first 24 hours of admission (42 CFR 482.24(4)(i)(B)). CMS rules specify that the history and physical examination be completed by the physician or another qualified individual who has medical staff privileges in accordance with state law and hospital policy. State licensure laws vary on the acceptable time frame for completion of the history and physical.

The Joint Commission requires the history and physical examination to be recorded and made part of the patient health record prior to any operative procedure. When the practitioner chooses to dictate the history and physical, the dictated report must be transcribed and attached to the chart before the procedure. When the report is dictated but not transcribed, a written preoperative note covering the history and physical is acceptable only in an emergency. The physician must write an explanation of the emergency circumstances (Joint Commission 2013).

The HIM professional is responsible for ensuring that the most stringent time requirements are followed so that the facility is in compliance with state and federal laws and regulations, licensure standards, CMS Conditions of Participation, and accreditation requirements for the specific type of facility. Table 4.2 shows the information usually documented in the report of a physical examination.

Table 4.2. Information usually documented in the report of a physical examination

Report components	Content
General condition	Apparent state of health, signs of distress, posture, weight, height, skin color, dress and personal hygiene, facial expression, manner, mood, state of awareness, speech
Vital signs	Pulse, respiration, blood pressure, temperature
Skin	Color, vascularity, lesions, edema, moisture, temperature, texture, thickness, mobility and turgor, nails
Head	Hair, scalp, skull, face
Eyes	Visual acuity and fields; position and alignment of the eyes, eyebrows, eyelids; lacrimal apparatus; conjunctivae; sclerae; corneas; irises; size, shape, equality, reaction to light, and accommodation of pupils; extraocular movements; ophthalmoscopic exam
Ears	Auricles, canals, tympanic membranes, hearing, discharge
Nose and sinuses	Airways, mucosa, septum, sinus tenderness, discharge, bleeding, smell
Mouth	Breath, lips, teeth, gums, tongue, salivary ducts
Throat	Tonsils, pharynx, palate, uvula, postnasal drip
Neck	Stiffness, thyroid, trachea, vessels, lymph nodes, salivary glands
Thorax, anterior	Shape, symmetry, respiration and posterior
Breasts	Masses, tenderness, discharge from nipples
Lungs	Fremitus, breath sounds, adventitious sounds, friction, spoken voice, whispered voice
Heart	Location and quality of apical impulse, trill, pulsation, rhythm, sounds, murmurs, friction rub, jugular venous pressure and pulse, carotid artery pulse
Abdomen	Contour, peristalsis, scars, rigidity, tenderness, spasm, masses, fluid, hernia, bowel sounds and bruits, palpable organs
Male genitourinary	Scars, lesions, discharge, penis, scrotum, organs epididymis, varicocele, hydrocele
Female reproductive	External genitalia, Skene's glands and organs Bartholin's glands, vagina, cervix, uterus, adnexa
Rectum	Fissure, fistula, hemorrhoids, sphincter tone, masses, prostate, seminal vesicles, feces
Musculoskeletal	Spine and extremities, deformities, swelling, system redness, tenderness, range of motion
Lymphatics	Palpable cervical, axillary, inguinal nodes; location; size; consistency; mobility and tenderness
Blood vessels	Pulses, color, temperature, vessel walls, veins
Neurological system	Cranial nerves, coordination, reflexes, biceps, triceps, patellar, Achilles, abdominal, cremasteric, Babinski, Romberg, gait, sensory, vibratory
Diagnosis(es)	

Diagnostic and Therapeutic Orders

Physicians or other credentialed practitioners generate orders which direct the healthcare team. Orders may be for treatments, ancillary medical services, laboratory tests, radiological procedures, medications, devices, related materials, restraint, or seclusion. Orders change according to the patient's needs and responses to previous treatment. In the case of medications, the physician orders a specific drug in a particular dosage stating how often the drug is to be given, by what means (orally, intravenously, or by other method), and for how long.

Orders for tests and services must demonstrate the medical necessity and explain the reason for the order. This explanation is required because payers may not reimburse the facility if the reason for the test or treatment is not properly documented.

The legibility of orders is important to ensure that they are clearly understood by the personnel who must carry them out. Some facilities use a **computerized provider order entry (CPOE) system** for providers to directly enter orders. CPOE systems allow practitioners to enter orders directly into the clinical information system.

Clinicians Authorized to Give and Receive Orders

Orders must be written by the physician or other credentialed practitioner or verbally communicated to persons qualified and authorized to receive and record verbal orders either in person or by telephone. For verbal orders, the person accepting the order should record the order, sign it, and give his or her title, such as RN, PT, LPN, as appropriate. In some states, certified registered nurse practitioners and physician assistants are allowed to write or give verbal orders (AHIMA 2009).

Medical staff policies and procedures must specifically state the categories of personnel authorized to accept and record orders. Verbal orders for medication are usually required to be given to, and to be accepted only by, nursing or pharmacy personnel. Some categories of personnel that may accept verbal or oral orders for services within the specific area of practice include physical therapists, registered nurse anesthetists, dietitians, and medical technologists. The Joint Commission requires that the hospital identifies in writing the staff who are authorized to receive and record verbal orders. This is typically included in the medical staff by-laws (Joint Commission 2013).

The time the order was given should be recorded in the health record. Some facilities do not allow verbal orders for treatments or procedures that might put the patient at risk. The Joint Commission requires the documentation of verbal orders to include the date and names of individuals who gave, received, and implemented the orders (Joint Commission 2013).

Signatures on Orders

Orders must be dated and authenticated manually or electronically by the treating practitioner responsible for the patient's care who gave the orders. In the case of verbal or telephone orders, the practitioner should sign them as soon as possible after giving them and within the timeframe specified by state law and regulations. Many facilities require the ordering practitioner to indicate that the telephone orders are accurate, complete, and final by authenticating them in writing or electronically within 24 hours. The timing requirements for signatures on orders are governed by state law, facility policy, accreditation standards, and government regulations and may vary from facility to facility.

A review of orders is part of the concurrent review process, namely while the patient is still hospitalized; thus, orders can be signed in a timely manner, and providers with patterns of unsigned orders can be detected. A comparison of orders to laboratory and other ancillary reports and to nursing documentation is another way to ensure that all orders are carried out.

Some facilities have developed standing, or standard, orders for certain procedures that all physicians can use when performing the particular procedure. Other facilities require an additional order to implement the standing orders, and still others allow a registered nurse to initiate the standing orders because the medical staff has previously approved them.

CMS regulations allow verbal (telephone or oral) orders to be signed by another provider responsible for the patient's care even if the order did not originate with that provider. The CMS rules retain the current requirements that the use of verbal orders should be infrequent and used only when the orders cannot be written or given electronically. The CMS regulations further state that verbal orders must only be accepted by persons authorized by hospital policies and procedures and state and federal law (42 CFR 482.24(3)(c)(2)).

Special Types of Orders Certain categories of medications, such as narcotics and sedatives, have an automatic time limit or stop order. This means that these medications will be discontinued unless the practitioner gives a specific order to continue the medication. This method prevents patients from receiving drugs for a longer period of time than is necessary.

Do not resuscitate (DNR) orders must contain documentation that the decision to withhold resuscitative services was discussed, when the decision was made, and who participated in the decision. This discussion is often documented in the progress notes. Generally, patients are presumed to have consented to CPR unless a DNR order is present in the record. Do not resuscitate orders may be part of the advance directives in the record. The Joint Commission offers guidance through standards pertaining to end of life care and patient decision making regarding withdrawing life-sustaining treatment and withholding resuscitative services (Joint Commission 2013).

Orders for seclusion and restraint, including drugs used for restraint, must comply with facility policies and CMS regulations, state laws, and Joint Commission standards. These should never be standing or as-needed orders; instead, such treatments must be ordered only when necessary to protect the patient or others from injury or harm. Specific time limits for these orders must be followed, and there must be continuous oversight of the patient under restraint or seclusion. The Joint Commission has a standard on documentation of the use of restraint and seclusion in patient care (Joint Commission 2013).

Discharge Orders Discharge orders for hospital patients must be in writing and can only be issued by a physician. When a patient leaves against medical advice, this fact should be noted in lieu of a discharge order because the patient was not actually discharged. In the case of death, some facilities require that a discharge to the morgue order be written.

Clinical Observations Clinical observations of the patient are documented in the health record in several areas, including areas of medical services, nursing services, ancillary services, surgical services, and organ transplantation.

Medical Services There are several areas where medical services are documented in the health record. Two primary areas include progress notes and consultation reports.

Progress Notes Progress notes are chronological statements about the patient's response to treatment during his or her stay in the facility. Facility procedures and policies must state exactly what categories of personnel are allowed to write or enter information into progress notes. Generally, these personnel include physicians, nurses, physical therapists, occupational therapists, respiratory therapists, social workers, case managers, registered dietitians (RDs), nurse anesthetists, pharmacists, radiologic technologists, speech therapists, and others providing direct treatment or consultation to the patient. Each person authorized to enter documentation into the progress notes must write or enter his or her own note, authenticate and date it, and indicate authorship by signing his or her full name and title. In some facilities, various practitioners record progress notes on a common form (integrated progress notes) while in other record formats there may be separate sections for physician, nursing, and therapy progress notes.

Each progress note should include changes in the patient's condition, findings based on the facts of the case, test results, and response to treatment, as well as an analysis of the findings. The final part of the note contains the decisions or actions planned for future care. When writing in a paper patient record, providers must avoid leaving blank spaces between progress notes to prevent information from being added out of sequence.

Flowcharts are another effective way to illustrate the patient's progress and can be computerized to demonstrate progress or to keep track of certain data. Many physicians and other providers use mobile devices to maintain ongoing flowchart information about patients, such as blood glucose levels over time.

The patient's condition dictates how often progress notes are recorded, and the frequency is generally established by the healthcare facility or payers of care. In a hospital, the physician primarily responsible for the patient's care is often required to write a progress note daily. Doing so shows the physician's involvement and that he or she is aware of changes in the patient's condition.

Consultation Reports Consultations are opinions of physicians with specialty training beyond general board certification such as oncologists, cardiologists, or dermatologists. If the attending physician requests that a specialist see the patient, the specialist prepares a consultation report, which is included in the health record. Each consultant is responsible for writing, dictating, or entering his or her own report. The report should show evidence of the consultant's review of the record; examination of the patient; and any pertinent findings, opinions, and recommendations. Moreover, the documentation should show that the physician requesting the consultation reviewed the report. Not all patients receive consultations, so a consultation report is not found in every health record.

Nursing Services Nursing personnel have the most frequent contact with patients, and their notes provide the complete record of the patients' progress and condition and demonstrate the continuity of care. Licensed registered nurses, licensed practical nurses (sometimes called licensed vocational nurses), and nursing assistants record the patient's vital signs and facts of the physician's orders being carried out; observe the patient's response to treatment interventions and nursing interventions; and describe the patient's condition and complaints as well as the outcome of care as reflected in the patient's status at discharge or termination of treatment. The method most commonly used by nurses to enter notes is detailed narrative documentation.

Nursing personnel begin recording information in the health record when the patient is admitted to the facility. They coordinate the patient's care to ensure that orders are carried out. The initial nursing assessment must summarize the date, time, and method of admission; the patient's condition, symptoms, and vital signs; and other information. Nurses may use a variation of the SOAP (subjective, objective, assessment, and plan) notes from the problem-oriented medical record format (discussed later in this chapter) when recording notes. All nursing notes must be signed by the individuals who provided the service or observed the patient's condition. Full names and titles are required with each entry.

Charting by exception, or focus charting, is a method of documenting only abnormal or unusual findings or deviations from the prescribed plan of care. A complete patient assessment is performed every shift. When events differ from the assessment or the expected norm for a particular patient, the notes should focus on that particular event and include the data, assessment, intervention, and response. Flow sheets and care plans may be used to illustrate changes in the patient's condition. The purpose of charting by exception is to reduce repetitive recordkeeping and documentation of normal events. Bedside terminals and direct input of monitoring information and other computerization of nursing observations and medication distribution save nurses a great deal of time because information does not have to be rewritten numerous times.

Medication administration records (MARs) are maintained by nursing staff for all patients and include medications given, time, form of administration, and dosage and strength. The records are updated each time the patient is given his or her medication. The health record must reflect when a medication is given in error, indicating what was done about it and the patient's response. Adverse drug reactions must be fully documented and reported to the provider and to the performance improvement or risk management program according to guidelines established by the facility.

Flow sheets are often used in addition to narrative notes for intake and output records showing how much fluid the patient consumed and how much was eliminated. In addition, blood glucose records are often flowcharted for ease of comparison. Degree of pain is another aspect of the patient's condition that is commonly flowcharted.

Nurses are responsible for maintaining records of patient transfers (to surgery, to another room, or to another level of care) as well as visits to physician or treatment offices and other locations outside the facility.

Case managers are nurses, social workers, or other personnel who are responsible for assisting the patient through the care process. The case management process improves quality of care because care is scheduled in an orderly way and fragmentation is reduced. Hospitals, managed care organizations, and other facilities use case managers to improve coordination of care, scheduling, and discharge planning. Many facilities use predetermined **care paths** that are specific to diagnoses or conditions; case managers ensure that patients receive care according to the care path. Care paths are also called clinical pathways, critical paths, and clinical algorithms.

Ancillary Services   Laboratory and radiology reports and reports from other ancillary services, such as electrocardiographs (EKGs) and electroencephalographs (EEGs), must be signed by the physician responsible for the interpretations. A pathologist is responsible for the work of the pathology laboratory; a radiologist is responsible for the work of the radiology department. The final interpretations of the radiology or other reports become part of the health record and are kept as long as the health records are kept.

Healthcare facility policies and procedures must state that the practitioner approved by the medical staff to interpret diagnostic procedures, such as nuclear medicine procedures, MRIs, EEGs, and EKGs, should sign and date his or her interpretations. The interpretations then become part of the

health record. Scans and videotapes, tracings, or other actual recordings are often COLD-fed directly into the hospital information system. Providers may view such recordings, but the recordings do not become part of the permanent record. It is important that all tests or procedures ordered have corresponding reports in the health record.

Orders and records of services rendered to patients from rehabilitation, physical therapy, occupational therapy, audiology, or speech pathology should be included in the record, as appropriate to the patient's condition. These reports must contain evaluations, recommendations, goals, course of treatment, and response to treatment. Nutritional care plans need to be developed in compliance with a physician order, and information on nutrition and diet should be included in the discharge plan and transfer orders.

Surgical Services   The operative section of the health record includes the anesthesia record, the intraoperative record, and the recovery record. The history and physical examination, informed consents signed by the patient or his or her authorized representative, and the postoperative progress note also are part of the documentation about the operative procedure. Every patient's record must include a complete history and physical examination prior to any surgery or invasive procedure unless there is an emergency. When the history and physical report is dictated, it must be included in the record. The Joint Commissions standards require that prior to high-risk procedures and those involving use of anesthesia of deep sedation, a provisional diagnosis is recorded by the licensed independent practitioner involved in the patient's care (Joint Commission 2013).

Moreover, the anesthesiologist or the certified registered nurse anesthetist must write a preanesthesia evaluation or an updated evaluation prior to surgery. This evaluation must cover information on the anesthesia to be used, risk factors, allergy and drug history, potential problems, and a general assessment of the patient's condition. An intraoperative anesthesia record must be maintained of all events during surgery, including complete information on the anesthesia administration, blood pressure, pulse, respiration, and other monitors of the patient's condition. Finally, after surgery, the appropriate anesthesia personnel must write a postoperative anesthesia follow-up report including any anesthetic complications. The Joint Commission requires that the health record contain postoperative information including the patient's vital signs and level of consciousness, any medication, including intravenous fluids and any administered blood, blood products and blood components; any unanticipated events or complications and the management of those events (Joint Commission 2013). Outpatient surgical cases also must include postanesthesia evaluations. CMS regulations state that any individual qualified to administer anesthesia can complete the postanesthesia evaluation rather than limiting the postanesthesia documentation completion to the individual who actually administered the patient's anesthesia (Joint Commission 2013).

The operative report must be documented either in writing or dictated by the surgeon immediately after surgery and must include the names of the surgeon and assistants, the name of the procedures performed, a description of the procedures, findings of the procedures, any specimens removed, any estimated blood loss, and the postoperative diagnosis. The surgeon must enter a brief operative progress note in the record immediately after surgery before the patient is transferred to the next level of care. The postoperative progress notes and completion of the operative reports must be carefully monitored to ensure that this documentation is placed in the health record in a timely manner.

Pathology reports are required for cases in which a surgical specimen is removed or expelled during a procedure. The medical staff and a pathologist must decide which specimens require both a microscopic and macroscopic (gross or with the naked eye) evaluation of the tissue and which require a gross examination only. These reports are part of the operative section of the health record and must be signed by the pathologist. The preoperative diagnosis and pathological diagnosis can then be compared for quality-of-care purposes.

Information on the patient's discharge from the postoperative or postanesthesia care unit must be documented and signed by the licensed independent practitioner responsible for the discharge or by the provider verifying that the patient is ready for discharge according to specific discharge criteria.

The operative section also will contain data on implants, including product numbers, and additional information for follow-up.

Organ Transplantation   CMS and the Joint Commission require hospitals to inform families of the opportunity to donate organs, tissues, or eyes. All patients meeting the United Network of Organ Sharing (UNOS) criteria must be evaluated and the documentation must be part of the health record. Facilities participating in the transplant program are required to share patient information and provide access to health records to representatives of approved organ procurement organizations (OPOs). Documentation showing that the organ procurement organization has been notified regarding a deceased patient or a patient near death must be included in the health record so that anatomical gifts can be preserved and used. Sample forms and other information are available on the UNOS website. The Joint Commission also requires that hospitals have a written agreement with at least one tissue bank and at least one eye bank (Joint Commission 2013).

Conclusions at Termination of Care

At the time of discharge, the physician must summarize the patient's condition at the beginning of treatment and basic information about tests, examinations, procedures, and results occurring during treatment. This conclusion at termination of care is called the discharge summary.

Discharge Summary

The **discharge summary**, also called the clinical resume, provides details about the patient's stay while in the facility and is the foundation for future treatment. It is prepared when the patient is discharged or transferred to another facility or when the patient expires. The summary states the patient's reason for hospitalization and gives a brief history explaining why he or she needed to be hospitalized. Pertinent laboratory, x-ray, consultation, and other significant findings, as well as the patient's response to treatment or procedures, are included. In addition to a description of the patient's condition at discharge, the discharge summary delineates specific instructions given to the patient or family for future care, including information on medications, referrals to other providers, diet, activities, follow-up visits to the physician, and the patient's final diagnoses. The discharge summary must be authenticated and dated by the physician.

When a patient expires in the hospital, the facility often requires the physician who pronounced death to write a note that gives the time and date of death. This documentation, in addition to the discharge summary, is required in all cases when a patient expires no matter how long the patient was in the facility. In some cases nurses are allowed to declare a patient dead and subsequently complete the necessary documentation.

A discharge summary is not typically required for patients who are in the hospital for 48 hours or less. Such patients usually have a short-stay or short-service record. This one-page form can be used to record the history and physical examination, the operative report, the discharge summary, and discharge instructions. A final discharge progress note may also suffice in these cases to provide a summary of the hospitalization at the patient's discharge. When the patient dies 48 hours or less after admission, the short-stay record is insufficient and a complete discharge summary must be prepared. Also, most facilities do not require a discharge summary for normal newborns and obstetrical cases without complications, as long as there is a final progress note.

Typically, the discharge summary must be completed within 30 days after discharge; however, facility policy may require a quicker completion date. When a patient is transferred, the physician should complete the discharge summary within 24 hours. The Joint Commission allows for a transfer summary when the patient is transferred to another level of care in the facility or the patient's care is transferred to another provider (Joint Commission 2013).

Healthcare facilities must determine what information goes with the patient when he or she is transferred to another level of care such as a rehabilitation or skilled nursing facility. When the transfer is to an affiliated institution that is part of the same healthcare system, the original patient record is transferred with the patient and new orders are written at the receiving institution to initiate care. A discharge summary is generally required.

Discharge Plan Discharge planning information regarding further treatment of the patient after discharge should be part of the acute-care health record. The discharge planning process begins at admission and must include information on the patient's ability to perform self-care as well as other services needed by the patient. The case manager, the social worker, utilization review personnel, or nursing personnel may write this plan.

Records Filed with the Health Record

In the past, there was much debate about whether or not patient records received from other facilities should be made part of the receiving facility's health record. HIPAA regulations now require that all information, including information from other facilities, is included as part of the health record when the information was used in treating the patient (HHS 2013). It is important for healthcare facilities to develop policies to determine exactly what health information mailed, faxed, delivered by mobile devices or personally brought to the facility by the patient or patient's family becomes part of the receiving facility's designated health record.

The Personal Health Record

Patients frequently maintain information about their own health as well as that of their families. Recently there has been a strong interest in **personal health records (PHRs)**. These records may consist of copies of information from providers, insurance companies, pharmacies, and hospitals as well as immunization records and allergy information. Mobile technology allows consumers to readily use technology to create patient information to share with providers. Electronic PHRs may consist of a web-based tool or a PHR offered by the patient's healthcare provider, which is referred to as a **patient/member web portal**. The patient portal allows a patient to access all or part of the health record that is maintained by the patient's provider. Some have limited ability to enter comments that are added to the provider-based record. HIM professionals must work with the medical staff to determine when and how to incorporate patient-created information into the facility's health record. Another issue for the health information professional is the access by patients to the facility's health record in order to download information for their own PHR. This creates new challenges for the HIM professional to interface with patients electronically to share information from the facility's systems (AHIMA 2010). Many people are using wellness trackers and other mobile devices to collect and share information for personal health monitoring. HIM professionals must determine how this patient-generated data is incorporated into the patient health record. (Refer to chapter 14 for more detail on PHRs, portals, and patient-generated health data.)

Social Media and Electronic Communication

Social media include media such as Twitter, Facebook, LinkedIn, blogs, YouTube, and such and provide a method of communication between organizations, patients, and consumers. For HIM professionals, these communication methods can pose a risk of privacy breaches, even if patient names are not used. It is important for facilities to have a policy on managing social media that includes who in the organization can access official social media for the organization. Policies are also needed on disciplinary actions to be taken for inappropriate use of social media. Since social media are used primarily for marketing and communications, their content does not become part of the legal health record.

E-mail may become part of the patient's record when it is used as a method of communicating healthcare information from the practitioner or facility to a patient. In such cases, e-mail may include information such as laboratory values and other protected health information. The health informa-tion professional must ensure that such communications are captured as a permanent part of the patient's health record. Other administrative uses of e-mail, such as verifying an appointment, would not be considered part of the legal record. It is important that the facility have policies indicating which e-mail should become part of the patient's record, how long it must be retained, and how it will be stored. Training staff and other users of e-mail regarding appropriate procedures is also an important role for the HIM professional (Backman et al. 2011).

Specialized Health Record Content

The content of the patient health record varies according to the type of care provided. When specialized services are provided to the patient, additional documentation is required, which may require special templates and custom forms. Joint Commission standards and regulations for the type of facility often specify particular content to include in the record, as do data sets specific to each setting. The following specialized services typically have additional patient records. Obstetrical care typically includes prenatal records including labor and delivery records. Records of newborns are typically separate health records from the mother's record

Emergency Care

Emergency health records may be filed separately or incorporated into the health record when the patient is admitted to the same facility. When the records are filed separately, the emergency record must be available when the patient is readmitted or seeks care in the future. Most of the demographic and clinical information in emergency situations is recorded on one sheet in a paper health record format. Additional sheets may include laboratory, radiology, and other tests; consent forms; and follow-up instructions.

The content of the emergency health record should include the following items:

- Identification data
- Time of arrival
- Means of arrival (by ambulance, private automobile, or police vehicle)

- Name of person or organization transporting patient to the emergency department
- Pertinent history, including chief complaint and onset of injury or illness
- Significant physical findings
- Laboratory, x-ray, and EKG findings
- Treatment rendered
- Conclusions at termination of treatment
- Disposition of patient, including whether sent home, transferred, or admitted
- Condition of the patient upon discharge or transfer
- Diagnosis upon discharge
- Instructions given to the patient or the family regarding further care and follow-up
- Signatures and titles of the patient's caregivers

When the patient leaves the emergency department before being seen or against medical advice (AMA), this fact should be noted on the emergency department form. Consent forms for treatment also must be included in the record. A copy of the emergency department record should be made available to the provider of follow-up care.

In addition to the emergency department record, most states require facilities to maintain a chronological record or log of all patients visiting the emergency department with name, date, time of arrival, and record number. This register also includes the names of patients who were dead on arrival.

Emergency patients must be made aware of their rights. Transfer and acceptance policies and procedures must be delineated to ensure that facilities comply with the **Emergency Medical Treatment and Labor Act (EMTALA)** and state regulations regarding transfers. EMTALA states that patients cannot be transferred or refused treatment for reasons related to ability to pay or source of payment nor can hospitals determine that space is unavailable based on ability to pay or source of payment (42 CFR parts 413, 482 and 489). Anyone who requests or requires an examination must be provided an appropriate medical screening examination by hospital staff to determine whether a medical emergency exists. Further, the hospital must stabilize the medical emergency by ensuring an airway and ventilation, by controlling hemorrhage, and by stabilizing or splinting fractures before a patient can be transferred. Appropriate transfer means that the receiving hospital agrees to receive the patient and provide appropriate medical treatment. Records must be provided to the receiving hospital, and the patient or responsible person must understand the medical necessity of the transfer.

For demonstrating compliance with EMTALA regulations, hospitals must maintain screening examinations for a minimal period of five years. Nonemergency patients presenting to the emergency department are typically examined by the triage nurse or other emergency department staff and referred to a minor medical clinic, a physician office, or another nonemergency patient care facility.

Ambulatory or Outpatient Care

Ambulatory or outpatient care means that patients move from location to location and do not stay overnight. Ambulatory or outpatient care may be given in a freestanding clinic, a clinic that is part of a larger hospital system, or a physician or other provider office. Traditionally, physician office records have been less comprehensive than hospital medical records. Physicians must develop standardized formats and comprehensive documentation practices.

When patients are in a clinic affiliated with a hospital, the entire health record from previous hospital care should be available. The Joint Commission requires ambulatory patients to have a summary list by the third visit that includes known diagnoses, conditions, procedures, drug allergies, and medications (Joint Commission 2013). Contents of the ambulatory care record vary depending on the treatment received. The Accreditation Association for Ambulatory Health Care (AAAHC) has additional requirements for the content of the ambulatory care record that are provided for ambulatory surgery centers, community health centers, health plans and medical homes, office-based surgery centers and primary care (AAAHC 2015).

Ambulatory facilities that only perform surgery are called ambulatory surgery centers (ASCs). Patients having surgery at any type of ambulatory facility must have a history and physical examination prior to surgery, consents, an operative note, a postoperative progress note, and the same anesthesia information as an operative patient in the hospital. In addition, the record must document instructions for postoperative care and postoperative follow-up. Clinics often call patients after surgery to check on their condition, and these calls should be documented in the record.

Behavioral Healthcare

Behavioral health records, also known as mental health records or psychiatric records, must include diagnostic and assessment information related to both the patient's mental condition and his or her physical health. The Medicare Conditions of Participation require that the inpatients within a psychiatric hospital receive a psychiatric evaluation (42 CFR 482.61).

Home Health Services

According to the National Association for Home Care and Hospice (NAHC), the term *home care* covers many types of services that are delivered at home to patients requiring a variety of medical, nursing, therapy, or other services (NAHC 2011). Physicians order home care services that may include visits from many types of healthcare practitioners, including physical and occupational therapists and nurses. Patient health records must contain a legible record of each visit describing what was done to or for the patient during the visit. The practitioners working with patients must develop and document periodic plans of care. Specific documentation required by CMS is included in the home care health record for the attending physician to document and update the plan of care. It is also necessary for the physician to certify the patient's need for the care, and recertification of the need must be documented periodically (NAHC 2011).

Hospice Care Services

The National Hospice and Palliative Care Organization (NHPCO) defines hospice care as a "team-oriented approach to expert medical care, pain management, and emotional and spiritual support expressly tailored to the patient's needs and wishes" (NHPCO 2015). Because hospice care is delivered to patients with all types of terminal illnesses, the family is involved in the care, and support is given by the hospice organization. Hospice and palliative care may also consist of pain management, grief counseling, financial planning, and other services provided to the family. Hospice services are provided in numerous types of settings, including homes, hospitals, and long-term care facilities. Special documentation for the election of hospice care is required for CMS to reimburse for services. This includes certification by the patient's attending physician and the hospice that the patient has a terminal illness. Unique documentation issues in hospice care include documentation by volunteers of all patient contacts as well as documentation by bereavement counselors of services provided to the family after the patient's death.

Rehabilitation Services

Rehabilitation covers a wide range of services provided to build or rebuild the patient's abilities to perform the usual activities of daily living. In the rehabilitation setting, the history and physical must include a functional history covering the patient's functional status before and after injury or onset of illness. Additionally, the history should describe the equipment the patient uses at home including orthotics and prosthetics. It is important that the physician outline the goals for the patient's care to coordinate the interdisciplinary team involved in the care.

Long-Term Care

Long-term care describes the care provided for extended periods of time to patients recovering from illness or injury. Long-term care facilities offer a combination of services, ranging from independent living to assisted living to skilled nursing care. Rehabilitation services are often part of the long-term care plan. The long-term care record must document a comprehensive assessment that includes items in the Minimum Data Set (MDS) to meet CMS requirements stated in 42 CFR 483.20 (2010).

In addition, long-term facilities must meet state requirements. Individualized patient care plans must be developed and included in the health record. These plans must cover the potential for rehabilitation, the ability to perform activities of daily living, medications prescribed, and other aspects of care.

Check Your Understanding 4.2

Instructions: **On a separate piece of paper, match the contents with the appropriate part of the record by placing the letter for the form in the blank preceding the description of the form's content.**

1. _____ Directions given for drugs, devices, and healthcare treatments

2. _____ Comprehensive assessment of patient to determine signs and symptoms

3. _____ Records maintained by physical therapists, speech therapists, respiratory therapists, and other providers of special services

4. _____ Protocol for the process of care

5. _____ Summary of background information about the patient's illness

6. _____ Statement of the patient's wishes or instructions for care

7. _____ Conclusions at the termination of care

8. _____ Observations of the patient's response to treatment

9. _____ Record that must contain the time and means of arrival and the name of the person transporting the patient to the facility

10. _____ Opinions of specialists

A. Care path
B. History
C. Physical examination
D. Orders
E. Consultations
F. Nursing notes
G. Advance directives
H. Emergency record
I. Discharge summary
J. Ancillary notes

Format of the Health Record

The term *format* refers to the organization of information in the health record. There are many possible formats, and most facilities use a combination of formats. During the patient care process, the paper-based health record is often in a different format than after the patient is discharged. This is especially true in facilities with a hybrid health record that in some cases scan the paper portions of the record after the discharge of the patient. Regardless of the media in which the health record is kept, a systematic format for the health record ensures all users of the health record can easily locate the patient information required for their needs.

Source-Oriented Health Records

The **source-oriented health record** is the conventional or traditional method of maintaining paper-based health records. In this method, health records are organized according to the source, or originating, department that rendered the service (for example, all lab reports are filed together, all radiological reports are filed together, and so on).

Many hybrid health record systems are source oriented and maintain the organization and format of the health record by scanning and indexing the forms based on the "tabs" from the paper-based health record.

Problem-Oriented Health Records

The **problem-oriented medical record** (POMR) was developed in the 1970s. The POMR is comprised of the problem list, the database (the history and physical examination and initial lab findings), the initial plan (tests, procedures, and other treatments), and progress notes organized so that every member of the healthcare team can easily follow the course of patient treatment (Weed 1970).

A distinctive feature of the POMR is the problem list, which serves as the record's table of contents. All relevant problems—medical, social, or other—that may have an impact on the patient are listed with a number. As problems are resolved, the resolution is noted on the list; new problems are added as they occur. The problem list serves as a permanent index that providers can quickly check to review the status of past and current problems. Entries in the record, such as orders and progress notes, include the number of the problem addressed as provided on the problem list.

The most recognizable component of the POMR is the SOAP format, which is a method for recording progress notes. SOAP is an easy acronym that helps providers remember the specific and systematic decision-making process being documented. *S* stands for subjective findings and includes statements from the patient's viewpoint such as symptoms. *O* stands for objective findings, such as laboratory and test results as well as observations and findings from the physical examination. *A* stands for assessment, which consists of appraisals and judgments based on the findings and observations. *P* stands for plan, which states the methods to be followed in addressing the problems identified. Although the full POMR has not been adopted universally, many providers routinely use the SOAP method, or an adaptation of it, to document progress notes and also include a problem list in the record.

Integrated Health Records

The content of the **integrated health record** is arranged in strict chronological order. The order of the record is determined by the date the information was entered, the date of the service, or the date the report was received, rather than by the source department; the record gives the sequence of the patient's care as delivered. Different types of information and sources of information are mixed together according to the dates on the entries. Although this system makes it difficult to find a particular document unless one knows the date, it does provide a better picture of the story of the patient's care. Physician offices often use this format.

Check Your Understanding 4.3

Instructions: **On a separate piece of paper, fill in the blanks with the appropriate terms.**

1. _____ This is the conventional or traditional method of maintaining paper-based health record.

2. _____ This type of record maintains the organization and format of the health record by scanning and indexing the forms based on the "tabs" from the paper-based health record.

3. _____ This record is maintained in strict chronological order.

4. _____ This record begins with a problem list that serves as the table of contents for the record.

5. _____ This is what the *P* in the SOAP records means

Management of Health Record Content

The HIM professional manages health record content through oversight responsibilities for medical transcription services to produce clinical reports that become part of the health record. The HIM responsibilities for incomplete records include analyzing and monitoring incomplete records to ensure that they are properly completed to meet facility standards and patient healthcare needs, as well as controlling the design and production of forms and electronic templates to ensure that all health records are in a standardized format.

Transcription

Completion of the health record is greatly enhanced by the sophisticated dictation and transcription methods and equipment in use today. Physicians and other providers first dictate the necessary reports, including, but not limited to, history and physical examinations, operative reports, discharge summaries, consultation reports, progress notes, clinic notes, pathology reports, and radiology reports. The dictated report then is transcribed to produce final printed output that can be filed or scanned into the EHR, COLD-fed into the electronic system, or directly transcribed into the EHR, to become a part of the legal health record. Personnel who type—that is, transcribe—the dictation are called medical transcriptionists. Facilities should encourage providers to dictate to enable reports to be retrieved electronically. With the growing use of electronic health records, documentation options beyond traditional transcription of dictation include the provider entering information directly into the EHR through narrative text or templates or the transcriptionist entering dictation directly into the EHR.

Components of a Transcription System

Digital dictation is the process by which voice sounds are recorded and converted into a digital format. The physician or provider begins the dictation process using a telephone, a microphone attached to a PC, or a hands-free microphone. The dictator enters digits to indicate certain basic information, such as identification of the dictator, identification of the patient, and the type of report to be dictated (a history and physical examination, a discharge summary, an operative report, and so on).

The dictator then speaks and the dictation is transmitted to a computer that digitizes the voice. After the voice sounds have been digitized, the dictation is accessed by the transcriptionist, who transcribes the report by listening to the voice and converting it to typed output. Special software features allow the transcriptionist to produce reports with as few keystrokes as possible, using techniques such as word expanders. Word expanders are shortened versions of phrases.

Planning for and Selecting Transcription Equipment

When purchasing or upgrading a dictation and transcription system, the HIM professional must be aware of the long-range consequences of this important decision. Equipment vendors can provide a wealth of information based on their experience working in various facilities. They can help the HIM department determine the number of ports, or entry points, that need to be available based on the number of dictators and transcriptionists requiring simultaneous access. The system needs to have sufficient accessibility to avoid collision, which would prevent a dictator or transcriptionist from gaining access to the system. Immediate access for all users, whether dictating or transcribing, is critical to the system's success. When dictators call in, a digital channel selector automatically selects an available line without input from the dictator.

The facility must have vendor support to ensure that the system is operational at all times. Transcription systems should be designed so that the transcriptionists can work independently if the general facility information system is not working. Although entering patient information without the connection to the general information system will require greater effort, the work can continue to be generated.

Transcription services may be centralized or decentralized. In a decentralized system, pathology, radiology, and other departments in addition to health information management may have their own transcriptionists. Some HIM departments have centralized transcription areas that transcribe reports for the entire facility or for all facilities in an integrated system. Moreover, some transcription departments perform work for physician offices in order to generate revenue. The transcription department must consider every possible customer and analyze every possible location for dedicated dictation stations, including nurses' stations, clinics, operative areas, and workrooms in the HIM department. Practitioners may use other phones to call into the dictation service however cell phones are discouraged from use since they can be intercepted and recorded by cell phone scanners.

The HIM professional must fully understand the dictation and transcription system application. A certified medical transcriptionist (CMT) may supervise the transcription area, but the manager of the HIM department is ultimately responsible for the work produced. Before purchasing any large system, the HIM professional should interview references and visit similar facilities to see the system in operation. Often the vendor will arrange these site visits. The HIM professional also might visit facilities that are using the equipment under consideration but have not been specifically recommended by the vendor. Further, he or she might attend trade shows and seminars and narrow the field of products to avoid confusion. In addition, he or she should include the people who will actually use the system in the decision-making process.

Speech and Voice Recognition

Speech or **voice recognition technology** is used increasingly as the accuracy of output improves. In voice recognition technology, the spoken word is transmitted immediately to a database and converted to typed output, which eliminates the need for the transcriptionist to listen to and type the information. The quality of the output is very dependent on the quality of the dictation. The speaker must speak clearly and distinctly. The role of the transcriptionist will change as this new technology increases in accuracy. In time, the transcriptionist will become primarily an editor and a proofreader.

Speech recognition technology may be utilized on the front end, where the person dictates through a microphone or headset apparatus connected to a computer. As the person dictates, the words appear on the screen and are corrected if they are not displayed correctly. The document is correct when completed and the dictator controls the entire process. The facility may still require the document to be sent to a transcriptionist or another person who controls its distribution. This method also requires training of the individual who is dictating, and the dictator may feel that this process is too slow and takes too much physician time. In back-end speech recognition, after the physician dictates in the usual manner, the audio is sent as a draft text along with the voice file to the transcriptionist—who serves as an editor—to listen to the audio in comparison with the displayed text and to make changes to the text document. This document then goes back to the dictating provider for approval. The advantage is that the person dictating does not have to change dictation behavior. Back-end speech recognition does not improve productivity because editing is as time consuming as transcribing. Radiology departments and other departments that have many repetitive reports have utilized speech recognition technology more effectively than the general facility (AHIMA e-HIM Work Group on Speech Recognition in the EHR 2003).

Evaluation of the Effectiveness and Efficiency of Transcription Services

The effectiveness and efficiency of transcription services are judged primarily by turnaround time and accuracy in typing the dictation. History and physical examinations and operative reports have time limitations set forth in Joint Commission regulations. Discharge summaries are valuable sources of information for coding, billing, and reimbursement. With EHR systems, the dictated information and transcribed documents are accessible to all providers and healthcare personnel who need to refer to them. The success of the transcription service depends on both the cooperation of the providers who dictate and the skills of the medical transcriptionists.

Abstracting

Abstracting is the compilation, usually in an electronic database, of pertinent information extracted from the patient record. The purpose of abstracting is to make information from the patient record readily available for internal and external reporting needs. Abstracting supports the secondary use of patient data for registries, public reporting, research, and other purposes. It is important for the HIM professional to understand the mission of the facility when determining both the amount of information to abstract from the health record and the appropriate staff required for the abstracting. The process of abstracting begins with defining the needs and the purposes for the abstracted information.

In a facility with paper-based and hybrid health records there are typically administrative systems for registration, coding, and billing and some clinical systems with electronic processes that require data input through an abstracting process. In these cases, the HIM professional may be required to abstract more information than in facilities with advanced electronic health record systems that provide electronic query functions. When obtaining information such as the treating physician and procedures performed, the information included may come from a combination of information from other systems that integrate into the system (Tegan et al. 2005).

Incomplete Record Control

Health records must be complete in order to provide all the information that is necessary for patient care, billing, and reimbursement. The HIM department must verify that all paper records are received from the nursing floor, including records of any previous admissions that were sent to the nursing unit. After the records arrive in the HIM department, their location must be carefully tracked until they reach final storage in the filing area or are scanned.

The business office notifies the HIM department of bills that are waiting for information from the physician so that the record can be coded and the bill prepared. The administration places a great deal of pressure on the HIM department to process bills in a timely manner so that revenue can be generated for the facility. In turn, the HIM professional must motivate physicians to provide the information the department needs to do its work. Incomplete records are less of a problem in most healthcare facilities with hybrid or electronic health records. However, monitoring incomplete health records is a constant challenge for the HIM professional.

Quantitative Analysis

Quantitative analysis, often called discharge analysis, is a review of the health record for completeness and accuracy. It is generally conducted retrospectively, that is, after the patient's discharge from the facility or at the conclusion of treatment. Quantitative analysis also may be done while the patient is in the facility, in which case it is referred to as concurrent review or concurrent analysis. Concurrent analysis means that the record is analyzed during the patient's stay in the healthcare facility. It has the advantage of HIM or other personnel being present on the floors where the physicians see patients. HIM personnel can remind providers to complete items in the record and to sign orders and progress notes. Some facilities have HIM personnel physically located on the nursing floors to monitor record completion closely. Other facilities have HIM personnel visit patient care areas to obtain signatures and ensure that loose reports are placed in the health record. Discharge analysis serves as an additional check to ensure that the record is complete and that all information belongs in the patient's record. The concurrent review and discharge analysis review typically analyze the health records for the same documentation.

Electronic health record systems facilitate the record completion process with workflows that notify providers when record entries require authentication. These systems can also be utilized to automate the division of work to the HIM personnel by routing specific record types to designated personnel for analysis, coding, and other HIM operations. These workflows can reduce the manpower requirements and shorten the record completion time.

One component of the discharge analysis process is to assemble the record, which is the arrangement of the forms in the paper-based health record in a standard permanent sequence for filing. The order of the forms in the record is unique to each hospital. This order also may differ from the sequencing of forms while patients are under active treatment when convenient reference to certain information is needed. When the patient is in active treatment in the hospital, for example, the record is often maintained in reverse chronological order, with the most recent information in the front of each record section. Tabs for each source allow easy reference to the grouped reports, enabling staff to quickly find the patient's response to treatment.

Any corrections or amendments to the record must be entered properly. In paper records, the provider should draw a single line through the error, add a note explaining the error, initial and date the error with the date it was discovered, and enter the correct information in chronological order. For electronic entries, a procedure should be followed that explains how to correct errors and enter addenda to the health record including the current date and reason for the information being added to the record (AHIMA 2009). In cases of medical identify theft, when someone presents using another's identity, the record must be identified as such so the appropriate health information is entered into the correct health record. This is a growing area of concern for the HIM professional, and procedures and guidance will continue to evolve until a standard of practice is established.

Criteria for Adequacy of Documentation
Documentation must reflect the care rendered to the patient and the patient's response to care. It must be timely and legible and authenticated by the person who wrote it. The health record is considered a legal document and a business record because it records events at or about the time they happen. Timeliness and legibility are two of the main areas of focus for accreditation and licensure bodies. Personnel in the HIM department analyze the health record for timeliness, accuracy, and completeness of entries in the health record. There are many patient safety concerns as discussed in chapter 21 of this text. However, one patient safety issue that relies on proper documentation is the use of abbreviations in the health record. The health record must be analyzed to ensure that symbols and abbreviations used in documentation have been approved by the medical staff and have only one clear meaning. The HIM department staff often analyze the health record for adequacy of documentation during (concurrent analysis) and after (discharge analysis) the patient's stay in the hospital.

Authentication of Health Record Entries
Authentication means to prove authorship and can be done in several ways. Signatures handwritten in ink are the most common method for signing paper-based health records. The Joint Commission allows rubber-stamp facsimile signatures when there is a statement verifying that the physician is the only one who will use the stamp and will maintain control of it (2013). CMS specifically forbids the use of rubber stamps as an authentication method (CMS 2015).

An electronic signature or e-signature is "any electronic process signifying an approval of terms, and/or documentation presented in electronic format" (AHIMA e-HIM Work Group Best Practices for Electronic Signature and Attestation 2009). Methods of electronically signing documentation include a digital signature, a digitized image of a signature, a biometric identifier such as fingerprint or retinal scan, or a code or password. If a password or code is used, a statement ensuring that the password or code is controlled and used only by the responsible provider should be required to protect patient confidentiality and to ensure that others do not use it. Password security is critical. In today's health record, electronic signatures are used more frequently as more documents in the record are produced by, and remain in, the system rather than becoming part of the paper record.

Authentication of record entries in teaching hospitals is especially important to show that the attending physician responsible for the patient is actively involved in the patient's care. Signatures by attending physicians are generally required on all reports completed by residents and medical students. In electronic signature programs, the attending physician's co-signature should be entered after the resident has reviewed and signed the report to confirm the attending physician's participation.

Record Completion Policies and Procedures

The health record is not complete until all its parts are assembled, organized, and authenticated. The HIM professional, the administration, and the medical staff must develop record completion policies and procedures and include them in the medical staff bylaws. Although the facility's governing body has overall responsibility for patient care, responsibility for the delivery and documentation of patient care is delegated to the medical staff. The medical staff and the individual physician have primary responsibility for completing the health record to document the process of care that was rendered.

The medical record committee chair may communicate directly with physicians or other medical staff members to solve problems related to record completion. The committee can be a valuable resource to the HIM professional because it has representation from every area that enters documents into the patient record. Committee members can often assist the HIM department in acquiring equipment and personnel needed to properly perform its responsibilities. The committee generally reports to the executive committee of the medical staff and makes recommendations for executive staff action to improve patient record services.

Qualitative Analysis

In **qualitative analysis**, HIM personnel carefully review the quality and adequacy of record documentation and ensure that it is in accordance with the policies, rules, and regulations established by the facility; the standards of licensing and accrediting bodies; and government requirements. Like quantitative analysis, qualitative analysis may be done concurrently or retrospectively.

Qualitative analysis is a more in-depth review of health records than quantitative analysis, although the processes may overlap somewhat, depending on the facility. When qualitative analysis is done

while the patient is in the facility or under active treatment, it is called **open-record review**, ongoing records review, point-of-care review, or continuous record review. Joint Commission requires an open-record review to ensure that its documentation standards are met at the point of care delivery (Joint Commission 2013). HIM personnel as well as case management personnel, nurses, physicians, and other providers should participate in the open-record review process. This review process looks at requirements such as presence of the history and physical examination prior to surgery, completion of the postoperative note, and many other aspects of the care process as documented in the health record. Open-record review should be done on a continuous basis.

Qualitative review also is performed on **closed records**, which are records of discharged patients. **Closed-record review** means that the qualitative review is done retrospectively following discharge or termination of treatment. The benefit of open-record review is that problems in the care process that are revealed through the review can be corrected immediately. Closed-record review is an important way to obtain information about trends and patterns of documentation.

Role of Health Information Management Professionals

CMS and state licensure standards require healthcare facilities to have an HIM department with a designated person having administrative responsibility for health records. This requirement includes having the staff, equipment, and policies and procedures to ensure that records are current and accurate and that information is accessible.

The HIM department works closely with the business department regarding record completion. The business department and the entire organization depend on the HIM staff to work with physicians and other healthcare professionals to provide the necessary information so that bills can be finalized in a timely manner. Bills are usually sent within two to three days after discharge. The health information manager receives daily notification of accounts that need information, and procedures must be established to expedite the flow of information for payment purposes.

Role of the Medical Staff

Role of the Medical Staff   Medical staff members are responsible for developing bylaws governing their operation. The requirements for documentation and completion of health records as well as penalties for not adhering to these rules are included in the medical staff bylaws. Each member of the medical staff signs a statement that he or she will abide by the bylaws, and each is responsible for documentation.

Management of Incomplete Records

The HIM professional is responsible for ensuring that health records, whether manual or electronic, are readily accessible and that adequate equipment and personnel are available to facilitate record completion. No matter how well staffed and well organized the HIM department is, it can only facilitate the process. The providers are responsible for the documentation and must dictate, authenticate, and otherwise complete the patient health record.

Storage, Retrieval, and Tracking of Incomplete Records

Storage, Retrieval, and Tracking of Incomplete Records   With the hybrid health record system, the paper-based portion of the record may be scanned at discharge of the patient into the HIS, and providers are allowed to electronically authenticate incomplete records. This method is convenient for the providers as deficient health records may be simultaneously routed to multiple providers via workflow software. It is more efficient than the paper-based routing of health records as it requires fewer HIM personnel to locate, transport, and refile the paper-based health record. It is also more efficient for the providers who may access, authenticate, and complete the hybrid or fully electronic health record remotely. Hybrid and electronic health record systems have decreased the health record delinquency rates in many facilities.

Policies and Procedures on Record Completion

Policies and Procedures on Record Completion   CMS, accrediting bodies, and state licensure standards require that the health record be completed in a timely manner. The completion time clock begins running when the patient is discharged, he or she expires, or treatment is terminated. Records are considered deficient or incomplete immediately at discharge. Some facilities choose to begin the time clock after the records are reviewed quantitatively by the HIM staff and made available to the providers; however, regulations and standards do not provide for extra time for analysis or transcription delays, computer system downtime, or physician unavailability. Healthcare facility policies and medical staff bylaws must define when incomplete or deficient records become delinquent.

Delinquent health records are those records that are not completed within the specified time frame, for example, within 14 days of discharge. The definition of a delinquent chart varies according to the facility, but most facilities require that records be completed within 30 days of discharge as mandated by CMS regulations and Joint Commission standards. Some facilities require a shorter time frame for completing records because of concerns about timely billing.

Numerous methods may be used to encourage the timely completion of records. The Joint Commission specifies that the number of delinquent records cannot exceed 50 percent of the average number of discharges, so keeping the number of delinquent charts as low as possible is a constant challenge for HIM staff (Joint Commission 2013). Concurrent analysis by HIM or other facility personnel can help speed up completion time. Using case managers to work with physicians on chart completion issues while the patient is in the facility, for example, helps reduce the burden on the HIM department. HIM professionals rely on medical staff committees, such as the health record committee, chiefs of medical services, and medical staff leaders, to motivate providers to complete records. As previously discussed, hybrid and electronic health records alleviate some of the past issues with completion of the health record.

Template (Forms) Design and Management

The management and design of forms used in the healthcare environment is a concern of all providers because well-designed forms and input screens can facilitate the documentation of care. Forms within the paper record must be developed and approved in a careful, systematic process to ensure that they meet facility standards, are compatible with imaging and microfilming systems, and do not duplicate information on existing forms. (Examples of commonly used health record forms are provided in appendix B of this book.) HIM department personnel must be constantly vigilant to ensure that only approved forms become part of the permanent health record. As health records move toward an electronic format, the forms design process becomes the process of designing computer views and templates for entry of data, but the principles of control still apply. Facilities with hybrid health records have to transition existing forms into templates for the EHR. This transition requires extensive input and expertise from the HIM professional. A well-designed form or template improves the reliability of the data entered on it. A form or template should be designed to collect information in a consistent way and to remind providers of information that needs to be included. Considerations include the number of clicks required to enter patient information into an electronic form or computer view.

Electronic Forms Management

Facilities must develop strict guidelines and processes for forms control. Forms control systems must

- Provide for the development of forms according to established guidelines
- Control the printing and use of paper forms and integration of new screen designs or electronic templates
- Guide providers in designing forms and templates according to established guidelines
- Prevent staff from changing or designing forms that duplicate existing forms or could be combined into other forms or templates

Forms control is critical to the transition toward hybrid and EHR systems. The transition to electronic records usually begins with creating a hybrid health record by using an imaging system to gather information about existing forms and to ensure that all forms can be properly scanned and indexed. Without indexing, the information cannot be easily retrieved.

Role for Data Recording During Systems Downtime

Paper forms are critical for data recording in the health record during system downtimes and outages. Forms should be made available for printing in the patient care areas in instances of systems downtime. This allows for easy access to the forms when necessary and also provides a mechanism to manage and update the forms and ensure that only approved forms are available for providers to enter documentation for the health record.

Check Your Understanding 4.4

Instructions: **Answer the following questions on a separate sheet of paper.**

1. How will speech recognition technology change the job of the medical transcriptionist?

2. How is the effectiveness and efficiency of transcription services measured?

3. Differentiate between quantitative analysis and qualitative analysis. What purpose do they serve?

4. How does concurrent review facilitate record completion?

5. Why is the finance department concerned about the timely completion of records?

6. What is the difference between an incomplete record and a delinquent record?

7. How does the HIM professional help providers to complete health records?

8. Describe the two methods facilities use to authenticate health records.

9. Why is it important for providers wanting a new form to go through the approval process?

10. How will the forms review process, including HIM oversight, change with implementation of electronic health records?

Health Record Life Cycle

Healthcare organizations need policies covering the distribution and storage of health records to ensure that the records can be located quickly when they are needed for patient care and other uses. Controlling the storage of health records is critical to patient care. The quality of patient care as well as the image and reputation of the HIM department may depend on the speed with which patient health information can be retrieved.

Management of health records includes three processes: creation and identification, storage and retrieval, and retention and disposition. This is a foundation for information governance.

Health Record Creation and Identification

As discussed earlier, the health record is created when the patient is first admitted to or treated in a healthcare facility. Every patient is assigned a specific identification number, and the health record is initiated with the collection of admission or registration information. As data and information about the patient's care and condition are documented, the record grows. The record remains in active use for the purposes of patient care, clinical coding, billing, statistical analysis, and other operational processes until the episode of care ends.

Health Record Identification Systems

For the correct health record to be quickly retrieved when it is needed, each record must be assigned a unique identifier. The choice of record identification system is tied to the organization's filing system and other core information systems.

Small healthcare facilities, such as physician offices, often use a simple alphabetical identifier: the patient's last and first names. This identifier is also used for filing of paper medical records in strict alphabetical order by the patient's last name. Alphabetical systems are more appropriate for facilities with a smaller number of records because of the problem of different patients with the same name. Most healthcare organizations use a record identification system that assigns a numerical identifier to each patient. A variety of methods is used in assigning these numbers and using them in filing the record.

Unit Numbering System   Most large facilities use a unit numbering system. In a **unit numbering system**, the patient is assigned a number during the first encounter for care and keeps it for all subsequent encounters. The number may be assigned automatically by a computer program.

Serial-Unit Numbering System   In a **serial-unit numbering system**, the patient is issued a different number for each admission or encounter for care and the records of past episodes of care are brought forward to be filed under the last number issued. This creates a unit record that contains information from all the patient's encounters. Because this system requires a great deal of shifting of records and changing of numbers, it is not as commonly used as the unit numbering system.

Health Record Filing Systems

Most healthcare facilities use numerical filing systems for permanent storage of paper-based health records. Small facilities, such as physician offices and clinics, often use alphabetic filing; larger facilities generally use numerical filing systems.

Straight Numeric Filing System   In a **straight numeric filing system**, records are filed in numerical order according to the number assigned. The major shortcoming of straight numeric filing is that most of the file activity is where the most recent numbers have been assigned since records of recent hospitalizations or visits are the ones most in use.

Terminal-Digit Filing System   In a **terminal-digit filing system**, records are filed according to a three-part number made up of two-digit pairs. The basic terminal-digit filing system contains

10,000 divisions, made up of 100 sections ranging from 00 to 99 with 100 divisions within each section ranging from 00 to 99. In a terminal-digit filing system, the shelving units (filing space) are equally divided into 100 sections.

In terminal-digit filing, the record number is placed into terminal-digit order when the health record is ready for filing. The number is broken down into two-digit pairs and is read from right to left. For example, the number 670144 would be written as 67-01-44. The first pair of digits on the right (44) is called the primary number or the terminal-digit number, the second pair of digits (01) is called the secondary number, and the third pair of digits (67) is called the tertiary or final number.

The primary number is considered first for filing. The primary numbers range from 00 to 99 and represent the 100 sections of the filing area. Because many records will be filed in each section, each section needs to be further subdivided, first according to the secondary number and then according to the tertiary number. As shown in figure 4.2, a record numbered 67-01-44 would be filed in section 44, in subsection 01, and then in numerical sequence for 67 (after 66-01-44 and before 68-01-44). All records with the tertiary and secondary numbers of 01 to 44 would be filed within this part of the file.

Another use of terminal-digit filing is for random distribution of voice files for transcription and health records for coding. The primary digits of the system are randomly assigned to staff so that

difficult-to-understand dictators and difficult-to-code records are randomly assigned. Terminal-digit filing concepts may also be utilized to evenly distribute loose paperwork filing and the doctors' incomplete area.

Patient Identity Management As healthcare delivery becomes more connected, correctly identifying patients and linking patient records is more important and has elevated the role of the HIM professional in patient identity management. HIM professionals have long been charged with the correct assignment of the medical record or health record number, which is used to assimilate, store, and access patient health records.

Master Patient Index The **master patient index (MPI)** is a permanent database including every patient ever admitted to or treated by the facility. Even though patient health records may be destroyed after legal retention periods have been met, the information contained in the MPI must be kept permanently. The MPI is also referred to as the master person index, master name file, enterprise master patient index (EMPI), regional master patient index (RMPI), and master patient database. Whatever it is called, the MPI is an important key to the health record because it contains the patient's identifying information including patient name and health record number.

Each facility has an MPI, which includes information for all patients who have been registered or treated at any location in the facility. The MPI can be a simple manual file containing cards with basic identification information about the patient, or it can be a sophisticated computerized system. Regardless of the format of the MPI, it associates the patient with the particular number under which patient treatment information can be located. The index also helps to control number assignments to ensure that former patients with unit numbers are not inadvertently assigned a new number.

The challenges in maintaining the master patient index are many. For example, patients may not remember previous admissions or may have been admitted under a different name. A person other than the patient may have provided incorrect

Figure 4.2. Filing of three consecutive patient records under the terminal-digit system

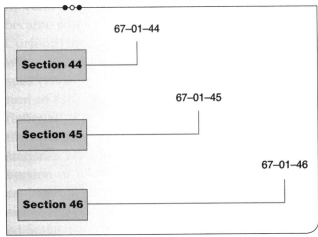

information, resulting in a new number being assigned when the patient returns for an appointment or is readmitted to the hospital. Sometimes patients use different middle initials or a nickname rather than a given name, or their names may have many possible spellings or may be hyphenated. Babies may have names changed, first and last names can be reversed, and outside laboratories may use different data. Basic demographic information such as addresses can be abbreviated incorrectly. In some cases, patients do not speak the same language as the clerk entering the information, resulting in miscommunication and incorrect data. Facilities that have either merged or separated must keep information on patients treated and often have problems combining information from two computer systems into one master patient index. Facilities may have manual card files that have been microfilmed in the past or may use a variety of formats over time, from index cards to microfilmed cards on rolls or microfiche to a computerized database.

The challenge for facilities is to maintain a correct and current MPI so that each patient has a unique identifier number. Duplication and overlays and overlaps are major problems. An **overlap** occurs when a patient has more than one medical record number assigned across more than one database. An **overlay** occurs when one patient record is overwritten with data from another patient's record. The goal is to have a true longitudinal record from birth to death, and the MPI serves as the link to information and certainty of identification that are critical to the quality and safety of patient care. Healthcare facilities have hired HIM professionals as EMPI coordinators or have hired consultants to clean and maintain EMPI systems to ensure that the correct information on the correct patient is available to the provider and others who need it. This has become even more important with the growth of electronic health records. With an EMPI, patient information is included from all entities within the enterprise and shared as needed. The sharing of data is a worthy goal, but incorrect information can adversely affect the quality and safety of care; thus, accuracy of the MPI is a critical issue. There has been some interest in a uniform

patient identifier that would be used nationwide, but action toward creating such a universal identifier has not progressed because of concerns about compromising patient confidentiality, identity theft, and medical identity theft.

The MPI usually includes the following information:

- Patient's full name and any other names the patient uses
- Patient's date of birth
- Patient's complete address
- Patient's phone numbers including cellular phone number
- Patient's health record number
- Patient's billing or account number
- Name of the attending physician
- Dates of the patient's admission and discharge or the date of the visit or encounter
- Patient's disposition at discharge or the conclusion of treatment
- Patient's marital status
- Patient's gender
- Patient's race
- Name of the patient's emergency contact

Other information may be included to further identify the patient and ensure that his or her name is linked to the proper record number. Some facilities include the mother's maiden name as another way to link the patient health record number and information to the proper patient. Many facilities develop a standard of five common fields to search for each new entry in the MPI and to review the MPI database for potential duplicate entries.

Controls for accuracy of the MPI include limiting access to the index and limiting the ability to make changes to a few key personnel. The first step in maintaining an accurate index is to obtain the correct information at admission or registration, but there are numerous problems, such as situations when the patient is unable to provide the correct information or when items are entered improperly. In the past, when only HIM personnel assigned numbers, there was more control; today, numbers are entered by many different personnel to patients entering the facility through many areas such as the emergency department, the inpatient admissions area, or the outpatient clinic. The more people involved in entering data, the greater the potential for error.

When a patient's record or healthcare information cannot be located, his or her care may be compromised. Without prior information, the physician and other providers might duplicate tests or treatments. A second record for the same patient is then created under a new number, which adds to the problem of bringing the parts of the patient record together. Research to "clean up" duplicate numbers and other errors is among the HIM professional's responsibilities.

As electronic information exchange becomes more prevalent, it is critical that the master patient indexing system correctly identifies the patient. One possible way to exchange healthcare information among facilities would be to utilize an MPI as an additional technical layer infrastructure serving as an umbrella to connect and provide access to electronic patient information at different facilities. Although the MPI consists of demographic information, it is the first step in ensuring that correct clinical information about the correct patient is shared. The MPI becomes the link among multiple computer systems that must be able to share information with each other. This process is complicated within one facility with many computer systems, but when multiple facilities try to share information, the EMPI or RMPI is a prerequisite to linking together the data within their various computer systems (AHIMA MPI Task Force 2004).

Health Record Storage and Retrieval

The HIM department is responsible for ensuring that the health record is available when needed by the provider for patient care. No matter how well organized and well managed the HIM department is, the timeliness of record delivery to providers is the measure of the quality of the department's services. The hybrid state of the health record makes reproduction of the health record more difficult since the health record may be stored in various formats within the same facility. Many facilities in-

cluding physician practices rely on paper records for part of the patient care process.

Health Record Storage

Storage is the application of efficient procedures for the use of physical filing equipment and storage media to keep records secure and available to those providers and other healthcare personnel authorized to access them. Record storage equipment can range from numerous types of file cabinets to open shelves of various heights and types.

Planning for health record storage is a major responsibility for the HIM professional. He or she must maintain a leadership role in ensuring that sufficient, conveniently accessible space is available for the storage of paper records. Ways must be provided to consistently maintain sufficient filing room by moving inactive records out of the main filing area or imaging records. With hybrid records in which some parts of the record are electronic, the paper sections of the record may be smaller and take less filing space than records that are entirely paper based.

Because space is expensive, administrators and facilities management personnel are always looking for ways to better use it. The HIM professional must make sure that paper health records are not located in poor environmental conditions where they can be either damaged or difficult to locate. For example, health records should not be stored in areas where pipes and flammable substances are located due to the danger of flooding or fire. Subbasements without proper flooring and temperature control, parking garages, and non–temperature-controlled commercial storage units are not appropriate storage locations for health records. Water, pests, and mold are all potential problems. Temperature and humidity control are important to prevent mold. The storage area must be clean and dust free and located away from food and trash in order to prevent bugs such as paper mites. Chemical treatments for mold and pests can cause problems for workers who must sort through and locate records for patient treatment. The HIM professional must be firm in the need to protect the original records for the duration of the legally required period. The potential need for the health records should be considered when deciding to send records to an off-site storage facility. Many companies specialize in the storage of vital records and provide the proper conditions for the protection of records as well as access to records.

HIM professionals have had to deal with the restoration of paper records damaged by water resulting from hurricanes, earthquakes, and tornadoes. There are companies that specialize in the restoration of records and can handle disaster recovery. Moreover, some companies negotiate contracts ensuring that the healthcare provider is first in line for recovery efforts should a disaster occur. Paper is extremely fragile when wet, and indirect circulation of air is critical; dehumidification and perhaps vacuum freezing are considerations in the restoration process. In a hybrid record where part of the record is in an electronic format, methods must be utilized to ensure the physical security of those parts of the record also (Burrington-Brown and Hughes 2010).

Health Record Retrieval

Retrieval is concerned with locating requested records and information. It involves signing out or checking out records from the filing area and tracking their location. Those that are not returned within the specified time period must be retrieved. A number of excellent software systems are available for tracking patient records.

HIM professionals are charged with safeguarding patient information by ensuring the person accessing the record has a need to know and an appropriate reason to access the patient record. In both paper and electronic retrievals, the HIM professional is responsible for ensuring that access was appropriate.

HIM personnel must be able to quickly determine the exact location of a specific health record at any time. Facilities should have strict policies and procedures in place that specify who is permitted to check out records from the filing area and for what time period. Past records are generally requested when patients are readmitted or appear for appointments. Large clinics create a lot of activity in the filing area because records must be pulled in advance for patient appointments.

The facility or provider is responsible for maintaining the health record. When the facility or provider cannot produce a record, it must be able to prove that the loss was unintentional.

Regardless of the filing system used, the filing area should be audited periodically to ensure that files are in correct order for rapid access and retrieval. Loose reports should be attached, and those awaiting attachment should be sorted and organized to facilitate retrieval. Audits of the record tracking system should be conducted to ensure that the health record is still under the responsibility of the person named in the system.

Health Record Filing and Storage Equipment

Filing equipment vendors are the HIM professional's best resource in planning a filing area that makes the best use of the available space. Open-shelf filing is the least expensive option for storage of paper health records. Shelves are usually arranged back to back just as shelving is in a library. Shelving uses space more efficiently than file cabinets because only 30 to 36 inches are needed for each aisle (ADA 2014). When standard file cabinets with drawers are used, aisles should be at least five feet wide to allow two facing file cabinets to be opened at the same time and to allow personnel who need to work in the same area to pass. Lateral files with drawers and doors also require sufficient aisle space for opening the individual drawers and allowing personnel to pass. Reference the American with Disabilities Act (ADA) Accessibility Guidelines for buildings and facilities for information related to accessible space requirements (ADA 2014).

Many facilities use open-shelf files mounted on tracks to conserve valuable space. These are referred to as movable files, and many different styles are available. With movable files mounted on tracks, more sections of files can be installed because the floor space for many fixed aisles is not needed. The files in a mobile unit can be opened one aisle at a time. With permanently installed open shelves, there are fixed aisles between each shelf. Another consideration is whether the files open electronically or manually to create the aisles. Whichever type of shelving is selected, the shelves must handle the heavy weight of paper-based health records, which may require reinforced flooring.

The estimated number of file shelves needed is based on several factors. One consideration is the average size of individual records. The volume of patients and the number of repeat visits or re-admissions affect the potential expansion of each individual patient record. The type of facility also affects the size of individual records. Acute-care facilities with extensive ancillary services and more acutely ill patients have larger individual patient records, as do facilities specializing in transplants, cancer, and other chronic diseases. When unit records are organized in a terminal-digit filing system, there must be adequate expansion space in each division of the filing area to allow for expansion of individual records. Hybrid records in which portions of the records are maintained solely in electronic format are smaller than totally paper-based records, so less filing space is needed. Electronic data has varying methods of storage requiring different considerations than paper. See chapter 12 for more information on electronic storage methods.

Health Record Retention and Disposition

Health records cannot be stored indefinitely because storage space is expensive. **Retention** involves determining the schedule to be followed to protect and preserve active and inactive records. **Disposition** involves the process of destroying the records once the end of the retention period has been reached. Establishing policies that incorporate state and federal laws and maintaining a disaster plan are part of the disposition process.

Accreditation and Legal Health Record Retention Requirements

The American Health Information Management Association (AHIMA) recommends that retention of health information be based on the needs and requirements of the facility, such as legal requirements, continued patient care, research, education, and other legitimate uses (AHIMA e-HIM Work Group on Maintaining the Legal EHR 2005). The Joint Commission asserts that the length of health

record retention depends on laws, regulations, and the use of health records for care and for other purposes such as research and education (Joint Commission 2013).

State laws, CMS regulations, and other federal regulations, accreditation standards, and facility policies and procedures must also be reviewed when establishing a retention schedule. The HIM professional must adhere to the strictest time limit if the recommended retention period varies among different laws and regulations. In addition to the length of time for maintaining health records, the HIM professional must consider the required length of retention for other documentation such as immunization records, mammography records, x-rays, and radiographs. It is important to realize that the retention periods are different for the records of minors and incompetent patients.

CMS requires health records to be maintained for at least five years, according to 42 CFR 482.24(b)(1). This requirement includes committee reports, physician certification and recertification reports, radiologist records (printouts, films, scans, and other images), home health agency records, long-term care records, laboratory records, and any other records that document information about claims. The Occupational Safety and Health Administration (OSHA) (29 CFR 1910.1020) requires records of employees with occupational exposure to be maintained for the duration of employment plus 30 years. The statutes of limitation (deadline for filing a lawsuit) in various types of legal actions are important considerations in developing a retention schedule.

Other departments rely on the expertise of the HIM professional to assist them in developing record retention procedures. A retention plan for the facility must be carefully written and included in the departmental policy and procedure manual to ensure that record destruction is part of the normal course of business and that no one particular health record or group of health records is singled out for destruction.

Retention Requirements for Ancillary Materials

E-mail messages and faxes are used for instructions, information about appointments, and the reporting of information. These must be printed or archived and included in the health record.

Images, such as complete readouts or "strips" from EEGs, EKGs, fetal monitors, Holter monitors, treadmill tests, electromyogram, echocardiograms, videotapes, and other imaging records, do not have to be kept within the physical health record but must be retrievable for as long as legally required. The original interpretations of the results must actually be part of the physical patient health record. Facilities may have computerized systems that COLD-feed the results into the imaging system so that the actual images are available to physicians and other providers. In some scanning systems, these images are not of adequate quality for use in diagnosis, so ancillary departments should maintain the original information for the appropriate retention period. State laws should be reviewed to determine the retention requirement of other images.

Fetal monitoring strips create storage problems for many HIM departments. They are part of the mother's record, but because the strips relate to the newborn, they should be maintained according to the length of time stipulated for a minor's records. Because these strips are not compatible with imaging systems, some facilities have digital systems software to maintain and store fetal monitoring strips within the labor and delivery area.

Magnetic tapes containing the digital versions of MRI and CT studies are not considered permanent health records as long as a hard copy of the final images (radiographic film) is placed in the patient's health record. The signed interpretation of the studies must be maintained in the record for the full retention period required by law. According to 21 CFR 900.12 (c)(4), mammograms must be maintained for 5 to 10 years, depending on whether or not additional mammograms are performed. State laws may require a retention period for mammograms of 20 to 30 years. This is another example of the HIM professional having to ensure that the longer time period is followed when retention schedules are determined.

Destruction and Transfer of Health Records

After time limits for retention have been reached, the HIM professional must decide on the destruction process for health records, which must ensure that health records are burned, shredded, or destroyed in such a way that protected health information is not revealed.

When the facility is closed or sold, its health records are transferred to the successor provider, meaning the entity or individual that purchases the facility. In ambulatory care settings or physician offices, patients are informed of their options to transfer their records to another provider of choice before their health records are transferred to the successor provider. When a physician leaves a group practice, patients should be given the choice to transfer their health records and move with the physician or to have the health records and the responsibility for care transferred to another provider in the group (AHIMA 2011).

Development of a Record Retention Program

Figure 4.3 lists the objectives of a record retention program. The program must ensure that current health records are retained; that inactive records are maintained; that retention is cost-effective in terms of storage space, equipment, and personnel; that a formal health record destruction process is in place; and that retention periods are established. A task force or committee might be established with representation from administration, medical staff, health information services, risk management, and legal counsel to give consideration to the needs of all groups who use patient health information. Figure 4.4 lists some of the elements to consider in a retention program. These include looking carefully at all of the record's uses and the cost of space.

The HIM director is generally responsible for implementing the retention program. However, other individuals may be charged with the shared responsibility of implementing the program in some facilities. Some facilities establish a task force to oversee the record retention program, sometimes chaired by an HIM professional.

Figure 4.3. Objectives of a record retention program

- To ensure retention and preservation of all valued health records
- To maintain noncurrent records of continuing value for uniform time periods and in designated locations
- To ensure cost-effectiveness in record storage space, equipment, and personnel
- To dispose of unnecessary records by developing an orderly, controlled, and confidential system of record destruction
- To establish record retention periods consistent with patient care, regulatory requirements, and other legal considerations

Figure 4.4. Elements to consider in the preservation of records

- Patient value for continued care
- Record usage in the facility as guided by the patient population and activity of its medical staff
- Legal value as determined by the statute of limitations
- Research value
- Historical value
- Volume and cost to maintain hard-copy storage versus microfilm, optical disk, or remote storage
- Storage and safety standards
- Contractual arrangements with payers

The steps in developing a record retention program include:

1. Conducting an inventory of the facility's records
2. Determining the format and location of record storage
3. Assigning each record a retention period
4. Destroying records that are no longer needed

Conducting an Inventory of Records The first step in establishing a record retention program is to carefully and completely inventory the records or categories of records that are maintained. In this phase, it is important to determine all the locations and formats of patient information, including images, videotapes, e-mails, tracings, computerized records, and other formats. The inventory also must include the records and registries maintained by all departments. Both primary and secondary records must be identified. A comprehensive list of all software and versions used also should be maintained so that health records, documents, and images can be retrieved in the future. Specialized computer systems used by individual departments should be included.

Determining Storage Format and Location Determining the format and location of storage is the second step in retention program development.

Facilities may choose to retain records in paper format or in hard copy and to store them either on-site or in off-site contract storage. Off-site contract storage should be located at a distance far enough away from the facility to ensure that a disaster affecting the facility will not also affect the storage location.

Another storage mechanism is optical **scanning**. Records can be scanned into optical scanning equipment or digitally transferred. The imaging process converts paper or microfilm documents into a computer-readable digital format. The facility must determine what information can be fed directly into the imaging system, for example, registration and face sheet, discharge summary, and all other dictated and transcribed reports. Digitized information, including that produced by laboratory and radiology, can be COLD-fed into the imaging system. COLD now refers to a variety of technologies related to digitized input and output. Optical scanning produces an image of the record that can be indexed and quickly retrieved and simultaneously viewed by many providers. This is not a true electronic record because the image cannot be changed after it has been permanently archived. Retrieval from images can be achieved at the report level, for example the history and physical, but more granular queries such as the patient's HbA1c level on a particular date are not possible.

Imaging involves preparing, or prepping, the documents, which must be done before the records are scanned. Staples must be removed, papers repaired, and each page checked to ensure the presence of a barcode on both the front and back of every form in the record. The scanning process involves inserting the paper into the optical scanner so that both the front and back of the forms are scanned at the same time. Two types of scanners are usually used for health records: flatbed scanners and automatic document-feed scanners. The type of scanner used depends on the volume to be scanned. Flatbed scanners are usually slower than automatic document-feed scanners but require less preparation of individual documents.

Indexing involves identifying each individual page according to the type of form such as discharge summary. Indexing is critical. If the image is not indexed to the appropriate patient and the correct form for that admission, the information cannot be retrieved. The scanner is the device that actually scans a human-readable document and uses software to make a picture of the document. After being scanned, records must be verified and generally are not submitted to the final stored archive until the physician completes them. Verifying that the image is clear and the indexing correct is important to make sure the image can be retrieved and used in the future. Facilities assign personnel to handle the tasks of preparation and scanning. Emergency department reports, outpatient reports, and reports submitted from physicians often do not have the correct patient numbers or encounter numbers, and all of this information must be entered so that each form in the record can be appropriately indexed and retrieved. A concern for HIM professionals is that scanning equipment from one vendor may not work with equipment from another vendor. The long-term storage capability of optical disk has not been evaluated for long-term quality because the technology is still evolving.

Beginning an imaging system requires detailed planning. Decisions must be made about converting existing records or whether only information from a certain date forward will be imaged. In addition, security backups of images should be available. Health records should be on the type of optical storage using WORM—write once, read

many—technology. This means that the data cannot be erased or altered. Rewritable or erasable **optical imaging technology** is not appropriate for health records. After records are archived in the imaging system, they cannot be changed. While waiting to be archived, images can be added or indexing changed, so it is important that any changes be made before archiving, if possible.

Although imaging has the advantages of rapid retrieval and simultaneous access, it is not an easy process to implement. Loose materials and late-arriving information still must be scanned and indexed. Moreover, problems still exist with recovering charts from the nursing areas after discharge and with unapproved forms being developed and included in the record that cannot be indexed because they do not have barcodes assigned. The HIM department still must perform open-record review and check forms for signatures. In other words, the traditional functions of the HIM department do not change. While the patient is in the facility or in active treatment, the record is paper. The imaging system does not convert the paper into images until after patient discharge or termination of treatment.

Imaging is a key part of the progression to an electronic document management system and ultimately to the electronic health record because it provides providers with quick access to pictures such as radiographs (x-rays), MRIs, and other digital images rather than having to wait for the paper copy. This type of quick access to images improves safety and quality of care.

Assigning a Retention Period After all departments have been inventoried, the third step is to assign a retention period for each type of record. The retention period should be defined as time in active files, time in inactive storage, and total time before destruction.

As discussed previously, state and federal laws and regulations must be reviewed to ensure that records are maintained for the longest length of time required. Many states recommend that patient health records be retained for 10 years following patient discharge or death. There are usually special requirements for minor patients. For example, the state of Minnesota requires that the records of minor patients be maintained for seven years following the age of majority. Therefore, the record of a newborn in Minnesota would be maintained until the patient reaches the age of majority, which is 18 years plus seven year or a total of 25 years (Office of the Revisor of Statutes 2015).

The retention period should reflect the scope and needs of the facility, along with the preliminary costs associated with imaging, microfilming, and other methods of maintaining and storing records. Storage mechanisms should be selected that protect records and provide ease of access and employee safety.

Protection of paper-based, hybrid, and electronic health records during the legally required retention period is extremely important and needs to be considered before a disaster occurs or a situation occurs where a health record in storage cannot be located or available.

Commercial storage vendors should be selected carefully to ensure that records are protected from unauthorized access. Policies for security of all satellite record storage areas must be developed and business associate agreements (discussed in chapter 11) signed regarding timely access to, and retrieval of, health records.

Destroying Unnecessary Records Destroying records that are not needed is the fourth step in developing a record retention program. In facilities utilizing an imaging system, the general rule is usually that paper records should be boxed up after all paper is scanned, indexed, and released in the electronic document management system (EDMS); stored for no longer than six months; and then destroyed. An organization may influence skeptics of destroying the paper by demonstrating quality processes on the front end—during scanning and indexing. The EDMS totally transitions a facility in terms of the legal medical record, and the legal definition is no longer based upon paper. There must be a rule that no patient health information can be destroyed without approval of the HIM director or other authorized committee or person, according to facility policy. The HIM professional must be alert to changes in departmental administration or departmental relocation or remodeling because departments often use these events to clean out files, which could result in the destruction of needed patient information.

The destruction of patient records must be done as part of the facility's usual business. When the required retention schedule has been satisfied, a complete list of records to be destroyed should be compiled and submitted to the individual designated to authorize the destruction. When paper records are scanned and no longer considered the legal record, they should be destroyed as per the organizational policy. Outsourcing of destruction to shredding companies should be carefully monitored to protect patient confidentiality. The destruction of electronic and digital records should follow security guidelines to ensure that the information is destroyed permanently. Facilities must maintain basic information about the patient in the MPI, which is maintained permanently even though the corresponding health record is destroyed.

AHIMA recommends that records be destroyed in such a way that the information cannot possibly be reconstructed (AHIMA 2011). The destruction should be documented, and the documentation should include the following:

- Date of destruction
- Method of destruction (shredding, burning, or other means)
- Description of the disposed record series of numbers or items
- Inclusive dates covered
- A statement that the records were destroyed in the normal course of business
- The signatures of the individuals supervising and witnessing the destruction

AHIMA further recommends that facilities maintain destruction certification documents permanently. Such certificates may be required as evidence that records were destroyed in the regular course of business (AHIMA 2011). When facilities fail to apply destruction policies uniformly or when destruction is contrary to policy, courts may allow a jury to infer that the facility destroyed its records to hide evidence.

Dealing with Outdated Media Dealing with various forms and sources of media is not new for HIM professionals and continues to evolve as technological changes impact healthcare delivery. The other side of advances with new media is the dilemma of dealing with outdated media as part of the record life cycle and retention program.

When determining whether or not to maintain records after the retention period has expired, the media type should be considered. As equipment ages and eventually becomes obsolete, the costs for retrieving that information can increase. This should become part of the decision-making process on record retention.

Check Your Understanding 4.5

Instructions: Answer the following questions on a separate piece of paper.

1. Why is the MPI considered the key index in the HIM department?

2. Why is accurate information critical for the MPI?

3. What are some of the reasons why incorrect information is obtained?

4. What is the consequence of a patient having duplicate health record numbers?

5. What are common attributes used to help correctly identify patients?

6. What is the difference between a serial-unit numbering system and a unit numbering system?

7. What are two advantages of terminal-digit filing over straight numerical filing?

8. What are the main factors in determining how long to maintain a health record?

9. What are the four primary steps in a record retention program?

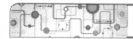

References

Accreditation Association for Ambulatory Health Care. 2015. *Accreditation Handbook for Ambulatory Health Care.* http://www.aaahc.org/en/accreditation/

AHIMA e-HIM Work Group Best Practices for Electronic Signature and Attestation. 2009 (Nov–Dec). Practice brief: Electronic Signature, Attestation and Authorship (Updated). *Journal of AHIMA* 9(11).

AHIMA e-HIM Work Group on Maintaining the Legal EHR. 2005 (Nov.–Dec.). Update: Maintaining a legally sound health record—paper and electronic. *Journal of AHIMA* 76(10):64A–L.

AHIMA e-HIM Work Group on Speech Recognition in the EHR. 2003 (Oct. 20). Practice brief: Speech recognition in the electronic health record. *Journal of AHIMA*–Web exclusive. http://library.ahima.org/xpedio/groups/public/documents/ahima/bok1_022107.hcsp?dDocNamebok1_022107

AHIMA MPI Task Force. 2004. Practice brief: Building an enterprise master person index. *Journal of AHIMA* 75(1):56A–56D.

American Health Information Management Association. 2011. Retention and Destruction of Health Information. http://library.ahima.org/xpedio/groups/public/documents/ahima/bok1_049252.hcsp?dDocNamebok1_049252

American Health Information Management Association. 2010. Role of the Personal Health Record in the EHR (Updated). http://library.ahima.org/xpedio/groups/public/docu-ments/ahima/bok1_048517.hcsp?dDocNamebok1_048517

American Health Information Management Association. 2009. Amendments, corrections and deletions in the electronic health record: an American Health Information Management Association Toolkit. http://library.ahima.org/xpedio/

groups/public/documents/ahima/bok1_044678. hcsp?dDocName=bok1_044678

Americans with Disabilities Act of 2010. 2014 (April 10). Accessibility Guidelines for buildings and facilities. Appendix A to Part 1191.

Backman, C., S. Dolack, D. Dunyak, L. Lutz, A. Tegen, and D. Warner. 2011. Social Media + Healthcare. *Journal of AHIMA* 82(3):20–25.

Burrington-Brown, J. and G. Hughes. 2010 (Dec.). Practice brief: Disaster planning for health information. *Journal of AHIMA*–Web exclusive. http://library.ahima.org/xpedio/groups/public/ documents/ahima/bok1_048638.hcsp?dDocName&#x F03D;bok1_048638

Centers for Medicare and Medicaid Services. 2015. Medicare Program Integrity Manual. Chapter 3: Verifying Potential Errors and Taking Corrective Actions. https://www.cms.gov/Regulations-and-Guidance/Guidance/Manuals/downloads/ pim83c03.pdf

Joint Commission. 2013. *Comprehensive Accreditation Manual for Hospitals.* Oak Brook Terrace, IL: Joint Commission.

National Association for Home Care and Hospice. 2011. http://www.nahc.org.

National Hospice and Palliative Care Organization. 2015 (July 23). http://www.nhpco.org/about/ hospitce-care

Office of the Revisor of Statutes. 2015. 2015 Minnesota statutes. https://www.revisor.mn.gov/ statutes/?id=145.32

Tegan, A., et al. 2005. Practice brief: The EHR's impact on HIM functions. *Journal of AHIMA* 76(5):56C–H.

US Department of Health and Human Services. 2013. HIPAA Administrative Simplification Regulation Text. http://www.hhs.gov/ocr/ privacy/hipaa/administrative/combined/hipaa-simplification-201303.pdf

Weed, L.L. 1970. *Medical Records, Medical Education, and Patient Care.* Cleveland, OH: Case Western Reserve University.

21 CFR 900.12 (c)(4): Mammography. 2012 (April 6).

29 CFR 1910.1020: Maintenance of and access to employee medical records. 1998 (June 16).

42 CFR 482.24: Conditions of participation: Medical record services. 2015 (Nov. 10).

42 CFR 482.61: Condition of participation. 2015 (Nov. 10).

42 CFR 483.20: Resident assessment. 2010 (Oct.1).

42 CFR 413, 482, and 489: Medicare program; clarifying policies related to the responsibilities of Medicare-participating hospitals in treating individuals with emergency medical conditions. 2002 (May 9).

5

Clinical Classifications, Vocabularies, Terminologies, and Standards

Brooke Palkie, EdD, RHIA

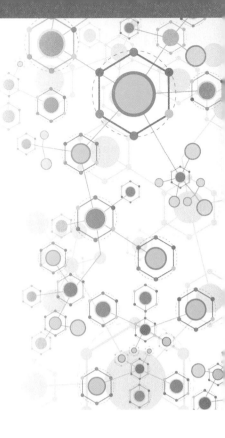

141

Clinical vocabulary
Concept
Continuity of care
  document (CCD)
Continuity of care record
  (CCR)
Current Dental Terminology
  (CDT)
Current Procedural Terminology
  (CPT)
Diagnostic and Statistical Manual
  of Mental Disorders, 5th edition
  (DSM-5)
Functional interoperability
Healthcare Common Procedure
  Coding System (HCPCS)
Interface terminology
International Classification of
  Diseases (ICD)
International Classification of
  Diseases, 10th Revision,
  Clinical Modification
  (ICD-10-CM)
International Classification of
  Diseases, 10th Revision,

Procedure Coding System
  (ICD-10-PCS)
International Classification
  of Diseases, 11th Revision
  (ICD-11)
International Classification of
  Diseases for Oncology, 3rd
  edition (ICD-O-3)
International Classification of
  Primary Care (ICPC-2)
International Classification on
  Functioning, Disability, and
  Health (ICF)
International Health Terminology
  Standards Development
  Organization (IHTSDO)
Interoperability
Lexicon
Logical Observation Identifiers
  Names and Codes
  (LOINC)
Mapping
MEDCIN
Medical Subject Headings database
  (MeSH)

Morphology
Multiaxial
National Drug Codes (NDC)
  directory
National Library of Medicine
  (NLM)
Nomenclature
Patient medical record information
  (PMRI)
Reference terminology
Relationship
RxNorm
Semantic interoperability
Systemized Nomenclature of
  Medicine–Clinical Terminology
  (SNOMED CT)
Systematized Nomenclature of
  Medicine–Reference Terminol-
  ogy (SNOMED RT)
Terminology
Topography
Transitions of care (ToC)
  initiative
Unified Medical Language System
  (UMLS)

Healthcare is faced with many challenges, including an aging population, the need to conserve resources, medical data that are increasing exponentially, and a consumer population that is technologically savvy. To meet these challenges, healthcare organizations must have the ability to operate effectively and efficiently using current medical data and knowledge. Although moving in the right direction, the healthcare industry in the United States has yet to fully agree on common terminologies that would allow healthcare facilities and practitioners throughout the country to exchange and use information reliably.

The quest to classify to establish common terminologies to classify morbidity and mortality is quite old. London parishes first began to keep death records in 1532. In the 1600s, Sir William Petty was able to extrapolate from mortality rates an estimate of community economic loss caused by deaths (Encyclopedia Britannica 2015). Two hundred years later, in *Notes on a Hospital*, Florence Nightingale wrote:

In attempting to arrive at the truth, I have applied everywhere for information, but in scarcely an instance have I been able to obtain hospital records fit for any purposes of comparison. If they could be obtained ... they would show subscribers how their money was being spent, what amount of good was really being done with it, or whether the money was not doing mischief rather than good. (Barnett et al. 1993, 1046)

Many of the issues with availability of information remain in healthcare today. It is vitally important to be able to compare data for outcomes measurement, quality improvement, resource utilization, best practices, medical research, and reimbursement purposes. These tasks can be accomplished only when healthcare has standardized terminology that is easily integrated into the electronic health record (EHR).

This chapter examines the history, current practices, and desired characteristics of classifications, terminologies, vocabularies, and standards in the healthcare industry.

Development of Classification Systems, Vocabularies, and Terminologies for Healthcare Data

As the discussion of classification systems, terminologies, and vocabularies for healthcare data begins, it is important to have an understanding of several terms related to clinical content representation. It is difficult to get standards developers to completely agree on definitions for even basic concepts; however, there are some commonly accepted definitions. Table 5.1 provides definitions and examples of classification system terms. A **clinical classification** is "a clinical vocabulary, terminology, or nomenclature that lists words or phrases with their meanings; provides for the proper use of clinical words as names or symbols; and facilitates mapping of standardized terms to broader classifications for administrative, regulatory, oversight, and fiscal requirements" (AHIMA 2011). A classification system provides easy storage, retrieval, and analysis of data for the purposes of transmitting and comparing data. A **nomenclature** is a recognized system of terms used in a science or an art that follows preestablished naming conventions (AHIMA 2011). The terms *classification* and *nomenclature* are often used interchangeably. However, the two can be distinguished: "classifications and nomenclatures can be more helpfully regarded as lying along a continuum, where the first categorizes and aggregates while the second supports detailed descriptions" (Chute 2000, 298). The International Classification of Diseases, 10th Revision is a classification system that organizes (categorizes) many of its disease entries by body system or etiology. For example, disorders related to the circulatory system are organized and classified within a single chapter. The Diagnostic Statistical Manual (DSM) is an example of a nomenclature that provides a listing of the terms and definitions (criteria) used to describe mental health disorders.

A **terminology** is "a set of terms representing a system of concepts" (Giannangelo 2015, 4). Another generic term often used when discussing terminologies is **lexicon**, which refers to the listings of words or expressions in a language (terminology) and information about the language such as definitions, related principles, and description of (grammatical) structure (NLM 2015a).

Table 5.1. Definitions and examples of classification system terms

Terms	Definition	Example
Clinical classification	A clinical vocabulary, terminology, or nomenclature that lists words or phrases with their meanings; provides for the proper use of clinical words as names or symbols; and facilitates mapping of standardized terms to broader classifications for administrative, regulatory, oversight, and fiscal requirements (AHIMA 2014).	ICD-10-CM
Nomenclature	A recognized system of terms used in a science or an art that follows preestablished naming conventions (AHIMA 2014).	DSM-5
Clinical terminology	A set of standardized terms and their synonyms that record patient findings, circumstances, events, and interventions with sufficient detail to support clinical care, decision support, outcomes research, and quality improvement (AMIA and AHIMA Terminology and Classification Policy Task Force 2007, 41).	SNOMED CT
Clinical vocabulary	A formally recognized list of preferred medical terms (AHIMA 2014, 34).	HL7 (in terms of structural vocabulary)

It is important to recognize that the problem of multiple definitions and names is endemic in the field of healthcare terminology. A **clinical terminology** is "a set of standardized terms and their synonyms that record patient findings, circumstances, events, and interventions with sufficient detail to support clinical care, decision support, outcomes research, and quality improvement" (AMIA and AHIMA Terminology and Classification Policy Task Force 2007, 41). A **clinical vocabulary** is "a formally recognized list of preferred medical terms" (AHIMA 2014, 34). The definition for the vocabulary is similar to that of terminology except that it includes the meanings or definitions of words. Because of their very similar meanings, the terms *clinical terminology* and *clinical vocabulary* are often used interchangeably in practice. To further complicate the issue, many working within the field also often use *terminology* to refer to the entire spectrum of issues related to clinical data representation from classifications and nomenclatures to clinical terminologies (Chute 2000, 299). The pyramid in figure 5.1 illustrates how these terms are all related. A nomenclature can be less specific than a terminology, which is less specific than a language. So while a classification or nomenclature categorizes and aggregates, a terminology represents the whole of a subject field. Each plays a specific yet interdependent role in data standardization.

Clinical classifications and terminologies do serve different functions. For example, the classification systems ICD-10-CM and ICD-10-PCS (Clinical Modification and Procedure Coding System) and Current Procedural Terminology (CPT) represent similar procedures and diagnoses with single codes. This broad categorization of information is useful for functions such as billing and monitoring resource utilization. In contrast, terminologies support the capture and representation of information collected within an EHR at the time of documentation (Bowman 2005). Terminologies exist to represent topics ranging from nursing documentation and laboratory data to medical devices. This detailed level of data capture is useful to support functions such as clinical decision support and clinical alerts.

Depending on the purpose of a given classification or terminology, differences are also seen at the level of granularity (detail) used to represent content. For example, the CPT classification system has a single code (86003 Allergen specific IgE: quantitative or semiquantitative, each allergen) to report a laboratory test to detect a specific allergen. The same code is used regardless of the allergen (for example, food, weeds, dust). On the other hand, Logical Observation Identifier Names and Codes (LOINC), a clinical terminology, provides a common language for clinical and laboratory observations (LOINC 2015b). LOINC provides many different codes (for example, 11195-5, 11196-3, 11197-1) to represent the test for each unique allergen (NLM 2015d). In this case, the LOINC representation of the allergen tests is more granular, that is, more specific. Granularity is important because it represents the degree to which a term specifies the concept it is representing.

Figure 5.1. Comparative level of detail in classifications, terminologies, vocabularies, and data standards

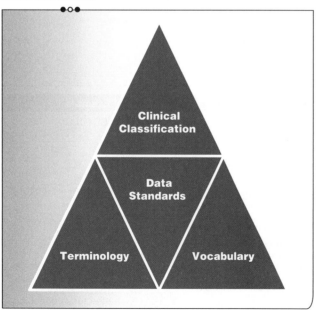

Check Your Understanding 5.1

Instructions: **Answer the following questions on a separate piece of paper.**

1. Define clinical classifications, vocabularies, and terminologies.

2. What are the general functions of clinical classifications, vocabularies, and terminologies?

3. Give one example of a classification and one example of a terminology.

4. When were the first known efforts to collect and use healthcare data and what was the purpose?

5. Why is it important to have standardization with healthcare data/information?

Common Healthcare Classifications and Code Sets

Systems for classifying diseases have progressed through various stages since the first classification system was developed in the late 19th century. The following section describes past, current, and near-future developments for a variety of classification systems.

International Classification of Diseases

The International Classification of Diseases (ICD) began as the Bertillon Classification of Diseases in 1893. In 1900, the French government convened an international meeting to update the Bertillon classification to the International List of Causes of Death (WHO 2015a). The goal was to develop a common system for describing the causes of mortality. The World Health Organization (WHO) became responsible for maintaining ICD in 1948. Currently, ICD is used by more than 100 countries worldwide to classify diseases and other health issues (WHO 2015a). The **International Classification of Diseases (ICD)** facilitates the storage and retrieval of diagnostic information and serves as the basis for compiling mortality and morbidity statistics reported by WHO members. The latest version of the International Classification of Diseases, the 10th edition (ICD-10), has been in use since 1994 by WHO members. In 1999, the United States began using ICD-10 to report mortality

statistics under its agreement with WHO. The United States, after several yearlong delays, transitioned to the clinical modification of ICD-10 (meaning capturing diseases or causes of illness—morbidity) in 2015. ICD-10 is routinely updated by WHO and allows for data comparability internationally. The development of an 11th edition of ICD integrates updated medical data that has been discovered since ICD-10 was published. ICD-11 still needs to be clinically modified for use in the United States. A significant difference in **International Classification of Diseases, 11th Revision (ICD-11)** is that it will be designed to include linkages to standardized healthcare terminologies to facilitate processing and use of the data for a variety of purposes such as research (WHO 2007). The process of transition from ICD-10 to ICD-11 will be much more efficient than the transition from ICD-9 to ICD-10. ICD-10 was structurally and significantly different than ICD-9; however, ICD-11 will be an update to ICD-10's current structure.

International Classification of Diseases, 10th Revision, Clinical Modification

The US government modified the **International Classification of Diseases, 10th Revision, Clinical Modification (ICD-10-CM)** for the reporting of morbidity data and reimbursement in the United States. In 2008, the Department of Health and Human Services (HHS) published a notice of proposed rulemaking that identified the replacement of ICD-9-CM with ICD-10-CM for diagnosis coding and ICD-10-PCS (International Classification of Diseases, 10th Revision, Procedure Coding System) for inpatient procedure coding (HHS 2008). In 2008, the Department of Health and Human Service (HHS) published a notice effective October 1, 2013. However, the implementation was delayed twice and the new effective date for ICD-10 was set as October 1, 2015.

When the United States modified ICD-9 to create ICD-9-CM more than 30 years ago, a third volume was added to capture procedure codes. However, instead of appending a short volume to ICD-10-CM, a complete classification, ICD-10-PCS, was developed. This procedure coding system is much more detailed and specific than the short volume of procedure codes included in ICD-9-CM (CMS 2015a).

The Centers for Medicare and Medicaid Services (CMS) (2015a) identifies ICD-10-CM as a system that consists of more than 86,000 diagnosis codes, compared to approximately 13,000 ICD-9-CM diagnosis codes. ICD-10-PCS consists of 87,000 procedure codes (CMS 2015a). Together, the ICD-10 codes have the potential to reveal more about quality of care so that data can be used in a more meaningful way to better understand complications, better design clinically robust algorithms, and better track the outcomes of care (CMS 2015a). ICD-10-CM and ICD-10-PCS incorporate greater specificity and clinical detail to provide information for clinical decision making and outcomes research. CMS defines ICD-10 as follows:

- ICD-10-CM is a US clinical modification of WHO's ICD-10 and is maintained by the National Center for Health Statistics (NCHS). It is a morbidity classification system that classifies diagnoses and other reasons for healthcare encounters. The code structure is alphanumeric, with codes comprised of three to seven characters.

- ICD-10-PCS is a procedure coding system developed under contract by the Centers for Medicare and Medicaid Services (CMS) as a replacement of the ICD-9-CM procedure coding system for hospital reporting

of inpatient procedures. It has a seven-character alphanumeric code structure. (CMS 2015a)

The value of transitioning to ICD-10-CM is broad and contains a substantial increase in content over ICD-9-CM. Improvements in the content and format of ICD-10-CM will result in the following:

- Additional information relevant to ambulatory care
- Expanded cause of injury codes
- New combination diagnosis/symptom codes to reduce the number of codes needed to fully describe a condition and reduce coding errors
- Greater specificity in code assignment
- Laterality information (right and left)
- Greater achievement of the benefits of an electronic health record
- Enhanced ability to meet the Health Insurance Portability and Accountability Act (HIPAA) electronic transaction/code set requirements
- Increased value in the US investment in Systematized Nomenclature of Medicine–Clinical Terminology (SNOMED CT)
- Use of seven-digit alphanumeric format, which facilitates expansion and revision of classification (space to accommodate future expansion) (CMS 2015a)

Figure 5.2 provides an example of an entry in the Tabular List of Diseases, ICD-10-CM. In the figure, the category level is flush with the left hand margin (T40) and subcategory level is indented once and bold (T40.0). This code itself is not a valid ICD-10-CM code. In this case, the coding note identifies that code T40.0 must include a seventh character; meaning, it will be seven character code (for example, T40.0X6A).

International Classification of Diseases, 10th Revision, Procedure Coding System

In the mid-1990s, CMS awarded a contract to the 3M Health Information Systems group to develop a new procedure coding system to replace

Figure 5.2. Example of an ICD-10-CM entry

T40	**Poisoning by, adverse effect of and underdosing of narcotics and psychodysleptics [hallucinogens]**
	Excludes2: drug dependence and related mental and behavioral disorders due to psychoactive substance use (F10.-F19.-)
	The appropriate seventh character is to be added to each code from category T40

A initial encounter
D subsequent encounter
S sequela

T40.0 Poisoning by, adverse effect of and underdosing of opium

T40.0X Poisoning by, adverse effect of and underdosing of opium

T40.0X1	**Poisoning by opium, accidental (unintentional)**
	Poisoning by opium NOS
T40.0X2	**Poisoning by opium, intentional self-harm**
T40.0X3	**Poisoning by opium, assault**
T40.0X4	**Poisoning by opium, undetermined**
T40.0X5	**Adverse effect of opium**
T40.0X6	**Underdosing of opium**

Source: CMS 2015b.

the Tabular List of Procedures, Volume 3 of ICD-9-CM. The classification developed the **International Classification of Diseases, 10th Revision, Procedure Coding System (ICD-10-PCS)**. It is considered an improvement over ICD-9-CM, Volume 3 for many reasons including the use of standardized definitions, ease of expandability, ease of use, and comprehensiveness. ICD-10-PCS uses very precise definitions. For example, a percutaneous approach is defined as "entry, by puncture or minor incision, of instrumentation through the skin or mucous membrane and any other body layers necessary to reach the site of the procedure" (CMS 2015c). This is a substantial improvement over ICD-9-CM in which a term could have a different meaning in different sections of the classification. For example, when referring to a percutaneous liver biopsy in ICD-9-CM, *percutaneous* means through the skin. However, percutaneous in the term *percutaneous coronary angioplasty* refers to an endoscopic percutaneous approach. The greater coverage of ICD-10-PCS is illustrated by the significantly larger number of codes. ICD-9-CM contains approximately 4,000 procedure codes and ICD-10-PCS contains over 86,000 (Averill et al. 2005; CMS 2015c).

ICD-10-PCS is composed of seven-character alphanumeric codes. Each character can be one of 34 values (numbers 0 through 9 and the letters of the alphabet excluding I and O). The classification is divided into 16 sections, each of which covers a specific diagnostic area (for example, medical and surgical, radiation oncology, and mental health). Depending on the requirements of each section, the seven characters are assigned different meanings. For example, in the medical and surgical section, the fourth character represents the body part or region involved in the procedure; in the placement section, it represents the body region or orifice; and in the chiropractic section, it represents the body region (CMS 2015a).

Figure 5.3 illustrates the meanings of each character of ICD-10-PCS codes in the medical surgical section of the classification.

Table 5.2 is an excerpt from a table used for code assignment in the medical and surgical section of ICD-10-PCS. All codes represented in the table begin with the three characters identified in the header and are completed with characters selected from each of the four columns depending upon the nature of the procedure being coded.

International Classification of Diseases for Oncology, 3rd Edition

The **International Classification of Diseases for Oncology (ICD-O-3)** is currently in its third edition via the World Health Organization (WHO). This classification is used for coding diagnoses of neoplasms in tumor and cancer registries and in pathology laboratories. The **topography** code describes the site of origin of the neoplasm and uses the same three- and four-character categories as in the neoplasm section of the second chapter of ICD-10. The morphology code describes the characteristics of the tumor itself, including cell type and biologic activity (Percy et al. 2000). The topography codes remain the same as in the previous edition, but the morphology codes have been thoroughly revised where necessary in the third edition.

To the greatest extent possible, ICD-O uses the nomenclature published in the WHO series, International Histological Classification of Tumors. ICD-O is under the purview of WHO Collaborating Centres for Classification of Disease (WHO 2015b).

International Classification on Functioning, Disability, and Health

The International Classification on Functioning, Disability, and Health (ICF) is a classification developed by the World Health Organization (WHO) of health and health-related domains that describe body functions and structures, activities, and participation. Three lists exist within ICF:

- Body functions and structure
- Domains of activity and participation
- Environmental factors that interact with all these components

ICD-10 and ICF are complementary, and users are encouraged to use them together to create a broader and more meaningful picture of the experience of health of individuals and populations (WHO 2015c). Table 5.3 provides examples of ICF self-care codes (WHO 2015d).

Healthcare Common Procedure Coding System

Healthcare Common Procedure Coding System (HCPCS) is used to report services and supplies primarily for reimbursement purposes in the outpatient or ambulatory setting. The system is divided into two sections referred to as levels. Level I of HCPCS is composed of the CPT codes as published by the AMA and represents medical services and procedures performed by physicians and other healthcare providers. Level II of HCPCS contains codes that represent products, supplies, and services not included in the CPT codes. The Level I (CPT) codes are five-digit numeric codes,

Figure 5.3.   ICD-10-PCS code structure

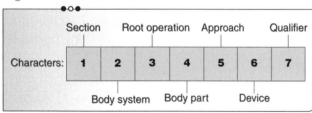

Source: CMS 2015f.

Table 5.2.   PCS table

Within a PCS table, valid codes include all combinations of choices in characters 4 through 7 contained in the same row of the table. In the following example, **0JHT3VZ** is a valid code, and 0JHW3VZ is *not* a valid code.

Section: 0 Medical and Surgical
Body System: J Subcutaneous Tissue and Fascia
Operation: H Insertion: Putting in a nonbiological appliance that monitors, assists, performs, or prevents a physiological function but does not physically take the place of a body part

Body part	Approach	Device	Qualifier
S Subcutaneous Tissue and Fascia, Head and Neck **V** Subcutaneous Tissue and Fascia, Upper Extremity **W** Subcutaneous Tissue and Fascia, Lower Extremity	**0** Open **3** Percutaneous	**1** Radioactive Element **3** Infusion Device	**Z** No Qualifier
T Subcutaneous Tissue and Fascia, Trunk	**0** Open **3** Percutaneous	**1** Radioactive Element **3** Infusion Device **V** Infusion Pump	**Z** No Qualifier

Source: CMS 2015d.

Table 5.3. Examples of ICF self-care codes 2010 version

Chapter	Description	Categories	Category description	Subcategories
Self-Care	This chapter is about caring for oneself; washing and drying oneself; caring for one's body and body parts; dressing, eating, and drinking; and looking after one's health	d530 Toileting	Planning and carrying out the elimination of human waste (menstruation, urination, and defecation) and cleaning oneself afterwards.	**d5300** Regulating urination **d5301** Regulating defecation **d5302** Menstrual care **d5308** Toileting, other specified **d5309** Toileting, unspecified
		d540 Dressing	Carrying out the coordinated actions of putting on and taking off clothes and footwear in sequence and in keeping with climatic and social conditions, such as by putting on, adjusting, and removing shirts, skirts, blouses, pants, undergarments, saris, kimono, tights, hats, gloves, coats, shoes, boots, sandals, and slippers.	**d5400** Putting on clothes **d5401** Taking off clothes **d5402** Putting on footwear **d5403** Taking off footwear **d5404** Choosing appropriate clothing **d5408** Dressing, other specified **d5409** Dressing, unspecified

Reprinted from the World Health Organization, ICF Browser, Copyright (2015).

whereas Level II codes are five-character alphanumeric codes. HCPCS codes may also be reported with two-character modifiers which provide further detail about the service or procedure.

HCPCS codes are updated every year on January 1. The HCPCS Level II codes can be downloaded from the HCPCS website. Table 5.4 contains examples of various types of HCPCS Level II codes (CMS 2015e).

Current Procedural Terminology

The American Medical Association (AMA) publishes the **Current Procedural Terminology (CPT)**. The purpose of CPT is "to provide a uniform language that accurately describes medical, surgical, and diagnostic services, and thereby serves as an effective means for reliable nationwide communication among physicians, patients, and third parties" (AMA 2015). CPT was first developed and published by the AMA in 1966. In 1983, the system was adopted by CMS as Level I of the Healthcare Common Procedure Coding System (HCPCS). HCPCS is has two identified subsections: Level I CPT and Level II is a standardized coding system to identify products, supplies, and services not included in CPT (CMS 2015e). Since that time, CPT has become widely used as a standard for outpatient and ambulatory care procedural coding in contexts related to reimbursement.

Table 5.4. Examples of HCPCS Level II codes

HCPCS Level II code	Code title
A0130	Non-emergency transportation: wheel-chair van
A4918	Venous pressure clamp, for hemodialysis, each
B4036	Enteral feeding supply kit; gravity fed, per day, includes but not limited to feeding/flushing syringe, administration set tubing, dressings, tape
E0619	Apnea monitor, with recording feature
J3370	Injection, vancomycin HCl, 500 mg
Q0480	Driver for use with pneumatic ventricular assist device, replacement only
S0274	Nurse practitioner visit, outside of a capitation arrangement

Source: CMS 2015e.

CPT is updated annually on January 1. The codebook is organized into chapters by specialty, body system, and service provided. The codes themselves consist of five digits, and the descriptions of the codes are often accompanied by inclusion and exclusion notes (for example, 90630 Intradermal Flu Shot). Modifiers to the five-digit codes also are used extensively as a way to offer additional information (for example, 19120-LT Extension of breast cyst—left). CPT also contains two supplemental sections. The first, Category II codes, contains optional codes used for performance measurement reporting purposes. The CPT Category III codes are temporary codes assigned to facilitate data collection for emerging technologies.

CPT is maintained by the CPT Editorial Panel, which is authorized to revise, update, and modify CPT. The majority of the panel are physicians, with the rest coming from industry and government. Supporting the work of the CPT Editorial Panel is the CPT Health Care Professionals Advisory Committee (HCPAC). The HCPAC includes participation in the CPT process from organizations representing licensed independent practitioners and allied health professionals.

The AMA is responsible for developing and publishing the official guidelines for CPT. The association provides support in several ways. It publishes *CPT Assistant*, a monthly newsletter, and offers CPT Information Services, a telephone service that provides users with expert advice on code use. The association also conducts an annual CPT coding symposium (AMA 2015).

Diagnostic and Statistical Manual of Mental Disorders

The **Diagnostic and Statistical Manual of Mental Disorders, 5th edition (DSM-5)** is the handbook used by healthcare professionals as a guide to diagnose mental disorders and was first published by the American Psychiatric Association (APA) in 1952. The fifth and most recent complete revision was published in 2013 and introduced in 2014 to replace the DSM-IV-TR (Fourth Edition, Text Revision) (APA 2015a).

The DSM-5 has transitioned away from the **multiaxial** (five axes) coding system for the documentation of diagnosis. DSM-5 has combined the former Axes I clinical disorders, II personality disorders, and III general medical conditions and has created a separate notation for psychosocial and contextual factors (formerly Axis IV), and for disability (formerly Axis V) (APA 2015b). The psychosocial and environmental elements are now captured with ICD-10-CM Z-codes. The Global Assessment of Functioning (GAF) (scale for level of functioning and formerly Axis V) was replaced with the WHO Disability Assessment Schedule (WHODAS), which is a scale developed by the World Health Organization (WHO) as the recommended best global measure of disability. The DSM-5 chapters have been restructured based on

disorders' apparent relatedness to one another (similarities in disorders' underlying symptom characteristics) that will eventually align with ICD-11.

The APA states two general uses for DSM: as a source of diagnostic information that enhances clinical practice, research, and education, and as a tool for collecting and communicating accurate public health statistics. The APA updates DSM information to correspond to the International Classification of Diseases (ICD) (APA 2015b). There are several differences among DSM-5 and ICD-10-CM. DSM-5 diagnoses are reclassified, criteria was clarified, not otherwise specified (NOS) designation was removed, and there is no longer the axis system. In comparison to ICD-10, at certain times different disorders or subtypes share the same diagnostic code. Behavioral health professionals must be fluent in both systems, focusing on the diagnostics sets that have the greatest differences. A strategy is in place to align the mental and behavioral disorders in ICD-11 and DSM-5. There is strong support from the ICD-DSM Harmonization Coordination Group formed by WHO for the harmonization effort of these two systems.

International Classification of Primary Care

The **International Classification of Primary Care (ICPC-2)** is a coding terminology for the classification of primary care developed by the World Organization of National Colleges, Academies, and Academic Associations of General Practitioners/ Family Physicians (WONCA) International Classification Committee (WHO 2015e). ICPC-2 has been developed as a tool for general practitioners and family doctors throughout the world. It has been mapped to ICD-10 so that conversion systems can be used (Wonca Global Family Doctor 2015). Extensive use has confirmed that it and ICD-10 are complementary. ICPC-2 includes a severity of illness checklist and functional status assessment charts (Wonca Global Family Doctor 2015). Table 5.5 depicts the four categories of diagnosis in primary care in ICPC.

Current Dental Terminology

The **Current Dental Terminology (CDT)** is a reference manual maintained and updated annually by the American Dental Association (ADA). Included in the manual is the Code on Dental Procedures

Table 5.5. ICPC-2: four categories of diagnosis in primary care

Category	Description	Examples
1. Aetiological and pathological	The diagnosis has proven pathology or aetiology	Appendicitis, acute myocardial infarction
2. Pathophysiological	The diagnosis has a proven pathophysiological substrate	Presbycusis, hypertension
3. Nosological	The diagnosis depends on a symptom complex based on consensus between physicians	Depression, irritable bowel syndrome
4. Symptom	A symptom or complaint is the best medical label for the episode	Fatigue, eye pain

Reprinted from International Classification of Primary Care, Second Edition (ICPC-2). 2015e. ©WHO 2016.

and Nomenclature (the Code), which is a classification system for dental treatment procedures and services. The Code has been designated as the national standard for reporting dental services by the federal government under the Health Insurance Portability and Accountability Act (HIPAA), and is recognized by third-party payers nationwide. The code set is organized into 12 categories of service, each with its own series of five-digit alphanumeric codes (see table 5.6). Each category of service is divided into subcategories of generally recognized related procedures (ADA 2015).

National Drug Codes

The Food and Drug Administration (FDA) developed the **National Drug Codes (NDC) directory** to

Table 5.6. Examples of CDT 2015 codes

Category of service	Code series	Example code	Nomenclature	Descriptor (if applicable)
I. Diagnostic	D0100– D0999	D0277	Vertical bitewings—7 to 8 films	This does not constitute a full mouth intraoral radiographic series
II. Preventive	D1000–D1999	D1320	Tobacco counseling for the control and prevention of oral disease	Tobacco prevention and cessation services reduce patient risks of developing tobacco-related oral diseases and conditions and improves prognosis for certain dental therapies
III. Restorative	D2000–D2999	D2390	Resin-based composite crown, anterior	Full resin-based composite coverage of tooth
IV. Endodontics	D3000–D3999	D3410	Apicoectomy/periradicular surgery—anterior	For surgery on root of anterior tooth. Does not include placement of retrograde filling material.
V. Periodontics	D4000–D4999	D4355	Full mouth debridement to enable comprehensive evaluation and diagnosis	The gross removal of plaque and calculus that interfere with the ability of the dentist to perform a comprehensive oral evaluation; this preliminary procedure does not preclude the need for additional procedures
VI. Prosthodontics, removable	D5000–D5899	D5110	Complete denture—maxillary	
VII. Maxillofacial Prosthetics	D5900–D5999	D5984	Radiation shield	Synonymous terminology: radiation stent, tongue protector, lead shield; an intraoral prosthesis designed to shield adjacent tissues from radiation during orthovoltage treatment of malignant lesions of the head and neck region
VIII. Implant Services	D6000–D6199	D6010	Surgical placement of implant body: endosteal implant	Includes second-stage surgery and placement of healing cap
IX. Prosthodontics, fixed	D6200–D6999	D6794	Crown—titanium	
X. Oral and Maxillofacial Surgery	D7000–D7999	D7220	Removal of impacted tooth—soft tissue	Occlusal surface of tooth covered by soft tissue; requires mucoperiosteal flap elevation.
XI. Orthodontics	D8000–D8999	D8691	Repair of orthodontic appliance	Does not include bracket and standard fixed ortho appliances. It does include functional appliances and palatal expanders.
XII. Adjunctive General Services	D9000–D9999	D9230	Inhalation of nitrous oxide/ anxiolysis, analgesia	

Source: ADA 2015.

serve as a universal product identifier for human drugs. It identifies the labeler/vendor, product, and trade package size. It is an approved HIPAA billing/financial transaction code set for reporting drugs and biologicals. In 2004, the NDCs were adopted as a federal healthcare information interoperability standard to enable the federal healthcare sector to share information regarding drug products (USHIK 2008).

Each drug product is assigned a unique 10-digit, 3-segment number. The three segments of an NDC represent the following:

- First segment—labeler code, assigned by the FDA. A labeler is a firm that manufactures, repacks, or distributes a drug product.

- Second segment—product code, identifies a specific strength, dose form, and formulation for a particular firm.

- Third segment—package code, identifies package sizes; both the product and package codes are assigned by the firm (FDA 2015).

Table 5.7. Examples of NDC codes

Drug	NDC code
Fluoxetine 100 mg Caps	00172-4363-70
Prenatal Plus Tab	0093-9111-01
Hydrocodone/APAP 7.5/500 mg Tab	00591-0385-05
Glycolax 3350 NF POW	62175-442-31
Flonase 0.05% Nasal Spray	00173-0453-01
Progesterone 600 mg Supp	51927-1046-00
Seraquel 100 mg Tab	00310-0271-10
Axert 12.5 mg Tab	00062-2085-06
Amitriptyline 25 mg Tab	00603-2213-32
Amoxicillin 400 mg/5 Susp	63304-0970-04

Source: FDA 2015.

The NDCs will be in one of the following configurations of digits in each segment: 4-4-2, 5-3-2, or 5-4-1 (see table 5.7). Each manufacturer defines the specific codes for its own products. Therefore, there is no uniform class hierarchy for the codes and codes may be reused at the manufacturer's discretion (Hammond and Cimino 2001).

Check Your Understanding 5.2

Instructions: **Answer the following questions on a separate piece of paper.**

1. Articulate the differences between ICD-10-CM and ICD-10-PCS.

2. Do ICD-10-CM and ICD-10-PCS codes apply for the inpatient or outpatient setting (identify each individually)?

3. Define the structure of HCPCS. What level within HCPCS defines CPT and what is the primary function of CPT? Do HCPCS and CPT codes apply within the inpatient or outpatient setting?

4. What are the major differences between DSM-5 and ICD-10 and what impact has utilizing two companion systems had on behavioral health providers?

5. What purpose does the National Drug Codes directory serve in healthcare?

6. Why was ICPC-2 developed?

Other Healthcare Terminologies, Vocabularies, and Classification Systems

Healthcare terminologies facilitate health information exchange by standardizing the data collected. Through this standard representation of data, terminologies provide shared meaning and a sense of context for the information being used. In simple terms, this ability to exchange information between computer systems is referred to as **interoperability**.

A more detailed definition for interoperability is

the ability to communicate and exchange data accurately, effectively, securely, and consistently with different information technology systems, software applications, and networks in various settings, and exchange data such that clinical or operational purpose and meaning of the data are preserved and unaltered (Bush 2006).

Many experts have identified a lack of interoperability as a major obstacle to realizing the full potential of EHR systems and the exchange of health information (AMIA and AHIMA Terminology and Classification Policy Task Force 2007; Ash and Bates 2005; NCVHS 2005).

The NCVHS has identified three levels of interoperability: basic, functional, and semantic. **Basic interoperability** relates to the ability to successfully transmit and receive data from one computer to another. The ability to understand or interpret the information being transmitted is not essential to basic interoperability. **Functional interoperability** refers to sending messages between computers with a shared understanding of the structure and format of the message. With functional interoperability, the receiving computer can store information in a similar data field because the nature (context) of the data being sent is understood. For example, the receiving computer could recognize that the information being sent is a lab result and store it accordingly. The NCVHS definition of **semantic interoperability** is similar to that of the Health Level Seven (HL7) EHR Interoperability Work Group, in which the information being transmitted is understood (EHR Interoperability Work Group 2007). Building on the previous example, the receiving system would not only recognize that what was being sent is a lab value but would also understand the method used to calculate the value and the reference ranges for a normal result. The use of clinical terminologies in EHRs to provide standardized data is essential to achieving semantic interoperability. Progress is being made in the incorporation of clinical terminologies into EHR systems.

There are different types of clinical terminologies, each of which serves unique purposes. A **reference terminology** for clinical data is defined as "a set of concepts and relationships that provides a common reference point for comparison and aggregation of data about the entire healthcare process, recorded by multiple different individuals, systems, or institutions" (Spackman et al. 1997). A reference terminology provides a common source to which data captured through other terminologies and classifications can be mapped. This linkage back to a common source facilitates aggregation and comparison of data. Systematized Nomenclature of Medicine–Clinical Terminology (SNOMED CT), a widely used reference terminology, is discussed later in this chapter. An **interface terminology** is concerned with facilitating clinician documentation within the standardized structure (for example, menus, drop-down boxes) needed for an EHR. An interface terminology provides a limited set of words and phrases in a manner that is consistent with a clinician's thought process used while documenting. Information represented by an interface terminology is often mapped to similar concepts in a comprehensive reference terminology. In this sense, the interface terminology serves as a conduit between the natural language expression of the healthcare provider and the data as they are represented by the reference terminology (Rosenbloom et al. 2006).

The following describes some of the terminologies being used more commonly in EHRs and their uses.

Systematized Nomenclature of Medicine—Clinical Terms

Systemized Nomenclature of Medicine—Clinical Terminology (SNOMED CT) is a comprehensive, multihierarchical, concept-oriented clinical terminology owned, maintained, and distributed by the **International Health Terminology Standards Development Organization (IHTSDO)**, an international nonprofit organization based in Denmark. Figure 5.4 lists the top-level hierarchies into which SNOMED CT is organized.

The size of the terminology conveys how extensive it is. SNOMED CT is updated and released every six months. As of publication, SNOMED CT includes more than 315,000 active concepts, 806,000 active descriptions, and 945,000 defining relationships (IHTSDO 2015a). A **concept** is the most granular unit within a terminology. In SNOMED CT, it is specifically defined as "a single clinical meaning identified by a unique numeric identifier" (College of American Pathologists 2008). Multiple descriptions are often assigned to a single concept. For example, the descriptions heart attack, myocardial infarction, and cardiac infarction would all be linked to a single concept (myocardial infarction 2298006). **Relationships** describe how the concepts within SNOMED CT are linked to one another. An example of a relationship is that the concept *diabetes mellitus* is an *endocrine disorder*, another concept with a broader meaning (IHTSDO 2015b).

The current terminology—SNOMED CT—is the result of the evolution and combination of various classifications and terminologies over the past several decades. SNOMED was originally built on the Systematized Nomenclature of Pathology (SNOP), which was introduced in 1965. Like SNOP, SNOMED uses an alphanumeric, multiaxial coding scheme (Kudla and Blakemore 2001). In 1997, the College of American Pathologists (CAP)

worked with a team of physicians and nurses from Kaiser Permanente to begin development of the **Systematized Nomenclature of Medicine—Reference Terminology (SNOMED RT)**. One of the ways that SNOMED RT came to be recognized as a reference terminology was by the inclusion of an elementary mapping to ICD-9-CM (Kudla and Blakemore 2001). SNOMED also worked with the Digital Imaging and Communications in Medicine (DICOM) community, the Logical Observation Identifiers Names and Codes (LOINC) system, and the various nursing vocabularies to further expand its content. In 2002, SNOMED RT and Clinical Terms, Version 3 (CTV3), also known as the Read Codes, merged to create the SNOMED–Clinical Terminology (CT) system. In 2007, the SNOMED CT intellectual property rights were transferred from the College of American Pathologists to IHTSDO.

The Department of Health and Human Services (HHS) recommended SNOMED CT as part of a core set of **patient medical record information (PMRI)** terminology in 2003 for the adoption of uniform data standards for patient medical record information and electronic information exchange (NCVHS 2003). Then in 2004, SNOMED CT was adopted as a federal information technology interoperability standard to:

- Describe specific nonlaboratory interventions and procedures performed or delivered
- Exchange results of laboratory tests between facilities
- Describe anatomical locations for clinical, surgical, pathological, and research purposes
- Define diagnosis and problem lists
- Define terminology of the delivery of nursing care (IHTSDO 2015d)

Tables 5.8 and 5.9 illustrate level of detail comparisons between SNOMED CT concepts and codes to ICD-10-CM and CPT, respectively.

Examples of Implementations of SNOMED CT

SNOMED CT is currently being used in EHR systems as a clinical reference terminology to

Figure 5.4. Example of SNOMED CT hierarchies

Clinical finding
- Finding *(Swelling of arm)*
- Disease *(Pneumonia)*

Procedure *(Biopsy of lung)*
Observable entity *(Tumor stage)*
Body structure *(Structure of thyroid)*
- Morphologically abnormal structure *(Granuloma)*

Substance *(Gastric acid)*
Pharmaceutical/biologic product *(Tamoxifen)*
Specimen *(Urine specimen)*
Qualifier value *(Right)*
Record artifact *(Death certificate)*
Physical object *(Suture needle)*
Physical force *(Friction)*
Environments/geographical locations *(Intensive care unit)*
Social context *(Organ donor)*
Situation with explicit content *(No nausea)*
Staging and scales *(Barthel index)*
Linkage concept
- Link assertion *(Has etiology)*
- Attributes *(Finding site)*

Special concept *(Inactive concept)*

Source: IHTSDO 2015c.

capture data for problem lists and patient assessments at the point of care. It also supports alerts, warnings, or reminders used for decision support. The Department of Veteran Affairs (VA) is using SNOMED CT for standardization of problem list entries, allergic reactions, and anatomy coding in autopsy reports. A subset of SNOMED CT terms that can be used to represent problem list entries documented within an EHR is available for download at the Unified Medical Language System's website. The list is being provided without any licensing or intellectual property restrictions in an effort to facilitate use of the SNOMED CT terms for problem list data representation (NLM 2015b). The incorporation of SNOMED CT into EHR applications is increasing (IHTSDO 2015b).

Table 5.8. SNOMED CT ICD clinical detail comparison

SNOMED CT	Description	ICD-10
49455004	Diabetic polyneuropathy (disorder)	E08.42 E09.42 E10.42 E11.42 E13.42
	One to many	
190502001	Pituitary-dependent Cushing's Disease (disorder)	E24.0
	Exact Match	
102572006	Ankle edema (finding)	R60.0
	Inexact Match	

Source: Steindel 2012.

Table 5.9. SNOMED CPT clinical detail comparison: Procedures

SNOMED CT	Description	CPT
	Total abdominal hysterectomy with or without removal of tubes, with or without removal of ovaries	58150
2795001	–total unilateral removal of ovary	
3154500	–with unilateral removal of tube	
59750000	–with unilateral removal of tube and ovary	

Adapted from UMLS 2015.

Logical Observation Identifiers Names and Codes

Development of the **Logical Observation Identifiers Names and Codes (LOINC)** began in February 1994. LOINC is the exchange standard for laboratory results. The Regenstrief Institute maintains the LOINC database and its supporting documentation. Most healthcare facilities and reference laboratories use their own protocols for storing lab test and result information. The goal for LOINC is not to replace the laboratory fields in facility databases but, rather, to provide a mapping mechanism. The LOINC committee hoped that laboratories would create fields in their master files for storing LOINC codes and names as attributes of their own data elements (Regenstrief Institute 2015). Each LOINC name identifies a distinct laboratory observation and is structured to contain up to six parts, including:

- Analyte/component (for example, potassium, hemoglobin)
- Kind of property measured or observed (for example, mass, mass concentration, enzyme concentration)
- Time aspect of the measurement or observation (a point in time versus an observation integrated over time)
- System and sample type (for example, urine, blood, serum)
- Type of measurement or observation scale (quantitative [a number] versus qualitative [a trait such as cloudy])
- Type of measurement or observation method used (for example, clean catch or catheter)

Table 5.10 provides an example of a LOINC code and the characteristics with its corresponding attributes.

The primary disadvantage to LOINC is that it may require significant modifications to work with a current laboratory information system that has been previously using its own protocols for lab data representation. A distinct advantage to using LOINC is that it enables the standardized communication of laboratory results. Large inte-

Table 5.10. Example of a LOINC code and its attributes

LOINC number	10968-6
Component/Analyte	Smudge cells/100 leukocytes
Property	NFr (number fraction)
Time aspect	Pt (point in time)
System (sample type)	Bld (whole blood)
Scale type	Qn (quantitative—continuous numeric scale)
Method type	Manual count

This material contains content from LOINC® (http://loinc.org). LOINC are copyright © 1995-2015, Regenstrief Institute, Inc.

grated delivery systems that have very diverse laboratory processing systems (the machines that perform the tests) will find it easier to maintain and use an EHR with LOINC-identified laboratory results.

LOINC is divided into two major sections: Lab LOINC and Clinical LOINC. Lab LOINC was established by the Regenstrief Institute (2015) to identify observations in HL7 messages as a universal standard for laboratory test names. Clinical LOINC includes entries for vital signs, intake/output, EKG, obstetric ultrasound, cardiac echo, urologic imaging, gastroendoscopic procedures, and other clinical observations (LOINC 2015c).

In 2003, LOINC was adopted as a federal health information interoperability standard for the electronic exchange of laboratory test orders and drug label section headers using Structured Product Labeling (SPL) (Regenstrief Institute 2015).

Examples of LOINC Implementations

LOINC has been implemented in a number of different healthcare settings. Many large commercial laboratories have adopted LOINC as an alternate format for reporting lab data. The Veterans Affairs (VA) has implemented Lab LOINC as their primary coding system for laboratory tests and HL7 messages. The Consolidated Health Informatics (CHI) initiative (collaborative to create and adopt health informatics standards by federal departments) recommended in May 2004 the use of Clinical LOINC to fully specify document titles in text-based documentation (HHS 2015). Several

healthcare facilities have reported successful use of LOINC to standardize the reporting of laboratory data (Baorto et al. 1998; Khan et al. 2006).

Clinical Care Classification

The **Clinical Care Classification (CCC)** system is two interrelated taxonomies, the CCC of Nursing Diagnoses and Outcomes and the CCC of Nursing Interventions and Actions that provide a standardized framework for documenting patient care in hospitals, home health agencies, ambulatory care clinics, and other healthcare settings (AHIMA 2014). This system increases the opportunities for health information and interoperability in the important area of nursing.

The CCC system can be used for a number of purposes. Primarily, it facilitates capturing standardized data with the electronic documentation of patient care at the point of care. It can be used to track nursing activities in patient care, clinical pathways, decision support, and the effect of nursing care on patient outcomes. Furthermore, it can be used to predict workload, assess resource needs, and determine costs of nursing care. This is difficult to capture without a standardized method for codifying nursing data.

The CCC also has applications in nursing education. It can be used to teach students how to document patient care electronically and the characteristics of a nursing terminology for documentation purposes.

Another important functionality the CCC provides is in the area of nursing research (table 5.11). It supports analysis and evaluation of patient outcomes, facilitates the design of expert systems, and advances nursing practice knowledge. The CCC's standardized terminology allows much higher quality data for the research. It also allows the data to be captured and reviewed more quickly than paper documentation. Thus, the knowledge gained can be utilized to improve the nursing care provided to patients at the point of care (Saba 2015).

RxNorm

RxNorm is a standardized nomenclature for clinical drugs that provides information on a drug's ingredients, strengths, and form in which it is to be administered or used. It is produced by the National Library of Medicine (NLM) and allows various systems using different drug nomenclatures to share data efficiently at the appropriate level of detail (NLM 2015c). RxNorm's standard names for clinical drugs are connected to the names of drugs present in many other controlled vocabularies, including those available in drug information sources today. These connections facilitate interoperability among the electronic health record systems that record or process data dealing with clinical drugs (NLM 2015d). Examples of the linkages provided through RxNorm include from brand-named and generic-named clinical drugs to their active ingredients, drug components, and related brand names. They can also be connected to the FDA's NDCs (refer to table 5.7) for specific drug products and many of the drug vocabularies commonly used in pharmacy management and drug interaction (NIST 2015). This nomenclature provides a detailed level of codified data that facilitates interoperability between pharmacy systems. It allows these systems to check for drug–drug or drug–allergy interactions so that providers can avoid prescribing certain drugs and to give them other prescription choices with no adverse effects. This functionality is available today on a limited basis for patients who are treated in both the VA and Department of Defense (DoD) medical treatment facilities. It has already been shown to significantly decrease medication errors, reduce duplicate prescriptions, and most importantly, improve patient safety.

MEDCIN

MEDCIN is a proprietary clinical terminology owned and maintained by Medicomp Systems. The system was initially developed by Peter Goltra in 1978 and has been updated regularly (NLM 2015g). Table 5.12 contains examples of a few of MEDCIN'S approximately 270,000 clinical elements

Table 5.11. Examples of CCC system nursing diagnoses

Code	Category	Diagnosis
A01.0	Activity Alteration	Change in or modification of energy used by the body
A01.1	Activity Intolerance	Incapacity to carry out physiological or psychological daily activities
A01.2	Activity Intolerance Risk	Increased chance of an incapacity to carry out physiological or psychological daily activities
O38.1	Activities of Daily Living (ADLs) Alteration	Change in modification of ability to maintain oneself
Q45.1	Acute Pain	Severe pain of limited duration.
E12.1	Adjustment Impairment	Inadequate adaptation to condition or change in health status
L26.1	Airway Clearance Impairment	Inability to clear secretions/obstructions in airway
N58.2	Alcohol Abuse	Excessive use of distilled liquors
P40.0	Anxiety	Feeling of distress or apprehension whose source is unknown
N33.1	Aspiration	Increased chance of material into trachea-bronchial passages

Source: "Table 8.6: Clinical Care Classification of 176 Nursing Diagnoses, Version 2.5 ©: Coded Alphabetically with Definitions" (pp.116-123), Copyright 2012. In, Saba, VK (2014). *Clinical Care Classification (CCC) System, Version 2.5: User's Guide.* New York: Springer.

Table 5.12. Examples of MEDCIN clinical elements

Code number	Clinical element
1931	Joint swelling, fingers, right hand
34183	Chronic interstitial cystitis
49339	Mechanical vitrectomy by pars plana approach
48618	Acetaminophen + Diphenhydramine
35034	Accident involving a motor vehicle, collision with another motor vehicle on the road

Source: Goltra 1997.

created with a strong focus on facilitating documentation by providing clinically relevant choices in a format that is consistent with the provider's clinical thought processes. Because of this feature, the system is considered to be an interface terminology (Bowman 2005; Fraser 2005). MEDCIN is licensed by EHR developers that incorporate the terminology into their EHR systems. For example, MEDCIN is the clinical terminology used by the DoD in its Armed Forces Health Longitudinal Technology Application (AHLTA) system. MEDCIN also identifies relationships through multiple hierarchies for each of its clinical elements. These linkages support other functionalities of the system such as clinical alerts, automated note generation, and computer-assisted coding for CPT evaluation and management codes (Goltra 1997; Medicomp Systems 2012).

Check Your Understanding 5.3

1. Define interoperability and describe how terminologies play a role in interoperability.

2. Provide a description of the intent of LOINC and identify the attributes of the LOINC codes.

3. Identify the appropriate classification, terminology, vocabulary, or standard that would be a good candidate to represent: (a) laboratory data, (b) nursing documentation, and (c) problem list documentation.

4. Identify the difference between a reference terminology and an interface terminology.

5. Identify the major difference between RxNorm and MEDCIN.

6. What do the terms *concept* and *relationship* mean in the context of SNOMED CT?

Emerging Healthcare Terminologies, Vocabularies, and Classifications

No single terminology, vocabulary, or classification has the depth and breadth to represent the broad spectrum of medical knowledge; thus, a core group of well-integrated, nonredundant methods will be needed to serve as the backbone of clinical information (Open Clinical 2012).

Table 5.13 provides a reference to many of the specialized terminologies, vocabularies, and classifications available for use in healthcare. Tables 5.14 through 5.18 provide examples of the coding methodologies for several of these systems.

Data Standardization

Data standardization exists to support different healthcare functions. Classifications are used to aggregate data for functions such as data analysis and reimbursement. Clinical terminologies play an essential role in capturing and sharing data in a manner that meets the requirements of semantic interoperability, which is essential for reliable health information exchange. **Mapping** is a function that allows for the reuse of data captured for one purpose to be used for other purposes. In order to reach the full potential of health information exchange, HIM professionals must participate in the development, implementation, and maintenance of information systems that use standards for collecting and reporting data.

As health information management (HIM) professionals search for ways to formalize the myriad types of data contained in EHRs, it helps to be able to evaluate the different classifications and terminologies. Certain characteristics are desirable. The characteristics are as follows:

Table 5.13. Emerging healthcare terminologies, vocabularies, and classifications

Name	Description
The National Cancer Institute (NCI) Thesaurus (table 5.13)	Contains the working vocabulary used in NCI data systems. It covers clinical, translational, and basic research as well as administrative terminology. In May 2004, the NCI Thesaurus was adopted as a federal healthcare information interoperability standard to describe anatomical locations for clinical, surgical, pathological, and research purposes (NCI 2015).
The Human Gene Nomenclature Committee (HGNC) (table 5.14)	Provides data for all human genes that have approved symbols. It is managed by the Human Genome Organisation (HUGO) Gene Nomenclature Committee (HGNC) as a confidential database containing over 16,000 records. Web data are integrated with other human gene databases, and approved gene symbols are carefully coordinated with the Mouse Genome Database (MGD). HUGN was adopted as a federal health information interoperability standard for exchanging information regarding the role of genes in biomedical research and healthcare (HGNC 2015).
The Global Medical Device Nomenclature (GMDN) (table 5.15)	Consists of medical devices such as home blood pressure monitors, blood glucose devices, and ventilators. A standard is needed to inventory devices, document their use by healthcare providers, and regulate their tions of devices as well as ensuring the safety and effectiveness of these products. GMDN is a collection of internationally recognized terms used to describe and catalogue medical devices and supplies. GMDN is currently divided into 12 categories that encompass all of these products (Table 5.15). It is strongly supported by the FDA for communicating these data. The agency also recommends that the GMDN eventually replace the FDA terminology for devices. The nomenclature is used extensively outside the United States and is recognized by the European Committee for Standardization (CEN) and other international bodies. The FDA and Emergency Care Research Institute (ECRI) are currently producing a map of UMDNS to GMDN to coordinate their practices leading to a merger between them. This should result in a terminology that enables the US federal system to utilize one set of medical device names, definitions, and codes. These identifiers may also be used to communicate with foreign entities.
The Universal Medical Device Nomenclature System (UMDNS)	Is a standard international nomenclature and computer coding system for medical devices. It facilitates identifying, processing, filing, storing, retrieving, transferring, and communicating data about medical devices. It is primarily used by healthcare institutions. It has been adopted by many nations, including the entire European Union (EU). It is used in applications ranging from hospital inventory and work-order controls to national agency medical device regulatory systems. It is incorporated into the UMLS. UMDNS has been merged with the GMDN.
The Environmental Protection Agency (EPA) Substance Registry System (SRS) (table 5.16)	Provides information on substances and how they are represented in the EPA's regulations and information systems. It provides a common basis for identification of chemicals, biological organisms, and other substances listed in EPA regulations and data systems, as well as substances of interest from other sources, such as publications. The EPA SRS was adopted as the federal health information interoperability standard for chemicals in May 2004 (EPA SRS 2015).
The Breast Imaging Reporting and Data System Atlas (BI-RADS) (table 5.17)	Is designed to serve as a comprehensive guide providing standardized breast imaging terminology, a report organization, an assessment structure, and a classification system for mammography, ultrasound, and MRI of the breast (ACS 2015). BI-RADS assessment categories are listed in table 5.17. BI-RADS is the product of a collaboration effort among members of various committees of the American College of Radiology with cooperation from the National Cancer Institute, the Centers for Disease Control and Prevention, the FDA, and the College of American Pathologists. Results are compiled in a standardized manner that permits the maintenance and collection analysis of demographic, mammographic, and outcome data (ACR 2015).
The Medical Dictionary for Regulatory Activities (MedDRA)	Is a medically valid terminology that has an emphasis on ease of use for data entry, retrieval, analysis, and display. It was developed by the International Conference on Harmonisation (ICH) to provide a single standardized international medical terminology. MedDRA terminology applies to all phases of drug development and also applies to the health effects and malfunction of devices. Those who should subscribe to MedDRA include: <ul><li>Pharmaceutical companies</li><li>Biotechnology companies</li><li>Device manufacturers</li><li>Regulatory authorities</li><li>Contract research organizations</li><li>Systems developers</li><li>Other support service organizations</li></ul>The Maintenance and Support Services Organization (MSSO) serves as the repository, maintainer, and distributor of MedDRA (MedDRA 2015).
The Systematized Nomenclature of Dentistry (SNODENT)	Is a clinical vocabulary developed by the American Dental Association (ADA) for data representation of clinical dentistry content. The need for interoperable dental information is increasing as the field of dentistry is moving more into the medical management of oral diseases. For example, dentists now sometimes perform saliva testing for the purpose of substance abuse and disease monitoring. This type of information may need to be shared with other healthcare providers.

Table 5.14. NCI Thesaurus taxonomy concept details

Identifiers:	
Name	Pancreas
Code	C12393
Relationships to other concepts:	
Anatomic_Structure_Has_Location	Epigastric Region
Anatomic_Structure_is_Physical_Part_of	Gastrointestinal System
Information about this concept:	
Display_Name	Pancreas
Mitelman_Code	218
Preferred_Name	Pancreas
Semantic_Type	Body Part, Organ, or Organ Component
Subsource	ICD
Subsource	LASH
Subsource	Mitelman
Unified Medical Language System	C0030274

Source: NCI 2015.

Table 5.15. Human genes with approved symbols: single-letter amino acid codes

Amino Acid	Three-Letter Symbol	One-Letter Symbol
Alanine	Ala	A
Arginine	Arg	R
Asparagine	Asn	N
Aspartic Acid	Asp	D
Cysteine	Cys	C
Glutamine	Gln	Q
Glutamic Acid	Glu	E
Valine	Val	V
Glycine	Gly	G

Source: HGNC 2015.

Table 5.16. GMDN device categories

The Standard allocates codes for a possible 20 categories. For this version of the GMDN 13 device categories are now established. These are:	
01	Active implantable devices
02	Anaesthetic and respiratory devices
03	Dental devices
04	Electro mechanical medical devices
05	Hospital hardware
06	In vitro diagnostic devices (IVD)
07	Nonactive implantable devices
08	Ophthalmic and optical devices
09	Reusable instruments
10	Single use devices
11	Technical aids for disabled persons
12	Diagnostic and therapeutic radiation devices
13	Obsolete terms
14	Vacant
15	Vacant
16	Vacant
17	Vacant
18	Vacant
19	Vacant
20	Vacant

Source: NCVHS 2012.

Table 5.17. Example of an EPA SRS substance list

Name	Liquid Nitrogen (Containing)
Molecular Formula	[No Criteria Specified]
Type	All
Classification	All
Display Option	Substance Name
Sort Option	Name
Systematic Name	Nitrogen
EPA Registry Name	Nitrogen
Classification	Chemical
CAS number	7727-37-9
TSN	
ICTV	
EPA ID	

Source: EPA SRS 2015.

- Content: The content of clinical classifications and terminologies should be determined by their intended use. It is wise to assume that the first identified need will never be the last or only need. It is far better to have too much content initially than to have too little to meet subsequent needs.

- Concept orientation: The content of terminologies and classifications should be oriented toward concepts rather than terms or code numbers. For example, "cold" can either be a disease such as chronic obstructive lung disease or the common cold or a feeling of temperature—these are three separate concepts.

- Concept permanence: Terminologies and classifications must be permanent if they are to

Table 5.18. BI-RADS mammography assessment categories

Assessment	Category
a. Mammographic Assessment is Incomplete	0: Need to review prior studies and/or complete additional imaging
b. Mammographic Assessment is Complete–Final Categories	1: Negative Continue routine screening
	2: Benign finding Continue routine screening
	3: Probably Benign Finding Short-term follow-up mammogram at 6 months, then every 6 to 12 months for 1 to 2 years
	4: Suspicious Abnormality Perform biopsy, preferably needle biopsy
	5: Highly Suggestive of Malignancy–Appropriate Action Should Be Taken (Biopsy and treatment, as necessary)
	6: Known Biopsy–Proven Malignancy–treatment pending (ensure that treatment is completed)

Source: ACR 2015.

be useful for longitudinal reporting. Concepts may be inactivated but must never be deleted.

- Nonsemantic concept identifier: No implicit or explicit meaning can be associated with the code numbers used in a classification system. Because primary healthcare systems are now computerized, the human ability to use a classification system without a computer is no longer necessary (Cimino 1998).

- Polyhierarchy: Multiple relationships should exist for every concept. For example, bacterial pneumonia is both a pulmonary disease and an infectious disease.

- Formal definitions: Standardized definitions are necessary to ensure comparability among terminologies and classifications. They also reduce confusion.

- Reject Not Elsewhere Classified: Not Elsewhere Classified (NEC) is not the same as Not Otherwise Specified (NOS). NOS means that there is no additional information. NEC means there is more information but no place to put it. It also means that any additional information will be lost forever if it is assigned the NEC label.

- Multiple granularities: Because classifications and terminologies must fulfill multiple purposes, the information in them may be specific or general so that all needs can be met.

- Multiple consistent views: Classifications and terminologies must accommodate more than one viewpoint to allow them to be multipurpose as well as to ensure continuity of care. When caring for the same patient, nurses want to use nurse speak and physicians want to use physician speak.

- Context representation: Words have different meanings when used in different contexts or as different grammatical parts of language. Context is determined by how the concepts relate to each other. For example, consider the term *cold*. In the phrase "the patient is cold," cold is how the patient feels. In the phrase "the patient has a cold," cold is a disease. The difference between the two phrases reflects the two different contexts of the word *cold* (Cimino 1998).

- Graceful evolution: The days of yearly updates need to end soon. Future updates will have to be made monthly or, more likely, weekly. The growth of medical knowledge is exponential; classification systems and terminologies must to be able to keep up (Cimino 1998).

- Recognized redundancy: Classifications and terminologies need to accommodate redundancy (Cimino 1998).

- Licensed and copyrighted: Terminologies and classifications need to be copyrighted and licensed to control local modifications, which result in semantic drift and produce incomparable data (Campbell et al. 1999).

- Vendor neutral: Classifications and terminologies must be vendor neutral so that they can be readily used as national standards by all vendors without conferring a competitive advantage to any one of them (Campbell et al. 1999).

- Scientifically valid: Terminologies and classifications should be understandable, reproducible, and useful and should reflect the current understanding of the science (Campbell et al. 1999).

- Adequate maintenance: A central authority that provides a rapid response to requests for new terms is essential to minimize the need for local enhancements and to keep terminologies and classifications current (Campbell et al. 1999).

- Self-sustaining: Classifications and terminologies should be supported by public or endowment funding. Alternatively, licensing fees should be proportional to the value the system provides to users (Campbell et al. 1999).

- Scalable infrastructure and process control: The tools and processes for maintaining a terminology or classification should be scalable, especially for a nationally standardized terminology (Campbell et al. 1999).

Several organizations are actively involved in developing standards for healthcare. See table 5.19 for examples of standards development organizations. Both private organizations and government agencies such as ONC, CSM, FDA, the Agency for Health Care Policy and Research, the Office of the Assistant Secretary for Planning and Evaluation, and the CDC work collaboratively in the development and maintenance of these standards.

The critical importance of healthcare information standards has been recognized in federal initiatives including the legislatively mandated Office of the National Coordinator of Health Information Technology (ONC) and the establishment of two official Department of Health and Human Services (HHS) advisory committees as a result of the Health Information Technology for Economic and Clinical Health (HITECH) Act, part of the American Recovery and Reinvestment Act of 2009 (ARRA). The Health Information Technology Standards Committee (HITSC) makes recommendations to the National Coordinator regarding "standards, implementation specifications, and certification criteria for the electronic exchange and use of health information for purposes of adoption, consistent with the implementation of the Federal

Health IT Strategic Plan, and in accordance with policies developed by the HIT Policy Committee" (HealthIT.gov 2015). In addition, the HITSC provides for the testing of these standards and specifications by the National Institute for Standards and Technology (NIST) (ONC 2011a).

One of the government's health outcomes policy priorities used to create the framework for Meaningful Use (MU) of EHRs is to improve care coordination. A key to interoperable electronic information exchange is having defined core data sets. ASTM International was instrumental in identifying a core data set for a patient's clinical summary with the publication in 2005 of ASTM E2369-05e2 Standard Specification for Continuity of Care Record (CCR). It was updated in 2013 to ASTM E2522-07 and is a health record standard specification. Another organization, Health Level Seven (HL7), developed the Clinical Document Architecture (CDA). The CDA provides an exchange model for clinical documents (such as discharge summaries and progress notes). ASTM International and HL7 combined their work to create the Continuity of Care Document (CCD). The CCD is an implementation guide for sharing CCR patient summary data using the CDA. The CCD was recognized as part of the first set of interoperability standards.

Continuing the work toward interoperability is the transitions of care (ToC) initiative, one of the projects of the Standards and Interoperability (S&I) Framework. According to the initiative's charter, "the exchange of clinical summaries is hampered by ambiguous common definitions of what data elements must at a minimum be exchanged, how they must be encoded, and how those common semantic elements map to MU specified formats (C32/CCD and CCR)" (S&I Framework 2011). An outcome of the initiative is a clinical information model (CIM) "consisting of unambiguous, clinically-relevant definitions of the core data elements that should be included in care transitions" (ONC 2011b).

National Library of Medicine's Role in Healthcare Terminologies

The National Library of Medicine (NLM) is the world's largest medical library. It collects materials

Table 5.19. Standards development organizations

Resource	Description	Source
AIIM	AIIM is an ANSI (American National Standards Institute) accredited standards development organization. AIIM also holds the Secretariat for the ISO (International Organization for Standardization) committee focused on information management compliance issues, TC171.	http://www.aiim.org
Accredited Standards Committee (ASC) X12	ASC X12 is a designated committee under the Designated Standard Maintenance Organization (DSMO), which develops uniform standards for cross-industry exchange of business transactions through electronic data interchange (EDI) standards. ASC X12 is an ANSI-accredited standards development organization	http://www.x12.org
American Dental Association (ADA)	The ADA is an ANSI-accredited standards developing organization that develops dental standards that promote safe and effective oral healthcare.	http://www.ada.org/ prof/resources/ standards/index.asp
ASTM International	Formerly the American Society for Testing and Materials, ASTM International is an ANSI-accredited standards development organization that develops standards for healthcare data security, standard record content, and protocols for exchange of laboratory data.	http://www.astm. org
European Committee for Standardization (CEN)	CEN contributes to the objectives of the European Union and European Economic Area with voluntary technical standards that promote free trade, the safety of workers and consumers, interoperability of networks, environmental protection, exploitation of research and development programs, and public procurement.	http://www.cenorm. be/cenorm/index. htm
Clinical and Laboratory Standards Institute (CLSI)	CLSI is a global, nonprofit, standards development organization that promotes the development and use of voluntary consensus standards and guidelines within the healthcare community. Its core business is the development of globally applicable voluntary consensus documents for healthcare testing.	http://www.clsi.org
Clinical Data Interchange Standards Consortium (CDISC)	CDISC is an open, multidisciplinary, nonprofit organization that has established worldwide industry standards to support the electronic acquisition, exchange, submission, and archiving of clinical trials data and metadata for medical and biopharmaceutical product development	http://www.cdisc. org
Designated Standard Maintenance Organization (DSMO)	The DSMO was established in the final HIPAA rule and is charged with maintaining the standards for electronic transactions, and developing or modifying an adopted standard.	http://www. hipaa-dsmo.org
Health Industry Business Communications Council (HIBCC)	HIBCC is an industry-sponsored and supported nonprofit organization. As an ANSI-accredited organization, its primary function is to facilitate electronic communications by developing standards for information exchange among healthcare trading partners.	http://www.hibcc. org
Health Level 7 (HL7)	HL7 is an ANSI-accredited standards development organization that develops messaging, data content, and document standards to support the exchange of clinical information.	http://www.hl7.org
Institute of Electrical and Electronic Engineers (IEEE)	IEEE is a national organization that develops standards for hospital system interface transactions, including links between critical care bedside instruments and clinical information systems.	http://www.ieee.org
International Organization for Standardization (ISO)	ISO is a nongovernmental organization and network of national standards institutes from 157 countries.	http://www.iso.org/ iso/en/ISOOline. frontpage
National Council for Prescription Drug Programs (NCPDP)	NCPDP is a designated committee under the Designated Standard Maintenance Organization (DSMO) that specializes in developing standards for exchanging prescription and payment information.	http://www.chpdp. org
National Information Standards Organization (NISO)	NISO is an ANSI-accredited, nonprofit association that identifies, develops, maintains, and publishes technical standards to manage information. NISO standards address areas of retrieval, repurposing, storage, metadata, and preservation	http://www.niso.org
National Uniform Billing Committee (NUBC)	NUBC is a designated committee under the Designated Standard Maintenance Organization (DSMO) that is responsible for identifying data elements and designing the CMS-1500.	http://www.nubc. org
National Uniform Claim Committee (NUCC)	NUCC is the national group that replaces the Uniform Claim Form Task Force in 1995 and developed a standard data set to be used in the transmission of noninstitutional provider claims to and from third-party payers.	http://www.nucc. org

Source: Giannangelo 2013, 209–210.

in all aspects of biomedicine and healthcare, as well as works on biomedical aspects of technology, the humanities, and the physical, life, and social sciences (NLM 2015g). It is a standards-supporting and promoting organization that explores the uses of computer and communication technologies to improve organizations and the use of biomedical information.

Medical Subject Headings

The **Medical Subject Headings database (MeSH)** is the NLM's controlled vocabulary thesaurus. It consists of terms naming descriptors in a hierarchical structure that permits searching at various levels of specificity (NLM 2015e). The descriptors exist in both alphabetic and hierarchical structures. It contains very broad headings, such as "Mental Disorders," and more specific levels, such as "Conduct Disorder." There are 22,568 descriptors in MeSH and more than 139,000 headings, called Supplementary Concept Records, within a separate thesaurus (UMLS 2012). Thousands of cross-references also exist. MeSH is used by the NLM for indexing articles from 4,600 of the world's leading biomedical journals for the MEDLINE/PubMed database. Each bibliographic reference is associated with a set of MeSH terms that describe the content of the item (UMLS 2012). Staff subject specialists are responsible for revising and updating the vocabulary on a continuous basis. MeSH is available in electronic format at no charge at the NLM website and a hard copy version is published each January (UMLS 2012).

Unified Medical Language System

The **Unified Medical Language System (UMLS)** is a government-funded project from the NLM that has been in development since 1986. The purpose of the UMLS is "to facilitate the development of computer systems that behave as if they 'understand' the meaning of the language of biomedicine and health…. The UMLS provides data for system developers as well as search and report functions for less technical users" (NLM 2015e). This goal is achieved through the three knowledge sources found in the UMLS:

- UMLS Metathesaurus: A list containing information on biomedical concepts and terms
- SPECIALIST Lexicon: An English language lexicon containing many biomedical terms
- UMLS Semantic Network: A consistent categorization of all concepts represented in the UMLS Metathesaurus

More information on the UMLS can be obtained from the NLM website. When looking in-depth at the UMLS, it is important to keep in mind that it has been designed for computer use; its layouts and other structures are meant to be read by machines. It is not structured to be readable by humans.

Examples of Unified Medical Language System Implementation The VA has used the UMLS Metathesaurus as a lookup tool for finding concepts, synonyms, and linkages to other terminologies in the data standardization of allergies data. It is also using the UMLS RxNorm for standardizing pharmacy data and are sharing those data with the Department of Defense. It has also been proposed to use UMLS as the mediation terminology for VA drug classes. Vanderbilt University has used the UMLS in its WizOrder order entry and decision support system.

If health professionals are to be able to send and receive data in an understandable and usable manner, both the sender and the receiver must have standardization for describing, classifying, and exchanging medical terms and concepts. Use of standardization facilitates electronic data collection at the point of care; retrieval of relevant data, information, and knowledge; and reuse of data for multiple purposes (Aspen et al. 2003).

Mapping Initiatives

As illustrated by descriptions of widely varying clinical classifications and terminologies, no single system meets all needs. "Mappings are sets of relationships of varying complexity established between two vocabularies in order to allow automated translation or connection between them. More specific concepts can generally be mapped accurately to more general concepts" (NLM 2015f). Maps that link related content in classifications and terminologies allow data collected for one purpose to be used for another. For example, a laboratory system that manages data using the LOINC terminology can map the LOINC terms to CPT codes to be used for billing purposes. The NLM, within the framework of the UMLS, contains many sets of mapping among terminologies including LOINC to CPT mapping and SNOMED CT to ICD-10-CM mapping (WHO 2015c). Many maps are created to support a specific use case. For example, the map created for a reimbursement use case might be very different from that for a public health use case. This is even true if the two use cases were mapping between the same two systems. Therefore, successful mapping requires a thorough understanding of the intended use of the map (use case), the structure and purpose of the source, and target terminologies (Foley et al. 2007).

Check Your Understanding 5.4

Instructions: **Answer the following questions on a separate piece of paper.**

1. Why is data standardization so important in healthcare today?

2. What are five desirable characteristics of terminologies and classifications for data standardization?

3. Generally, who develops and maintains healthcare data standards?

4. What are the names of the federal initiatives that recognize healthcare information standards?

5. How can HIM professionals play a role in health informatics and data standardization?

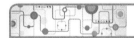 # References

American Cancer Society (ACS). 2015. BI-RADS. http://www.cancer.org/treatment/understandingyourdiagnosis/examsandtestdescriptions/mammogramsandotherbreastimagingprocedures/mammograms-and-other-breast-imaging-procedures-mammo-report

American College of Radiology (ACR). 2015. *BI-RADS Atlas*. http://www.acr.org

American Dental Association. 2015. Current Dental Terminology. http://www.ada.org/en/publications/cdt/

American Health Information Management Association. 2011. *Pocket Glossary of Health Information Management and Technology*, Fourth Edition. Chicago: AHIMA Press.

American Health Information Management Association. 2014. Health Data Analysis Toolkit. http://library.ahima.org/xpedio/groups/public/documents/ahima/bok1_048618.pdf

American Medical Association. 2015. CPT (Current Procedural Terminology). http://www.ama-assn.org/ama/pub/physician-resources/solutions-managing-your-practice/coding-billing-insurance/cpt/cpt-process-faq/code-becomes-cpt.page

American Medical Informatics Association and American Health Information Management Association Terminology and Classification Policy Task Force. 2007 (June 27). Healthcare terminologies and classifications: An action agenda for the United States. *Perspectives in Health Information Management*. http://library.ahima.org/xpedio/groups/public/documents/ahima/bok1_032401.html

American Psychiatric Association. 2015a. DSM-5 Development. http://psychiatryonline.org.akin.css.edu

American Psychiatric Association. 2015b. Diagnostic and Statistical Manual. http://dsm.psychiatryonline.org.akin.css.edu/doi/full/10.1176/appi.books.9780890425596.Introduction

Ash, J.S. and D.W. Bates. 2005. Factors and forces affecting EHR system adoption: Report of a 2004

ACMI discussion. *Journal of the American Medical Informatics Association* 12(1):8–12.

Aspen, P., J.M. Corrigan, J. Wolcott, and S.M. Erickson. 2002. *Patient Safety: Achieving a New Standard of Care.* Institute of Medicine of the National Academies Committee on Data Standards for Patient Safety. Washington, D.C: Institute of Medicine of the National.

ASTM E2522-07. (2013), Standard Guide for Quality Indicators for Health Classifications, ASTM International, West Conshohocken, PA: www.astm.org

Averill, R.F., R.L. Mullin, B.A. Steinbeck, N.I. Goldfield, T.M. Grant, and R.R. Butler. 2005. *Development of the ICD-10 Procedure Coding System (ICD-10-PCS).* 3M HIS Research Report 1-05. St. Paul, MN: 3M.

Baorto, D.M., J.J. Cimino, C.A. Parvin, and M.G. Kahn. 1998. Combining laboratory data sets from multiple institutions using the Logical Observation Identifier Names and Codes (LOINC). *International Journal of Medical Informatics* 51(1):29–37.

Barnett, O.G., et al. 1993. The computer-based clinical record: Where do we stand? *Annals of Internal Medicine* 119(10):1046–1048.

Bowman, S. 2005 (Spring). Coordination of SNOMED-CT and ICD-10: Getting the most out of electronic health record systems. *Perspectives in Health Information Management.* Chicago: AHIMA.

Bush, G.W. 2006. Executive Order: Promoting quality and efficient health care in federal government administered or sponsored health care programs. Washington, DC: White House.

Campbell, K.E., B. Hochhalter, J. Slaughter, and J. Mattison. 1999. *Enterprise Issues Pertaining to Implementing Controlled Terminologies. IMIA Conference Proceedings.* Edmonton, AB: IMIA.

Centers for Medicare and Medicaid Services. 2015a. The ICD-10 Transition: An Introduction. http://www.cms.gov/Medicare/Coding/ICD10/Downloads/ICD10Introduction20140819.pdf

Centers for Medicare and Medicaid Services. 2015b. CMS ICD-10-CM 2015 Official Code Set. http://www.cms.gov/Medicare/Coding/ICD10/2015-ICD-10-CM-and-GEMs.html

Centers for Medicare and Medicaid Services. 2015c. ICD-10-PCS 2015 Version: What's New in this Release. http://www.cms.gov/Medicare/Coding/ICD10/Downloads/2015-pcs-whats-new.pdf

Centers for Medicare and Medicaid Services. 2015d. CMS ICD-10-PCS 2015 Official Coding Guidelines.

http://www.cms.gov/Medicare/Coding/ICD10/2015-ICD-10-PCS-and-GEMs.html

Centers for Medicare and Medicaid Services. 2015e. HCPCS General Information. http://www.cms.gov/Medicare/Coding/HCPCSReleaseCodeSets/Alpha-Numeric-HCPCS.html?DLSort=0&DLEntries=10&DLPage=1&DLSortDir=descending

Centers for Medicare and Medicaid Services. 2015f. ICD-10-PCS Reference Manual. https://www.cms.gov/Medicare/Coding/ICD10/downloads//pcs_refman.pdf

Chute, C.G. 2000. Clinical classification and terminology: Some history and current observations. *Journal of the American Medical Informatics Association* 70(3):298–303.

Cimino, J.J. 1998. Desiderata for controlled medical vocabularies in the twenty-first century. *Methods of Information in Medicine* 37:394–403.

Clinical Care Classification System. 2015. Terminology Tables. http://www.sabacare.com/Tables/Diagnoses.html?SF=DiagCode&SO=Asc

College of American Pathologists. 2008. SNOMED Terminology Solutions. http://www.cap.org/apps/cap.portal?_nfpb=true&_pageLabel=snomed_page

Department of Health and Human Services. 2015. Office of the National Coordinator for Health Information Technology: Consolidated Health Informatics. http://www.healthit.gov/policy-researchers-implementers/glossary

Department of Health and Human Services. 2008. HIPAA administrative simplification: Modifications to medical data code set standards to adopt ICD-10CM and ICD-10-PCS. *Federal Register* 73(164):49796–49832.

EHR Interoperability Work Group. 2007. *Coming to Terms: Scoping Interoperability for Health Care.* Ann Arbor, MI: HL7. Health Level Seven.

Encyclopedia Britannica. 2015. Sir William Petty. http://www.britannica.com/EBchecked/topic/454631/Sir-William-Petty

Environmental Protection Agency Substance Registry Services (EPA SRS). 2015. Substance Details. http://iaspub.epa.gov/sor_internet/registry/substreg/searchandretrieve/substancesearch/search.do?details=displayDetails

Foley, M.M., C. Hall, K. Perron, and R. D'Andrea. 2007. Translation please: Mapping translates clinical data between the many languages that document it. *Journal of AHIMA* 78(2):34–38.

Fraser, G. 2005. Problem list coding in e-HIM. *Journal of AHIMA* 76(7):68–70.

Giannangelo, K. 2015. *Healthcare Code Sets, Clinical Terminologies, and Classification Systems*. Chicago: AHIMA.

Giannangelo, K. 2013. Health informatics standards. Chapter 8 in *Health Information Management: Concepts, Principles and Practice*, 4th ed. Edited by LaTour, K.M., S. Eichenwald Maki, and P. Oachs. Chicago: AHIMA.

Goltra, P.S. 1997. *MEDCIN: A New Nomenclature for Clinical Medicine*. New York: Springer-Verlag.

Hammond, W.E. and J.J. Cimino. 2001. Standards in medical informatics. In *Health Informatics.* Edited by K.J. Hannah and M.J. Ball. New York: Springer-Verlag.

HealthIT.gov. 2015. Health IT Standards Committee. https://www.healthit.gov/facas/health-it-standards-committee

Human Gene Nomenclature Committee (HGNC). 2015. http://www.genenames.org

International Health Terminology Standards Development Organisation. 2015a. About SNOMED CT. http://www.ihtsdo.org/snomed-ct/what-is-snomed-ct

International Health Terminology Standards Development Organisation. 2015b. Who Is Using SNOMED-CT? http://www.ihtsdo.org/snomed-ct/mapping-to-other-terminologies

International Health Terminology Standards Development Organisation. 2015c. *SNOMED CT Browser—2015 United States Release*. http://browser.ihtsdotools.org/

International Health Terminology Standards Development Organization. 2015d. Why SNOMED CT? http://www.ihtsdo.org/snomed-ct/why-should-i-get-snomed-ct

Khan, A.N., S.P. Griffith, C. Moore, D. Russell, A.C. Rosario, Jr., and J. Bertolli. 2006. Standardizing laboratory data by mapping to LOINC. *Journal of the American Medical Informatics Association* 13(3):353–355.

Kudla, K.M. and M. Blakemore. 2001. SNOMED takes the next step. *Journal of AHIMA* 72(7):62–68.

Logical Observation Identifiers Names and Codes. 2015a. https://search.loinc.org.

Logical Observation Identifiers Names and Codes. 2015b. About LOINC. https://loinc.org/background

Logical Observation Identifiers Names and Codes. 2015c. Scope of LOINC. http://loinc.org/get-started/04.html

Medical Dictionary for Regulatory Activities (MedDRA) 2015. http://www.meddra.org/about-meddra

Medicomp Systems, Inc. 2012. *MEDCIN*. http://www.medicomp.com/products/medcinengine/

National Cancer Institute. 2015. NCI Thesaurus (NCIT). http://ncit.nci.nih.gov/ncitbrowser/ConceptReport.jsp?dictionary=NCI%20Thesaurus&code=C12393

National Committee on Vital and Health Statistics. 2012. The Global Medical Device Nomenclature. http://www.ncvhs.hhs.gov/030819p2.pdf

National Committee on Vital and Health Statistics. 2005. NCVHS Subcommittee on Standards and Security. http://www.ncvhs.hhs.gov/stdschrg.htm

National Committee on Vital and Health Statistics (NCVHS). 2003. Recommendations for PMRI Terminology Standards. http://www.ncvhs.hhs.gov/wp-content/uploads/2014/05/031105lt3.pdf

National Institute of Standards and Technology. 2015. HIT Implementation Support and Testing. http://healthcare.nist.gov/testing_infrastructure/index.html

National Library of Medicine. 2015a. Unified Medical Language System Glossary. http://www.nlm.nih.gov/research/umls/new_users/glossary.html

National Library of Medicine. 2015b. UMLS enhanced VA/KP problem list subset of SNOMED CT. http://www.nlm.nih.gov/research/umls/licensedcontent/vakpproblemlist.html

National Library of Medicine. 2015c. RxNorm Overview. http://www.nlm.nih.gov/research/umls/rxnorm/overview.html

National Library of Medicine. 2015d. UMLS Knowledge Source Server Mappings: Draft LNC215 to CPT2005 Mapping. http://www.nlm.nih.gov/research/umls/mapping_projects/loinc_to_cpt_map.html

National Library of Medicine. 2015e. UMLS Metathesaurus Fact Sheet. http://www.nlm.nih.gov/pubs/factsheets/umlsmeta.html

National Library of Medicine. 2015f. Basic Mapping Project Assumptions. http://www.nlm.nih.gov/research/umls/mapping_projects/mapping_assumptions.html

National Library of Medicine. 2015g. Collection Development Manual. https://www.nlm.nih.gov/tsd/acquisitions/cdm/collections.html

Office of the National Coordinator for Health Information Technology. 2011a. Health IT Standards Committee. http://healthit.hhs.gov/portal/server.pt/community/healthit_hhs_gov__health_it_standards_committee/1271

Office of the National Coordinator for Health Information Technology. 2011b. HITSC—Standards and Implementation: Update on Standards Effort. http://healthit.hhs.gov/portal/server.pt/gateway/

PTARGS_0_16869_955993_0_0_18/HITSC_StandardsUpdate102111.pdf

Open Clinical. 2012. Medical Terminologies, Nomenclatures, Coding and Classification Systems: An Introduction. http://www.openclinical.org/medicalterminologies.html

Percy, C., A. Fritz, A. Jack, S. Shanmugarathan, L. Sobin, D.M. Parkin, and S. Whelan. 2000. *International Classification of Diseases for Oncology (ICD-O)*, 3rd ed. World Health Organization.

Regenstrief Institute, Inc. 2015. Logical Observation Identifiers Names and Codes. http://loinc.org

Rosenbloom, S.T., R.A. Miller, K.B. Johnson, P.L. Elkin, and S.H. Brown. 2006. Interface terminologies: Facilitating direct entry of clinical data into electronic health record systems. *Journal of the American Informatics Association* 13(3):277–288.

S&I Framework. 2011. Transitions of Care Overview. http://wiki.siframework.org/ Transitions +of+Care+Overview

Saba. 2015. About Clinical Care Classification System. http://www.sabacare.com/About/

Spackman, K.A., K.E. Campbell, and R.A. Cote. 1997. SNOMED RT: A reference terminology for health care. *Proceedings/AMIA Annual Fall Symposium* 640:4.

Steindel, S.J. 2012. A comparison between a SNOMED CT problem list and the ICD-10-CM/PCS HIPAA code sets. Online Research Journal Perspectives in Health Information Management. http://perspectives.ahima.org/index.php?option=com_content&view=article&id=231:a-comparison-between-a-snomed-ct-problem-list-and-the-icd-10-cmpcs-hipaa-code-sets&catid=45:icd-9icd-10&Itemid=93

Unified Medical Language System. 2015. SNOMED CT Browsers. https://www.nlm.nih.gov/research/umls/Snomed/snomed_browsers.html

Unified Medical Language System. 2012. RxNorm. http://www.nlm.nih.gov/research/umls/rxnorm/

United States Health Information Knowledgebase. 2008. Consolidated Health Informatics. http://www.dcg.dnsalias.net/chi

US Food and Drug Administration (FDA). 2015. http://www.fda.gov/Drugs/InformationOnDrugs/ucm142438.htm

Wonca Global Family Doctor. 2015. Evidence & Guidelines. http://www.globalfamilydoctor.com/Resources/Evidenceandguidelines.aspx

World Health Organization. 2015a. History of ICD. http://www.who.int/classifications/icd/en/HistoryOfICD.pdf

World Health Organization. 2015b. International Classification of Diseases for Oncology, 3rd Edition. http://www.who.int/classifications/icd/adaptations/oncology/en/

World Health Organization. 2015c. SNOMED CT to ICD-10 Cross Map Release. http:www.who.int/classifications/icd/snomedCTTOICD10Maps/en/

World Health Organization. 2015d. ICF Browser Self-Care Codes. http://apps.who.int/classifications/icfbrowser/

World Health Organization. 2015e. International Classification of Primary Care, Second Edition (ICPC-2). http://www.who.int/classifications/icd/adaptations/icpc2/en/

World Health Organization. 2007. Production of ICD-11: The Overall Revision Process. http://www.who.int/classifications/icd/ICDRevision.pdf

6

Data Management

Marcia Y. Sharp, EdD, RHIA, and Charisse Madlock-Brown, PhD

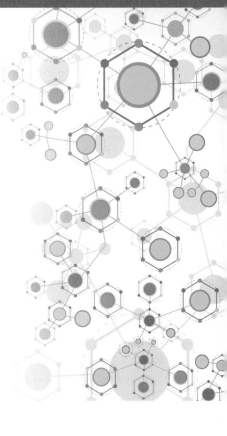

Learning Objectives

- Distinguish between primary and secondary data and between patient-identifiable and aggregate data
- Identify the internal and external users of secondary data
- Compare the facility-specific indexes commonly found in hospitals
- Describe the registries used in hospitals according to purpose, methods of case definition and case finding, data collection methods, reporting and follow-up, and pertinent laws and regulations affecting registry operations

- Distinguish among healthcare databases in terms of purpose and content
- Compare manual and automated methods of data collection
- Compare the use of vendor registries with facility-specific registries
- Describe database design, development, and use
- Describe AHIMA's data quality model and explain its elements
- Identify the role of the health information management professional in creating and maintaining secondary records

Key Terms

Abbreviated Injury Scale (AIS)
Abstracting
Accession number
Accession registry
Agency for Healthcare Research and Quality (AHRQ)
Aggregate data
Attributes
Cancer staging
Cardinality

Case definition
Case finding
Clinical trial
Collaborative Stage Data Set
Data dictionary
Data modeling
Database management system (DBMS)
Disease index
Entity relationship diagram (ERD)

Entity
Facility-based registry
Health services research
Healthcare Cost and Utilization Project (HCUP)
Healthcare Integrity and Protection Data Bank (HIPDB)
Index
Injury Severity Score (ISS)
Master patient index (MPI)

Medical Literature, Analysis, and Retrieval System Online (MED-LINE)

Medicare Provider Analysis and Review (MEDPAR)

National Center for Health Statistics (NCHS)

National Health Care Survey

National Practitioner Data Bank (NPDB)

NoSQL

Normalization

Operation index

Patient-identifiable data

Physician index

Population-based registry

Primary data source

Protocol

Public health

Registry

Relational database

Relationships

Schema mapping

Secondary data source

Staging system

Structured Query Language (SQL)

Traumatic injury

Unified Medical Language System (UMLS)

Vital statistics

As a rich source of data about an individual patient, the health record fulfills the uses of patient care and reimbursement for individual encounters. However, it is not easy to see trends in a population of patients by looking at individual records. For this purpose, data must be extracted from individual records and entered into specialized databases that support analysis across individual records. A database is an organized collection of data typically stored in a structured format in a computer system. These data may be used in a facility-specific or population-based registry for research and improvement in patient care. In addition, they may be reported to the state and become part of state- and federal-level databases that are used to set health policy and improve healthcare.

The health information management (HIM) professional can play a variety of roles in managing secondary records and databases. He or she plays a key role in helping to set up databases. This task includes determining the content of the database or registry and ensuring compliance with the laws, regulations, and accrediting standards that affect the content and use of the registry or database. All data elements included in the database or registry must be defined in a data dictionary. In this role, the HIM professional may oversee the completeness and accuracy of the data abstracted for inclusion in the database or registry.

This chapter explains the difference between primary and secondary data sources and their uses. It also offers an in-depth look at various types of secondary databases and how they are processed and maintained, as well as indexes and registries and their functions. The chapter examines relational and NoSQL database management systems, and explores data quality standards, models, and requirements.

Data and Data Sources

The health record is considered a **primary data source** because it contains information about a patient that has been documented by the professionals who provided care or services to that patient. Data taken from the primary health record and entered into registries and databases are considered a **secondary data source**.

Data also are categorized as either patient-identifiable data or aggregate data. The health record consists entirely of **patient-identifiable data**. In other words, every fact recorded in the record relates to a particular patient. Secondary data also may be patient identifiable. In some instances, data are entered into a database, along with information such as the patient's name, and maintained in an identifiable form. Registries are an example of patient-identifiable data on groups of patients.

More often, however, secondary data are considered aggregate data. **Aggregate data** include data on groups of people or patients without identifying any particular patient individually. Examples of aggregate data are statistics on the average length of stay (ALOS) for patients discharged within a particular diagnosis-related group (DRG).

Secondary data sources consist of facility-specific indexes; registries, either facility or population based; and other healthcare databases. Healthcare organizations maintain those indexes, registries, and databases that are relevant to their specific operations. States as well as the federal government also maintain databases to assess the health and wellness of their populations.

Secondary data sources provide information that is not easily available by looking at individual health records. With a diagnosis index, the task would involve simply looking at the list of diagnoses in numerical order and selecting those with the appropriate diagnosis code for, say, myocardial infarction for inclusion in a study.

Data extracted from health records and entered into disease-oriented databases can, for example, help researchers determine the effectiveness of alternate treatment methods. They also can quickly demonstrate survival rates at different stages of disease.

Internal users of secondary data are individuals located within the healthcare facility including medical staff and administrative and management staff. Secondary data enable these users to identify patterns and trends that are helpful in patient care, long-range planning, budgeting, and benchmarking with other facilities. External users of patient data are individuals and institutions outside the facility like state data banks and federal agencies. States have laws that mandate cases of patients with diseases such as tuberculosis and AIDS be reported to the state department of health. Moreover, the federal government collects data from the states on vital events such as births and deaths. The secondary data provided to external users is generally aggregate data and not patient-identifiable data. Thus, these data can be used as needed without risking breaches of confidentiality.

Check Your Understanding 6.1

Instructions: **Answer the following questions on a separate piece of paper.**

1. What is the difference between a primary data source and a secondary data source?
2. What is the difference between an internal and external user of secondary data sources?
3. Why are secondary data sources developed?
4. What is the difference between patient-identifiable data and aggregate data?
5. Who are the internal users within a healthcare facility?

Facility-Specific Indexes

The secondary data sources that have been in existence the longest are the indexes that have been developed within facilities to meet their individual needs. An **index** is simply a report from a database that enables health records to be located by diagnosis, procedure, or physician. Prior to extensive computerization in healthcare, these indexes were kept on cards with handwritten data. Now, indexes are computerized reports available from data included in databases routinely maintained in the healthcare facility. Most acute-care facilities maintain indexes described in the following sections.

Master Patient Index

The **master patient index (MPI)**, which is sometimes called the master person index, contains patient-identifiable data such as name, address, date of birth, dates of hospitalizations or encounters, name of attending physician, and health record number. The MPI is an important source of patient health record numbers. These numbers enable the facility to quickly retrieve health information for specific patients.

Hospitals with a unit numbering system also depend on the MPI to determine whether or not a patient has been seen in the facility before and, therefore, has an existing medical record number. Having this information in the MPI helps to avoid issuance of duplicate record numbers. (Refer to chapter 4 for more information on unit numbering and duplicate record numbers.) Most of the information in the MPI is entered into the facility database at the time of the admission, preadmission, or registration process.

Disease and Operation Indexes

In an acute care setting, the **disease index** is a listing in diagnosis code number order for patients discharged from the facility during a particular time period. Each patient's diagnoses are converted from a verbal description to a numerical code, usually using a coding system such as the International Classification of Diseases (ICD). In most cases, patient diagnosis codes are entered into the facility health information system as part of the discharge processing of the patient health record. The index always includes the patient's health record number as well as the diagnosis codes so that records can be retrieved by diagnosis. Because each patient is listed with the health record number, the disease

index is considered patient-identifiable data. The disease index also may include other information such as the attending physician's name or the date of discharge. In nonacute settings, the disease index might be generated to reflect patients currently receiving services in the facility.

The **operation index** is similar to the disease index except that it is arranged in numerical order by the patient's procedure code(s), usually using ICD or Current Procedural Terminology (CPT) codes. The other information listed in the operation index is generally the same as that listed in the disease index except that the surgeon may be listed in addition to, or instead of, the attending physician.

In many cases, facilities no longer have an actual listing for the diagnosis and operation indexes. Instead, they query the health information system utilizing the diagnosis or procedure code needed.

Physician Index

The **physician index** is a listing of cases in order by physician name or physician identification number. It also includes the patient's health record number and may include other information, such as date of discharge. The physician index enables users to retrieve information about a particular physician, including the number of cases seen during a particular time period. As with the disease and operation indexes, facilities generally query the health information system (HIS) to obtain physician data.

 ## Check Your Understanding 6.2

Instructions: **Answer the following questions on a separate piece of paper.**

1. How do HIM departments use facility-specific indexes?

2. What is the purpose of the master patient index? What types of information does it include?

3. What is an index?

4. What is the purpose of disease and operation indexes? What types of information do they include?

5. What is the purpose of the physician index? What types of information does it include?

Registries

Registries are different from indexes in that they contain more extensive data. Index reports can usually be produced using data from the facility's existing databases. Registries often require more extensive data from the patient record. Each registry must define the cases that are to be included. This process is called case definition. In a trauma registry, for example, the case definition might be all patients admitted with a diagnosis falling into ICD-10 code numbers S00 through S99, the trauma diagnosis codes.

After the cases to be included have been determined through the case definition process, the next step in collecting data is usually case finding. Case finding includes the methods used to identify the patients who have been seen and treated in the facility for the particular disease or condition of interest to the registry. After cases have been identified, extensive information is abstracted from the patient record into the registry database or fed from other databases and entered into the registry database.

The sole purpose of some registries is to collect data from the patient health record and to make them available to users. Other registries take further steps to enter additional information in the registry database, such as routine follow-up of patients at specified intervals. Follow-up might include rate and duration of survival and quality-of-life issues over time.

Cancer Registries

Cancer registries have a long history in healthcare. According to the National Cancer Registrars Association (NCRA), the first hospital registry was founded in 1926 at Yale-New Haven Hospital (NCRA 2014a). Aggregate clinical information is needed to improve the diagnosis and treatment of cancer. Cancer registries were developed as an organized method to collect these data. The registry may be a facility-based registry (located within a facility such as a hospital or clinic) or a population-based registry (gathering information from more than one facility within a geographic area such as a state or region).

The data from facility-based registries are used to provide information for the improved understanding of cancer, including its causes and methods of diagnosis and treatment. The data collected also may provide comparisons in survival rates and quality of life for patients with different treatments and at different stages of cancer at the time of diagnosis. In population-based registries, emphasis is on identifying trends and changes in the incidence (new cases) of cancer within the area covered by the registry.

The Cancer Registries Amendment Act of 1992 provided funding for a national program of cancer registries with population-based registries in each state. According to the law, these registries were mandated to collect data such as:

- Demographic information about each case of cancer
- Information on the industrial or occupational history of the individuals with the cancers (to the extent such information is available from the same record)
- Administrative information, including date of diagnosis and source of information
- Pathological data characterizing the cancer including site, stage of neoplasm, incidence, and type of treatment (CDC 2012)

Case Definition and Case Finding in the Cancer Registry

Case definition is the process of deciding what cases should be entered in the registry. In a cancer registry, for example, all cancer cases except certain skin cancers might meet the definition for the cases to be included. Skin cancers such as basal cell carcinomas might be excluded because they do not metastasize and do not require the follow-up necessary for other cancers included in the registry. Data on benign and borderline brain or central nervous system tumors must be collected according to the National Program of Cancer Registries (CDC 2015a).

In the facility-based cancer registry, the first step is case finding. One way to find cases is through the discharge process in the HIM department. During the discharge process, coders or HIM professionals can easily identify cases of patients with cancer for inclusion in the registry. Another case-finding method is to use the facility-specific disease indexes or the health information system to identify patients with diagnoses of cancer. Additional methods may include reviews of pathology reports and lists of patients receiving radiation therapy or other cancer treatments to determine cases that have not been found by other methods.

Population-based registries usually depend on hospitals, physician offices, radiation facilities, ambulatory surgery centers (ASCs), and pathology laboratories to identify and report cases to the central registry. The population-based registry has a responsibility to ensure that all cases of cancer in the target area have been identified and reported to the central registry. All cancer registry data is formally reported to the state central registry and the Centers for Disease Control (CDC 2015a)

Data Collection for the Cancer Registry

When a case is first entered in the registry, an accession number is assigned; this number is used to identify the patient. The accession number consists of the first digits of the year the patient was first seen at the facility, with the remaining digits assigned sequentially throughout the year. The first case in 2017, for example, might be 17-0001. The accession number may be assigned manually or by the automated cancer database used by the organization. An accession registry of all cases can be kept manually or provided as a report by the database software. This listing of patients in accession number order provides a way to monitor that all cases have been entered into the registry.

Data collection methods vary between facility-based registries and population-based registries. In a facility-based registry, data are initially obtained by reviewing and collecting them from the patient's health record. In addition to demographic information (such as name, health record number, address), patient data in a cancer registry include:

- Type and site of the cancer
- Diagnostic methodologies

- Treatment methodologies
- Stage at the time of diagnosis

Cancer staging is the process of determining the size and extent of spread of the tumor throughout the body. Historically, several different staging systems have been used. A staging system is a classification system that describes the extent of cancer within a patient. The American Joint Committee on Cancer (AJCC) through its Collaborative Stage Task Force has worked with other organizations with staging systems to develop a standardized data set called the Collaborative Stage Data Set, which uses computer algorithms to describe how far a cancer has spread (AJCC 2015).

Frequently, the population-based registry only collects information when the patient is diagnosed. Sometimes, however, it receives follow-up information from its reporting entities. These entities usually submit the information to the central registry electronically.

Reporting and Follow-up for Cancer Registry Data

Formal reporting of cancer registry data is done through an annual report which goes to the state central cancer registry and the Centers for Disease Control (CDC 2015a). The annual report includes aggregate data on the number of cases in the past year by site and type of cancer. It also may include information on patients by gender, age, and ethnic group. Often a particular site or type of cancer is featured with more in-depth data provided.

Other reports are provided as needed. Data from the cancer registry are frequently used in the quality assessment process for a facility as well as in research. Data on survival rates by site of cancer and methods of treatment, for example, would be helpful in researching the most effective treatment for a type of cancer.

Another activity of the cancer registry is patient follow-up. On an annual basis, the registry attempts to obtain information about each patient in the registry, including whether he or she is still alive, status of the cancer, and treatment received during the period. Various methods are used to obtain this information. For a facility-based registry, the facility's patient health records may be checked for return hospitalizations or visits for treatment. The patient's physician also may be contacted to determine whether the patient is still living and to obtain information about the cancer.

When patient status cannot be determined through these methods, an attempt may be made to contact the patient directly, using information in the registry such as address and telephone number of the patient and other contacts. In addition, contact information from the patient's health record may be used to request information from the patient's relatives. Other methods used include using the Internet to locate patients through sites such as the Social Security Death Index and online telephone books. The information obtained through follow-up is important to allow the registry to develop statistics on survival rates for particular cancers and different treatment methodologies.

Population-based registries do not always include follow-up information on the patients in their databases. They may, however, receive the information from the reporting entities such as hospitals, physician offices, and other organizations providing follow-up care.

Standards and Approval Agencies for Cancer Registries

Several organizations have developed standards or approval processes for cancer programs (see table 6.1). The American College of Surgeons (ACS) Commission on Cancer has an approval process for cancer programs. One of the requirements of this process is the existence of a cancer registry as part of the program. The ACS standards are published in the Cancer Program Standards (ACS 2012). When the ACS surveys the cancer program, part of the survey process is a review of cancer registry activities.

Table 6.1. Standard-setting or approval agencies for cancer registries

Agency	Type of registry
American College of Surgeons (ACS)	Facility based
North American Association of Central Cancer Registries (NAACCR)	Population based
Centers for Disease Control and Prevention (CDC)	Population based

The North American Association of Central Cancer Registries (NAACCR) has a certification program for state population-based registries. Certification is based on the quality of data collected and reported by the state registry. The NAACCR has developed standards for data quality and format, and it works with other cancer organizations to align their various standards sets (NAACCR 2015).

The Centers for Disease Control and Prevention (CDC) also has national standards regarding completeness, timeliness, and quality of cancer registry data from state registries through the National Program of Cancer Registries (NPCR) (CDC 2015b). The NPCR was developed as a result of the Cancer Registries Amendment Act of 1992. The CDC collects data from the NPCR state registries.

Education and Certification for Cancer Registrars

Traditionally, cancer registrars have been trained through on-the-job training and professional workshops and seminars. The National Cancer Registrar's Association (NCRA) has worked with colleges to develop formal educational programs for cancer registrars either through a certificate or an associate's degree program. A cancer registrar may become certified as a certified tumor registrar (CTR) by passing an examination provided by the National Cancer Registrars Association's certification board. Eligibility requirements for the certification examination include a combination of experience and education (NCRA 2014b).

Trauma Registries

Trauma registries maintain databases on patients with severe traumatic injuries. A **traumatic injury** is a wound or another injury caused by an external physical force such as an automobile accident, a shooting, a stabbing, or a fall. Examples of such injuries would include fractures, burns, and lacerations. Information collected by the trauma registry may be used for performance improvement and research in the area of trauma care. Trauma registries are usually facility-based but in some cases may include data for a region or state.

Case Definition and Case Finding for Trauma Registries

The case definition for the trauma registry varies from registry to registry. To find cases with trauma diagnoses, the trauma registrar may query the facility's health information system looking for cases with codes in the trauma section of ICD-10-CM. In addition, the registrar may look at deaths in services with frequent trauma diagnoses such as trauma, neurosurgery, orthopedics, and plastic surgery to find additional cases.

Data Collection for Trauma Registries

After the cases have been identified, information is abstracted from the health records of the injured patients and entered into the trauma registry database. The data elements collected in the abstracting process vary from registry to registry but usually include the following:

- Demographic information on the patient
- Information on the injury
- Care the patient received before hospitalization (such as care at another transferring hospital or care from an emergency medical technician who provided care at the scene of the accident or in transport from the accident site to the hospital)
- Status of the patient at the time of admission
- Patient's course in the hospital
- ICD diagnosis and procedure codes
- Abbreviated Injury Scale (AIS)
- Injury Severity Score (ISS)

The **Abbreviated Injury Scale** (AIS) reflects the nature of the injury and the severity (threat to life) by body system. It may be assigned manually by the registrar or generated as part of the database from data entered by the registrar. The **Injury Severity Score** (ISS) is an overall severity measurement calculated from the AIS scores for the three most severe injuries of the patient (Trauma.org 2008). The AIS and ISS classify and describe the severity of injuries and can be used for reporting registry activity.

Reporting and Follow-up for Trauma Registries

Reporting varies among trauma registries. An annual report is often developed to show the activity of the trauma registry. Other reports may be generated as part of the performance improvement process, such as self-extubation (patients removing their own tubes) and delays in abdominal surgery or patient complications. Some hospitals report data to the National Trauma Data Bank, a large database of aggregate data on trauma cases (ACS 2015). An example of the use of such population data is the number of head injuries from motorcycle accidents in a state to encourage passage of a helmet law.

Trauma registries may or may not do follow-up of the patients entered in the registry. When follow-up is done, emphasis is frequently on the patient's quality of life after a period of time. Unlike cancer, where physician follow-up is crucial to detect recurrence, many traumatic injuries do not require continued patient care over time. Thus, follow-up is often not given the same emphasis receives in cancer registries.

Standards and Agencies for Approval of Trauma Registries

The American College of Surgeons certifies levels I, II, III, and IV trauma centers. As part of its certification requirements, the ACS states that the level I trauma center, the type of center receiving the most serious cases and providing the highest level of trauma service, must have a trauma registry (ACS 2015). Refer to table 6.2 for a description of each trauma center level.

Education and Certification of Trauma Registrars

Trauma registrars may be registered health information technicians (RHITs), registered health information administrators (RHIAs), registered nurses (RNs), licensed practical nurses (LPNs), emergency medical technicians (EMTs), or other health professionals. Training for trauma registrars is accomplished through workshops and on-the-job training. The American Trauma Society (ATS), for example, provides core and advanced workshops for trauma registrars and also provides a certification examination for trauma registrars through its Registrar Certification Board. Certified trauma registrars have earned the certified specialist in trauma registry (CSTR) credential (ATS 2015).

Table 6.2. Trauma center levels and definitions

Trauma center level	Description
Level I	Able to provide total care for every aspect of injury from prevention through rehabilitation
Level II	Able to initiate definitive care for all injured patients
Level III	Able to provide prompt assessment, resuscitation, surgery, intensive care, and stabilization of injured patients and emergency operations
Level IV	Able to provide advanced trauma life support (ATLS) prior to transfer of patients to a higher level trauma center; provides evaluation, stabilization, and diagnostic capabilities for injured patients
Level V	Able to provide initial evaluation, stabilization, and diagnostic capabilities and prepares patients for transfer to higher levels of care

Source: ATS 2015.

Birth Defects Registries

Birth defects registries collect information on newborns with birth defects. Often population based, these registries serve a variety of purposes. For example, they provide information on the incidence of birth defects to study causes and prevention of birth defects, to monitor trends in birth defects to improve medical care for children with birth defects, and to target interventions for preventable birth defects such as folic acid to prevent neural tube defects.

In some cases, registries have been developed after specific events have put a spotlight on birth defects. After the initial Persian Gulf War, for example, some feared an increased incidence of birth defects among the children of Gulf War veterans. The Department of Defense subsequently started a birth defects registry to collect data on the children of these veterans to determine whether any pattern could be detected.

Case Definition and Case Finding for Birth Defects Registries

Birth defects registries use a variety of criteria to determine which cases to include in the registry. Some registries limit cases to those birth defects found within the first year of life. Others include those children with a major defect that occurred in the first year of life and was discovered within the first five years of life. Still other registries include only children who were liveborn or stillborn babies with discernible birth defects.

Cases may be detected in a variety of ways, including review of disease indexes, labor and delivery logs, pathology and autopsy reports, ultrasound reports, and cytogenetic reports. In addition to information from hospitals and physicians, cases may be identified from rehabilitation centers and children's hospitals and from vital records such as birth, death, and fetal death certificates.

Data Collection for Birth Defects Registries

A variety of information is abstracted for the birth defects registry, including:

- Demographics
- Codes for diagnoses
- Birth weight
- Status at birth, including liveborn, stillborn, aborted
- Autopsy
- Cytogenetics results
- Whether the infant was a single or multiple birth
- Mother's use of alcohol, tobacco, or illicit drugs
- Father's use of drugs and alcohol
- Family history of birth defects

Thus, these items are essential for tracking and trending birth anomalies.

Diabetes Registries

Diabetes registries collect data about patients with diabetes for the purpose of assistance in managing care as well as for research. Patients whose diabetes is not well managed frequently have numerous complications. The diabetes registry can keep up with whether the patient has been seen by a physician in an effort to prevent complications.

Case Definition and Case Finding for Diabetes Registries

There are two types of diabetes mellitus: insulin-dependent diabetes (type I) and non–insulin-dependent diabetes (type II). Registries sometimes limit their cases by type of diabetes. In some instances, there may be further definition by age; for example, some diabetes registries only include children with diabetes.

Case finding includes the review of health records of patients with diabetes. Other case-finding methods include the reviews of the following types of information:

- ICD diagnostic codes
- Billing data
- Medication lists
- Physician identification
- Health plans

Although facility-based registries for cancer and trauma are usually hospital based, facility-based diabetes registries are often maintained by physician offices and clinics because they are the main location for diabetes care. Thus, the data about the patient to be entered into the registry are available at these sites rather than at the hospital. Patient health records of diabetes patients in the physician practice may be identified through ICD-10 code numbers for diabetes, billing data for diabetes-related services, medication lists for patients on diabetic medications, or identification of patients as the physician sees them.

Health plans also are interested in optimal care for their enrollees because diabetes can have serious complications when not managed correctly. They may provide information to the office or clinic on diabetic enrollees in the health plan.

Data Collection for Diabetes Registries

In addition to demographic information about the cases, other data collected may include laboratory values such as HbA1c. This test is used to determine the patient's blood glucose level for a period of approximately 60 days prior to the time of the test. Moreover, facility registries may track patient visits to follow up with patients who have not been seen in the past year.

Reporting and Follow-up for Diabetes Registries

A variety of reports may be developed from the diabetes registry. For facility-based registries, one report may keep up with laboratory monitoring of the patient's diabetes to allow intensive intervention with patients whose diabetes is not well controlled. Another report might be of patients who have not been tested within a year or who have not had a primary care provider visit within a year.

Population-based diabetes registries might provide reporting on the incidence of diabetes for the geographic area covered by the registry. Registry data also may be used to investigate risk factors for diabetes.

Follow-up is aimed primarily at ensuring that the diabetic is seen by the physician at appropriate intervals to prevent complications.

Implant Registries

An implant is a material or substance inserted in the body, such as breast implants, heart valves, and pacemakers. Implant registries have been developed for the purpose of tracking the performance of implants, including complications, deaths, and defects resulting from implants, as well as longevity.

In the past, the safety of implants was an issue in a number of highly publicized cases. In some cases, implant registries have been developed in response to such events. For example, there have been questions from concerned citizens about the safety of silicone breast implants and temporomandibular joint implants. When such cases arise, it has often been difficult to ensure that all patients with the implant have been notified of safety concerns.

A number of federal laws have been enacted to regulate medical devices, including implants. These devices were first covered under Section 15 of the Food, Drug, and Cosmetic Act. The Safe Medical Devices Act of 1990 was passed and then amended through the Medical Device Amendments of 1992. These acts required facilities to report deaths and severe complications thought to be due to a device to the manufacturer and the Food and Drug Administration (FDA) through its MedWatch reporting system (FDA 2015; 2008). Implant registries can help in complying with the legal requirement for reporting for the sample of facilities required to report.

Data Collection for Implant Registries

Demographic data on patients receiving implants are included in the registry. The FDA requires that all reportable events involving medical devices include information on the following:

- User facility report number
- Name and address of the device manufacturer
- Device brand name and common name
- Product model, catalog, and serial and lot number
- Brief description of the event reported to the manufacturer or the FDA (FDA 2008)

Thus, these data items also should be included in the implant registry to facilitate reporting.

Reporting and Follow-up for Implant Registries

Data from the implant registry may be used to report to the FDA and the manufacturer when devices cause death or serious illness or injury. Follow-up is important to track the performance of the implant. When patients are tracked through the registry, they can be easily notified of product failures, recalls, or upgrades.

Transplant Registries

Transplant registries may have varied purposes. Some organ transplant registries maintain databases of patients who need organs. When an organ becomes available, an equitable way then may be used to allocate the organ to the patient with the highest priority. In other cases, the purpose of the registry is to provide a database of potential donors for transplants using live donors, such as bone marrow transplants. Posttransplant information also is kept on organ recipients and donors.

Because transplant registries are used to match donor organs with recipients, they are often national or even international in scope. Examples of national registries include the UNet of the United Network for Organ Sharing (UNOS) and the registry of the National Marrow Donor Program (NMDP).

Data collected in the transplant registry also may be used for research, policy analysis, and quality control projects.

Case Definition and Case Finding for Transplant Registries

Physicians identify patients needing transplants and information about the patient is provided to the registry. When an organ becomes available, information about it is matched with potential donors. For donor registries, donors are often solicited through community outreach efforts similar to those carried out by blood banks to encourage blood donations.

Data Collection for Transplant Registries

The type of information collected varies according to the type of registry. Pretransplant data about the recipient include:

- Demographics
- Patient's diagnosis
- Patient's status codes regarding medical urgency
- Patient's functional status
- Whether the patient is on life support
- Previous transplantations

Information on donors varies according to whether the donor is living. For organs harvested from patients who have died, information is collected on the following:

- Cause and circumstances of the death
- Organ procurement and consent process
- Medications the donor was taking
- Other donor history

For a living donor, information includes relationship of the donor to the recipient (if any), clinical information, and information on organ recovery.

Data collection is an integral component of transplant registries.

Reporting and Follow-up for Transplant Registries

Reporting includes information on donors and recipients as well as survival rates, length of time on the waiting list for an organ, and death rates. Follow-up information is collected for recipients as well as living donors. For living donors, the information collected might include complications of the procedure and length of stay (LOS) in the hospital. Follow-up information about recipients includes information on status at the time of follow-up (for example, living, dead, lost to follow-up), functional status, graft status, and treatment, such as immunosuppressive drugs. Follow-up is carried out at intervals throughout the first year after the transplant and then annually after that.

Immunization Registries

Children are encouraged to receive a large number of immunizations during the first six years of life. These immunizations are so important that the federal government has set several objectives related to immunizations in Healthy People 2020, a set of health goals for the nation (HHS 2016). These include increasing the proportion of children and adolescents who are fully immunized and increasing the proportion of children in population-based immunization registries.

Immunization registries usually have the purpose of increasing the number of infants and children who receive proper immunizations at the proper intervals. To accomplish this goal, they collect information within a particular geographic area about children and their immunization status. They also help by maintaining a central source of information for a particular child's immunization history, even when the child has received immunizations from a variety of providers. This central location for immunization data also relieves parents of the responsibility of maintaining immunization records for their own children.

Case Definition and Case Finding for Immunization Registries

All children in the population area served by the registry should be included in the registry. Some registries limit their inclusion of patients to those seen at public clinics, excluding those seen exclusively by private practitioners. Although children are usually targeted in immunization registries, some registries do include information on adults for influenza and pneumonia vaccines.

Children are often entered in the registry at birth. Registry personnel may review birth and death certificates and adoption records to determine what children to include and what children to exclude because they died after birth. In some cases, children are entered electronically through a connection with an electronic birth record system. Accuracy and completeness of the data in the registry are dependent on the thoroughness of the submitters in reporting immunizations.

Data Collection for Immunization Registries

The National Immunization Program at the CDC has worked with the National Vaccine Advisory Committee (NVAC) to develop a set of core immunization data elements to be included in all immunization registries. The data elements are divided into required and optional. The required data elements include (CDC 2015c):

- Patient's name (first, middle, and last)
- Patient's birth date
- Patient's sex
- Patient's birth state and country
- Mother's name (first, middle, last, and maiden)
- Vaccine type
- Vaccine manufacturer
- Vaccination date
- Vaccine lot number

Other optional items may be included, as needed, by the individual registry.

Reporting and Follow-up for Immunization Registries

Because the purpose of the immunization registry is to increase the number of children who receive immunizations in a timely manner, reporting should emphasize immunization rates, especially changes in rates in target areas. Immunization registries also can provide automatic reporting of children's immunization to schools to check the immunization status of their students.

Follow-up is directed toward reminding parents that it is time for immunizations as well as seeing whether the parents do not bring the child in for the immunization after a reminder. Moreover, registries must decide how frequently to follow up with parents who do not bring their children for immunization. Maintaining up-to-date addresses and telephone numbers is an important factor in providing follow-up. Registries may allow parents to opt out of the registry if they prefer not to be reminded.

Standards and Agencies for Approval of Immunization Registries

The CDC, through its National Immunization Program, provides funding for some population-based immunization registries. The CDC has identified 12 minimum functional standards for population-based immunization registries, including the following:

- Electronically store data on all NVAC-approved core data elements
- Establish a registry record within six weeks of birth for each newborn child born in the geographic area
- Enable access to and retrieval of immunization information in the registry at the time of the encounter
- Receive and process immunization information within one month of vaccine administration
- Protect the confidentiality of healthcare information
- Ensure the security of healthcare information
- Exchange immunization records using Health Level Seven (HL7) standards
- Automatically determine the routine childhood immunization(s) needed, in compliance with current Advisory Committee on Immunization Practices (ACIP) recommendations, when an individual presents for a scheduled immunization
- Automatically identify individuals due or late for an immunization(s) to enable the production of reminder or recall notifications
- Automatically produce immunization coverage reports by providers, age groups, and geographic areas
- Produce official immunization records
- Promote the accuracy and completeness of registry data (CDC 2015c)

The CDC provides funding for population-based immunization registries.

Other Registries

Registries may be developed for any type of disease or condition. Examples of other types of registries that are commonly kept include HIV/AIDS and cardiac registries.

In 2007, the state of Nebraska initiated a partnership within the state called the Nebraska Registry Partnership (NRP) to introduce, sustain, and gradually expand a registry for chronic disease management for cardiovascular diseases and diabetes care improvement for patients seen in rural health clinics.

In addition, the American Gastroenterological Association (AGA) sponsors the AGA Registry. The AGA Registry is the only gastroenterology registry sponsored by the Centers for Medicare and Medicaid Services (CMS), enabling practices to directly submit data for the CMS Physician Quality Reporting System (AGA 2011). It is a national outcomes-driven registry that allows clinicians to monitor and improve patient care while generating data to compare the efficacy of treatments.

A registry used to track cases of sudden unexpected infant deaths (SUIDs) represents a collaboration between the Centers for Disease Control and Prevention and the National Center for Child Death Review. The SUID Registry aims to improve knowledge of factors surrounding SUID events, create prevention strategies and interventions, and ultimately reduce SUIDs and injury-related infant deaths (Shapiro-Mendoza et al. 2012).

Registries may be developed for administrative purposes also. The National Provider Identifier (NPI) Registry is an example of an administrative registry. The NPI Registry enables users to search for a provider's national plan and provider enumeration system information, including the national provider identification number. The NPI number is a 10-digit unique identification number assigned to healthcare providers in the United States. There is no charge to use the registry, and it is updated daily. Data collected for healthcare administrative purposes are also discussed in the next section.

There is also a registry of patient registries. The Registry of Patient Registries (RoPR) is a database of registry specific information intended to promote collaboration, reduce redundancy, and improve transparency. The Agency for Healthcare Research and Quality (AHRQ) has designed and deployed the RoPR system to complement ClinicalTrials.gov by providing additional registry-specific data elements (RoPR 2015).

Check Your Understanding 6.3

Instructions: **Answer the following questions on a separate piece of paper.**

1. What is a registry? What is the purpose of a registry?

2. What is the difference between a facility-based registry and a population-based registry?

3. How is case definition different from case finding?

Answer questions 4 through 10 for each of the following registries: cancer, trauma, birth defects, diabetes, implant, transplant, and immunization.

4. What methods are used for case definition and case finding?

5. What methods of data collection are used?

6. What methods of reporting are used?

7. What methods of follow-up are used?

8. What standards are applicable, and what agencies approve or accredit the registry?

9. What education is required for registrars?

10. What certification is available for registrars? What agency or organization provides certification? What are the certification requirements?

Database Management and Design

Information retrieval and storage are at the heart of medical activities. Databases contain patient demographics, financial, and health-related data. They store information about supplies, staff, and system use. **Database management systems (DBMS)** are software tools used to store, analyze, modify, and access data.

Relational Databases

There are several types of database systems and DBMS can be characterized by the way they model data. **Relational databases** are the most widely used in numerous industries, including healthcare. This model consists of a database with a set of formally described tables, related (linked) to each other by a shared reference (Pratt and Adamski 2011). It is widely used because it offers a simple, yet powerful view of stored information. Developers can easily understand how information is organized and users can create their own interactive queries. It is flexible enough that databases can be simple or complex, and yet each part has an easy to understand representation. There are three steps to database design: conceptual, logical, and physical design. Figure 6.1 details the processes for each design phase.

Entity Relationship Modeling

The process of formalizing data requirements and the structure used to organize data is called **data modeling**. The most widely used form of data

Figure 6.1. Database design process

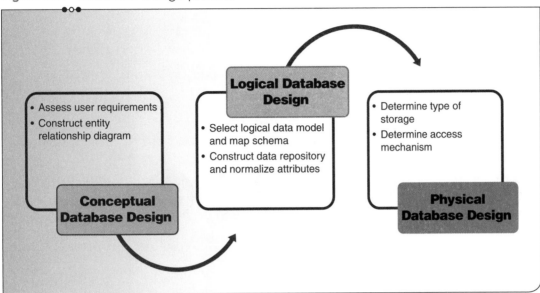

modeling is the entity relationship. It visually represents and defines groupings of data and their relationships to each other. It combines semantic modeling with object-oriented modeling (Sikha and Earp 2011). Semantic modeling is used by linguists to represent the meaning of words. Object-oriented modeling is used by computer programmers to develop systems that are analogous to the real world by formalizing concepts such as objects, their functions, and relationships. An **entity relationship diagram (ERD)** has three basic graphical symbols. First, there are entities, which are data objects represented as rectangles. An **entity** can be thought of as a class of objects that exist in the real world and have related properties. Entities can be a type of person, place, or thing. Second, there are **attributes**, which describe characteristics and are represented as circles. Third, there are **relationships**, which describe associations between entities and are represented with diamonds.

Entity relationship modeling is a type of conceptual modeling. Conceptual models are abstract and encourage high-level problem structuring; they help establish a common ground for communication between users and developers. They also help developers understand how an existing model can be modified. ERDs are used often in conceptual design; an example of an entity relationship is displayed in figure 6.2.

ERDs are converted into tables by a process called **schema mapping** (Sikha and Earp 2011). There are a few simple rules used for mapping. The main rule used to determine table structure is based on the **cardinality** of the relationship (the maximum number of occurrences of each entity that occurrences of other entities can link to). For example, if a patient can have only one doctor, the mapping would be different from a model where the patient can link to multiple doctors. The type of relationship and the unique identifier (for example, patient ID and visit ID in figure 6.2) for each entity further determine how tables will be arranged.

Entity relationship diagramming is a very useful process because it helps reduce errors. Intrinsic to the process is **normalization**, which eliminates errors associated with updates, deletions, and insertions of data into the database. This reduces redundancy and improves data quality. Mapping and normalization is done as a part of the logical database design.

Database Implementation

Implementing the database using a specific DBMS is the goal of the physical design phase. In this phase, designers select a storage system, translate the data model from the logical design phase into a physical representation, create indexes for ease

Figure 6.2. Example of an entity relationship

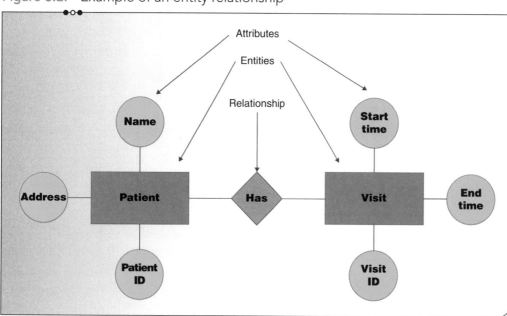

of access, and grant user access rights (Pratt and Adamski 2011). Designers must make decisions based on the specific type of DBMS used. The most popular type of DBMS is the relational database management system (RDBMS). RDBMS follow a set of integrity rules that ensure accuracy and accessibility.

Structured Query Language

Structured Query Language (SQL) is the formal language used to retrieve information stored in relational databases. SQL defines a number of operations, or activities, which can be used to access data across tables based on a set of conditionals (Pratt and Adamski 2011). The following example shows a query to select patient names from a patient table where the gender is female:

> SELECT patient_name FROM patients WHERE gender='f';

In this example, the operator "select" indicates what data to get. The keyword "from" specifies the table or tables to access. The "where" keyword indicates the criteria for selection, in this case gender='f'. The above example is a simple one. SQL's syntax consists of many operators and conditionals. It is a flexible language that can be used for almost any Information need.

NoSQL Data Model and Use

Though relational databases are an industry standard, there have been several other DBMS through the years. The most recent model to increase in use is **NoSQL** (or not only SQL) database management system (Leavitt 2010). It differs from the relational model in that it does not provide a table-based representation. It uses either a document or graph-oriented model. It has two main advantages over other DBMS. First, it has a fast response time for large datasets. This is in part due to the fact that it does not distribute data across tables but holds data in one central place. Second, it scales out rather than up (Pokorny 2013). In this context, scaling out means that as the DBMS needs more storage space, new machines can be bought to link to existing DBMS storage machines without the need to migrate the entire database. Relational DBMS scale up, which means that when there is a need for more storage, a new larger machine must be acquired that can store all data in the DBMS. This can be costly and time-consuming.

Despite the advantages listed, NoSQL is not as useful for critical data. Relational databases have a predefined schema design to reduce errors while NoSQL databases have dynamic schemas for less well-structured data. Relational databases also allow for more complex queries. There are, however, several use-cases in healthcare settings where a NoSQL database would be useful in conjunction with relational databases. For example, clinical data is heterogeneous, often disjoined, and stored on a large scale, making access to pertinent patient information sometimes difficult and frequently time-consuming (Wasan et al. 2006). NoSQL can be used to generate aggregated views of patient data in one place in less time than a relational database (Lee et al. 2013). Additionally, real-time analytics and visualizations are easier to achieve for patient trend analysis and hospital statistics because the data model is less rigid (Mazurek 2014).

Check Your Understanding 6.4

Instructions: Answer the following questions on a separate piece of paper.

1. What are the three phases of database design?

2. What are the advantages of entity-relationship modeling?

3. What advantages do NoSQL databases have over relational databases?

4. What advantage does a relational database have over a NoSQL database?

5. What does SQL stand for?

Healthcare Databases

Databases may be developed for a variety of purposes. The federal government, for example, has developed a wide variety of databases to enable it to carry out surveillance, improvement, and prevention duties. Health information managers may provide information for these databases through data abstraction or from data reported by a facility to state and local entities. They also may use these data to do research or work with other researchers on issues related to reimbursement and health status.

There are concerns about collecting healthcare data in an environment without clear guidance about ownership of secondary data, unauthorized reuse of data, and spotty confidentiality and security regulations. Patients have concerns that secondary data collected about them may adversely affect their employment or ability to obtain health insurance. It is much more difficult for patients to determine what information about them is maintained in secondary databases than it is to view their primary health records. Although facilities utilize secondary data under the "healthcare operations" section of the Health Insurance Portability and Accountability Act (HIPAA), patients must be made aware of this practice through the Notification of Privacy Practices.

National and State Administrative Databases

Some databases are established for administrative rather than disease-oriented reasons. Data banks are developed, for example, for claims data submitted on Medicare claims. Other administrative databases assist in the credentialing and privileging of health practitioners.

Medicare Provider Analysis and Review File

The **Medicare Provider Analysis and Review** (**MEDPAR**) file is made up of acute-care hospital and skilled nursing facility (SNF) claims data for all Medicare claims. It consists of the following types of data:

- Demographic data on the patient
- Data on the provider
- Information on Medicare coverage for the claim
- Total charges
- Charges broken down by specific types of services, such as operating room, physical therapy, and pharmacy charges
- ICD-10-CM diagnosis and procedure codes
- DRGs

The MEDPAR file is frequently used for research on topics such as charges for particular types of care and analysis by DRG. The limitation of the MEDPAR data for research purposes is that it only contains data about Medicare patients.

National Practitioner Data Bank

The **National Practitioner Data Bank (NPDB)** was mandated under the Health Care Quality Improvement Act of 1986 to provide a database of medical malpractice payments; adverse licensure actions including revocations, suspensions, reprimands, censures, probations, and surrenders of licenses for quality-of-care purposes only; and certain professional review actions (such as denial of medical staff privileges) taken by healthcare entities such as hospitals against physicians, dentists, and other healthcare providers (NPDB 2006). The NPDB was developed to address the lack of information on malpractice decisions, denial of medical staff privileges, or loss of medical license. Because these data were not widely available, physicians could move to another state or another facility and begin practicing again with the current state or facility unaware of the previous actions against the physician.

Information in the NPDB is provided through a required reporting mechanism. Entities making malpractice payments, including insurance companies, boards of medical examiners, and entities such as hospitals and professional societies, must report to the NPDB. The information to be reported includes information on the practitioner, the

reporting entity, and the judgment or settlement. Information on physicians must be reported. The law requires entities such as private accrediting organizations and peer review organizations to report adverse actions to the data bank (NPDB 2006). In addition, adverse licensure and other actions against any healthcare entity must be reported, not just physicians and dentists. Monetary penalties may be assessed for failure to report.

The law requires healthcare facilities to query the NPDB as part of the credentialing process when a physician initially applies for medical staff privileges and every two years thereafter (NPDB 2006). (See chapter 21 for more detail on the physician credentialing process.)

Healthcare Integrity and Protection Data Bank

Part of HIPAA mandated the collection of information on healthcare fraud and abuse because there was no central place to obtain this information. As a result, the national **Healthcare Integrity and Protection Data Bank (HIPDB)** was developed. The types of items that must be reported to the data bank include reportable final adverse actions such as:

- Federal or state licensing and certification actions, including revocations, reprimands, censures, probations, suspensions, and any other loss of license; or the right to apply for or renew a license, whether by voluntary surrender, non-renewability, or otherwise
- Exclusions from participation in federal or state healthcare programs
- Any other adjudicated actions or decisions defined in the HIPDB regulations (HHS 2008)

There may be some overlap with the National Practitioner Data Bank, so a single report is made and then sorted to the appropriate data bank. Information to be reported includes information on the healthcare provider, supplier, or practitioner that is the subject of the final adverse action, the nature of the act, and a description of the actions on which the decision was based. Only federal and state government agencies and health plans are required to report, and access to the data bank is limited to these organizations and to practitioners, providers, and suppliers who may only query about themselves.

State Administrative Data Banks

States also frequently have health-related administrative databases. Many states, for example, collect either Uniform Hospital Discharge Data Set (UHDDS) or UB-04 data on patients discharged from hospitals located within their area. The State-wide Planning and Research Cooperative System (SPARCS) in New York is an example of this type of administrative database. It combines UB-04 data with data required by the state of New York.

National, State, and County Public Health Databases

Public health is the area of healthcare dealing with the health of populations in geographic areas such as states or counties. Publicly reported healthcare data vary from quality and patient safety measurement data to patient satisfaction results. The aggregated data range from a local to national perspective, such as state-specific public health conditions to national morbidity and mortality statistics. In addition, consumers are becoming more actively involved in their healthcare. Publicly reported data may be presented for consumer use through various star ratings on different quality measures via organizations such as the Leapfrog Group, HealthGrades, or Hospital Compare. One of the duties of public health agencies is the surveillance of health status within their jurisdiction.

Databases developed by public health departments provide information on the incidence and prevalence of diseases, possible high-risk populations, survival statistics, and trends over time. Data for these databases may be collected using a variety of methods including interviews, physical examination of individuals, and review of health records. At the national level, the **National Center for Health Statistics (NCHS)** has responsibility for these databases. NCHS provides a database of statistical health information to guide public health action and health policy making. Their website provides information on population health status and trends in health status and care delivery (CDC 2015d).

National Health Care Survey

One of the major national public health surveys is the **National Health Care Survey**. To a large extent, it relies on data from patient health records. It consists of a number of databases, including:

- National Hospital Care Survey
- National Survey of Ambulatory Surgery
- National Nursing Home Survey
- National Home and Hospice Care Survey

Table 6.3 lists the component databases of the National Health Care Survey (NHCS), along with their corresponding data sources.

The National Health Care Survey combines the National Hospital Discharge Survey (NHDS) and the National Hospital Ambulatory Medical Care Survey (NHAMCS). The integration of the two surveys allows for examination of care provided across treatment settings. Information on the utilization of healthcare provided in inpatient settings, emergency departments, outpatient departments, and ambulatory surgery centers are collected in one place.

Data for the National Survey of Ambulatory Surgery are collected on a representative sample of hospital-based and freestanding ambulatory surgery centers. Data include patient demographic characteristics, source of payment, information on anesthesia given, the diagnoses, and the surgical and nonsurgical procedures on patient visits to hospital-based and freestanding ambulatory surgery centers. The survey consists of a mailed survey about the facility and abstracts of patient data.

The National Nursing Home Survey provides data on the facility, current residents, and discharged residents. Information is gathered through an interview process. The administrator or designee provides information about the facility. For information on the residents, the nursing staff member most familiar with the resident's care is interviewed. The staff member uses the resident's health record for reference in the interview. Data collected on the facility include information on ownership, size, certification status, admissions, services, full-time equivalent employees, and basic charges. Both the current and discharged resident interviews provide demographic information

Table 6.3. Components of the National Health Care Survey

Database	Type of setting	Content	Data source	Method of data collection
National Hospital Care Survey (NHCS)	Inpatient, emergency, outpatient, ambulatory surgery centers	Uniform Hospital Discharge Data Set and data on the patient and the visit	Discharged patient records	Abstract
National Survey of Ambulatory Surgery	Hospital-based and freestanding ambulatory surgery centers	Data on the facility and patients	Facility response to survey and patient records	Survey and abstract
National Nursing Home Survey	Nursing home	Data on the facility and current and discharged residents	Administrator; nurse caregiver	Interview
National Home and Hospice Care Survey	Home health and hospice	Facility data and patient data	Administrator; caregiver	Interview

on the resident as well as length of stay, diagnoses, level of care received, activities of daily living (ADLs), and charges.

For the National Home and Hospice Care Survey, data are collected on the home health or hospice agency as well as on its current and discharged patients. Data include referral and length of service, diagnoses, number of visits, patient charges, health status, reason for discharge, and types of services provided. Facility data are obtained through an interview with the administrator or designee. Patient information is obtained from the caregiver most familiar with the patient's care. The caregiver may use the patient's health record in answering the interview questions.

Other national public health databases include the National Health Interview Survey, which is used to monitor the health status of the population of the United States, and the National Immunization Survey, which collects data on the immunization status of children between the ages of 19 months and 35 months living in the United States.

State and local public health departments also develop databases as needed to perform their duties of health surveillance, disease prevention, and research. An example of a state database is the infectious and notifiable disease database. Each state has a list of diseases that must be reported to the state—such as AIDS, measles, and syphilis—so that containment and prevention measures may be taken to avoid large outbreaks. These state and local reporting systems will be connected with the CDC through National Electronic Disease Surveillance System (NEDSS) to evaluate trends in disease

outbreaks. Statewide databases and registries also may collect extensive information on particular diseases and conditions such as birth defects, immunization, and cancer.

Because of bioterrorism scares in recent years, the CDC developed the NEDSS, which serves as a major part of the Public Health Information Network (PHIN). It provides a national surveillance system by connecting the CDC with local and state public health partners. This integrated system allows the CDC to monitor trends from disease reporting at the local and state level to look for possible bioterrorism incidents.

Vital Statistics

Vital statistics include data on births, deaths, fetal deaths, marriages, and divorces. Responsibility for the collection of vital statistics rests with the states and then the states share information with NCHS. The actual collection of the information is carried out at the local level. For example, birth certificates are completed at the facility where the birth occurred and are then sent to the state. The state serves as the official repository for the certificates and provides vital statistics information to NCHS. From the vital statistics collected, states and the national government develop a variety of databases and statistics about vital events in the state or country.

One vital statistics database at the national level is the Linked Birth and Infant Death Data Set. In this database, the information from birth certificates is compared to death certificates for infants who die under one year of age. This database provides data to conduct analyses for patterns of infant death. Other national programs that use vital statistics data include the National Mortality Followback Survey, the National Survey of Family Growth, and the National Death Index (CDC 2015e). In some of these databases, such as the National Mortality Followback Survey, additional information is collected on deaths originally identified through the vital statistics system.

Similar databases using vital statistics data as a basis are found at the state level. Birth defects registries, for example, frequently use vital records data with information on the birth defect as part of their data collection process.

Clinical Trials Databases

A clinical trial is a research project in which new treatments and tests are investigated to determine whether they are safe and effective. The trial proceeds according to a protocol, which is the list of rules and procedures to be followed. Clinical trials databases have been developed to allow physicians and patients to find clinical trials. For example, a patient with cancer or AIDS might be interested in participating in a clinical trial but not know how to locate one applicable to his or her type of disease. Clinical trials databases provide the data to enable patients and practitioners to determine what clinical trials are available and applicable to the patient.

The Food and Drug Administration Modernization Act of 1997 mandated that a clinical trials database be developed. The National Library of Medicine has developed the database, called ClinicalTrials.gov, which is available on the Internet for use by both patients and practitioners (NLM 2008). Information in the database includes the following:

- Abstracts of clinical study protocols
- Summary of the purpose of the study
- Recruiting status
- Criteria for patient participation
- Location of the trial and specific contact information

- Additional information (may help a patient decide whether or not to consider a particular trial)
- Research study design
- Phase of the trial
- Disease or condition and drug or therapy under study

Each data element has been defined. For example, the brief summary gives an overview of the treatments being studied and types of patients to be included. The location of the trial tells where the trial is being carried out so that patients can select trials in convenient locations. Recruitment status indicates whether subjects are currently being entered in the trial or will be in the future or whether the trial is closed to new subjects. Eligibility criteria include information on the type of condition to be studied, in some cases the stage of the disease, and what other treatments are allowed during the trial or must have been completed before entering the trial. Age is also a frequent eligibility criterion. Study types include diagnostic, genetic, monitoring, natural history, prevention, screening, supportive care, training, and treatment (McCray and Ide 2000, 316). Study design includes the research design being followed.

A clinical trial consists of four study phases.

- Phase I studies—Research the safety of the treatment in a small group of people
- Phase II studies—Determine the treatment's effectiveness and further investigate safety
- Phase III studies—Look at effectiveness and side effects and make comparisons to other available treatments in larger populations
- Phase IV studies—Look at the treatment after it has entered the market

Some clinical trials databases concentrate on a particular disease. The National Cancer Institute sponsors the Physician Data Query (PDQ), a database for cancer clinical trials. These databases contain information similar to ClinicalTrials.gov. Although ClinicalTrials.gov has been set up for use by both patients and health practitioners, some databases are more oriented to practitioners.

Health Services Research Databases

Health services research is research concerning healthcare delivery systems, including organization and delivery and care effectiveness and efficiency. Within the federal government, the organization most involved in health services research is the Agency for Healthcare Research and Quality (AHRQ). AHRQ looks at issues related to the efficiency and effectiveness of the healthcare delivery system, disease protocols, and guidelines for improved disease outcomes. AHRQ also provides access to different types of data that are primarily used for quality and utilization management purposes.

A major initiative for AHRQ has been the Healthcare Cost and Utilization Project (HCUP). HCUP uses data collected at the state level from either claims data from the UB-04 or discharge-abstracted data, including UHDDS items reported by individual hospitals and, in some cases, by freestanding ambulatory care centers. Which data are reported depends on the individual state. Data may be reported by the facilities to a state agency or to the state hospital association, depending on state regulations. The data are then reported from the state to AHRQ, where they become part of the HCUP databases.

HCUP consists of the following set of databases:

- Nationwide Inpatient Sample (NIS) consists of inpatient discharge data from a sample of hospitals in 35 states throughout the United States

- State Inpatient Database (SID) includes data collected by states on hospital discharges

- State Ambulatory Surgery Databases (SASD) include information from a sample of states on hospital-affiliated ASCs and, from some states, data from freestanding surgery centers

- State Emergency Department Databases include data from hospital-affiliated emergency departments (EDs)

- Abstracts for visits that do not result in a hospitalization

- Kids Inpatient Database (KID) is made up of inpatient discharge data on children younger than 19 years

These databases are unique because they include data on inpatients whose care is paid for by all types of payers including Medicare, Medicaid, and private insurance as well as by self-paying and uninsured patients. Data elements include demographic information, information on diagnoses and procedures, admission and discharge status, payment sources, total charges, length of stay, and information on the hospital or freestanding ambulatory surgery center. Researchers may use these databases to look at issues such as those related to the costs of treating particular diseases, the extent to which treatments are used, and differences in outcomes and cost for alternative treatments.

National Library of Medicine

The National Library of Medicine produces two databases of special interest to the HIM professional: MEDLINE and UMLS.

Medical Literature, Analysis, and Retrieval System Online

Medical Literature, Analysis, and Retrieval System Online (MEDLINE) is the best-known database from the National Library of Medicine. It includes bibliographic listings for publications in the areas of medicine, dentistry, nursing, pharmacy, allied health, and veterinary medicine. HIM professionals use MEDLINE to locate articles on HIM issues as well as articles on medical topics necessary to carry out quality improvement and medical research activities.

Unified Medical Language System

The Unified Medical Language System (UMLS) provides a way to integrate biomedical concepts from a variety of sources to show their relationships. This process allows links to be made between different information systems for purposes such as the electronic health record. UMLS is of particular interest to the HIM professional because medical classifications such as ICD-10-CM, CPT, and the Healthcare Common Procedure Coding System (HCPCS) are among the items included. UMLS is covered in more detail in chapter 5.

Check Your Understanding 6.5

***Instructions:* Answer the following questions on a separate piece of paper.**

1. What information is included in the Medicare Provider Analysis and Review file?

2. What limitations are encountered when using MEDPAR data in research?

3. What types of information must be reported to the National Practitioner Data Bank and the Healthcare Integrity and Protection Data Bank? Do the two data banks overlap in any way?

4. Why is the UMLS of interest to HIM professionals?

5. How do healthcare organizations use the National Practitioner Data Bank? Who may use the HIPDB?

6. What is included in the Medical Literature, Analysis, and Retrieval System Online (MEDLINE)?

7. What is the source of data for the Healthcare Cost and Utilization Project?

8. Why was the National Practitioner Data Bank developed? What law requires its use?

9. Why was the Healthcare Integrity and Protection Data Bank developed? What law requires its use?

Processing and Maintenance of Secondary Databases

Several issues surround the processing and maintenance of secondary databases. HIM professionals are often involved in decisions concerning these issues.

Manual Versus Automated Methods of Data Collection

Although registries and databases are almost universally computerized, data collection is sometimes done manually. The most frequent method is **abstracting**, the process of reviewing the patient health record and entering the required data elements into the database. In some cases, the abstracting may initially be done on an abstract form. The data then would be entered into the database from the form. In many cases, it is done directly from the primary patient health record into a data collection screen in the computerized database system.

Not all data collection is done manually. In some cases, data can be downloaded directly from other electronic systems. Birth defects registries, for example, often download information on births and birth defects from the vital records system. In some cases, providers such as hospitals and physicians send information in electronic format to the registry or database. The National Hospital Care Survey from the National Center for Health Statistics uses information in electronic format from state databases. As the electronic health record (EHR) develops further, less and less data will need to be manually abstracted since it will be available electronically through the EHR.

Vendor Systems Versus Facility-Specific Systems

Each registry must determine what information technology solution best meets its needs. In some cases that will be a vendor-created product specifically for registries. In other cases, the registry system may be part of an overall facility health information system. It is important that either type of product is able to incorporate demographic and other pertinent information from the facility health information system. In this way, time is saved and data integrity between the registry information and the health information system is maintained. If registries utilize registry applications as part of a facility-wide health information system, it is important that the registry manager be included in the decision of which health information system to purchase for the facility as well as in pertinent training and implementation decisions.

Data Security and Confidentiality Issues

For HIPAA-covered entities, the data collection done by registries is considered part of healthcare operations. The patient does not, therefore, have to sign an authorization for release of protected health information (PHI) to be included in the registry. Reporting of notifiable diseases to the state falls under "required reporting" and does not require patient authorization for release (AHIMA 2003, 7). Release of information to requestors other than the state will depend on the requestor. Data may be released to internal users, such as physicians for research, without the patient's consent as well because research also comes under healthcare operations. External users, such as the American College of Surgeons, collect aggregate data from facilities so individual patient authorization is not required. Information about patients that may be included in registries or other secondary data sources and reported to outside entities must be included in the facility's Notice of Privacy Practices given to each patient on his or her initial encounter. Through this mechanism, patients are made aware that data about them may be reported to outside entities.

HIPAA security regulations also apply to data in registries and indexes. These regulations require policies in the areas of administrative, technical, and physical security, which are discussed here. (See chapter 11 for further discussion of privacy, security, and confidentiality.)

Not all registries and databases are covered under HIPAA if they do not bill for patient care services. Central registries would be an example of a registry that is not covered under HIPAA. In such cases, the general norms for data security and confidentiality should be followed.

Data Security

Registries and secondary databases must ensure the security of the information that they maintain. A number of methods such as passwords and role-based access may be used to ensure that only authorized people have access to patient data in the facility's computer system. Loss of data is another important consideration in data security that could severely affect registries and secondary data sources. Although data sometimes are lost as a result of unauthorized access, more often they are lost in more routine ways such as computer malfunction or computer viruses that can cause data to be erased or lost.

Data Privacy and Confidentiality

Maintaining the privacy and confidentiality of health data is a traditional role of HIM professionals. When looking at methods to protect secondary records, patient-specific information requires more control than secondary databases that include only aggregate data because individual patients cannot be identified in aggregate data. Policies on who may access the data provide the basic protection for confidentiality.

The type of data maintained also may affect policies on confidentiality. For many of the government databases discussed previously, the information is aggregate and the data are readily available to any interested users. For example, public health data are frequently published in many formats, including printed reports, Internet access, and direct computer access.

As is true of all employees working with patient data, employees working with data in indexes, registries, and databases should receive training on confidentiality. Further, they should be required to sign a yearly statement indicating that they have received the training and understand the implications of failure to maintain confidentiality of the data. (Refer to chapter 11 for more information in these areas.)

Trends in the Collection of Secondary Data

The most significant trend in collecting secondary data is the increased use of automated data entry. Registries and databases are more commonly using data already available in electronic form rather than manually abstracting all data. As the EHR becomes more common, the need for separate databases for various diseases and conditions such as cancer, diabetes, and trauma is becoming unnecessary. The patient health record itself is shifting into a database that can be queried for information currently obtained from specialized registries.

Since not all data can currently be entered through automated means, other facilities are using existing technologies such as point-of-care data collection at the patient's bedside using wireless technology (Free et al. 2013). Finally, secondary data collection is becoming more common and more secondary data are being collected about patients. Because of this fact, national stakeholders such as the American Medical Informatics Association (AMIA) and the National Center for Vital and Health Statistics (NCVHS) are becoming more involved in setting national policy related to secondary data. One of the issues of concern is the ownership of secondary data. As stated in an AHIMA practice brief, "'Who can do what to which data and under which circumstances' is really the central question that must be asked in determining the rights and responsibilities of each stakeholder" (Burrington-Brown and Hjort 2007). Stakeholders include patients, health facilities, HIE organizations, vendors, governmental agencies, employers, and researchers. There is currently no clear-cut guidance on the sometimes conflicting rights and responsibilities of each stakeholder of the data.

As more secondary data are collected, the role of the HIM professional remains that of data steward. According to AMIA, data stewardship "encompasses the responsibilities and accountabilities associated with managing, collecting, viewing, storing, sharing, disclosing, or otherwise making use of personal health information" (AMIA 2006). These are traditional roles for the HIM professional in relationship to primary data. It will be necessary for these roles to be expanded to encompass secondary data.

Check Your Understanding 6.6

Instructions: **Answer the following questions on a separate piece of paper.**

1. What trends are evident in the collection of secondary data?
2. What is abstracting?
3. What is data stewardship?
4. Give an example of data collected electronically.
5. Into what format is the patient health record shifting?

Data Quality

Healthcare delivery systems are increasingly using quality metrics to benchmark and assess quality of care, and inform improvement initiatives. Effectively data management requires attention to data quality, otherwise data comparison and aggregation are not possible, and effective measurement cannot be done.

Data Quality Standards

For quality measurements to be constructive, data must conform to recognized standards. However, there are no universally accepted set of healthcare quality guidelines, which hinders health information managers from ensuring data quality. One reason for this is that the quality of the data needed in any situation is driven by how the data or the information that comes from the data will be used. For example, in a patient care setting the margin of error for critical lab tests must be zero or patient safety is in jeopardy. However, a larger margin of error may be acceptable in census counts or discharge statistics. Healthcare organizations must establish data quality standards specific to the intended use of the data or resulting information.

Although no universally adopted healthcare data standards exist, two organizations have published guidance that can assist healthcare organizations in establishing their own data quality standards. In *Healthcare Documentation: A Report on Information Capture and Report Generation,* the Medical Records Institute (MRI; 2002, 9) has published a set of "essential principles of healthcare documentation," and the American Health Information Management Association (AHIMA) has published the data quality management model (Wager et al. 2005).

MRI Principles of Healthcare Documentation

AHIMA defines documentation as "the methods and activities of collecting, coding, ordering, storing, and retrieving information to fulfill future tasks" (AHIMA e-HIM Workgroup of Assessing and Improving Healthcare Data Quality in the EHR 2007, 66). The MRI report states that many steps must be taken to ensure the quality of healthcare documentation (and, thus, the quality of healthcare data). It lists the essential principles to which healthcare organizations should adhere as they establish healthcare documentation and information systems (and their accompanying policies). (See figure 6.3.) The MRI recommends that these principles be uniformly adopted by healthcare organizations. It is noteworthy that the MRI takes the position that when practitioners interact with electronic resources, their ability to adhere to these principles is increased. All documentation records data and information, which need to be retrieved in order to be used. The MRI argues that all healthcare information should be indexed "to facilitate both clinical and administrative retrieval" (MRI 2002, 16). This is difficult to do with unstructured, free text, such as handwriting, e-mails, and transcription. As electronic medical records are implemented and information capture methods become more

interactive. The ability to retrieve information will improve. Figure 6.3 details documentation systems components and major information capture.

AHIMA Data Quality Model

AHIMA Data Quality Management Task Force (2012) has published a data quality model and an accompanying set of general data characteristics. The model is used as a framework for the design and management process and data quality measures. There are some similarities between the AHIMA characteristics and the MRI essential principles (refer to figures 6.4 and 6.3 respectively). However, one difference is that AHIMA strives to include all healthcare data and limits characteristics to clinical documentation. Figure 6.4 illustrates AHIMA's data quality model.

Data Quality Requirements for Information Systems

In addition to the 10 characteristics of data quality, AHIMA has published data quality best practices:

- Access permissions: Define and enforce access to data.
- Data dictionary: A data dictionary exists and each data element is defined. The definitions are communicated to all staff.
- Standardized format: Use a standardized format to ensure consistency.
- State and federal laws: All laws, regulations, accreditation standards, and policies are followed.
- Data Integrity: Implement policies and procedures throughout the patient encounter to ensure data integrity (AHIMA e-HIM Workgroup of Assessing and Improving Healthcare Data Quality in the EHR 2007).

Users must be involved in defining their information needs and designing information systems. One of the first steps in systems analysis is to identify the users' specific data needs. As part of this process, it is important to identify the level of quality the user requires for each data element. Another way to view this is to evaluation the use of the data along the AHIMA model's 10 characteristics of data quality. This evaluation eventually will

Figure 6.3. MRI Consensus Workgroup essential principles of healthcare documentation

Unique identification of patient

Systems, policies, and practices should:
• Provide unique patient identification at the time of recording or accessing information

Provide within and across organizations:
• Simple and easy methods to identify individuals and correct duplicate identities methods to distinguish between individuals
• Linkages between different identifications of the same individual

Accuracy

Systems, policies, and practices should:
• Promote accuracy of information throughout all information process
• Require review to assure accuracy prior to record insertion

• Include a means to append correction without altering the original
• Require the use of standard terminology so as to diminish misinterpretations

Completeness

Systems, policies, and practices should:
• Identify minimum set of information required to describe an incident, observation, or intent.
• Provide means to ensure information meets legal, regulatory, institutional, and other policies

• Discourage nonrelevant and excessive documentation
• Link to amendments to the original document
• Discourage duplication of informationv

Timeliness

Systems, policies, and practices should:
• Require and facilitate that healthcare documentation be done during or immediately following healthcare event
• Promote rapid system response time for entry as well as retrievability

Provide for automatic, unalterable time, date, and place stamp of each:
• Documentation entry
• Documentation access
• Documentation Transmittal

Interoperability

Systems, policies, and practices should:
• Provide highest level of interoperability
• Enable authorized practitioners to capture, share, and report healthcare information from any system

• Support ways to document healthcare information so that it can be correctly read, integrated, and supplemented within any other system in the same or another organization

Figure 6.3. Continued.

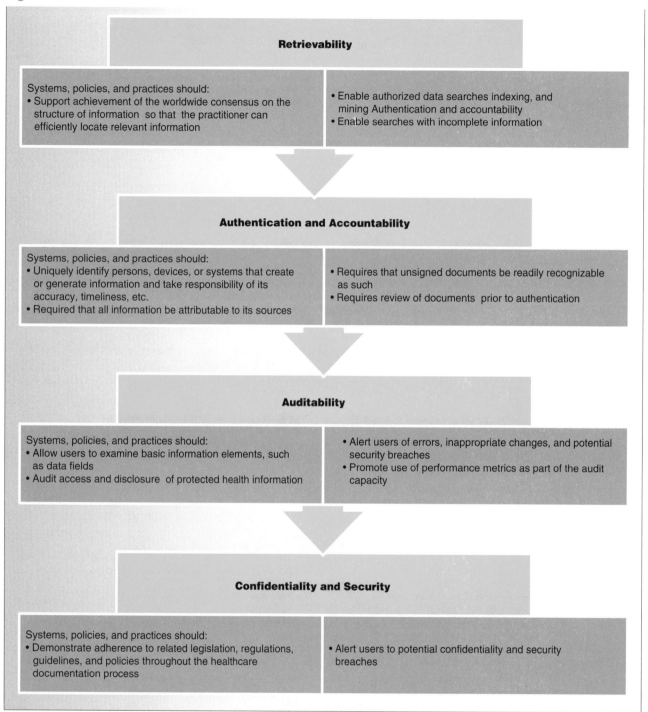

Source: Waegemann et al. 2002.

be translated into technical performance requirements for the information system (IS).

Types of Data Dictionaries

A **data dictionary** is a set of descriptions of data items in a data model for reference for systems users. There are two general types of data dictionaries: the database management system data dictionary and the organizational-wide data dictionary.

The DBMS data dictionary is developed in conjunction with development of a specific database. Modern DBMS's have built-in data dictionaries that go beyond data definitions and store information about tables and data relationships. These integrated

Figure 6.4.   AHIMA characteristics of data quality

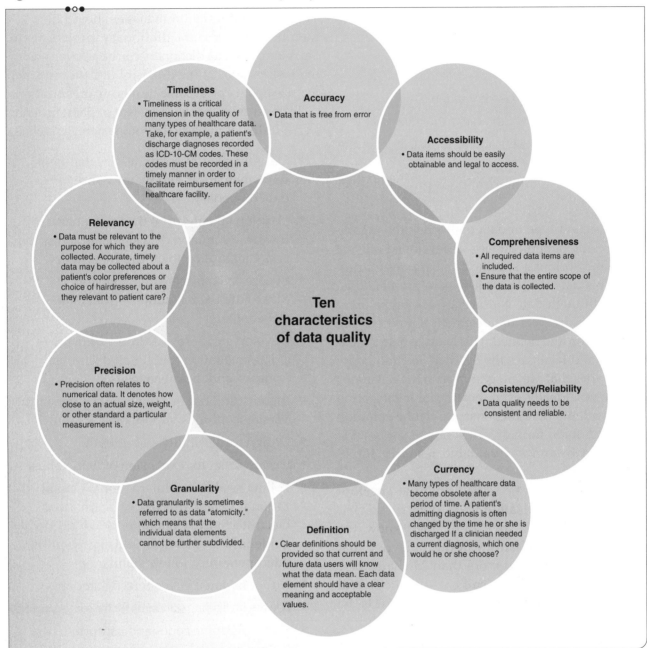

Source: AHIMA Data Quality Management Task Force 2012.

data dictionaries are sometimes referred to as system catalogs, reflecting their technical nature. A typical data dictionary associated with a DBMS allows for at least documentation of the following:

- Table names
- All attribute or field names
- A description of each attribute
- The data type of the attribute (text, number, date, and so on)

- The format of each attribute, such as DD_MM_YYYY
- The size of the each attribute, such as 12 characters in a phone number with dashes
- An appropriate range of values, such as integers 100000–999999 for the health record number
- Whether the attribute is required
- Relationships among attributes

Other descriptions that might be stored in the data dictionary associated with a database include:

- Who created the database
- When the database was created
- Where the database is located
- What programs can access the database
- Who the end users and administrators of the database are
- How access authorization is provided to all users

The second type of data dictionary, the organization-wide data dictionary, is developed outside the framework of a specific database design process. This data dictionary serves to promote data quality through data consistency across the organization. Individual data element definitions are agreed upon and defined. This leads to better quality data and facilitates the detailed, technical data dictionaries that are integrated with the databases themselves. Ideally, every healthcare organization will develop a data dictionary to define common data and their formats. This organization-wide document becomes a valuable resource for IS development.

Many issues can be settled with the development of an organization-wide data dictionary. Although everyone may think they know the definition of a last name, can they all agree that it will be stored as no more than 25 characters? How should the middle name be handled? Will it be the maiden name for married women? Is the medical record number to be stored with leading zeros?

Another challenge for healthcare managers results from interorganizational projects or the merger of healthcare organizations. Suppose a multifacility organization wanted to merge its MPI systems. Imagine the challenges involved not only in defining data elements but also in uncovering existing definitions. If the organizations in question built other systems based on internal MPI definitions, all of these systems would need to be analyzed and changed.

Development of Data Dictionaries

The health information manager should be a key member of any data dictionary project team. Developing a data dictionary can be an overwhelming task in light of the diversity of data users and the size and scope of some healthcare organizations.

To assist with the development of data dictionaries, AHIMA has published recommended guidelines.

- Design a plan: Preplan the development, implementation, and maintenance of the data dictionary.
- Develop an enterprise data dictionary: Integrate common data elements across the entire institution to ensure consistency.
- Ensure collaborative involvement: Make sure there is support from all key stakeholders.
- Develop an approvals process: Ensure a documentation trail for all decisions, updates, and maintenance.
- Identify and retain details of data versions: Version control is important.
- Design for flexibility and growth.
- Design room for expansion of field values.
- Follow established International Organization for Standards (ISO)/International Electrotechnical Commission (IEC) 11179 guidelines for metadata registry: To promote interoperability, follow standards.
- Adopt nationally recognized standards.
- Beware of differing standards for the same concepts.
- Use geographic codes and conform to the National Spatial Data Infrastructure and the Federal Geographic Data Committee.
- Test the information system: Develop a test plan to ensure the system supports the data dictionary.
- Provide ongoing education and training.
- Assess the extent to which the data elements maintain consistency and avoid duplication. (AHIMA e-HIM Workgroup on EHR Data Content 2006)

Data dictionaries support medical professionals in exchanging accurate information linked across various clinical systems through data standardization. Standardized clinical data supports interoperability and ensures consistent use. Health information managers are increasingly inundated with complex information requests and data standardization can help provide the structure to enable decision support, reporting, and information retrieval.

Check Your Understanding 6.7

Instructions: **Answer the following questions on a separate piece of paper.**

1. What data quality characteristics are listed in both AHIMA's data quality model and the MRI essential principles of documentation?

2. What is the major difference between AHIMA's data quality model and the MRI essential principles of documentation? Are they compatible with one another?

3. List the 10 characteristics of data quality.

4. What is a data dictionary? What is its importance in ensuring data quality?

5. What type of information would be listed in an organization-wide or enterprise-wide data dictionary?

6. What are AHIMA's recommended guidelines for development of data dictionaries?

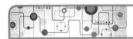

References

AHIMA Data Quality Management Task Force. 2012. Practice brief: data quality management model. *Journal of AHIMA* 83(7).

AHIMA e-HIM Workgroup of Assessing and Improving Healthcare Data Quality in the EHR. 2007. Practice brief: Assessing and improving EHR data quality. *Journal of AHIMA* 78(3):69–72.

AHIMA e-HIM Workgroup on EHR Data Content. 2006. Practice brief: Guidelines for developing a data dictionary. *Journal of AHIMA* 77(2):64A–D.

American College of Surgeons. 2015. Trauma Programs. http://www.facs.org/quality-programs/trauma

American College of Surgeons. 2012. Commission on Cancer. http://www.facs.org/quality-programs/cancer/coc/standards

American Gastroenterological Association. 2011. AGA Digestive Health Outcomes Registry. http://www.gastro.org/practice/digestive-health-outcomes-registry

American Health Information Management Association. 2003. Handling cancer registry requests for information. *In Confidence* 11(5):7.

American Joint Committee on Cancer. 2015. http://www.cancerstaging.org

American Medical Informatics Association. 2006. *Toward a National Framework for the Secondary Use of Health Data*. Bethesda, MD: American Medical Informatics Association.

American Trauma Society. 2015. http://www.amtrauma.org/

Burrington-Brown, J. and B. Hjort. 2007. Health data access, use and control. *Journal of AHIMA* 78(5):63–66.

Centers for Disease Control and Prevention. 2015a. How Cancer Registries Work. http://www.cdc.gov/cancer/npcr/value/registries.htm

Centers for Disease Control and Prevention. 2015b. National Data Quality Standard. http://www.cdc.gov/cancer/npcr/standards.htm

Centers for Disease Control and Prevention. 2015c. National Immunization Program. http://www.cdc.gov/vaccines/programs/iis/core-data-elements.html

Centers for Disease Control and Prevention. 2015d. National Center for Health Statistics. http://www.cdc.gov/nchs/

Centers for Disease Control and Prevention. 2015e. National Vital Statistics System. http://www.cdc.gov/nchs/nvss/about_nvss.htm

Centers for Disease Control and Prevention. 2012. National Program of Cancer Registries. http://www.cdc.gov/cancer/npcr/amendmentact.htm

Department of Health and Human Services. 2016. Healthy People 2020. http://www.healthypeople.gov/

Department of Health and Human Services. 2008. Fact sheet on the Healthcare Protection and Integrity Data Bank. https://www.ire.org/media/uploads/files/datalibrary/npdb/factsheet.pdf

Food and Drug Administration. 2015. Medical Device Reporting (MDR). http://www.fda.gov/MedicalDevices/Safety/ReportaProblem/default.htm

Food and Drug Administration. 2008. Medical Device Reporting for User Facilities. http://www.fda.gov/downloads/MedicalDevices/DeviceRegulationandGuidance/GuidanceDocuments/UCM095266.pdf

Free, C., G. Phillips, L. Watson, L. Galli, L. Felix, P. Edwards, and A. Haines. 2013. The effectiveness of mobile-health technologies to improve health care service delivery processes: a systematic review and meta-analysis. *PLoS Med* 10(1):e1001363.

Leavitt, N. 2010. Will NoSQL databases live up to their promise? *Computer* 43(2):12–14.

Lee, K.K.-Y., W-C. Tang, and K-S. Choi. 2013. Alternatives to relational database: Comparison of NoSQL and XML approaches for clinical data storage. *Computer Methods and Programs in Biomedicine* 110(1):99–109.

Mazurek, M. 2014. Applying NoSQL Databases for Operationalizing Clinical Data Mining Models. In Beyond Databases, Architectures, and Structures. 11th International Conference, BDAS 2015, Ustroń, Poland, New York: Springer.

McCray, A. and N.C. Ide. 2000. Design and implementation of a national clinical trials registry. *Journal of the American Medical Informatics Association* 7(3):313–323.

Medical Records Institute. 2002. *Healthcare Documentation: A Report on Information Capture and Report Generation.* Boston: Medical Records Institute.

National Cancer Registrars Association. 2014a. History of Cancer Registries. http://www.ncra-usa.org/i4a/pages/index.cfm?pageid=3873

National Cancer Registrars Association. 2014b. Education. http://www.ncra-usa.org/i4a/pages/index.cfm?pageid=3865

National Library of Medicine. 2008. http://www.clinicaltrials.gov

National Practitioner Data Bank. 2006 (Mar 21). National Practitioner Data Bank for adverse information on physicians and other health care practitioners: Reporting on adverse and negative actions. *Federal Register* 71 FR 14135.

North American Association of Central Cancer Registries. 2015. http://www.naaccr.org/AboutNAACCR/NAACCRMission.aspx

Pokorny, J. 2013. NoSQL databases: A step to database scalability in web environment. *International Journal of Web Information Systems* 9(1):69–82.

Pratt, P. and J. Adamski. 2011. *Concepts of Database Management,* 7th ed. Boston: Course Technology.

Registry of Patient Registries. 2015. https://patientregistry.ahrq.gov/

Shapiro-Mendoza, C.K., L.T. Camperlengo, S.Y. Kim, and T. Covington. 2012. The sudden unexpected infant death case registry: A method to improve surveillance. *Pediatrics* 129(2):e486–492. http://pediatrics.aappublications.org/content/129/2/e486

Sikha, B. and R. Earp. 2011. *Database Design Using Entity-Relationship Diagrams,* 2nd ed. Boca Raton, FL: Auerbach Publications.

Trauma.org. 2008. http://www.trauma.org

Waegemann, C.P., C. Tessier, A. Barbash, B.H. Blumenfeld, J. Borden, and R.M. Brinson. 2002. Healthcare documentation: A report on information capture and report generation. Consensus Workgroup on Health Information Capture and Report Generation. Newton, MA: Medical Records Institute.

Wager, K.A., R.W. Lee, and J.P. Glaser. 2005. *Managing Health Care Information Systems: A Practical Approach for Health Care Executives.* San Francisco: Jossey-Bass.

Wasan, S.K., V. Bhatnagar, and H. Kaur. 2006. The impact of data mining techniques on medical diagnostics. *Data Science Journal* 5:119–126.

PART II
Revenue Management and Compliance

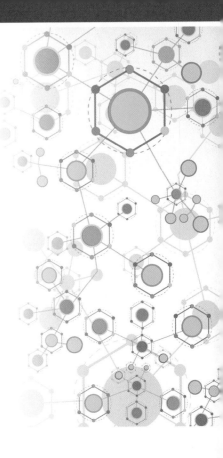

7

Reimbursement Methodologies

Anita C. Hazelwood, MLS, RHIA, FAHIMA and
Carol A. Venable, MPH, RHIA, FAHIMA

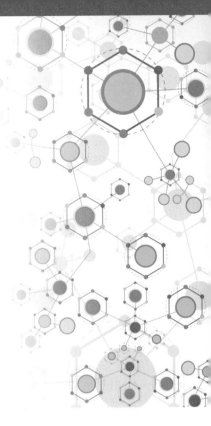

Learning Objectives

- Assess current reimbursement processes and support practices for healthcare reimbursement
- Determine the difference between private health insurance plans and employer self-insurance plans
- Outline the purpose and basic benefits of the following government-sponsored health programs: Medicare Part A, Medicare Part B, Medicare Advantage, Medicaid, CHAMPVA, TRICARE, IHS, TANF, PACE, CHIP, workers' compensation, and FECA
- Examine the concept of managed care and provide examples of different types of managed care organizations
- Compare the different types of fee-for-service reimbursement methods
- Classify ambulatory surgery center rates
- Analyze prospective payment systems for various types of healthcare facilities and services

Key Terms

Acute-care prospective payment system

Administrative services only (ASO) contract

Ambulatory surgery center (ASC)

Balanced Budget Refinement Act (BBRA) of 1999

Capitation

Case-mix groups (CMGs)

Case-mix group (CMG) relative weight

Case-mix index

Categorically needy eligibility group

Children's Health Insurance Program (CHIP)

Civilian Health and Medical Program—Uniformed Services (CHAMPUS)

Civilian Health and Medical Program—Veterans Administration (CHAMPVA)

Claim

Comorbidity

Complication

Coordination of benefits (COB) transaction

Cost outlier

Cost outlier adjustment

Diagnosis-related group (DRG)

Discounting

Employer-based self-insurance

Episode-of-care (EOC) reimbursement

Exclusive provider organization (EPO)

Explanation of benefits (EOB)

Fee-for-service reimbursement

Geographic practice cost index (GPCI)
Global payment
Global surgery payment
Group model HMO
Group practice without walls (GPWW)
Health maintenance organization (HMO)
Home Assessment Validation and Entry (HAVEN)
Home health agency (HHA)
Home health resource group (HHRG)
Hospice
Hospital-acquired conditions (HAC)
Independent practice association (IPA)
Indian Health Service (IHS)
Inpatient Rehabilitation Validation and Entry (IRVEN) system
Integrated delivery system (IDS)
Integrated provider organization (IPO)
Long-term care hospital (LTCH)
Low-utilization payment adjustment (LUPA)
Major diagnostic category (MDC)

Managed care
Management service organization (MSO)
Medicaid
Medical foundation
Medical home
Medically needy option
Medicare
Medicare administrative contractor (MAC)
Medicare Advantage plan
Medicare fee schedule (MFS)
Medicare severity diagnosis-related groups (MS-DRGs)
Medicare summary notice (MSN)
Medigap
Minimum Data Set 3.0 (MDS)
National conversion factor (CF)
Network model HMO
Network provider
Omnibus Budget Reconciliation Act (OBRA)
Outcome and Assessment Information Set (OASIS)
Outpatient code editor (OCE)
Outpatient prospective payment system (OPPS)
Packaging
Partial hospitalization

Payment status indicator (PSI)
Physician–hospital organization (PHO)
Point-of-service (POS) plan
Preferred provider organization (PPO)
Premium
Present on admission (POA)
Primary care physician (PCP)
Principal diagnosis
Programs of All-Inclusive Care for the Elderly (PACE)
Prospective payment system (PPS)
Relative value unit (RVU)
Remittance advice (RA)
Resident Assessment Validation and Entry (RAVEN)
Resource-based relative value scale (RBRVS)
Resource Utilization Groups, Version IV (RUG-IV)
Respite care
Retrospective payment system
Skilled nursing facility prospective payment system (SNF PPS)
Staff model HMO
Tax Equity and Fiscal Responsibility Act of 1982 (TEFRA)
TRICARE
Workers' compensation

In the United States, very complex systems are used to pay healthcare organizations and individual healthcare professionals for the services they provide. This complexity is due in part to the variety of reimbursement methods in use today as well as the strict requirements for detailed documentation to support medical claims. The government and other third-party payers also are concerned about potential fraud and abuse in claims processing. Therefore, ensuring that bills and claims are accurate and correctly presented is an important focus of healthcare compliance.

A reimbursement **claim** is a statement of services submitted by a healthcare provider (for example, a physician or a hospital) to a third-party payer (for example, an insurance company or Medicare). The claim documents the medical and surgical services provided to a specific patient during a specific period of care. Accurate reimbursement is critical to the operational and financial health of healthcare organizations. In most healthcare organizations, health insurance specialists process reimbursement claims. Health information management (HIM) professionals also play an important role in healthcare reimbursement by:

- Ensuring that health record documentation supports services billed

- Assigning diagnosis and procedural codes according to patient record documentation

- Applying coding guidelines and edits when assigning codes or auditing for coding quality and accuracy

- Appealing insurance claims denials

This chapter explains the different reimbursement systems commonly used since the adoption of various types of prospective payment systems. It then discusses a variety of healthcare reimbursement methodologies with a focus on Medicare prospective payment systems. Finally, it explains how reimbursement claims are processed and the support processes involved.

Healthcare Reimbursement Systems

Before the widespread availability of health insurance coverage, individuals were assured access to healthcare only when they were able to pay for the services themselves. They paid cash for services on a retrospective fee-for-service basis in which the patient was expected to pay the healthcare provider the amount of the billed charges after a service was rendered. Until the advent of managed care, capitation, and other prospective payment systems (PPS), private insurance plans and government-sponsored programs also reimbursed providers on a retrospective fee-for-service basis.

Fee-for-service reimbursement is now rare for most types of medical services. Today, most Americans are covered by some form of health insurance, and most health insurance plans compensate providers according to predetermined discounted rates rather than fee-for-service charges. However, some types of care are not covered by most health insurance plans and are still paid for directly by patients on a fee-for-service basis. Cosmetic surgery is one example of a medical service that is not considered medically necessary and so is not covered by most insurance plans.

Commercial Insurance

Most Americans are covered by private group insurance plans tied to their employment. Typically, employers and employees share the cost of such plans. Two types of commercial insurance are commonly available—private insurance and employer-based self-insurance.

Private Health Insurance Plans

Private commercial insurance plans are financed through the payment of premiums. Each covered individual or family pays a pre-established amount (usually monthly) called a premium, and the insurance company sets aside the premiums from all the people covered by the plan in a special fund. When a claim for medical care is submitted to the insurance company, the claim is paid out of the fund's reserves.

Before payment is made, the insurance company reviews every claim to determine whether the services described on the claim are covered by the patient's policy. The company also reviews the claim to ensure that the services provided were medically necessary. Payment then is made to either the provider or the policyholder.

When purchasing an insurance policy, the policyholder receives written confirmation from the insurance company when the insurance goes into effect. This confirmation document usually includes a policy number and a telephone number to be called in case of medical emergency. An insurance policy represents a legal contract for services between the insured and the insurance company.

Most insurance policies include the following information:

- What medical services the company will cover
- When the company will pay for medical services
- How much and for how long the company will pay for covered services
- What process is to be followed to ensure that covered medical expenses are paid

Employer-Based Self-Insurance Plans

During the 1970s, a number of large companies discovered that they could save money by self-insuring their employee health plans (employer-based self-insurance) rather than purchasing coverage from private insurers. Large companies have large workforces, and so aggregate (total) employee medical experiences and associated expenses vary only slightly from one year to the next. The companies understood that it was in their best interest to self-insure their health plans because yearly expenses could be predicted with relative accuracy.

The cost of self-insurance funding is lower than the cost of paying premiums to private insurers because the premiums reflect more than the actual cost of the services provided to beneficiaries. Private insurers build additional fees into premiums to compensate them for assuming the risk of providing insurance coverage. In self-insured plans, the employer assumes the risk. By budgeting a certain amount to pay its employees' medical claims, the employer retains control over the funds until the time when group medical claims need to be paid.

Employer-based self-insurance has become a common form of group health insurance coverage. Many employers enter into **administrative services only (ASO) contracts** with private insurers and fund the plans themselves. An administrative services only contract is an agreement between an employer and an insurance organization to administer the employer's self insurance health plan. The private insurers administer self-insurance plans on behalf of the employers.

Blue Cross and Blue Shield Plans

Blue Cross and Blue Shield (BCBS) plans were the first prepaid health plans in the United States. Originally, Blue Cross plans covered hospital care and Blue Shield plans covered physicians' services.

The first Blue Cross plan was created in 1929 (Wellmark 2015). In 1939, a commission of the American Hospital Association (AHA) adopted the Blue Cross national emblem for plans that met specific guidelines (BCBS of Minnesota 2015). The Blue Cross Association was created in 1960, and the relationship with the AHA ended in 1972 (East Coast Health Insurance 2015).

The first Blue Shield plan was created in 1939, and the Associated Medical Care Plans (later known as the National Association of Blue Shield Plans) adopted the Blue Shield symbol in 1948 (East Coast Health Insurance 2015). In 1982, the Blue Cross Association and the National Association of Blue Shield Plans merged to create the Blue Cross and Blue Shield Association (Wellmark 2015).

Today, the Blue Cross and Blue Shield Association includes over 36 independent, locally operated companies with plans in 50 states, the District of Columbia, and Puerto Rico. BCBS offers health insurance to individuals, small businesses, seniors, and large employer groups (BCBS 2015).

Government-Sponsored Healthcare Programs

The federal government administers several healthcare programs. The best known are Medicare and Medicaid. The **Medicare** program pays for the healthcare services provided to Social Security beneficiaries age 65 and older as well as permanently disabled people, people with end-stage renal disease, and certain other groups of individuals. State governments work with the federal **Medicaid** program to provide healthcare coverage to low-income individuals and families.

In addition, the federal government offers three health programs to address the needs of military personnel and their dependents as well as Native Americans. The Civilian Health and Medical Program–Veterans Administration (CHAMPVA) provides healthcare services for dependents and survivors of disabled veterans, survivors of veterans who died from service-related conditions, and survivors of military personnel who died in the line of duty. TRICARE (formerly CHAMPUS, the Civilian Health and Medical Program of the Uniformed Services) provides coverage for the dependents of armed forces personnel and retirees receiving care outside a military treatment facility. The Indian Health Service (IHS) provides federal health services to American Indians and Alaska Natives.

Medicare

The original Medicare program was implemented on July 1, 1966. In 1973, Medicare benefits were expanded to include individuals of any age who suffered from a permanent disability or end-stage renal disease.

For Americans receiving Social Security benefits, Medicare automatically provides hospitalization insurance (HI) (Medicare Part A). It also offers voluntary supplemental medical insurance (SMI) (Medicare Part B) to help pay for physicians' services, medical services, and medical–surgical supplies not covered by the hospitalization plan. Enrollees pay extra for Part B benefits. To fill gaps in Medicare coverage, most Medicare enrollees also supplement their benefits with private insurance policies. These private policies are referred to as Medigap or supplemental insurance. The Medicare Advantage plan (a type of supplemental plan) was established by the Balanced Budget Act (BBA) of 1997 to expand the options for participation in private healthcare plans. Established in 2003, Medicare Part D covers prescription drugs.

According to CMS, approximately 19 million Americans were enrolled in the Medicare program in 1966. In 2008, approximately 45 million people were enrolled in Parts A or B (or both) of the Medicare program. In 2013 this number increased to approximately 52.3 million (CMS 2013; Henry J. Kaiser Family Foundation n.d.). By 2013, 14.4 million of the enrollees participated in a Medicare Advantage plan (Henry J. Kaiser Family Foundation 2013).

Medicare Part A Medicare Part A is generally provided free of charge to individuals age 65 and over who are eligible for Social Security or Railroad Retirement benefits. Individuals who do not claim their monthly cash benefits are still eligible for Medicare. In addition, workers (and their spouses) who have been employed in federal, state, or local government for a sufficient period of time qualify for Medicare coverage beginning at age 65.

Similarly, individuals who have been entitled to Social Security or Railroad Retirement disability benefits for at least 24 months and government employees with Medicare coverage who have been disabled for more than 29 months are entitled to Part A benefits. This coverage also is provided to insured workers (and their spouses) with end-stage renal disease as well as to children with end-stage renal disease. In addition, some otherwise-ineligible aged and disabled beneficiaries who voluntarily pay a monthly premium for their coverage are eligible for Medicare Part A (CMS 2015a).

The following healthcare services are covered under Medicare Part A: inpatient hospital care, skilled nursing facility (SNF) care, home healthcare, hospice care, and inpatient care in a religious non-medical healthcare institution. (See table 7.1.) Medicare Part A pays for inpatient hospital care and skilled nursing care when such care is medically necessary. An initial deductible payment is required for each hospital admission, plus copayments for all hospital days following day 60 within a benefit period.

Table 7.1. Medicare Part A benefit period, beneficiary deductibles and copayments, and Medicare payment responsibilities according to healthcare setting

Healthcare setting	Benefit period	Patient's responsibility	Medicare payments
Hospital (inpatient)	First 60 days Days 61–90 Days 91–150 (these reserve days can be used only once in the patient's lifetime) Beyond 150 days	$1,260 annual deductible, $315 per day $630 per day All costs	All but $1,260 All but $315/day All but $630/day Nothing
Skilled nursing facility	First 20 days Days 21–100 Beyond 100 days	Nothing $157.50 per day All costs	100% approved amount All but $157.50 per day Nothing
Home healthcare	For as long as patient meets Medicare medical necessity criteria	Nothing for services, but 20% of approved amount for durable medical equipment (DME)	100% of the approved amount, and 80% of the approved amount for DME
Hospice care	For as long as physician certifies need for care	Limited costs for outpatient drugs and inpatient respite care ($5 per outpatient prescription and 5% for respite care)	All but limited costs for outpatient drugs and inpatient respite care
Blood banks	Unlimited if medical necessity criteria are met	First three pints unless patient or someone else donates blood to replace what patient uses	All but first three pints per calendar year

Source: CMS 2015b.

Each benefit period begins the day the Medicare beneficiary is admitted to the hospital and ends when he or she has not been hospitalized for a period of 60 consecutive days. Inpatient hospital care is usually limited to 90 days during each benefit period. There is no limit to the number of benefit periods covered by Medicare hospital insurance during a beneficiary's lifetime. However, copayment requirements apply to days 61 through 90. When a beneficiary exhausts the 90 days of inpatient hospital care available during a benefit period, a nonrenewable lifetime reserve of up to a total of 60 additional days of inpatient hospital care can be used. Copayments are required for such additional days.

SNF care is covered when it occurs within 30 days of a three-day-long or longer hospitalization and is certified as medically necessary. The number of SNF days provided under Medicare is limited to 100 days per benefit period, with a copayment required for days 21 through 100. Medicare Part A does not cover SNF care when the patient does not require skilled nursing care or skilled rehabilitation services (CMS 2015b).

Care provided by a **home health agency (HHA)**, a program or organization that provides a blend of home-based medical and social services to homebound patients and their families, may be furnished part-time in the residence of a homebound beneficiary when intermittent or part-time skilled nursing or certain other therapy or rehabilitation care is needed. Certain medical supplies and durable medical equipment (DME) also may be paid for under the Medicare home health benefit.

The Medicare program requires the HHA to develop a treatment plan that is periodically reviewed by a physician. Home healthcare under Medicare Part A has no limitations on duration, no copayments, and no deductibles. For DME, beneficiaries must pay 20 percent coinsurance, as required under Medicare Part B.

Terminally ill persons whose life expectancies are six months or less may elect to receive hospice services. **Hospice** is an interdisciplinary program of palliative care and supportive services that addresses the physical, spiritual, social, and economic needs of terminally ill patients and their families. To qualify for Medicare reimbursement for hospice care, patients must elect to forgo standard Medicare benefits for treatment of their illnesses and agree to receive only hospice care. When a hospice patient requires treatment for a condition that is not related to his or her terminal illness, however, Medicare does pay for all covered services necessary for that condition. The Medicare beneficiary pays no deductible for hospice coverage but does pay coinsurance amounts for drugs and inpatient respite care. **Respite care** is any inpatient care provided to the hospice patient for the purpose of giving primary caregivers a break from their caregiving responsibilities.

Medicare Part B   Medicare Part B (supplemental medical insurance) covers the following services and supplies:

- Physicians' and surgeons' services, including some covered services furnished by chiropractors, podiatrists, dentists, and optometrists; and services provided by the following Medicare-approved practitioners who are not physicians such as certified registered nurse anesthetists, clinical psychologists, clinical social workers (other than those employed by a hospital or an SNF), physician assistants, nurse practitioners, and clinical nurse specialists working in collaboration with a physician

- Services in an emergency department or outpatient clinic, including same-day surgery and ambulance services

- Home healthcare not covered under Medicare Part A

- Laboratory tests, x-rays, and other diagnostic radiology services, as well as certain preventive care screening tests

- Ambulatory surgery center (ASC) services in Medicare-approved facilities

- Most physical and occupational therapy and speech pathology services

- Comprehensive outpatient rehabilitation facility services and mental healthcare provided as part of a partial hospitalization psychiatric program when a physician certifies that inpatient treatment would be required without the partial hospitalization services; a **partial hospitalization** program offers intensive psychiatric treatment on an outpatient basis to psychiatric patients, with an expectation that the patient's psychiatric condition and level of functioning will improve and that relapse will be prevented so that rehospitalization can be avoided

- Radiation therapy, renal dialysis and kidney transplants, and heart and liver transplants under certain limited conditions

- Durable medical equipment (DME) approved for home use, such as oxygen equipment; wheelchairs; prosthetic devices; surgical dressings, splints, and casts; walkers; and hospital beds needed for use in the home

- Drugs and biologicals that cannot be self-administered, such as hepatitis B vaccines and transplant and immunosuppressive drugs (plus certain self-administered anticancer drugs)

- Preventive services such as bone mass measurements, cardiovascular screening blood tests, colorectal cancer screening, diabetes services, glaucoma testing, Pap test and pelvic exam, prostate cancer screening, screening mammograms, and vaccinations (flu, pneumococcal, hepatitis B) (CMS 2015a)

To be covered, all Medicare Part B services must be either documented as medically necessary or covered as one of several prescribed preventive benefits. Also, Part B services are generally subject to deductibles and coinsurance payments. (See table 7.2.) Certain medical services and related care are subject to special payment rules, for example:

- Deductibles for administration of blood and blood products

- Maximum approved amounts for Medicare-approved physical or occupational therapy services performed in settings other than hospitals

- Higher cost-sharing requirements, such as those for outpatient psychiatric care

Table 7.2. Medicare Part B benefit deductibles and copayments and Medicare payment responsibilities according to type of service

Type of service	Benefit	Deductible and copayment	Medicare payment
Medical expense	Physicians' services, inpatient and outpatient medical and surgical services and supplies, and durable medical equipment (DME)	$147 annual deductible, plus 20% of approved amount after deductible has been met, except in outpatient setting	80% of approved amount (after patient has paid $147 deductible)
	Mental healthcare	20% of most outpatient care	80% of most outpatient care
Clinical laboratory services	Blood tests, urinalysis, and more	Nothing	100% of approved amount
Home healthcare	Intermittent skilled care, home health aid services, DME and supplies, and other services	Nothing for home care service, 20% of approved amount for DME	100% of approved amount 80% of approved amount for DME
Outpatient hospital services	Services for diagnosis and treatment of an illness or injury	A coinsurance (for doctors' services) or a copayment amount for most outpatient hospital services; the copayment for a single service cannot be more than the amount of the inpatient hospital deductible Charges for items or services that Medicare does not cover	Payment based on ambulatory patient classifications and outpatient prospective payment system
Blood	Unlimited if medical necessity criteria are met	First three pints or have blood donated by someone else (if met under Part B, does not have to be met again under Part A)	All but first three pints

Source: CMS 2015b.

It should be noted that some healthcare services are usually not covered by Medicare Part A or B and are only covered by private health plans, for example, long-term nursing care, cosmetic surgery, dentures and dental care, acupuncture, and hearing aids and exams for fitting hearing aids.

Medicare Advantage   Medicare Advantage provides expanded coverage of many healthcare services. Although any Medicare beneficiary may receive benefits through the original fee-for-service program (Parts A and B), some beneficiaries choose to participate in a Medicare Advantage plan instead.

Primary Medicare Advantage products include the following types of plans:

- *Health maintenance organization (HMO) plans:* In most HMOs, the patient can only go to doctors, other healthcare providers, or hospitals on the plan's list, except in an emergency. You may also need to get a referral from your primary care doctor.

- *Preferred provider organization (PPO) plans:* In a PPO plan, patients use doctors, specialists, and hospitals in the plan's network and can go to doctors and hospitals not on the list, usually at an additional cost. Patients do not need referrals to see doctors or go to hospitals that are not part of the plan's network and may pay lower copayments and receive extra benefits.

- *Private fee-for-service plans:* A private fee-for-service plan is similar to original Medicare in that the patient can generally go to any doctor, other healthcare provider, or hospital as long as they agree to treat you. This plan determines how much it will pay doctors, other healthcare providers, and hospitals and how much you must pay when you get care.

- *Special needs plans:* Special needs plans provide focused and specialized healthcare for specific groups of people, such as those who have both Medicare and Medicaid, who live in a nursing home, or who have certain chronic medical conditions.

- *HMO point-of-service (HMOPOS) plans:* These are HMO plans that may allow the patient to get some services out-of-network for a higher copayment or coinsurance.

- *Medical savings account (MSA) plans:* MSA plans combine a high-deductible health plan with a bank account. Medicare deposits money into the account (usually less than the deductible) and the patient can use the money to pay for healthcare services during the year (CMS 2015a).

Medicare Prescription Drug Improvement and Modernization Act   The Medicare Prescription Drug Improvement and Modernization Act, also known as the Medicare Reform Bill, was signed into law by President George W. Bush in December 2003. This legislation provides seniors and individuals with disabilities with a prescription drug benefit, more choices, and better benefits under Medicare. Medicare drug plans are run by insurance companies and other private companies approved by Medicare. Each plan can vary in cost and drugs covered, and beneficiaries select their preferred plan.

Out-of-Pocket Expenses and Medigap Insurance   Medicare beneficiaries who elect the fee-for-service option are responsible for charges not covered by the Medicare program and for various cost-sharing aspects of Parts A and B. These liabilities may be paid by the Medicare beneficiary; by a third party, such as an employer-sponsored health plan or private Medigap insurance; or by Medicaid, when the person is eligible.

Medigap, or supplemental insurance, is private health insurance that pays, within limits, most of the healthcare service charges not covered by Medicare Parts A or B. These policies must meet federal and state laws.

Medicaid

Title XIX of the Social Security Act enacted Medicaid in 1965. The Medicaid program pays for medical assistance provided to individuals and families with low incomes and limited financial resources. Individual states must meet broad national guidelines established by federal statutes, regulations, and policies to qualify for federal matching grants under the Medicaid program. Individual state medical assistance agencies, however, establish the Medicaid eligibility standards for residents of their states. The states also determine the type, amount, duration, and scope of covered services; calculate the rate of payment for covered services; and administer local programs.

Medicaid policies on eligibility, services, and payment are complex and vary considerably among states, even among states of similar size or geographic proximity. Therefore, an individual who is eligible for Medicaid in one state may not be eligible in another. In addition, the amount, duration, and scope of care provided vary considerably from state to state. Moreover, Medicaid eligibility and services within a state can change from year to year.

Medicaid Eligibility Criteria   Low income is only one measure for Medicaid eligibility. Other financial resources also are compared against eligibility standards. Each state determines these standards according to federal guidelines.

Generally, each state can determine which groups Medicaid will cover. Each state also establishes its own financial criteria for Medicaid eligibility. However, to be eligible for federal funds, states are required to provide Medicaid coverage to certain individuals. These individuals include recipients of federally assisted income maintenance payments as well as related groups of individuals who do not receive cash payments. The federal **categorically needy eligibility groups** (categories of individuals to whom states must provide coverage under the federal Medicaid program) include the following:

- Families who meet states' Aid to Families with Dependent Children (AFDC) eligibility requirements in effect on July 16, 1996
- Children ages 6 to 19 with family income up to 100 percent of the federal poverty level

- Pregnant women and children under age 6 whose family income is at or below 133 percent of the federal poverty level
- Caretakers (relatives or legal guardians who take care of children under age 18, or 19 if still in high school)
- Supplemental security income (SSI) recipients (or, in certain states, aged, blind, and disabled people who meet requirements that are more restrictive than those of the SSI program)
- Individuals and couples who are living in medical institutions and who have monthly income up to 300 percent of the SSI income standard federal benefit rate (CMS 2005)

States also have the option of providing Medicaid coverage to other categorically related groups. Categorically related groups share the characteristics of the eligible groups (that is, they fall within defined categories), but the eligibility criteria are somewhat more liberally defined. A **medically needy option** also allows states to extend Medicaid eligibility to persons who would be eligible for Medicaid under one of the mandatory or optional groups except that their income and resources are above the eligibility level set by their state. Individuals may qualify immediately or may "spend down" by incurring medical expenses that reduce their income to or below their state's income level for the medically needy.

In 1996, Congress passed the Personal Responsibility and Work Opportunity Reconciliation Act (also known as welfare reform). The act made restrictive changes in the eligibility requirements for SSI coverage. These changes also affected eligibility for participation in the Medicaid program.

The welfare reform act also affected a number of disabled children. Many lost their SSI benefits as a result of the restrictive changes. However, their eligibility for Medicaid was reinstituted by the BBA.

In addition, the welfare reform act repealed the open-ended federal entitlement program known as Aid to Families with Dependent Children (AFDC). Temporary Assistance for Needy Families (TANF), which replaced AFDC, provides states with grant money to be used for time-limited cash assistance.

A family's lifetime cash welfare benefits are generally limited to a maximum of five years. Individual states also are allowed to impose other eligibility restrictions.

The Affordable Care Act, enacted in 2014, expanded coverage for low-income Americans by creating an opportunity for states to provide Medicaid eligibility for individuals under 65 years of age with income up to 133 percent of the federal poverty level. States can provide Medicaid coverage for low-income adults and children and be guaranteed coverage through Medicaid in every state without need for a waiver (CMS 2015c).

Medicaid Services   To be eligible for federal matching funds, each state's Medicaid program must offer medical assistance for the following basic services:

- Inpatient hospital services
- Outpatient hospital services
- Emergency services
- Prenatal care and delivery services
- Vaccines for children
- Physicians' services
- Skilled nursing facility (SNF) services for persons age 21 or older
- Family planning services and supplies
- Rural health clinic services
- Home healthcare for persons eligible for skilled nursing services
- Laboratory and x-ray services
- Medical and surgical services of a dentist
- Pediatric and family nurse practitioner services
- Nurse-midwife services
- Federally qualified health center (FQHC) services and ambulatory services performed at the FQHC that would be available in other settings
- Early and periodic screening and diagnostic and therapeutic services for children under age 21 (CMS 2015c)

States also may receive federal matching funds to provide some of the optional services, the most common being:

- Diagnostic services
- Clinic services
- Prescription drugs and prosthetic devices
- Transportation services
- Rehabilitation and physical therapy services
- Prosthetic devices
- Home care and community-based care services for persons with chronic impairments

The BBA also called for implementation of a state option called **Programs of All-Inclusive Care for the Elderly (PACE)**. PACE provides an alternative to institutional care for individuals age 55 or older who require a level of care usually provided at nursing facilities. It offers and manages all of the health, medical, and social services needed by a beneficiary and mobilizes other services, as needed, to provide preventive, rehabilitative, curative, and supportive care.

PACE services can be provided in day healthcare centers, homes, hospitals, and nursing homes. The program helps its beneficiaries to maintain their independence, dignity, and quality of life. PACE also functions within the Medicare program. Individuals enrolled in PACE receive benefits solely through the PACE program.

Medicaid–Medicare Relationship   Medicare beneficiaries who have low incomes and limited financial resources also may receive help from the Medicaid program. For persons eligible for full Medicaid coverage, Medicare coverage is supplemented by services that are available under their state's Medicaid program according to their eligibility category. Additional services may include, for example, nursing facility care beyond the 100-day limit covered by Medicare, prescription drugs, eyeglasses, and hearing aids. For those enrolled in both programs, any services covered by Medicare are paid for by the Medicare program before any payments are made by the Medicaid program because Medicaid is always the payer of last resort (Social Security Administration 2004). Table 7.3 provides a comparison of the Medicare and Medicaid programs.

Table 7.3. Comparison of Medicare and Medicaid programs

Medicare	Medicaid
Health insurance for people age 65 and older, or people under 65 who are entitled to Medicare because of disability or are receiving dialysis for permanent kidney failure	Health assistance for people of any age
Administered through fiscal intermediaries, insurance companies under contract to the government to process Medicare claims	Administered by the federal government through state and local governments following federal and state guidelines
Medicare regulations are the same in all states	Medicaid regulations vary from state to state
Financed by monthly premiums paid by the beneficiary and by payroll tax deductions	Financed by federal, state, and county tax dollars
For people age 65 and over, eligibility is based on Social Security or Railroad Retirement participation; For people under age 65, eligibility is based on disability For people who undergo kidney dialysis, eligibility is not dependent on age	Eligibility based on financial need
Beneficiary responsible for paying deductibles, coinsurance or copayments, and Part B premiums	Medicaid can help pay Medicare deductible, coinsurance or copayment, and premiums
Hospital and medical benefits; preventive care and long-term care benefits are limited	Comprehensive benefits include hospital, preventive care, long-term care, and other services not covered under Medicare such as dental work, prescriptions, transportation, eyeglasses, and hearing aids

Children's Health Insurance Program   The Children's Health Insurance Program (CHIP) (Title XXI of the Social Security Act) is a program initiated by the BBA. CHIP allows states to expand existing insurance programs to cover children up to age 19. It provides additional federal funds to states so that Medicaid eligibility can be expanded to include a greater number of children.

CHIP became available in October 1997 and is jointly funded by the federal government and the states. Following broad federal guidelines, states establish eligibility and coverage guidelines and have flexibility in the way they provide services. Recipients in all states must meet three eligibility criteria:

- They must come from low-income families.
- They must be otherwise ineligible for Medicaid.
- They must be uninsured.

States are required to offer the following services: inpatient hospital services; outpatient hospital services; physicians' surgical and medical services; laboratory and x-ray services; and well-baby and child care services, including age-appropriate immunizations (Healthcare.gov 2015).

TRICARE

TRICARE is a healthcare program for active-duty members of the military and other qualified family members. Eligible retirees and their family members, as well as eligible survivors of members of the uniformed services, also are eligible for TRICARE.

The idea of medical care for the families of active-duty members of the uniformed military services dates back to the late 1700s. It was not until 1884, however, that Congress directed Army medical officers and contract surgeons to care for the families of military personnel free of charge.

There was very little change in the provision of medical care to members of the military and their families until the World War II, when the military was made up mostly of young men who had wives of childbearing age. The military medical care system could not handle the large number of births or the care of young children. In 1943, Congress authorized the Emergency Maternal and Infant Care (EMIC) Program to assist.

During the early 1950s, the Korean conflict also strained the capabilities of the military healthcare system. As a result, the Dependents Medical Care Act was signed into law in 1956. Amendments to the act created the **Civilian Health and Medical Program—Uniformed Services (CHAMPUS)** in 1966. CHAMPUS is defined as a federal program supplying supplementary civilian-sector hospital and medical services, beyond that which is available in military dependents, and certain others.

During the 1980s, the search for ways to improve access to top-quality medical care and control costs at the same time led to implementation of CHAMPUS demonstration projects in various parts of the country. The most successful of these projects was the CHAMPUS Reform Initiative (CRI) in California and Hawaii. Initiated in 1988, the CRI offered military service families a choice in the way their military healthcare benefits could be used. Five years of successful operation and high levels of patient satisfaction persuaded Department of Defense officials that they should extend and improve the CRI concepts as a uniform program nationwide.

The new program, known as TRICARE, was phased in nationally by 1998. TRICARE offers three options: TRICARE Prime, TRICARE Extra, and TRICARE Standard.

TRICARE Prime Of the three options, TRICARE Prime provides the most comprehensive healthcare benefits at the lowest cost. Military treatment facilities, such as military base hospitals, serve as the principal source of healthcare and a primary care manager (PCM) is assigned to each enrollee.

Two specialized programs supplement TRICARE Prime. TRICARE Prime Remote provides healthcare services to active-duty military personnel stationed in the United States in areas not served by the traditional military healthcare system. (Active-duty personnel include members of the Army, Navy, Marine Corps, Air Force, Coast Guard, and active National Guard.) TRICARE Senior Prime is a managed care demonstration program designed to serve the medical needs of military retirees who are age 65 or older, as well as their dependents and survivors.

TRICARE Extra TRICARE Extra is a cost-effective preferred provider network (PPN) option. Healthcare

costs in TRICARE Extra are lower than for TRICARE Standard because beneficiaries must select physicians and medical specialists from a network of civilian healthcare professionals working under contract with TRICARE. The healthcare professionals who participate in TRICARE Extra agree to charge a pre-established discounted rate for the medical treatments and procedures provided to participants in the plan.

TRICARE Standard TRICARE Standard incorporates the services previously provided by CHAMPUS. TRICARE Standard allows eligible beneficiaries to choose any physician or healthcare provider. It pays a set percentage of the providers' fees, and the enrollee pays the rest. This option permits the most flexibility but may be the most expensive for the enrollee, particularly when the provider's charges are higher than the amounts allowed by the program.

CHAMPVA

The **Civilian Health and Medical Program–Veterans Administration (CHAMPVA)** is a healthcare program for dependents and survivors of permanently and totally disabled veterans, survivors of veterans who died from service-related conditions, and survivors of military personnel who died in the line of duty. CHAMPVA is a voluntary program that allows beneficiaries to be treated for free at participating VA healthcare facilities, with the VA sharing the cost of covered healthcare services and supplies. Because of the similarity between CHAMPVA and TRICARE, people sometimes confuse the two programs. However, CHAMPVA is separate from TRICARE, and there are distinct differences between them. TRICARE is for individuals currently serving in the armed forces, and CHAMPVA is for retired military personnel.

Indian Health Service

The provision of health services to Native Americans originally developed from the relationship between the federal government and federally recognized Indian tribes established in 1787. It is based on Article I, Section 8, of the US Constitution and has been given form and substance by numerous treaties, laws, Supreme Court decisions, and executive orders.

The **Indian Health Service (IHS)** is an agency within the HHS. It is responsible for providing healthcare services to American Indians and Alaska Natives. The American Indians and Alaska Natives served by the IHS receive preventive healthcare services, primary medical services (hospital and ambulatory care), community health services, substance abuse treatment services, and rehabilitative services. Secondary medical care, highly specialized medical services, and other rehabilitative care are provided by IHS staff or by private healthcare professionals working under contract with the IHS.

A system of acute- and ambulatory care facilities operates on Indian reservations and in Indian and Alaska Native communities. In locations where the IHS does not have its own facilities or is not equipped to provide a needed service, it contracts with local hospitals, state and local healthcare agencies, tribal health institutions, and individual healthcare providers.

Workers' Compensation

Most employees are eligible for some type of workers' compensation insurance. **Workers' compensation** programs cover healthcare costs and lost income associated with work-related injuries and illnesses. Federal government employees are covered by the Federal Employees' Compensation Act (FECA). Individual states pass legislation that addresses workers' compensation coverage for nonfederal government employees. Some states exclude certain workers, for example, business owners, independent contractors, farm workers, and so on. Texas employers are not required to provide workers' compensation coverage.

Federal Workers' Compensation Funds

In 1908, President Theodore Roosevelt signed legislation to provide workers' compensation for certain federal employees in unusually hazardous jobs. The scope of the law was narrow and its benefits were limited. This law represented the first workers' compensation program to pass the test of constitutionality applied by the US Supreme Court.

FECA replaced the statute in 1916. Under FECA, civilian employees of the federal government are provided medical care, survivors' benefits, and compensation for lost wages. The Office of Workers' Compensation Programs (OWCP) administers FECA as well as the Longshore and Harbor Workers' Compensation Act of 1927 and the Black Lung Benefits Reform Act of 1977.

FECA also provides vocational rehabilitation services to partially disabled employees. Employees who fully or partially recover from their injuries are expected to return to work. FECA does not provide retirement benefits.

State Workers' Compensation Funds

According to the American Association of State Compensation Insurance Funds (AASCIF), state workers' compensation insurance was developed in response to the concerns of employers (AASCIF 2015). Before state workers' compensation programs became widely available, employers faced the possibility of going out of business when insurance companies refused to provide coverage or charged excessive premiums. Legislators in most states have addressed these concerns by establishing state workers' compensation insurance funds that provide a stable source of insurance coverage and serve to protect employers from uncertainties about the continuing availability of coverage. Because state funds are provided on a nonprofit basis, the premiums can be kept low. In addition, the funds provide only one type of insurance: workers' compensation. This specialization allows the funds to concentrate resources, knowledge, and expertise in a single field of insurance.

State workers' compensation insurance funds do not operate at taxpayer expense because, by law, the funds support themselves through income derived from premiums and investments. As nonprofit departments of the state or as independent nonprofit companies, they return surplus assets to policyholders as dividends or safety refunds. This system reduces the overall cost of state-level workers' compensation insurance. Numerous court decisions have determined that the assets, reserves, and surplus of the funds are not public funds but, instead, the property of the employers insured by the funds.

In states where state funds have not been mandated, employers purchase workers' compensation coverage from private carriers or provide self-insurance coverage.

Managed Care

Healthcare costs in the United States rose dramatically during the 1970s and 1980s. As a result, the federal government, employers, and other third-party payers began investigating more cost-effective healthcare delivery systems. The federal government decided to move toward PPSs for the Medicare program in the mid-1980s. Prospective payment as a reimbursement methodology is discussed later in this chapter. Commercial insurance providers looked to managed care.

Managed care is the generic term for prepaid health plans that integrate the financial and delivery aspects of healthcare services. In other words, managed care organizations work to control the cost of, and access to, healthcare services at the same time that they strive to meet high-quality standards. They manage healthcare costs by negotiating discounted providers' fees and controlling patients' access to expensive healthcare services. In managed care plans, services are carefully coordinated to ensure that they are medically appropriate and needed.

The cost of providing appropriate services is also monitored continuously to determine whether the services are being delivered in the most efficient and cost-effective way possible.

Since 1973, several pieces of federal legislation have been passed with the goal of encouraging the development of managed healthcare systems. (See table 7.4.) The Health Maintenance Organization Assistance Act of 1973 authorized federal grants and loans to private organizations that wished to develop health maintenance organizations (HMOs). Another important advancement in managed care was development of the Healthcare Effectiveness Data and Information Set (HEDIS) by the National Committee for Quality Assurance (NCQA).

The NCQA is a private, not-for-profit organization that accredits, assesses, and reports on the quality of managed care plans in the United States.

It worked with public and private healthcare purchasers, health plans, researchers, and consumer advocates to develop HEDIS in 1989. HEDIS (formerly known as the Health Plan Employer Data and Information Set) is a set of standardized measures used to compare managed care plans in terms of the quality of services they provide. The standards cover areas such as plan membership, utilization of and access to services, and financial indicators. The goals of the program include:

- Helping beneficiaries make informed choices among the numerous managed care plans available
- Improving the quality of care provided by managed care plans
- Helping the government and other third-party payers make informed purchasing decisions

Health Maintenance Organizations

A health maintenance organization (HMO) is a prepaid voluntary health plan that provides healthcare services in return for the payment of a monthly membership premium. HMO premiums are based on a projection of the costs that are likely to be involved in treating the plan's average enrollee over a specified period of time. If the actual cost per enrollee were to exceed the projected cost, the HMO would experience a financial loss. If the actual cost per enrollee turned out to be lower than the projection, the HMO would show a profit. Because most HMOs are for-profit organizations, they emphasize cost control and preventive medicine.

The benefit to third-party payers and enrollees alike is cost savings. Most HMO enrollees have significantly lower out-of-pocket expenses than enrollees of traditional fee-for-service and other types of managed care plans. The HMO premiums shared by employers and enrollees also are lower than the premiums for other types of healthcare plans.

HMOs can be organized in several different ways, including the group model HMO, the independent practice association (IPA), the network model HMO, and the staff model HMO, or there

Table 7.4. Federal legislation relevant to managed care

Year	Legislative title	Legislative summary
1973	Federal Health Maintenance Organization Assistance Act of 1973 (HMO Act of 1973)	• Authorized grants and loans to develop HMOs under private sponsorship • Defined a federally qualified HMO (certified to provide healthcare services to Medicare and Medicaid enrollees) as one that has applied for and met federal standards established in the HMO Act of 1973 • Required most employers with more than 25 employees to offer HMO coverage when local plans were available
1974	Employee Retirement Income Security Act of 1974 (ERISA)	• Mandated reporting and disclosure requirements for group life and health plans (including managed care plans) • Permitted large employers to self-insure employee healthcare benefits • Exempted large employers from taxes on health insurance premiums
1981	Omnibus Budget Reconciliation Act of 1981 (OBRA)	• Provided states with flexibility to establish HMOs for Medicare and Medicaid programs • Resulted in increased enrollment
1982	Tax Equity and Fiscal Responsibility Act of 1982 (TEFRA)	• Modified the HMO Act of 1973 • Created Medicare risk programs, which allowed federally qualified HMOs and competitive medical plans that met specified Medicare requirements to provide Medicare-covered services under a risk contract • Defined risk contract as an arrangement among providers to provide capitated (fixed, prepaid basis) healthcare services to Medicare beneficiaries • Defined competitive medical plan (CMP) as an HMO that meets federal eligibility requirements for a Medicare risk contract but is not licensed as a federally qualified plan
1985	Preferred Provider Health Care Act of 1985	• Eased restrictions on preferred provider organizations • Allowed subscribers to seek healthcare from providers outside the PPO
1985	Consolidated Omnibus Budget Reconciliation Act of 1985 (COBRA)	• Established an employee's right to continue healthcare coverage beyond scheduled benefit termination date (including HMO coverage)
1988	Amendment to the HMO Act of 1973	• Allowed federally qualified HMOs to permit members to occasionally use non-HMO physicians and be partially reimbursed
1989	Healthcare Effectiveness Data and Information Set (HEDIS)—developed by National Committee for Quality Assurance (NCQA)	• Created standards to assess managed care systems in terms of membership, utilization of services, quality, access, health plan management and activities, and financial indicators
1994	HCFA's Office of Managed Care established	• Facilitated innovation and competition among Medicare HMOs
2010	Patient Protection and Affordable Care Act	• Individual mandate requirements; expansion of public programs; health insurance exchanges; changes to private insurance; employer requirements; and cost and coverage estimates

can also be a combination of the staff, group, and network models.

Group Model HMOs In the **group model HMO**, the HMO enters into a contract with an independent multispecialty physician group to provide medical services to members of the plan. The providers usually agree to devote a fixed percentage of their practice time to the HMO. Alternatively, the HMO may own or directly manage the physician group, in which case the physicians and their support staff would be considered its employees.

Group model HMOs are closed-panel arrangements. In other words, the physicians are not allowed to treat patients from other managed care plans. Enrollees of group model HMOs are required to seek services from the designated physician group.

Independent Practice Associations In an **independent practice association (IPA)** model, the HMO enters into a contract with an organized group of physicians who join together for purposes of fulfilling the HMO contract but retain their individual practices. The IPA serves as an intermediary during contract negotiations. It also manages the premiums from the HMO and pays individual physicians as appropriate. The physicians are not considered employees of the HMO. They work from their own private offices and continue to see other patients. The HMO usually pays the IPA according to a prenegotiated list of discounted fees. Alternatively, physicians may agree to provide services to HMO members for a set prepaid capitated payment for a specified period of time. Capitation is discussed later in this chapter.

The IPA is an open-panel HMO, which means that the physicians are free to treat patients from other plans. Enrollees of such HMOs are required to seek services from the designated physician group.

Network Model HMOs

Network Model HMOs Network model HMOs are similar to group model HMOs except that the HMO contracts for services with two or more multispecialty group practices instead of just one practice. Members of network model HMOs receive a list of all the physicians on the approved panel and are required to select providers from the list.

Staff Model HMOs

Staff Model HMOs Staff model HMOs directly employ physicians and other healthcare professionals to provide medical services to members. Members of the salaried medical staff are considered employees of the HMO rather than independent practitioners. Premiums are paid directly to the HMO, and ambulatory care services are usually provided within the HMO's corporate facilities. The staff model HMO is a closed-panel arrangement.

Preferred Provider Organizations

Preferred provider organizations (PPOs) represent contractual agreements between healthcare providers and a self-insured employer or a health insurance carrier. Beneficiaries of PPOs select providers such as physicians or hospitals from a list of participating providers who have agreed to furnish healthcare services to the covered population. Beneficiaries may elect to receive services from

nonparticipating providers but must pay a greater portion of the cost (in other words, higher deductibles and copayments). Providers are usually reimbursed on a discounted fee-for-service basis.

Point-of-Service Plans

Point-of-service (POS) plans are similar to HMOs in that subscribers must select a primary care physician (PCP) from a network of participating physicians. The PCP is usually a family or general practice physician or an internal medicine specialist. The PCP acts as a service gatekeeper to control the patient's access to specialty, surgical, and hospital care as well as expensive diagnostic services.

POS plans are different from HMOs in that subscribers are allowed to seek care from providers outside the network. However, the subscribers must pay a greater share of the charges for out-of-network services. POS plans were created to increase the flexibility of managed care plans and to allow patients more choice in providers.

Exclusive Provider Organizations

Exclusive provider organizations (EPOs) are similar to PPOs except that EPOs provide benefits to enrollees only when the enrollees receive healthcare services from network providers, healthcare professionals who are members of a managed care network. In other words, EPO beneficiaries do not receive reimbursement for services furnished by nonparticipating providers. In addition, healthcare services must be coordinated by a PCP. EPOs are regulated by state insurance departments. By contrast, HMOs are regulated by state departments of commerce or departments of incorporation.

Integrated Delivery Systems

An integrated delivery system (IDS) is a healthcare provider consisting of a number of associated medical facilities that furnish coordinated healthcare services. Most IDSs include a number of facilities that provide services along the continuum of care, for example, ambulatory surgery centers, physicians' office practices, outpatient clinics, acute-care hospitals, SNFs, and so on.

Integrated delivery systems can be structured according to several different models, including:

- Group practices without walls (GPWWs)
- Integrated provider organizations (IPOs)
- Management service organizations (MSOs)
- Medical foundations
- Physician–hospital organizations (PHOs)

Group Practices without Walls Group practices without walls (GPWWs) is an arrangement that allows physicians to maintain their own offices but to share administrative, management, and marketing services (for example, medical transcription and billing) for the purpose of fulfilling contracts with managed care organizations.

Integrated Provider Organizations Integrated provider organizations (IPOs) manage and coordinate the delivery of healthcare services performed by a number of healthcare professionals and facilities. IPOs typically provide acute-care (hospital) services, physicians' services, ambulatory care services, and skilled nursing services. The physicians working in an IPO are salaried employees. IPOs are sometimes referred to as delivery systems, horizontally integrated systems, health delivery networks, accountable health plans, integrated service networks (ISNs), vertically integrated plans (VIPs), and vertically integrated systems.

Management Service Organizations Management service organizations (MSOs) provide practice management (administrative and support) services to individual physicians' practices. They are usually owned by a group of physicians or a hospital.

Medical Foundations Medical foundations are nonprofit organizations that enter into contracts with physicians to manage the physicians' practices. The typical medical foundation owns clinical and business resources and makes them available to the participating physicians. Clinical assets include medical equipment and supplies as well as treatment facilities. Business assets include billing and administrative support systems.

Physician–Hospital Organizations Physician–Hospital Organizations (PHOs), previously known as medical staff–hospital organizations, provide healthcare services through a contractual arrangement between physicians and hospital(s). PHO arrangements make it possible for the managed care market to view the hospital(s) and physicians as a single entity for the purpose of establishing a contract for services.

Check Your Understanding 7.1

Instructions: Answer the following questions on a separate piece of paper.

1. What services are covered under Part B of Medicare?

2. State the differences between the Tricare options (that is, Tricare Prime, Tricare Extra, and Tricare Standard).

3. What federal law established an employee's right to continue healthcare coverage beyond the benefit termination date?

4. Which HMO model directly employs physicians and other healthcare professionals to provide medical services to members?

5. Describe the difference between private health insurance plans and employer-based self-insurance plans.

6. How do exclusive provider organizations differ from preferred provider organizations?

Healthcare Reimbursement Methodologies

Most healthcare expenses in the United States are reimbursed through third-party payers rather than by the actual recipients of the services. The recipients can be considered the first parties and the providers the second parties. Third-party payers include commercial for-profit insurance companies, nonprofit Blue Cross and Blue Shield organizations, self-insured employers, federal programs (Medicare, Medicaid, CHIP, TRICARE, CHAMPVA, and IHS), and workers' compensation programs.

Providers charge their own determined amounts for services rendered. However, providers are rarely reimbursed this full amount because third-party payers may have a unique reimbursement methodology. For example, commercial insurance plans usually reimburse healthcare providers under some type of retrospective payment system. In retrospective payment systems, the exact amount of the payment is determined after the service has been delivered. In a prospective payment system (PPS), the exact amount of the payment is determined before the service is delivered. The federal Medicare program uses PPSs.

Fee-for-Service Reimbursement Methodologies

Fee-for-service reimbursement methodologies issue payments to healthcare providers on the basis of the charges assigned to each of the separate services that were performed for the patient. The total bill for an episode of care represents the sum of all the itemized charges for every element of care provided. Independent clinical professionals such as physicians and psychologists who are not employees of the facility issue separate itemized bills to cover their services after the services are completed or on a monthly basis when the services are ongoing.

Before prepaid insurance plans became common in the 1950s and the Medicare and Medicaid programs were developed in the 1960s, health-care providers sent itemized bills directly to their patients. Patients were held responsible for paying their own medical bills. When prepaid health plans and the Medicare and Medicaid programs were originally developed, they also based reimbursement on itemized fees.

Traditional Fee-for-Service Reimbursement

In traditional fee-for-service (FFS) reimbursement systems, third-party payers or patients issue payments to healthcare providers after healthcare services have been provided (for example, after the patient has been discharged from the hospital). Payments are based on the specific services delivered. The fees charged for services vary considerably by the type of services provided, the resources required, and the type and number of healthcare professionals involved. Payments can be calculated on the basis of actual billed charges, discounted charges, pre-negotiated rate schedules, or the usual or customary charges in a specific community.

For example, some third-party payers pay only the maximum allowable charges as determined by the plan. Maximum allowable charges may be significantly lower than the provider's billed charges. Some payers issue payments on the basis of usual, customary, and reasonable (UCR) charges. Commercial insurance and BCBS plans often issue payments based on pre-negotiated discount rates and contractual cost-sharing arrangements with the patient.

For many plans, the health plan and the patient share costs on an 80/20 percent arrangement. The portion of the claim covered by the patient's insurance plan would be 80 percent of allowable charges. After the third-party payer transmits its payment to the provider, the provider's billing department issues a final statement to the patient. The statement shows the amount for which the patient is responsible (in this example, 20 percent of allowable charges).

The traditional FFS reimbursement methodology is still used by many commercial insurance companies for visits to physicians' offices.

Managed Fee-for-Service Reimbursement

Managed FFS reimbursement is similar to traditional FFS reimbursement except that managed care plans control costs primarily by managing their members' use of healthcare services. Most managed care plans also negotiate with providers to develop discounted fee schedules. Managed FFS reimbursement is common for inpatient hospital care. In some areas of the country, however, it also is applied to outpatient and ambulatory services, surgical procedures, high-cost diagnostic procedures, and physicians' services.

Utilization controls include the prospective and retrospective review of the healthcare services planned for, or provided to, patients. For example, a prospective utilization review of a plan to hospitalize a patient for minor surgery might determine that the surgery could be safely performed less expensively in an outpatient setting. Prospective utilization review is sometimes called precertification.

In a retrospective utilization review, the plan might determine that part or all of the services provided to a patient were not medically necessary or were not covered by the plan. In such cases, the plan would disallow part or all of the provider's charges and the patient would be responsible for paying the provider's outstanding charges.

Discharge planning also can be considered a type of utilization control. The managed care plan may be able to move the patient to a less intensive, and therefore less expensive, care setting as soon as possible by coordinating his or her discharge from inpatient care.

Episode-of-Care Reimbursement Methodologies

Plans that use **episode-of-care (EOC) reimbursement** methods issue lump-sum payments to providers to compensate them for all the healthcare services delivered to a patient for a specific illness or over a specific period of time. EOC payments also are called bundled payments. Bundled payments cover multiple services and also may involve multiple providers of care. EOC reimbursement methods include capitated payments,

global payments, global surgery payments, Medicare ambulatory surgery center rates, and Medicare PPSs.

Capitation

Capitation is based on per person premiums or membership fees rather than on itemized per procedure or per service charges. The capitated managed care plan negotiates a contract with an employer or a government agency representing a specific group of individuals. According to the contract, the managed care organization agrees to provide all the contracted healthcare services that the covered individuals need over a specified period of time (usually one year). In exchange, the individual enrollee or third-party payer agrees to pay a fixed premium for the covered group. Like other insurance plans, a capitated insurance contract stipulates as part of the contract exactly which healthcare services are covered and which ones are not.

Capitated premiums are calculated on the projected cost of providing covered services per patient per month (PPPM) or per member per month (PMPM). The capitated premium for an individual member of a plan includes all the services covered by the plan, regardless of the number of services actually provided during the period or their cost. If the average member of the plan actually used more services than originally assumed in the PPPM calculation, the plan would show a loss for the period. If the average member actually used fewer services, the plan would show a profit.

The purchasers of capitated coverage (usually the member's employer) pay monthly premiums to the managed care plan. The individual enrollees usually pay part of the premium as well. The plan then compensates the providers who actually furnished the services. In some arrangements, the managed care plan accepts all the risk involved in the contract. In others, some of the risk is passed on to the PCPs who agreed to act as gatekeepers for the plan.

The capitated managed care organization may own or operate some or all of the healthcare facilities that provide care to members and directly employ clinical professionals. Staff model HMOs operate in this way. Alternatively, the capitated managed care organization may purchase services from independent physicians and facilities, as do group model HMOs.

Global Payment

Global payment methodology is sometimes applied to radiological and similar types of procedures that involve professional and technical components. **Global payments** are lump-sum payments distributed among the physicians who performed the procedure or interpreted its results and the healthcare facility that provided the equipment, supplies, and technical support required. The procedure's professional component is supplied by physicians (for example, radiologists), and its technical component (for example, radiological supplies, equipment, and support services) is supplied by a hospital or free-standing diagnostic or surgical center. For example:

> Larry Timber underwent a scheduled carotid angiogram as a hospital outpatient. He had complained of ringing in his ears and dizziness, and his physician scheduled the procedure to determine whether there was a blockage in one of Larry's carotid arteries. The procedure required a surgeon to inject radiopaque contrast material through a catheter into Larry's left carotid artery. A radiological technician then took an x-ray of Larry's neck. The technician was supervised by a radiologist and both were employees of the hospital.
>
> *Professional component:* Injection of radiopaque contrast material by the surgeon
> *Technical component:* X-ray of the neck region
> *Global payment:* The facility received a lump-sum payment for the procedure and paid for the services of the surgeon from that payment.

Global Surgery Payments

A single **global surgery payment** covers all the healthcare services entailed in planning and completing a specific surgical procedure. In other words, every element of the procedure from the treatment decision through normal postoperative patient care is covered by a single bundled payment. For example:

> Tammy Murdock received from Dr. Thomas Michaels all the prenatal, perinatal, and postnatal care involved in the birth of her daughter. She received one bill from the physician for a total of $2,200. The bill represented the total charges for the obstetrical services associated with her pregnancy. However, the two-day inpatient hospital stay for the normal delivery was not included in the global payment, nor were the laboratory services she received during her hospital stay. Tammy received a separate bill for these services. In addition, if she had suffered a postdelivery complication (for example, a wound infection) or an unrelated medical problem, the physician and hospital services required to treat the complication would not have been covered by the global surgical payment.

The Medical Home

One of the newest concepts in managed care is that of the **medical home**. According to the Patient-Centered Primary Care Collaborative a medical home is "best described as a model or philosophy of primary care that is patient-centered, comprehensive, team-based, coordinated, accessible, and focused on quality and safety. It has become a widely accepted model for how primary care should be organized and delivered through the healthcare system" (PCPCC 2015).

 Check Your Understanding 7.2

Instructions: **Answer the following questions on a separate piece of paper.**

1. Describe the fee-for-service reimbursement methodology.
2. How is discharge planning used as a type of utilization control?
3. What are global payments?
4. What are episode-of-care payments and how do they relate to bundle payments?
5. What is a capitated managed care plan?

Medicare's Prospective Payment Systems

Congress enacted the first Medicare prospective payment system in 1983 as a cost-cutting measure. Implementation of the acute-care prospective payment system, which is the reimbursement system for inpatient hospital services provided to Medicare and Medicaid beneficiaries that is based on the use of diagnosis-related groups as a classification tool, resulted in a shift of clinical services and expenditures away from the inpatient hospital setting to outpatient settings. As a result of the cost containment efforts in the acute-care setting, spending on nonacute care exploded.

Congress responded by passing the Omnibus Budget Reconciliation Act (OBRA) of 1986, which mandated that CMS develop a prospective system for hospital-based outpatient services provided to Medicare beneficiaries. In subsequent years, Congress mandated the development of PPSs for other healthcare providers.

Medicare's Acute-Care Prospective Payment System

Prior to 1983, Medicare Part A payments to hospitals were determined on a traditional FFS reimbursement methodology. Payment was based on the cost of services provided, and reasonable cost or per diem costs were used to determine payment.

During the late 1960s, just a few years after the Medicare and Medicaid health programs were implemented, Congress authorized a group at Yale University to develop a system for monitoring quality of care and utilization of services. This system was known as diagnosis-related groups (DRGs). A DRG is a unit of case-mix classification adopted by the federal government and some other payers as a prospective payment mechanism for hospital inpatients in which diseases are placed into groups because related diseases and treatments tend to consume similar amounts of healthcare resources and incur similar amounts of cost. DRGs were implemented on an experimental basis by the New Jersey Department of Health in the late 1970s as a way to predetermine reimbursement for hospital inpatient stays.

At the conclusion of the New Jersey DRG experiment, Congress passed the Tax Equity and Fiscal Responsibility Act of 1982 (TEFRA). TEFRA modified Medicare's retrospective reimbursement system for inpatient hospital stays by requiring implementation of the DRG PPS in 1983. Under DRGs, Medicare paid most hospitals for inpatient hospital services according to a predetermined rate for each discharge. Very simply, the DRG system was a way of classifying patients on the basis of diagnosis. Patients within each DRG were said to be "medically meaningful"—that is, patients within a group were expected to evoke a set of clinical responses that statistically would result in an approximately equal use of hospital resources. On October 1, 2007, the DRG system became known as the Medicare severity diagnosis-related groups (MS-DRGs), which better accounts for severity of illness and resource consumption.

To determine the appropriate MS-DRG, a claim for a healthcare encounter is first classified into one of 25 major diagnostic categories (MDCs). Most MDCs are based on body systems and include diseases and disorders relating to a particular system. However, some MDCs include disorders and diseases involving multiple organ systems (for example, burns). The number of MS-DRGs within a particular MDC varies.

The principal diagnosis is defined as the condition that, after study, is determined to have caused the admission of the patient to the hospital for care, and it determines the MDC assignment. Within each MDC, decision trees are used to determine the correct MS-DRG. Within most MDCs, cases are divided into surgical MS-DRGs (based on a surgical hierarchy that orders individual procedures or groups of procedures by resource intensity) and medical MS-DRGs. Medical MS-DRGs generally are differentiated on the basis of diagnosis and age. Some surgical and medical MS-DRGs are further differentiated on the basis of the presence or absence of complications or comorbidities (CCs).

A **complication** is a secondary condition that arises during hospitalization and is thought to increase the length of stay by at least one day for approximately 75 percent of patients. A **comorbidity** is a condition that existed at admission and is thought to increase the length of stay at least one day for approximately 75 percent of patients. During the initial years of DRGs, there was a standard list of diagnoses that were considered CCs. Each year new CCs are added and others deleted from the CC list.

Each base MS-DRG can be subdivided in one of three possible alternatives:

- MS-DRGs with three subgroups (Major Complication/Comorbidity [MCC, CC, and non-CC; referred to as: with MCC, with CC, and w/o CC/MCC])
  - MS-DRG 682 Renal Failure with MCC
  - MS-DRG 683 Renal Failure with CC
  - MS-DRG 684 Renal Failure w/o CC/MCC
- MS-DRGs with two subgroups (MCC and CC/non-CC; referred to as: with MCC and w/o MCC)
  - MS-DRG 725 Benign Prostatic Hypertrophy with MCC
  - MS-DRG 726 Benign Prostatic Hypertrophy w/o MCC
- MS-DRGs with two subgroups (non-CC and CC/MCC; referred to as: with CC/MCC and w/o CC/MCC)
  - MS-DRG 294 Deep Vein Thrombophlebitis with CC/MCC
  - MS-DRG 295 Deep Vein Thrombophlebitis w/o CC/MCC

The increased number of classifications is intended to differentiate between the levels of resource consumption within a base MS-DRG group.

Under the acute-care prospective payment system, a predetermined rate based on the MS-DRG assigned to each case (only one is assigned per case) is used to reimburse hospitals for inpatient care provided to Medicare and TRICARE beneficiaries. Hospitals determine MS-DRGs by assigning ICD-10-CM/PCS codes to each patient's principal diagnosis, comorbidities, complications, major complications, principal procedure, and secondary procedures. These code numbers and other information on the patient (age, gender, and discharge status) are entered into a grouper. A MS-DRG grouper is a computer software program that assigns appropriate MS-DRGs according to the information provided for each episode of care.

Reimbursement for each episode of care is based on the MS-DRG assigned. Different diagnoses require different levels of care and expenditures of resources. Therefore, each MS-DRG is assigned a different level of payment that reflects the average amount of resources required to treat a patient assigned to that MS-DRG. Each MS-DRG is associated with a description, a relative weight, a geometric mean length of stay (LOS), and an arithmetic mean LOS. The relative weight represents the average resources required to care for cases in that particular MS-DRG relative to the national average of resources used to treat all Medicare patients. A MS-DRG with a relative weight of 2.000, on average, requires twice as many resources as a MS-DRG with a relative weight of 1.000. The geometric mean LOS is defined as the total days of service, excluding any outliers or transfers, divided by the total number of patients; the arithmetic mean LOS is defined as the total days of service divided by the total number of patients.

For example, MS-DRG 1, organized within MDC 01, is described as heart transplant or implant of heart assist system with MCC and has a relative weight of 25.3518, a geometric mean LOS of 28.3, and an arithmetic mean LOS of 35.9.

CMS adjusts the Medicare MS-DRG list and reimbursement rates every fiscal year (October 1 through September 30). There are currently 758 MS-DRGs (CMS 2015d).

In some cases, the MS-DRG payment received by the hospital may be lower than the actual cost of providing Medicare Part A inpatient services. In such cases, the hospital must absorb the loss. In other cases, the cost of providing care is lower than the MS-DRG payment, and the hospital may receive a payment for more than its actual cost and, therefore, make a profit.

Special circumstances can also apply to inpatient cases and result in an outlier payment to the hospital. An outlier case results in exceptionally high costs when compared with other cases in the same DRG. To qualify for a **cost outlier,** a hospital's charges for a case (adjusted to cost) must exceed the payment rate for the MS-DRG by a fixed dollar amount, which changes each year. The additional payment amount is equal to 80 percent of the difference between the hospital's entire cost for the stay and the threshold amount.

There can be further hospital-specific adjustments resulting in add-on payments:

- *Disproportionate share hospital (DSH):* If the hospital treats a high percentage of low-income patients, it receives a percentage add-on payment applied to the MS-DRG-adjusted base payment rate.

- *Indirect medical education (IME):* If the hospital is an approved teaching hospital, it receives a percentage add-on payment for each case paid under MS-DRGs. This percentage varies depending on the ratio of residents to beds.

- *New technologies:* If the hospital can demonstrate the use of a new technology that is a substantial clinical improvement over available existing technologies and the new technology is approved, additional payments are made. Hospitals must submit a formal request to CMS with a significant sample of data to demonstrate that the technology meets the high-cost threshold.

The MS-DRG system creates a hospital's **case-mix index** (types or categories of patients treated by the hospital) based on the relative weights of the MS-DRG. The case-mix index can be figured by multiplying the relative weight of each MS-DRG by the number of discharges within that MS-DRG. This provides the total weight for each MS-DRG. The sum of all total weights divided by the sum of total patient discharges equals the case-mix index. A hospital may relate its case-mix index to the costs incurred for inpatient care. This information allows the hospital to make administrative decisions about services to be offered to its patient population. For example:

The hospital's case-mix report indicated that a small population of patients was receiving obstetrical services, but that the costs associated with providing such services was disproportionately high. This report along with other data might result in the hospital's administrative decision to discontinue its obstetrical services department.

Hospital-Acquired Conditions and Present on Admission Indicator Reporting

The Deficit Reduction Act of 2005 (DRA) mandated a quality adjustment in the MS-DRG payments for certain hospital-acquired conditions. CMS titled the program "Hospital-Acquired Conditions and Present on Admission Indicator Reporting" (HAC and POA). The following hospitals are exempt from the POA indicator requirement: critical access hospitals, long-term care hospitals, Maryland waiver hospitals, cancer hospitals, children's inpatient facilities, inpatient rehabilitation facilities, and psychiatric hospitals.

Present on admission (POA) is defined as a condition present at the time the order for inpatient admission occurs—conditions that develop during an outpatient encounter, including in the emergency department, observation, or outpatient surgery, are considered as present on admission. A POA indicator is assigned to principal and secondary diagnoses and the external cause of injury codes. The reporting options that are available are:

- Y = Yes, diagnosis was present at the time of inpatient admission.

- N = No, diagnosis was not present at the time of inpatient admission.

- U = Unknown, documentation is insufficient to determine if condition was present at the time of inpatient admission.

- W = Clinically undetermined. The provider is unable to clinically determine whether the condition was present at the time of admission.

- 1 = Unreported/not used = Exempt from POA reporting.

Complete guidelines with examples are part of the *ICD-10-CM Official Guidelines for Coding and Reporting* and should be reviewed.

CMS identified eight **hospital-acquired conditions (HACs)** (not present on admission) as "reasonably preventable," and hospitals will not receive additional payment for cases in which one of the eight selected conditions was not present on admission. This is termed the HAC payment provision. The eight originally selected conditions include:

- Foreign object retained after surgery
- Air embolism
- Blood incompatibility
- Stage III and IV pressure ulcers
- Falls and trauma
- Catheter-associated urinary tract infection
- Vascular catheter-associated infection
- Surgical site infection—mediastinitis after coronary artery bypass graft

Additional conditions were added in 2010 and remain in effect:

- Surgical site infections following certain orthopedic procedures
- Surgical site infections following bariatric surgery
- Manifestations of poor glycemic control
- Deep vein thrombosis (DVT)/pulmonary embolism (PE) following certain orthopedic procedures
- Iatrogenic pneumothorax with venous catheterization
- Surgical site infection following cardiac implantable electronic devices (CIED)

Resource-Based Relative Value Scale System

In 1992, CMS implemented the **resource-based relative value scale (RBRVS)** system for physician's services such as office visits covered under Medicare Part B. The system reimburses physicians according to a fee schedule based on predetermined values assigned to specific services.

The **Medicare fee schedule (MFS)** is the listing of allowed charges that are reimbursable to physicians under Medicare. Each year's MFS is published by CMS in the *Federal Register*.

To calculate fee schedule amounts, Medicare uses a formula that incorporates the following **relative value units (RVUs)** for:

- Physician work (RVUw)
- Practice expenses (RVUpe)
- Malpractice costs (RVUm)

RVUs are a measurement that represents the value of the work involved in providing a specific professional medical service in relation to the value of the work involved in providing other medical services. Sample RVUs for selected Healthcare Common Procedure Coding System (HCPCS) codes are shown in table 7.5.

Payment localities are adjusted according to three geographic practice cost indices (GPCIs):

- Physician work (GPCIw)
- Practice expenses (GPCIpe)
- Malpractice costs (GPCIm)

Sample GPCIs for selected US cities are shown in table 7.6.

Table 7.5. Sample 2015 RVUs for selected HCPCS codes

HCPCS Code	Description	Work RVU	Facility practice expense RVU	Malpractice expense RVU
99203	Office visit	1.42	0.6	0.15
99204	Office visit	2.43	1.02	0.22
11010	Debridement skin at fracture site	4.19	3.11	0.74
45380	Colonoscopy with biopsy	4.43	2.31	0.66
52601	TURP, complete	15.26	7.3	1.7

Source: CMS 2015e.

Table 7.6. Sample GPCIs for selected US cities

City	Work GPCI	Practice expense GPCI	Malpractice expense GPCI
Baltimore	1.023	1.097	1.181
Dallas	1.018	1.009	0.772
Miami	1.000	1.033	2.49
New Orleans	1.000	0.983	1.39

Source: CMS 2015e.

A **geographic practice cost index** is a number used to multiply each RVU so that it better reflects a geographical area's relative costs. For example, costs of office rental prices, local taxes, average salaries, and malpractice costs are all affected by geography.

A **national conversion factor (CF)** converts the RVUs into payments. In 2015, the CF was $35.8013 (ASCRS 2015).

The RBRVS fee schedule uses the following formula:

$$[(RVUw \times GPCIw) + (RVUpe \times GPCIpe) + (RVUm \times GPCIm)] \times CF = Payment$$

As an example, payment for performing a repair of a nail bed (code 11760) in Birmingham, Alabama, can be calculated. RVU values include:

- RVUw = 1.63
- RVUpe = 1.91
- RVUm = 0.22

GPCI values include:

- GPCIw = 1.00
- GPCIpe = 0.850
- GPCIm = 0. 617
- National CF = $35.8013

The calculation is as follows:

$$(1.63 \times 1.00) + (1.91 \times 0.850) +$$
$$(0.22 \times 0.617) \times \$35.8013$$
$$1.63 + 1.6235 + 0.13574$$
$$3.38924 \times \$35.8013$$

Fee schedule payment of $121.3391

Medicare Skilled Nursing Facility Prospective Payment System

The Balanced Budget Act (BBA) mandated implementation of a **skilled nursing facility prospective payment system (SNF PPS)**. A SNF PPS is defined as a per diem reimbursement system for all costs (routine, ancillary, and capital) associated with covered SNF services furnished to Medicare Part A beneficiaries. Certain educational activities were exempt from the new system.

The SNF PPS was implemented on July 1, 1998. Under the PPS, SNFs are no longer paid under a system based on reasonable costs. Instead, they are paid according to a per-diem PPS based on case mix–adjusted payment rates. Per diem rates range from a high of over $750 to a low of about $200 (CMS 2015f).

Medicare Part A covers posthospital SNF services and all items and services paid under Medicare Part B before July 1, 1998 (other than physician and certain other services specifically excluded under the BBA). Major elements of the SNF PPS include rates, coverage, transition, and consolidated billing. OBRA required CMS to develop an assessment instrument to standardize the collection of SNF patient data. That document is called the **Minimum Data Set 3.0 (MDS)**. The MDS is the minimum core of defined and categorized patient assessment data that serves as the basis for documentation and reimbursement in an SNF. The MDS form contains a face sheet for documentation of resident identification information, demographic information, and the patient's customary routine.

Resource Utilization Groups

SNF reimbursement rates are paid according to **Resource Utilization Groups, Version IV (RUG-IV)**, a case mix–adjusted resident classification system based on the MDS used in skilled nursing facilities for resident assessments.

The RUG-IV classification system uses resident assessment data from the MDS collected by SNFs to assign residents to one of 66 groups.

Resident Assessment Validation and Entry

CMS developed a computerized data-entry system for skilled nursing facilities that offers users the ability to collect MDS assessments in a database and transmit them in CMS-standard format to their state database. The data-entry software is entitled **Resident Assessment Validation and Entry (RAVEN)**. RAVEN imports and exports data in standard MDS record format; maintains facility, resident, and employee information; enforces data integrity via rigorous edit checks; and provides comprehensive online help. It includes a data dictionary and a RUG calculator.

Consolidated Billing Provision

The BBA includes a billing provision that requires an SNF to submit consolidated Medicare bills for its residents for services covered under either Part A or Part B except for a limited number of specifically excluded services. For example, when a physician provides a diagnostic radiology service to an SNF patient, the SNF must bill for the technical component of the radiology service because this is included in the SNF consolidated billing payment. The rendering physician must develop a business relationship with the SNF in order to receive payment from the SNF for the services he or she rendered. The professional component of the physicians' services is excluded from SNF consolidated billing and must be billed separately to the Medicare administrative contractor. There are, of course, other exclusions to this provision, including physician assistant services, nurse practitioner services, and clinical nurse specialist services when these individuals are working under the supervision of, or in collaboration with, a physician, certified midwife services, qualified psychologist services, and certified registered nurse anesthetist services. Other exclusions include hospice care, maintenance dialysis, selected services furnished on an outpatient basis such as cardiac catheterization services, CT elsewhere scans and MRIs, radiation therapy, and ambulance services. In addition, SNFs report Healthcare Common Procedure Coding System (HCPCS) codes on all Part B bills.

Medicare and Medicaid Outpatient Prospective Payment System

The **outpatient prospective payment system (OPPS)** was first implemented for services furnished on or after August 1, 2000. OPPS is the Medicare prospective payment system used for hospital-based outpatient services and procedures that is determined from the assignment of ambulatory payment classifications. Under the OPPS, the federal government pays for hospital outpatient services on a rate-per-service basis that varies according to the ambulatory payment classification (APC) group to which the service is assigned. The HCPCS identifies and groups the services within

each APC group. Services included under APCs follow:

- Surgical procedures
- Radiology including radiation therapy
- Clinic visits (evaluation and management, or E/M)
- Emergency room visits
- Partial hospitalization services for the mentally ill
- Chemotherapy
- Preventive services and screening exams
- Dialysis for other than end-stage renal disease
- Vaccines, splints, casts, and antigens
- Certain implantable items

The OPPS does not apply to critical access hospitals (CAHs), hospitals in Maryland that are excluded, IHS hospitals, or hospitals outside the 50 states, the District of Columbia, and Puerto Rico.

The calculation of payment for services under the OPPS is based on the categorization of outpatient services into APC groups according to Current Procedural Terminology (CPT)/HCPCS codes. ICD-10-CM/PCS coding is not utilized in the selection of APCs. The APCs are categorized into significant procedure APCs, radiology and other diagnostic APCs, medical visit APCs, and a partial hospitalization APCs. Services within an APC are similar, both clinically and with regard to resource consumption, and each APC is assigned a fixed payment rate for the facility fee or technical component of the outpatient visit. Payment rates are also adjusted according to the hospital's wage index. Multiple APCs may be appropriate for a single episode of care as the patient may receive various types of services such as radiology or surgical procedures.

The OPPS **payment status indicators (PSIs)** that are assigned to each HCPCS code and APCs play an important role in determining payment for services under the OPPS. They indicate whether a service represented by a HCPCS code is payable under the OPPS or another payment system and also whether particular OPPS policies apply to the code. Status indicator "C", for example, is used to show that a procedure is performed on an inpatient basis only. This inpatient only list is updated each year.

Other notable payment status indicators include:

- A Fee schedule payment
- F Reasonable cost payment
- G Pass-through payment
- K APC payment
- S APC payment
- T APC payment

Status indicator "N" refers to items and services that are "packaged" into APC rates. **Packaging** means that payment for that service is packaged into payment for other services and, therefore, there is no separate APC payment. Packaged services might include minor ancillary services, inexpensive drugs, medical supplies, and implantable devices (Casto and Forrestal 2015).

Discounting applies to multiple surgical procedures furnished during the same operative session. For discounted procedures, the full APC rate is paid for the surgical procedure with the highest rate, and other surgical procedures performed at the same time are reimbursed at 50 percent of the APC rate. When a surgical procedure is terminated after a patient is prepared for surgery but before induction of anesthesia, the facility is reimbursed at 50 percent of the APC rate. Modifier 73 should be appended to the procedure code indicating that the procedure was discontinued. Modifier 74 is appended to the procedure code when a procedure is interrupted after its initiation or the administration of anesthesia. The facility receives the full APC payment.

The OPPS does pay outlier payments on a service-by-service basis when the cost of furnishing a service or procedure by a hospital exceeds 1.75 times the APC payment amount and exceeds the APC payment rate plus a fixed-dollar threshold. If a provider meets both of these conditions, the outlier payment is calculated as 50 percent of the amount by which the cost of furnishing the service exceeds 1.75 times the APC payment rate. The fixed-dollar threshold changes each year.

Special payments are also made for new technology in one of two ways. Transitional pass-through payments are temporary additional payments that are made when certain drugs, biological agents, brachytherapy devices, and other expensive medical devices new to medicine are used. These new technology APCs were created to allow new procedures and services to enter the OPPS quickly even though their complete costs and payment information are not known. New technology APCs house modern procedures and services until enough data are collected to properly place the new procedure in an existing APC or to create a new APC for the service or procedure. Coding for E/M medical visits is difficult under the APC system. CMS states that each facility should develop a system for mapping the provided services furnished to the different levels of effort represented by E/M codes. As long as services furnished are documented and medically necessary and the facility is following its own system, which reasonably relates the intensity of hospital resources to the different levels of codes, CMS assumes that the hospital is in compliance with its reporting requirements.

Ambulatory Surgery Centers

For Medicare purposes, an **ambulatory surgery center (ASC)** is a distinct entity that operates exclusively for the purpose of furnishing outpatient surgical services to patients. An ASC is either independent or operated by a hospital. If it is operated by a hospital, it has the option of being covered under Medicare as an ASC or can continue to be covered as an outpatient surgery department. To be considered an ASC of a hospital it has to be a separately identifiable entity physically, administratively, and financially.

The Medicare Modernization Act (MMA) of 2003 extensively revised the ASC payment system with changes going into effect on January 1, 2008. The system is called the ambulatory surgery center prospective payment system (ASC PPS).

ASCs must accept assignment as payment in full. Eighty percent of the payment comes from the government and 20 percent from the beneficiary. Under the ASC payment system, Medicare will make payments to ASCs only for services on the ASC list of covered procedures. The surgical procedures included in the list are those that have been determined to pose no significant risk to beneficiaries when furnished in an ASC. The ASC payment includes services such as medical and surgical supplies, nursing services, surgical dressings, implanted prosthetic devices not on a pass-through list, and splints and casts. Examples of services not included in the ASC payment are brachytherapy, procurement of corneal tissue, and certain drugs and biologicals.

The payment rates for most covered ASC procedures and covered ancillary services are established prospectively based on a percentage of the OPPS payment rates while a small number of services are contractor based, such as the pass-through items.

The HCPCS code is used as the basis for payment. Each HCPCS code falls into one of more than 1,500 ASC groups, with each group having a unique payment. Medicare pays 80 percent of the wage-adjusted rate, and the beneficiary is responsible for the other 20 percent. Similar to the OPPS, each HCPCS has a payment indicator that determines whether the surgical procedure is on the ASC list (A2); device-intensive procedure paid at adjusted rate (J8); or packaged service or item for which no separate payment is made (N1). These are just a few examples of some of the payment indicators; there are others.

Again, like the OPPS, there are guidelines for payment of terminated procedures. The following rules apply:

1. 0 percent payment for procedures terminated for unforeseen circumstances before the ASC has expended substantial resources
2. 50 percent payment for procedures that are terminated due to medical complications prior to anesthesia
3. 100 percent payment for procedures that have started but are terminated after anesthesia is induced

Home Health Prospective Payment System

The BBA called for the development and implementation of a home health prospective payment system (HHPPS) for reimbursement of services provided to Medicare beneficiaries. The PPS for HHAs was implemented on October 1, 2000. Extensive changes were made in 2008. The following are components of this PPS.

OASIS and HAVEN

HHAs use the OASIS data set and HAVEN data-entry software to conduct all patient assessments, not just the assessments for Medicare beneficiaries. The **Outcome and Assessment Information Set (OASIS)** consists of data elements that (1) represent core items for the comprehensive assessment of an adult home care patient and (2) form the basis for measuring patient outcomes for the purpose of outcome-based quality improvement (OBQI). OASIS is a key component of Medicare's partnership with the home care industry to foster and monitor improved home healthcare outcomes. The Conditions of Participation for HHAs require that HHAs electronically report all OASIS data (Casto and Forrestal 2015).

CMS also developed the OASIS data-entry system called **HAVEN (Home Assessment Validation and Entry)**. HAVEN is available to HHAs at no charge through CMS's website. HAVEN offers users the ability to collect OASIS data in a database and transmit them in a standard format to state databases. The data-entry software imports and exports data in standard OASIS record format; maintains agency, patient, and employee information; maintains data integrity through rigorous edit checks; and provides comprehensive online help.

Home Health Resource Groups

Home health resource groups (HHRGs) represent the classification system established for the prospective reimbursement of covered home care services to Medicare beneficiaries during a 60-day episode of care. Covered services include skilled nursing visits, home health aide visits, therapy services (for example, physical, occupational, and speech therapy), medical social services, and non-routine medical supplies. DME is excluded from the episode-of-care payment and is reimbursed under the DME fee schedule.

The classification of a patient into 1 of 153 HHRGs is based on OASIS data, which establish the severity of clinical and functional needs and services utilized. Grouper software is used to determine the appropriate HHRG (see table 7.7). For example:

> OASIS data collected on a 76-year-old male home care patient resulted in an HHRG of C2, F3, and S2. This HHRG is interpreted as a clinical domain of low severity, a functional domain of moderate severity, and a service utilization domain of low utilization.

The HHRG assigned as well as the type of supplies provided and the number of home health visits comprise the Health Insurance Prospective Payment System (HIPPS) code, which is the unit of payment for the episode of care.

Episode-of-care reimbursements vary and are affected by treatment level and regional wage differentials. There is no limit to the number of 60-day episodes of care that a patient may receive as long as Medicare coverage criteria are met.

Low Utilization and Outlier Payments

When a patient receives fewer than four home care visits during a 60-day episode, an alternate (reduced) payment, or **low-utilization payment adjustment (LUPA)**, is made instead of the full HHRG reimbursement rate. HHAs are eligible for a **cost outlier adjustment**, which is a payment for certain high-cost home care patients whose costs are in excess of a threshold amount for each HHRG. The threshold is the 60-day episode

Table 7.7. HHRG severity levels in three domains: clinical, functional, and service utilization

Domain	Score	Severity level
Clinical	C1	Minimum severity
	C2	Low severity
	C3	Moderate severity
Functional	F1	Minimum severity
	F2	Low severity
	F3	Moderate severity
Service utilization	S1	Minimum utilization
	S2	Low utilization
	S3	Moderate utilization
	S4	High utilization
	S5	Maximum utilization

Source: CMS 2015g.

payment plus a fixed-dollar loss that is constant across the HHRGs.

Ambulance Fee Schedule

A Medicare payment system for medically necessary transports effective for services provided on or after April 1, 2002, was included as part of the BBA. The payment system applies to all ambulance services including volunteer, municipal, private, independent, and institutional providers (hospitals, critical access hospitals, SNFs, and HHAs).

Ambulance services are reported on claims using HCPCS codes that reflect the seven categories of ground service and two categories of air service. Mandatory assignment is required for all ambulance service providers.

The seven categories of ground (land and water) ambulance services include basic life support, advanced life support (level 1), advanced life support (level 2), specialty care transport, paramedic intercept, fixed wing air ambulance and rotary wing air ambulance (Casto and Forrestal 2015).

Inpatient Rehabilitation Facility Prospective Payment System

The BBA (as amended by the Balanced Budget Refinement Act of 1999) authorized implementation of a per discharge PPS for care provided to Medicare beneficiaries by inpatient rehabilitation hospitals and rehabilitation units, referred to as inpatient rehabilitation facilities (IRFs). The PPS for IRFs became effective on January 1, 2002.

IRFs must meet the regulatory requirements to be classified as a rehabilitation hospital or rehabilitation unit that is excluded from the PPS for inpatient acute-care services. To meet the criteria, an IRF must operate as a hospital. Requirements state that during the most recent, consecutive, and appropriate 12-month time period, the hospital will have treated an inpatient population of whom at least 75 percent required intensive rehabilitative services for treatment of conditions such as stroke, spinal cord injury, congenital deformity, amputation, major multiple trauma, fracture of femur, brain injuries, neurological disorders, burns, rheumatoid arthritis, osteoarthritis, polyarthritis, systemic vasculitides, or knee or hip replacement (Casto and Forrestal 2015).

Patient Assessment Instrument

IRFs are required by CMS to complete a patient assessment instrument (PAI) upon each patient's admission and also discharge from the facility. CMS provides facilities with the **Inpatient Rehabilitation Validation and Entry (IRVEN) system** to collect the IRF-PAI in a database that can be transmitted electronically to the IRF-PAI national database. These data are used in assessing clinical characteristics of patients in rehabilitation settings. Ultimately, they can be used to provide survey agencies with a means to objectively measure and compare facility performance and quality and to allow researchers to develop improved standards of care.

The IRF PPS uses information from the IRF-PAI to classify patients into distinct groups on the basis of clinical characteristics and expected resource needs. Data used to construct these groups, called **case-mix groups (CMGs)**, include rehabilitation impairment categories (RICs), functional status (both motor and cognitive), age, comorbidities, and other factors deemed appropriate to improve the explanatory power of the groups.

Case-Mix Group Relative Weight

An appropriate weight, called the **case-mix group (CMG) relative weight**, is assigned to each case-mix group and measures the relative difference in facility resource intensity among the various groups. Separate payments are calculated for each group, including the application of case- and facility-level adjustments. Facility-level adjustments include wage-index adjustments, low-income patient adjustments, and rural facility adjustments. Case-level adjustments include transfer adjustments, interrupted-stay adjustments, and cost outlier adjustments.

Long-Term Care Hospital Prospective Payment System

The **Balanced Budget Refinement Act (BBRA) of 1999** amended by the Benefits Improvement Act of 2000 mandated the establishment of a per discharge, DRG-based PPS for longer-term care hospitals beginning October 1, 2002.

Long-term care hospitals (LTCHs) are defined as having an average inpatient LOS greater than 25 days (Casto and Forrestal 2015). Typically, patients with the following conditions are treated in LTCHs:

- chronic cardiac disorders;
- neuromuscular and neurovascular diseases such as after-effects of strokes or Parkinson's disease;
- infectious conditions requiring long-term care such as methicillin-resistant *Staphylococcus aureus*;
- complex orthopedic conditions such as pelvic fractures or complicated hip fractures;
- wound care complications;
- multisystem organ failure;
- immunosuppressed conditions;
- respiratory failure and ventilation management and weaning;
- dysphagia management;
- postoperative complications;
- multiple intravenous therapies;
- chemotherapy;
- pre- and postoperative organ transplant care;
- chronic nutritional problems and total parenteral nutrition issues;
- spinal cord injuries;
- burns;
- and head injuries.

MS-LTC-DRGs

Patients are classified into distinct diagnosis groups based on clinical characteristics and expected resource use. These groups are based on the current inpatient MS-DRGs. The payment system includes the following three primary elements: (1) patient classification into a MS-LTC-DRG weight; (2) relative weight of the MS-LTC-DRG, as the weights reflect the variation in cost per discharge as they take into account the utilization for each diagnosis; and (3) federal payment rate. Payment is made at a predetermined per-discharge amount for each MS-LTC-DRG.

Adjustments The PPS does provide for case (patient)–level adjustments such as short-stay outliers, interrupted stays, and high-cost outliers. Facility-wide adjustments include area wage index and cost of living adjustments.

A short-stay outlier is an adjustment to the payment rate for stays that are considerably shorter than the average length of stay (ALOS) for a particular MS-LTC-DRG. A case would qualify for short-stay outlier status when the LOS is between one day and up to and including five-sixths of the ALOS for the MS-LTC-DRG. Both the ALOS and the five-sixths of the ALOS periods are published in the *Federal Register*. Payment under the short-stay outlier is made using different payment methodologies. (See table 7.8 for examples of MS-LTC-DRGs and the ALOS for each.)

An interrupted stay occurs when a patient is discharged from the long-term care hospital and then is readmitted to the same facility for further treatment after a specific number of days away from the facility. There are different policies if the patient is readmitted to the facility within three days (called three-day or less interrupted-stay policy) or if the patient is away from the facility more than three days (called the greater than three-day interrupted-stay policy).

A high-cost outlier is an adjustment to the payment rate for a patient when the costs are unusually high and exceed the typical costs associated with a MS-LTC-DRG. High-cost outlier payments reduce the facility's potential financial losses that can result from treating patients who require more costly care than is normal. A case qualifies for a high-cost outlier payment when the estimated cost of care exceeds the high-cost outlier threshold, which is updated each year.

Inpatient Psychiatric Facilities Prospective Payment System

The Balanced Budget Refinement Act of 1999 mandated the development of a per diem PPS for inpatient psychiatric services furnished in hospitals and exempt units. The PPS became effective on January 1, 2005, establishing a standardized per diem rate to inpatient psychiatric facilities (IPFs) based on the national average of operating, ancillary, and capital costs for each patient day of care in the IPF. The system uses the same MS-DRGs as the acute-care hospital inpatient system.

Adjustments

Patient-level or case-level adjustments are provided for age, specified MS-DRGs, and certain comorbidity categories. Payment adjustments are made for eight age categories beginning with age 45 at which point, statistically, costs are increased as the patient ages.

The IPF receives an MS-DRG payment adjustment for a principal diagnosis that groups to 1 of 17 psychiatric MS-DRGs. (See table 7.9.) Fifteen comorbidity categories that require comparatively more costly treatment during an inpatient stay also generate a payment adjustment.

In addition, there is a variable per diem adjustment to recognize higher costs in the early days of a psychiatric stay.

The IPF PPS also includes an outlier policy for those patients who require more expensive care

Table 7.8. Examples of MS-LTC-DRGs, relative weights, and geometric ALOS

MS-LTC-DRG	Description	Relative weight	Geometric ALOS
28	Spinal procedures with MCC	1.635	34.5
114	Orbital procedures w/o CC/MCC	0.4959	17.7
132	Cranial/facial procedure w/o CC/MCC	0.5373	16.4
150	Epistaxis with MCC	0.7584	21.4
163	Major chest procedure with MCC	2.2257	37.3
181	Respiratory neoplasm with CC	0.6214	20.3
194	Simple pneumonia and pleurisy with MCC	0.5959	17.9

Source: CMS 2015h.

Table 7.9.   Psychiatric DRGs

MS-DRG	MS-DRG description
056	Degenerative nervous system disorders with MCC
057	Degenerative nervous system disorders w/o MCC
080	Nontraumatic stupor and coma with MCC
081	Nontraumatic stupor and coma w/o MCC
876	OR procedure with principal diagnoses of mental illness
880	Acute adjustment reaction and psychosocial dysfunction
881	Depressive neuroses
882	Neuroses except depressive
883	Disorders of personality and impulse control
884	Organic disturbances and mental retardation
885	Psychoses
886	Behavioral and developmental disorders
887	Other mental disorder diagnoses
894	Alcohol/drug abuse or dependence, left Against Medical Advice (AMA)
895	Alcohol/drug abuse or dependence with rehabilitation therapy
896	Alcohol/drug abuse or dependence w/o rehabilitation therapy with MCC
897	Alcohol/drug abuse or dependence w/o rehabilitation therapy w/o MCC

Source: CMS 2015i.

than expected in an effort to minimize the financial risk to the IPF. Although the basis of the system is a per diem rate, outlier payments are made on a per case basis rather than on the per diem basis. Payment is also adjusted for patients who are given electroconvulsive therapy (ECT).

The PPS also includes regulations on payments when there is an interrupted stay, meaning the patient is discharged from an IPF and returns to the same or another facility before midnight on the third consecutive day. The intent of the policy is to prevent a facility from prematurely discharging a patient after the maximum payment is received and subsequently readmitting the patient.

Facility adjustments include a wage-index adjustment, a rural location adjustment, a teaching status adjustment, a cost-of-living adjustment for Alaska and Hawaii, and a qualifying emergency department adjustment.

Check Your Understanding 7.3

Instructions: **Answer the following questions on a separate piece of paper.**

1. What does case-mix index refer to?

2. Describe the major components of the resource-based relative value scale.

3. What concept is applied when multiple surgical procedures are furnished during the same operative session?

4. What must the average length of stay be to meet the definition of a long-term care hospital?

5. What other PPSs use the MS-DRGs currently used for inpatient hospitals?

Processing of Reimbursement Claims

Understanding payment mechanisms is an important foundation for accurately processing claims forms. However, it is not enough just to understand payment mechanisms.

A facility's patient accounts department is responsible for billing third-party payers, processing accounts receivable, monitoring payments from third-party payers, and verifying insurance coverage. Medicare administrative contractors (MACs) contract with CMS to serve as the financial agent between providers and the federal government to locally administer Medicare's Part A and Part B.

Coordination of Benefits

In many instances, patients have more than one insurance policy, and the determination of which policy is primary and which is secondary is necessary so that there is no duplication of benefits paid. This process is called the coordination of benefits (COB) or the **coordination of benefits transaction**. The monies collected from third-party payers cannot be greater than the amount of the provider's charges.

Submission of Claims

According to a report by America's Health Insurance Plans, more than 96 percent of hospital claims are submitted electronically to Medicare (AHIP 2013). The Administrative Simplification Compliance Act (ASCA), which was part of the Health Insurance Portability and Accountability Act (HIPAA), mandated the electronic submission of all healthcare claims with a few exceptions.

Healthcare facilities submit claims via the 837I electronic format, which replaces the UB-04 (CMS-1450) paper billing form. Physicians submit claims via the 837P electronic format, which takes the place of the CMS-1500 billing form. For those healthcare facilities with a waiver of the ASCA requirements, UB-04 and CMS-1500 are used.

Explanation of Benefits, Medicare Summary Notice, and Remittance Advice

An **explanation of benefits (EOB)** is a statement sent by a third-party payer to the patient to explain services provided, amounts billed, and payments made by the health plan. Medicare sends a **Medicare summary notice (MSN)** to a beneficiary to show how much the provider billed, how much Medicare reimbursed the provider, and what the patient must pay the provider by way of deductible and copayments.

A **remittance advice (RA)** is sent to the provider to explain payments made by third-party payers. Payments are typically sent in batches with the RA sent to the facility and payments electronically transferred to the provider's bank.

Medicare Administrative Contractors

A **Medicare Administrative Contractor (MAC)** is "a private healthcare insurer that has been awarded a geographic jurisdiction to process Medicare Part A and Part B (A/B) medical claims or Durable Medical Equipment (DME) claims for Medicare Fee-For-Service (FFS) beneficiaries" (CMS 2015j). A network of MACs serve as the primary operational contact between the Medicare FFS program and the healthcare providers enrolled in the program. "MACs are multistate, regional contractors responsible for administering both Medicare Part A and Medicare Part B claims. MACs perform many activities including:

- Process Medicare FFS claims
- Make and account for Medicare FFS payments
- Enroll providers in the Medicare FFS program
- Handle provider reimbursement services and audit institutional provider cost reports
- Handle redetermination requests (1st stage appeals process)

- Respond to provider inquiries
- Educate providers about Medicare FFS billing requirements
- Establish local coverage determinations (LCDs)
- Review medical records for selected claims
- Coordinate with CMS and other FFS contractors" (CMS 2015j)

National Correct Coding Initiative

CMS implemented the National Correct Coding Initiative (NCCI) in 1996 to develop correct coding methodologies to improve the appropriate payment of Medicare Part B claims.

NCCI policies are based on:

- Coding conventions defined in the CPT codebooks
- National and local policies and coding edits
- Analysis of standard medical and surgical practice
- Review of current coding practices

The NCCI edits explain what procedures and services cannot be billed together on the same day of service for a patient. The mutually exclusive edit applies to improbable or impossible combinations of codes. For example, code 58940, Oophorectomy, partial or total, unilateral or bilateral, would never be used with code 58150, Total abdominal hysterectomy (corpus and cervix), with or without removal of tube(s), with or without removal of ovary(s). Modifiers may be used to indicate circumstances in which the NCCI edits should not be applied and payment should be made as requested. Modifier-59, for example, is used when circumstances require that certain procedures or services be reported together even though they usually are not.

Portions of the NCCI are incorporated into the **outpatient code editor (OCE)**, against which all ambulatory claims are reviewed. The OCE also applies a set of logical rules to determine whether various combinations of codes are correct and appropriately represent services provided. Billing issues generated from these NCCI and OCE edits often result in claim denials.

 Check Your Understanding 7.4

Instructions: **Answer the following questions on a separate piece of paper.**

1. What is a COB transaction, and what is its purpose?
2. What purpose does the remittance advice serve? What purpose does the EOB serve?
3. What is the Medicare summary notice?
4. Differentiate between the 837I and the 837P.
5. What is a Medicare administrative contractor and what do they do?

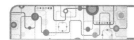 References

American Association of State Compensation Insurance Funds. 2015. History. http://www.aascif.org/index.php?page=histroy

American Society of Cataract and Refractive Surgery. 2015. 2015 Medicare Physician Fee Schedule (MPFS) Final Rule Released. http://www.ascrs.org/node/20577

America's Health Insurance Plans. 2013. An Updated Survey of Health Insurance Claims Receipt and Processing Times. **www.ahip.org/**SurveyHealthCare-January2013

BlueCross BlueShield. 2015. About Blue Cross Blue Shield Association. http://www.bcbs.com/about-the-association/

BlueCross BlueShield of Minnesota. 2015. 80 Years of Innovation. https://mktg.bluecrossmn.com/timeline/bcbsmn/

Casto, A. and E. Forrestal. 2015. *Principles of Healthcare Reimbursement*, 5th ed. Chicago: AHIMA.

Centers for Medicare and Medicaid Services. 2015a. Medicare and You 2016. https://www.medicare.gov/Pubs/pdf/10050.pdf

Centers for Medicare and Medicaid Services. 2015b. Medicare 2015 and 2016 Costs at a Glance. https://www.medicare.gov/your-medicare-costs/costs-at-a-glance/costs-at-glance.html

Centers for Medicare and Medicaid Services. 2015c. Eligibility. http://www.medicaid.gov/affordablecareact/provisions/eligibility.html

Centers for Medicare and Medicaid Services. 2015d. Details for title: CMS-1632-F and IFC, CMS-1632-CN2. https://www.cms.gov/Medicare/Medicare-Fee-for-Service-Payment/AcuteInpatientPPS/FY2016-IPPS-Final-Rule-Home-Page-Items/FY2016-IPPS-Final-Rule-Regulations.html

Centers for Medicare and Medicaid Services. 2015e. PFS Relative Value Files. https://www.cms.gov/Medicare/Medicare-Fee-for-Service-Payment/PhysicianFeeSched/PFS-Relative-Value-Files-Items/RVU15A.html?DLPage=1&DLEntries=10&DLSort=0&DLSortDir=descending

Centers for Medicare and Medicaid Services. 2015f. Details for title: CMS-1622-P. https://www.cms.gov/Medicare/Medicare-Fee-for-Service-Payment/SNFPPS/List-of-SNF-Federal-Regulations-Items/CMS-1622-P.html

Centers for Medicare and Medicaid Services. 2015g. Medicare and Medicaid Programs; CY 2016 Home Health Prospective Payment System Rate Update; Home Health Value-Based Purchasing Model; and Home Health Quality Reporting Requirements. *Federal Register*. http://federalregister.gov/a/2015-27931

Centers for Medicare and Medicaid Services. 2015h. MS-LTC-DRG Files FY 2016. https://www.cms.gov/Medicare/Medicare-Fee-for-Service-Payment/LongTermCareHospitalPPS/LTCHPPS-Regulations-and-Notices-Items/LTCH-PPS-CMS-1632-F.html?DLPage=1&DLEntries=10&DLSort=3&DLSortDir=descending

Centers for Medicare and Medicaid Services. 2015i. Medicare Program; Inpatient Psychiatric Facilities Prospective Payment System-Update for Fiscal Year Beginning October 1, 2015 (FY 2016). Federal Register. https://federalregister.gov/a/2015-18903

Centers for Medicare and Medicaid Services. 2015j. Medicare Administrative Contractors (MACs) as of December 2015. https://www.cms.gov/Medicare/Medicare-Contracting/Medicare-Administrative-Contractors/Downloads/MACs-By-State-Dec-2015.pdf

Centers for Medicare and Medicaid Services. 2013. Medicare Enrollment: Hospital Insurance and/or Supplemental Medical Insurance Programs for Total, Fee-for-Service and Managed Care Enrollees as of July 1, 2011: Selected Calendar Years 1966–2011; 2012–2013, HHS Budget in Brief, FY2014.

Centers for Medicare and Medicaid Services. 2005. Medicaid At-a-Glance 2005: A Medicaid Information Source. https://downloads.cms.gov/cmsgov/archived-downloads/MedicaidGenInfo/downloads/medicaidataglance2005.pdf

East Coast Health Insurance. 2015. Blue Cross Blue Shield Association Plans. http://echealthinsurance.com/companies/blue-cross-blue-shield-association/

Healthcare.gov. 2015. The Children's Health Insurance Program (CHIP). https://www.healthcare.gov/medicaid-chip/childrens-health-insurance-program/

Henry J. Kaiser Family Foundation. n.d. Medicare Enrollment, 1966–2013. http://kff.org/medicare/slide/medicare-enrollment-1966-2013/

Henry J. Kaiser Family Foundation. 2013. Medicare Advantage 2013 Spotlight: Enrollment Update. https://kaiserfamilyfoundation.files.wordpress.com/2013/06/8448.pdf

Patient-Centered Primary Care Collaborative. 2015. Defining the Medical Home. https://www.pcpcc.org/about/medical-home

Social Security Administration. 2004. Annual Statistical Supplement. https://www.ssa.gov/policy/docs/statcomps/supplement/2004/prog_desc.pdf

Wellmark. 2015. History. https://www.wellmark.com/AboutWellmark/CompanyInformation/History.aspx

8

Revenue Cycle Management

Colleen Malmgren, MS, RHIA, and
C. Jeanne Solberg, MA, RHIA, FAHIMA

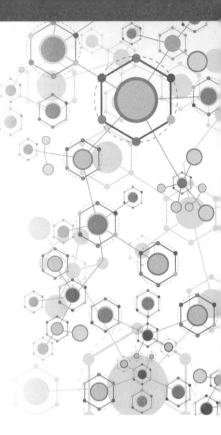

Learning Objectives

- Examine revenue cycle management's key phases
- Utilize key performance indicators to compare performance among peers within the industry
- Identify critical points in the revenue cycle processes
- Analyze the key functions in each phase of the revenue life cycle from point-of-service collections to claims adjudication
- Evaluate the impact of a clinical documentation improvement program on the revenue cycle
- Evaluate the impact of case management and utilization management on the revenue cycle
- Analyze and correct issues at the source of denial
- Recommend proper claims denial management tactics
- Build a successful denial management team

Key Terms

Accounts receivable (A/R) days
Adverse determination
Bill hold period
Case management
Case manager
Case-mix index (CMI)
Charge capture
Charge description master (CDM)
Charity care
Claims scrubber software

Clean claim
Denial
Discharged, no final bill (DNFB)
Facility charge
Financial counselor
Hospital-issued notice of noncoverage (HINN)
Insurance verification
Key performance indicator (KPI)

Local coverage determination (LCD)
MAP key
Medical necessity
National coverage determination (NCD)
Point-of-service (POS) collection
Preauthorization
Revenue cycle
Utilization management

There is significant financial pressure on healthcare organizations to manage their costs as consumers of services take on an increased financial responsibility for their healthcare costs. The **revenue cycle** is the process that begins when a patient comes to a healthcare system for services and includes those activities that have to occur in order for a provider of the care to bill at the end of the patient's service encounter. The healthcare revenue cycle encompasses people, tools, methodologies, and techniques that medical institutions use to manage their patients' financial responsibility. Revenue cycle management is a complex process that involves balancing people, processes, technology, and the environment in which the processes take place.

The revenue management life cycle can be broken down into three phases—the front-end, middle, and back-end (see figure 8.1). The front-end of the revenue cycle includes patient access functions such as scheduling the patient for services, registration of the patient, prior or preauthorization for services, insurance verification, service estimates, and financial counseling. During this phase, healthcare organizations need to ascertain the source of payment for the service, follow requirements specified by the payer, accurately collect the patient's demographic information, and ensure a positive patient experience. Contract negotiations and renegotiations with third-party payers impact the front-end process. Specific contract terms negotiated with payers drive patient services covered for reimbursement. These terms need to be defined and understood by staff to properly support the front-end of the revenue cycle.

The middle process of the revenue cycle includes case management, capture of charges for the services rendered, and coding for those services based on clinical documentation. The key objectives in this phase are to manage clinical practice according to accepted medical guidelines, identify reimbursable services and ensure that documentation supports those services, and ensure accurate and complete coding of the documented services.

The back end of the revenue cycle is the business office or patient financial service process and includes claims processing and payment posting, follow-up, customer service, collections of unpaid bills, and denial management (HIMSS 2010). In this phase, organizations focus on releasing claims to the payers as quickly as possible after service is rendered and generating accurate and complete claims resulting in reimbursement of the amount expected by the payer.

Figure 8.1. Revenue management life cycle

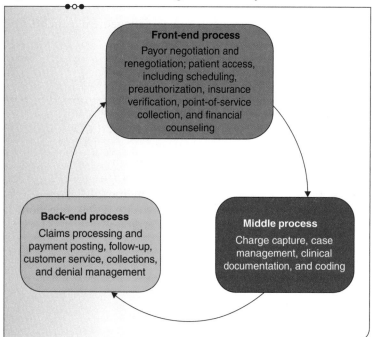

Revenue Cycle Front-End Process

The front end of the healthcare revenue cycle starts at the point of scheduling a patient for healthcare services, or when the patient presents for services if not previously scheduled. Revenue cycle staff ascertain the source of payment for the service, accurately collect patient demographic information, and ensure an excellent patient experience with the front-end process. Healthcare organizations have the best opportunity to improve the overall revenue cycle process during the front-end process by accurately identifying, scheduling, and registering patients (Llewellyn and Moore 2014).

Scheduling and Registration

The scheduling of patient visits requires optimal assignment of patients to the available healthcare resources. Accuracy of information captured in this stage is vital to many of the processes occurring later in the revenue cycle, and the goal is to continuously improve data collection and accuracy.

Staff responsible for scheduling and registration functions requires a significant amount of knowledge regarding the medical services provided, insurance carrier requirements, provider preferences, and operational hours of services to be rendered. The registration staff is tasked with gathering and entering the required patient demographic and financial information. This staff also takes an active role in promoting positive public relations with patients to increase community trust in the facility. Examples of demographic data collected include name, date of birth, residence, sex, marital status, race and ethnicity, employer, insurance carrier, and guarantor. Incomplete or inaccurate information can delay care and negatively impact the revenue cycle (Corrigan 2009). When a patient arrives for services, the registration staff is responsible for validating the patient's identity, for example by

photo identification; obtaining copies of insurance card(s); and obtaining patient (responsible party) signatures for insurance payment and release of medical information.

Initiating patient registration at the time of scheduling saves time and is more user-friendly for patients when they arrive for services. Each time a patient presents for clinical services, the prior collected data need to be verified for accuracy and updated with any changes.

The most common registration errors that affect the revenue cycle are noted in figure 8.2.

Insurance Verification

Insurance verification is a vital component of the prearrival process for scheduled patients. Verification of the patient's insurance for unscheduled patients occurs at the time of their registration for clinical services or shortly thereafter. The verification process entails validating that the patient is a member of the insurance plan given and is covered for the scheduled service date. It is also important to validate whether the patient's insurance plan is in-network versus out-of-network, whether the scheduled service expenses will be covered, whether a referral or an authorization is required prior to the service being rendered, and whether the patient will incur an out-of-pocket expense (Langford et al. 2010). The validation of insurance coverage occurs through either electronic or telephonic communication with insurers.

Patient demographic and insurance information needs to be complete and correct. In the absence of proper eligibility determination, payment for services may be delayed or denied; claims may need to be reprocessed or reworked, adding delays in receiving payment for services; and patients may become dissatisfied due to late statements and increased financial responsibility for services (Llewellyn and Moore 2014).

Figure 8.2.   Most common registration errors

- Incorrect insurance plan listed
- Policy number or group number missing or invalid
- Patient not eligible on date of service
- Patient with insurance listed as private pay
- Medicare listed when plan is Medicare health maintenance organization (HMO)
- Medicare listed as primary when should be secondary
- Minors listed as guarantors
- More than one medical record number per patient
- Accident claims without occurrence codes
- Patient relationship to insurance subscriber code errors
- Failure to list medical necessity
- Missing guarantor or employer information
- Physician orders incomplete or missing

- Internal coding mismatches (for example, financial class to patient type to stay type to service code to admit code)
- Missing prior authorization or precertification required for service provided
- Transposed digits: Social Security number, date of birth, policy number, group number
- Invalid punctuation in specified text fields
- Misspelled name
- Insurance eligibility verification failure
- Address verification failure (returned mail cost)
- Observation patient with inpatient stay type
- Point-of-service collection failure
- Incomplete or inaccurate Medicare secondary payer questionnaire

Source: Shorrosh 2011.

Preauthorization

Preauthorization is the requirement that a healthcare provider obtain permission from the health insurer prior to predefined services being provided to the patients. Preauthorization may also be referred to as prior approval, authorization, precertification, or predetermination. Insurers have established more stringent approval guidelines due to the increase in high-technology and high-cost procedures and tests. For example, if a physician orders a fluorodeoxyglucose positron emission tomography (FDG-PET) scan for a Medicare patient, the Center for Medicare and Medicaid Services (CMS) provides a list of oncological conditions that must be present to receive payment for the FDG-PET service (CMS 2014a).

Scheduling or preauthorization teams need to understand medical procedures and tests, initial diagnoses, and scheduled treatments in order to obtain the necessary preauthorization by the insurance company. There is a wide variation in prior authorization requirements and criteria among payers (HASC Summit 2009). It is important for healthcare providers to have current lists of procedures and tests requiring prior authorization from all health insurers and have processes in place to obtain the authorization prior to services being rendered. Reimbursement for services without preauthorization is often denied by insurers and

results in significant negative financial impact to the healthcare organization (Bendix 2013).

Financial Counseling

A healthcare organization needs to ensure the patient understands the financial aspects of his or her encounter of care and the process for resolving any fiscal responsibility. **Financial counselors** are staff dedicated to helping patients and physicians determine sources of reimbursement for healthcare services. The counselors are responsible for identifying and verifying the method of payment and debt resolution for services rendered to patients. Counselors need to understand a patient's financial assets and discuss payment alternatives with patients. Some patients are eligible for **charity care**, which is defined as healthcare services that have been or will be provided but are never expected to result in cash inflows. Charity care results from a provider's policy to provide healthcare services free or at a discount to individuals who meet the established criteria (HFMA 2016). The counselors can establish payment options such as credit card payments, bank loans, and interest-bearing, hospital-funded payment arrangements as necessary.

Strategies for financial counselors can include the ability to provide discounts on hospital bills for patients who do not have health insurance and who meet certain eligibility criteria. The amount of the discount is determined after an assessment of the patient's or a family's financial need and is typically based on current federal poverty guidelines. Incentives for prompt-payment discounts can also be offered to patients. Healthcare facilities need to follow consistent procedures and steps to obtain appropriate payment and to enhance revenue cycle processes (Butcher 2014).

Point of Service Collection

Patients have taken on an increasing amount of financial responsibility for their healthcare costs. Insurance companies determine that the annual copayments and deductibles for which the patient is responsible account for approximately 5 percent of total net revenue and more than 40 percent of outstanding receivables (Advisory Board Company 2015). Point-of-service (POS) collection is the collection of the portion of the bill that is the patient's responsibility to pay prior to the provision of service being rendered. POS collection works well with scheduled and nonemergent patient visits. Access to billing data from both payers and the healthcare's own system is needed to be able to estimate what a patient owes at the point of service. Revenue cycle staff needs to communicate with the patient to set expectations regarding the cost of the services, insurance coverage, and the expected payment at the time of service. It is also important that community healthcare providers and clinical leadership be educated about the POS policy and procedures within the healthcare organization so they understand and support the process (Brzon 2011).

Medical Necessity Coverage Issues

Health insurance companies provide coverage only for health-related services that they define or determine to be medically necessary. Medicare defines medical necessity as a determination that a service is reasonable and necessary for the related diagnosis or treatment of illness or injury.

The American College of Medical Quality (ACMQ) is an organization whose focus is providing leadership and education in healthcare quality management.

ACMQ defines the application of appropriate services and supplies as those that are neither more nor less than what the patient requires at a specific point in time. The ACMQ (2015) has also adopted nine principles as part of their policy related to the application of medical necessity (see figure 8.3).

Medicare's national coverage policies are known as national coverage determinations (NCDs), and local fiscal intermediary policies are known as local coverage determinations (LCDs). These policies define the specific diagnosis and procedure codes that support medical necessity for many services provided. There are not NCD or LCD policies for every type of procedure or service that could be provided for a patient, so healthcare organizations must remain current with the regulatory requirements and revisions in order to reduce billing denials and ensure that payment is received for the services rendered. Resources to support specific requirements include payer billing manuals, Medicare billing manuals, local fiscal intermediary policies and local Part B Medicare carrier policies.

Pre-Encounter Services

Many healthcare facilities have combined staff resources related to the revenue cycle front-end process and developed pre-encounter service centers for patients. The centers handle preregistration, insurance eligibility and benefit verification, payer authorizations, and preservice collections for all scheduled diagnostic testing and surgery patients. Healthcare organizations have developed the following performance characteristics to support the front-end processes:

- Ninety-five percent of all scheduled services will be preregistered.
- All areas performing registration functions will be guided by the same operating characteristics.
- Procedures will be standardized and all staff will be trained accordingly.
- Lack of preregistration will not contribute to treatment delays.
- Insurance clearance processes will drive a decrease in payer denials.

Figure 8.3. Definition and application of medical necessity

1. Determinations of medical necessity must adhere to the standard of care that applies to the actual direct care and treatment of the patient.
2. Medical necessity is the standard terminology that all healthcare professionals and entities will use in the review process when determining if medical care is appropriate and essential.
3. Determinations of medical necessity must reflect the efficient and cost-effective application of patient care including, but not limited to, diagnostic testing, therapies (including activity restriction, after-care instructions, and prescriptions), disability ratings, rehabilitating an illness, injury, disease or its associated symptoms, impairments or functional limitations, procedures, psychiatric care, levels of hospital care, extended care, long-term care, hospice care, and home healthcare.
4. Determinations of medical necessity made in a concurrent review should include discussions with the attending provider regarding the current medical condition of the patient whenever possible. A physician advisor or reviewer can make a positive determination regarding medical necessity without necessarily speaking with the treating provider if the advisor has enough available information to make an appropriate medical decision. A physician advisor cannot decide to deny care as not medically necessary without speaking to the treating provider and these discussions must be clearly documented.
5. Determinations of medical necessity must be unrelated to payers' monetary benefit.
6. Determinations of medical necessity must always be made on a case-by-case basis consistent with the applicable standard of care and must be available for peer review.
7. Recommendations approving medical necessity may be made by a nonphysician reviewer. Negative determinations for the initial review regarding medical necessity must be made by a physician advisor who has the clinical training to review the particular clinical problem (clinically matched) under review. A physician reviewer or advisor must not delegate his or her review decisions to a nonphysician reviewer.
8. The process to be used in evaluating medical necessity should be made known to the patient.
9. All medical review organizations involved in determining medical necessity shall have uniform, written procedures for appeals of negative determinations that services or supplies are not medically necessary.

Source: ACMQ 2015.

- Patient payment expectations will be communicated to the patients and (except for emergency department services) will be collected prior to or at the time of service.

- All uninsured patients will be offered a self-pay discount package or will be screened for either medical assistance or charity care, or both.

- Quality monitoring will be performed on a monthly basis with feedback to the employees.

- Physician offices will be notified of any non-covered services to make decisions regarding continuing with services.

- Denials will be work-listed for identification and resolution.

- Preregistration and financial clearance of scheduled services will be completed five days before the patient's appointment.

- Staff will use automated credit-scoring and address-checking software to identify a patient's potential to pay and potential eligibility for charity care (Butcher 2012).

Results from combining the front-end processes have eliminated last-minute cancellations of scheduled services, improved patient flow, and increased patient satisfaction.

Contract Management

The management of contracts is an integral part of the revenue cycle. Healthcare facilities negotiate contract terms with third-party insurers for payment of services rendered to patients. This is where allowable costs, chargeable services, and supplies provided by a hospital or physician that qualify as covered expenses are defined. The contract terms need to benefit and be cost-effective for the facility, its patients, and the insurer.

Contract management has its own life cycle and contract managers need to have an understanding of competitor and local market rates in order to negotiate reasonable reimbursement rates that cover the healthcare organization's expenses, while remaining competitive. It is important to track variances from contract terms and understand the root cause and responsible party of the variances. Variance may be caused from the healthcare organization's internal processes, from a payer's contract term setup in their computer system or from a payer's or provider's a lack of understanding of the contract terms negotiated. Routine meeting with payers often help resolve variances and improve the revenue cycle performance (Emdeon 2015).

Technology Tools

Hospitals and healthcare systems need to accurately forecast, calculate, and capture all net revenue contractually owed to them from payers and patients. Contract management technology can assist with understanding the expected net revenue of every patient at discharge regardless of payer. Contract management software systems enable organizations to coordinate all phases of contracted payer business (negotiations, payment compliance, performance review); recover prior contract management underpayments by identifying payment variances; ensure proper payments on all subsequent claims as the system accurately calculates expected reimbursement; model complex contracts with multiple reimbursement formulas in a simple and timely manner; and take appropriate action when expected results are not achieved.

Technology tools used in the front-end revenue cycle process are important to support quality of work and enhance the productivity of staff. Tools identified by the 2008–2009 HIMSS Revenue Cycle Improvement Task Force to support the front-end process include:

- Enterprise-wide scheduling system that allows patients to scheduled inpatient or outpatient services throughout an entire healthcare system.

- Order tracking and management system is tracking technology that identifies when an order is placed and then received by the processing department, such as laboratory or radiology; scheduling of the patient; actual test performed, and eventually reports the results of the test.

- Telephony system in order to measure call activity such as calls received, the amount of time to answer a call, or measurement of time to transmit a fax.

- Registration quality assurance tools such as electronic advanced beneficiary notification, which specifics which medical tests or procedures Medicare will not cover. If a Medicare patient continues to desire to have a test or procedure after being notified that it is not covered, a notice would be given to the patient stating they are responsible for the payment of the service, if rendered.

- Online third-party eligibility and coverage limitations is a system that allows healthcare staff to validate the third-party insurance coverage provided by the patient and identify any limitations in the healthcare coverage terms.

- Workflow drivers to ensure all financial clearance functions are completed.

- Estimation tools for patient out-of-pocket financial responsibility that calculate the expected patient payment based on the terms of their specific healthcare insurance.

- Electronic financial assistance applications is an electronic format for requesting financial assistance for healthcare expenses (HIMSS 2010).

Check Your Understanding 8.1

Instructions: Answer the following questions on a separate piece of paper

1. Name the Medicare coverage policies that list diagnoses supporting medical necessity?

2. What strategies are employed by the financial counseling staff to obtain appropriate payment for services provided to the patient?

3. List five common registration errors that affect the revenue cycle.

4. What information does the scheduling staff need in order to obtain authorization prior to services being rendered?

5. Identify five principles related to the application of medical necessity.

Revenue Cycle Middle Process

The middle section of the healthcare revenue cycle represents the intersection of clinical practice and documentation charge capture and billing for services. The key objectives are to "manage clinical practice and charging within accepted guidelines to ensure reimbursement, document services completely and accurately, and ensure coding of documented services is complete and accurate" (HIMSS 2010).

Case and Utilization Management

The Case Management Society of America (CMSA) defines **case management** as "a collaborative process of assessment, planning, facilitation, care coordination, evaluation, and advocacy for options and services to meet an individual's and family's comprehensive health needs through communication and available resources to promote quality cost effective outcomes" (CMSA 2015). The American Case Management Association (ACMA) defines case management as:

> A collaborative practice model including patients, nurses, social workers, physicians, other practitioners, caregivers, and the community. The case management process encompasses communication and facilitates care along a continuum through effective resource coordination. The goals of case management include the achievement of optimal health, access to care, and appropriate utilization of resources, balanced with the patient's right to self-determination. (ACMA 2012)

Both organizations support professionals, called **case managers**, who evaluate the appropriateness of hospital admissions according to pre-established criteria.

Case managers' responsibilities were initially to manage and ensure the appropriate utilization of acute care resources with a focus on improving quality and reducing costs. The case manager role has evolved further and involves:

- Partnering with physicians during rounds to participate in treatment plan progress reporting

- Questioning duplicative interventions or interventions that may be contrary to evidence-based protocols

- Collaborating with the nurses to identify any obstacles to move the treatment plan forward and bring that information to the bedside to resolve with the physician

- Facilitating communication among attending physicians and consultants

- Advocating for the patient and family to ensure that prescribed interventions are suitable to the patient's preferences and economic circumstances

- Prompting a planning discussion for transitioning patients from one level of care to another—whether from a critical care area to a medical unit or from a medical unit to the patient's home (Daniels and Frater 2011)

These responsibilities allow the case managers to quickly identify barriers that may impede the efficient progression of the patient through the healthcare service process. Unexpected delays in care or discharge can be prevented, and unnecessary consumption of resources such as additional patient days can be avoided (Daniels 2007). The case manager can have a positive impact on the revenue cycle by avoiding the delays, navigating the patient through the healthcare process, and acting as an advocate for the patient resulting in higher patient satisfaction with the healthcare facility (Miodonski 2011).

Utilization management works in conjunction with case management and, at times, the terms and responsibilities are used interchangeably. Health **utilization management** (UM) is the "evaluation of the medical necessity, appropriateness, and efficiency of the use of healthcare services, procedures, and facilities under the provisions of the applicable health benefits plan" (URAC 2015). The UM staff is responsible for the day-to-day provisions of the hospital's utilization plan as required by the Medicare Conditions of Participation. Utilization staff responsibilities include:

- Reviewing the health record to extract information required to make utilization associated decisions
- Using pre-established criteria to evaluate the appropriateness of admissions, continued stay, level of care, and discharge readiness
- Acting as a resource to hospital departments 24 hours a day, 7 days a week
- Screening all inpatient admissions or observation stays within 24 hours of the event
- Reviewing conversions from inpatient to observation and observation to inpatient to assure compliance to pre-established criteria
- Applying utilization criteria to all admissions regardless of the third party payer
- Reviewing inpatient continued stays on a routine and consistent basis, but minimally every three days or sooner
- Screening the patient's health record for timeliness, appropriateness and safety of services or resources being provided
- Organizing weekly meetings with the patient's care team to solve identified problems for complex cases with high-dollar or long length of stays
- Following Utilization Management Committee's direction, perform retrospective or focused reviews (McLean 2011a)

The UM staff works with external quality improvement organizations under the direction of the Centers for Medicare and Medicaid Services, to support the quality of patient care and services. They also work with third-party reviewers to provide requested clinical information, facilitate health record access, supervise external insurance reviewers, and ensure communication to patients and their families resulting from the external review organization communications.

According to the Centers for Medicare and Medicaid Services (CMS 2014a), hospitals have the responsibility to issue **hospital-issued notices of noncoverage (HINNs)** to Medicare beneficiaries prior to admission, at admission, or at any point during an inpatient stay if the hospital determines that the care the beneficiary is receiving, or is about to receive, is not covered because it:

- is not medically necessary,
- is not delivered in the most appropriate setting, or
- is custodial in nature.

Medicaid requirements vary from state to state for notification of denial of care or termination of benefits. The healthcare facility's utilization plan should include the state's specific requirements associated with denial or termination of benefits coverage (McLean 2011b).

Commercial payers are responsible for providing written documentation to the patient or the patient's family, attending physician, and facility of an **adverse determination**. Adverse determinations are when a healthcare insurer denies payment for proposed or already rendered healthcare service. Payers work with the hospital department responsible for utilization management to communicate the decision. Utilization personnel take an active role in monitoring, reporting, and communicating adverse determination to patients and their families and ensuring all procedures are followed in rendering the communication. These procedures are important to ensure financial responsibility of services provided and are important in a well-managed revenue cycle process (McLean 2011b).

Charge Capture

Charge capture is a method of recording services and supplies or items delivered to the patient and directing them to be billed on a claim form. It is the process of documenting, posting, and reconciling the charges for services rendered to patients. Organizational success is directly dependent upon accurately documenting and reporting charges in a timely manner; and the aim is to have policies, procedures, and resources in place to ensure quality charge capture that enhances revenue and adheres to compliance and other standards.

Quality charge capture is critical for the following reasons:

- Payments are often related to charges; reimbursement for outpatient services is often driven by the specific charges along with Current Procedural Terminology (CPT) and Healthcare Common Procedure Coding System (HCPCS) codes listed on the claim.

- Charges drive prices and rates for reimbursement; payment rates established for diagnosis-related groups (DRGs) and ambulatory patient classifications (APCs) are determined by analyzing historical cost data; if true, costs are not being reflected, reimbursement rates are set too low.

- Charges reflect resource utilization; this allows analysis and comparison of the resources used for patients with similar diagnoses treated in similar service lines or receiving similar treatments.

- Charges help in the measurement of labor cost and productivity; this assists the organization in monitoring the cost of doing business and determining staffing needs.

- Errors in charge capture create significant rework and billing delays; errors may also go undetected and result in loss of revenue or put the organization at risk by not meeting regulatory requirements.

A variety of charge capture mechanisms may be in place to get charges entered into the billing system. Charges may be entered from paper or electronic charge tickets or encounter forms, or they may be interfaced from source systems used in areas such as a lab or pharmacy that submit large volumes of charges. Electronic health record systems may also be configured to apply charges to patient accounts, and health information management coding staff often has responsibility for some charge entry based on clinical documentation. Regardless of the mechanism for charge entry, it is important to verify the accuracy of the charge codes being entered and to ensure they are posted to the correct patient accounts for the correct dates of service.

The primary responsibility for charge capture is assigned to staff in the departments providing the services; but there are complex regulatory requirements surrounding compliant charge capture, so ongoing charge capture education with well-documented policies and procedures is vital.

Organizations may utilize internal billing system edits designed to detect and correct charge capture errors before claims are submitted to the third-party payers. They may also utilize APC grouper software or Medicare **claims scrubber software** designed to detect errors that would result in payer denials, Common edits include a male patient with charges for a procedure that could only be performed on a female, or reporting charges for a blood transfusion, without any charges for the blood product transfused. As errors are detected, they should appear on reports or in electronic record work queues that are reviewed by the appropriate staff. Charge corrections can then be made and issues or problems can be detected and resolved.

Timely submission of charges is also critical for revenue cycle success. Each facility has a defined number of days during the **bill hold period**. These are the number of days in which accounts will be held from billing so charges can be entered after the patient is discharged. Bill hold assumes that there will be a delay in accumulating the charges incurred by a patient. By incorporating this predicted delay into normal operations, the facility creates a preventive control to avoid under billing or having to submit late charges to the payer. Charges added after this bill hold (typically two to five days) are considered late charges.

Third-party payers generally will not reimburse a claim that does not include the clinical diagnostic and procedural codes. This is true whether the reimbursement is based on a prospective payment system (PPS), actual charges, or some other method. For this reason, the patient accounts department cannot drop a bill until the patient record has been coded. Therefore, timely, accurate coding is critical to the reimbursement process and directly affects the facility's cash flow.

An additional responsibility in revenue cycle management is determining items or services that are not separately billable. Routine supplies are commonly defined by CMS as a supply used as part of the normal course of service where the care is delivered, given to most patients treated in a particular setting or incidental to the procedure, or inherent to a procedure (CMS 2016c). These supplies are not billable and are considered part of the room and board charge for a hospital or an overhead cost for the healthcare facility. Examples of routine supplies include specimen collection containers, syringes, needles, gloves, pillows, sponges, heating pads, and irrigation solutions. Equipment available to all patients in an area or commonly used during a procedure is also considered not separately billable. Examples of equipment not separately billable include cardiac monitors, blood pressure monitors, wall suction units, and intravenous pumps.

Another important aspect of charge capture includes the facility charge for outpatient clinic and emergency department visits. Initially on April 7, 2000, CMS had instructed hospitals to report resources utilized for hospital clinic outpatient visits and Emergency Department visits using the CPT evaluation and management (E/M) codes (CMS 2008). The **facility charge** allows capture of an E/M charge that represents resources not included with the CPT code for the clinic environment. Hospitals were also instructed to develop internal hospital guidelines for reporting the appropriate visit level. Three options were outlined to allow for capture of the facility evaluation and management charge:

- Guidelines based on the number or type of staff interventions
  - Number and type of interventions
  - Based upon diagnosis—evaluating most common versus extreme trauma
  - Interventions not identified by CPT
- Guidelines based on the time that nonphysician staff spent with the patient
  - Nursing time spent with patient
- Guidelines based on a point system
  - Resource intensity points
  - Severity acuity based upon patient complexity (CMS 2008)

CMS never developed national guidelines but set the expectation for hospitals to establish internal guidelines to follow the principles listed here.

1. The coding guidelines should follow the intent of the CPT code descriptor in that the guidelines should be designed to reasonably relate the intensity of hospital resources to the different levels of effort represented by the code (65 FR 18451).
2. The coding guidelines should be based on hospital facility resources. The guidelines should not be based on physician resources (67 FR 66792).
3. The coding guidelines should be clear to facilitate accurate payments and be usable for compliance purposes and audits (67 FR 66792).
4. The coding guidelines should meet the Health Insurance Portability and Accountability Act (HIPAA) requirements (67 FR 66792).
5. The coding guidelines should only require documentation that is clinically necessary for patient care.
6. The coding guidelines should not facilitate upcoding or gaming (67 FR 66792).
7. The coding guidelines should be written or recorded, be well documented, and provide the basis for selection of a specific code.
8. The coding guidelines should be applied consistently across patients in the clinic or emergency department to which they apply.
9. The coding guidelines should not change with great frequency.
10. The coding guidelines should be readily available for fiscal intermediary (or, if applicable, Medicare administrative contractor) review.
11. The coding guidelines should result in coding decisions that could be verified by other hospital staff as well as outside sources. (CMS 2008)

CMS provided additional clarification surrounding some of the principles.

- The first principle states coding guidelines should follow the intent of the CPT code descriptor to relate to the intensity of resources to different levels of effort represented by the code, not that the hospital's guidelines need to specifically consider the three factors included in the CPT E/M codes for consideration regarding physician visit reporting.

- Regarding principle two, hospitals are responsible for reporting the CPT E/M visit code that appropriately represents the resources utilized by the hospital rather than the resources utilized by the physician. This does not preclude the hospital from using or adapting the physician guidelines if the hospital believes that such guidelines adequately describe hospital resources.

- In principle eight, a hospital with multiple clinics (for example, primary care, oncology, wound care, and such) may have different coding guidelines for each clinic, but the guidelines must be applied uniformly within each separate clinic. The hospital's various sets of internal guidelines must measure resource use in a relative manner in relation to each other. For example, resources required for a Level 3 established patient visit under one set of guidelines should be comparable to the resources required for a Level 3 established patient visit under all other sets of clinic visit guidelines used by the hospital.

- Regarding principle nine, CMS would generally expect hospitals to adjust their guidelines less frequently than every few months, and CMS believes it would be reasonable for hospitals to adjust their guidelines annually, if necessary.

- Regarding the tenth principle, hospitals should use their judgment to ensure that coding guidelines are readily available in an appropriate and reasonable format. CMS would encourage fiscal intermediaries and Medicare administrative contractors to review a hospital's internal guidelines when an audit occurs.

- Regarding the eleventh principle, hospitals should use their judgment to ensure that

their coding guidelines can produce results that are reproducible by others. In the absence of national visit guidelines, hospitals have the flexibility to determine whether or not to include separately payable services as a proxy to measure hospital resource use that is not associated with those separately payable services. The costs of hospital resource use associated with those separately payable services would be paid through separate outpatient PPS payment for the other services (Bowman 2008).

In order to be paid for outpatient Medicare claims, healthcare facilities must also make the determination as to whether the patient is new or established. CMS stated:

> …the meanings of new and established pertain to whether or not the patient has been registered as an inpatient or outpatient of the hospital within the past three years. If a patient has been registered as an outpatient in a hospital's off-campus provider-based clinic or emergency department within the past three years, that patient would still be considered an established patient to the hospital for an on-campus or off-campus clinic visit even if the medical record was initially created by the hospital prior to the past three years. (CMS 2008)

In January 2014, CMS published the OPPS/ASC final rule creating a new policy of using a HCPCS code (G0463—Hospital outpatient clinic visit for assessment and management of a patient) for hospitals to represent all clinic visits and also eliminate the new versus established patient designation, while continuing to use the five-level coding structure for emergency department visits (CMS 2016b). While the changes directly impact Medicare patient reimbursement, other third party payers continue to use the E/M codes for clinic facility resource (charge) capture and reimbursement of services.

Charge Description Master

The **charge description master (CDM)** is an electronic file that represents a master list of all services, supplies, devices, and medications charged for

Table 8.1.   Sample charge description master

Charge code	Charge code description	CPT/HCPCS code	Modifier	Revenue code	Price
2721159	CATHETER, DRAINAGE			0272	79.00
2786337	CATHETER, HEMODIALYSIS LONG TERM	C1750		0278	438.00
3008423	DRUG SCREEN ONE/MULT CLASS	80303		0300	41.00
3007215	CBC COMPLETE, WITH DIFFERENTIAL	85025		0300	123.00
3207721	VENOGRAM EXTREMITY BILATERAL	75822		0320	1,320.00
3406973	PARATHYROID SCAN	78070		0340	798.00
3618306	DRAINAGE OF HEMATOMA/SEROMA	10140		0361	1,517.00
3612905	INJECTION SACROILIAC JOINT	G0259		0361	786.00
4245986	PHYSICAL THERAPY EVALUATION	97001	GP	0424	196.00
4302398	OCCUPATIONAL THERAPY RE-EVALUATION	97004	GO	0430	134.00
4802563	ECHO TRANSTHORACIC, CONGENITAL W/ CONTRAST	93303		0480	1,232.00

inpatient or outpatient services (see table 8.1). The CDM contains the basic elements for identifying, coding, and billing items and services provided to patients, and it is the mechanism for representing captured charges on the billing claim.

Each billable service or supply is set up in the CDM and assigned an internal charge code number, which links it to the various data elements necessary for billing and for tracking charge activity within the organization. All charges that are set up in charging source systems or charges that are listed on paper or electronic charge tickets must be identical to those set up in the CDM file in the billing system.

The CDM contains the following general data elements:

- *Charge code*—a unique identifier to identify and represent each billable service or supply. The number is meaningful only to the organization and does not appear on the billing claim.

- *Charge code description*—a narrative description of the service or supply. It does not appear on the billing claim but would be available on an itemized patient statement.

- *CPT or HCPCS code*—a nationally recognized five-digit code. Not all CDM line items have a CPT or HCPCS code because there are services and supplies for which no code has been developed. These charges are represented on the claim using only the revenue code. When a CPT or HCPCS code does exist to represent a chargemaster line item, it is reported on the outpatient billing claim.

- *Modifiers*—two-digit numeric or alphanumeric extensions that are added to the CPT or HCPCS codes to provide further information about the code. The claim form allows room for one or two modifiers to be attached to a CPT or HCPCS code.

- *Revenue code*—a nationally recognized four-digit code that provides a general identification of what the line item charge represents. There are more than 500 revenue codes that represent categories like room and board, lab services, radiology services, pharmacy items, therapy services, supply items, and surgical procedures. The revenue code and its description are required on each line item of a billing claim for both inpatients and outpatients.

- *Price*—the charge that is established for the line item service, item, or supply. Factors that may determine the price that is established include:
  - The Medicare and Medicaid reimbursement rates (set by federal and state government agencies)
  - Reimbursement provided by other third-party payers (set by contract negotiations with the payers)

○ Cost information that is calculated by the accounting or finance area (the cost to the organization to provide that service, such as supplies, equipment, and labor)

○ Standard markup rates for services or supplies (to factor in indirect costs to the organization or discount rates that are negotiated with the third-party payers)

○ Benchmark data on pricing in comparable organizations

○ Market competitive services

Organizations typically establish different prices based on where the services were provided, so the same CPT code would generate a different price based on whether it was performed in a hospital setting or in a freestanding clinic setting. Organizations with multiple hospitals may also establish price variation for each hospital, based on the costs associated with the separate facilities. All established prices should be reviewed and updated at least annually.

Additional CDM data elements may include the date the charge code was created or made active; the date the charge code was deactivated; a code that uniquely identifies the department cost center that uses the code; and payer-specific requirements for reporting the charge, for example, a different CPT, HCPCS, or modifier that needs to be reported to the payer for the charge submitted. These additional data elements allow the CDM to be used as a tool to collect data to evaluate costs related to resources, to prepare departmental budgets, and to provide information necessary in contract negotiations with managed care payers.

The chargemaster must continually be updated to ensure that it represents all billable services and supplies and to keep up with changes in CPT or HCPCS codes, revenue code assignment, and payer-specific requirements. Any number of events may trigger a need for CDM modifications. Examples include:

1. Regulatory changes such as CPT or HCPCS code changes
2. Changes in CMS reimbursement guidelines
3. New department services
4. New product lines
5. Identification that the existing code does not match the service being provided
6. Recurring claim scrubber or APC edits identifying inappropriate setup in the CDM
7. Payer denials identifying inappropriate revenue code or CPT or HCPCS code assignment in the CDM (HFMA 2007)

A variety of resources are used to support the maintenance of the CDM and are listed in figure 8.4.

Many larger organizations use a software system to assist with maintenance of the CDM and to view items that are set up in a department or cost center's chargemaster. The software is primarily designed to continuously apply edits that point out compliance issues, validity of elements such as CPT codes and revenue codes, and identification of items priced below national reimbursement levels.

Maintenance of the CDM is a multidisciplinary activity. Proper chargemaster maintenance requires expertise in coding, clinical procedures, health record or clinical documentation, and billing

Figure 8.4.   CDM resources

- Medicare contractor bulletins and advisories
- Medicare manuals
  ○ Claims Processing Manual (combination of the old hospital, intermediary, and carrier manuals)
  ○ Benefit Policy Manual
  ○ Provider Reimbursement Manual
  ○ National Coverage Determinations Manual
- Transmittals related to:
  ○ Hospital OPPS
  ○ Fraud and abuse
  ○ Coverage determinations
  ○ Durable medical equipment regional carriers (DMERCs)
  ○ Orthotics, prosthetics, and supplies
  ○ Ambulance billing
  ○ HIPAA
  ○ Clarifications of previous transmittals
- Office of Inspector General
- National Correct Coding Initiative (NCCI) edits
- Medicare Addendum B

Source: Shuler 2011.

regulations. For example, the health information management (HIM) department is knowledgeable of the codes, the patient accounts department knows the general ledger codes, the pharmacy department is familiar with the drugs and their costs, and the finance or revenue integrity department knows the associated charge formulas. Pharmacy cannot realistically update radiology's data nor can finance update charges without knowledge of underlying costs and input from the specific department (OptumInsight 2011).

Representatives from various areas that impact the revenue life cycle are critical to the success of the team. It is equally beneficial to include representatives from those departments that capture and generate charges; additional representatives may be included depending upon the facility structure. Department representation typically includes the chargemaster coordinator; patient access including admitting, registration, and scheduling; compliance; revenue integrity; patient financial service (billing department); contracting; finance; information services; HIM; ancillary departments such as radiology, laboratory, surgery, or pharmacy; and physicians as needed.

Responsibilities of the CDM committee include oversight for:

- Developing policies and procedures for the chargemaster review process
- Reviewing the CDM at least annually and when new CPT and HCPCS codes are available or changes are made throughout the year
- Attending to key elements of the annual chargemaster review, including:
  o Reviewing all CPT and HCPCS codes for accuracy, validity, and relationship to charge description number
  o Reviewing all charge descriptions for accuracy and clinical appropriateness
  o Reviewing all revenue codes for accuracy and linkage to charge description numbers
- Ensuring that the usage of all CPT, HCPCS, and revenue codes are in compliance with Medicare guidelines or other existing payer contracts
- Reviewing all charge dollar amounts for appropriateness by payer
- Reviewing all charge codes for uniqueness and validity
- Reviewing all department code numbers for uniqueness and validity
- Performing ongoing chargemaster maintenance as the facility adds or deletes new procedures, updates technology, or changes services provided
- Ensuring that all necessary maintenance to systems affected by changes to the chargemaster (such as order entry feeder systems, charge tickets, and interfaces) is performed when chargemaster maintenance is performed
- Performing tests to make sure that changes to the chargemaster result in the desired outcome
- Educating all clinical department directors on the chargemaster and the effect of the chargemaster on corporate compliance
- Establishing a procedure to allow clinical department directors to submit chargemaster change requests for new, deleted, or revised procedures or services
- Ensuring there is no duplication of code assignment by coders and chargemaster-assigned codes in any department (for example, interventional radiology or cardiology catheterization laboratory)
- Reviewing all charge ticket and order entry screens for accuracy against the chargemaster and appropriate mapping to CPT or HCPCS codes when required
- Reviewing and complying with directives in Medicare transmittals, Medicare manual updates, and official coding guidelines
- Complying with guidelines in the National Correct Coding Initiative, Outpatient Code Editor edits, and any other coding or bundling edits
- Considering carefully any application that involves one charge description number that expands into more than one CPT or HCPCS code to prevent inadvertent

unbundling and unearned reimbursement for services

- Reviewing and taking action on all remittance advice denials involving HCPCS or CPT coding rules and guidelines or CMS payer rules

- Educating all staff affected by changes to the chargemaster in a timely fashion (AHIMA 2010)

The CDM staff must also communicate with staff that negotiates commercial and managed care contracts for the hospital to ensure that data elements meet specific payer requirements. Chargemaster maintenance also involves good communication with the billing staff with regard to payment denials related to an incorrect revenue code or CPT or HCPCS code, so that necessary changes get made to the chargemaster.

Consequences of an improperly maintained or inaccurate chargemaster are the following:

- Services are provided, but associated charges are not set up in the CDM, so the organization is unable to bill and is providing free service.

- If a charge is not set up in the CDM until after the service is provided, the charge might not get posted to the patient's account during the bill hold time.

- When all services are not set up in the CDM, the department is only capturing part of its charges, and the result is reduced revenue.

- If charges are not set up in the CDM or if there are errors in the way they are set up, billing edits and APC edits may be generated, holding up processing of the claim. All billing delays result in increased accounts receivable (A/R) days.

- APC and billing edits result in multiple individuals investigating the issues and making necessary changes, which results in increased cost to the organization.

An up-to-date, complete, and well-maintained chargemaster is a significant financial, operational, and compliance asset to a healthcare organization.

Clinical Documentation

Complete, accurate, and timely documentation of patient history, assessment, surgical and procedure notes, and clinical plan are important aspects of the revenue cycle. Clinicians need to document the services that are performed and the medical necessity of the services, and staff needs to verify the charges are matching the services that are being performed prior to bill submission. CMS regulations require documentation to support the care provided to the patient (CMS 2014b). In order to comply with these regulations, hospitals have placed an increased focus on clinical documentation management and coding practices due to their direct impact on the healthcare facility's revenue.

Hospitals have invested in clinical documentation improvement (CDI) programs to assure the health record accurately reflects the actual condition of the patient. A focus on appropriate clinical documentation can reduce the risks from incomplete and unclear documentation resulting in lost revenue for the healthcare facility. Accurate and thorough clinical documentation that is properly coded and billed to payers results in benefits such as increased third-party payer billing compliance, improved quality reporting to external parties, and increased revenues by coding the most appropriate DRG and minimizing denials. Refer to chapter 9 for more detail on clinical documentation improvement and coding compliance.

Coding

The HIM professional performs a variety of functions, but the primary one related to the revenue cycle is code assignment. Upon a patient's discharge, the clinical documentation is reviewed and ICD diagnosis codes are assigned for inpatient and outpatient claims, and CPT or HCPCS codes are assigned only for outpatient claims. It is very important to have experienced, well-trained coders in order to ensure accurate and complete code assignment and optimum reimbursement. Coders must be skilled at reading through documentation on a variety of different forms and formats and interpreting that documentation to arrive at the correct code assignment. When documentation is vague or ambiguous, they may need to query the physician for clarification. The physician query process can create significant delays in the revenue cycle when the coder is waiting for the physician response and cannot complete the coding until it is received.

A bill cannot be generated until the coding is complete, so organizations routinely monitor the discharged, no final bill (DNFB) days. Generally this is done by reviewing the DNFB report that includes all patients who have been discharged from the facility, but for whom the billing process is not complete. The goal for an efficient revenue cycle is to eliminate any backlog of uncoded charts and to complete the coding process within the time frame of the bill hold days that have been established for the organization.

The hospital's **case-mix index (CMI)** is also measured and analyzed. The case-mix index allows an organization to compare its cost of providing care to its DRG mix of patients in relation to other hospitals. The DRG weights do not reflect an individual hospital's costs relative to another hospital or peer group. The CMI is calculated by summing the Medicare DRG weight for every inpatient discharge and dividing by the number of discharges. Medicare DRG weights are used and applied to patients within all payers. The accuracy of clinical documentation and of code assignment can influence a facility's case-mix index. By missing diagnoses or procedures that should be coded, or failing to assign the most specific coding possible, the coding staff can cause the case-mix index to be lower than it should be.

Technology Tools

Similar to the front-end process of the revenue cycle, technology tools play a vital role in the efficiency and quality of work produced by healthcare staff. The following tools and techniques were identified by the HIMSS Revenue Cycle Improvement Task Force to support the middle process:

- Clinical documentation may first originate as written text, dictation, or text keyed directly to the system. Ultimately, clinical documentation must result in codified procedures and diagnoses to support billing.

- Charge capture may be completed with a mix of forms, online entry (keyed or scanned), and automatic triggering.

- Electronic or e-tools help with maintenance of chargemasters. Optimal software packages include online reference tools that compile the latest coding and regulatory information, a complete and active code book feature, and a browser-based, cross-reference toolkit enabling users to research coding, regulations, and pricing information.

- HIM processes are dependent on access to all clinical documentation and any precoded data. Reference materials may be required to support the coding process; once determined, coded values must be input into systems for inclusion in claims processing. Automated edits may be imbedded in transactions systems to identify discrepancies at the time of entry (prior to submission into the claim cycle). Final coded records must be submitted through DRG tools to calculate and assign DRGs. Systems tools may include a mix of health information system (HIS) applications or an HIM-specific application that is integrated with other HIS applications (HIMSS 2010).

Check Your Understanding 8.2

Instructions: Answer the following questions on a separate piece of paper.

1. What effect does the charge capture process have on the reimbursement received for services?

2. To ensure appropriate and effective resource coordination, what roles should be performed by the case managers or utilization management staff?

3. How is the hospital case-mix index calculated?

4. To ensure multidisciplinary representation, what areas should be involved in the chargemaster committee?

5. What is the relationship between charging source systems and the CDM?

Revenue Cycle Back-End Process

The back-end of the revenue cycle process begins with billing and claims submission of the patient care services and carries through to payment or settlement of the healthcare services rendered to the patient.

Claims Processing

Claims processing involves accumulating charges for services, submitting claims for reimbursement, and ensuring that claims are satisfied. The patient financial services or billing area has the responsibility for the collection of revenue for the patient encounter. Once a patient has been discharged, the goal is to get a complete and accurate claim generated and submitted for payment as quickly as possible. Organizations routinely measure **accounts receivable (A/R) days**—the average number of days between the discharge date and the receipt of payment for services rendered as a measure of how successful the revenue cycle is. An efficient revenue cycle helps the organization lower the A/R days, which in turn improves cash flow.

Claims processing is sometimes outsourced in nonhospital ambulatory care because physician offices and other small facilities often do not have the resources to perform this complex activity effectively. The activity of submitting a claim is often called dropping a bill. Because reimbursement for clinical services provided is the healthcare facility's largest source of revenue, timely and accurate claims processing is necessary.

Most billing systems are programmed to automatically submit claims to the payers (after the bill hold time frame) if the account is not being held for any type of edit resolution; these are often referred to as **clean claims**. Because there are so many complex rules and edits, manual intervention is required for many claims, but the goal is to continually increase the percentage of clean claims that can be billed with no intervention. The sophistication level of the organization's billing system determines how much is able to be programmed into the system versus how much has to be handled manually by the billing staff.

America's Health Insurance Plans, an association representing the health insurance industry, released a study to show the percentage of claims received electronically was 94 percent in 2011, up from 82 percent in 2009 and 44 percent in 2006 (AHIP 2013). The study also shows an increase from 58 to 66 percent in the number of claims submitted to health insurance plans within two weeks of the date of patient service. Sixteen percent of claims received from healthcare providers were greater than 30 days after the date of patient service, and 12 percent of claims were received more than 60 days after the date of the patient's service. The 2011 survey also showed health insurance plans processed 98 percent of claims within 30 days, and 99 percent within 60 days (AHIP 2013).

Payment Posting

Payment is received from third-party payers and patients in various ways, and the payments must be posted to the correct individual patient accounts. Internally, some allocation of the revenue must be made to the various areas that provided services. This process is established by the organization's financial accounting area, and the methods of allocation may vary. Since payment received usually does not equal the amount that was billed, it is a complex process to determine the correct allocations and to post the necessary payments, adjustments, and discounts to the correct accounts. Ultimately, the balance on each patient's account must equal zero (Nelson 2011). There are instances when too many payments are posted to the accounts because there can be multiple payments from one or more insurance companies and copayment or coinsurance payments received from the patient. In these cases, the account has a negative balance, and it must be determined where the overpayments occurred so funds can be refunded to the correct payer or to the patient.

Follow-up

Once payment is received from third-party payers and the discounts and adjustments are applied to the balance on the account, there may still be a portion that is due from the patient (related to deductibles, coinsurance, and copayments). The patient financial services staff works to collect this portion from the patient and to appropriately refer patients to medical assistance or other programs or apply charge discounts as appropriate.

Organizations may also utilize third-party collection agencies to assist with collection of payment on problem accounts. These engagements may also necessitate a relationship with a third-party collection attorney and an internal legal review team that reviews all accounts prior to legal collection.

Denial Management

Denials may simply be defined as a payer's refusal to provide payment. According to the Advisory Board Company, the nation's largest hospital research organization, the cost of denials to healthcare organizations ranges from 1.4 to 2 percent of net outstanding revenue (Advisory Board Company 2013). Approximately 90 percent of denials are preventable and 67 percent are recoverable (Haines 2014). The most common reasons for the denials include:

- Beneficiary not covered
- Lack of medical necessity—not reasonable or necessary
- Lack of precertification
- Inappropriate utilization
- Noncovered services
  - Incorrect charging—unbundled code
  - Incorrect coding
  - Procedure code does not match patient sex
  - Diagnosis procedure code does not match service provided
  - Procedure code inconsistent with modifier used
  - Procedure code inconsistent with place of service
  - Diagnosis inconsistent with age, sex, and procedure
  - Modifier not provided
  - Late charges or untimely filing (Haines 2014)

A denial management program requires facilities to seek both prevention and recovery. Denial management requires a cross-functional team to evaluate reasons for the denials and to facilitate changes in work processes to prevent further denials from occurring. Denial team stakeholders often include staff or managers from departments such as patient financial services or billing; health information management; compliance; revenue integrity or chargemaster; patient access, including registration, admissions, and surgery scheduling; utilization or case management; contracting; finance; and various ancillary services and clinics where the denials may be occurring. A successful denial management program includes the following:

- Focus on recovery of lost reimbursement and prevention of further denials
- Teamwork to manage the denials
- Need to appropriately value the staff and provide appropriate and clear work guidelines, standards, and expectations
- Investment in staff training and education
- Utilization of technology to assist with processes
- Creation of a departmental dashboard to monitor progress of team efforts used to
  - Measure individual departments against a benchmark
  - Compare individual departments against the organization as a whole
  - Trend success within a department
- Denial tracking by payer
- Identification, quantification, and sorting by carrier
- Identification of trends that are not "true" denials but potential stall tactics
- Sharing of specific examples with managed care or contracting departments (Dunn 2009)

A successful denial management program requires consistent focus and evaluation of denial trends. Denials should be addressed within one week of receiving the denial from the insurer. Findings from trends or patterns identified need to be shared on a routine basis with denial management stakeholders. Edits or rules for certain payers may be set up in a claim scrubber to assist with managing claims prior to sending them to an insurer. For example, if Medicare does not pay for a certain drug but other payers do, a rule can be built to write-off the charge if it is a Medicare patient but bill all other payers. The rule would prevent further denials from Medicare.

Revenue Audit and Recovery

After payment has been received, it is audited against the terms of the contract to determine whether the organization has received the correct reimbursement. Since the terms of payer contracts are usually very complex, the revenue audit and recovery function is greatly enhanced by the use of software systems that model the contracts and produce reports of accounts with variation to the expected reimbursement.

To achieve optimum benefit, audits should occur for all payment relationships that can be modeled. The government payers and most commercial payers have fairly straightforward terms of reimbursement without a lot of specific language. Those payers that negotiate specific terms of a contract with the organization's contracting team usually have more complex terms of payment and variations for differing plans or products offered by their company. It is particularly helpful to model the specific terms of these contracts in a software system in order to detect variation in payment.

In organizations utilizing modeling software, the information about expected reimbursement is calculated after all charges have been posted to the account and the bill has been submitted to the payer. The level of detail specified in negotiated contracts requires the software modeling programs to create a hierarchy when there are multiple types of services provided to the patient. Once payment is received and the reimbursement amounts are posted to the account, the software system generates a weekly or monthly report of all accounts with payment variation. A threshold is usually established for the percentage of variation that must exist in order for an account to be included on the variation report. The number of accounts may be too high to enable a 100 percent review, so guidelines should be established to determine which accounts will be reviewed. Reports can be generated to allow review of accounts by a specific payer, a payer plan, inpatients versus outpatients, accounts with high dollar amount, and others.

Payments are examined against the Explanation of Benefits (EOB) to see if specific items were paid, if they were considered to be bundled services, were denied, or returned to the provider for correction. Payment audits may detect errors in the modeling that was applied or errors in insurance assignment at the time of registration. This provides an opportunity to offer feedback and further educate staff. Audits can detect patterns of underpayments or overpayments, so the organization can initiate a focus on accounts with similar charges and may reveal the need to make revisions to the chargemaster set up, or to prices established in the fee schedules. They may also identify the need to evaluate the quality of documentation and coding, or to implement or enforce compliance standards.

Technology Tools

The following tools and techniques were identified by the HIMSS Revenue Cycle Improvement Task Force (2009) to support the back-end revenue cycle process:

- Workflow claims management system for follow-up that validates all required electronic and paper documents are captured.
- Denial management system permits for tracking of denial types, reasons, and payment discrepancies.
- Contract management system that manages terms of the contract between the healthcare organization and the payer, such as payment for service or diagnosis.
- Claims editing system that reviews claims prior to the submission to a payer by reviewing

- requirements by the payer or to assure all information on the claim is complete.
- Integration to payers for automated claims status and cash posting allows the healthcare organization and payers to partner on managing claim status such as receipt through payment along with cash payment posting of services provided.
- Telephony system in order to measure call activity such as number of calls and time it takes to answer a call.

- Electronic financial assistance application is an electronic format for requesting financial assistance for healthcare expenses.

Similar to the front-end and middle process of the revenue cycle, technology tools play a vital role in the back-end revenue cycle process by providing consistent workflow practices; evaluating the complete and accuracy of work, such as claims, to avoid denials; and providing the capability of consistent data collection.

Check Your Understanding 8.3

Instructions: Answer the following questions on a separate piece of paper

1. How is an organization's accounts receivable days impacted by their bill hold days and their percentage of clean claim submission?

2. What factors can cause a patient account balance to display a negative amount?

3. What are four of the most common reasons for billing denials?

4. What criteria are used to select claims that should be audited to determine whether proper reimbursement has been received?

5. Explain how you measure account receivable days.

Quality Measures for Improvement

Increasing revenue cycle performance can have a positive impact on a healthcare organization's financial bottom line (see table 8.2). Measuring the various processes of the revenue cycle against established benchmarks provides an opportunity for organizations to focus on areas to improve. Influences such as geographical location, bed size, payer mix, net patient revenue, and the mix of inpatient, outpatient, and emergency room visits can impact the revenue cycle (HFMA 2011). The Healthcare Financial Management Association (HFMA) defined key measures to evaluate revenue cycle performance. The tool allows hospitals to track its

revenue cycle performance using industry-standard metrics and to compare the results with peer groups based on the previously mentioned influences (table 8.3).

Key performance indicators (KPIs) allow healthcare facilities to measure and benchmark their data against best practice. The KPIs were developed by the HFMA based upon research from HFMA publications, forums, and website; the American Health Information Management Association publications and website; accounting firms; vendor internal standards and client data; and hospital accounts receivable analysis report standards (Hammer 2009).

Table 8.2.   Benchmarking

Use of benchmarking can drive significant improvements			
Key performance indicator	**Top quartile**	**Median**	**Difference**
Days in A/R	37.7	43.1	5.4
Point-of-service cash collection	46%	30%	16%

Source: HFMA 2011.

Table 8.3.   HFMA denial key performance indicators

Denial type	Percent
Overall initial denials rate (percentage of gross revenue)	≤4
Clinical initial denials rate (percentage of gross revenue)	≤5
Technical initial denials rate (percentage of gross revenue)	≤3
Underpayments additional collection rate	≤75
Appealed denials overturned rate	40–60
Electronic eligibility rate	≥75
Physician precertification double-check rate	100
Case managers' time spent securing authorization	≥20
Total denial reason codes	≥25
Scheduling	**Percent**
Overall scheduling rate of potentially eligible patients	100
Scheduling rate for elective and urgent inpatients	100
Scheduling rate for ambulatory surgery patients	100
Scheduling rate for high-dollar outpatient diagnostic patients	100
Scheduled patients' preregistration rate	98
Registration/Preregistration	**Percent**
Overall preregistration rate of scheduled patients	≥98
Overall insurance verification rate of preregistered patients	≥98
Data quality compared with pre-established department standards	≥99
Health information	**Measure**
Copies of medical records pursuant to payers' requests	≥2 days
Potential "over codes" beyond 75th percentile	≥2%
Potential "under codes" below 10th percentile	≥2%
Data quality compared with pre-established department standards	≥99%
Chargemaster	**Percent**
Chargemaster duplicate items	0
Chargemaster incorrect or missing HCPCS/CPT-4 codes	0
Chargemaster incorrect or invalid revenue codes	0
Chargemaster revenue code lacks necessary HCPCS/CPT-4 code	0
Chargemaster item has invalid or incorrect modifier	0
Chargemaster item has missing modifier	0
Chargemaster item description is "miscellaneous"	0

Source: HIMSS 2010.

In addition to measuring key revenue cycle tasks, there are seven additional strategies for revenue cycle success including:

- The need to focus on revenue cycle improvement and a dedicated team to maintain the focus.
- The use of metrics to conduct root cause analysis to facilitate changes throughout the healthcare system.
- The need for a shared sense of accountability for revenue cycle performance.
- Collaboration with other departments to enhance the revenue cycle performance focus.
- Development of a comprehensive approach to address uncompensated care.
- The identification of innovative ways to enhance customer service.
- The focus on improving the total patient experience (Williams 2011).

Revenue cycle management success is dependent on multiple processes, people, and technology. Effective management requires identification of trends and then adjustment to processes and procedures and, at times, software technology updates. The revenue cycle could be considered the heart of the organization as it impacts patients and their families; physicians and other providers of care; ancillary departments such as radiology and laboratory; support departments such as scheduling and registration; finance; health information management; clinical documentation; patient financial services; and information technology. Combining efforts across departments and staff members to improve the revenue cycle processes and establishing performance expectations will lead to a successful revenue cycle program

HFMA developed additional indicators to consistently measure the key performance indicators known as **MAP keys**. The purpose was to develop the standard for revenue cycle excellence (HFMA 2010). Each MAP key measures a specific revenue cycle function and provides the purpose for the measurement, the value of the measure, and the specific equation (numerator and denominator) to consistently calculate the measure. Examples of MAP keys are found in table 8.4.

Table 8.4. Examples of MAP keys

Measure	Purpose	Value	Equation*
Point-of-service cash collections	Trending indicator of point-of-service collection efforts	Indicates revenue cycle efficiency and effectiveness	N: Number of patient encounters preregistered D: Number of scheduled patient encounters
Preregistration rate	Trending indicator that patient access processes are timely, accurate, and efficient	Indicates revenue cycle efficiency and effectiveness	N: Number of patient encounters preregistered D: Number of scheduled patient encounters
Insurance verification rate	Trending indicator that patient access functions are timely, accurate, and efficient	Indicates revenue cycle process efficiency and effectiveness	N: Total number of verified encounters D: Total number of registered encounters
Service authorization rate	Trending indicator that patient access functions are timely, accurate, and efficient	Indicates revenue cycle process efficiency and effectiveness	N: Number of encounters authorized D: Number of encounters requiring authorization
Days in total discharged, no final bill (DNFB)	Trending indicator of claims generation process	Indicates revenue cycle performance and can identify performance issues impacting cash flow	N: Gross dollars in A/R (no final billed) D: Average daily gross revenue
Days in total discharged, not submitted to payer (DNSP)	Trending indicator of total claims generation and submission process	Indicates revenue cycle performance and can identify performance issues impacting cash flow	N: gross dollars in DNFB + gross dollars in FBNS D: Average daily gross revenue

Table 8.4. Continued.

Measure	Purpose	Value	Equation*
Late charges as percentage of total charges	Measure of revenue capture efficiency	Indicates revenue cycle performance and can identify performance issues impacting cash flow	N: Charges with post date greater than three days from last service date D: Total gross charges
Net days revenue in credit balance	Trending indicator to accurately report account values, ensure compliance with regulatory requirements, and monitor overall payment system effectiveness	Indicates whether credit balances are being managed to appropriate levels and are compliant with regulatory requirements	N: Dollars in credit balance D: Average daily net patient services revenue

*N = Numerator, D = Denominator.
Source: HFMA 2016a.

Check Your Understanding 8.4

Instructions: Answer the following questions on a separate piece of paper

1. Name four key strategies of success for the revenue cycle.

2. How do are late charges measured as a percent of total charges?

3. What is the purpose of MAP keys?

4. What is the purpose of key performance indicators?

5. What is the map key formula to determine the Insurance Verification Rate?

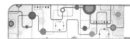

References

Advisory Board Company. 2015. Driving Next-Generation Patient Access Performance. https://www.advisory.com/solutions/revenue-cycle-solutions/driving-next-generation-patient-access-performance

Advisory Board Company. 2013. Results from the 2013 National Survey of Hospital Revenue Cycle Operations. https://www.advisory.com/sitecore%20modules/web/research/financial-leadership-council/studies/2013/benchmarking-revenue-cycle-performance/key-findings/denials-and-uncompensated-care

American Case Management Association. 2012. Definition of Case Management. http://acmaweb.org/section.aspx?mn=mn1&sn=sn1&wpg=mh.&sid=4

American College of Medical Quality. 2015. Policy 8—Definition and Application of Medical Necessity. http://www.acmq.org/policies/policy8.pdf

American Health Information Management Association. 2010. Care and Maintenance of

Chargemasters (Updated). Chicago: AHIMA. http://library.ahima.org/xpedio/groups/public/documents/ahima/bok1_047258.hcsp?dDocName=bok1_047258

America's Health Insurance Plans Center for Policy and Research. 2013. An Updated Survey of Health Care Claims Receipt and Processing Times. 2011. http://www.ahip.org/AHIPResearch/

Bendix, J. 2013. Curing the Prior Authorization Headache. Medical Economics. http://medicaleconomics.modernmedicine.com/medical-economics/content/tags/americas-health-insurance-plans/curing-prior-authorization-headache

Bowman, S. 2008. Analysis of Final Rule for 2008 Revisions to the Medicare Hospital Outpatient Prospective Payment System. Chicago: AHIMA. http://library.ahima.org/xpedio/groups/public/documents/ahima/bok1_044014.pdf

Brzon, L. 2011. Point-of-Service Collections for Scheduled, Nonurgent Services. http://www.hfma.org/Content.aspx?id=4124

Butcher, L. 2014. Pre-pay Discounts Offer Advantages to Patients and Providers. Healthcare Financial Management Association. http://www.hfma.org/Content.aspx?id=22680

Butcher, L. 2012. Centralizing Registration Boosts Collections, Patient Experience at Crozer-Keystone. Healthcare Financial Management Association. http://www.hfma.org/Content.aspx?id=1829

Case Management Society of America. 2015. What Is Case Management? http://cmsa.org/Home/CMSA/WhatisaCaseManager/tabid/224/Default.aspx

Centers for Medicare and Medicaid Services. 2016a. FFS HINNs. http://www.cms.gov/Medicare/Medicare-General-Information/BNI/HINNs.html

Centers for Medicare and Medicaid Services. 2016b. OPPS Final Rule http://www.cms.gov/Medicare/Medicare-Fee-for-Service-Payment/HospitalOutpatientPPS/Hospital-Outpatient-Regulations-and-Notices-Items/CMS-1601-FC-.html

Centers for Medicare and Medicaid Services. 2016c. Medicare Benefit Policy Manual. https://www.cms.gov/Regulations-and-Guidance/Guidance/Manuals/downloads/bp102c07.pdf

Centers for Medicare and Medicaid Services. 2014a. CMS Manual, Transmittal 168. https://www.cms.gov/Regulations-and-Guidance/Guidance/Transmittals/Downloads/R168NCD.pdf

Center for Medicare and Medicaid Services. 2014b Complying with Medical Record Documentation Requirements. https://www.cms.gov/Outreach-and-Education/Medicare-Learning-Network-MLN/MLNProducts/Downloads/CERTMedRecDoc-FactSheet-ICN909160.pdf

Centers for Medicare and Medicaid Services. 2008. Final Changes to the Hospital Outpatient Prospective Payment System and CY 2008 Payment Rates. https://www.cms.gov/Medicare/Medicare-Fee-for-Service-Payment/HospitalOutpatientPPS/Hospital-Outpatient-Regulations-and-Notices-Items/CMS1204971.html

Corrigan, J. 2009. Improving Patient Access. Healthcare Financial Management Association. http://www.highbeam.com/doc/1G1-206388294.html

Daniels, S. 2007. The Business Case for Hospital Case Management. http://healthleadersmedia.com/content/HOM-87605/The-Business-Case-for-Hospital-Case-Management.html

Daniels, S. and J. Frater. 2011. Hospital Case Management and Progression of Care. Healthcare Financial Management Association. http://www.readperiodicals.com/201108/2436166681.html

Dunn, R. 2009. Improving cash flow in a down economy: How HIM can help reduce denial. *Journal of AHIMA* 80(3).

Emdeon. 2015. Partnering with Payers to Optimize the Revenue Cycle. http://www.hfma.org/Content.aspx?id=28682

Hammer, D. 2009. Using Key Performance Indicators to Prepare for Contract Renegotiation. Northeast New York HFMA Education Session. http://www.powershow.com/view/128264-Yjk2Y/Using_Key_Performance_Indicators_to_Prepare_for_Contract_Renegotiation_powerpoint_ppt_presentation

Haines, M. 2014. An Ounce of Prevention Pays Off: 90% of Denials are Preventable. https://www.advisory.com/research/financial-leadership-council/at-the-margins/2014/12/denials-management

HASC Summit on Administrative Simplification Final Report. 2009. Bringing Better Value: Recommendations to Address the Costs and Causes of Administrative Complexity in the Nation's Healthcare System. www.hfma.org/DownloadAsset.aspx?id=21761

Healthcare Financial Management Association. 2016. Principles and Practices Board Statements and Publications: Sample 501(c)(3) Hospital Charity Care & Financial Assistance Policy & Procedures. http://www.hfma.org/Content.aspx?id=1069

Healthcare Financial Management Association. 2011. Research Shows Path to Revenue Cycle Gains through Effective Benchmarking. Special Research Report. http://www.hfma.org/Content.aspx?id=3070

Healthcare Financial Management Association. 2010. Mapkeys. http://www.hfma.org/MAP/MapKeys/

Healthcare Financial Management Association. 2007 (June). Missed Opportunities—Your Strategy for Correct—and Complete—Charge Capture. Educational Report. http://www.highbeam.com/doc/1G1-165165026.html HFMA

Healthcare Information Management Systems Society. 2010. Revenue Cycle Management: A Life Cycle Approach for Performance Measurement and System Justification. http://www.himss.org/ResourceLibrary/ResourceDetail.aspx?ItemNumber=10794

Langford, A., L. Dye, J. Moresco, and D. Riefner. 2010. Improving the Revenue Cycle by Taking the Patient's Perspective. Healthcare Financial Management Association. http://www.hfma.org/Content.aspx?id=2794

Llewellyn, R. and K. Moore. 2014. Best Practice Concepts in Revenue Cycle Management. https://www.ruralcenter.org/sites/default/files/rhpi/hit-guides/Best%20Practices%20in%20Revenue%20Cycle%20Management.pdf

McLean, D. 2011a. Authority and Responsibility for the Utilization Management (UM) Plan. RACmonitor. http://racmonitor.com/news/33-top-stories/696-authority-and-responsibility-for-the-utilization-management-um-plan.html

McLean, D. 2011b. The Essential Requirements for Effective Utilization Review. RACmonitor. http://racmonitor.com/news/27-rac-enews/724-the-essential-requirements-for-effective-utilization-review.html

Miodonski, K. 2011. The Role of Case Managers in Controlling Hospital Costs. Fierce Health Finance. http://www.fiercehealthfinance.com/story/role-case-managers-controlling-hospital-costs/2011-05-31

Nelson, R. 2011. What's This About Revenue Cycle Management? http://www.medpagetoday.com/Columns/PracticePointers/24796

OptumInsight. 2011. Hospital Chargemaster Guide. Real life applications. http://static1.1.sqspcdn.com/static/f/547060/18389092/1337865979687/01%20User's%20Guide.pdf)

Shorrosh, P. 2011. The Hidden KPI: Registration Accuracy. Healthcare Financial Management Association. http://www.hfma.org/Content.aspx?id=3084

Shuler, G. 2011. "Chargemaster 101—Let's Start at the Beginning." Paper provided at the Minnesota Hospital Association Education Program. St. Paul, MN. August 2011.

Utilization Review Accreditation Commission. 2015. What Is Health Utilization Management? https://www.urac.org/accreditation-and-measurement/accreditation-programs/all-programs/health-utilization-management/

Williams, J. 2011. Mapping Out Strategies for Improving Value in the Revenue Cycle. Healthcare Financial Management Association. http://www.hfma.org/Content.aspx?id=2778

9

Clinical Documentation Improvement and Coding Compliance

T.J. Hunt, PhD, RHIA, FAHIMA

Learning Objectives

- Determine processes for compliance with laws and standards related to coding and revenue cycle
- Develop methods to ensure the accuracy of coded data based on established guidelines
- Determine processes to monitor healthcare fraud and abuse
- Develop methods to manage elements of the clinical documentation improvement process

Key Terms

Abuse
Benchmarks
Case mix
Case-mix index
Clinical
Clinical documentation improvement (CDI)
Compliance

Computer-assisted coding
Concurrent review
Extrapolation method
Federal False Claims Act
Fraud
Maximization
Optimization

Physician champion
Query
Qui tam relators
Retrospective review
Unbundling
Upcoding
Utilization management
Whistleblowing

For as long as the patient health record has existed, it has been a central hub for communication between healthcare providers. The first widely-known reference regarding health records, *Manual for Medical Records Librarians*, was authored in 1941 by health information management (HIM) pioneer Edna Huffman. It was in print as the recognized authority on the profession for over 50 years. She defines the complete health record as consisting of "sufficient data written in sequence of events to justify the diagnosis and warrant the treatment and end results" (Huffman 1941, 21).

The format of patient records has evolved in the last century. They have been paper-based, ranging from basic to complex; have been scanned to microfilm, microfiche, and electronic mediums; have operated in a hybrid record in which information is both scanned and directly entered into electronic systems; and today seeks to be almost completely paperless. However, the purpose is still the same. Today the information justifying the diagnosis, warranting the treatment, and detailing the progress and end result for the patient are utilized for patient care, future quality improvement, research, provider payment, decision making, and more. See chapter 4 for additional uses of the patient record. It is the legal business record of the care provider (AHIMA 2011).

In many ways, the record can be compared to an itemized receipt for services. It communicates what was done and why it was necessary. The clinical documentation inside the record has been referred to as the "cornerstone of recording a patient's condition, relevant diagnoses, and communication between physicians" (Rosenbaum et al. 2014). The term *clinical* refers to work done with real patients, about or relating to the medical treatment that is given to patients in facilities such as hospitals and clinics. Documentation regarding the clinical evaluation and treatment of the patient is the core of the medical record in paper, scanned, or electronic form. Further functions of the patient health record are to facilitate the care and treatment of patients, serve as a communication method between caregivers and organizations, be a resource for clinical and organizational decision making, and provide information for research and quality improvement.

Information found in the patient health record is the foundation on which decision making is based. The many functions and uses of the record drive the need for accuracy. Accurate clinical documentation is an important organizational asset in the healthcare industry. Incomplete, inaccurate, or nonspecific information in the record have negative consequences on all of the functions of the record listed here. This is why many healthcare organizations have formalized clinical documentation improvement processes.

Clinical Documentation Improvement

There are many examples in healthcare where improved documentation will benefit both patients and providers. **Clinical documentation improvement** is a process to facilitate the accurate representation of a patient's clinical status in the patient health record that is then transformed into coded data (AHIMA 2015). Information is collected from the patient health record and recorded as codes representing the diagnoses and procedures performed. This information is then utilized for many purposes in healthcare.

The first and ultimate reason for excellent documentation is improved patient care through clear communication between providers and an accurate picture of the patient's medical situation and course of treatment. Additional examples are for more accurate reimbursement and data reporting through programs dependent on diagnosis and procedure codes such as:

- Medicare severity diagnosis-related groups (MS-DRG)
- Value-based purchasing (VBP)
- Quality of care measures including inpatient quality reporting (IQR)
- Severity of illness (SOI)
- Expected risk of mortality (ROM)
- Present on admission (POA) or hospital-acquired condition (HAC) reporting
- Patient safety measures
- Utilization of resource measures such as case-mix and medical necessity
- Protection from liability
- Public health monitoring (AHIMA 2014a; Roat 2014).

In addition, these measures may also be used as a comparison with peers for both physicians and facilities (Rosenbaum et al. 2014). The benefit of better documentation has been apparent for over 100 years, articulated in one example in the foreword of *Manual for Medical Records Librarians*:

> Meagre information other than nurses' notes was to be found in the medical records of most hospitals when the American College of Surgeons initiated its program of Hospital Standardization in 1918.... Many a surgeon, wishing to become a Fellow of the College, could not qualify because acceptable records of the operations he had performed were not obtainable.... Better medical records have had a share in, and will continue to affect, medical progress. (Huffman 1941)

While HIM professionals had been reviewing documentation even before the *Manual for Medical Record Librarians* was published, the increased need for information about the care provided to the patient from all of these programs and functions made the existence of clinical documentation improvement (CDI) programs shift from a program for improvement used by some providers to a standard function in many healthcare organizations (Rollins 2009). The transition to the ICD-10-CM/PCS coding system in 2015 that now requires a higher level of specificity is one major factor in the growth (Butler 2014). CDI professionals are "tasked with obtaining appropriate clinical documentation to ensure the level of service rendered to the patient and the clinical complexity of the patient's condition are completely and accurately documented" (Barnhouse and Rudman 2013). The end result of improving clinical documentation is not to amass *more*, but to produce *better* documentation that easily communicates what patient care was delivered and the reason for the treatment.

Documentation for Coded Data

Many of the reporting and communication needs of healthcare that are dependent on documentation are accomplished through the use of coded data. See chapter 5 for the transformation of documentation into coded data. In October 2015, the United States transitioned to the International Classification of Diseases, 10th Revision Clinical Modification (ICD-10-CM) and the ICD-10 Procedural Coding System (ICD-10-PCS). The ninth revision (ICD-9) had been in effect since 1979. The new system has greater capability to learn more specific detail about the care provided—this includes ensuring higher quality information to make decisions about patient care, offering more accurate reimbursement to providers, and benefiting from improved data for information needs. The challenge continues to be ensuring that detailed clinical documentation matches the detailed capability of the ICD-10-CM coding system. In some cases, the documentation that sufficed for assigning codes in ICD-9-CM in the 36 years from 1979 to 2015 is not detailed enough to successfully capture data in ICD-10-CM (DeAlmeida et al. 2014; Hinkle-Azzara and Carr 2014).

The need for a CDI process in these cases not only impacts the accuracy and detail of diagnosis and procedure codes, but perhaps even the ability to assign a code at all. For example, laterality of a disease or procedure was not a detail captured in ICD-9; however, in ICD-10 knowing if the condition or procedure affects the right or left eye is an essential piece to assigning a code. Without the needed documentation there will be delays in the completion of coding for the care encounter resulting in delayed action on all processes in which coded information is needed, including financial functions.

CDI Goals

The American Health Information Management Association (AHIMA) states the purpose of a CDI program is to "initiate concurrent and, as appropriate, retrospective reviews of health records for conflicting, incomplete, or nonspecific provider documentation" (AHIMA 2014a). **Concurrent review** of the record occurs while the patient care is ongoing, often the reviewers are alongside the healthcare providers on the patient care units to facilitate communication. **Retrospective review** occurs later after that patient has been discharged.

The goals of the reviews should be clearly defined by the organization embarking on the CDI process. Key stakeholders need to be involved for a successful program and need to be part of the goal-setting process. Examples of key stakeholders in an acute-care or integrated organization are displayed in table 9.1.

The range of stakeholders is wide because the information from a patient record is used for multiple functions throughout a healthcare organization. The clinical documentation is generated by healthcare providers, which then has a domino effect on many other functions related to patient care such as communication between caregivers. Goals of a CDI program include:

- Obtain clinical documentation that captures the patient severity of illness and risk of mortality

- Identify and clarify missing, conflicting, or nonspecific physician documentation related to diagnoses and procedures

- Support accurate diagnostic and procedural coding, and MS-DRG assignment, leading to appropriate reimbursement

- Promote health record completion during the patient's course of care, which promotes patient safety

- Provide awareness and education

- Improve documentation to reflect quality and outcome scores

- Improve coders' clinical knowledge (AHIMA 2014a)

Overarching themes in a CDI program are identifying areas of documentation deficiencies, improving documentation to be more specific or clear, and providing ongoing education for future excellence. An initial gap assessment indicating a need for CDI and the service areas in which it is required

Table 9.1. List of key CDI stakeholders

Executive leadership	Medical staff
Health information management/coding	Compliance
Risk management	Finance/revenue cycle
Utilization management	Nursing
Case management	Quality improvement
Patient financial services/billing	Ethics

Source: AHIMA 2014a.

is an important benchmark at the beginning of a CDI process.

Operational Considerations

The AHIMA CDI Toolkit suggests the following decisions must be made before implementing a CDI program to ensure the right people, processes, and technology are in place:

- Composition of the CDI staff

- Alignment of the CDI program

- Identification of the types of records to review

- Frequency of chart reviews

- Budget

- Training needs

- Reporting and performance monitoring (AHIMA 2014a)

Each facility or organization can use this list as a starting point in creating their CDI process. It is a roadmap including topics of discussion and investigation for planning a successful CDI implementation.

Interdisciplinary Team

The many uses and users of information derived from clinical documentation support the need for an interdisciplinary approach to CDI. Each organization or healthcare provider is unique and may have a different mix of people that contribute to a successful program (AHIMA 2014b). While there are multiple stakeholders involved in the planning of goals for the CDI process, the team performing the review functions should include physicians, other healthcare providers, and coding professionals. Formal concurrent review documentation improvement teams can use a single discipline model (teams consisting of all nurses, HIM professionals, or physicians) or a hybrid staffing model utilizing the skills from combination of disciplines (AHIMA 2010c). Employer polls relating to CDI specialist education levels report hiring a mix of educational backgrounds (Buttner et al. 2014). This suggests that organizations have evolved to the point of using an interdisciplinary approach.

As previously mentioned, the health information management staff has been performing retrospective quantitative and qualitative analysis for many years. **Utilization management** is a planned, systematic review of patients in a healthcare facility against care criteria for admission, continued stay, and discharge. Utilization management (UM) professionals review documentation concurrently for specific indicators and criteria related to the appropriate and resource-efficient care of the patient. CDI teams throughout the development of the process have sometimes incorporated already existing HIM and UM functions versus creating a completely new process.

One approach to CDI involves using only physician reviewers to communicate findings peer-to-peer with other physicians. While this can have advantages in relationship building between CDI programs and physicians, not all organizations have the ability to devote full-time physician resources to the process. Even when the CDI team is comprised of other healthcare professionals, a physician champion is often included to assist in communicating with their peers. The **physician champion**, also known in some organizations as the physician advisor, is an individual who assists in communicating with and educating medical staff in areas such as documentation procedures for accurate billing and EHR procedures. Another approach to clinical review is to use only clinical staff such as nursing professionals who are familiar with the patient care unit and working with clinicians to treat patients. This has benefits in regard to communication and strong relationships; but if the team lacks knowledge of documentation requirements for coding compliance, reimbursement, and other uses of coded data, the CDI program still struggles. Many CDI teams have incorporated the best of these approaches, with one or more physician champions and a mix of reviewers, some with a clinical background and others with a HIM or coding background (AHIMA 2013c). This interdisciplinary approach makes the documentation review, communication of findings, and education more effective by including talent from those who are users of clinical documentation.

Regardless of the professional background, those performing CDI must be able to work with a wide variety of team members. Treating each discipline, department, and individual with respect is important in the support and success of a CDI process. Cultural compatibility with the organization, leadership, and communication skills, and the ability to succeed in the complex healthcare environment are all important aspects to consider (AHIMA 2010c, 2013c). Reviewers must have a mix of knowledge regarding the uses of documentation and coded data internally for the organization and externally for government, regulatory, and quality purposes. A survey of organizations in 2014 indicated most CDI professionals have an associate or bachelor's degree, while 17 percent have a master's degree, and 7 percent of the reviewers are physicians (Buttner et al. 2014). Recruitment for people who can fit this dynamic role often start with professionals working in HIM and coding, quality improvement (QI), UM, nursing, or case management departments.

Clinical Documentation Improvement Professional (CDIP) Certification

AHIMA's Commission on Certification for Health Informatics and Information Management (CCHIIM) developed the Clinical Documentation Improvement Professional (CDIP) credential in response to the demand for professionals who have the needed skillset. Healthcare organizations seeking CDI staff may want to seek candidates who have passed the exam indicating they are:

- distinguished as knowledgeable and competent in clinical documentation in patient health records,
- ready for leadership roles in the health informatics and information management community, and
- able to demonstrate competency in capturing documentation necessary to fully communicate patients' health status and conditions (AHIMA 2015).

In order to qualify for the exam, candidates must be an RHIA, RHIT, CCS, CCS-P, RN, MD, or DO and have two years' experience in clinical documentation improvement; or have earned an associate's degree or higher and three years of experience in clinical documentation improvement (candidates must also have completed coursework in medical terminology and anatomy and physiology) (AHIMA 2015). This certification can offer employers seeking CDI staff some evidence of the applicant's baseline knowledge and can be a component of the organizational or departmental compliance plan in hiring qualified CDI professionals.

The CDIP exam covers content including knowledge of clinical coding practice, leadership, record review and document clarification, CDI metrics and statistics, research, and education. According to AHIMA, CDI professionals are able to:

- Identify opportunities for documentation improvement by ensuring that diagnoses and procedures are documented to the highest level of specificity
- Query providers in an ethical manner to avoid potential fraud or compliance issues
- Formulate queries to providers to clarify conflicting diagnoses
- Ensure provider query response is documented in the medical record
- Formulate queries to providers to clarify the clinical significance of abnormal findings identified in the record
- Track responses to queries and interact with providers to obtain query responses
- Interact with providers to clarify present on admission (POA) indicators
- Identify post-discharge query opportunities that will affect severity of illness (SOI), risk of mortality (ROM), and, ultimately, case weight
- Collaborate with the case management and utilization management staff to affect change in documentation
- Interact with providers to clarify hospital-acquired conditions (HAC)
- Interact with providers to clarify the documentation of core measures
- Interact with providers to clarify patient safety indicators (PSI)

- Determine facility requirements for documentation of query responses in the record to establish official policy and procedures related to CDI query activities
- Develop policies regarding various stages of the query process and time frames to avoid compliance risk (AHIMA 2015).

The entire CDI team must carry out these actions in an ethical manner following industry recognized best practices and facility policies and procedures. AHIMA has also developed the Ethical Standards for Clinical Documentation Improvement (CDI) Professionals to guide CDI planning, decision making, and creation of procedures. CDI professionals will:

1. Facilitate accurate, complete, and consistent clinical documentation within the health record to support coding and reporting of high-quality healthcare data.
2. Support the reporting of all healthcare data elements (for example, diagnosis and procedure codes, and present on admission indicator) required for external reporting purposes (for example, reimbursement and other administrative uses, population health, quality and patient safety measurement, and research) completely and accurately, in accordance with regulatory and documentation standards and requirements and applicable official coding conventions, rules, and guidelines.
3. Query provider (physician or other qualified healthcare practitioner), whether verbal or written, for clarification and additional documentation when there is conflicting, incomplete, or ambiguous information in the health record regarding a significant reportable condition or procedure or other reportable data element dependent on health record documentation (for example, present on admission indicator).
4. Refuse to participate in or support documentation practices intended to inappropriately increase payment, qualify for insurance policy coverage, or distort data by means that do not comply with federal and state statutes, regulations, and official rules and guidelines.

5. Facilitate interdisciplinary collaboration in situations supporting proper reporting practices.
6. Advance professional knowledge and practice through continuing education.
7. Refuse to participate in or conceal unethical reporting practices.
8. Protect the confidentiality of the health record at all times and refuse to access protected health information not required for job-related activities.
9. Demonstrate behavior that reflects integrity, shows a commitment to ethical and legal reporting practices, and fosters trust in professional activities (AHIMA 2010b).

AHIMA's CDIP certification supports a healthcare organization's CDI process. In the hiring process, the CDIP certification can be helpful in assessing what knowledge the applicants bring in addition to any potential skill-based assessments during the hiring process. It is a development goal requiring continued education and growth to achieve the certification for professionals working in the CDI process who are not certified, and gives job-seekers an advantage in obtaining a CDI position.

Alignment

A CDI program may be housed in various areas of the organization such as corporate compliance, health information management, or quality improvement; however, each organization must evaluate where it fits best. Many organizations have a dedicated CDI manager and staff structure. In addition to a specific division or department being responsible for the CDI process, an inclusive CDI oversight committee is a beneficial group in bringing together the multiple stakeholders identified in the previous section, including executive administration and medical staff leadership (Gold and Kuehn 2011).

The administration of the organization as well as the medical staff need to support documentation improvement efforts. The support of top level administration is required as it would be for any organizational change, and documentation processes and practices affect the organization in every area of patient care.

Support of the medical staff leadership is a key driver of success. Depending on the medical staff model used, physicians and physician leaders are not necessarily employees of the healthcare organization; although they work in tandem with healthcare professionals to provide care regardless of the model. This can be described as the dual-pyramid organization of healthcare facilities (Liebler and McConnell 2012). The responsibility and authority structure of the medical staff functions alongside the administrative functions of executives, directors, and managers in hospitals and health systems. Depending on size and type of facility and the medical staff bylaws, a chief of staff, medical director, or corresponding position is responsible as a counterpart to the hospital chief executive officer. Physicians who are not directly hired as employees wishing to practice at the facility apply for clinical privileges to practice there and report to the chief of staff or to a departmental physician lead or chairperson who ultimately reports to the chief of staff or medical director. CDI teams will need to know what type of physician model and reporting structure is utilized in seeking the support of medical staff. Even though the CDI process may not be initiated by a particular physician, service, or office, the support of the medical staff and leadership are just as important as support from hospital administration.

An AHIMA practice brief regarding CDI reinforces physician leadership and involvement is an essential component in a successful and sustainable CDI program, and gives the recommendation that the physician advisor or champion be a full-time employee of the hospital or healthcare organization (AHIMA 2014c). In some organizations, that may not be possible; however, regardless of the status of the one or multiple physician supporters of CDI, it is important that they are able to connect with peers regarding the benefits of improved documentation to both the facility and physicians.

The physician advisor or champion role is essential to the success of the CDI process. As noted earlier, the physician advisor carries a responsibility to communicate, educate, and build or maintain respectful relationships with peers in improving documentation practices. The physician advisor is involved with CDI and HIM staff on a routine basis as the medical expert regarding clinical documentation. CDI teams without physician champions miss out on a valuable resource. The physician advisor is involved in the education of fellow physicians and the education plans for specific medical departments that may have unique areas of opportunity and needs for improvement (AHIMA 2010c). The physician advisor role is an active participant and is tasked with devoting time to:

- Educating providers on the importance of documentation
- Planning education for different medical departments
- Communicating with the medical staff regarding CDI (via newsletters, website, presentations, and such)
- Participating in investigating admission denials, DRG changes, Medicare core measures documentation
- Assisting in formulating clinically appropriate and compliant queries for physicians to clarify documentation (AHIMA 2014a)

Physician CDI advisors should be selected based on their medical experience, ability to plan and provide education both in groups and individually, and ability to communicate to peers the needs of CDI in a positive manner while working as a problem-solver (Gold and Kuehn 2011). They should be respected by the members of the medical staff and be able to influence their peers (Huff et al. 2014). Even in programs where all or the majority of the documentation review is being performed by nonphysician CDI professionals, the physician component for reviewer support and peer-to-peer communication and education is essential. The physician advisor cannot be the leader in name or on paper only but is actively influential in successful CDI programs.

Record Review

In many cases, reviewing every record concurrently is not a feasible undertaking for the CDI team. Selecting the priority areas of service, patient care units, type of insurance, or other criteria that is high impact is often needed to direct the process. It is important to remember that more accurate reimbursement is a benefit of a successful CDI program; however, focusing only on maximizing reimbursement may expose risks of penalties (Buttner et al. 2014). The goal is to obtain the most accurate clinical documentation that represents the patient medical status and treatment received, not to target or exploit reimbursement programs. A survey of providers in 2014 indicated over 80 percent looked at a variety of payers and insurance types, possibly indicating CDI programs are indeed evolving to perform more than reimbursement functions and are aiming at a whole spectrum of outcomes including quality measures and patient safety. Of those organizations with CDI programs, 88 percent of them review only inpatient records in the documentation improvement process (Buttner et al. 2014). Benchmarking information relating to what types of records and how many to review is limited; however, it is expected to grow as CDI programs become more commonplace than in the past. Reviewing every record before discharge is a difficult task. Organizations need to select the areas and types of records to focus on based in their needs.

Further consideration for record review comes with ICD-10-CM/PCS regarding documentation gaps that may occur as coding requirements require more detail than in the past. Initial studies have indicated some potential areas for documentation gaps (displayed in table 9.2), as reviews of actual patient records have been missing the details needed in these cases. These diagnoses and procedures require detailed documentation such as type, site, laterality, or stage in order to assign the most accurate codes.

As for the actual documentation review, seven items that a CDI professional will often need to obtain more specific documentation in order to meet the needs of accurate coding are suggested:

- Disease type
  - The inclusion of descriptors is needed for the most accurate code and often needed before any code can be assigned.

Is a fracture traumatic or pathological, or a tumor malignant or benign?

- Disease acuity
  - o Is the disease chronic, acute, or subacute?
- Site specificity
  - o Does the most accurate code require location such as a specific lobe, or distal, proximal, superior, or inferior location?
- Disease stage
  - o How severe or advanced is the disease?
- Laterality
  - o Specifying the left or right eye, ear, or limb
- Details needed to assign a combination code
  - o Many diseases and conditions are related and could be communicated with one code instead of multiple if specified as related in the documentation such as diabetic complications, while others can be assumed related unless specified otherwise like hypertension and kidney disease
- Documentation missing completely (Hinkle-Azzara and Carr 2014)

Not all documentation issues are related to the transition to ICD-10-CM/PCS. Many potential weaknesses in documentation that existed when using ICD-9-CM still exist using ICD-10-CM/PCS. Conditions such as respiratory failure, pressure ulcer, coma, and pregnancy that have detailed coding requirements have been areas in which CDI has the potential to make the most difference even when using the previous coding system. They will continue to be potential focus areas due to the complex nature and many clinical factors that need to be considered and documented (AHIMA 2015).

In addition to potential code–system documentation gaps, another potential area to begin with record review includes diagnoses that can make a difference in the organization's case mix under Medicare severity diagnosis-related groups (MS-DRG) (AHIMA 2014c). **Case mix** is a description of a patient population based on characteristics including age, gender, type of insurance, diagnosis, risk factors, treatment received, and resources used (Hazelwood and Venable 2011). Healthcare facilities review the **case-mix index** (CMI) by averaging the MS-DRG relative weights of each inpatient treated, which reflects the resource intensity and clinical severity of that group of patients. The focus in looking at the MS-DRG is not to aggressively maximize payment from insurers but to work toward the most accurate payment that the provider is justly and legally entitled to receive (AHIMA House of Delegates 2008). In 1997, an Office of the Inspector General (OIG) investigation found upcoding done to manipulate DRGs had resulted in millions of dollars being inappropriately paid to providers (Butler 2014). Upcoding is the practice of assigning diagnostic or procedural codes that represent higher payment rates than the services that were provided. The resulting legal action for fraud has proved a lesson and guide for CDI programs to focus on accurate, quality data as opposed to only payment; and it is one reason AHIMA has developed the Ethical Standards for Clinical Documentation Improvement (CDI) Professionals (AHIMA 2010b). (Refer to online appendix C to review these ethical standards.) In addition, the

Table 9.2. Potential areas for documentation gaps in the health record

Diabetes mellitus	Neoplasms	Heart disease
Injuries	Pregnancy	Pneumonia
Drug under- or overdose	Respiratory/ventilators	Ear disorders
Cerebral infarction	Rehabilitation	Eye disorders
Acute myocardial infarction	Musculoskeletal conditions	Atrial fibrillation
Procedures with contrasts	Transfusions	All ICD-10-PCS

Sources: Moczygemba and Fenton 2012; DeAlmeida et al. 2014; Hinkle-Azzara and Carr 2014.

case mix is used for a myriad of other patient severity measures. The multiple comorbidities and complications (CC) and major comorbidities and complications (MCC) that impact the organization the most in regard to differences in MS-DRG assignment are good targets for record review. More information about MS-DRG and case mix can be found in chapter 7.

Each organization may have its own need to focus on a specific set of records as well. Factors such as past results of external reviews such as Recovery Audit Contractor (RAC) audits, Program for Evaluation Payment Patterns Electronic Reports (PEPPER), or types of services that have had claims denials or rejections are also a good indicator of where to begin reviewing.

In many cases, even missing a small detail can delay the coding process while further clarification is sought. In the example of the ICD-10-PCS system, missing information to determine even one of the seven characters representing different aspects of the procedure will prevent code assignment. This is one of the reasons concurrent review is preferred, both to obtain more accurate documentation in a timely manner, but also to facilitate communication with providers during the care episode. Working for improved documentation during the episode of care has quality of care and safety benefits for the patient. Retrospective reviews do have value and are useful for identifying trends and gathering data for decisions; however as far as improved documentation for communication, retrospective review is not as helpful. The patient has already been discharged (thus the opportunity to provide care has passed) and if clarification is needed, waiting until after discharge delays the coding and claims process.

Determining where to start when planning a CDI process can be difficult. One strategy is to identify the top 5 to 10 MS-DRGs and surgeries occurring in the organization. From there define the documentation requirements needed for ICD-10-CM and PCS coding, identify the current weaknesses through record review, and develop a plan for documentation improvement starting with these areas (AHIMA 2014a).

Frequency and Number of Record Reviews

The organization will have to determine how many records are reasonable to be reviewed depending on the size of the CDI team and complexity of records reviewed, as well as the types of records to be reviewed in the target areas. As mentioned, in most cases 100 percent review is not possible. The frequency of record review is also a consideration. In concurrent review, the records continue to grow as the patient stay progresses; one record may need to be reviewed multiple times throughout the stay whether that be on a daily basis or every other day. Another plan is to review upon admission and day of expected discharge then an alternating schedule in between. The frequency of record review depends on the individual organization.

Budget

Any program, process, or department's success is dependent on access to the appropriate resources. The budget is a tool to be used both for planning and controlling (Liebler and McConnell 2012). Budgetary needs for hiring staff; providing education; utilizing communication tools; and measuring, tracking, and reporting should be considered. The composition of the CDI team, number and type of records to be reviewed, methods of education, communication needs, and information and results tracking will vary between organizations. The number and types of records requiring review and frequency of desired review also impacts the budget for personnel and hours. Regardless of the final dollar figure, the budget should provide enough resources to complete the essential functions of CDI. Adequate resources are required to allow the CDI leader to accomplish the goals of organization.

CDI Staff Training

Both physicians and the CDI team need continuous education to stay current in regulatory, legal, coding, and external reporting trends. Because CDI professionals come from a variety of healthcare backgrounds and bring strengths in different areas (clinical, coding, quality, legal, and others), it may also be beneficial to have a common orientation program for new team members to ensure everyone has the same understanding of documentation issues and considerations. Specific education may be required for CDI staff who are very strong in some areas but lack experience in others. For example, a CDI team member with a clinical background may need further knowledge in coding guidelines, or a professional with a coding background may need more orientation on completing concurrent reviews on the patient unit.

CDI Medical Staff and Physician Training

The physician education component should increase awareness of documentation issues. This includes the many uses and impacts of documentation and coded data, where areas of improvement are to be found, and feedback on the quality of documentation and what improvements and benefits have been discovered. One of the benefits of having a physician advisor for CDI is peer-to-peer insight in planning and facilitating training sessions. While everyone on the CDI team should be comfortable speaking with physicians and building respectful working relationships, the physician advisor(s) can be a great asset in both group sessions and individual meetings with physicians about specific documentation issues. Education before the CDI program begins and continuously afterward can be a tool to reduce tension and misunderstanding about CDI (Lo 2014).

While most physicians are not experts in the method of determining facility reimbursement or the acuity and severity of the patients that the hospital serves (Rosenbaum et al. 2014), documentation and the resulting coded data are used for much more than hospital reimbursement. Data collected are used for multiple purposes including many that reflect upon the physician's medical practices. Topics include physician profiling and public reporting, quality assessment including mortality and surgical complications, credentialing and reappointment, peer review, and performance improvement (Pinson and Tang 2008). Better documentation can also help physician reimbursement for their professional services. Third-party reimbursement systems for physicians also use coded data that is based on clinical documentation.

It is suggested that short education sessions to change documentation practices be provided incrementally over time rather than attempting to schedule and conduct one or a few exhaustive sessions (AHIMA 2013a). Short sessions, even by department or specialty, could give an opportunity to tailor the message specifically to different groups of physicians. The following methods may be used to facilitate effective training sessions:

- Utilize real, practical examples of actual documentation from the facility or physician in CDI review
- Communicate the specific documentation needs of the ICD-10-CM/PCS system
- Create templates for diagnoses, procedures, or services needing improvement in documentation
- Distribute handouts as communication tools
- Leverage newsletters
- Display posters or signage to increase awareness
- Utilize "pocket cards" for quick reference (AHIMA 2013a)

Multiple methods can be used to communicate, educate, and remind those who document in the health record regarding the CDI process. As with any change, more communication, even in a small or short message, is better than less.

Administrative Reports and Performance Monitoring Metrics

Metrics and statistics are about decision making (Horton 2012). Data regarding the success of the program are essential components not only to support the decision to continue CDI, but to identify continuing areas of improvement. Metrics are important for knowing what is working, how well it is working, and what is not working. Measuring performance and being able to use that feedback for either correction or further improvement is part of the management function of controlling (Liebler and McConnell 2012). See chapter 25 for more information in this topic. Multiple sources indicate the need for some essential measurements to assist in the development and continuing improvement of the CDI process. Metrics are identified in figure 9.1.

Figure 9.1. Basic metrics for CDI program evaluation

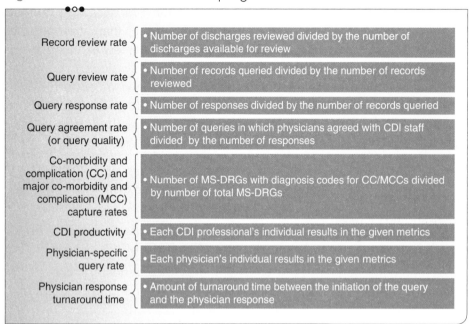

Record review rate	• Number of discharges reviewed divided by the number of discharges available for review
Query review rate	• Number of records queried divided by the number of records reviewed
Query response rate	• Number of responses divided by the number of records queried
Query agreement rate (or query quality)	• Number of queries in which physicians agreed with CDI staff divided by the number of responses
Co-morbidity and complication (CC) and major co-morbidity and complication (MCC) capture rates	• Number of MS-DRGs with diagnosis codes for CC/MCCs divided by number of total MS-DRGs
CDI productivity	• Each CDI professional's individual results in the given metrics
Physician-specific query rate	• Each physician's individual results in the given metrics
Physician response turnaround time	• Amount of turnaround time between the initiation of the query and the physician response

Sources: Buttner et al. 2014; AHIMA 2014a; Gold and Kuehn 2011; Russo 2008.

Each specific organization may have differing data reporting needs. The end goal of metrics is not simply to collect data, but to use the data to evaluate and improve the organization and CDI process. It may be useful to utilize a dashboard or scorecard as in figure 9.2 to assist stakeholders in keeping aware of progress and making decisions regarding strategy, policy, and processes (AHIMA 2014a).

CDI Benchmarks

Benchmarks for measures and performance statistics are a comparison of one's own results with the results of other individuals, departments, or organizations (Liebler and McConnell 2012). The purpose is to identify and compare best practices of organizations with similar characteristics to assist in improving performance. Because each organization is different, national industry benchmarks are not always the best measure; however, some examples of benchmarks for CDI metrics (AHIMA 2014a) are found in figure 9.3.

Benchmarks are tools for performance improvement. Measurements provide important feedback regarding the outcomes of the CDI program and identify successes as well as areas for improvement. Achieving a certain score or number is not the

most important consideration—the overall goal of these metrics is the accuracy of information, ultimately leading to better patient care.

Query Process

Successful communication between the CDI team and the healthcare providers who are documenting care is identified as a key element to success (AHIMA 2014a). One form of communication is the process of asking questions of providers for clarification on documentation. While there is much variation to the methods of communication, there are some essential components. A sender must initiate and transmit the message, and a recipient must understand the message and acknowledge the receipt for both parties to be successful in the process. Both CDI professionals and physicians in the documentation improvement process must be senders and receivers to be successful. In cases where a CDI specialist or coder needs to ask a physician a question regarding documentation, it is referred to as a query. A **query** is a routine communication and education tool used to advocate for complete and compliant documentation (AHIMA 2010c). This includes communication for the purpose of correct code assignment (AHIMA 2013b).

Figure 9.2. Example of a CDI dashboard

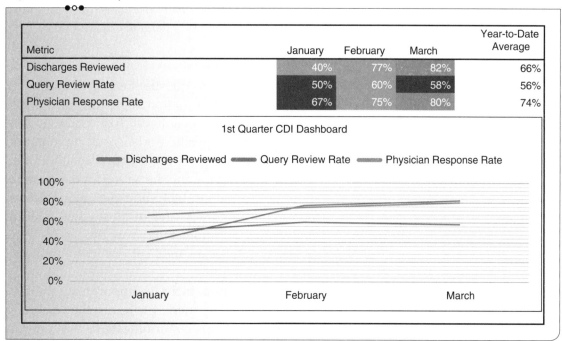

Figure 9.3. Sample CDI benchmarks

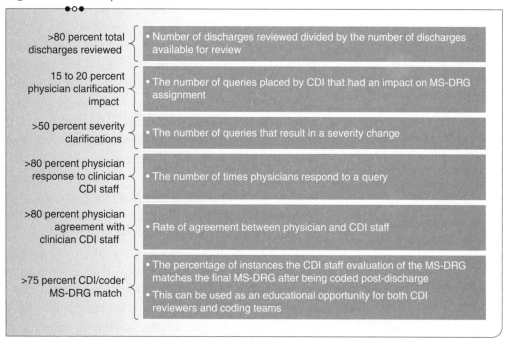

The intent is to clarify what has been recorded, not to call into question the provider's clinical judgment or medical expertise. For that reason, some organizations have chosen to title the specific communication a clarification rather than query in an effort to avoid being perceived as questioning a provider's judgment (Gold and Kuehn 2011).

Regardless of naming convention, the query process as well as physician feedback about the process are essential pieces of communication. One of the roles of the CDI physician advisor is to assist and intervene when queries are lacking responses, or when misunderstandings occur in the process (Huff et al. 2014).

As CDI staff review documentation, situations where a query may be necessary include when documentation:

- is conflicting, imprecise, incomplete, illegible, ambiguous or inconsistent;
- describes clinical indicators without a definitive relationship to an underlying diagnosis;
- includes clinical indicators, diagnostic evaluation, or treatment not related to a specific condition or procedure;
- provides a diagnosis without supporting clinical validation; or
- is unclear for present on admission indicator assignment (AHIMA 2013b).

Some circumstances require additional specific information in order to assign the proper ICD-10-CM or ICD-10-PCS code. It is important to understand that the exact term is not required to be used in the documentation if the meaning and description of treatment is clear. In this case, a query is not necessary simply to have the matching term recorded. For coding accuracy, the ICD-10-PCS Official Guidelines for Coding and Reporting indicates:

> Many of the terms used to construct PCS codes are defined within the system. It is the coder's responsibility to determine what the documentation in the medical record equates to in the PCS definitions. The physician is not expected to use the terms used in PCS code descriptions, nor is the coder required to query the physician when the correlation between the documentation and the defined PCS terms is clear. (CMS 2014, A11)

Coding professionals are not qualified to diagnose patients or perform procedures; however the Centers for Medicare and Medicaid Services (CMS) do not expect physicians to be experts in ICD-10-PCS terminology and language either. CDI and coding professionals do not need to ask the physician to document the exact phrasing contained in the ICD-10-PCS coding system if the documentation in the health record supports the code assigned based on PCS guidance. This CMS determination should be part of the education and training of both CDI staff and physicians as well as in policy for guidance to CDI and coding professionals. This will avoid needless queries to physicians.

Developing a Query

When formulating a question about the specificity or clarity of the information in the record, multiple factors should be considered. Just as the goal of CDI is accurate, specific, and clear documentation in the record, the query to the provider should also be easily understood and the reason for the question should be apparent. Including clinical indicators, focusing on accuracy, and in most cases creating open-ended questions that allow the results to be driven by physician medical expertise are some methods to employ.

It is important to include support from the documentation in the query. Including the reasoning for the query helps communicate to the clinician why they are being asked to clarify and what pieces of information are or are not already specified in the record. It assists the clinician in reviewing the request and gives justification for the query.

Reimbursement impact should not be the focus of the query. The goal is to achieve the greatest amount of specificity and accuracy, not always the highest severity condition to obtain increased reimbursement (Brown et al. 2009). Inclusion of the reimbursement impact also confuses the motive of better communication and patient care with a monetary goal. It can also be viewed as a leading question to provide clinical indicators directing the response to a specific diagnosis or procedure that carries higher reimbursement.

It is wise to determine if open- or closed-ended questions are most appropriate. Some situations are acceptable for closed-ended, yes or no type questions, such as clarifying a cause and effect relationship between diagnosis, seeking agreement or clarification between clinicians or reports, confirming details regarding established diagnosis, and determining if a diagnosis was present on admission. Looking at potential new diagnoses that are not already specified in the record could be viewed as attempting to lead a clinician to a particular diagnosis when presenting clinical support for only one diagnosis followed by only yes or no options. A better format in this case is an open-ended question asking if further detail can be provided or multiple-choice structure to allow for the most accurate response. Regardless of format, the query should not be formulated to lead the physician's response (AHIMA 2013b).

Documentation of Queries

The documentation as a result of the query should be included in the patient record to communicate to other providers and support the patient's course of treatment. This is often recorded in the progress notes, discharge summary, or addendum to the documentation. Each organization will need to determine if the actual query is part of the permanent patient record or retained in other administrative records. Policy and procedure should be created to indicate if the query is a part of the medical record where is it located and how long it is retained. Involvement of compliance and legal departments can aid in determining the policy for each institution (AHIMA 2014a). Refer to chapter 10 for more information on compliance and risk in the healthcare setting. Any information affecting the billed services obtained after the physician's documentation was completed must be included in accordance with accepted standards for amending the medical record (AHIMA 2011). During concurrent review, CDI professionals may have the opportunity to verbally communicate with physicians to clarify documentation. These queries and interactions should also be recorded to capture the impact of the CDI process. While not every verbal communication between CDI and physicians is always an official query for clarification, instances where information that would have been communicated through a paper or electronic communication has been discussed face-to-face should be recorded as a query.

Format of Queries

Although the content of the question is more important than the format, some uniform format guidelines have been suggested:

- Patient name
- Admission date and time

- Account number
- Medical record number
- Date the query is initiated
- Contact information of the CDI reviewer
- Individualized diagnosis-specific information relevant to the patient (AHIMA 2013b)

In addition to the format or template of the query, other operational considerations need to be determined. Items such as:

- where in the record queries are placed;
- the process for notifying a physician that there is a query;
- standard procedures for how long a query is left open or unanswered before following up;
- what happens to an open query after the patient is discharged;
- who will monitor the unanswered queries; and
- feedback or corrective action to be taken and who will undertake it (AHIMA 2013b).

Figures 9.4 and 9.5 provide examples of a physician queries. Each situation will require different documentation considerations depending on the method of communication—paper, electronic, or verbal.

Open-ended questions can also be an effective method of querying physicians, as noted in the situations of figure 9.5.

Technology Considerations

The meaningful use of technology has expanded in healthcare to provide many advances in treating patients and making recordkeeping and administrative functions more efficient. While technology such as the electronic health record (EHR) with the ability to integrate clinical pathways and provide real-time reminders to clinicians is helpful, it is not an automatic fix to documentation deficiencies. In some cases, facilities have developed or used documentation templates that are specific to particular diagnoses, procedures, or services and can be very useful to help capture relevant and required details for ICD-10-CM/PCS coding, core measures, and other quality indicators. If the

Figure 9.4. Examples of closed-ended queries

Compliant Example 1

Clinical scenario: In the impression of the pathology report, ovarian cancer is documented; however, only ovarian mass is documented in the final discharge statement by the provider.

Query: Do you agree with the pathology report specifying the "ovarian mass" as an "ovarian cancer"? Please document your response in the health record or below.

Yes _____
No _____
Other _____
Clinically Undetermined _____
Name: _____ Date: _____

Rationale: This yes/no query involves confirming a diagnosis that is already present as an interpretation of a pathology specimen in the health record.

Compliant Example 2

Clinical scenario: Consulting pulmonologist documents pneumonia as an impression based on the chest x-ray. However, the attending physician documents bronchitis throughout the record, including in the discharge summary.

Query: Do you agree with the pulmonologist's impression that the patient has pneumonia? Please document your response in the health record or below.

Yes _____
No _____
Other _____
Clinically Undetermined _____
Name: _____ Date: _____

Rationale: This is an example of a yes/no query resolving conflicting practitioner documentation.

Source: AHIMA 2013b.

Figure 9.5. Example of an open-ended query

A patient is admitted with pneumonia. The admitting H&P examination reveals WBC of 14,000; a respiratory rate of 24; a temperature of 102 degrees; heart rate of 120; hypotension; and altered mental status. The patient is administered an IV antibiotic and IV fluid resuscitation.

Leading: The patient has elevated WBCs, tachycardia, and is given an IV antibiotic for *Pseudomonas* cultured from the blood. Are you treating for sepsis?

Nonleading: Based on your clinical judgment, can you provide a diagnosis that represents the below-listed clinical indicators?

In this patient admitted with pneumonia, the admitting history and physical examination reveals the following:

• WBC 14,000
• Respiratory rate 24
• Temperature 102°F
• Heart rate 120
• Hypotension
• Altered mental status
• IV antibiotic administration
• IV fluid resuscitation

Please document the condition and the causative organism (if known) in the medical record.

Source: AHIMA 2010c.

query templates being used were created before the transition to ICD-10-CM/PCS, they need to be reviewed to ensure they are still helpful in capturing needed details. Such reviews should be conducted each year as changes in coding and quality reporting occur (AHIMA 2013a). Even if edits and prompts can be built into the EHR system, they should not be depended on as the sole method of documentation improvement (Buttner et al. 2014).

Computer-assisted coding (CAC) is also an emerging technology being utilized in the coding process. CAC is a tool intended for improved efficiency of the coding and claims submission process. While CAC can be useful in settings where documentation is structured and has a limited vocabulary, it is critical to remember that specific and accurate documentation is the underlying resource for technologic advances relating to patient records, medical coding, and quality improvement. As healthcare continues to advance technologically, the content, including documentation of patient treatment, inside the software and hardware utilized provides the real benefit to patient care and the processes that support it.

Supporting the CDI Process

In the end, the overarching goal of CDI is to ensure specific and accurate documentation that reflects the "true cost of care, severity of illness, complexity of care, and resource utilization" (Pinson and Tang 2008). The process does not necessarily seek more documentation from physicians, but specific documentation that clearly indicates what treatment was undertaken and the reason for it. In order to be successful, the organization needs to understand the:

- many uses of clinical documentation;
- benefit of specific and accurate documentation;
- need for multiple stakeholder involvement;
- need for talented interdisciplinary CDI staff;
- required resources for success;
- need for predetermined policies and procedures for record review and queries; and
- metrics for building the business case for CDI initiatives.

Success depends on utilizing the right people, processes, and technologies (Buttner et al. 2014). That mix involves respect, communication, and relationships between coding professionals, CDI staff, and physicians with the support of leadership from administration and medical staff (AHIMA 2014c). Clinical documentation should match the diagnosis and procedure codes and should match the claim; looking at any of the three should give a uniform picture of the patient's severity and course of treatment.

Check Your Understanding 9.1

Instructions: **Answer the following questions on a separate piece of paper.**

1. What is clinical documentation improvement (CDI)?

2. What is the aim of the CDI process?

3. Why is clinical documentation important?

4. Why is it important to have a CDI physician champion/advisor?

5. What elements of a CDI program need to be considered during the planning process?

Coding Compliance

Compliance means complying with rules, laws, standards, or regulations (see chapter 10). Following the required rules and expected practices in regard to coding is of particular interest since coded data is used for so many purposes, including being the data on which most payment and reimbursement decisions are made in the American healthcare system. This includes the federal Medicare and state Medicaid programs for which the discrepancy between submitted coded data and the actual service provided is an area often reviewed for fraud (Scichilone 2008). Government investigators have the authority to examine claims for payment from any organization or provider who delivers services or treatments to Medicare beneficiaries (AHIMA 2011). Professional ethics and accepted practice are to comply with the rules of programs in which the healthcare provider participates; this is because the "collection of accurate and complete coded data is critical to healthcare delivery, research, public reporting, reimbursement, and policy making" (AHIMA 2007, 1). In addition to the inherent benefits of ensuring accurately coded data, the risk of negative consequences is also a driver for coding compliance plans.

There are numerous factors that could result in organizational harm due to incorrect coded data on claims for reimbursement. *Fraud* and *abuse* are two terms often used to describe a provider or organization collecting undeserved payments. **Fraud** is an intentional or deliberate deception or misrepresentation that an individual makes in order to receive additional benefits, and **abuse** describes practices or incidents that are not done deliberately even though they may result in improper payments from Medicare (Hazelwood 2008).

Fraudulent activities misrepresent the care that actually took place. Billing for services that were not provided or providing a lesser service than what is reported is an example of fraud. Other examples are billing for new equipment while providing the patient with used or old equipment, reporting that services were completed at a different site than they were in reality, or misrepresenting which practitioner provided the service. There are many more ways fraudulent requests for payment using coded data could occur, all of them involving a misrepresentation.

Abuse is defined as unintentional; however, the idea that the person or organization "knows or should know better" applies when determining the difference between fraud and abuse (Hazelwood 2008). No proof of intent is required, if a person or organization acts in deliberate ignorance of the truth or acts in reckless disregard their actions can still be seen as fraud (Burke et al. 2009). Examples of abuse include unintentional unbundling of codes or mistakenly reporting the wrong place of service or discharge status. By submitting a claim for payment, the provider is certifying they have earned the requested payment and complied with all requirements to receive it. If the provider or organization knew or should have known the claim for payment was false, they are in violation (CMS 2014). Penalties apply under federal and state law for both fraud and abuse, intentional or unintentional, which is why compliance programs are essential.

Regulation

Many laws apply to healthcare fraud and abuse. For example, the federal False Claims Act, Civil Money Penalties Act, Health Insurance Portability and Accountability Act (HIPAA), Balance Budget Act of 1997, Tax Relief and Health Care Act of 2006, and others have aspects or outline programs specifically dealing with coded data used for financial purposes. The Deficit Reduction Act of 2005 necessitated that compliance programs by healthcare providers shift from voluntary to a mandatory practice (Burke et al. 2009). Continuing awareness of new and changing legislation and regulation is important for health information management professionals.

Federal False Claims Act

Even if there is not intent to defraud the government; a provider, organization, or individual can be found in violation (Williams 2008). The **Federal False Claims Act** is a federal law that seeks to protect governmental programs from fraud by individuals and companies. It outlines how both deliberate ignorance and reckless disregard to the truth or falsity of a claim are included with having knowledge of the false information (Department of Justice 2011). A coding compliance plan will work to eliminate the ignorance or indifference throughout the organization regarding inaccurate data on claims. The civil False Claims Act was originally enacted during the American Civil War to prevent government contractors from collecting money for services or goods not actually provided, or misrepresenting what was provided in the claim to the government. In 1986, the Act was amended and one of the most significant updates included the provision to allow involvement of qui tam relators, or those acting on behalf of the government. This is sometimes referred to as "whistleblowing," where anyone—including employees, patients, and competitors—can bring lawsuits based on their knowledge of fraud (Enriquez 2011). Qui tam relators receive a minimum of 15 percent of the fraudulent monies recovered by the government.

Deficit Reduction Act of 2005

The Deficit Reduction Act of 2005 is multifaceted law concerning the nation's budget. One section specifically aims at fighting Medicaid fraud and abuse. The act requires any program that receives or makes payments of over $5,000,000 annually to provide education to employees regarding the False Claims Act (CMS n.d.). The Act requires written policies for anyone working with claims including contractors to communicate to employees details of the False Claims Act including the organizational process for reporting and correcting inaccuracies; whistleblower protections; the prevention and detection of waste, fraud, and abuse; as well as related laws (Burke et al. 2009). It also allocated further resources to identifying Medicare fraud and abuse.

Health Insurance Portability and Accountability Act

The Health Insurance Portability and Accountability Act (HIPAA) enacted in 1996 is a law regarding many aspects of the healthcare system. There has been considerable attention paid to the patient privacy and information security aspects in the administrative simplification section, although there are pieces that relate to coding compliance as well. Preventing healthcare fraud and abuse is a major focus of the legislation. Providing medically unnecessary services, billing for services that were not provided, and misrepresentations in coding practices are examples that HIPAA outlines as fraud and abuse (Enriquez 2011). Unbundling and upcoding are types of coding misrepresentations that lead to inaccurate and undeserved reimbursement. Both are practices that are investigated by the Department of Health and Human Services (HHS) Office of the Inspector General (OIG).

Governmental Programs

There are many different audit programs regarding the accuracy of coded data submitted to federal agencies. The reviews typically include reviewing the documentation in the patient record and comparing it to the codes submitted on a claim for payment. Some examples are listed in figure 9.6 (AHIMA 2011).

Exclusion from Federal Programs

Those found to be fraudulent or abusive in receiving payments from the government can be excluded from being allowed to participate in Medicare and any other federal government programs. Exclusion is significant as the government is the largest purchaser and provider of services in the country (Hazelwood and Venable 2011). Any provider or supplier who has been convicted of Medicare fraud or other healthcare fraud, theft, or financial misconduct is required to be excluded from any federal healthcare program (CMS 2014).

In addition to the examples of governmental programs related to fraud, private insurers also administer audits and reviews. This is to ensure both quality and efficient care by providers and that appropriate payment by the insurer is provided for the privately insured population.

Advances in technology are also making the need for compliance plans apparent (Williams 2008). More sophisticated tools and data analysis

Figure 9.6.   Governmental agencies and programs

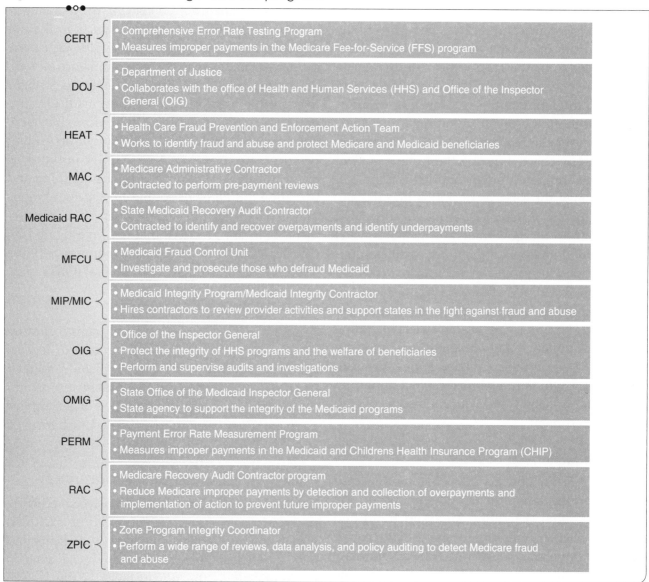

CERT	• Comprehensive Error Rate Testing Program • Measures improper payments in the Medicare Fee-for-Service (FFS) program
DOJ	• Department of Justice • Collaborates with the office of Health and Human Services (HHS) and Office of the Inspector General (OIG)
HEAT	• Health Care Fraud Prevention and Enforcement Action Team • Works to identify fraud and abuse and protect Medicare and Medicaid beneficiaries
MAC	• Medicare Administrative Contractor • Contracted to perform pre-payment reviews
Medicaid RAC	• State Medicaid Recovery Audit Contractor • Contracted to identify and recover overpayments and identify underpayments
MFCU	• Medicaid Fraud Control Unit • Investigate and prosecute those who defraud Medicaid
MIP/MIC	• Medicaid Integrity Program/Medicaid Integrity Contractor • Hires contractors to review provider activities and support states in the fight against fraud and abuse
OIG	• Office of the Inspector General • Protect the integrity of HHS programs and the welfare of beneficiaries • Perform and supervise audits and investigations
OMIG	• State Office of the Medicaid Inspector General • State agency to support the integrity of the Medicaid programs
PERM	• Payment Error Rate Measurement Program • Measures improper payments in the Medicaid and Childrens Health Insurance Program (CHIP)
RAC	• Medicare Recovery Audit Contractor program • Reduce Medicare improper payments by detection and collection of overpayments and implementation of action to prevent future improper payments
ZPIC	• Zone Program Integrity Coordinator • Perform a wide range of reviews, data analysis, and policy auditing to detect Medicare fraud and abuse

allow government entities and private insurers to identify trends in provider claims and more easily benchmark and compare data among similar providers. HIM professionals need to engage in continuing education throughout their career to keep aware of new and changing programs and agencies both governmental and nongovernmental.

Auditing

When an auditor of a governmental agency or third-party payer is preparing to review records on-site or through remote access, a notification of what records are needed and the method of review is provided. In some cases, the auditors will select many records for review and in others a smaller sample. Audits can be performed for many reasons reviewing quality indicators, compliance with regulations, reimbursement for services, and more. When the audit is for reimbursement purposes any over- or underpayments might be corrected on only the accounts reviewed. Another method of adjustment is referred to as the extrapolation method. The extrapolation method of auditing claims looks at a small sample of records and applies the correction in payment/reimbursement across a large number of claims in a time period or service area. One strategy for healthcare providers in preparation for the audit is to review the selected records beforehand, once the sample has been selected by the auditing agency or team (AHIMA 2011). The purpose is not to make changes or alter ahead of time, but to be able to estimate any potential change in retroactive reimbursement and begin to prepare financially for any anticipated adjustments.

OIG Compliance Guidance

The Office of the Inspector General (OIG) was created in 1976 with the mission to "protect the integrity of the Health and Human Services (HHS) programs as well as the health and welfare of program beneficiaries" (OIG 2015). Different departments of the government have their own investigatory agencies, although the HHS OIG is larger than any other governmental OIG. The OIG gives advice to organizations seeking guidance, although the specific recommendations they suggest are not mandatory as the OIG realizes every provider is different and each specific item may not apply to every organization (Burke et al. 2009). Guidance to hospitals, nursing facilities, researchers, ambulance suppliers, pharmaceutical manufacturers, physicians, clinical laboratories, third-party billing agencies, Medicare+Choice programs, and durable equipment companies can be found on the OIG website. Some foundational guidelines provided by the OIG are:

- The development and distribution of written standards of conduct, as well as written policies and procedures that promote the hospital's commitment to compliance (for example, by including adherence to compliance as an element in evaluating managers and employees);

- The designation of a chief compliance officer and other appropriate bodies, for example, a corporate compliance committee charged with the responsibility of operating and monitoring the compliance program and who report directly to the CEO and the governing body;

- The development and implementation of regular, effective education and training programs for all affected employees;

- The maintenance of a process, such as a hotline, to receive complaints, and the adoption of procedures to protect the anonymity of complainants and to protect whistleblowers from retaliation;

- The development of a system to respond to allegations of improper or illegal activities and the enforcement of appropriate disciplinary action against employees who have violated internal compliance policies, applicable statutes, regulations or federal healthcare program requirements;

- The use of audits and/or other evaluation techniques to monitor compliance and assist in the reduction of identified problem areas; and

- The investigation and remediation of identified systemic problems and the development of policies addressing the non-employment or retention of sanctioned individuals (OIG 2005).

Benchmarking, longitudinal studies, and regular reporting are elements supported by the OIG as the essential components of an overall compliance plan (Schedel and Parker 2006). This can include both internal self-audits as well as external reviewers with the aim to identify weaknesses and improve practices on a voluntary basis. The best practice for internal audits is to avoid having the same people review records who are responsible for the coding initially. Many healthcare organizations have a coding compliance reviewer separate from the HIM coding department. External reviewers are often consultants or agencies also designed to give outside, unbiased advice based on results of record review, coded data, and claims reviews. The goal is to prevent any practices that may not meet the standards of federal and state laws, as well as other accreditation or regulatory practices. While prevention is the best outcome, identification and correction of issues also fall within the realm of compliance.

Target Areas and OIG Workplan

Each year the HHS OIG publishes the projects that are planned and the areas identified for review. These published workplans cover CMS and the Administrations for Children and Families and

Administration on Aging. The workplan can be found on the HHS OIG website. It is advisable to include the OIG workplan items that may be applicable to an organization in the compliance plan, as well as addressing other high-risk areas for review including billing for noncovered services, inaccurate claim forms, duplicate billing, correction of overpayments, unbundling, overcoding, or upcoding (Burke et al. 2009).

During the process of reviewing the medical record for code assignment, unbundling and upcoding are practices that would be identified as fraud and abuse. Unbundling is the reporting of multiple codes to describe a service or procedure when according to coding conventions, one code would accurately describe the procedure. Unbundling often results in additional reimbursement as if the provider performed various smaller procedures separately when in actuality the procedure is intended to include all of the essential components bundled together. Upcoding describes using diagnosis or procedure codes that are selected specifically because they result in higher payment from third-party payers. Unbundling and upcoding are examples of attempts to maximize reimbursement to the highest possible amount through coded data, or maximization. This practice puts an organization or provider at risk of violating the previously mentioned federal and state laws. A better focus is the intent of coding optimization. Optimization seeks the most accurate documentation, coded data, and resulting payment in the amount the provider is rightly and legally entitled to receive (AHIMA 2010b). Clinical documentation improvement and coding compliance programs support coding optimization.

Developing a Coding Compliance Plan

While compliance in general refers to meeting the requirements of laws and regulations, a specific compliance plan related to coding is beneficial to healthcare organizations because of the relationship of coded data to financial reimbursement for services. Organizational compliance programs are addressed in chapter 10. Formal policies and procedures must be in place to provide instruction in the entire process from the provision of care through to the submission of claims (AHIMA 2010a). The coding compliance plan should include the following components:

- Policy statement regarding the commitment of the organization to correctly assign and report codes
- The source of official coding guidelines used to direct code selection
- Identification of who is responsible for code selection
- The procedure to follow when clinical information is not clear or specific enough to assign the correct code
- Specification of policies and procedures by care setting (ER, OP, IP)
- Applicable reporting requirements mandated by specific agencies, including where payer-specific instructions can be found
- Procedures for correction of inaccurate code assignments
- Areas of risk that have been identified through audits and monitoring, a defined plan for audit and review, and corrective actions outlined for identified problems
- Identification of essential coding resources available to and used by coding professionals
- A process for coding new procedures or unusual diagnoses
- A procedure to identify any optional codes gathered for statistical purposes by the facility and clarification of the appropriate use of external cause codes
- Appropriate methods for resolving coding or documentation disputes with physicians
- A procedure for processing claim rejections
- A statement regarding "codes will not be assigned, modified, or excluded solely for the purpose of maximizing reimbursement or avoiding reduced payment. Clinical codes will not be changed or amended merely because of either physician or patient request

to have the service in question covered by insurance. If the initial code assignment did not reflect actual services, codes may be revised on the basis of documentation" (AHIMA 2010a, 3)

- Statement on the use and reliance on encoding software; coding staff will be skilled in the review of records and proper assignment of diagnostic and procedural codes, not dependent or relying solely on coding software

- Medical records are analyzed and codes selected only with complete and appropriate physician documentation available; official coding guidelines state codes are not assigned without supporting documentation from the provider and the entire record should be reviewed (AHIMA 2010a)

In addition to policies and procedures, the individuals completing the coding function should have guidance as to the correct and ethical method of medical coding. The "most important part of a coding compliance plan are the standards supporting it" (Hanna 2002, 1). All coding compliance plans should reference AHIMA's Standards of Ethical Coding (AHIMA 2010a). (Refer to online appendix C.) The guides used to determine coding process should be American Hospital Association (AHA) *Coding Clinic*, AHA *HCPCS Clinic*, American Medical Association (AMA) *CPT Assistant*, and additional guidance from CMS.

Key Clinical Documents

The official coding guidelines indicate complete and appropriate documentation be reviewed when assigning diagnostic and procedural codes. No external rule or regulation exists that outlines or defines specific documents required to be complete or appropriate for coding (Scichilone 2008). As part of the compliance plan the organization should define what key clinical documents are required based on the care setting and type of record (Cassidy 2012). A policy should identify what documents are considered mandatory in the organization to be available and reviewed before assigning diagnostic or procedural codes. This can reduce the pressure to code an encounter without the complete documentation needed in order to expedite the claims submission process. The required set also gives new and experienced coders a facility- and service-specific guide as to what documentation to review. The documents listed in figure 9.7 are suggested as a guide when defining the core designated clinical documentation set for coding compliance (Cassidy 2012).

The identification of these documents can also assist in the successful implementation of electronic processes, including accurate CAC. Requiring any CAC process to include a specific and complete set of information allows the process to stay on track with the compliance plan (Cassidy 2012) and can help prevent variance and error before it occurs as part of a well-developed coding process (Scichilone 2008).

Figure 9.7. Core clinical documents for coding

Inpatient Coding	Outpatient/Ambulatory Surgery Coding	Observation Coding	Emergency Department Coding	Outpatient/Ancillary Coding
• Face sheet (or similar document organization-specific) • Progress notes • History and physical • Discharge summary • Consultation report • Operative reports • Pathology reports • Laboratory • Radiology • Physician's orders • Nutritional assessments	• History and physical • Results of previous diagnostics tests related to the encounter • Operative/procedure report • Pathology report • Medication list	• History and physical • Progress notes • Physician orders (both for admission to observation and for treatment) • Clinical observations • Final progress note/summary	• Emergency department report • Initial encounter • Diagnostic interventions • Treatment interventions • Nursing notes • Physician's orders • Progress notes with principal diagnosis	• Authenticated physician order for services • Clinician visit notes • Diagnosis/reason the service was ordered • Test results • Therapies if applicable to the service • Problem list if applicable to the service • Medication list if applicable to the service

Coding Compliance Education

Ongoing education for everyone from providers to claims submission staff is an integral part of the prevention of fraud and abuse. Even before a coding compliance education program is implemented, it has been a longstanding practice that formal policies and job descriptions outline that those hired to coding positions have the appropriate training, experience, and credentials to successfully perform the job (Prophet and Hammen 1998). It is common for employers to require coding applicants to also pass an assessment for hire even if the candidate possesses coding credentials or certifications. Coding compliance training beyond the general orientation for anyone newly hired who is responsible for assigning codes is recommended, as well as ongoing regular education (Burke et al. 2009; Enriquez 2011). The content should ensure employees understand the organization's compliance plan and the need to comply based on laws and regulations. Some education can be in conjunction with CDI training sessions to foster communication and collaboration between clinicians, CDI professionals, and coders; other sessions can be coding specific. Topics for ongoing coding compliance education include:

- Yearly updates to ICD, CPT, and HCPCS coding systems
- New guidance from the AHA ICD-10 Coding Clinic, AHA HCPCS Clinic, and AMA CPT Assistant

- OIG workplan
- Review of ICD-10-CM/PCS Official Guidelines for Coding and Reporting
- Present on admission (POA) reporting
- Complicated areas of coding depending on setting, such as modifiers, global surgery package, add-on codes, evaluation and management (E&M) codes
- Changes in reimbursement systems
- Uses of coded data—severity of illness, mortality, and case-mix index
- Organizational processes for reporting and resolving potential compliance violations (OIG 2011)

The education sessions should be documented with attendance recorded. Ongoing training needs to be a requirement of employment and testing is encouraged to measure the success of the training (OIG 2011). Referring to the definitions of fraud and abuse, the idea of what providers and organizations know or should know about coded data and billing practices should be the aim of ongoing education. Prevention, detection, and correction are the goals of a successful coding compliance program. See chapter 24 for more detail on employee training and development.

Check Your Understanding 9.2

Instructions: **Answer the following questions on a separate piece of paper.**

1. What does compliance mean?

2. What is healthcare fraud and abuse?

3. What is the difference between optimization versus maximization in regard to coding and reimbursement?

4. What resources and organizations should be consulted for coding compliance guidance?

5. Why is exclusion from Medicare or other federal programs significant?

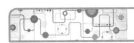

References

AHIMA House of Delegates. 2008. *American Health Information Management Association standards for ethical coding.* Chicago: AHIMA. http://library.ahima.org/xpedio/groups/public/documents/ahima/bok2_001166.hcsp?dDocName=bok2_001166

American Health Information Management Association. 2015. Certified Documentation Improvement Practitioner (CDIP®). http://www.ahima.org/certification/cdip

American Health Information Management Association. 2014a. *AHIMA Clinical Documentation Improvement Toolkit.* Chicago: AHIMA.

American Health Information Management Association. 2014b. Appropriate Use of the Copy and Paste Functionality in Electronic Health Record. http://library.ahima.org/xpedio/groups/public/documents/ahima/bok1_050621.pdf

American Health Information Management Association. 2014c. Clinical documentation guidance for ICD-10-CM/PCS. *Journal of AHIMA* 85(7):52–55.

American Health Information Management Association. 2013a. Using CDI programs to improve acute care documentation in preparation for ICD-10-CM/PCS. *Journal of AHIMA* 84(6):56–61.

American Health Information Management Association. 2013b. Guidelines for achieving a compliant query practice. *Journal of AHIMA* 84(2):50–53.

American Health Information Management Association. 2013c. Recruitment, selection, and orientation for CDI specialists. *Journal of AHIMA* 84(7):58–62.

American Health Information Management Association. 2011. Understanding governmental audits. *Journal of AHIMA* 82(7):50–55.

American Health Information Management Association. 2010a. Developing a coding compliance policy document (updated). *Journal of AHIMA* 81(3).

American Health Information Management Association. 2010b. *Ethical standards for clinical documentation improvement (CDI) professionals.* Chicago: AHIMA. *http://library.ahima.org/xpedio/groups/public/documents/ahima/bok1_047843.pdf*

American Health Information Management Association. 2010c. Guidance for clinical documentation improvement programs. *Journal of AHIMA* 81(5).

American Health Information Management Association. 2007 (Dec.). Statement on Consistency of Healthcare Diagnostic and Procedural Coding. AHIMA position statement. http://library.ahima.org/xpedio/groups/public/documents/ahima/bok1_036177.hcsp?dDocName=bok1_036177

Barnhouse, T. and W. Rudman. 2013. The growth in the clinical documentation specialist profession. *Educational Perspectives in Health Information Management* Summer:1–7.

Brown, M., J.S. Kennedy, M. Kruse, and L. Spryszak. 2009. *Physician Queries Handbook: Guide to Compliant and Effective Communication.* Danvers, MA: HCPro.

Burke, D.D., D. Wilkinson, and S. Bowman. 2009. Compliance. In *Fundamentals of Law for Health Informatics and Information Management.* Edited by Brodnik, M.S., M.C. McCain, L.A. Rinehart-Thompson, and B.B. Reynolds. Chicago: AHIMA.

Butler, M. 2014. Reinventing CDI. *Journal of AHIMA* 85(7):24–29.

Buttner, P., A. Comfort, J. Devrick, M. Endicott, D. Kohn, W. Lo, M. Ward, L.A. Wiedemann, and A. Zender. 2014. Leading the documentation journey: A report from the AHIMA 2014 clinical documentation improvement summit. *Perspectives in Health Information Management* Fall:1–9.

Cassidy. B. 2012. AHIMA Thought Leadership Series: Defining the Core Clinical Documentation Set for Coding Compliance. http://library.ahima.org/xpedio/groups/public/documents/ahima/bok1_049822.pdf

Centers for Medicare and Medicaid Services. 2014 (July). Avoiding Medicare Fraud and Abuse: A Roadmap for Physicians. http://www.cms.gov/outreach-and-education/medicare-learning-network-mln/mlnproducts/downloads/avoiding_medicare_fanda_physicians_factsheet_905645.pdf

Centers for Medicare and Medicaid Services. n.d. The Deficit Reduction Act: Important Facts for State Government Officials. https://www.cms.gov/Regulations-and-Guidance/Legislation/DeficitReductionAct/downloads/checklist1.pdf

DeAlmeida, D.R., V.J. Watzlaf, P. Anania-Firouzan, O. Salguero, E. Rubinstein, M. Abdelhak, and B. Parmanto. 2014. Evaluation of inpatient clinical documentation readiness for ICD-10-CM. *Perspectives in Health Information Management* Winter:1–16.

Enriquez, K.D. 2011. Compliance. In *Effective Management of Coding Services*, 4th ed. Edited by Schraffenberger, L.A. and L. Kuehn. Chicago: AHIMA.

Gold, R.S., and L. Kuehn. 2011. Clinical documentation improvement. In *Effective Management of Coding Services*, 4th ed. Edited by Schraffenberger, L.A. and L. Kuehn. Chicago: AHIMA.

Hanna, J. 2002. Constructing a coding compliance plan. *Journal of AHIMA* 73(7):48–56.

Hazelwood, A. 2008. Challenges of Compliance and Ethical Coding in Physician Practices. http://campus.ahima.org/audio/fastfacts/FRB0802.pdf

Hazelwood, A. and C. Venable. 2011. Reimbursement Methodologies. In *Health Information Management: Concepts, Principles, and Practices*, 4th ed. Edited by LaTour, K.M., S.E. Eichenwald Maki, and P.K. Oachs. Chicago: AHIMA.

Hinkle-Azzara, B. and K.J. Carr. 2014. Bird's eye view of ICD-10 documentation gaps. *Journal of AHIMA* 85(6):34–38.

Horton, L.A. 2012. *Calculating and Reporting Healthcare Statistics*, 4th ed. Chicago: AHIMA.

Huff, G.L, J.P. Fee, W. Clesi, J. Perry, and M. Rajappan 2014. Selecting the ideal CDI physician advisor. *Journal of AHIMA* 85(7):30–35.

Huffman, E.K. 1941. *Manual for Medical Record Librarians*. Chicago: Physicians' Record Company.

Liebler, J.G. and C.R. McConnell. 2012. *Management Principles for Health Professionals*, 6th ed. Sudbury, MA: Jones and Bartlett.

Lo, W. 2014. Document like this, not that. *Journal of AHIMA* 85(7):36–40.

Moczygemba, J. and S.H. Fenton. 2012. Lessons learned from an ICD-10-CM clinical documentation pilot study. *Perspectives in Health Information Management* Winter:1–11.

Office of the Inspector General. 2015. https://oig.hhs.gov/about-oig/about-us/index.asp

Office of the Inspector General. 2011. Operating an

Effective Compliance Program. https://oig.hhs.gov/compliance/provider-compliance-training/files/OperatinganEffectiveComplianceProgramFinalBR508.pdf

Office of the Inspector General. 2005, January 1. *Federal Register* 70(4858).

Pinson, R.D. and C.L. Tang. 2008. Comprehensive CDI: Making it happen. In *2008 AHIMA Convention Proceedings*.

Prophet, S. and C. Hammen. 1998. Coding compliance: Practical strategies for success. *Journal of AHIMA* 69(1):50–61.

Roat, L. 2014. Linking quality of care to clinical data integrity. *Journal of AHIMA* 85(1):56–57.

Rollins, G. 2009. Clinical documentation improvement: Gauging the need, starting off right. *Journal of AHIMA* 80(9):24–29.

Rosenbaum, B.P., R.R. Lorenz, R.B. Luther, L. Knowles-Ward, D.L. Kelly, and R.J. Weil. 2014. Improving and measuring inpatient documentation of medical care within the MS-DRG system: Education, monitoring, and normalized case mix index. *Perspectives in Health Information Management* Summer:1–11.

Russo, R. 2008. *A Compelling Case for Clinical Documentation: Use the CAMP Method to Improve Clinical Documentation Quality*, Vol. 2. Bethlehem PA: DJ Iber.

Scichilone, R.A. 2008. Enhanced compliance results by improving the code assignment process. *Journal of Health Care Compliance* 10(4):63–66.

Schedel, E. and B. Parker. 2006. Compliance and Operations: Can the Marriage Survive? *AHIMA's 78th National Convention and Exhibit Proceedings*.

US Department of Justice. 2011. *The False Claims Act: A Primer* [Fact sheet]. http://www.justice.gov/sites/default/files/civil/legacy/2011/04/22/C-FRAUDS_FCA_Primer.pdf

Williams, V.J. 2008. Walking the Tightrope—Coding Compliance in the Electronic Age. *AHIMA Convention Proceedings*.

10

Organizational Compliance and Risk

Brooke Palkie, EdD, RHIA

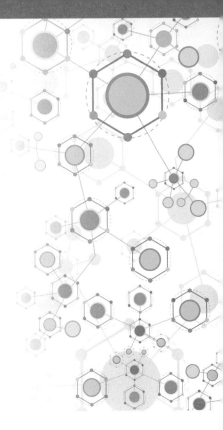

Learning Objectives

- Demonstrate a working knowledge of the function of a healthcare corporate compliance program
- Identify the key elements in the development, management, monitoring, evaluation, and enhancement of a compliance program
- Assess the importance of the OIG workplan to organize compliance
- Demonstrate knowledge of the elements of the Federal Sentencing Guidelines, False Claims Act, Anti-Kickback Statute, EMTALA, and Stark Law and apply to the healthcare industry
- Apply risk management principles
- Distinguish between identity theft and medical identity theft
- Analyze the regulations addressing identity theft
- Demonstrate knowledge of contingency planning and disaster recovery

Key Terms

Abuse
Anti-Kickback Statute (AKS)
Centers for Medicare and Medicaid Services (CMS)
Civil Monetary Penalties Law
Contingency planning
Corporate integrity agreement (CIA)
Emergency Medical Treatment and Active Labor Act (EMTALA)
Exclusion Provisions
False Claims Act (FCA)
Fraud
Health Care Fraud Statute
Identity theft
Medical identity theft
Office of the Inspector General (OIG)
OIG workplan
Potentially compensable event (PCE)
Red Flags Rule
Risk management
Stark Law
Waste
Whistleblowers

Regulatory compliance is viewed as an organization's adherence to rules, laws, regulations, guidelines, and specifications. In developing compliance program guidance, the Centers for Medicare and Medicaid (CMS) and the Office of the Inspector General (OIG) have relied primarily on the Federal Sentencing Guidelines brought forth by the US Sentencing Commission. The Federal Sentencing Guidelines require that "organizational defendants exercise due diligence in the design and implementation of a compliance program intended to detect and deter fraud, waste and abuse" (US Sentencing Commission 2013a). In the current regulatory environment within healthcare, corporate compliance programs are essential now more than ever.

Corporate Compliance

A corporate compliance program is designed to help detect and prevent the violations of fraud, waste, and abuse. Along with assuring the employees adhere to ethical conduct, corporate compliance programs conform to the goals of the OIG. The mission of the Office of the Inspector General (OIG) is to protect the integrity of Department of Health and Human Services (HHS) programs, operations, and the health and well-being of the people served. The OIG's strategic plan includes the following four goals:

- fight fraud, waste, and abuse;
- promote quality and safety;
- secure the future; and
- advance innovation (OIG 2015a).

The OIG's work consists of auditing and evaluating its annual workplan. The OIG workplan "sets forth various projects to be addressed during the fiscal year by the Office of Audit Services, Office of Evaluation and Inspections, Office of Investigations, and Office of Counsel" to the Inspector General including projects planned by CMS (OIG 2015b).

The Centers for Medicare and Medicaid Services (CMS) is an agency of the Department of Health and Human Services (HHS). Similar to the OIG, CMS develops compliance program guidance specific to Medicare fee-for-service contractors to promote adherence to all Medicare statutory and regulatory requirements (CMS 2015a). According to both CMS and the OIG, effective healthcare compliance programs are based on seven fundamental elements. These elements include:

- Enforcing policies, procedures, and standards of conduct
- Establishing a formalized compliance committee and designating a compliance officer
- Regularly conducting, reviewing, and updating trainings
- Maintaining open lines of communication
- Continuously measuring effectiveness through ongoing internal monitoring and audits
- Enforcing standards though established guidelines
- Providing a swift response to any and all compliance issues (CMS 2015a; OIG 2015c).

In the United States, noncompliance in healthcare can lead to civil or criminal penalties. It is important to understand the minimum general corporate compliance program elements to help establish a culture that promotes prevention, detection, and appropriate resolution of conduct that does not conform to federal and state laws and healthcare program requirements. Table 10.1 provides an overview of the general compliance content areas that help organizations to establish this type of culture.

Standards of conduct should exist as written policy. Compliance officers are ultimately responsible for making sure employees adhere to the code of conduct and to provide timely reporting

Table 10.1. Corporate compliance attributes

Topic area	Topic area content
Laws vs. regulations	• Laws are federally enforceable • Regulations are implementation details of the law and also legally enforceable
Objectives of a compliance program (US Sentencing Commission 2013b)	• To reduce the risk of or prevent criminal or unethical conduct • To be compliant with laws and regulations • To follow US Sentencing Commission Guidelines

Attributes of a compliance program
(US Sentencing Commission 2013b)
	• Established written policies and procedures for crime prevention
	• Organizational support of the compliance program through
	  ○ Visibility to the governing authority
	  ○ Executive management support of compliance resources
	  ○ Dedicated staff to daily compliance
	• Maintain ethical staff in management and executive positions
	  ○ All management and above staff have clear criminal records
	• Education of staff on policies and procedures through:
	  ○ Annual and periodic reminders on compliance
	  ○ Annual training sessions
	• Ensured proper functioning of compliance program
	  ○ Monitoring and auditing of activity
	  ○ Periodic evaluation of program effectiveness
	  ○ Promote and publicize anonymous communication channels for compliance complaints
	• Appropriate measures to ensure compliance
	  ○ Incentives for compliance
	  ○ Disciplinary actions for noncompliance
	• Responses to criminal conduct, including:
	  ○ Disciplinary actions
	  ○ Prevention measures

What could happen if the organization has criminal conduct per US Sentencing Guidelines? (US Sentencing Commission 2013b)	• Office of the Inspector General investigation • Would need to remedy the problem • May need to pay restitution • Will have to notify all victims • Fines will be levied against the organization
What are the US Sentencing Commission Guidelines?	• Defines individual and organizational criminal conduct • Defines sentencing and fines guidelines for individual and organizational criminal conduct • Provides compliance guidelines for reducing or preventing criminal conduct

Source: Ziemba 2015.

of compliance violations. Although a distinction exists between unintentional mistakes and fraud, sound prevention and detection processes should be incorporated into compliance plans. The compliance officer is responsible for identifying and locating primary law sources to assist in this process (table 10.2). Primary sources should always be sought for review and to base recommendations; including citing the sources to validate recommendations. The main themes from the code of conduct include healthcare fraud, abuse, and waste.

Table 10.2.   Fraud and abuse statutes

Statute	Reference*
Civil FCA	http://www.gpo.gov/fdsys/pkg/USCODE-2012- title31/pdf/USCODE-2012-title31-subtitleIII-chap37-subchapIII.pdf
Criminal FCA	http://www.gpo.gov/fdsys/pkg/USCODE-2012-title18/pdf/USCODE-2012-title18-partI-chap15-sec287.pdf
Anti-Kickback Statute	http://www.gpo.gov/fdsys/pkg/USCODE-2012-title42/pdf/USCODE-2012-title42-chap7-subchapXI-partA-sec1320a-7b.pdf
Regulatory Safe Harbors	http://www.gpo.gov/fdsys/pkg/CFR-2013-title42-vol5/pdf/CFR-2013-title42-vol5-sec1001-952.pdf
Stark (Physician Self-Referral Law)	http://www.gpo.gov/fdsys/pkg/USCODE-2012-title42/pdf/USCODE-2012-title42-chap7-subchapXVIII-partE-sec1395nn.pdf
Criminal Health Care Fraud	http://www.gpo.gov/fdsys/pkg/USCODE-2012-title18/pdf/USCODE-2012-title18-partI-chap63-sec1347.pdf
Exclusions and Civil Monetary Penalties Law (CMPL)	http://www.gpo.gov/fdsys/pkg/USCODE-2012-title42/pdf/USCODE-2012-title42-chap7-subchapXI-partA-sec1320a-7.pdf

* The websites listed here were current and valid as of publication. However, webpage addresses and the information on them may change at any time. *Source*: CMS 2014.

Fraud

A variety of federal and state laws exist to punish (civil and criminal) and deter fraud (CMS 2015b):

- Health Care Fraud Statute (criminal)
  - 18 US Code § 1347, 1349
- False Claims Act
  - Statute: 31 USC §§ 3729–3733
- Red Flags Rule
  - FCRA §§ 615(e)(1)(A)–(B); 15 USC 1681m(e)(1)(A)–(B)
- Exclusion Provisions
  - Statutes: 42 USC §§ 1320a–7, 1320c–5
  - Sate Regulations: 42 CFR pts. 1001 (OIG) and 1002
- Civil Monetary Penalties Law
  - Statute: 42 USC § 1320a–7a
  - Regulations: 42 CFR pt. 1003

Health Care Fraud Statute

The criminal Health Care Fraud Statute identifies that it is illegal to defraud any healthcare benefit program or to obtain fraudulent funds or property by any of the healthcare benefit programs (CMS 2014). Fraud consists of submitting false statements or misrepresenting facts, such as falsifying records or billing for services at a level of complexity higher than that what was rendered.

Fraud also consists of purposefully rewarding referrals or making prohibited referrals reimbursed by CMS. Fraud ranges in scale from solo ventures to broad operations instituted by organizations. CMS defines fraud as "an intentional deception or misrepresentation made by a person with the knowledge that the deception could result in some unauthorized benefit to himself or some other person. It includes any act that constitutes fraud under applicable federal or state law" (42 CFR 455.2).

False Claims Act

The False Claims Act (FCA) imposes liability on any person who submits a claim to the federal government that he or she knows (or should know) is false (CMS 2015c). The FCA prosecutes healthcare providers who demonstrate a pattern of coding for overcharging claims for payment to CMS. A false claims statute also protects whistleblowers. Under Section 3730(h) of the False Claims Act, the following whistleblower protections are provided to employees who are:

- Discharged
- Demoted
- Harassed
- Or otherwise discriminated against (Whistleblowerlaws 2015).

The False Claims Act has a strong whistleblower protection provision. In qui tam actions, under the False Claims Act, "any persons or entities with evidence of fraud against federal programs or contracts may file a qui tam lawsuit on behalf of the US government" (NWC 2015). Many states have implemented versions of the False Claims Act to help deter fraud at the state level.

Identity Theft

Another component of fraud in healthcare is identity theft. **Identity theft** is "a fraud attempted or committed using identifying information of another person without authority" (FTC 2015a). When identity theft occurs in the context of medical care, it is known as medical identity theft. According to the Federal Trade Commission (FTC), **medical identity theft** "occurs when someone uses another person's name or insurance information to get medical treatment, prescription drugs, surgery, or even healthcare organizations using another person's information to submit false bills to insurance companies" (FTC 2015a). In order to help fight identity theft, the FTC enforces the Red Flags Rule requirements.

Red Flags Rule

The **Red Flags Rule** requires many businesses and organizations to implement a written identity theft prevention program designed to detect the "red flags" of identity theft in day to day operations, take steps to prevent the crime, and mitigate its damage (FTC 2015b). The intent is to deter identity theft and have a plan in place for quick detection if suspicious activity is suspected. The Red Flags Rule requires organizations to implement four basic identity theft elements:

1. Include reasonable policies and procedures to identify the red flags of identity theft
2. Design the program to be able to detect red flags that have been identified in step 1
3. Detail appropriate actions when red flags are detected
4. Detail how to keep the plan current and to reflect new and emerging threats (FTC 2015b)

Although policy is a very important approach to identity theft, the most important component of prevention is an organization's plan on how to incorporate these elements in day-to-day activities by alerting staff to watch for red flags such as suspicious personal identifying information. An example of suspicious activity could be inconsistencies such a Social Security number used that is listed on the Social Security Administrations Death list (FTC 2015a). Finally, conducting risk assessments are an important activity to proactively determine potential risks. Risk assessment is also covered in chapter 11 of the text.

Exclusion Provisions and Civil Monetary Penalties Law

The **Exclusion Provisions**, a component of the Social Security Act, indicates that the OIG has the authority to "exclude individuals from participating in federal healthcare programs and will not pay for items or services furnished by an excluded individual or entity" (Social Security Act 2015). The **Civil Monetary Penalties Law** provides punitive fines imposed by a civil court to organizations that profit from illegal or unethical activities (OIG 2015d). Depending upon the extent and intent of the fraudulent activity, one or both of these sanctions can be applied. An example would be billing for services that were not medically necessary, which is classified as healthcare abuse.

Abuse

Any practice that creates unnecessary cost to federal healthcare programs is considered abuse. This includes both direct and indirect practices. A common example of abuse is billing for services that are not consistent with the standards of medical necessity. CMS defines **abuse** as provider practices that are inconsistent with sound fiscal, business, or medical practices, and result in an unnecessary cost to the Medicaid program, or in reimbursement for services that are not medically necessary or that fail to meet professionally recognized standards for healthcare. It also includes beneficiary practices that result in unnecessary cost to the Medicaid program (42 CFR 455.2).

Similar to fraud, abuse laws exists to deter waste and include:

- Anti-Kickback Statute
  - Statute: 42 USC § 1320a–7b(b)
  - Safe Harbor Regulations: 42 CFR 1001.952
- Stark Law (also referred to as the Physician Self-Referral Law)
  - (42 USC § 1395nn)
- EMTALA
  - 42 USC §1395dd, 42 CFR Parts 413, 482, and 489

Anti-Kickback Statute

The **Anti-Kickback Statute (AKS)** makes knowingly offering, paying, soliciting, or receiving any remuneration that rewards referrals for services reimbursable by a federal program a criminal offense (CMS 2015d). The only exception to the statute is the Safe Harbor Regulations that describe various payment and business practices that shall not be treated as a criminal offense under the anti-kickback statutes and serve as an exclusion, such as an investment interest (42 CFR 1001.952). In these cases, AKS will not treat the arrangements as offenses.

Stark Law

The **Stark Law** (or Physician Self-Referral Law) prohibits a physician from referring certain health service to "an entity in which the physician (or member of immediate family) has an ownership or investment or with which the physician has a compensation arrangement, unless an exception applies" (CMS 2015d). CMS allows an additional avenue for physician self-referral disclosures for noncompliance through the Medicare self-referral disclosure protocol.

Emergency Medical Treatment and Labor Act

The **Emergency Medical Treatment and Labor Act (EMTALA)**, otherwise known as the patient antidumping statute, was enacted by congress in 1986 as part of the Consolidated Omnibus Budget Reconciliation Act (COBRA) (CMS 2015c). EMTALA is a component of the Social Security Act that imposes obligations on hospitals (including critical access hospitals) that offer emergency department (ED) services. "The obligations concern individuals who come to a hospital emergency department and request examination or treatment for medical conditions, and apply to all individuals, regardless of whether or not they are beneficiaries of any program under the Act" (HHS 2015a). This ensures public access to emergency services regardless of the ability to pay. The components of the obligation include medical screening examinations (MSE), stabilization treatment, and transferring patients (to another organization or released from the ED). Under the EMTALA statute, "all participating hospitals with an emergency department would be required to provide an appropriate medical screening examination to determine whether an emergency medical condition exists or if the patient is in active labor" (HHS 2015a). Stabilization treatment for emergency medical conditions includes stabilizing the medical condition or transferring the patient to another medical facility only when the transfer is appropriate and when medical benefits outweigh the risks. The enforcement of EMTALA is initiated by a complaint. If the hospital did violate EMTALA, they may be subject to a civil monetary penalty or termination from a participation agreement with CMS.

Waste

Although waste is not a legally defined term, CMS identifies **waste** as "overutilization, underutilization, or misuse of resources" (CMS 2015d). Waste is typically not intentional or criminal in nature; however, waste does have a financial impact on services. An example of overutilization includes repeat lab tests; underutilization includes bypassing preventative screenings; and an example of misuse includes using a CT scan for a mammography when not warranted.

Check Your Understanding 10.1

Instructions: **Answer the following questions on a separate piece of paper.**

1. What are the four compliance goals as identified by the Office of the Inspector General (OIG)?

2. What are the differences between healthcare fraud, abuse, and waste?

3. Why was the Emergency Medical Treatment and Labor Act (EMTALA) enacted and what are the components of EMTALA?

4. What are the seven fundamental elements of a compliance program?

5. What rule was enforced to help combat identity theft?

Fraud Surveillance

Fraud, abuse, and waste divert significant resources away from needed healthcare services. Both state and federal initiatives have implemented steps against healthcare fraud. One important example of an antifraud effort is CMS's Center for Program Integrity (CPI). CPI serves as the central point for CMS's program integrity mission (CMS 2015e). In addition to CMS, the US Office of the Inspector General (OIG) issues annual guidelines for compliance to healthcare providers. The OIG protects the integrity of HHS programs, including CMS. OIG workplans are issued at the beginning of each fiscal year and provide for new and ongoing reviews or audits in programs administered by HHS. The goals of the reviews are to protect the integrity of both state and federal programs by:

- detecting and preventing fraud, waste, and abuse;
- identifying opportunities for improvement in economy, efficiency, and effectiveness; and
- holding accountable those who do not meet program requirements or violate federal laws (OIG 2015b).

Healthcare organizations should carefully study the OIG workplan each year to ensure that they are in compliance with specifically targeted areas. The increased attention on investigating, preventing, and prosecuting fraud and abuse in healthcare was apparent in 1996 with passage of the Health Insurance Portability and Accountability Act (HIPAA). HIPAA expanded the role of the OIG to include private insurance programs as well as federally funded programs.

The OIG negotiates **corporate integrity agreements (CIAs)** with healthcare providers and other entities. "As part of the settlement of federal healthcare program investigations, providers or entities agree to the obligations in exchange for the OIG to not seek their exclusion from participation in federal healthcare programs" (OIG 2015e). CIAs may last for many years and are imposed when serious misconduct (fraud and abuse) is discovered through an audit or self-disclosure. Remediation initiatives, such as training or designation of a compliance officer, are part of the CIA. Remediation activities are intended to offer providers another chance to prove they are worthy of participating in federal healthcare programs (OIG 2015e). CIAs generally do not result from unintentional errors and are imposed where there is evidence of intentional fraud.

As a preventative measure, the US Sentencing Commission has developed key criteria for establishing an effective compliance and ethics program and includes:

- Standards and procedures to prevent and detect criminal conduct
- Oversight by high-level personnel
- Due care in delegating substantial discretionary authority
- Effective communication to all levels of employees
- Reasonable steps to achieve compliance, which include systems for monitoring, auditing, and reporting suspected wrongdoing without fear of reprisal
- Consistent enforcement of compliance standards including disciplinary mechanisms
- Reasonable steps to respond to and prevent further similar offenses upon detection of a violation (US Sentencing Commission 2013a)

These initiatives are designed to ensure that fraudulent activities do not occur.

External Drivers

External fraud surveillance approaches include whistleblower incentives, data mining and data validation, working with CMS federal contractors (RACs), and other audits such as those for complaints. Some of the commonly known government auditors in healthcare include:

- HEAT (Health Care Fraud Prevention and Enforcement Action Team): Identify fraud perpetrators and those preying on Medicare and Medicaid beneficiaries
- MACs (Medicare Administrative Contractors): Perform prepayment reviews to ensure services provided Medicare beneficiaries are covered and medically necessary
- MICs (Medicaid Integrity Contractors): Review Medicaid claims to determine potential provider waste or abuse, identify overpayments, and provide education to

providers on payment integrity and quality of care issues
- RACs (Recovery Audit Contractors): Work with a mission of reducing Medicare improper payments through detection and collection of overpayments, the identification of underpayments, and the implementation of actions that will prevent future improper payments (Quinsey 2013)

External audits are conducted by both the state and federal governments to combat fraud and abuse, as well as to focus on improving government programs and services.

Internal Drivers

Building fraud and abuse controls and cost-effective performance monitoring in all organization functional areas will help provide a process of continuous improvement and eliminate waste. In order to operate an effective compliance program, it is important to have internal monitoring measures. These measures include:

- continually reviewing fraud and abuse surveillance plans;
- maintaining system hardware and software upgrades;
- conducting risk assessments;
- monitoring marketing practices;
- enforcing polices and procedures; and
- providing prompt response to compliance issues such as reporting and findings from compliance reviews and audits (OIG 2015f).

Another internal driver of compliance is the proactive review of coding, contracts, repayment and post-payment, and the monitoring of third party transactions. See chapter 9 for a full description of assessing a coding compliance program.

Check Your Understanding 10.2

Instructions: **Answer the following questions on a separate piece of paper.**

1. Describe the role of ethics and integrity within a compliance program.

2. What are the identified key criteria for establishing an effective compliance and ethics program?

3. Identify three examples of fraud surveillance approaches from the external audit perspective.

4. Identify three examples of fraud surveillance approaches from the internal audit perspective.

5. What is the intent of the OIG corporate integrity agreements?

Risk Management

Risk is the possibility of a bad or good event occurring. It is important to understand and clarify the different terms when discussing risk assessment processes within an organization. Assessment is a method for evaluating performance or a judgment based on evaluating and understanding a specific scenario. Analysis is a process of examining a system or application to understand how it works and determine conclusions. **Risk management** is the process of planning, organizing, directing, and controlling resources to achieve given objectives when events are possible (Head 2009). The purpose of a risk management program is to protect an organization and its assets against negative risks (loss), including accidental losses. This is done by seeking and preventing **potentially compensable events** (PCE) and reducing the liability from injuries or accidents. A PCE is an event (for example, an injury, accident, or medical error) that may result in financial liability for a healthcare organization (AHIMA 2014).

Organizations that have effective policies and procedures for reporting accidents and injuries (or near-accidents and injuries) have the opportunity to correct system problems before a major incident occurs, potentially saving a patient from an accident, injury, or even death. This can save the organization from negative financial impacts and may preserve the reputation of the organization in the community by avoiding legal action and potentially damaging related publicity (Quinsey 2013).

Insurance carriers for both liability and healthcare require risk management programs to be in place. Federal and state governments also require risk management activities aimed at patient safety and reducing and preventing injuries or accidents in healthcare facilities.

Traditional risk management has now expanded beyond just preserving assets to the concept of enterprise risk management, which looks to create value and optimize risk opportunities. This includes investigative and compliance strategies focused on reducing risk, expanding profitability, and increasing revenue. The eight categories of risk include:

- Operational: Healthcare should follow the Institute of Medicine's (IOM's) six aims for healthcare (delivery of care that is safe, timely, effective, efficient, equitable, and patient-centered). Operational risks can result from inadequate or failed internal processes.

- Clinical/patient safety: Risks can include failure to follow evidence-based practice and errors such as medication-related mistakes, hospital-acquired conditions, and serious safety events.

- Strategic: Risks are associated with the strategic direction of the organization. Risks include failure to adapt, health reform, customer priorities, conflicts of interest, marketing and sales, media relations, mergers, affiliations, and such.

- Financial: The focus is on financial sustainability. Risks include malpractice, litigation, insurance credit, growth, billing, and collections.

- Human capital: Risks are associated with workforce including retention and turnover, workers' compensation, and productivity.

- Legal/regulatory: Risks include failure to identify and manage legal, regulatory, and statutory mandates on the local, state, and federal levels.

- Technology: Risks include those related to hardware, software, use of technology for clinical diagnosis and treatment, and information storage and retrieval (that is, electronic health records [EHR]).

- Hazard: There are risks to assets such as facility management, parking, or natural disasters (ASHRM 2014).

Once an organization identifies risk, the next steps are to analyze and take action by implementing a risk response strategy. In order to implement the most appropriate strategy, a cost-benefit analysis should be conducted to identify the total anticipated cost of the strategy as well as analysis of data analytics to help drive decisions and improve the overall outcomes.

Incident Reporting

The promptness of reporting an unplanned occurrence is critical to a successful risk management plan. An incident report is a form used to record these unplanned or unusual occurrences in detail. It is important to capture any dates, times, and locations of incident occurrences. Each incident report can be reviewed individually or used to create report data that is tabulated and analyzed to help identify trends and establish probable cause. Tabulated incident report data can include types of occurrences, severity of the injuries, frequencies and patterns, demographics, and effectiveness of corrective measures. The risk management department should develop policies and procedures around incident reporting guidelines. This includes the types of events that should be reported, the reporting process, and identification of the reporting channels. While there are many types of incidents

that are reported, typical reportable events include patient complaints, medication errors, security incidents, and adverse events. Some incidents require risk management plans at the hospital strategic level, known as contingency planning.

Business Continuity and Contingency Planning

Contingency planning "is one component of a much broader emergency preparedness process that includes items such as business practices, operational continuity, and disaster recovery planning" (HHS 2015b). A comprehensive contingency plan needs to highlight potential vulnerabilities and threats as well as to identify the approaches to either prevent them or at least minimize the impact. There are three major categories or types of threats:

- Natural threats (for example, floods or earthquakes)

- Technical/manmade (that is, mechanical, biological, or the like)

- Intentional acts (namely, terrorism, computer security, and such) (HHS 2015b)

The key is to be prepared for any type of emergency situation. Contingency planning includes plans to be followed in order to continue normal business operations. The National Institute of Standards and Technology (NIST) Special Publication SP800-34 defines seven components to a viable contingency planning program. HHS identifies that the following NIST steps are "to be integrated throughout a project's life cycle to help guide stakeholders in the planning, development, implementation, key success factors and maintenance of contingency plans" (2015b):

1. Identify specific regulatory requirements related to contingency planning
2. Conduct a business impact analysis to prioritize critical systems, business processes, and components
3. Identify and implement preventive controls and measures
4. Develop recovery strategies
5. Develop contingency plans with guidance and procedures

6. Plan and implement testing and training to both validate and identify gaps, as well as prepare staff

7. Maintain contingency plans, updating regularly

The goal is to become a resilient organization that can continue its mission essential functions during any type of disruption. NIST provides a list of various types of contingency and continuity plans as identified in table 10.3.

Specific to health information management (HIM), the core principles of managing records, disclosing health information, retention, and confidentiality are at risk during disasters (AHIMA 2013). One key component of planning for a disaster includes the development of a business continuity plan. This plan needs to identify how to:

- Protect patient safety;
- Secure health information from damage;
- Ensure stability in continuity of care activities; and
- Provide for recovery of information (AHIMA 2013).

This plan covers downtimes, disaster recovery, and backup procedures as addressed in table 10.4. The overall goal of the plan is to reduce interruptions while lessening the impact on the organization and to remain in compliance with laws and regulations.

The key elements in implementing the continuity plans include:

- a proactive governance process to define and align plans with strategic priorities;
- the use of data to understand risks and measure their impacts (business impact analysis);
- a plan, design, and integration of the strategies (HHS 2015b).

It is important to continually educate and train on the business continuity plan (BCP) through practice drills. The results of drills will help to prepare staff and resources as well as to identify gaps. With these strategies, organizations should be able to avoid interruptions to care, financial losses, regulatory fines, and damage to property and equipment.

Implications for Health Informatics and Information Management (HIIM)

Compliance remains one of the greatest challenges for healthcare organizations today. Health information management (HIM) professionals have long been responsible for the privacy and security of patient information. However, the HIM professional is well positioned to organize, manage, and assess all corporate compliance functions. Adding on to the legal requirements, technology provides a new set of challenges in managing the dynamic information infrastructure

Table 10.3.   NIST-identified contingent and continuity plans

Plan	Purpose of procedure
Business continuity plan	For sustaining business operations
Continuity of operations plan	For sustaining an organization's mission essential functions (alternate site)
Crisis communications plan	For disseminating internal and external communications
Critical infrastructure protection plan	For protection of critical infrastructure components that are supported by an agency (risk management plan that supports continuity of operations plan)
Cyber incident response plan	For mitigating a system cyber attack
Disaster recovery plan	For relocating information systems operations to an alternate site
Information system contingency plan	For recovering an information system
Occupant emergency plan	For minimizing loss of life or injury and protecting property from a physical threat

Source: Swanson n.d.

Table 10.4. AHIMA business continuity plan (BCP) elements for an organizational policy

Areas covered in a BCP	Description
Risk assessment and analysis	• Must be completed prior to the BCP • The intent is to review and prepare for potential disasters • HIPAA includes requirements for risk assessments and is covered in chapter 11 of the textbook
Downtime and contingency planning	• The focus is on sustaining business functions during short interruptions • The intent is to list the various types of potential disasters whether they are manmade or natural along with the department's core processes • A contingency should be developed for each possible disaster and core process
Disaster recovery	• Unlike routine or regular downtime, the focus here is for major or catastrophic events with extended downtimes • This plan needs to be aligned to the institution's overall disaster plan • The intent is to provide criteria to determine how crucial decisions will be reached (for example, when visits are back-loaded into the master patient index [MPI])
Data backup	• Addresses data availability and integrity for protecting health information • The intent is to have a documented backup plan for applications and information systems • Security and data recovery are also vital focus areas of this plan
Emergency mode operations	• This is also considered the crisis management plan • The operations of this plan runs from declaration of the disaster until the organization fully returns to its predisaster operational status • The intent is to provide workflows, security, change controls, reports, inventory control, and such within the emergency mode; some example elements of this mode include a communications plan, minimal documentation requirements, emergency registrations, and use of emergency paper charts

Source: AHIMA 2013.

of healthcare enterprise and healthcare consumer information. The Office of the National Coordinator (ONC) has been driving the escalation of technology through its National Strategic Framework requirement of mandating the implementation of EHRs and toward the acceleration of Health Information Exchange (HIE) (Thompson and Brailer 2004). The strategic framework is being driven through Meaningful Use (MU), which uses certified electronic health record technology to:

- Improve quality, safety, efficiency, equitable care

- Engage patients

- Improve the coordination of care

- Maintain the privacy and security of health information (healthIT.gov 2015)

The compliance of MU will result in better and improved outcomes as well as more robust data to help make informed health decisions. MU identifies set criteria for eligible professionals (EPs) and hospitals to meet the CMS incentive programs. There are three stages identified within the CMS incentive program and includes: stage 1 (2011–2012), which focuses criteria to meet data capture and sharing; stage 2 (2014), which focuses on advanced clinical processes; and stage 3 (2016), which focuses on improved outcomes (healthIT.gov 2015). CMS provides specification sheets to both the EPs and hospitals to identify the criteria each would need to attest to (called attestation) meaningfully using a certified EHR. As the industry continues to change, HIM professionals are positioned to grow in leadership roles related to policy, compliance, privacy, security, and the national HIT initiatives to promote an interoperable health information infrastructure.

Check Your Understanding 10.3

Instructions: **Answer the following questions on a separate piece of paper.**

1. What is risk management and what is its purpose?

2. What are the eight categories of risk?

3. What is an incident report?

4. Identify three examples of reportable events on an incident report.

5. Why is it important to capture incident reports?

6. What is contingency planning?

7. What are the three major categories of types of threats?

8. What are the major risks to an organization lacking solid continuity plans?

9. Identify the seven components defined by NIST to a viable contingency planning program.

10. Describe how HIM professionals are positioned to lead in the roles of compliance, risk management, and business continuity planning?

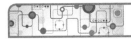

References

American Health Information Management Association. 2014. *Pocket Glossary of Health Information Management and Technology.* Chicago: AHIMA.

American Health Information Management Association. 2013. Disaster Planned and Recovery Toolkit. http://library.ahima.org/xpedio/groups/secure/documents/ahima/bok1_050296.pdf

American Society for Healthcare Risk Management. 2014. Executive Summary of Risks-Rewards. http://www.ashrm.org/pubs/files/white_papers/Executive-Summary_Risks-Rewards-Healthcare-Reform_FINAL2.pdf

Centers for Medicare and Medicaid Services. 2015a. Compliance Program Guidance for Medicare Fee-For-Service Contractors. https://www.cms.gov/Medicare/Medicare-Contracting/Medicare-Administrative-Contractors/Downloads/compliance.pdf

Centers for Medicare and Medicaid Services. 2015b. Emergency Medical Treatment and Labor Act. https://www.cms.gov/Regulations-and-Guidance/Legislation/EMTALA/index.html?redirect=/EMTALA/

Centers for Medicare and Medicaid Services. 2015c. False Claim Act. http://downloads.cms.gov/cmsgov/archived-downloads/SMDL/downloads/smd032207att2.pdf

Centers for Medicare and Medicaid Services. 2015d. Fraud, Waste, and Abuse Toolkit. https://www.cms.gov/Medicare-Medicaid-Coordination/Fraud-Prevention/Medicaid-Integrity-Education/Downloads/fwa-overview-booklet.pdf

Centers for Medicare and Medicaid Services. 2015e. Center for Program Integrity. https://www.cms.gov/About-CMS/Agency-Information/CMSLeadership/Office_CPI.html

Centers for Medicare and Medicaid Services. 2014. Medicare Fraud and Abuse. http://www.cms.gov/Outreach-and-Education/Medicare-Learning-Network-MLN/MLNProducts/downloads/Fraud_and_Abuse.pdf

Federal Trade Commission. 2015a. Medical Identity Theft. https://www.ftc.gov/tips-advice/business-center/guidance/medical-identity-theft-faqs-health-care-providers-health-plans

Federal Trade Commission. 2015b. Red Flags Rule. https://www.ftc.gov/tips-advice/business-center/guidance/fighting-identity-theft-red-flags-rule-how-guide-business

Head, G.L. 2009. Risk Management Why and How: An Illustrative Introduction to Risk Management for Business Executives. International Risk Management

Institute, Inc. http://www.irmi.com/online/riskmgmt/risk-management-why-and-how.pdf

HealthIT.gov. 2015. Meaningful Use Definition and Objectives. https://www.healthit.gov/providers-professionals/meaningful-use-definition-objectives

National Whistleblowers Center. 2015. False Claims Act/Qui Tam FAQ. http://www.whistleblowers.org/index.php?Itemid=64

Office of the Inspector General. 2015a. http://oig.hhs.gov/reports-and-publications/strategic-plan/index.asp

Office of the Inspector General. 2015b. http://oig.hhs.gov/reports-and-publications/workplan/index.asp

Office of the Inspector General. 2015c. OIG Operating an Effective Compliance Plan. http://oig.hhs.gov/compliance/provider-compliance-training/files/OperatinganEffectiveComplianceProgramFinalBR508.pdf

Office of the Inspector General. 2015d. Civil Monetary Penalties and Affirmative Exclusions. http://oig.hhs.gov/fraud/enforcement/cmp/

Office of the Inspector General. 2015e. Corporate Integrity Agreements. http://oig.hhs.gov/compliance/corporate-integrity-agreements/index.asp

Office of the Inspector General. 2015f. Compliance Education Materials. http://oig.hhs.gov/compliance/101/

Quinsey, C.A. 2013. Managing Organizational Compliance and Risk. Chapter 28 in *Health Information Management: Concepts, Principles and Practice*, 4th ed. Edited by LaTour, K.M., S. Eichenwald Maki, and P. Oachs. Chicago: AHIMA.

Social Security Act. 2015. § 1128: Exclusion of Certain Individuals and Entities from Participation in Medicare and State Health Care Programs. http://www.ssa.gov/OP_Home/ssact/title11/1128.htm

Swanson, M. n.d. NIST SP 800-34, Revision 1–Contingency Planning Guide for Federal Information Systems. http://csrc.nist.gov/news_events/HIPAA-May2010_workshop/presentations/2-2b-contingency-planning-swanson-nist.pdf

Thompson, T.G. and D.J. Brailer. 2004 (July 21). The Decade of Health Information Technology: Delivering Consumer-centric and Information-rich Health Care: Framework for Strategic Action. Office of the National Coordinator for Health Information Technology. http://www.providersedge.com/ehdocs/ehr_articles/the_decade_of_hit-delivering_customer-centric_and_info-rich_hc.pdf

US Department of Health and Human Services. 2015a. Guidance on 42 CFR Parts 413, 482, and 489. https://www.cms.gov/Regulations-and-Guidance/Legislation/EMTALA/downloads/cms-1063-f.pdf

US Department of Health and Human Services. 2015b. Practices Guide: Contingency Plan. http://www.hhs.gov/ocio/eplc/EPLC%20Archive%20Documents/36-Contingency-Disaster%20Recovery%20Plan/eplc_contingency_plan_practices_guide.pdf

US Sentencing Commission. 2013a. Effective Compliance and Ethics Program. http://www.ussc.gov/guidelines-manual/2013/2013-8b21

US Sentencing Commission. 2013b. Federal Sentencing Guidelines Manual. §8A1.2, Application Note (k),

Whistleblowerlaws. 2015. False Claims Act. http://www.whistleblowerlaws.com/false-claims-act/

Ziemba, W. Corporate Compliance Content. HIM6545 Blackboard Course. Duluth, MN. July 30, 2015.

42 CFR 455.2: Definitions. 2015.

42 CFR 1001.952: Safe Harbor Regulations. 2015.

11

Data Privacy, Confidentiality, and Security

Danika Brinda, PhD, RHIA, CHPS, HCISPP, and
Amy Watters, EdD, RHIA, FAHIMA

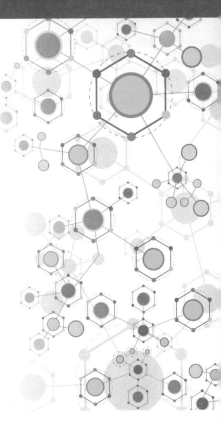

Learning Objectives

- Interpret the privacy, security, and breach notification requirements of the Health Insurance Portability and Accountability Act (HIPAA) of 1996
- Differentiate between privacy, confidentiality, and security
- Identify the requirements of the Breach Notification Rule
- Demonstrate the appropriate uses and disclosures of health information
- Identify when an authorization is or is not needed for disclosure, and when the patient has the right to object
- Utilize the basic steps of risk analysis and risk management
- Identify best practices for privacy and security in health information exchange
- Apply security measures to safeguard information being accessed on mobile technology
- Apply the HIPAA workforce training requirement and strategies

Key Terms

Accept the risk
Accounting of disclosure
Addressable standards
Administrative safeguards
Assessment
Audit
Audit log
Authorization
Biometric authentication
Breach
Breach notification
Breach Notification Rule
Bring your own device

Business associate
Business associate agreement (BAA)
Cipher text
Compound authorization
Confidentiality
Contingency plan
Contrary
Covered entity
Criticality analysis
Cryptographic key
Data at rest
Data backup plan
Data in motion

Data security
Decryption
Deidentification
Designated record set
Disaster recovery plan
Disclosure
Emergency mode operation plan
Encryption
Expert determination method
Health information exchange
Health Insurance Portability and
Accountability Act (HIPAA)
of 1996

HITECH-HIPAA Omnibus
   Privacy Act
Individually identifiable health
   information
Logic bombs
Malware
Minimum necessary
Mitigate the risk
Notice of privacy practices (NPP)
Organizational safeguards
Physical safeguards
Plaintext

Privacy
Privacy Rule
Protected health information (PHI)
Reasonable cause
Reidentification
Required standards
Residual risk
Risk analysis
Risk management
Rootkit
Safe harbor method
Secure information

Security
Security Rule
Stringent
Technical safeguards
Transfer the risk
Trojan horse
Use
User authentication
Virus
Willful neglect
Worm

Effective healthcare requires trusting relationships between patients and their healthcare providers. As the use of health information technology continues to grow, it has the potential to improve healthcare delivery and decision making, as well as reduce costs, but that can only happen if patients trust in the confidentiality and accuracy of their health information. If patients are concerned about the privacy, confidentiality, and security of their information, they may not disclose their health information to their healthcare provider, which can impact patient care or even have life-threatening consequences (ONC 2015).

Protecting patient information is a core responsibility of health information management (HIM) professionals. By maintaining knowledge of rules and regulations, establishing and overseeing policies and procedures, and reporting any violations to the proper authorities, HIM professionals ensure that patient privacy is maintained, confidential information is protected, and security measures are implemented to prevent unauthorized access to information (Harman 2013, 343).

The terms *privacy*, *confidentiality*, and *security* are often used interchangeably; however, there are some important distinctions among them:

- **Privacy** is "the right of an individual to be let alone. It includes freedom from observation or intrusion into one's private affairs and the right to maintain control over certain personal and health information" (Harman 2006, 634). In the context of health information, privacy refers to who should have access, what constitutes the patient's rights to confidentiality, and what constitutes inappropriate access to health records (Minnesota Administrative Uniformity Committee n.d.).

- **Confidentiality** means that data or information is not made available or disclosed to unauthorized persons or processes, and establishes how the records (or the systems that hold those records) should be protected from inappropriate access (Minnesota Administrative Uniformity Committee n.d.). Confidentiality carries "the responsibility for limiting disclosure of private matters. It includes the responsibility to use, disclose, or release such information only with the knowledge and consent of the individual" (Harman 2006, 627–628).

- **Security** is the means by which the privacy and confidentiality of information is maintained (Minnesota Administrative Uniformity Committee n.d.). Security includes "physical and electronic protection of the integrity, availability, and confidentiality of computer-based information and the resources used to enter, store, process, and communicate it; and the means to control access and protect information from accidental or intentional disclosure" (Harman 2013, 343; 2006, 635).

In order to maintain the privacy, confidentiality, and security of patient information, HIM professionals must be knowledgeable of the applicable standards, rules, and regulations, both at the state and national levels.

The Health Insurance Portability and Accountability Act (HIPAA) of 1996

Over the years, the right to privacy and the establishment of requirements to maintain patient confidentiality have been addressed by various state and federal rulings and legislation (refer to chapter 2). The **Health Insurance Portability and Accountability Act (HIPAA) of 1996** was originally established to ensure health insurance continuity (also known as portability), set standards for electronic claims and national identifiers, and protect against fraud and abuse. It was subsequently expanded to establish national standards for the protection of privacy and the assurance of the security of health information, which was a significant moment for the healthcare industry. It has had a major impact on the collection and dissemination of information, and it will continue to have this impact long into the future as healthcare organizations ensure compliance with the rules in an increasingly complex electronic environment. This chapter focuses on three of the regulations that provide federal protections for patient health information and give patient's rights with respect to that information—the Privacy Rule, the Security Rule, and the Breach Notification Rule, all of which are housed within Title II of HIPAA, known as the Administrative Simplification provisions (ONC 2015).

HIPAA's Privacy and Security Rules are focused on assuring the privacy and security of **protected health information (PHI)** (referred to as ePHI when it is in electronic form), which is individually identifiable health information held or transmitted by a covered entity or business associate (HHS 2013). **Individually identifiable health information** is information that identifies the individual or there is reasonable belief that it can be used to identify the individual, and relates to:

- the individual's past, present, or future physical or mental health or condition;
- the provision of healthcare to the individual; or

- the past, present, or future payment for the provision of healthcare to the individual (ONC 2015).

Any documentation that includes a patient's name or any other identifying information would be considered PHI, such as a radiology report, a hospital bill, or an email communication to a healthcare provider.

Part of the impetus for HIPAA was the development of the electronic health record (EHR). As patient information has moved to the electronic medium, integrated systems across the continuum of care have been developed; thus, standardized federal legislation became imperative as patient information was used and disclosed to many people and organizations needing access to it. HIPAA was designed to guarantee that information transferred and exchanged in this way would be protected. In an electronic environment, protecting privacy has become extremely difficult and patients have become increasingly concerned about the privacy and security of their information. More and more, patients are seeking ways to control the dissemination of their information by requesting anonymity and addressing their desires regarding the use and disclosure of their health information, such as how it is used in the hospital directory, for notification purposes such as disasters; and for other disclosures required by law such as public health (Harman 2013, 344).

HIPAA applies to specific organizations referred to as covered entities and business associates. A **covered entity (CE)** is defined as a "health plan, healthcare clearinghouse, or healthcare provider that transmits information in electronic form in connection with a transaction" (HHS 2013). A **business associate (BA)** is a "person or entity that performs certain functions or activities that involve the use or disclosure of protected health information on behalf of, or provides services to, a covered entity" (HHS 2013). Whether patient health information is electronic, on paper, or in any other media, providers are responsible for safeguarding the information by meeting the requirements of the HIPAA Rules (ONC 2015). HIPAA provides only the minimum requirements regarding privacy and security. States are free to adopt more stringent regulations, making it essential that HIM professionals have knowledge of both federal and state requirements in order to maintain compliance.

The Privacy Rule

The Standards for Privacy of Individually Identifiable Health Information, commonly known as the **Privacy Rule** (45 CFR Part 160 and Subparts A and E of Part 164), was established to assure the protection of health information. Specifically, the goal of the Privacy Rule is "to assure that individuals' health information is properly protected while allowing the flow of health information needed to provide and promote high quality healthcare and to protect the public's health and well-being" (HHS 2013). The Privacy Rule was established with three major purposes:

1. to protect and enhance the rights of healthcare consumers by providing them access to their health information and ensure the appropriate use of that information;
2. to improve the quality of healthcare in the United States by restoring trust in the healthcare system; and
3. to improve the efficiency and effectiveness of healthcare delivery by creating a national framework for privacy protection that builds on the efforts of states, health systems and organizations, and individuals (HHS 2013).

The Privacy Rule can be broken into eight primary sections:

1. Uses and disclosures of protected health information: General rules (45 CFR 164.502 through 164.512): Identifies how and for what purposes PHI can be used and disclosed, and identifies requirements for authorizations. It also establishes the **minimum necessary** standard that requires that a covered entity or business associate make "reasonable efforts to limit protected health information to

the minimum necessary to accomplish the intended purpose of the use, disclosure, or request" (HHS 2013). This standard is meant to limit unnecessary or inappropriate access to and disclosure of PHI so that it is only used or disclosed to carry out necessary functions for treatment, payment, and healthcare operations.

2. Uses and disclosures: Organizational requirements (45 CFR 45 164.504): Establishes requirements for business associates and **business associate agreements (BAA)**, which are contracts between a covered entity and a business associate that establish the permitted and required uses and disclosures of PHI by the business associate (45 CFR 164.504). Examples of scenarios that require a BAA include an attorney providing legal services that require access to PHI, an independent consultant providing services to a facility, or a third party that processes claims for an organization.

3. Notice of privacy practices for protected health information (45 CFR 164.520): Requires the establishment and dissemination of a **notice of privacy practices (NPP)**, which healthcare providers and health plans must give to patients to inform them of how they may use and share the patient's health information and how patients can exercise their health privacy rights (see appendix B) (HHS n.d.(a)).

4. Rights to request privacy protection for protected health information (45 CFR 164.522): Establishes patients' rights to request alternative means of communication and restrictions for the use and disclosure of their PHI.

5. Access of individuals to protected health information (45 CFR 164.524): Establishes patients' rights to access their health information by allowing them to inspect and obtain a copy of their PHI in a designated record set, which is the group of records maintained by or for a covered entity (HHS 2013).

6. Amendment of protected health information (45 CFR 164.526): Establishes patients'

rights to request that a covered entity make an amendment to the PHI in the designated record set.

7. Accounting of disclosures of protected health information (45 CFR 164.528): Establishes a patient's right to receive an accounting of disclosures of their PHI made by a covered entity.

8. Administrative requirements (45 CFR 164.530): Requirements for covered entities related to the designation of a privacy official, training of the workforce, the implementation of privacy safeguards, the process for individuals to make complaints, and the establishment of anti-retaliatory standards to ensure there is no intimidation or retaliation for filing a complaint.

As indicated in the Privacy Rule's Administrative Requirements (45 CFR 164.530), organizations "must implement policies and procedures" to address each standard as well as implementing a process to ensure that those policies and procedures are being followed (HHS 2013).

The Security Rule

The purpose of the Security Standards for the Protection of Electronic Protected Health Information, or the **Security Rule** (45 CFR Part 160 and Subparts A and C of Part 164), is to operationalize the protections identified in the Privacy Rule by addressing the technical and nontechnical safeguards that covered entities must put in place to secure individuals' electronic PHI (ePHI) (HHS 2013). The Security Rule specifies "a series of administrative, technical, and physical security procedures for covered entities to use to assure the confidentiality, integrity, and availability of e-PHI" (HHS 2013). It identifies four specific types of safeguards that organizations must have in place:

1. **administrative safeguards**, such as policies and procedures, to manage administrative actions, policies, and procedures to prevent, detect, contain, and correct security violations (ONC 2015);

2. **physical safeguards**, such as surveillance cameras and identification badges, to identify measures to protect information systems, buildings, and equipment from natural and environmental hazards;

3. **technical safeguards**, such as automatic log-off and unique user identification, to protect access and control of ePHI; and

4. **organizational safeguards**, such as BAAs, so that arrangements are made to protect ePHI between organizations (KHA n.d.).

All of these safeguards are intended to protect the privacy of health information as covered entities continue to adopt new and evolving technologies to improve patient care.

The Security Rule contains two different types of standards—required and addressable. **Required standards** are standards that are mandated and the organization must implement them as written by the HIPAA Security Rule. **Addressable standards** provide flexibility to the covered entity and business associate by allowing the organization to implement the standard based on:

- The size and complexity of the covered entity or business associate
- The organization's technical infrastructure, hardware, and software security capabilities
- The costs of security measures
- The probability and criticality of potential risks to ePHI (HHS 2013).

If an organization decides to not implement an addressable standard as written in the regulation, documentation must exist on why the decision was made to implement the standard in a different manner including what other safeguards the organization has implemented to protect ePHI (HHS 2013).

The HITECH-HIPAA Omnibus Privacy Act

Although organizations were required to be in compliance with the Privacy and Security Rules in 2003 and 2005, respectively, they were impacted in 2009 when the Health Information Technology for Economic and Clinical Health (HITECH) Act was enacted to promote the adoption and meaningful use of health information technology as part of the American Recovery and Reinvestment Act (ARRA). The HITECH Act established more detailed provisions and strengthened the requirements included in the HIPAA Privacy and Security Rules by establishing:

- Mandatory reporting requirements and penalties in the event of a breach
- New enforcement responsibilities
- New privacy requirements such as new accounting requirements for the EHR
- Extended requirements to the business associates of covered entities (KHA n.d.)

In response, the US Department of Health and Human Services (HHS) Office for Civil Rights (OCR) published the final omnibus rules in 2013 to address many of the HITECH requirements. The rule is officially titled "Modifications to the HIPAA Privacy, Security, Enforcement, and Breach Notification Rule Under the Health Information Technology for Economic and Clinical Health Act, and the Genetic Information Nondiscrimination Act; Other Modifications to the HIPAA Rule," but is often referred to as the **HITECH-HIPAA Omnibus Privacy Act**, or the Omnibus Rule.

The Omnibus Rule includes some of the most significant changes to patient privacy since HIPAA was first enacted in 2003. It went into effect on March 26, 2013, and covered entities were to ensure compliance by September 23, 2013 (AHIMA 2013a). The Omnibus Rule strengthens the privacy and security of patient health information, modifies the Breach Notification Rule, strengthens privacy protections for genetic information by prohibiting health plans from using or disclosing such information for underwriting, makes business associates of HIPAA-covered entities liable for compliance, strengthens limitations on the use and disclosure of PHI for marketing, research and fundraising, and allows patients increased restriction rights (KHA n.d.).

The OCR indicates that more provisions will be established in the future. The Omnibus Rule does not address all of the HITECH privacy requirements such as the requirement for accounting of disclosures and access to EHR audit logs. It is anticipated

that the OCR will release provisions related to this and other requirements at a later date.

The Breach Notification Rule

One of the largest regulation provisions to privacy and security under the HITECH Act were the new requirements related to **breach notification**, which entails notifying patients if their PHI has been breached (Quinsey 2013, 855). Unauthorized uses and disclosures of any PHI at any time may be considered a data breach under the updated regulations. The breach notification regulation created a new process for covered entities and business associates to investigate and evaluate if a breach occurred for an unauthorized use or disclosure of PHI. The regulation also created a short timeline for investigation, conclusion, and notification of the potential breach (Dimick 2010; Kempfert and Reed 2011).

The final HITECH-HIPAA Omnibus Act of 2013, defined a **breach** as:

> An impermissible use or disclosure under the Privacy Rule that compromises the security or privacy of the protected health information. An impermissible use or disclosure of protected health information is presumed to be a breach unless the covered entity or business associate, as applicable, demonstrates that there is a low probability that the protected health information has been compromised based on a risk assessment. (Kastel 2013)

A risk assessment should be conducted to determine if a breach has occurred. The risk assessment should address the following factors at minimum:

1. The nature and extent of the PHI involved in the data breach, including the types of identifiers and likelihood of the reidentification
2. The unauthorized person (people) who used the PHI or to whom it was disclosed
3. Whether the PHI was viewed, acquired, or redisclosed
4. The extent to which the risk to the PHI has been mitigated (Kastel 2013)

The **Breach Notification Rule** requires covered entities and business associates to establish policies and procedures to investigate an unauthorized use or disclosure of PHI to determine if a breach occurred, conclude the investigation, and to notify affected individuals and the secretary of the Department of Health and Human Services within 60 days of date of discovery of the breach (Kempfert and Reed 2011). Based on the findings of the investigation into the potential breach, an organization will make a determination regarding whether or not the incident falls into the breach notification process and will take the proper steps to notify the affected. If the number of individuals impacted by the breach exceeds 500, a healthcare organization must notify and report the incident to the local media as well as the individuals impacted by the breach and the secretary of the Department of Health and Human Services (Dimick 2010). The Omnibus Rule defines three exceptions to the Breach Notification Rule requirement.

1. The PHI disclosure was not intentional and the individual or individuals that received the information have the requirement to keep the information confidential.

2. The access to the PHI was unintentional by a workforce member and the person or persons receiving the information has a right to keep the information confidential.

3. The healthcare organization believes in good faith that the protected health information could not have been retained by the person receiving it (Kempfert and Reed 2011).

If the investigation finds any of these to be true, it can be concluded that a data breach did not occur and the notification requirements of the Breach Notification Rule would not be necessary.

HIPAA Enforcement Under the Omnibus Rule

Included in the HIPAA regulation is the Enforcement Rule, which contains provisions relating to compliance, investigations, penalties for violations, and procedures for hearings (HHS n.d.(b)) If any person or organization believes that a covered entity or a business associate is violating the HIPAA Privacy or Security Regulations, a complaint may be filed to the Secretary of HHS. The Office of Civil Rights (OCR) is the enforcement body of HIPAA and is responsible for reviewing all complaints and conducting investigations as necessary. Additionally, the OCR can open an investigation based on any data breaches that have been reported by the covered entity or business associate. Based on the findings of the investigation conducted by the OCR, the covered entity or business associate may be subject to a corrective action plan (CAP) that may include a civil monetary penalty (CMP).

The Omnibus Rule created a new fine structure for CMP based on a four-tier system for HIPAA violations that occurred after February 18, 2009 (see table 11.1). Tier 1 is the lowest tier and is used for minor violations that have given a CMP. Tier 2 is based on reasonable cause, which was further defined within the HIPAA Omnibus Rule. **Reasonable cause** is "an act or omission in which a covered entity or business associate knew, or by exercising reasonable diligence would have known, that the act or omission violated an administrative simplification provision, but in which the covered entity or business associate did not act with willful neglect" (HHS 2013, 23).

Tier 3 and Tier 4 are based on violations that have been determined to be due to willful neglect. **Willful neglect** is defined as "conscious,

Table 11.1. Categories of violations and respective penalty amounts available

Violation category—45 CFR 160.404	Each violation	All such violations of an identical provision in a calendar year
Tier 1 (A) Did not know	$100–$50,000	$1,500,000
Tier 2 (B) Reasonable cause	$1,000–$50,000	$1,500,000
Tier 3 (C)(i) Willful neglect—corrected	$10,000–$50,000	$1,500,000
Tier 4 (C)(ii) Willful neglect–not corrected	$50,000	$1,500,000

Source: AHIMA 2013b, 9.

intentional failure or reckless indifference to the obligation to comply with the administrative simplification provision violated" (HHS 2013, 23). The difference between falling into a Tier 3 or Tier 4 CMP is based on when the violation was corrected after the covered entity of business associate became aware of the violation. If the data breach caused by willful neglect is corrected within 30 days from the date of the covered entity or business associate becoming aware of it, it would fall into Tier 3. If the data breach wasn't corrected within 30 days of discovery and was due to willful neglect, it would fall into Tier 4 (AHIMA 2013b).

The Omnibus Rule also defined the factors that will be considered for applying a CMP when evaluating a violation of the HIPAA Privacy and Security Regulations. The CMP will be based on:

- Nature and extent of the violation (number of individual affected and time period during which the violation occurred)

- Nature and extent of the harm resulting from the violation (physical harm, financial harm, or reputational harm)

- Covered entity or business associates prior compliance with the HIPAA regulations (previous violations, previous CAP, response to correct the violation)

- Financial condition of the covered entity or business associate (financial difficulties affecting ability to comply, imposition of CMP would jeopardize the ability to continue business, size of the organization)

- Other such matters as justice may require (HHS 2013).

The OCR will evaluate each violation separately and determine the best CAP, which may include a CMP or just changes in policies, procedures, and practices within the organization. Since February 2009, the OCR has initiated 26 CMPs for noncompliance with HIPAA resulting in approximately $27 million (HHS 2015a).

The final Omnibus Rule also amended a few other important elements within the HIPAA enforcement regulations. If the OCR determined that the covered entity or business associate was not aware of the violation and had been following smart business practices for compliance with the HIPAA regulations, the Secretary of HHS may apply a waiver to the penalty (HHS 2013). The new regulations under enforcement were created to make the process more streamlined and transparent for consumers, covered entities, business associates, and HHS.

 ## Check Your Understanding 11.1

Instructions: **Answer the following questions on a separate piece of paper.**

1. What are the main sections of the HIPAA Security Rule?
   A. Technical, administrative, physical, and system-wide safeguards
   B. Physical, technical, administrative, and organizational safeguards
   C. Administrative, organizational, technical, and privacy safeguards
   D. Organizational, technical, physical, and system-wide safeguards

2. True or false: One purpose of establishing the Privacy Rule was to protect and enhance the rights of healthcare consumers by providing them access to their health information and ensure the appropriate use of that information.

3. Describe the difference between privacy, confidentiality, and security.

4. True or false: The minimum necessary standard requires a covered entity or business associate to make reasonable efforts to limit protected health information to the minimum necessary to accomplish the intended purpose of the use, disclosure, or request.

5. The Breach Notification Rule requires covered entities to do which of the following?
   A. Establish a process for investigating whether a breach occurred
   B. Notify affected individuals when a breach occurs
   C. Establish a policy on minimum necessary
   D. Both a and b

Privacy and Security Requirements for Disclosure Management

Use and disclosure of patient information is a necessity for day-to-day operations within a healthcare organization. HIPAA distinctly defines the difference between the use and disclosure of PHI. **Use** is defined as the sharing, employment, application, utilization, examination, or analysis within a covered entity that creates and maintains the PHI. **Disclosure** is the release, transfer, provision of access to, or divulging in any manner of information outside the entity holding the information (HHS 2013). HIPAA provides specific requirements regarding when protected health information can be used or disclosed with and without a signed authorization form by the patient. An **authorization** is a document that gives covered entities permission to use protected health information for specified purposes or to disclose protected health information to a third party specified by the individual. All covered entities and business associates should assure they have established policies and procedures to manage and govern the use and disclosures of protected health information.

One of the foundational elements to the use and disclosure of PHI is the definition of the organization's designated record set. The HIPAA Privacy Rule (45 CFR 164.501) defines a **designated record set** as:

> A group of records maintained by or for a covered entity that may include patient medical and billing records; the enrollment, payment, claims, adjudication, and cases or medical management record systems maintained by or for a health plan; or information used in whole or in part to make care-related decisions. (45 CFR 164.501)

The designated record set is used to support a variety of patients' rights under the HIPAA Privacy Rule such as patients' access to PHI, electronic copy of PHI, and amendment of a record (HHS 2013).

Use and Disclosure of Patient Information with Patient Authorization

A valid authorization for use and disclosure of protected health information is needed prior to releasing the information unless it is permitted without an authorization under the HIPAA privacy regulation (45 CFR 164.508(a)(1)). A valid authorization of disclosure of health information must be reviewed and evaluated for each specific request received at a covered entity. The HIPAA Privacy Rule requires a valid authorization be completed for disclosure of information for the following:

- Disclosure of PHI not permitted to be released without an authorization (45 CFR 164.508(a)(1))
- Psychotherapy notes (45 CFR 164.508(a)(2))
- Marketing (45 CFR 164.508(a)(3))
- Sale of protected health information (45 CFR 164.508(a)(4))

Table 11.2 defines the core elements and statements that must be included on an authorization for uses and disclosures of protected health information.

Additionally, the authorization must be written in plain language and the covered entity must provide a copy of the authorization for disclosure to the individual (45 CFR 164.508(3))(45 CFR 164.508(4)). All of these elements must be present in order for the disclosure of protected health information to be valid. A covered entity has 30 days to respond and disclose the information from the date the authorization was received (45 CFR 164.524(b)). Prior to the release of any information, all authorizations should be evaluated by the healthcare organization to assure that all required pieces of information are present and appropriate.

An authorization is considered to be defective under the HIPAA Privacy Rule if any of the following scenarios are true:

- The expiration date has passed or the expiration event has occurred
- The authorization is not completely filled out
- The authorization has been revoked
- Any required elements defined here are missing
- The authorization is combined with any other documentation to create a compound authorization except where permitted
- The facility knows that the material information included in the authorization is false (HHS 2013).

In the event that an authorization is considered defective, the requestor of the information should be notified in writing, indicating why the authorization is defective and the process for correcting and resubmitting the authorization for disclosure.

Although patient authorization is required for research, the HIPAA Omnibus Rule changed the regulations to strike a better balance between maintaining patient privacy and allowing access to enough information for effective research to occur. The change to the regulation allows for authorization of future research studies with an appropriate and adequate description of how the PHI will be used in the future research through compound authorizations. **Compound authorizations** com-bine the use and disclosure of PHI with other legal permissions such as consent for treatment, which is prohibited by the current HIPAA Privacy Rule. However, this provision was amended by the Omnibus Rule, which permits combining an authorization for the use and disclosure of PHI for a research study with authorization for other permissions for the same study, including informed consent to participate in the study. The Omnibus Rule allows authorization for both conditioned and unconditioned research on one form. This means authorization for multiple research studies may exist on the same form as long as the authorization form clearly differentiates between the studies and allows the individual to opt in to the unconditioned research activities. A conditioned authorization is used for an individual to consent into the main research study; whereas, an unconditioned authorization is used for the individual to consent into additional research studies if the patient elects to be involved. For example, a patient may authorize to be part of a breast cancer research study as the main research study and also may elect to be in an additional study on tissue, based on the specific diagnosis of breast cancer. The conditioned authorization would be the consent to participate in the main breast cancer study and the unconditioned authorization would be the tissue research study. In addition, the authorization must give participants

Table 11.2. Authorizations for uses and disclosures: required elements and statements

Core Elements (45 CFR 164.508(c)(1)): A valid authorization must contain at least the following elements:	Required Statements (45 CFR 164.508(c)(2)): In addition to the core elements, a valid authorization must contain statements notifying individuals of:

• A description of the information to be used or disclosed that identifies the information in a specific and meaningful way.
• The name or other specific identification of the person(s), or class of persons, authorized to make the requested use or disclosure.
• The name or other specific identification of the person(s), or class of persons, to whom the covered entity may make the requested use or disclosure.
• A description of each purpose of the requested use or disclosure.
• An expiration date or an expiration event that relates to the individual or the purpose of the use or disclosure.
• Signature of the individual and date.
	• The individual's right to revoke the authorization in writing, and either:
	  ○ The exceptions to the right to revoke and a description of how the individual may revoke the authorization; or
	  ○ The extent to which the information is included in the notice of privacy practices
	• The ability or inability for the authorization to place conditions on the treatment, payment, enrollment or eligibility for benefits.
	• The potential for information disclosed pursuant to the authorization to be subject to redisclosure by the recipient and no longer be protected by this subpart.

Source: HHS 2013.

an opt-in option; combined authorizations that only allow the individual to opt-out of the unconditioned research are not permitted. This provision applies to all types of research studies except for authorization to use and disclose psychotherapy notes which may not be combined with any other authorization (AHIMA 2013b).

For compliance with the rules around use and disclosure, a covered entity should have clear policies and procedures that define the requirements for disclosures, when an authorization is needed, when an authorization is valid, signatures and personal representatives, and administrative information such as requiring authorizations be maintained for a minimum of six years (45 CFR 164.530(j)).

Use and Disclosure of Patient Information without Patient Authorization

The HIPAA Privacy Rule allows covered entities to use and disclose protected health information for the purpose of treatment, payments, or healthcare operations (TPO) (45 CFR 164.506(a)). Covered entities should clearly define what uses and disclosures of PHI fall into these categories to assure proper adherence to the regulations. The following are examples of uses and disclosures of PHI where an authorization is not needed:

- Uses and disclosures to business associates
- Uses and disclosures required by law
- Uses and disclosures for public health reporting, and other public health activities
- Disclosures about victims of abuse, neglect, or domestic violence
- Uses and disclosures for health oversight activities such as audits, investigations, and inspections
- Disclosures for judicial and administrative proceedings
- Disclosures for law enforcement purposes
- Uses and disclosures to coroners, medical examiners, and funeral directors
- Uses and disclosures for organ, eye, or tissue donation

- Uses and disclosures for research purposes
- Uses and disclosures to avert a serious threat to health or safety
- Uses and disclosures for specified government functions including: military and veterans activities, national security and intelligence activities, protective services for the President and others, medical suitability determinations, and correctional institutions
- Disclosures for workers' compensation (HHS 2013)

Any request for information that falls into these categories should be individually evaluated to verify that it does in fact meet the criteria of one of the given categories. In addition to having clear guidelines and procedures for releasing information without authorization, healthcare organizations and business associates must assure that they have a process to account for these types of disclosures. Under the HIPAA Privacy Rule, a patient has a right to receive an **accounting of disclosures** for the past six years at any time, which is information that describes a covered entity's disclosures of PHI other than for treatment, payment, and healthcare operations; disclosures made with authorization; and certain other limited disclosures (45 CFR 164.528). The accounting must include all disclosures made by the covered entity or business associate, except if the account falls into one of these categories:

- To carry out treatment, payment and healthcare operations
- To individuals receiving their own protected health information
- Incident to a use or disclosure otherwise permitted or required by the use and disclosure requirements
- Pursuant to an authorization
- For the facility's directory or to persons involved in the individual's care or other notification purposes
- For national security or intelligence purposes
- To correctional institutions or law enforcement officials

- As part of a limited data set
- That occurred prior to the compliance date for the covered entity (45 CFR 164.528(a)(1)).

If a patient requests an accounting of disclosures, the covered entity must respond within 60 days. The accounting report must include (1) date of disclosures, (2) name or entity that received the PHI, (3) a brief description of the PHI, and (4) a brief statement of the purpose of the disclosure (45 CFR 164.528(b)(2)). If during the request time of the accounting, a disclosure was made multiple times to the same recipient for the same purpose, rather than listing each individual disclosure, a covered entity may list the disclosure one time on the report with the addition of the frequency of the disclosures, number of disclosures and the date of the last disclosure (45 CFR 164.528(b)(3)). A major change from the HIPAA Privacy Rule of 2003 to the final Omnibus Rule of 2013 was that any accounting of disclosures made by a business associate must also be included in the report for accounting of disclosures provided by the covered entity (HHS 2013).

A majority of the disclosures being made within healthcare organizations are being made from electronic health records, which have the capability to track and create a disclosure management log. Since many healthcare organizations still manage and use paper medical records, policies and procedures should be established to document the process for disclosures of the paper medical records and electronic tracking of the disclosures.

Deidentification of Health Information

PHI can be used and disclosed without permission of the patient if the PHI is deidentified. Under HIPAA, **deidentification** refers to health information that has had identifiers removed so there is not the capability to reasonably identify the individual to which the information belongs (45 CFR 164.514(a)). The HIPAA regulations define two methods in which information can be deidentified to meet the standard. The first method is using the **expert determination method**. In this method, data elements that could identify an individual are removed from the data and then an expert, such as a statistician, applies scientific methodology to determine the likelihood of identification of the individual. The expert that the

organization hires to statistically analyze the information provides documentation of the probability that the information would be identified. If there is low probability that the information can be identified, the information is considered to be deidentified (HHS 2013). If there is a high probability that the information could be identified, further evaluation of removal of data elements should occur.

The second method of deidentification is the **safe harbor method**. The safe harbor method requires the covered entity or business associate to remove 18 data elements from the health information. The data elements are defined as the following:

- Names
- All geographic subdivision smaller than state (street address, city, county, precinct, zip code, and any other equivalent geocodes)
- All elements of dates excluding year (birth date, admission date, discharge date, death date); if over 89 years of age, all elements of dates including year
- Telephone number(s)
- Fax number(s)
- Social Security Number
- Medical record number
- Health plan beneficiary numbers (insurance information)
- Account numbers
- Certificate/license numbers
- Vehicle identification numbers and series numbers (example: license plate numbers)
- Device numbers or identifiers
- Web universal resource locator (URL)
- Internet protocol (IP) address
- Biometric identifiers (fingerprints, voice recognition, palm reading)
- Full face photographs
- Any other unique identifiable number, characteristic, or code (HHS 2013)

All of these data elements must be removed from all the health information that is being deidentified. Challenges arise with this method to assure that all data elements are removed from the entire record. If the organization that is deidentifying the information wants to be able to reidentify the information for some reason, they are allowed to create a **reidentification** method. For reidentification, an organization can apply a specific code, or other means, to the data for future reidentification purposes; however, the specific code cannot be derived from any type of data elements that come from the patient's health information. The information regarding reidentification needs to be kept separate from the deidentified data and should have proper safeguards such as limited access and secure storage to prevent unauthorized re-identification (HHS 2013).

Use and Disclosure Requiring an Opportunity to Object

A covered entity has the right to use and disclose protected health information for healthcare operations, which can include utilization review, quality improvement, and accreditation activities; however, the Privacy Rule allows the patient to agree or object to disclosure of PHI within the facility directory. For this specific requirement for use and disclosure of PHI, a written authorization is not required as oral acceptance or objection is acceptable (45 CFR 164.510). A covered entity must inform a patient that PHI may be included in the directory and they may disclose the directory PHI to individuals such as clergy. The patient may orally agree to the PHI in the directory or object to the information in the directory. If the patient allows the information to be within the directory, the only PHI that may be allowed and disclosed in the directory is (1) patient name, (2) the individual's location in the covered healthcare provider's facility, (3) individual's condition described in general terms that does not communicate specific medical information about the individual, and (4) religious affiliation. The disclosure of this information can only be for the purpose of releasing the information to clergy or to an individual who asks for the person by name. A clear process should be established to assure all patients are given the right to object to PHI being entered in the directory (45 CFR 164.510).

In some cases the patient is unable to object to the directory information due to being incapacitated or due to another emergency situation. In these scenarios, the covered entity may disclose the information as long as it is consistent with the patient's previously expressed preferences or it is in the best interest of the patient based on professional judgment (45 CFR 164.510(a)(3)). A covered entity should assure that a process regarding the use and disclosure of patient directory information is addressed in their policy and procedure.

Patient Identity Management for Use and Disclosures of PHI

When managing the use and disclosures of PHI within a covered entity or business associate, ensuring that the correct patient's information is being used or disclosed is a vital step to prevent data breaches and unauthorized uses and disclosures of protected health information. Policies and procedures created by the covered entity or business associate to manage the use and disclosures of PHI should address the process for patient identification, including verification of the individual or personal representatives. A clearly defined data dictionary can help establish the basic input of patient demographic information to create consistency for input and creation of patients. Basic demographic identifiers include patient name, medical record number, gender, date of birth, social security number, address, city, state, zip code, and telephone number (HIMSS 2011). With consistent data input and data collection, the identification of a patient can be made easier to assure the right patient and the right information is being used or disclosed.

When verifying the identity of a patient, the Joint Commission recommends verification of a minimum of two different data elements (Joint Commission 2015). Best practice recommends that multiple elements are checked with the patient or patient representation. An example of patient identity verification can be four elements such as name, date of birth, address and last four digits of a social security number (HIMSS 2011). While this process can be seen as challenging and cumbersome, the process for investigating an unauthorized use or disclosure of PHI or fixing a patient record in which there is incorrect documentation is even more challenging and causes patient safety issues and concerns. Taking the time to verify a patient's identify up front can save a lot of rework,

Table 11.3. Techniques to verify requestors

Requestor of protected health information	Suggested verification documentation
Patient	Personal identification: driver's license, passport, state-issued identification
Power of attorney	Power of attorney documentation and personal identification
Court-appointed guardians	Court paperwork for appointment of guardianship and personal identification
Attorney	Request on letterhead, business card, and personal identification
Executor of the estate	Legal documentation showing appointment of executor of the estate, personal identification
Spouse	Marriage license and personal identification

reduce the likelihood of a data breach, and reduce patient safety issues.

Under the HIPAA Privacy Rule, verification of requestor identity must be completed prior to disclosing any patient information in any format. Verification may come in a variety of different formats such as requesting a driver's license of the patient, verification of pertinent data elements such as name and date of birth, verification of the requestor such as a business card with identification, or verification of a fax number prior to faxing patient information (45 CFR 164.504). Table 11.3 provides some common techniques to verify requestors of health information.

Clearly defined processes for the purpose of patient verification and request verification should be addressed within written policies and procedures for disclosure management within an organization.

State Privacy and Security Laws

One of the challenges of compliance with privacy and security regulations is navigating between adhering to federal regulations, such as HIPAA, or state law requirements. HIPAA establishes the minimum requirements for application of privacy and security standards under state law. Many states have laws and regulations that are more stringent than HIPAA. This requires a covered entity to evaluate and apply the regulations based on both federal and state privacy, security, and breach notification requirements for protected health information.

HIPAA requirements state that covered entities and business associates must comply with both the federal privacy and security regulations as well as state privacy and security regulations (Dinh 2010). Preemption is defined as the principle that a statute at one level supersedes or is applied over the same or similar statute at a lower level (45 CFR 160.202). When both laws are unable to be properly complied with, the state law is either considered to be contrary or more stringent. State law is considered to be **contrary** when (1) a covered entity determines that

it is impossible to comply with both the federal and state privacy regulations; or (2) compliance with the state law would create a barrier to compliance with the federal regulations under HIPAA (Dinh 2010). In the event that a state regulation is considered to be contrary to the HIPAA regulations, a request to accept a provision of state law can be submitted to the secretary of Health and Human Services (HHS) from an elected official or designee (AHIMA 2013a).

In some cases, state laws are considered to be more stringent that federal laws. Under HIPAA, state law is considered more **stringent** if the law prohibits or restricts use or disclosure in circumstances under which such use or disclosure would be permitted under federal law. State law is considered to be more stringent if it:

- Gives an individual greater rights to acquire, copy, or amend their PHI
- Further prohibits the use and disclosure of protected health information
- Provides the individual greater rights of access to the information

- Requires greater authorization requirements for compliance
- Requires more privacy protections
- Requires greater protection with sensitive notes such as mental health or HIV/AIDS (HHS 2013).

For example, under the Minnesota Health Record Act, a patient must provide authorization to release patient information for the purposes of treatment, payment, and healthcare operations (TPO). While HIPAA states that information can be shared for the purposes of TPO, Minnesota law is stricter and requires a signature for the release of information for the purpose of TPO (Revisor of Statutes, State of Minnesota 2015). Covered entities and business associates need to do due diligence to understand both state law and federal law to assure they are adequately complying with privacy and security regulations.

Check Your Understanding 11.2

Instructions: **Answer the following questions on a separate piece of paper.**

1. If state law mandated more requirements on an authorization that the HIPAA regulations, the state law is considered to be
   A. Strict
   B. Contrary
   C. Conflicting
   D. Stringent

2. How many identifiers are required to be removed during deidentifcation under the safe harbor method?
   A. 14
   B. 17
   C. 18
   D. 20

3. True or false: If a patient requests that his or her name is removed from the hospital directory, the hospital must comply and remove the patient's name.

4. True or false: PHI can be used and disclosed without permission of the patient if the PHI is deidentified.

5. If an attorney comes in to request medical records for a malpractice case that he or she is assigned to, what documentation requirements are necessary to release the records, and what type of verification should be completed prior to releasing the records?

Managing an Effective Security Program

Managing all the patient data and information that a healthcare organization creates, receives, maintains, or transmits can be a challenge; however, it is a necessity to ensure the confidentiality, integrity, and availability of health information. The HIPAA Security Rule requires organizations to implement a variety of physical, technical, and administrative safeguards to protect patient data.

The Office for the National Coordinator for Health Information Technology created the *Guide to Privacy and Security of Health Information* to guide healthcare organizations through the establishment and creation of a privacy and security compliance program within their organization. The guide reinforces the importance of the establishment and creation of a security management process within a healthcare organization (ONC 2015). A seven-step approach for creation of an effective security program within the guide provides the following steps:

- Step 1: Lead your culture, select your team, and learn
- Step 2: Document your process, findings, and actions
- Step 3: Review existing security of ePHI
- Step 4: Develop an action plan
- Step 5: Manage and mitigate risks
- Step 6: Attest for Meaningful Use security-related objects (if applicable)
- Step 7: Monitor, audit, and update security on an ongoing basis (ONC 2015).

Policies and procedures are an effective part of governance to create consistency in processes across the organization. Supporting the organization's goals and objectives and properly creating policies and procedures that directly link the organization's objectives and mission are key steps toward building an effective security management program (Thakkar and Davis 2006). In addition, they assist in the creation of the basic understanding and uniformity for an organization, supporting the information security governance model being designed. It is a necessary part of the oversight and governance structure of security management that the policies and procedures are evaluated and monitored on a regular basis to assure compliance and enforcement within an organization (Thakkar and Davis 2006; Walsh 2013a).

Risk Analysis and Risk Management

Under HIPAA, healthcare organizations and business associates must execute a risk analysis by conducting a complete and accurate **assessment** of the potential risks and vulnerabilities to the confidentiality, integrity, and availability of electronic protected health information (ePHI) (45 CFR 164.308(a)(1)(ii)(A); Walsh 2013a; CMS 2007a). A **risk analysis** is a systemic process for reviewing all systems, applications, and processes to identify potential threats and vulnerabilities, document current controls, and understand the likelihood of the impact (Walsh 2013a).

HIPAA does not define the methodology for how to conduct the risk analysis due to the vast difference in healthcare organizations and covered entities, nor does the regulation define how often a risk analysis needs to be completed. It is up to each individual covered entity and business associate to create and establish a policy, procedure, and process for regularly conducting a risk analysis. A common methodology for risk analysis is based on the framework defined by the National Institute of Standards and Technology (NIST):

- System characterization
- Threat identification
- Control assessment
- Vulnerability identification
- Likelihood determination
- Impact analysis
- Risk determination
- Recommendation for controls
- Results documentation (NIST 2012)

In addition to conducting a risk analysis, a plan should be established for the **risk management** component of the HIPAA requirements that requires covered entities and business associates to implement security measures sufficient to reduce risks and vulnerabilities to a reasonable level (45 CFR 164.308(a)(1)(ii)(B)) (see table 11.4 for the five security components for risk management). Based on the findings from the risk analysis, covered entities and business associates need to evaluate and implement adequate and appropriate security measures and controls that will sufficiently reduce or eliminate the risks and vulnerabilities to an organization. When addressing risks, three basic methods to address the risk exist. The first method is to **mitigate the risk**, which refers to the process of reducing or eliminating the risk by implementing a control. The next method is to **transfer the risk** by outsourcing or insuring the risk against any potential loss to the organization. The last method is to **accept the risk**, understanding that **residual risk** will exist as no additional controls would be implemented leaving some risk to the organization (Walsh

Table 11.4.   Five security components for risk management

Security component	Examples of vulnerabilities	Examples of security mitigation strategies
Administrative safeguards	• No security officer is designated • Workforce is not trained or is unaware of privacy and security issues	• Security officer is designated and publicized • Workforce training begins at hire and is conducted on a regular and frequent basis • Security risk analysis is performed periodically and when a change occurs in the practice or the technology
Physical safeguards	• Facility has insufficient locks and other barriers to patient data access • Computer equipment is easily accessible by the public • Portable devices are not tracked or not locked up when not in use	• Building alarm systems are installed • Officers are locked
Technical safeguards	• Poor controls allow inappropriate access to EHR • Audit logs are not used enough to monitor users and other EHR activities • No measures are in place to keep electronic patient data from improper changes • No contingency plan exists • Electronic exchanges of patient information are not encrypted or otherwise secured	• Secure user IDs, passwords, and appropriate role-based access are used • Routine audits of access and changes to EHR are conducted • Anti-hacking and anti-malware software is installed • Contingency plans and data backup plans are in place • Data is encrypted
Organizational standards	• No breach notification and associated policies exist • Business associate (BA) agreements have not been updated in several years	• Regular reviews of agreements are conducted and updated made accordingly
Policies and procedures	• Generic written policies and procedures to ensure HIPAA security compliance were purchased but not followed • The manager performs ad hoc security measures	• Written policies and procedures are implemented and staff is trained • Security team conducts monthly review of user activities • Routine updates are made to document security measures

Source: ONC 2015.

2013a). No risks should be left unaddressed or unevaluated. Each risk should be evaluated and fall into one of the categories noted.

The EHR incentive program, or Meaningful Use, has returned the focus to HIPAA risk analysis and risk management through the requirements of the programs. Stage 1 and 2 of Meaningful Use both require covered entities to protect ePHI stored, maintained, and transmitted in an EHR by conducting a risk analysis in accordance with the HIPAA regulation and mitigate all risks identified, as appropriate. This requirement of the EHR incentive program is the first time that a requirement regarding the frequency of conducting a risk analysis has been established through federal legislation. An eligible hospital or eligible provider must conduct or update the HIPAA risk analysis for each time (attestation period) that they attest for Meaningful Use (Walsh 2013a). The risk analysis and risk management process must be conducted in the year that the attestation took place and prior to the end of the attestation period. It is important to have clearly written risk analysis reports and risk management documentation that show supporting dates and evidence that the work was completed prior to the end of a specific attestation period. Refer to chapter 1 for more information on Meaningful Use.

Audit Logs and Monitoring

As data becomes more electronic, the HIPAA regulations play an important part in the safe keeping of information. After the implementation of an EHR, a process for regular security audits should be implemented. The HIPAA Security Rule requires an organization to (1) implement a process for regular review of system activity, and (2) implement hardware, software, and such to allow the ability to track and review activity on an information system (45 CFR 164.308(a)(1)(ii)(D)). Reviewing electronic systems and activities to test the adequacy and effectiveness of data security by conducting security **audits** can help a healthcare organization proactively assure that the information they store and maintain is only being accessed for the normal course of business. To be a certified EHR for Meaningful Use, EHR vendors must be able to provide an **audit log**, a chronological record of electronic system activities (AHIMA 2014b) of individual user activity over a period of time, as well as record different actions that a user takes within the system (AHIMA 2011). The core steps of an effective audit and monitoring program are:

- Determine what systems produce audit logs
- Establish a process and document a procedure
- Define and determine who and what will be audited
- Create and implement effective audit tools
- Define and determine who will conduct the audits and the frequency
- Define the process for confronting employees when audits determine a potential breach
- Define and document the process for documenting audits and how long the data will be kept

By establishing an effective program, an organization can assure they are protecting patient information and meeting the requirements of HIPAA.

Another area in which HIPAA mandates monitoring is login monitoring (45 CFR 164.308(a)(5)(ii)(C; CMS 2007a). Covered entities and business associates must assure that procedures are established for review of system logins and that a process exists for reporting and reviewing any potential discrepancies. Some systems are set up with capabilities to produce alerts or warnings when a number of failed logins have occurred. In other cases, a user may be locked out of the system or require a password reset if they fail a login for a predetermined amount of times (CMS 2007a). Clear policies and procedures should be written to address how login discrepancies will be reviewed and evaluated.

In 2015, many large scale data breaches were reported due to hacking into systems with user names and passwords of credentialed people. Evaluation from these large data breaches indicates that many systems and servers are not equipped with robust log file audit reports and software that helps to assist and manage login monitoring. While these systems may not be able to block hackers and malware that get access to the system, they will assist in the identification of suspicious activity based on logins and potential activity happening (Tittel and Follis 2015). They can assist in an early detection of a potential security incident or data breach.

Contingency Planning

A **contingency plan**, also known as a disaster plan, prepares organizations for an event that may happen that could impact the ability to access patient information, the integrity of the information, or the confidentiality of information. The contingency plan requires all covered entities and business associates to adequately plan in case of an event that disrupts normal day-to-day operations (45 CFR 164.308(a)(7); CMS 2007a). In recent years there have been many cases across the United States where contingency planning needed to be established, such as the flooding and Hurricane Katrina in New Orleans, LA, and the F5 tornado in Joplin, MO. The HIPAA Security Rule requires healthcare organization to create a contingency plan in the case of such events so that there is a strategy in place to assure ePHI is available when needed. Refer to chapter 10 for information on organizational contingency planning.

Data Backups

The first requirement under the contingency planning regulation is data backup (45 CFR 164.308(a)(7)(ii)(A)). This HIPAA requirement mandates that organizations create and store exact copies of electronic protected health information (CMS 2007a). This requirement exists to assure that in the event of a loss of data, the data will be able to be restored to support continuity of care and business operations. Healthcare organizations need to ensure that all data are being backed up, not just the data in the electronic health record. For example, on a daily basis, the server that houses the EHR, file system, and PACs system is backed up to a cloud-based server that allows for an exact retrievable copy. It is important to evaluate the organization to know all existing systems that store and maintain protected health information to properly understand backup processes. Each of the electronic systems should have a documented **data backup plan** that defines how the system is being backed up, the method of backing up the data, location of the backup, frequency of the backup, and testing of the backup (AHIMA 2013c). Table 11.5 represents an example of documentation that should be maintained as part of a data backup plan.

Backup storage needs to be taken into consideration for all backup systems. There have been numerous data breaches reported due to lost and stolen backup tapes. Additionally, healthcare organizations should evaluate the process of encrypting backup media to know that they are properly secured in the event of lost or stolen backup (AHIMA 2013c). An example of a data breach occurring with unencrypted backups occurred in 2011. A data breach was reported impacting approximately 1.6 million patients due to the loss of unencrypted computer data backups that contained patient billing information. The data breach could have been prevented if the backups were encrypted, which would verify the information unreadable and indecipherable (Healthcare Informatics 2011). Healthcare organizations should make certain that only authorized staff have access to the data backups (AHIMA 2013c). To support the backup process, AHIMA recommends a functional backup plan that includes the following:

- Processes for backing up all data on all systems, as well as steps for recreating all components of the health information system

- Description and location of all components of the electronic, hybrid, or paper records, and the configuration of any networked device including hardware and software deployed

- Processes for recreating data tables, contracts, licenses, and policies and procedures

- Assignment of responsibility for each component that identifies backup personnel if key individuals are inaccessible or incapacitated

- An estimate of how long the organization or provider can continue to function at various stages of recovery (AHIMA 2013c, 8).

Table 11.5. Examples of data backup documentation

System name	Purpose of system	Location of system	Backup process	Backup location	Frequency of backup	Testing frequency
ABC Health System	Electronic health record	Onsite Server #1A	Backup Cloud System–Cloud Based	Cloud-Based System in Austin, TX	Continuous backup	Data tested monthly
ABC Health System	Lab information system	Onsite Server #2A	Weekly Tape BackUp	On-site Backup, stored in fireproof safe in the Ambulance Garage	Weekly backup	Data tested monthly

Source: AHIMA 2013c.

A well-defined data backup plan with well-established physical controls is critical to helping an organization restore data in the event of an emergency.

Disaster Recovery Plan

The second requirement of the contingency planning regulation is that covered entities and business associates should have a **disaster recovery plan** that defines the processes for recovery of data in the event of a disaster. Stated in 45 CFR 164.308(a)(7)(ii)(B), procedures should be created to restore any loss of data that may have occurred (CMS 2007a). The disaster recovery plan should be specific to each hospital unit or clinical location and allow guidance and support for decision-making processes regarding the data created during a disaster (AHIMA 2013c).

The disaster recovery plan should also address how the data that are created during a downtime will be restored in the electronic format. When defining data restoration, healthcare organizations need to address what information will be back-entered into the electronic system, the steps and processes for entering data, including sequence of events, communication regarding data restoration, and verification and checks on the integrity of the restored data (AHIMA 2013c; CMS 2007a). With the system being unavailable, most of the documentation will be done in a paper format. An organization should evaluate what information will be entered into the system, or back-entered when the system is available again and what information will be scanned into the system. The back-entered information will be based on patient care needs, reimbursement requirements, and organization workflow. A clearly defined plan for the restoration of data should be documented and kept within the contingency planning documentation.

Emergency Mode Operation Plan

As part of contingency planning, all covered entities and business associates need to create a plan on how they will run and operate day-to-day operations in the event of an emergency (45 CFR 164.308(a)(7)(ii)(C)). An **emergency mode operation plan** creates processes and procedures to support the continuation of critical business and patient care operations while protecting the security of ePHI in the event of a disaster (CMS 2007a). Important areas to cover within the emergency operation plan are how the covered entity or business associate will protect the confidentiality, integrity, and accessibility of the ePHI; what additional security measures need to be implemented to provide protection; processes and procedures for collection of data and protection of the data; and contact information for key people involved in the emergency mode operations plan (CMS 2007a). The plan should be easily accessible to all of those who need it in the event of an emergency.

The emergency mode plan may include the following:

- Detailed communication plan including scope of disaster, extent of resources disabled, and recovery and restoration process as it occurs
- Documentation requirements needed at a minimum
- Emergency registration sets including patient identification
- Emergency paper chart
- Downtime procedures for paper documentation
- Stickers or other processes for alerts of allergies
- Filing procedures that will allow information to be accessed a later date and time (AHIMA 2013c).

Creating a plan and training staff on this process is essential. During an emergency, the day-to-day operations can become frantic. With proper planning and preparing of the emergency plan, the workforce of an organization will feel confident and the likelihood of ePHI being mishandled will be reduced.

Emergency Access

Another area that needs to be addressed within a contingency plan is how the organization will manage and provide emergency access into systems (45 CFR 164.312(a)(2)(ii)). Covered entities and business associates should ensure that procedures exist for obtaining access to the necessary ePHI in the event of an emergency situation. This requirement defines instructions and practices for providing and obtaining access to pertinent ePHI in the event of an emergency (CMS 2007b). The procedures should evaluate different emergency scenarios, determine what workforce members might need access to ePHI, what ePHI they will need access to, how the access will be obtained, and who is responsible for providing access (CMS 2007b).

Software Criticality Analysis

Under the HIPAA Security Rule, covered entities and business associates should assess all current systems and applications that interact with patient information and are defined in the contingency plan and conduct a criticality analysis for each individual application (45 CFR 164.308(a)(7)(ii)(E); CMS 2007a). A **criticality analysis** consists of evaluating each of the different systems of the organization to determine how crucial the information in the system is to day-to-day healthcare operations and patient care (CMS 2007a). The goal of this addressable requirement is to create a listing that prioritizes all systems to allow for the successful restoration of critical systems more efficiently after an unexpected or expected downtime. Having clear, established processes in the event of a disaster or interruption to system is critical to data management.

Data Security Methods

Data security is the process in which organizations implement different tools that help protect and safeguard protected health information. The Security Rule allows for healthcare organizations to be flexible with the implementation of different data security methods depending on the needs of the organization. Common types of data security methods include authentication, malicious software protection and evaluation, data encryption, and other methods. Chapter 12 provides addition information regarding data security methodology on specific technologies.

Authentication

User authentication is the front-line process for protecting sensitive information that an organization has ownership over. **User authentication** is the process where an end user logs into an electronic system using specific credentials defined by the organization. Whether it is information about a patient's personal health information or sensitive business information, it is important to create a process to govern how authentication processes will be used and deployed within an organization. Some common forms of authentication are a username and password, a user name and personal identification number, and biometrics log-in. The most common use of authentication in healthcare is username and password. Through the push of government regulations, password management is becoming a requirement and allows for organizations to focus attention and funding on managing passwords. For most computer systems, the user identification (ID) and password is the first step in the authentication process to access a network (Weirich and Sasse 2002). Knowing that password authentication is a commonly used mechanism for organizations, user IDs and passwords remain the most vulnerable to an organization's security as they are the easiest to hack and gain access to a system (Holt 2011). With the user ID and password being used to access all information on an information network, organizations must assure they are effectively and efficiently managing passwords within their organization.

The first step to building an effective password management process within an organization is to create a systemwide policy that defines password management. The policy should include standards regarding the length of the password, what type of characters need to be included in the password, the process of password expiration, the process of password reuse, sharing of passwords, and potential sanctions or penalties (AHIMA e-HIM Workgroup 2009). With a standard policy used systemwide, organizations have the ability to better govern and use passwords within their systems and protect their information against hackers.

Password strength is an important factor for effective password management. It is always encouraged that users use passwords that are unique and not predictable. While password length alone is not the determination of a strong password, it is recommended that password be eight characters in length at a minimum (Holt 2011). In addition to password length, strong passwords also consist of three of the four from the following categories: numeric, alphabetic, capitals, and symbols (Zhang et al. 2010). A common way to create a strong password is to determine what a password is and make it more secure by adding symbols and numbers. For example, the password "SummerTime-Sunshine," it becomes more secure and meets best practices by changing some characters to "$ummerT!meSun$h1ne." By implementing and increasing password strength, the ability to guess a password and hack into a system decreases.

Another important process for password management is requiring that passwords expire regularly. The regular expiration of passwords allows for organizations to properly reduce the ability for hackers to gain and maintain access to systems with proprietary and personal information (Mercuri 2004). Best practice in the industry suggests that passwords change every 120 to 180 days. Many organizations are implementing self-service password reset software that will remove some of the costs of having to staff and maintain a robust help desk for password management reset (Holt 2011). With the regular changing of passwords, information becomes more secure and less likely that a hacker will be able to access it.

The use of a username and a PIN is also a form of authentication. This process is very similar to the strategy of using a username and password; however, the password is replaced with a PIN. In some cases, PINs are selected by the user and do not change each time the individual logs in to the system. In other cases, the PIN is a generated code from an alternate device such as a token or a text message. When a code is autogenerated, the PIN will only be valid for a specific length of time to provide added security to the authentication process (McKay 2014).

Another form of authentication is the use of biometric identifiers. **Biometric authentication** allows a user to be uniquely identified and access the system based on one or more biometric traits such as fingerprints, hand geometry, retinal pattern, or voice waves. The most common and oldest form of biometrics is fingerprint recognition. It is also

the most cost effective biometric authentication process that is available. Not only are the devices for the scanning of the fingerprint more reasonably priced, the storage space needed to store the data and information regarding the fingerprint doesn't require a lot of space (PBWorks 2007). The technology is designed to read the specific ridges and characteristics that make up a person's fingerprint. Since the fingerprint is unique and detailed to each specific person, it is difficult to duplicate (Zorkadis and Donos 2004). In addition to the use of fingerprint technology, other biometric technology is also starting to emerge.

Another biometric technology that continues to become popular in authentication is voice recognition technology. Voice recognition technology is based on different vocal characteristics that individuals possess. Like fingerprint technology, voice recognition technology is relatively cost effective and nonintrusive to the end users. A disadvantage with voice recognition technology is that it is easier to hack and has a low reliability standard (Zorkadis and Donos 2004). Organizations that implement voice recognition should have a good security and governance structure to manage and protect the data files containing the voice recognition.

The highest reliability for biometric use today is retina scan technology. While this technology tends to cost the most due to the storage space required to store the data and the cameras that are needed to take the scan of the retina, it has the lowest acceptability among end users as it is the most invasive biometric technology (Zorkadis and Donos 2004). Since it is the highest cost and the most challenging to convince people to use, it is least common type of biometric use for authentication purposes.

Encryption and Decryption of ePHI

Under HIPAA, encryption of data is defined in two separate requirements: the encryption of data at rest and the encryption of data in motion (45 CFR 164.312(a)(2)(iv); 45 CFR 164.312(e)(2)(ii)). **Data at rest** is when the data are in storage within a database or on a server and are no longer being used or access. **Data in motion** are data in the process of being transmitted from one location to another location such as an e-mail. Both of the requirements under HIPAA are addressable requirements, which allows the covered entity and business associate to evaluate and determine if they are going to implement the technical safeguard. If the covered entity chooses not to implement the encryption safeguards, other safeguards to protect the information need to be documented, including the reason for not implementing the encryption (CMS 2007b).

Encryption is defined as a mathematical method for the transformation of data from plaintext into cipher text, allowing no individual or machine to get access and decipher the original information (45 CFR 164.304). Plaintext is the original text that has not been altered and cipher text is unreadable or indecipherable text due to encryption. The process of transforming the information from cipher text to plaintext is referred to as decryption (Stine and Dang 2011). In order to encrypt the information, the plaintext is changed into cipher text using a cryptographic key. A cryptographic key is the tool applied to the data in order to turn the information into cipher text as well as converting the data from cipher text back to plaintext (Stine and Dang 2011). Figure 11.1 depicts the process when data is encrypted and when the data is decrypted.

Under the final HIPAA Omnibus Rule, information is considered to be secure information if it is encrypted. Secure information is considered unreadable, unusable, and indecipherable (Stine and Dang 2011). Under the Breach Notification Rule, if the information is considered secure PHI, then an investigation does not need to take place and the determination that a breach did not occur can be applied to most scenarios. Essentially, encryption allows the assumption that the data is secured and therefore no risk to the data or patient has occurred (Butler 2015). The final HIPAA Omnibus Rule of 2013 also added a few standards regarding encryption into the regulations. While it did not change any of the regulations from the HIPAA Security Rule, it did call out a few examples of use of encryption. The HIPAA Final Omnibus Rule of 2013 allows for patients to get access to PHI in an electronic format if the PHI is part of the organization's designated record set and stored in an electronic format. While encryption of the medium used to provide the electronic copy is not required, covered entities should implement proper safeguards to ensure the ePHI are in place, including encryption of information (AHIMA 2013b). E-mail is an acceptable method for producing the electronic copy of information; however, if the covered entity is using unencrypted e-mail, the patient must be advised and agree to the risks to the data while being sent in an unencrypted format (AHIMA 2013b). Covered entities should create a policy and procedure for electronic access to ePHI to address this requirement and establish how the information will be protected.

Stage 2 Meaningful Use also adds encryption into different areas of its requirements. Under stage 2 Meaningful Use, eligible providers and eligible hospitals must "protect electronic health information created or maintained by the Certified EHR Technology through the implementation of appropriate technical capabilities" (Walsh 2013b, 7). This process happens by conducting a

Figure 11.1. The process of data encryption and data decryption

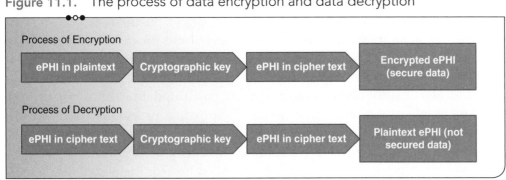

Source: Stine and Dang 2011.

risk analysis and risk management processes in accordance with HIPAA. The difference between the risk analysis requirement under stage 1 and stage 2 of Meaningful Use is that under stage 2, eligible providers and eligible hospitals must address the encryption and security of data at rest within the risk analysis (Walsh 2013b). This should be clearly defined within the risk analysis report and addressed within the risk mitigation plan depending on the findings.

From 2014 to 2015, covered entities and business associates saw a spike in the number of data breaches due to hacking into systems, as well as lost and stolen devices. Twenty-one data breaches occurred involving hacking and information technology (IT) incidents in 2014. In 2015, the number of data breaches involving hacking and IT incidents increased to 48. Anthem, Inc. reported the largest data breach in the history of the Breach Notification Rule due to hacking in 2015. This data breach impacted approximately 78,000,000 individuals (HHS 2015b). With the implementation of encryption technology of laptops and other portable media, some of the large-scale data breaches could have been prevented as the data would have been secured and not able to be accessed or used (Butler 2015). One of the best tools for preventing and fighting data breaches is the implementation of encryption of data at rest and data in motion. Evaluation of all ePHI should be defined and evaluated to determine if encryption is appropriate to protect data.

Malicious Software Management

HIPAA requires covered entities and business associates to protect all ePHI from malicious software, also known as malware, by implementing policies and procedures for the guarding against, detecting, and reporting malicious software within their organization (45 CFR 164.308(a)(5)(ii)(B)). **Malware** is any program that causes harm to systems by unauthorized access, unauthorized disclosure, destruction, or loss of integrity of any information.

There are many types of malware that can get into systems. Some of the common types of malware that healthcare organizations obtain are:

- **Viruses**: Programs that search out other programs and infect them by embedding a copy of itself. This type of malware has the capability to spread to other computers by attaching itself to programs shared through a network.

- **Worms**: Programs that reproduce on their own that have no need for a host application, they are self-contained programs.

- **Trojan horses**: Programs that are disguised as a normal program to trick users to download the file.

- **Logic bombs**: Malware that will execute a program, or a string of code, when a certain event happens.

- **Rootkit**: Type of malicious software that will remotely access or control a computer without being detected by users or security programs (Vericode 2012).

Malware gets into systems through a variety of different methods. Some frequent methods of infiltration of malware are through e-mail attachments, downloaded programs, social media sites, inappropriate websites, and lack of updating security patches (CMS 2007a). The challenges that healthcare organizations face in regard to malware and the impact on ePHI are:

- Data breaches
- Unauthorized access or disclosure of ePHI
- Increased central processing unit (CPU) use
- Slowed computer response time
- Modified or deleted files
- Additions or changes to ePHI being stored (Vericode 2012).

Covered entities and business associates need to establish policies and procedures for the management of malware within the organization. At a minimum, the policies and procedures should define security patch updating, antivirus process and review, reporting processes for malware infestations, containment and removal processes, verification of integrity of ePHI after a malware attached, and education for the workforce on malware (CMS 2007a). Written policies and procedures help to create consistent management over malware within organizations.

The patch management process includes ensuring the application of security patches for operating systems on all computers, servers, and applications within an organization. Organizations should create a process that when security updates are released to hardware or software, they should be tested and applied as soon as possible to prevent malware from being implemented on the organization's network. In addition, antivirus software should be applied to all hardware within the organization (Walsh 2013b). Antivirus software reviews and checks all the files on the computer or server to ensure there is no malware that can be identified within the system. Antivirus software can also provide real-time evaluation and blocking of potential threatening software from being applied to a computer or server. Additionally, organizations should ensure a process of security verification of all attachments received through e-mail. Some systems can be applied to e-mail that will scan the attachment for potential threats prior to downloading. These systems will alert the end user that there is potential harm if the attachment is downloaded. Staff training is crucial for ensuring that malware is not able to get into an organization's network.

In 2014, Anchorage Community Mental Health Services was fined $150,000 due to a data breach that was caused by malware accessing and compromising security to ePHI due to a data breach that occurred in 2012. In March 2012, the ePHI of 2,700 individuals was compromised when malware was able to get into the network and access ePHI stored in this organization (HHS 2014). The organization had a policy and procedure established for the management of malware and patch management within the organization; however, the policy and procedure was not being properly followed. In addition, security updates were not being implementing in a timely fashion, which caused the data breach to occur (HHS 2014). This was the first fine applied to an organization regarding malware management within an organization.

Check Your Understanding 11.3

Instructions: **Answer the following questions on a separate piece of paper.**

1. What are the three basic methods to address risk after a HIPAA risk analysis?
   A. Mitigate, transfer, accept
   B. Transfer, accept, delete
   C. Residual, transfer, delete
   D. Transfer, accept, residual

2. True or false: The HIPAA Security Rule requires an organization to review system activity only when a security breach occurs.

3. When establishing an audit and monitoring program, the first step is:
   A. Evaluate who should be audited and when
   B. Determine which systems produce audit logs
   C. Create a plan when a discrepancy arises
   D. Train staff on audit process

4. True or false: Data in motion are data stored within a database or on a server where it is no longer being used or access.

5. Which of the following is a potential impact of a virus getting onto an end-user device?
   A. Modified or deleted files
   B. Merging of user accounts
   C. Additional safeguards created
   D. Automatic saving of information

6. The process of an end user logging into an electronic system using specific credentials defined by the organization is called:

   A. Malware detection

   B. Encryption of data

   C. Verification of integrity of data

   D. User authentication

7. Define and explain the basic steps in the process of encryption of health data from plaintext to cipher text.

Management of Privacy and Security in Health Information Exchange

Health information exchange (HIE) is the process of electronic exchange of patient-specific information between two separate healthcare organizations (Kern and Kaushal 2007; Rhodes and Scichilone 2012). HIE can assist with the ability to improve quality of care and reduce healthcare costs for the patient and healthcare organization. With a combination of mandates and financial incentives from the government and the desire to improve patient care, many healthcare organizations want to be able to electronically exchange information; however, HIE does come with some concerns regarding the privacy and security of patient information.

A properly established health information exchange allows for many benefits to the patient as well as the healthcare organization. If the information is available electronically, it can help "to provide safer, more timely, efficient, effective, and patient-centered care" (AHIMA 2007, 3). The United States has a fragmented method of storing electronic health information. Many different types of electronic health records exist that do not have the capability to communicate with one another (Rhodes 2013). Pursuing health information exchange requires that organizations evaluate the benefits and risks to the organization. With the implementation of a HIE, covered entities need to evaluate current HIPAA privacy and security practices to assure adequate safeguards are established to control access to the information and provide adequate security.

One of the first challenges the healthcare community faces with a health information exchange is the assurance of the correct patient identity. Many groups continue to create and enhance a wide variety of technology solutions to help the matching of patients within a health information exchange; however, there is not one method that is 100 percent accurate and guarantees a match (AHIMA 2014a).

With the challenge of patient matching, advances in technology have created additional methods for patient matching within health information exchange, which include:

- Advanced algorithm methods
- Plastic identification cards
- Subscriber identity models for mobile phones and electronic passports
- Biometric identification (fingerprint, facial recognition, iris scanning, voice recognition)

The challenge with the advanced technology is there is a greater cost to the healthcare industry to implement (AHIMA 2014a). Additionally, if not all healthcare organizations can implement the technology; it reduces the ability for the technology to become effective in patient matching.

Another issue that challenges health information exchange is to ensure consumer privacy for information that is being exchanged in the HIE.

HIPAA provides regulations regarding patients' rights to information, patient restriction of information, and adequate privacy safeguards to protecting patient information. AHIMA and HIMSS (2011) conducted a gap analysis on HIE related to privacy and security. Two gaps were identified in regard to consumer privacy:

- Patient consent and authorization—ensuring adequate authorizations and consents are established to engage in HIE

- Restriction of sensitive information—potentially unable to protect sensitive health information such as behavioral health, drug abuse, and other sensitive diagnoses

Healthcare organizations must establish adequate processes to help reduce the risk to consumer security when it comes to health information exchange (AHIMA and HIMSS 2011).

HIEs bring many challenges to the compliance of the HIPAA security regulations. One of the basic steps to ensure adequate security safeguards are established for health information exchange is to conduct a risk analysis on the HIE. This should include analysis of all potential risks associated with the confidentiality, integrity, and accessibility of the data transmitted and stored in the HIE (AHIMA and HIMSS 2011). Some common areas of risk documented from the gap analysis performed for the HIE are as follows:

- Implementation of unique user identification
- Limitation of access to information needed for purpose of use of data
- Authentication processes
- Oversight and management of access management
- Evaluation of audit trails
- Management of failed logins
- Continuous technical evaluation (AHIMA and HIMSS 2011)

Without the establishment of basic principles that align with the HIPAA security regulations, HIE can be an easy target for unauthorized use and disclosure of protected health information management.

AHIMA and HIMSS (2011) recommend the following steps to manage and reduce risks to the privacy and security of patient information during health information exchange. The first step in the successful implementation of a HIE is to conduct a risk analysis to evaluate the potential risks to the organization and the data. All risks should be identified and a risk management plan created to help reduce or eliminate the risks associated with the HIE (AHIMA and HIMSS 2011). This will help to eliminate potential risks and reduce those that are able to be managed through implemented security controls.

In addition to mitigating the risks identified in the security risk analysis, a healthcare organization should create a policy and procedure to manage HIE within their organization. The policy and procedure should create consistent practices across the organization for access and use of the HIE and how information will be implemented and used for current care practices. At a minimum, the policy and procedure should define:

- Consent and authorization processes
- Patient identification and matching processes
- User access management processes
- Termination of user processes
- Access of patient information processes
- Breach notification processes if through HIE
- Secondary use of HIE data into the organization's record
- Audit trail review process and functionality
- Business associate agreement processes
- Data integrity management processes (AHIMA and HIMSS 2011; Landsbach and Just 2013)

Having clearly defined processes can help create a HIE governance structure within an organization that clearly identifies how and when the HIE is to be used, and protects the confidentiality, integrity, and accessibility of the information.

Another recommendation for managing privacy and security of HIE is to have a dedicated person or team responsible for the internal management of the HIE. Assigning a dedicated individual to manage the internal processes of when, how, and by whom the data in the HIE can be used will help alleviate some of the challenges and stresses that come with no oversight and management of a system (AHIMA and HIMSS 2011; Landsbach and Just 2013). This individual and team should be responsible for the creation of the policy and procedure, access management, review of audit trails, user termination processes, and overall evaluation of the use of HIE within the organization. By having dedicated individual(s) to manage the process and the development of a clear governance structure, the ability to successfully implement and manage HIE privacy and security within an organization is more easily attained.

The last recommendation for best practice of HIE is education of the workforce. Proper education should be provided to those individuals who will be using or interacting with the HIE or the data from the HIE in any manner to meet the requirements of their job responsibilities (AHIMA and HIMSS 2011). At minimum, training should cover the following areas:

- Process for consent and authorization
- Process for education to patients and families
- Process for adequate patient searching and patient matching
- Process for assurance of selection of the correct patient
- Process for patient information to be utilized to support care
- Process for processing patient information if used to support care
- Process for reporting any issues or concerns with the HIE and data being used
- Information regarding organization's evaluation of audit trails and supporting of patient care for accessing PHI in the HIE (AHIMA and HIMSS 2011).

Regular ongoing training should be a requirement. If there are concerns and issues with the way that the HIE is being utilized for supporting patient care, additional education should be provided.

Mobile Health Technology and HIPAA

With the increased use of technology within our healthcare organizations, health data is on the move now more than ever. To encourage the implementation and use of health information technology, many different mobile devices are being used within healthcare organizations. Common types of mobile devices being used include laptop computers, tablets, smart phones, USB drives, wearable technology, and external hard drives (Herzig 2012). The current term with mobile technology is **bring your own device** (BYOD), which refers to personal devices that are allowed to be used within a healthcare organization and interact with ePHI (Herzig 2012). As more mobile devices are being used in healthcare, risks emerge that impact the privacy and security of PHI and ePHI. If organizations are choosing to implement and use mobile technology, proper safeguards should be established for the management of mobile technology, compliance with HIPAA, and

protection of the security and privacy of patient information.

Healthcare organizations should evaluate and implement proper security measures to safeguard information being accessed on mobile technology. Best practices for the use of mobile technology within a healthcare organization or business associate include:

- Identification of device ownership
- Personal device use within the organization
- Required authorization for mobile technology use
- Conditions under which ePHI is allowed on mobile devices
- Acceptable behaviors and use of ePHI on mobile technology
- Safeguards and techniques for adequate protection of ePHI (encryption, access

management, remote wiping of data, data storage, and others)

- Procedures for reporting of a lost or stolen devices

- Evaluation and scanning of mobile technology on regular basis (Herzig 2012)

Policies and procedures should be established to help safeguard the mobile technology being used within the organization. The security management measures discussed earlier in this chapter should also be evaluated and implemented to mobile technology, as appropriate, to protect ePHI. In addition, regular employee education should be conducted to provide adequate awareness of the risks of mobile technology, including the processes and safeguards implemented to manage mobile technology use in the organization.

Check Your Understanding 11.4

Instructions: Answer the following questions on a separate piece of paper.

1. True or false: A healthcare organization should not be concerned if a workforce member uses a personal device to access patient information.

2. Which of the following is an example of a safeguard that can be implemented to protect patient information for health information exchange?
   A. Personal device use
   B. Unique user identification
   C. Malware detection
   D. Network access points

3. True or false: It is recommended that a dedicated person or team be assigned responsibility for the internal management of a HIE.

4. Best practices for the use of mobile technology include which of the following?
   A. Identifying device ownership
   B. Regular evaluation of mobile devices
   C. Required authorization for mobile technology use
   D. All of the above

5. Describe the areas that should be covered when educating the workforce about HIE.

Workforce Training

The HIPAA Privacy and Security Rules require formal education and training of the workforce to ensure ongoing accountability for the privacy and security of PHI. The Privacy Rule defines the workforce as "employees, volunteers, trainees, and other persons whose conduct in the performance of work for a covered entity is under the direct control of such entity, whether or not they are paid by the covered entity" (HHS 2013). The Omnibus Rule modified this definition to include business associates:

Employees, volunteers, trainees, and other persons whose conduct, in the performance of work for a covered entity or business associate, is under the direct control of such covered entity or business associate, whether or not they are paid by the covered entity or business associate. (AHIMA 2013a)

Although covered entities are not responsible for training the workforce of business associates, they should work closely with business associates to ensure all privacy and security training has been completed and documented (AHIMA 2013a). The Security Rule indicates that training must be applied to "all members of its workforce (including management)" (HHS 2013). The Rules independently address training requirements, and are nonprescriptive, giving organizations flexibility in implementation (AHIMA 2013a). The training component of HIPAA may be one of the largest and most important tasks in achieving compliance, as well as the most expensive and least effective if not performed properly (Amatayakul and Johns 2002). Therefore, it is especially important to examine the Privacy and Security Rules before planning a training program to gain a comprehensive understanding of the requirements needed to create a compliant training program in the most efficient manner possible.

The Privacy Rule requires that:

> A covered entity must train all members of its workforce on the policies and procedures with respect to protected health information required by this subpart, as necessary and appropriate for the members of the workforce to carry out their function within the covered entity. (HHS 2013)

This includes general training of HIPAA concepts and job specific training for new employees, as well as ongoing training for established employees, particularly for those whose job functions are affected by a change in policy or procedure.

The Security Rule mandates that entities "implement a security awareness and training program for all members of its workforce (including management)" (HHS 2013). Although this portion of the Security Rule is more abstract than the Privacy Rule, the underlying message is the same—the workforce must be trained effectively on the entity's policies and procedures as they relate to HIPAA, and the entity must have a program in place to address this on an ongoing basis. The security awareness and training standard identifies four addressable topics:

1. Security reminders: Implementing periodic security updates and reminders to the workforce. These can be done in many different mediums. Evidence of the reminders should

always be documented, including when they were done and what medium was used.

2. Protection from malicious software: Specifications on how the workforce is responsible for detecting, preventing, and reporting malicious software as well as system protection capabilities.

3. Login monitoring: Monitoring login attempts and the process for reporting discrepancies.

4. Password management: Procedures for creating, changing, and safeguarding passwords (AHIMA 2013a; KHA n.d.).

Between the Privacy Rule and the Security Rule, it is made clear that an entity must have a training program that is presented to all members of the workforce. The training program must cover information about privacy and security, how the two concepts relate to the employee's job and their workplace, and how they are addressed in the organization's policies and procedures. The program must also provide training on an ongoing basis and all of this must be documented by the entity. HIPAA asks that entities use a reasonable approach to achieving compliance, and that the efforts should reflect the size and scope of the business (Nutten 2003). The entity needs to use its best judgment to decide what is "reasonable" for them and what type of training program will work for their organization.

HIPAA Training Components

The Privacy and Security Rules can be further broken down to discern three distinct components of a compliant HIPAA training program. First, a program for training new employees should be in place. The Privacy Rule indicates that training on policies and procedures related to protected health information (PHI) needs to take place "within a reasonable period of time after the person joins the covered entity's workforce" (HHS 2013); and although the Security Rule does not specify a timeframe or impetus for training, one can infer that the training of new employees on security policies and procedures is required and expected to be done within a "reasonable period of time" from employment as well. This first category of training should include core training of general privacy and security principles such as purpose, background, and definitions (Gue 2003). It should also include information on the entity's particular policies and procedures regarding PHI and system security. Then, specific training should be provided based on the employee's job "as necessary and appropriate for the members of the workforce to carry out their function within the covered entity" (HHS 2013).

The second component of a HIPAA training program includes ongoing training and awareness-building. The Security Rule specifies "awareness" as a requirement of a training program that although not specified in the Privacy Rule, should be expanded to include privacy for continued workforce compliance (HHS 2013). The ongoing awareness and training on privacy and security should include everything that was addressed in initial training which includes core concepts, policies and procedures, and job specific information. This ongoing portion of the training program will reinforce the initial training and ensure that the behaviors expected by the workforce will become an automatic part of their daily activities.

The third component of a HIPAA training program addresses the inevitable changes that occur in any organization on a regular basis. As new laws and regulations are enacted, reorganization occurs and job duties change, or employees move into different roles within the organization, retraining needs to take place (Gue 2003). Furthermore, policies and procedures are continually being evaluated and changed, and new policies emerge. The Privacy Rule requires that as policies and procedures change over time, employees be kept apprised of these changes. In addition, employees are required to be trained on how the changes affect their job functions. Although this specification is not made in the Security Rule, one can deduce that retraining of the workforce on changing policies and procedures and the effects on job-specific functions is a requirement of ongoing compliance with the Security Rule as well.

The HIPAA Privacy Rule requires that "a covered entity must document that the training...has been provided" (HHS 2013). The Security Rule requires the maintenance of policies and procedures as necessary to comply with the standards. It further states, "if an action, activity, or assessment is required by this subpart to be documented, maintain a written (which may be electronic) record of the action, activity, or assessment" (AHIMA 2013a).

HIPAA Training Principles and Strategies

The HIPAA Privacy and Security Rules address minimum training standards that require scalability. Organizations can and should customize their programs to fit their operational needs as well as specific job responsibilities (AHIMA 2013a). Some of the privacy and security standards apply to a universal audience; however, other portions of the Rules may not. Taking the time to develop a comprehensive HIPAA training program can reduce the cost and administration of training by addressing audience overlap, reducing redundancies, and preventing multiple or conflicting messages. One approach to HIPAA workforce training is to consider creating levels of training. For example, level 1 would address the topics that are universal to the entire workforce, while level 2 would include training on topics that are specific to a role or job position. The training process should be prioritized so those who require training most urgently receive it as soon as possible. For example, workforce members who handle a large volume of PHI, such as nurses, would require more immediate training than those who have minimal access to PHI, such as building maintenance staff (AHIMA 2013a).

The following best practice guidance is recommended regarding HIPAA privacy and security training procedures:

- Provide general training for all workforce members, including contract workers.
- Establish timelines for training new employees according to their date of hire before the employee's first day of work in the department.
- Require annual training for all employees.
- Develop a training and awareness program that becomes part of the culture of the organization.

- Include in-depth education and ongoing awareness that includes training on PHI in all forms, including verbal, written, and electronic.
- Develop a regular communication process to address questions that arise after training and on an ongoing basis.
- Develop continuously updated reference materials of policies and procedures.
- Develop a procedure for evaluating training program effectiveness, reliability, and validity.
- Develop a process to verify that employees have completed privacy and security training before they receive access to paper and electronic PHI (AHIMA 2013a).

See chapter 24 for more information on effective training methods.

An important aspect of workforce training is documenting that such training has occurred. The documentation should include content, training dates, and attendee names (AHIMA 2013a).

Methods of documenting privacy and security training may include:

- Training program attendance sheets
- Signed statements acknowledging receipt and understanding of the training
- Electronic tracking of computer-based training or quiz and assessment results
- Training handouts, aids, and minutes
- E-mail communications
- A training database to record training activities such as e-mails, flier distribution, launching of screen savers or banners, or other organizational displays

It is essential that covered entities and business associates ensure that training and program assessments are documented on an ongoing basis. Revisions to training programs and methods should occur regularly and be based on assessment results, and all documents created should be maintained in accordance with HIPAA's retention requirement of six years (AHIMA 2013a).

Check Your Understanding 11.5

Instructions: **Answer the following questions on a separate piece of paper.**

1. True or false: HIPAA defines *workforce* as only those individuals that are paid by a covered entity.

2. What is the best timeframe to provide HIPAA education to the workforce?
    A. Only upon hire and policy changes
    B. Upon hire, after HIPAA policy changes, and when new regulations are implemented
    C. Upon hire, annual education, periodically throughout the year, and when policies change
    D. Annual education and periodically throughout the year

3. Under the HIPAA regulations, training of the workforce is defined in which of the following regulations?
    A. HIPAA Privacy Rule and Breach Notification Rule
    B. HIPAA Security Rule and Breach Notification Rule
    C. HIPAA Privacy Rule and Security Rule
    D. HIPAA Privacy Rule, Security Rule, and Breach Notification Rule

4. True or false: Covered entities are not responsible for training the workforce of business associates.

5. True or false: The HIPAA Privacy Rule requires that a covered entity document that HIPAA training has been provided to the workforce.

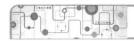

References

AHIMA and HIMSS. 2011. The Privacy and Security Gaps in Health Information Exchange. http://library.ahima.org/xpedio/groups/public/documents/ahima/bok1_049023.pdf

AHIMA e-HIM Workgroup. 2009. Best practices for electronic signature and attestation. *Journal of AHIMA* 80(11). http://library.ahima.org/xpedio/groups/public/documents/ahima/bok1_045551.hcsp?dDocName=bok1_045551

Amatayakul, M. and M.L. Johns. 2002. Compliance in the crosshairs: Targeting your training. *Journal of AHIMA* 73:16A-F.

American Health Information Management Association. 2014a. Managing the integrity of patient identity in health information exchange (updated). *Journal of AHIMA* 85(5):60–65.

American Health Information Management Association. 2014b. *Pocket Glossary of Health Information Management and Technology.* Chicago: AHIMA.

American Health Information Management Association. 2013a. Privacy and security training (updated). *Journal of AHIMA* 84(10). http://library.ahima.org/xpedio/groups/public/documents/ahima/ bok1_050439.hcsp?dDocName=bok1_050439

American Health Information Management Association. 2013b. Analysis of modification to the HIPAA privacy, security, enforcement, and breach notification rules under the Health Information Technology for Economic and Clinical Health Act and the Genetic Information Nondiscrimination Act; Other modifications to the HIPAA rules. http://library.ahima.org/xpedio/groups/public/documents/ahima/bok1_050067.pdf

American Health Information Management Association. 2013c. Disaster Planning and Recovery. http://library.ahima.org/xpedio/groups/secure/documents/ahima/bok1_050296.pdf

American Health Information Management Association. 2011. Security audits of electronic health information (updated). *Journal of AHIMA* 82(3):46–50. http://library.ahima.org/xpedio/groups/public/documents/ahima/bok1_048702.hcsp?dDocName=bok1_048702

American Health Information Management Association. 2007. HIM principles in health information exchange. *Journal of AHIMA* 78(7):1–9. http://library.ahima.org/xpedio/groups/public/documents/ahima/bok1_035095.hcsp?dDocName=bok1_035095

Butler, M. 2015. Cracking encryption: Despite benefits, technology still not widely used to combat multi-million dollar breaches. *Journal of AHIMA* 86(4):18–23. http://library.ahima.org/xpedio/groups/public/documents/ahima/bok1_050870.hcsp?dDocName=bok1_050870

Centers for Medicare and Medicaid Services. 2007a. HIPAA Security Series: Security Standards: Administrative Safeguards. http://www.hhs.gov/ocr/privacy/hipaa/administrative/securityrule/adminsafeguards.pdf

Centers for Medicare and Medicaid Services. 2007b. HIPAA Security Series: Security Standards: Technical Safeguards. http://www.hhs.gov/ocr/privacy/hipaa/administrative/securityrule/techsafeguards.pdf

Dimick, C. 2010. No harm done? Assessing risk of harm under the federal breach notification rule. *Journal of AHIMA* 81(8):20–25. http://library.ahima.org/xpedio/groups/public/documents/ahima/bok1_047857.hcsp?dDocName=bok1_047857

Dinh, A. 2010. Preemption of the HIPAA privacy rule (Updated). *Journal of AHIMA. http://library.ahima.org/xpedio/groups/public/documents/ahima/bok1_048022.hcsp?dDocName=bok1_048022*

Gue, D.G. 2003. Training—The First and Last Word in Privacy Compliance. http://www.hipaadvisory.com/action/awareness/privacytraining.htm

Harman, L.B. 2013. Ethical Issues in Health Information Management. Chapter 13 in *Health Information Management: Concepts, Principles and Practice*, 4th ed. Edited by LaTour, K.M., S. Eichenwald Maki, and P. Oachs. Chicago: AHIMA.

Harman, L.B., ed. 2006. *Ethical Challenges in the Management of Health Information*, 2nd ed. Sudbury, MA: Jones and Bartlett.

Health Information Management Systems Society. 2011. Patient Identity Integrity Toolkit: Model Data Practices. http://www.himss.org/ResourceLibrary/genResourceDetailPDF.aspx?ItemNumber=27736

Healthcare Informatics. 2011 (October 12). Nemours Health System Reports Data Breach. http://www.healthcare-informatics.com/news-item/nemours-health-system-reports-data-breach

Herzig, T.W. 2012. Mobile device security (updated). *Journal of AHIMA* 83(4):50–55. http://library.ahima.org/xpedio/groups/public/documents/ahima/bok1_049463.hcsp?dDocName=bok1_049463

Holt, L. 2011. Increasing real-world security of users IDs and passwords. *Proceedings of the 2011 Information Security Curriculum Development Conference*, 34–41.

Joint Commission. 2015. National Patient Safety Goals. http://www.jointcommission.org/assets/1/6/2015_NPSG_HAP.pdf

Kastel, G.M. 2013. HITECH Final Rule results in Significant Changes to HIPAA Provisions. Faegre Baker Daniels. http://www.faegrebd.com/19470

Kempfert, A. and B. Reed 2011. Health care reform in the United States: HITECH act and HIPAA privacy, security, and enforcement issues. *FDCC Quarterly* 61(3):240–273. http://www.thefederation.org/documents/Quarterly_V61N3.pdf

Kern, L. and R. Kaushal. 2007. Health information technology and health information exchange in New York state: New initiatives in implementation and evaluation. *Journal of Biomedical Informatics* 40(6):S17–S20.

Key Health Alliance. n.d. Healthcare Data Analytics Portal. Key Health Alliance. https://http://www.khareach.org/portal/data-analytics

Landsbach, G. and B.H. Just. 2013. Five risky HIE practices that threaten data integrity. *Journal of AHIMA* 84(11):40–42. http://library.ahima.org/xpedio/groups/public/documents/ahima/bok1_050474.hcsp?dDocName=bok1_050474

McKay, T. 2014. Who are you? Authentication consumer identity is becoming increasingly important in healthcare. *Journal of AHIMA* 85(9):32–37.

Minnesota Administrative Uniformity Committee. n.d. Security Standards. http://www.health.state.mn.us/auc/security.htm

Mercuri, R. 2004. The HIPAA-potamus in health care data security. *Communications of the ACM* 47(7):27–28. http://ezproxy.library.capella.edu/login?url=http://search.ebscohost.com/login.aspx?direct=true&db=iih&AN=13581634&site=ehost-live&scope=site

National Institute of Standards and Technology. 2012. Guide for Conducting Risk Assessments. NIST Special Publication 800-30 Revision 1. http://csrc.nist.gov/publications/nistpubs/800-30-rev1/sp800_30_r1.pdf

Nutten, S. 2003. Tackling the training mandate: How to get your work force privacy training under control and under way. *Journal of AHIMA* 74:22-25.

Office of the National Coordinator for Health Information Technology (ONC). 2015. Guide to Privacy and Security of Electronic Health Information. http://www.healthit.gov/sites/default/files/pdf/privacy/privacy-and-security-guide.pdf

PBWorks. 2007. Advantages and Disadvantages of Technology. http://biometrics.pbworks.com/w/page/14811349/Advantages%20and%20disadvantages%20of%20technologies

Quinsey, C.A. 2013. Managing Organizational Compliance and Risk. Chapter 28 in *Health Information Management: Concepts, Principles and Practice*, 4th ed. Edited by LaTour, K.M., S. Eichenwald Maki, and P. Oachs. Chicago: AHIMA.

Revisor of Statutes, State of Minnesota. 2015. Minnesota Health Record Act 144.293: Release and Disclosure of Health records. https://www.revisor.mn.gov/statutes/?id=144.293&format=pdf

Rhodes, H. 2013. Seven unintended consequences of electronic HIE. *Journal of AHIMA* http://journal.ahima.org/2013/08/01/seven-unintended-consequences-of-electronic-hie/

Rhodes, H. and R. Scichilone. 2012. Guidance for assessing critical success factors influencing adoption of health information exchange solutions. *Perspectives in Health Information Management*, 1–14. http://perspectives.ahima.org/guidance-for-assessing-critical-success-factors-influencing-adoption-of-health-information-exchange-solutions/

Stine, K and Q. Dang. 2011. Encryption basics. *Journal of AHIMA* 82(5):44–46. http://library.ahima.org/xpedio/groups/public/documents/ahima/bok1_048923.hcsp?dDocName=bok1_048923

Thakkar, M. and Davis, D. 2006. Risks, barriers, and benefits of EHR systems: A comparative study based on size of hospital. *Perspectives in Health Information Management* 3(5):1–19. http://perspectives.ahima.org/PDF/Finished/bok1_031769.pdf

Tittel, E. and Follis, E. 2015 (Feb. 24). How better log Monitoring Can Prevent Data Breaches. http://www.cio.com/article/2887924/security0/how-better-log-monitoring-can-prevent-data-breaches.html?page=2

US Department of Health and Human Services (HHS). 2015a. Case Examples and Resolution Agreements. http://www.hhs.gov/ocr/privacy/hipaa/enforcement/examples/

US Department of Health and Human Services (HHS). 2015b. Breach Portal: Notice to the Secretary of HHS Breach of Unsecured Protected Health Information. https://ocrportal.hhs.gov/ocr/breach/breach_report.jsf

US Department of Health and Human Services (HHS). 2014. Bulletin: HIPAA Settlement Underscores the Vulnerability of Unpatched and Unsupported Software. http://www.hhs.gov/ocr/privacy/hipaa/enforcement/examples/acmhs/acmhsbulletin.pdf

US Department of Health and Human Services (HHS). 2013. HIPAA Administrative Simplification Regulation Text. http://www.hhs.gov/ocr/privacy/hipaa/administrative/combined/hipaa-simplification-201303.pdf

US Department of Health and Human Services (HHS). n.d.(a) Notice of Privacy Practices. http://www.hhs.gov/ocr/privacy/hipaa/understanding/consumers/noticepp.html

US Department of Health and Human Services (HHS). n.d.(b) The HIPAA Enforcement Rule. http://www.hhs.gov/ocr/privacy/hipaa/administrative/enforcementrule/index.html

Vericode. 2012 (Oct. 12). Common Malware Types: Cybersecurity 101. https://www.veracode.com/blog/2012/10/common-malware-types-cybersecurity-101

Walsh, T. 2013a. Security risk analysis and management: An overview (updated). *Journal of AHIMA* 84(11). http://library.ahima.org/xpedio/groups/public/documents/ahima/bok1_048622.hcsp?dDocName=bok1_048622

Walsh, T. 2013b. The 10 security domains (updated 2013). *Journal of AHIMA* 84(10). http://library.ahima.org/xpedio/groups/public/documents/ahima/bok1_050430.hcsp?dDocName=bok1_050430

Weirich, D. and Sasse. M. 2002. Pretty good persuasion: A first step towards effective password security in the real world. *Proceedings of the 2001 workshop on New Security Paradigms*, 137-143.

Zhang, Y., F. Monrose, and M. Reiter. 2010. The security of modern password expiration: An algorithmic framework and empirical analysis. *Proceedings of the 17th ACM conference on Computer and communications security*, 176–186.

Zorkadis, V. and P. Donos. 2004. On biometrics-based authentication and identification from a privacy-protection perspective: Deriving privacy-enhancing requirements. *Information Management & Computer Security* 12(1):125–137.

45 CFR 160.202: Preemption definitions. 2013 (Jan 25).

45 CFR 164.308: Administrative safeguards. 2013 (Jan 25)..

45 CFR 164.312: Technical safeguards. 2013 (Jan 25).

45 CFR 164.501: Privacy of individually identifiable health information definitions. 2013 (Jan 25).

45 CFR 164.502: Uses and disclosures of protected health information: General rules. 2013 (Jan 25).

45 CFR 164.504: Uses and disclosures: Organizational requirements. 2013 (Jan 25).

45 CFR 164.506: Uses and disclosures to carry out treatment, payment, or health care operations. 2013 (Jan 25).

45 CFR 164.508: Uses and disclosures for which an authorization is required. 2013 (Jan 25).

45 CFR 164.510: Uses and disclosures requiring an opportunity for the individual to agree or to object. 2013 (Jan 25).

45 CFR 164.512: Uses and disclosures for which an authorization or opportunity to agree or object is not required. 2013 (Jan 25).

45 CFR 164.514: Other requirements relating to uses and disclosures of protected health information. 2013 (Jan 25).

45 CFR 164.520: Notice of privacy practices for protected health information. 2013 (Jan 25).

45 CFR 164.522: Rights to request privacy protection for protected health information. 2013 (Jan 25).

45 CFR 164.524: Access of individuals to protected health information. 2013 (Jan 25).

45 CFR 164.526: Amendment of protected health information. 2013 (Jan 25).

45 CFR 164.528: Accounting of disclosures of protected health information. 2013 (Jan 25).

45 CFR 164.530: Administrative requirements. 2013 (Jan 25).http://dx.doi.org/10.1108%2F09685220410518883

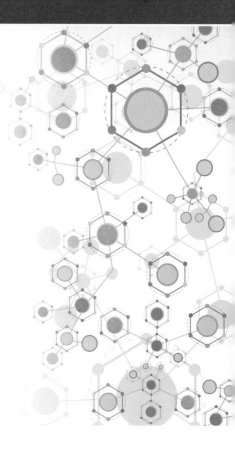

PART III
Healthcare
Informatics

12

Health Information Technologies

Ryan H. Sandefer, MA, CPHIT

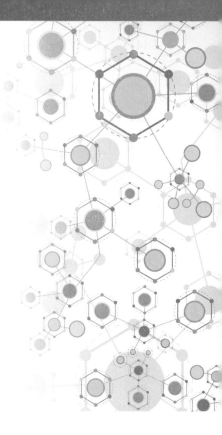

Electronic health record (EHR)
Electronic medical record (EMR)
Electronic records management technology
Encryption
Enterprise master patient index (EMPI)
ERx (e-prescribing)
Extranet
Firewall
Gesture recognition technology
Healthcare informatics
Information management
Intelligent document recognition (IDR) technology
Interoperability
Intranet

Master patient index (MPI)
Metadata
Multimedia
Natural language processing (NLP) technology
Neural network
Open source technology
Optical character recognition (OCR) technology
Patient/member web portals
Physiological signal processing system
Picture archiving and communication systems (PACS)
Point-of-care information system
Public key infrastructure (PKI)
Radio frequency identification (RFID)

Redundancy
Software as a Service (SaaS)
Source systems
Speech recognition technology
Structured data
Telemedicine/telehealth
Text mining
Two-factor authentication
Unstructured data
Usability
Vector graphic data
Virtualization
Web content management system
Web portal
Web service
Wireless systems
Workflow technology

Healthcare organizations are under increased pressure to control costs and improve efficiency. At the same time, they are experiencing increased demands to ensure patient safety, reduce medical errors, improve the quality of care, promote access, and ensure compliance with privacy and security regulations. Many healthcare organizations are looking to informatics to help them respond to these pressures and provide high-quality services in a more cost-effective manner. The use of computer technology to manage data and information means that well-trained and skilled individuals with knowledge about both healthcare and computerized information technologies are needed to manage (design, develop, select, and maintain) health data and information systems. It also means that healthcare organizations must prioritize the computer technologies and information systems (IS) to deploy in their institution.

This chapter introduces the field of informatics as it is currently being applied in the healthcare industry. Also, it describes the current and emerging technologies used to support the delivery of healthcare and the management and communication of patient information.

The Field of Informatics

Informatics is the science of information management. It uses computers to manage data and information and support decision-making activities. In short, informatics can be summarized by the following statement: "A person working in partnership with an information resource is 'better' than a person unassisted" (Friedman 2009, 169). **Information management** includes the generation, collection, organization, validation, analysis, storage, and integration of data, as well as the dissemination, communication, presentation, utilization, transmission, and safeguarding of information.

The healthcare industry is information intensive. The largest percentage of healthcare professional activities relates to managing massive amounts of data and information. This includes obtaining and documenting information about patients, consulting with colleagues, staying abreast of the current literature, determining strategies for patient care, interpreting laboratory data and test results, and conducting research. **Healthcare informatics** is the field of information science concerned with the management of all aspects of health data and information through the application of computers and computer technologies.

Historically, the healthcare industry has not valued informatics to the same degree that other industries have. The healthcare industry has been slow to both understand computerized information management and to incorporate it effectively into the work environment. Perhaps this is because the data and information requirements of the healthcare industry are more demanding than those of other industries in a number of areas. These areas include "implications of violations of privacy, support for personal values, responsibility for public health, complexity of the knowledge base and terminology, perception of high risk and pressure to make critical decisions rapidly, poorly defined outcomes, and support for the diffusion of power" (Stead and Lorenzi 1999, 343).

The use of information technologies to improve the healthcare delivery system gained attention in the early 1990s through the early 2000s with the publication of several reports from the Institute of Medicine that highlighted patient safety concerns and discussed how health information technologies can be used to improve care delivery (Kohn et al. 2001; 2000; Wunderlich and Kohler 2001). Momentum was gained with the establishment of the Office of the National Coordinator for Health Information Technology (ONC) in 2004. In 2008, the ONC published the Federal Health Information Technology Strategic Plan, which defined a number of goals, objectives, and strategies that bring together all federal efforts in health information technology (IT) in a coordinated fashion. The purpose of the plan was to guide the advancement of health IT throughout the federal government through 2012. The ONC has continued its federal health IT efforts and published an updated strategic plan for 2015 through 2020.

The Health Information Technology for Economic and Clinical Health (HITECH) provision of the American Recovery and Reinvestment Act of 2009 (ARRA) authorized the Centers for Medicare and Medicaid Services (CMS) to provide reimbursement incentives for eligible professionals and hospitals who are successful in becoming "meaningful users" of certified electronic health record (EHR) technology.

Examples of healthcare informatics successes are steadily growing. Charge collection and billing, automated laboratory testing and reporting, clinical documentation, computerized provider order entry (CPOE), patient and provider scheduling, diagnostic imaging, and secondary data use make up a distinguished list of healthcare informatics successes, proving what is doable and supporting further investment. Today's task for informatics is to design, develop, and implement computer information systems that enable healthcare organizations to accomplish visions for providing the highest-quality care in the most effective way.

Check Your Understanding 12.1

Instructions: **Answer the following questions on a separate piece of paper.**

1. How are the disciplines of information management and informatics related? How are they different?

2. Why are data and information so crucial to a healthcare professional's daily work?

3. Why is the healthcare industry perceived as being less proactive than other industries in the area of computerized information systems? How can this perception be changed?

4. The HITECH Act was a provision of which of the following:
   A. ONC
   B. CPOE
   C. ARRA
   D. Federal Register

5. True or False: The Office of the National Coordinator does not update its strategic plan.

Current and Emerging Information Technologies in Healthcare

To examine the information resources and systems that enable healthcare organizations to accomplish their visions in the most effective way, HIM professionals must possess fundamental knowledge of the components of computer-based information systems. This includes possessing knowledge of system hardware, software, and service components; communication and networking components; the Internet and its derived technologies; and system architectures.

Next, it is appropriate that HIM professionals review some of the current and emerging information technologies used to specifically support the delivery of healthcare as well as the management and communication of health data and information within the healthcare setting. To do this, four categories of current and emerging technologies in healthcare are discussed in this chapter:

- Supporting capture of various types of data and formats
- Supporting efficient access to and flow of data and information
- Supporting diagnosis, treatment, and care of patients
- Supporting security of data and information

Technologies Supporting the Capture of Different Types of Data and Formats

The information technologies currently in use for healthcare applications, as well as the new technologies being developed, support the capture of many different data types and formats that are all used to support the clinical services and administrative functions performed in every healthcare setting. Figure 12.1 shows the different types of data and their sources found in an EHR.

Data formats may be structured or unstructured. For example, the data elements in a patient's laboratory order, result, or demographic or financial information system are coded and alphanumeric. The fields are predefined and limited. In other words, the type of data is discrete, and the format is structured. Consequently, when a healthcare professional searches a database for one or more coded, discrete data elements based on the search parameters, the search engine can easily find, retrieve, and manipulate the element. However, the format of the data contained in a patient's transcribed radiology or pathology result, history and physical (H&P), or narrative clinical note is unstructured. Free-text data, as opposed to discrete, structured data, are not predefined and limited. Therefore, data embedded in unstructured text are not easily retrieved by the search engine.

Diagnostic image data, such as a digital chest x-ray or a computed tomography (CT) scan can be stored in a diagnostic image management system and represent a different type of data called bitmapped data. The format of bitmapped data also is unstructured. Saving each bit of the original image creates the image file.

Some diagnostic image data are based on analog, photographic films, such as an analog chest x-ray. These analog films must be digitally scanned, using film digitizers, to digitize the data. Other diagnostic image data are based on digital modalities, such as computed radiography (CR), CT, magnetic resonance (MR), or nuclear medicine.

Document image data are yet another type of data that are bit mapped and the format of which is unstructured. These data are based on analog paper documents or on analog photographic film documents. Most often, analog paper-based documents

Figure 12.1. EHR data types and their sources

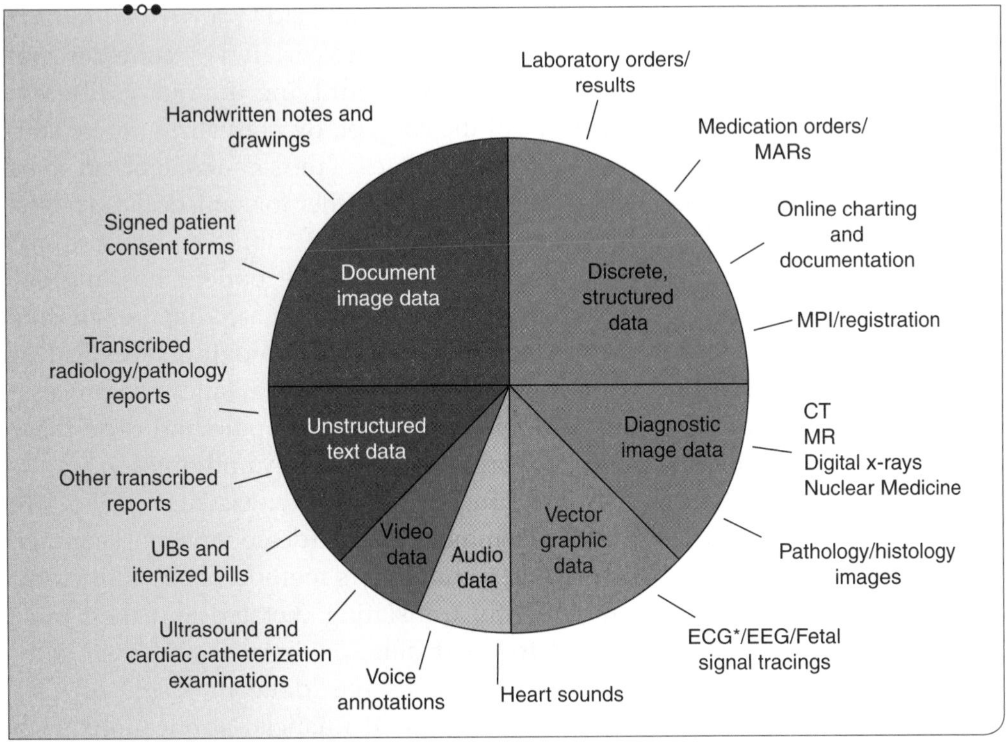

*ECG is the more correct term, but EKG is more widely used.
© Deborah Kohn 2001.

contain handwritten notes, marks, or signatures. However, such documents can include preprinted documents (such as forms), photocopies of original documents, or computer-generated documents. Analog photographic film-based documents (that is, photographs) are processed using an analog camera and film, similar to analog chest x-rays. Therefore, both the analog paper-based and the photographic film-based documents must be digitally scanned, using scanning devices that are similar to facsimile machines.

In addition, the EHR system's component information systems and technologies consist of other data types, the formats of which are also unstructured. Real audio data consist of sound bytes, such as digital heart sounds. Motion or streaming video/frame data, such as cardiac catheterizations, consist of digital film attributes such as fast forwarding. The files that consist of vector graphic (or signal tracing) data are created by saving lines plotted between a series of points, accounting for electrocardiograms (ECGs), electroencephalograms (EEGs), and fetal heart rate (FHR) tracings.

When more than one unstructured data type is present in an information system, the data and system they represent are referred to as **multimedia**. The EHR system is multimedia.

Speech Recognition Technology

For more than 20 years, the concept of generating an immediately available, legible, final, signed note or report based on computer speech input has been the catalyst for the development and application of different forms of speech recognition technology in healthcare (Nuance Communications 2008).

Today, **speech recognition technology** is speaker independent with continuous speech input. Speaker independence does not require extensive training. The software is already trained to recognize generic speech and speech patterns. **Continuous speech input** does not require the user to pause between words to let the computer distinguish between the beginning and ending of words. However, the user is required to be careful in the enunciation of words.

Although speech recognition vocabularies are expanding due to faster and more powerful computer hardware, only limited clinical vocabularies have been developed. Limited vocabulary-based speech recognition systems require the user to say words that are known or taught to the system. In healthcare, limited clinical vocabulary–based specialties such as radiology, emergency medicine, and psychiatry have realized significant benefits for dictation from the technology.

The ultimate goal in speech recognition technology is to be able to talk to a computer's central processor and rapidly create vocabularies for applications without collecting any speech samples (in other words, without training). It includes being able to talk at natural speed and tone and in no specific manner. It also includes having the computer understand what the user wants to say (the context of the word or words) and then apply the correct commands or words as coded data in a structured format. Finally, it includes identifying a user's voice and encrypting the voiceprint. Over the next years and decades, clinical vocabularies and algorithms will continue to improve, true speaker independence will be achieved, and natural language understanding will ultimately make structured dictation a reality.

Natural Language Processing Technology

Natural language processing (NLP) technology considers sentence structure (syntax), meaning (semantics), and context to accurately process and extract free-text data, including speech data for application purposes. As such, it differs from simple Boolean word search programs (simply combining search terms with *and*, *or*, *not*, or *near*) that often complement speech recognition technology–based systems. For example, the narratives "no shortness of breath, chest pain aggravated by exercise" and "no chest pain, shortness of breath aggravated by exercise" look the same to a Boolean word search engine when looking for occurrences of *chest* and *pain* in the same sentence.

On the other hand, natural language processing technology knows the difference in the narratives' meanings. For example, for health record coding

applications, it teaches computers to understand English well enough to "read" transcribed reports and notes and then find certain key concepts (not merely words) by identifying the many different phrasings of the concept. By normalizing these concepts, different phrases of the same content can all be compared with one another for statistical purposes. For example, "the patient thinks he has angina" and "the doctor thinks the patient has angina" have different meanings from a coding perspective (Schnitzer 2000, 96). By employing statistical or rules-based algorithms, natural language processing technology can then compare and code these similar expressions accurately and quickly.

Autocoding and **computer-assisted coding** are the terms commonly used to describe natural language processing technology's method of extracting and subsequently translating dictated and then transcribed free-text data, or dictated and then computer-generated discrete data, into ICD or CPT codes for clinical and financial applications such as patient billing and health record coding. **Text mining** and data mining are the terms commonly used to describe the process of extracting and then quantifying and filtering free-text data and discrete data, respectively.

Early results of several formative studies suggest that natural language processing technology improves health record coding productivity and consistency without sacrificing quality (Warner 2000, 78). Studies suggest that accuracy of natural language processing varies across applications and it is critical to have processes defined to review, edit, approve, and finalize (AHIMA 2011a). Despite the studies' outcomes, vendors continue to integrate natural language processing technology within health record coding reference tools, coding guidelines, drug databases, and legacy information systems to provide complete patient billing, health record coding, and other applications with little or no human intervention.

Electronic Document and Content Management Systems

Many care delivery organizations use bridge technology to enhance access to patient information when they do not have a full complement of source systems or have source systems that are not sufficient to support the major clinical components of an EHR. In some cases, clinicians interact fairly well with the bridge technology applications and in other cases the applications primarily enhance financial and administrative processes.

Electronic document management (EDM) systems greatly improve financial and administrative processes after discharge, where many departments need access to the patient's chart, where there are record completion responsibilities for several providers, and where access to clinical information may be needed in immediate outpatient or emergency department follow-up. It is also possible to add workflow technology to these systems, which can be used to queue work among staff or between departments. Other EDM systems, often then called enterprise (or electronic) content and record management (ECRM) systems, also enable digital documents—such as e-mails, e-faxes, transcription files, voice files (from digital and/or speech dictation), and wave forms—to be electronically fed (a process formerly referred to as computer output to laser disk [COLD]) into a repository for viewing via the ECRM system (Strong 2008). Natural language processing (NLP) is still in its infancy with respect to being able to parse all unstructured data in an EHR and create structured data from it. However, in the NLP form used in Discourse Representation Theory (DRT), templates guide the data to be dictated so that structured data fields are populated. If used in real time, clinician decision making can be supported. If not used in real time, the clinical decision support element is missing, but the structured data are still useful for analysis and reporting.

A document is any analog or digital, formatted, and preserved "container" of data or information, collectively referred to as content. The document is a well-worn and very useful human construct, but unless data contained within documents are formatted and accompanied by print-like qualities, such as headings or bolding, data are difficult to interpret. It is for this reason that documents and not data are required for evidentiary disclosure and discovery purposes. To settle legal disputes, the transaction *presentation*, not *representation*, is required for all business record documents. In healthcare organizations, this involves the retrieval of the bill document, the consultation report document, the photograph document, the image document, and so on.

An **electronic document/content management (ED/CM) system** is any electronic system that manages an organization's analog and digital documents and content (that is, not just the data) to realize significant improvements in business work processes. Like most information systems, the ED/CM system consists of a number of component technologies that support both digital and analog document and content management. These component technologies are discussed in the following sections.

Document Imaging Technology

Document imaging technology is one of the many ED/CM system component technologies. This technology electronically captures, stores, identifies, retrieves, and distributes documents that are not generated digitally or are generated digitally but are stored on paper for distribution purposes. Currently, in healthcare provider organizations, documents that typically are not generated in a digital format, are stored on paper and are candidates for this technology. They include handwritten physician problem lists and notes; "fill-in-the-blank" typeset nursing forms; preprinted Conditions of Treatment forms; and external documents (documents from the outside).

By digitally scanning the documents, the technology converts the analog data on the document into digital, bitmapped, document images. As more and more documents are created, distributed, and stored digitally, the dependence on, and use of, this technology decreases.

Document Management Technology

For every type of document as well as for every section or part of a document, **document management technology** automatically organizes, assembles, secures, and shares documents. Some of the more common document management technology functions include document version control, check in–check out control, document access control, and text and word searches.

Electronic Records Management Technology

Business records are bound by legal and regulatory requirements. Consequently, formats for long-term preservation, storage media for long-term viability, and strategies for record migration and accessibility are required. **Electronic records management technology** includes components that ensure the authenticity, security, and reliability of an organization's electronic records. Mass storage is required for the massive amounts of structured and unstructured data as well as the large number and variety of documents stored in ED/CM systems.

In addition, ED/CM system records must be properly classified using appropriate categories so that applicable legal and regulatory retention rules can be applied. These records must be identified so they can be deleted, purged, or destroyed at a defined point in their life cycle (Kohn 2003).

Workflow and Business Process Management Technology

Business process management (BPM) technology allows computers to add and extract value from document content as the documents move throughout an organization. The documents can be assigned, routed, activated, and managed through system-controlled rules that mirror business operations and decisions. For example, in healthcare organizations, **workflow technology** automatically routes electronic documents into electronic in-boxes of its department staff for work assignment (Kohn 2003).

Computer Output Laser Disk/Enterprise Report Management Technology

Computer output laser disk/enterprise report management (COLD/ERM) technology electronically stores, manages, and distributes documents that are generated in a digital format and whose output data are report formatted and print-stream originated. Unfortunately, documents that are candidates for this technology too often are printed to paper or microform for distribution and storage purposes. COLD/ERM technology not only electronically stores the report-formatted documents but also distributes them with fax, e-mail, web, and traditional hard-copy print processes.

One of the more recent trends for ERM is to store the coded, report-formatted output data natively and convert the data to Extensible Markup Language (XML) or HyperText Markup Language (HTML) when needed. In healthcare provider organizations, such documents generated by COLD/ERM technology typically include "green bar" financial system reports, Uniform Bills (UBs)/CMS 1500s, laboratory cumulative result summary reports, and transcribed word-processed medical reports.

Automated Forms-Processing Technology

Automated forms-processing (e-forms) technology allows users to electronically enter data into online forms and electronically extract the data from the online forms for various data-manipulation purposes. Powerful contextual verification processes have made such operations highly accurate. In addition, the form document is stored in a form format, as the user sees it on the screen, for ease of interpretation.

Digital Signature Management Technology

Digital signature management technology offers both signer and document authentication for analog or digital documents. Signer authentication is the ability to identify the person who digitally signed the document. Implementation of the technology is such that any unauthorized person will not be able to use the digital signature. Document authentication ensures that the document and the signature cannot be altered (unless both the original document and the change document are shown). As such, document authentication prevents the document signer from repudiating that fact.

Diagnostic Imaging Technologies

Diagnostic imaging technology (medical imaging) consists of using tools to capture images of the human body that can be used for clinical decision making. Picture archiving and communication systems (PACS) provide one example of diagnostic imaging technology where images taken from multiple sources (CT scans or MRIs, for example) are archived electronically for organizational access. Ultrasound technology, such as that used for echocardiography, is also considered imaging technology.

Instructions: **Answer the following questions on a separate piece of paper.**

1. What are the similarities and differences between a diagnostic image and a document image?

2. What is an EDM system?

3. What is the difference between (a) speech recognition technology and natural language processing technology, and (b) natural language processing searching and Boolean searching?

4. Provide a healthcare example for each of the following data types: real audio data, motion or streaming data, and signal or vector graphic data.

5. Explain the value of the following technologies: document imaging technology, workflow and BPM technology, COLD/ERM technology, automated forms technology, and digital signature management technology.

Technologies Supporting Efficient Access to and Flow of Data and Information

There are many current and emerging information technologies used to support efficient access to and flow of healthcare data and information. For purposes of this chapter, the following technologies are highlighted:

- Automatic recognition technologies
- Enterprise master patient indices and identity management
- Electronic data interchange (EDI) and e-commerce
- Secure messaging systems
- Web-derived technologies and applications

Automatic Recognition Technologies

Several technologies are used in healthcare to recognize analog items automatically, such as tangible materials or documents, or to recognize characters and symbols from analog items. Character and symbol recognition technologies recognize electronically scanned characters or symbols from analog items, enabling the identified data to be quickly, accurately, and automatically entered into digital systems. Other recognition technologies identify the actual items.

Character and Symbol Recognition Technologies

Character and symbol recognition technologies include bar-coding, optical character recognition (OCR), and gesture recognition technologies.

Barcoding Technology

Almost three decades ago, the barcode symbol was standardized for the healthcare industry, making it easier to adopt barcoding technology and to realize its potential. Since then, bar-coding applications have been adopted for labels, patient wristbands, specimen containers, business/employee/patient records, library reference materials, medication packages, dietary items, paper documents, and more. Benefits have been realized by the uniform consistency in the development of commercially available software systems, fewer procedural variations in healthcare organizations using the technology, and the flexibility to adopt standard specifications for functions while retaining current systems. Because virtually every tangible item in the clinical setting, including the patient, can be assigned a barcode with an associated meaning, it is not surprising to find barcoding as the primary tracking, identification, inventory data-capture, and even patient safety medium in healthcare organizations.

With bar-coding technology, an individual's computer data-entry rate can be increased in applications such as patient medication tracking, supply requisitioning, or chart/film tracking. In addition to eliminating time spent, bar-coding technology eliminates most of the mounds of paperwork (worksheets, count sheets, identification sheets, and the like) that are still associated with traditional computer keyboard entry. When bar-coding systems are interfaced to these types of healthcare information systems, the barcode can be used to enter the data, especially repetitive data, saving additional processing time and paper generation.

More importantly, the data input error rates with barcoding are as close to zero as most IT professionals think is possible. For all intents and purposes, bar-coded data, with an error rate of approximately three transactions in 1 million, can be considered error free. Thus, it is a most effective remedy for medication errors when used to ensure that the right medication dose is administered to the right patient.

Optical Character Recognition Technology

Like barcoding, **optical character recognition (OCR) technology** was invented to reduce manual data input, or hand-keying. OCR technology recognizes machine-generated characters (for example, pre-printed numbers and letters) by interpreting the scanned, bitmapped shapes of the characters' images and then converting the characters into computer-processable codes. OCR technology was initially used to automatically identify financial accounts consisting of preprinted Arabic numbers and Roman letters using a standardized font on thousands of paper-based documents, such as bank checks.

OCR has since been perfected to recognize the full set of preprinted typeset fonts as well as point sizes. The best OCR systems compensate for imperfectly formed characters and scanned pages by employing characteristics such as deskewing, broken character repair, and redaction. Deskewing "straightens" oblique characters, broken character

repair "fixes" incomplete characters, and redaction "hides" superfluous characters. OCR is used to perform everything from indexing scanned documents to digitizing full text. Its ability to dramatically reduce manual data input, or hand-keying, while increasing input speed represents the best aspect of this technology.

Unfortunately, like other technologies, OCR has been perfected but is not perfect. The high recognition rate realized by OCR systems may not be sufficient for the kind of text recognition applications OCR software is designed to perform. In addition, after an analog document is scanned by OCR technology, the data become unstructured, free-text data. As with all unstructured text data, when a healthcare professional needs to search the text, the search engine cannot easily find, retrieve, and manipulate one or more data elements embedded in text.

Gesture Recognition Technology

The recognition of constrained or unconstrained, handwritten, English language free text (print or cursive, upper- or lower-case, characters or symbols) typically stored on paper-based, analog documents is known as intelligent character recognition (ICR) technology. The recognition of hand-marked characters in defined areas of, typically, paper-based analog documents is known as mark sense technology. Collectively, these technologies are referred to as **gesture recognition technologies**.

Mark sense technology detects the presence or absence of hand-marked characters on analog documents. Consequently, it is used for processing analog questionnaires, surveys, and tests, such as filled-in circles by number 2 pencils on standardized exams.

ICR technology is quite an elaborate information-processing technique. An operation such as the detection of lines or the beginnings of words in sections of handwritten text can be accomplished with relative ease in the normal case. However, subsequent tasks turn out to be extraordinarily complicated. These include segmentation of the words into individual characters and assignment of the individual characters to a definite class of characters, such as words. Consequently, ICR error rates remain high. As such, ICR technology is being adopted slowly, primarily into the data-entry activities of certain types of pen-based computer devices, such as handheld devices.

Neural networks remain the leading ICR technology. These networks are modeled on the way synapses work in the brain: processing information by recognizing patterns of signals. As such, they adapt themselves into shifting configurations based on what they encounter. In other words, they change as they grow and learn.

Consequently, for each handwritten character or symbol recognized by ICR technology, a confidence level is expressed internally as a percentage and a user picks the threshold below which he or she wants to flag uncertain characters or symbols. Like speech recognition technology, a training or setup period is required for this emerging technology.

Other Recognition Technologies

Automatic recognition technologies that identify actual items include radio frequency identification (RFID) and intelligent document recognition (IDR) technologies.

Radio Frequency Identification Technology

Radio frequency identification (RFID) technology works in the following manner: Chips that emit radio signals are embedded in analog items and products. The signals are read and captured by receivers. The receivers act as data collectors and send the signals to PCs on a network, allowing the items and products to be tracked.

RFID's applicability in the healthcare industry is limited only by the imagination. Like barcodes, it is being used to track moveable patients, clinicians, medications, and equipment. As such, in a wireless environment, conceivably, RFID could replace barcodes for these applications. The greatest challenges regarding RFID technology are cost and privacy and security concerns.

Intelligent Document Recognition Technology

Recently, an automatic recognition technology has been developed to recognize types of analog documents or forms, eliminating the need for barcodes or other characters and symbols that identify the documents or forms. **Intelligent document recognition (IDR) technology** trains itself to identify document or form types and to sort the information accordingly for subsequent data entry. This training process requires a period of continuously scanning each type of document or form. As such, the pattern of document and form layouts and information locations educates the system to recognize the document or form for future recognition situations.

Enterprise Master Patient Indexes and Identity Management

Too often, breakdowns in patient identification cause patient record errors that threaten data integrity. The most common error occurs when healthcare provider organization registration personnel fail to locate existing patient information in the organization's **master patient index (MPI)**, including the patient's unique identification number. The patient is then assigned another record (in other words, a duplicate record) and a new file is created in the database. When this error occurs, it is unclear into which database file the patient's data should be entered. This often results in unnecessary duplicate tests, billing problems, and increased legal exposure in the case of adverse treatment outcomes.

Another common error occurs when registration personnel incorrectly register a patient under another person's existing, unique identification number. This error of overlay results in the merging of two different patients' data into one file. The clinical risks are significant.

As healthcare organizations continue to come together into integrated delivery networks (IDNs), the probability increases that information about a patient is spread across multiple databases and in multiple formats. In addition, the information is updated and accessed by multiple transaction processing systems and personnel. This causes problems when the IDN begins to assemble information about a patient in order to deliver care across diverse systems and encounters. Longitudinal applications, such as the EHR system, cannot be successful.

Consequently, healthcare provider organizations are developing strategic initiatives for **enterprise** master patient indices (EMPIs). In the broad sense, this involves the increasingly important service referred to as identity management.

EMPIs provide access to multiple repositories of information from overlapping patient populations that are maintained in separate systems and databases. This occurs through an indexing scheme to all unique patient identification numbers and information in all the organizations' databases. As such, EMPIs become the cornerstones of healthcare system integration projects.

EMPIs work in two ways. At the back end, EMPIs coordinate recordkeeping. The indices receive information from multiple systems that need no modification. The receiving is often performed through an integration gateway or engine. The enterprise index tests to see whether the patient is identified in all of the systems; if not, it may assign a unique identification number or other, related identifier as well as correlate records throughout the enterprise.

At the front end, EMPIs receive requests from existing registration systems to send data to these systems. Usually, these existing registration systems need some reprogramming to enable them to request and receive data from the EMPI. Currently, there is no consistent accepted trigger event and standard data format to do this.

EMPI building is complex. Variations in information systems, data capture, and organizational goals and objectives present multiple challenges to integrating patient data. For example, EMPI building involves a multitude of decision points. These include deciding whether to employ centralized or distributed data storage; whether to maintain limited, additional information such as allergies and encounter histories or robust information such as problem lists; and whether to establish batch processing or real-time communication between the registration system and the EMPI.

In addition, EMPIs include complex capabilities. These capabilities include merging records pertaining to the same person using probabilistic matching and algorithms, maintaining source systems' pointers, removing duplicate records, and providing a common user interface. Finally, after technical and organizational issues are overcome, the purely operational tasks of linking patients across multiple entities and episodes of care and maintaining these linkages are difficult and can be costly.

Electronic Data Interchange and E-Commerce

Electronic data interchange (EDI) allows the transfer (incoming and outgoing) of information directly from one computer to another by using flexible, standard formats. These formats function as a common language among many different healthcare trading or business partners (payers, government agencies, financial institutions, employer groups, healthcare providers, suppliers, and claims processors) who have agreed to exchange the information electronically but use a wide variety of application software with incompatible native formats. In the healthcare industry, with its traditionally strong reliance on paper-intensive processes, the goal of EDI is to eliminate the administrative nightmares of transferring paper documents back and forth between these partners and then hand-keying the information into the partners' disparate computer systems.

With widespread acceptance of the Internet and its derived technologies, such as the web, the term **e-commerce** began to replace the term EDI. Today, e-commerce is used to describe the integration of all aspects of business-to-business (B2B) and business-to-consumer (B2C) activities, processes, and communications, including EDI.

In addition, the term **e-health** is now used to describe the application of e-commerce in the healthcare industry. Several principles and concepts of e-health directly relate to EDI principles and concepts. These include the links among the healthcare trading and business partners; the links to healthcare equipment and supply vendors, providers, and health plans; and the transactions for exchanging data on healthcare eligibility, referrals, claims, and so forth.

Web-Derived Technologies and Applications

There are a variety of health information technologies that are accessed solely through the Internet.

This section will provide detailed information on a variety of these technologies.

Web Portals

No one information system (IS) can provide all the applications, data types, and data formats needed by all of the healthcare industry's diverse healthcare organizations and users. Consequently, most healthcare provider organizations maintain multiple, disparate feeder applications for their data repositories. Depending on their size and systems acquisition philosophies, some healthcare provider organizations maintain and often integrate large numbers of disparate feeder applications, and others maintain and integrate at least two or three.

Each disparate feeder application for the repository has a unique user interface, uses different data nomenclature, and takes limited advantage of data standards. Therefore, it is not only difficult to integrate the information from the disparate systems into the repositories, but it is also difficult for the organizations' users to learn and interact with the different systems.

Today, the term **clinical workstation** is still used to describe the presentation of healthcare data and the launching of applications in the most effective way for healthcare providers. However, for all intents and purposes, the concept of web-based, clinician/physician portals has replaced the concept of the clinical workstation.

A **web portal** is a single point of personalized access (an entryway) through which one can find and deliver information (content), applications, and services. Web portals began in the consumer market as an integration strategy rather than a solution. Portals offered users of the large, public, online Internet service provider websites fast, centralized access (via a web browser) to an array of Internet services and information found on those websites.

Consequently, like clinical workstations, **clinician/physician web portals** first were seen as a way for clinicians to easily access (via a web browser) the healthcare provider organizations' multiple sources of structured and unstructured data from any network-connected device. Like clinical workstations, clinician/physician web portals evolved into an effective medium for providing access to multiple applications as well as the data. And because clinician/physician portals are based on Internet technologies, they became the access points to sources of data and applications both internal and external to the organization.

In addition, clinician/physician web portals provide simplified, automated methods of creating taxonomy, or classifying data. As an example, consumer portals like Yahoo.com organize files and data corresponding to food, fashion, and travel for easy access. Finally, true clinician/physician web portals have at least one search engine and allow customization at the role and individual level. Search engines must be able to search e-mails, file servers, web servers, and databases; and customization must allow users to create individual, relevant views.

With the success of clinician/physician web portals and the trend toward improving patient engagement in healthcare through technology, a growing number of healthcare provider and payer organizations have established web portals for their patients/members. Each participant receives an account on the web portal with a unique login and password. Typical payer-based portal uses include accessing membership information and choosing a primary care physician. Typical provider-based portal uses include requesting prescription renewals, scheduling appointments, and asking questions of providers via secure messaging. Increasingly, **patient/member web portals** are allowing patients to pay their bills online and to securely view all or portions of their provider-based, electronic health record, such as current medical conditions, medications, allergies, and test results.

Although patients/members access the portals over the Internet, all the information including the secure messaging applications resides on the provider's or payer's secured servers. As such, these portals dovetail well with privacy and security regulations, which empower patients/consumers with the authority to determine who can have access to their healthcare information. Also, patients can use the portal to notify providers if their EHR is incorrect. As consumers seek to take a larger role in their healthcare, such patient/member "entryways" to information (content), applications, and services are expected to become more common.

Intranets and Extranets

Web-based information systems and applications cannot continue to proliferate without creating web-based **intranets** designed to enhance communication among an organization's internal employees and facilities; and web-based **extranets** designed to enhance communication among an organization's external business partners. This is true because intranets link every employee within an organization via an easy-to-navigate, comprehensive network devoted to internal business operations, while extranets link an organization's external business partners with the same comprehensive network but one that is devoted to external business operations. For example, private, secure networks provide every healthcare organization employee with basic information such as message boards, employee handbooks, manuals, mail, cafeteria menus, newsletters, directories, and contact lists. Also, they are used for the development of the organization's EHR. Restricted access to intranets by authorized users provides assurances that the general Internet public cannot access this private, secure network. However, through its intranet, a healthcare organization can access the Internet's servers for general Internet mail and messaging.

Extranets connect intranets that exist outside an organization's firewall. For example, typically, an IDN's autonomous care facilities (for example, acute care, long-term care, home healthcare), each with its own intranet, need to communicate between and among themselves via secure e-mail or other collaboration tools. The facilities connect the various intranets and form an extranet.

Web Content Management Systems

Web content management systems label and track the information that is placed on a website so that the information can be easily located, modified, and reused. These systems are a critical component in personalizing an organization's web-based intranet and extranet, web portal, and page content for site users and visitors. They also provide crucial versioning and globalization capabilities. Versioning enables each of the website's content components to be tracked individually. Then, as the content changes, each version of the content can be identified and the overall website can be recreated as it existed at any specific point in time. Globalization enables the look and feel of an organization's website to be managed centrally, while specific content is managed for local requirements.

Web Services

Web services technology is a platform for software applications (or services) whose basic communication mechanism is XML, the universal language of the web and the accepted format for data exchange over the Internet. In addition, web services technology utilizes web-based infrastructure protocols, such as HTTP and transmission control protocol/ Internet protocol (TCP/IP). As such, web services technology allows programs written in different languages and on different operating systems to communicate with each other in a standards-based way. In short, web services technology is an open, standardized way of integrating disparate, web browser–based and other applications.

By using XML messages to format and tag data, web services technology allows for data interchange without the need for translation. In addition, the messages use system-independent vocabularies and protocols, such as simple object access protocols (SOAP) to transfer the data; universal description, discovery, and integration (UDDI) to list what services are available; and web services description language (WSDL) to describe the services available. Healthcare organizations have been gradually installing web services to ease integration of disparate web-based and legacy applications, often written in incompatible languages. This ensures that the organizations' applications interoperate and that healthcare organizations can more easily choose tools for important interorganizational and regional data sharing. (See figure 12.2.)

Open Source Technology

Open source software products are applications whose source (human-readable) code is freely available to anyone who is interested in downloading the code. Advantages of **open source technology** include its availability, it extensibility to be customized, and the collaborative nature of the product in which a community of developers and users can interact, review, and improve upon each other's ideas.

Figure 12.2.   Web services

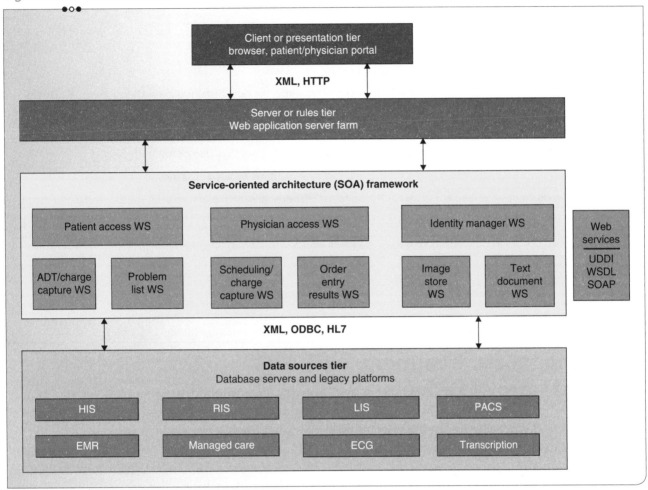

© Deborah Kohn 2005.

Ten criteria must be met to qualify a software program as open source.

- *Free redistribution*: Free redistribution is allowed and royalty payments are prohibited

- *Source code*: The program must include source code

- *Derived works*: Modifications and derived works are allowed

- *Integrity of author's source code*: The integrity of the original source code must be preserved

- *No discrimination against any person or groups*: The license must not discriminate against any person or group

- *No discrimination against fields of endeavor*: The license must not restrict anyone from making use of the program in a specific field of endeavor

- *Distribution of license*: The license remains with the program even if it is redistributed

- *License must not be specific to a product*: The rights attached to the program must not depend on the program's being part of a particular software distribution

- *License must not restrict other software*: The license must not insist that all other programs distributed on the same medium be open source software

- *License must be technology neutral*: No provision of the license may be predicated on any individual technology or style of interface (Open Source Initiative 2012)

Disadvantages of open source technology include the need for skilled developers within an organization to take advantage of the benefits noted earlier as well as a lack of dependable technical support.

Check Your Understanding 12.3

Instructions: **Answer the following questions on a separate piece of paper.**

1. How are the concepts of EDI, e-commerce, and e-health interrelated?

2. What is driving the heightened interest in EMPI technology within the healthcare industry?

3. Provide a healthcare example for each of the following automatic recognition technologies: barcoding, OCR, ICR, RFID, and IDR.

4. What is the primary purpose of the clinical workstation and the clinician/physician portal?

5. Explain why secure clinical messaging is often preferred over real-time tools such as instant messaging or chats.

6. What is the difference between an intranet and an extranet? Provide an example of how each can be used in healthcare.

7. Describe the benefits and drawbacks of open source technology.

8. How do web portals established by providers or payers assist consumers in taking a larger role in their healthcare?

Technologies Supporting the Diagnosis, Treatment, and Care of Patients

Many current and emerging information technologies are used to support the diagnosis, treatment, and care of patients. For the purposes of this chapter, the following technologies are highlighted:

- Physiological signal processing systems
- Point-of-care information systems
- Mobile and wireless technology and devices
- Automated care plans, clinical practice guidelines, clinical pathways, and protocols
- Telemedicine/telehealth
- EHR systems

Physiological Signal Processing Systems

The human body is a rich source of signals that carry vital information about underlying physiological processes. Traditionally, such signals have been used in clinical diagnosis as well as in the study of the functional behavior of internal organs.

Physiological signal processing systems, such as ECG, EEG, and FHR tracing systems, store data based on the body's signals and create output based on the lines plotted between the signals' points. The data type used by these systems is referred to as signal tracing or **vector graphic data**.

Physiological signal processing systems measure biological signals. Also, they help to integrate the medical science of analyzing the signals with such disciplines as biomedical engineering, computer graphics, mathematics, diagnostic image processing, computer vision, and pattern recognition. The integration of these disciplines allows these systems to electronically compile measurement equations, estimate the signals' parameters, and characterize the feedback elements. For example, the computer-based analysis of the neuromuscular system, the definition of cardiovascular system models, the control of cardiac pacemakers, the regulation of blood sugar levels, and the development of artificial organs not only serve patient diagnostic and care purposes but also support the development and simulation of instrumentation for physiological research and clinical investigation.

Point-of-Care Information Systems

Point-of-care information systems allow healthcare providers to capture and retrieve data and information at the location where the healthcare service is performed. These systems have come a long way since hardwired computer terminals with green screens were first placed at the patient's bedside more than 25 years ago. Functionally, almost every type of patient clinical and administrative application has been introduced to provide care services at the bedside, in the exam room, at the home, or even on the patient, as in medical monitoring. Technologically, massive changes have occurred in these systems' platforms, footprints, and networking capabilities.

For example, many acute-care facilities have installed clinical point-of-care information systems that, among other services, provide online medication order entry, profiles, administration schedules, and records. The records include information about medications not given (with reasons) as well as related information such as fluid balances, physical assessments, laboratory test results, and vital signs. All medications, including unit doses, are barcoded and scanned at or near the patient's bedside along with the patient's wristband and the caregiver's identification badge. This prompts a safety edit, documents administration of the medication, and generates the charge. Other acute-care facilities have installed administrative point-of-care (or service) systems that have eliminated admitting areas. Inpatients are greeted at the door with their room assignments, and roving admissions representatives visit patients in the assigned rooms to complete all the admission procedures.

Typically, point-of-care information systems use portable, handheld, wireless devices to enable entry of the data by a barcode scanner, keypad, or touch screen. Also, the devices are used to upload and download information to and from hardwired workstations. Retrieval of the data occurs at the wireless device or on wall-mounted or portable, cart-based computers. The data also can be entered and retrieved on hardwired workstations located in areas outside the point of care, such as central areas at patient care units, back offices, central or satellite pharmacies, and physician lounges, homes, and offices.

Mobile and Wireless Technology and Devices

Perhaps the biggest influence on, as well as challenge for, point-of-care information systems and

their use comes from significant advances in wireless technology and smaller, mobile devices. For the healthcare industry, the successful integration of wireless technology and smaller, mobile devices with point-of-care software supports and enhances the clinician's decision-making processes.

True **wireless systems** use wireless networks and wireless devices to access and transmit data in real time. At the basic level, wireless technology is based on the use of radio waves.

For years, healthcare organizations have used in-building wireless point-of-care information systems, such as telemetry systems. These systems were based on existing technologies and use a portion of the radio spectrum reserved for industrial, scientific, and medical purposes (ISM band). Individual licenses are not required for these types of systems.

Also, provider organizations have long used wide-area wireless technology to support information systems, such as point-of-care systems. This technology involves microwave systems that are based on fixed, point-to-point wireless technology used to connect buildings in a campus network. Microwave systems are regulated and require licenses and compliance with Federal Trade Commission (FTC) procedures.

Until recently, most in-building wireless systems were proprietary. However, adoption of the Institute of Electrical and Electronic Engineers wireless technology standard (IEEE 802.11) has begun to provide a reasonable level of standardization. The IEEE 802.11 standard allows data transmission speeds of up to 11 megabits per second, is relatively low power, and does not require licenses for installation and use. The IEEE 802.11b is an international standard that provides a method for wireless connectivity to fixed and portable devices within a local area. As such, this standard allows interoperability among multiple vendor products (IEEE 2015).

It is the widespread adoption of cellular telephone technology that has significantly advanced the development of wireless technology and, consequently, its support for point-of-care systems. A brief look at healthcare organizations today shows mobile phones, two-way pagers, Internet-enabled telephones (also known as smart phones), and tablets.

Mobile devices improve point-of-care systems by allowing clinicians to use a device personalized to their individual workflows, such as clinical (for example, e-prescribing), dictation, and billing workflows, not functions. In addition, mobile devices provide clinicians the information they need anytime, anywhere, and on any network-addressable device.

Automated Clinical Care Plans, Practice Guidelines, Pathways, and Protocols

The terms used to describe clinical practice mandates, care process guides or pathways, disease management protocols, and decision algorithms are not well standardized. They tend to be used informally and interchangeably, often resulting in miscommunication among healthcare professionals.

Consequently, when clinical care plans, practice guidelines, pathways, and protocols are automated and used by multidisciplinary teams, patient care can be adversely affected unless the definitions of these various terms are clearly understood by all. For example:

- Clinical care plans are created for individual patients by healthcare providers for a specific time period. Typically, clinical care plans are based on the clinician's training, and include a unique course of action given the patient's diagnoses, history, and needs.

- Clinical practice guidelines are recommendations based on systematic statements or clinical algorithms of proven care options. Often professional organizations and associations, health plans, and government agencies such as the Agency for Healthcare Research and Quality (AHRQ) develop these guidelines.

- Clinical (or critical) pathways (CareMaps) delineate standardized, day-to-day courses of care for a group of patients with the same diagnosis or procedure to achieve consistent outcomes. Typically, pathways (CareMaps) are developed by the local healthcare organization or health plan.

- Clinicians often use the term *protocol* to refer to the written documents that guide or specify a practice, including clinical practice guidelines and clinical pathways. Strictly speaking, however, protocols are more detailed care plans for individual patients based on investigations performed by professional societies, drug companies, or individual researchers (Bufton 1999, 258).

Providers now recognize the enormous variation that exists in how they diagnose, treat, and care for patients. Consequently, there is a trend to use guidelines, formalized pathways, and protocols that have emerged from clinical research (evidence-based medicine) in order to reduce variation and improve care outcomes. Automating these guidelines, pathways, and protocols for easier access by healthcare providers is a first step. As automated clinical documentation systems are implemented, there is a trend to incorporate automated clinical pathways and care plans into providers' notes.

In short, clinical care plans, guidelines, pathways, and protocols, as well as drug formularies and other clinical knowledge bases, are becoming automated for easier access and use by healthcare providers, as well as for easier updating and maintenance. Many healthcare organizations purchase subscriptions from agencies, societies, or research companies to gain access to peer-reviewed libraries of clinical practice guidelines and clinical knowledge bases. They do so in order to efficiently download periodic updates of this content into their transaction-based or analytic systems.

The challenge for automated care plans, practice guidelines, pathways, and protocols is that, like clinical workstations and web portals, no one form of clinical documentation or one view of the information suits everyone or all situations. Therefore, automated plans, guidelines, pathways, and protocols require customization capabilities to help individuals and groups better share knowledge to reach similar decisions about patient care. Automated drawing tools and anatomical diagrams are other documentation options.

Telemedicine/Telehealth

Interactive, patient–provider consultations across gulfs of time and space represent what is often referred to as classic telemedicine or telehealth. However, the field has always encompassed a multitude of strategies for moving clinical knowledge and expertise instead of moving people. As such, telemedicine/telehealth systems, like EHR systems, are concepts made up of several cost-effective technologies used to bridge geographic gaps between patients and providers.

In other words, telemedicine/telehealth is not videoconferencing technology. Rather, **telemedi-. cine/telehealth** is clinically adequate, interactive media conferencing (for example, video conferencing) integrated with other technologies. It can be dynamic and include interactive (or real-time processing) technology, or it can be static and include store-and-forward (or batch processing) technology. It includes telecommunications and remote control–based biomedical technologies. It utilizes in-room systems, mobile systems, desktop systems, and handheld units. Often it is integrated with component technologies of the EHR system and derived technologies of the Internet. The access and ability to transmit patient records and the integration with reference databases on the Internet all play into the telemedicine/telehealth model.

Telemedicine/telehealth takes existing ways of delivering healthcare and enhances them, such as enhancing patient–provider consultations via "electronic house calls." It extends care to underserved populations, whether they are located in rural or urban areas, and redefines the healthcare organization's community. It transfers clinical information between places of lesser and greater medical capability and expertise.

Like medicine in general, telemedicine/telehealth technology is made up of a number of specialties and subspecialties. Some examples include telecardiology, teledermatology, telesurgery, telepsychiatry, teleradiology, and telepathology, among many others.

The telemedicine/telehealth specialty that has been around for the longest time and, perhaps, is the most notable is teleradiology. Even today, spurred by a rising demand for sophisticated imaging tests as well as a smaller pool of radiologists from which to recruit, teleradiology is taking advantage of the speedy Internet transfer of medical data to outsourced radiologists who provide preliminary interpretations of scans during their normal business hours. In addition, since the early 1990s, the University of Pittsburgh Medical Center, the Mayo Clinic, and other prestigious provider organizations have employed dynamic telepathology interactions. Teleradiology and telepathology specialties are considered first-generation telemedicine/telehealth systems and services because they do not rely on patient interaction.

The second-generation telemedicine/telehealth systems and services involve those specialties relying on patient interaction and consultations. These include teleophthalmology, telepsychiatry, telehome healthcare, and so on.

The latest generation of telemedicine/telehealth systems and services involves patient interaction beyond the consultation. For example, in October 2001, telesurgeons in New York City performed the world's first complete (that is, from start to finish) telesurgery by successfully operating on the gallbladder of a patient in France. This was accomplished by sending high-speed signals through fiber-optic cables across the Atlantic Ocean to robots in a Strasbourg clinic. There have been numerous advances in the application of telemedicine/telehealth since the first telesurgery. The use of telehealth/telemedicine centers on "education, consultation (including decision support), psychosocial/cognitive behavioral therapy (including problem solving training), social support, data collection and monitoring, and clinical care delivery" (Chi and Demiris 2015, 37).

As both a clinical and technological endeavor, telemedicine/telehealth plays a key role in the integration of managing patient care and in the more efficient management of the information systems that support it. However, overcoming multiple technical challenges remains a concern. These challenges include the lack of systems interoperability and network integration as well as metropolitan broad bandwidth limitations. Other challenges that require overcoming complex behavioral, economic, and ethical constraints are physician resistance; lack of consistent, proven cost-effectiveness;

lack of consistent, proven medical effectiveness; concerns for safety; and challenges related to reimbursement for services provided.

Electronic Health Record Systems

An EHR is a concept that consists of a host of integrated, component information systems and technologies. The concept of the EHR has been around since the late 1960s; however, it has only been recently that most provider organizations have gotten serious about fully implementing and adopting EHRs. The intent of EHR technology is to capture clinical data from multiple sources for use at the point of care in clinical decision making and to exchange such data across the continuum of care for care coordination.

As originally described in its landmark work on patient records, the Institute of Medicine (IOM) defined what is today referred to as the EHR as a record

> that resides in a system specifically designed to support users by providing accessibility to complete and accurate data, alerts, reminders, clinical decision support systems, links to medical knowledge, and other aids. This definition encompasses a broader view of the patient record than is current today, moving from the notion of a location or device for keeping track of patient care events to a resource with much enhanced utility in patient care (including the ability to provide an accurate, longitudinal account of care—meaning that information is available about all of the patient's health conditions over a lifetime), in management of the healthcare system, and in extension of knowledge. (IOM 1991)

In addition, the IOM provided the caveat that "merely automating the form, content, and procedures of current patient records will perpetuate their deficiencies and will be insufficient to meet emerging user needs" (IOM 1991, reaffirmed by the IOM in a 1997 update to its original patient record study). EHR implementation, use, and optimization of workflow provides an opportunity for greatly improved patient care; not just automation of existing paper records and documentation.

As with any revolutionary system, the EHR has suffered somewhat from multiple different interpretations and rapid development of products that may not have fully met the vision. In fact, some of them were so disappointing or cumbersome to use that they may have discouraged potential users to such an extent that they may be unwilling to try again. While much has improved, a National Academy of Sciences/IOM study conducted in 2009 examined eight organizations acknowledged as leaders in applying IT to healthcare to assess the current state of affairs. While they identified a number of successes, they also found that EHRs were "rarely well integrated into clinical practice" (Stead and Lin 2009). Care providers felt they were spending a lot of time entering data, but doing so to meet reimbursement requirements or as a defense against potential lawsuits. The report further noted that this state of affairs "does not reflect incompetence on the part of healthcare professionals" but is a "consequence of the intellectual complexity of healthcare and an environment that has not been adequately structured to help clinicians avoid mistakes or to systematically improve their decision making and practice" (Stead and Lin 2009). Consistent with the IOM's Quality Chasm reports focused on quality of care in the United States, the 2009 National Academy of Sciences/IOM study concluded that the "nation faces a healthcare IT chasm" (Stead and Lin 2009).

Ultimately, the EHR should be able to:

- Improve the quality of healthcare through data availability and links to knowledge sources

- Enhance patient safety with context-sensitive reminders and alerts, clinical decision support, automated surveillance, chronic disease management, and drug and device recall capability

- Support health maintenance, preventive care, and wellness through patient reminders, health summaries, tailored instructions, educational materials, and home monitoring and tracking capability

- Increase productivity through data capture and reporting formats tailored to the user; streamlined workflow support; and patient-specific care plans, guidelines, and protocols

- Reduce hassle factors and improve satisfaction for clinicians, consumers, and caregivers by managing scheduling, registration, referrals, medication refills, and work queues and by automatically generating administrative data

- Support revenue enhancement through accurate and timely eligibility and benefit information, timely claims adjudication, cost-efficacy analysis, clinical trials recruitment, rules-driven coding assistance, external accountability reporting and outcomes measures, and contract management

- Support predictive modeling and contribute to development of evidence-based healthcare guidance

- Maintain patient confidentiality and exchange data securely among all stakeholders (Institute of Medicine 1991)

Overall, the EHR should assist clinicians and other healthcare professionals provide safer, more efficient, and more cost effective care by providing information and decision support to end users.

EHR Terms

As the EHR has evolved, a variety of terms have been used to describe what today the federal government is calling the EHR. In fact, there has been considerable confusion between electronic *health* record and electronic *medical* record (EMR). Hospitals sometimes describe that they have both an EMR, which is an electronic document management system, and an EHR, which is composed of applications used by clinicians at the point of care.

In 2008, the federal government asked the National Alliance for Health Information Technology (NAHIT) to develop a set of terms and definitions to help the industry avoid confusion and achieve consensus on terminology. While NAHIT no longer exists, the definitions it published serve as the foundation for the government's adoption of the term *EHR* and are distinguished as follows:

- **Electronic health record (EHR)** is defined as "an electronic record of health-related information on an individual that conforms to nationally recognized interoperability standards and that can be created, managed, and consulted by authorized clinicians and staff across more than one healthcare organization" (NAHIT 2008).

- **Electronic medical record (EMR)** is defined as "an electronic record of health-related information on an individual that can be created, gathered, managed, and consulted by authorized clinicians and staff within one healthcare organization" (NAHIT 2008).

The key difference between the terms *EHR* and *EMR* as suggested by NAHIT is in EHR being interoperable and EMR not. **Interoperability** refers to the ability of two different systems to exchange data with each other. Unfortunately, many care delivery organizations are challenged with systems not being as interoperable as desired within their own organization, let alone with other organizations.

Neither of NAHIT's definitions of EHR or EMR addresses the functionality that contributes to enhanced utility beyond that of paper-based records that the IOM originally envisioned in 1991 or which it supplied in its 2003 letter report to the secretary of Health and Human Services (HHS) (IOM 2003). In 2004, the standards development organization Health Level Seven (HL7) also helped overcome the lack of a comprehensive description of the EHR in its EHR-System Functional Model, which described a highly functional and interoperable system. However, the Health Information Management and Systems Society (HIMSS) continues to use the term *EMR* in its HIMSS Analytics™ EMR Adoption Model℠ (HIMSS Analytics 2010). This model is widely referenced as it provides a quarterly survey report on the cumulative capabilities of EHRs in hospitals.

EHR Complexity

The EHR remains a complex system to implement. It is a system of many elements that must work together to achieve specific goals. For an EHR, these system elements must include not only hardware and software but also attention to people, policy, and process. In fact, David Blumenthal, MD, national coordinator in the Office of the National Coordinator for Health Information Technology (ONC) from 2009 to 2011, observed the following in discussing the EHR:

> It's not the technology that's important, but its effect. Meaningful use is not a technology project, but a change management project. Components of meaningful use include sociology, psychology, behavior change, and the mobilization of levers to change complex systems and improve their performance. (Blumenthal 2009)

People are hugely impacted by the EHR. Even for clinicians who use computers frequently, the EHR represents a significantly different way of practicing their professional skills. For instance, most clinicians are taught to quickly assess a patient, take immediate action to stabilize a patient in an emergency, and then gather further information about the patient—through referencing previous records of care, interviewing the patient, and obtaining data diagnostic studies. Only after much of the fact finding is completed is information documented in narrative. As a result, the documentation is largely a summary of findings. Furthermore, where clinicians are generally expected to document an assessment and plan of care, and ideally should engage the patient in making clinical decisions about his or her ongoing care, the result often is simply the recording of a differential or final diagnosis and orders for any additional studies and treatments. Diagnostic studies and treatments are largely based on the provider's training and experience (Ball and Bierstock 2007) rather than evidence from (new) scientific research—although professional judgment must be applied to such evidence (Tonelli 2006).

When the EHR is introduced, the clinician is expected to document and even practice in very different ways. Data are to be entered as captured at the point of care, and in standardized and structured form rather than **unstructured data** or narrative form, often taking longer to enter than the typical dictation of a report and without the ability to express nuances important to clinicians (Resnik et al. 2008). The result of this **structured data** (data that can be captured in a fixed field) often is a bulleted list of findings that clinicians do not find very user friendly. The clinician is expected to receive and be guided by clinical decision support (CDS) systems that process the structured data against a drug knowledge database (DKB) and other evidence-based medicine (EBM) into alerts, reminders, and context-sensitive templates for data capture, although often the volume of such "incessant warnings" (Pulley 2010), as some consider these, are frequently ignored. Giving the patient a health summary, supporting a patient in compiling a personal health record (PHR), or accepting information from a PHR (Witry et al. 2010) are new concepts for many physicians, who in the past shied away from providing patients with access to their health information. In fact, not providing access to a person's health information is one of the top five Privacy Rule complaints levied against physician practices according to the Office for Civil Rights (OCR 2011).

Check Your Understanding 12.4

Instructions: **Answer the following questions on a separate piece of paper.**

1. Provide at least five distinct examples of diagnostic tests that involve physiological signal processing.

2. What patient data are typically collected and viewed (accessed) by care providers using point-of-care systems?

3. Describe how second- and third-generation telehealth applications differ in functionality from first-generation applications such as teleradiology.

4. What is driving the increased use of computerized care protocols in healthcare?

5 What is the key difference between the definition of EHR and EMR?

Technologies Supporting the Security of Data and Information

Many current and emerging information technologies are used to support the security of healthcare data and information. They are the same technologies used to support the security of data and information in most market industries. What sets the healthcare market industry apart is the application of the technologies according to the second portion (Title II) of the Health Insurance Portability and Accountability Act (HIPAA), which mandates the protection of health information.

For the purposes of this chapter, the following technologies are highlighted:

- Encryption and cryptography
- Biometrics technology
- Firewall systems
- Audit trails

Encryption and Cryptography

Computer technology's greatest strengths also are its greatest weaknesses. For example, computer technology, especially the Internet and its derived technologies, allows anyone to send and receive information. However, it also easily allows individuals to intercept transmissions.

Cryptography is an applied science in which mathematics transforms intelligible data and information into unintelligible strings of characters and back again. **Encryption** technology uses cryptography to code digital data and information. This is so that the information can be transmitted over communications media and the sender of the information can be sure that only a recipient who has an authorized decoding "key" can make sense of the information.

There are two broad categories of encryption. The first category is symmetric or single-key encryption. Here, each computer uses software that assigns a secret key or code. One computer uses the key to code the message, and the other computer uses the same key to decode the message before the recipient can read it. This form of encryption requires both computers to have the same key.

The second category is asymmetric or **public key infrastructure (PKI)** encryption. PKI does not require that both computers have the same key to decode messages. A private key is known to one computer, which gives a public key to the other computer with which it wants to exchange encrypted data. The public key can be stored anywhere it is convenient, such as on a website or within an e-mail. The second computer decodes the encrypted message by using the public key and its own private key.

To prevent abuse, some type of authority is needed to serve as a trusted third party. A certification authority (CA) is an independent licensing agency that vouches for the individual's identity and relationship to the individual's public key. A CA verifies and stores a sender's public and private encryption keys and issues a digital certificate or "seal of authenticity" to the recipient.

These keys come in various strengths or levels of security. The strengths vary not only according to the algorithm that codes the data but also on how well the encoding and decoding keys are maintained. The more bits a key has, the harder it is to break the code without massive computer assistance.

For Internet sites, the use of private and public keys is handled behind the scenes by users' computer browsers and the web servers for the sites. For example, when a healthcare Internet user performs an online, interactive business transaction, a secure socket layer (SSL) PKI is used to exchange sensitive healthcare data and information.

PKI is becoming the de facto encryption technology for secure data transfers and online authentication. As such, its use will enable healthcare organizations to meet HIPAA's regulations concerning the security of data and electronic signatures.

Biometrics Technology

Biometrics technology verifies a person's identity by measuring (comparing different mathematical representations of) biological and physical features or traits unique to the individual. For example, in signature verification technology, the biometrics of a handwritten signature are measured to confirm the identity of an individual. In data access technology, the biometrics of a hand (hand geometry), fingerprint (fingerprint matching), eye (iris or retinal scanning), voice (voice verification), or facial feature (facial image recognition) are measured to confirm the individual's identity.

Unique, positive identification or verification without the fear of replication or duplication for access to confidential health information is critical. As such, HIPAA requires a mechanism to ensure the authentication of the user and to restrict the user only to those systems that he or she is authorized to access. Because positive identification is reliable as a personal identifier, individuals might feel that their privacy is threatened or compromised.

Fingerprint matching is the oldest and most popular type of biometrics technology. Everyone has unique, immutable fingerprints made of a series of ridges, furrows, and minute points or contours on the surface of the finger that form a pattern. Retinal scanning is quite accurate because it involves analyzing the layer of blood vessels at the back of the eye. But it is not as popular an identification technology because of the close contact users must make with a scanning device and thus is unfriendly for users wearing eyeglasses or contact lenses. Iris scanning is less intrusive than retinal scanning but is considered clumsy to use.

Facial image recognition requires an unobtrusive, digital camera to develop a dynamic, facial image of the user. Unfortunately, matching dynamic images is not as easy as matching static images, such as two or more fingerprints or iris scans. Therefore, positive identification based on multiple biometrics technologies currently has the most promising potential for authentication purposes.

Firewall Systems

Firewalls are hardware and software security devices situated between the routers of a private and public network. They are designed to protect computer networks from unauthorized outsiders. However, they also can be used to protect entities within a single network, for example, to block laboratory technicians from getting into payroll records. Without firewalls, IT departments would have to deploy multiple-enterprise security programs that would soon become difficult to manage and maintain.

Firewalls originated during the 1980s and were used to screen a network's incoming data from unwanted, outside addresses. At that time, networks were not large and complicated and firewalls were easy to circumvent.

By contrast, today's massive and complex networks demand firewall systems fortified with software applications that, for example, authenticate users, encrypt messages, scan for viruses and spyware, and produce audit trails. Technically, most firewalls are made up of proxy and filtering services. Proxy services are special-purpose programs allowing network administrators to permit or deny specific applications or features of applications. They screen user names and all information that attempts to enter or leave the private network. Filtering allows the routers to permit or deny decisions for each piece of information that attempts to enter or leave the private network.

Firewalls are based on pre-established rules that allow or deny access to the network or exchange of information between the networks. Firewalls enforce security policies so that everything not explicitly permitted is denied. For example, firewall systems determine which inside services may be accessed from the outside, which outsiders are permitted access to the permitted inside services, and which outside services may be accessed by insiders. For a firewall to be effective, all traffic to and from the networks must pass through the firewall, where it can be inspected.

The firewall itself must be immune to penetration. Unfortunately, a firewall cannot offer protection after an attacker has gotten through or around it.

Audit Trails

Audit trails are chronological sets of records that provide evidence of computer system utilization. Data are collected about every system event, such as logins, logouts, file accesses, and data extractions. Audit trails are used to facilitate the determination of security violations and to identify areas for improvement. Their usefulness is enhanced when they include trigger flags for automatic, intensified review.

Today, audit trails serve as strong impediments to computer data abuse. For example, the presence of these tools promotes awareness that people who access confidential information can be tracked and held accountable.

Care must be taken to determine which audited data elements are required by law or which ones are exceptions. Following are some suggested data elements to track activity in healthcare information system audit trails:

- Date and time of event
- Patient identification
- User identification
- Access device used
- Type of action (view or read, print, update or add)

- Identification of patient data access by a category of content
- Source of access and software application used
- Reason for access by category (patient care, research, billing)

Practical issues concerning the use of audit trails involve trust. For example, healthcare organizations must be able to distinguish between users who access patient records for patient care and those who access them for unauthorized purposes. Frequent sampling by organizational managers is one way to determine system usage within an environment of trust. Delegating to users the responsibility to examine their own audit histories is another way to determine this. It is recommended that the results of audit trails be published and included in employee performance reviews.

Check Your Understanding 12.5

Instructions: **Answer the following questions on a separate piece of paper.**

1. What is cryptography and why is it important for health information technology?

2. What are the benefits and drawbacks of using each of the following human features for authentication purposes: fingerprints, iris images, and facial images?

3. What are two practical ways to instill user trust in healthcare organizations when deploying IS audit trails?

4. Firewalls protect network access by employing proxy and filtering services. What are proxy services and filtering services?

5. What is public key infrastructure, and why is it receiving so much attention within the healthcare industry?

EHR Functionality and Technology

An EHR is not a single application or computer device but a complex set of software and hardware. Figure 12.3 displays a conceptual model that depicts these components.

Source Systems

An important element of the EHR includes the ability to communicate data with multiple sources; hence there must be information systems in many,

if not all, hospital departments. Although physician practices will have fewer systems with which they must communicate, such systems may more commonly be external to the practice. Collectively these are called **source systems**, and there are several types.

Financial and Administrative Systems

Hospitals have numerous financial and administrative applications, and they are no longer solely the

Figure 12.3. EHR system technical components

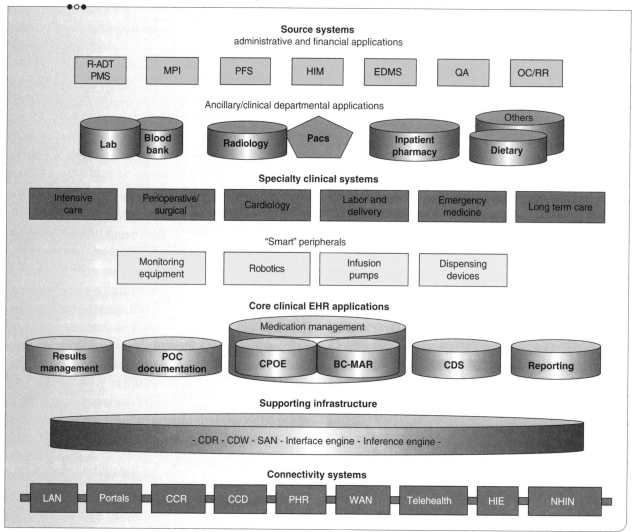

Source: Amatayakul 2013.

domain of the finance department or patient financial services. HIM professionals have long provided input via diagnostic and procedural codes and sometimes chargemaster management to the revenue cycle management (RCM) process, which includes creating, submitting, analyzing, and obtaining payment for healthcare services (TripleTree 2006). This link and more direct ties to clinical systems are becoming more and more important as there is increasing convergence of claims data (information required to be reported on a healthcare claim for service reimbursement) with health data. As claims data and clinical data are used together, healthcare quality and cost (value) improvements can be made, and improved business intelligence (BI) is available to support better decisions by both the administrative and clinical leadership of health-

care organizations. For example, with more complete clinical information available at the time of admission, a hospital is able to better verify a patient's eligibility for health plan benefits so that it is not faced with a denied claim later. An order placed for a potentially duplicate diagnostic study or therapy can be flagged for physician review, potentially displaying the previous study results simultaneously. While this may appear to be reducing hospital revenue, conducting a duplicate study or treatment is potentially hazardous for the patient and costly to the healthcare delivery system overall. Hospitals will save money and potentially increase their revenues if they are able to demonstrate their quality and cost-effectiveness measures when negotiating discounted fee-for-service contracts with payers. Often it requires staff with clinical backgrounds to aid in understanding where a duplicate test or therapy is effective and where it is not. Information that shows the hospital how many and what types of patients are readmitted within 30 days of discharge for the same condition is another example that will enable a hospital to take proactive measures to monitor these patients more closely after discharge and reduce the risk of not being reimbursed by Medicare for the admission.

Financial systems include both general accounting systems (such as general ledger, accounts payable, contract management, procurement, and others) as well as systems specific to patient accounting, often called patient financial services (PFS) systems. RCM starts with eligibility verification to determine if a patient's health plan will provide reimbursement for services to be performed. Sometimes prior authorization is required by health plans to review and approve a procedure (or referral) before performing the service. Once patient care commences, charge capture collects information from ancillary systems and the EHR about services performed; and claims are generated for reimbursement. Documents may need to be attached to the claim to support the claim. Checking claims status, posting remittance advice reflecting actual fees reimbursed to the organization, receiving electronic funds transfers (EFTs), sending explanations of benefits (EOBs) to patients, challenging denials, and managing collection are all RCM functions after claims have been sent. See chapter 8 for more details on the revenue cycle. Many of these processes utilize standard transaction and code sets (TCSs) mandated under the HIPAA's administrative simplification requirements. Under additional administrative simplification provisions of the Affordable Care Act (ACA) of 2010, some of these processes are just being implemented or are being enhanced with standard operating rules that will significantly reduce the thousands of companion guides, or unique paper rules, that have been used in the past.

Administrative applications that must also connect to EHR systems include admission, discharge, transfer (R-ADT); enterprise master patient index or master patient index (EMPI or MPI); encoders, chart tracking, chart deficiency management, release of information; order communication/results reporting (OC/RR); quality assurance (QA), including core measures abstracting (which pulls specified, quality-related data from health records for reporting to the Joint Commission and Centers for Medicare and Medicaid Services); and many others. Physician practices may have a practice management system (PMS) that provides patient registration, appointment scheduling, and all of the same patient financial services that a hospital performs.

Ancillary or Clinical Departmental Applications

Ancillary systems (clinical department applications) include laboratory information systems (LISs), radiology information systems (RISs), pharmacy information systems, and others. As migration toward an EHR is considered, it is important to recognize the primary purpose of ancillary systems—to help manage the operations of the departments in which they are used. For example, while LISs produce lab results, they do many other things in order to produce the results. They must receive the order for the test, assign an accession number to the order and specimen if the specimen accompanies the order, generate a specimen collection list and barcode labels for the specimen collection vials, schedule phlebotomists to collect the specimens from the patient, and interface with auto analyzers that run the tests to download the results. Once the results of the tests are available and quality checked, the system prints results or otherwise makes the results available for viewing by the ordering provider. In addition to these basic features, LISs manage workload balancing; supplies inventories; Medicare medical necessity checking, billing, and public health reporting; and generate custom reports for clinical or quality management. RISs perform equivalent functions for the radiology department. While the clinical pharmacy in a hospital does not produce diagnostic studies results as do the LIS and RIS, it must receive orders for medications, track and maintain inventory, perform quality checks, manage staff, and perform other departmental management functions. In addition, there are other departments that may have their own applications, such as a blood bank, nutrition and food services, housekeeping, and others. These may all ultimately have a connection to the EHR through ordering meals, special services, or other functions.

Large physician practices may have an LIS and/or RIS, as well as some other departmental systems. Small practices are likely to use the laboratory and radiology services of the hospital at which the physicians have medical staff privileges, or use commercial labs or imaging centers. Although physician practices may keep some drug samples they give selected patients, they do not maintain a clinical pharmacy. Rather, prescriptions must be written for a retail pharmacy to dispense.

A special type of system, **picture archiving and communication systems (PACS)**, digitizes medical images. PACS is "an integrated computer system that obtains, stores, retrieves, and displays digital images (in healthcare, radiological images)" (AHIMA 2011b). These are becoming increasingly popular in both hospital and physician practice environments. Some vendors offer free PACS viewer software to enable physicians who do not do their own imaging to view images from other sources.

Specialty Clinical Systems and Smart Peripherals

In addition to ancillary systems, there are specialty clinical applications. These include many systems for hospitals, but also some for physician practices. Examples include intensive care, perioperative or surgical services, cardiology, oncology, emergency medicine, labor and delivery, infection control, behavioral health, dentistry, and others.

Hospitals and physician practices are also acquiring smart peripherals, which are medical instruments that have information processing components including auto analyzers for lab testing, medication dispensing devices, robotics, smart infusion pumps, and vital signs monitoring equipment.

Core Clinical EHR Applications

Core clinical EHR applications are those used directly by clinicians at the point of care. Although there may be many specific applications, there are five major categories of these applications—results management, point-of-care documentation, medication management, clinical decision support, and reporting.

Results Management

Results management systems are applications that enable diagnostic studies results to be processed according to the needs of the users. In the past, results review systems enabled clinicians to view lab results. These were generally presented in print file format. While abnormal results were flagged in these reports, the data were not structured, so they could not be graphed or processed in other ways or with other data. Results management assumes that lab results are in structured form, ideally encoded using a standard vocabulary such as Logical Observation Identifiers Names and Codes (LOINC) (a data standard for laboratory data), and placed into a clinical data repository with other clinical data. The results management functionality then enables graphing of lab results over time and against medications, vital signs, and other data.

Point-of-Care Documentation

Also called point-of-care (POC) patient charting, POC documentation applications guide the user through the necessary data to collect in the context of the specific patient (often using context-sensitive templates that react to the nature of the data being entered and that tailor the template to the specific data entry needs). Hospitals often initiate POC charting with nursing documentation, such as admission assessments, care planning, nurses notes, vital signs documentation (if not coming directly from a monitoring device), intake/output records, and other documentation. As with lab results, nurse charting is aided by standard vocabularies, such as NANDA International for nursing diagnoses, and others (Lundberg et al. 2008); although none are required for the MU incentives at this time.

Physician documentation in a hospital remains largely performed by dictation of history and physical exams, consultations, operative reports, and discharge summaries with typed or dictated progress notes and structured problem lists. In order to earn the MU incentives, physicians must enter problems on the problem list using either ICD-10-CM or SNOMED-CT to achieve standardization of terminology. In physician practices with an EHR, however, physicians are much more apt to use the

EHR for most documentation, utilizing dictation primarily for complicated cases.

POC documentation is intended to capture more complete and accurate data and to avoid duplicative data entry. For example, a nursing admission assessment may include as many as 10 or 11 different forms. Although nurses sometimes find that automated nursing documentation does not save time, it is acknowledged that better information is valuable and it can be expected that there is downstream time savings from having such better information. Physicians in their practice also find similar results with POC documentation. Even though initial use of the system takes longer, most physicians are able to return to a normal documentation time or even gain some time after the learning curve.

Medication Management

Applications that support the closed-loop medication management process, where patient safety is ensured through proper drug ordering, dispensing, administering, and monitoring of reactions are special forms of POC documentation. These systems include CPOE, e-Rx as a special type of CPOE, electronic (EMAR) or barcode medication administration record (BCMAR), medication reconciliation systems, and automated drug dispensing. Although there is no required sequence for implementing these systems, many hospitals have implemented CPOE last because it is difficult to get physicians to use such systems in the hospital. This is changing as MU incentives require use of a CPOE system (although not EMAR or BCMAR systems at this time). In the ambulatory setting, e-prescribing (e-Rx) has sometimes been implemented as a standalone system before an EHR (and its CPOE functionality) because some insurers and Medicare were providing incentives for its use.

Computerized Provider Order Entry Computerized provider order entry (CPOE) systems enable ordering of everything from patient admission, laboratory tests, x-rays and other diagnostic studies, dietary/food and nutrition, therapies, nursing services, and consults to discharge of patient, referrals, and even building personal task lists, as well as entering orders for medications. In the past, physicians typically handwrote these orders, which were then faxed to the respective departments or transcribed by nursing personnel into an order communication system. The order communication system, however, only enabled transmission of the order to various departments' information systems. There was no CDS in the order communication system. CPOE systems today have at a minimum drug-allergy checking and drug-drug contraindication checking.

Physicians may dislike CPOE systems, at least initially, because they view order entry as a clerical task. Initial implementations also did not do a very good job of setting the sensitivity of alerts, so alert fatigue was often the result of an excessive amount of alerts that were then ignored. Another concern with CPOE systems is that they are based on standard order sets. These order sets reflect the current thinking about patient care from research, referred to as evidence-based medicine (EBM). Despite that EBM may reflect the best scientific evidence on how to treat a patient with a specific condition, there is rarely "one size fits all" for human beings (Cerrato 2012). A patient with a specific condition frequently has other conditions that may not have been taken into account when the research study was performed. As a result, most standard orders need to be modified for each patient. In haste, a physician may accept the standard orders or may make an error in modifying them—which may result in unintended consequences.

e-Prescribing E-Rx (e-prescribing) is a special type of CPOE application used to write prescriptions and transmit them to retail pharmacies via the National Council for Prescription Drug Programs (NCPDP) SCRIPT standard that is sent through a pharmacy information exchange. E-Rx is used in physician practice as well as when a patient is discharged from the hospital or emergency service with a prescription and in hospital outpatient departments or clinics. The e-Rx system includes medication alerts and reminders just as the hospital-based CPOE system, but it also includes formulary information from Pharmacy Benefit Managers (PBMs) that identifies whether the patient's health plan covers the cost of a drug and what copay may be required. Physicians find benefits from e-Rx systems as a result of availability of a medication list, fewer calls from pharmacies not able to read their handwriting or needing to advise them that a drug ordered is off formulary for a patient, and being able to receive electronic communications from retail pharmacies for renewal approvals.

Electronic Medication Administration Record

The medication administration record is used by nurses in a hospital to document the giving of drugs to patients. The frequency and care that must be taken to ensure that a nurse administers the right drug is critical to avoid medication errors. As a result, computerized systems have been created. Early electronic medication administration record (EMAR) systems were simply electronically generated paper lists of medications from the pharmacy information system after it processed physician orders. Later, the lists were retained on the computer and nurses were expected to post the date and time of medication administration to the computer. Any exceptions to or issues with medication administration, however, were still included in handwritten nurses' notes. Most importantly, these systems, while providing a legible list of medications, did not fully address the medication five rights—right patient, drug, dose, route, and time.

Today, many hospitals are moving to BCMAR systems. These require the hospital to have each patient identified with a barcode (usually on a wrist band) and to package (or buy prepackaged) drugs in unit dose form, each with a barcode or radio frequency identification (RFID) tag that identifies the drug, dose, and intended route of administration. At the time the drug is to be administered to a patient, the nurse logs onto the BCMAR system and scans the patient's wrist band and unit dose package. The system automatically dates and time-stamps the entry made through this process. As a result, the medication five rights have been followed. Most BCMAR systems also enable notes to describe exceptions, such as the fact that the patient was in surgery at the time the next dose was to

be administered. BCMAR systems provide some CDS, as do CPOE systems, often including links to additional information about drugs.

Although nurses value the more legible medication lists and patient safety assurances that are part of EMAR or BCMAR, there are issues to be overcome, just as with getting physicians to use CPOE. One issue is that to use a BCMAR system, nurses must bring a computer, barcode device, and medication to the patient's bedside. Some hospitals use wireless workstations on wheels (WOWs) that include these devices as well as a drug dispensing drawer (and a long-life battery). These can be heavy to push once fully loaded. An alternative is to carry, sometimes via a sling, a tablet computer that may be outfitted with a wanding device. Walking around all day with such equipment on one's person, however, is also not comfortable. Another alternative is bedside terminals, although many hospitals express privacy concerns with respect to implementing these. Still another issue with BCMAR in general is that the bags that contain specially compounded drugs administered intravenously require special labels, which not all hospital pharmacy information systems can accommodate, resulting in a patient safety gap.

A medication list is generated from the closed-loop medication management applications. The MU incentive program requires that the medications be documented using an RxNorm terminology. While this is a standard expression of drug names in clinical form, pharmacy information systems typically utilize the National Drug Code (NDC), which is an inventory coding system. (For example, a drug may be described in the NDC with respect to its package size, such as 100 bottles of 100 pills per bottle, information not relevant in clinical administration of the drug.) It is essential that translations are able to be made throughout the closed-loop medication management process so that drug naming conventions are followed appropriately.

Medication Reconciliation   The medication reconciliation process also can be automated, although not as easily as the other elements of medication management. Each time a patient is transferred across levels of care—when admitted, transferred into an intensive care unit, sent to surgery, and so on—a special review of medications needs to be performed. This is because very often certain medications must be discontinued or a dose changed as a result of the change in level of care. In addition, the clinicians working with the patient are different at different levels of care. Connecting all the systems at the different levels of care has been a challenge that only a few hospitals have been able to fully achieve as yet.

Automated Drug Dispensing Finally with respect to medication management, **automated drug dispensing machines** are available that are secure and make drugs specific to patient orders readily available to nursing staff. These machines are typically filled by pharmacy department staff based on the physician orders.

Clinical Decision Support

Clinical decision support (CDS) is perhaps the most important reason for documenting at the point of care and is the functionality that most clearly distinguishes an EHR from paper records. **CDS systems** are interactive programs designed to assist clinicians in making patient care decisions.

The most common CDS systems are those that are knowledge based. These are composed of four components:

- A knowledge-based system that provides facts, or evidence, concerning a domain of practice, such as drug knowledge
- Production rules that are a generic set of "if...then..." structures, or rules that draw from the knowledge base
- An inference engine, which is the software that controls how the rules are applied to specific facts (about the patient)
- The user interface, which is the presentation of the specific findings relative to application of a rule; this may include a set of questions or template on which to enter data, a process that checks responses for legal answers, a means to supply the user's responses to the inference engine, and alerts or reminders to the user (Friedlin et al. 2007)

There are also non–knowledge-based CDS systems. These use a form of artificial intelligence (such as artificial neural networks or genetic algorithms) rather than a knowledge base, enabling the computer to learn from past patterns of clinical data. Non–knowledge-based CDS systems are less frequently found in healthcare for a number of reasons, including that use of systems to capture data (that is, EHRs) is still very new by clinicians. Even if a hospital or physician practice has used an EHR for a long time, the volume of data upon which to create an accurate pattern is often insufficient. Finally, as the name implies, knowledge from clinical trials, experts, and other sources is not included in the CDS provided. Just the same, non–knowledge-based techniques can aid in the system learning practice patterns that may help data entry, such as the system learning "favorite" medications to display first.

CDS is frequently embedded as an integral part of CPOE, e-Rx, EMAR/BCMAR, point-of-care patient charting, and other applications, such as in a pharmacy information system that provides the pharmacy staff with information on potential drug contraindications (not providing a medication to a patient due to potential harm). In addition to the CDS that may exist in any one application, more robust CDS applications, often called CDS utilities, are available that can be added to these applications and work with data supplied from multiple applications in an integrated manner. For example, there are companies that are devoted to researching and using clinical evidence to build order sets, nurse care plans, quality forecasters, and practice guidelines (Versel 2011). Researchers identified a taxonomy of six major categories of CDS capabilities, with a total of 53 unique features across the capabilities:

1. Medication dosing
2. Order facilitators
3. POC alerts/reminders
4. Relevant information display
5. Expert systems
6. Workflow support (Wright et al. 2011)

The same researchers used this taxonomy to compare commercial vendor and homegrown EHR products on what features they integrated into their products. Commercial vendors surveyed ranged widely in the features they accommodated, from 28 percent for one vendor to 94 percent to another vendor (Wright et al. 2011). In this survey, researchers also found that medication dosing features were most common (86 percent of vendors had these features) while expert systems were least common (36 percent of vendors had these features)(Wright et al. 2011). Homegrown products had slight differences but were not significantly different.

Tracking the latest scientific information in making patient care decisions is critical. However, while the rewards of CDS use are great, it must be implemented carefully and must be maintained on an ongoing basis. CDS can contribute to EHR user satisfaction because users know there are controls built in to help them apply their professional knowledge in effective and efficient ways. There are also CDS utilities that can be invoked only on demand. Autopsy studies have shown that physicians misdiagnose fatal illnesses about 20 percent of the time, and in fact one such situation led to the creation of a differential diagnosis CDS utility that can scan reams of medical literature much more quickly than a human could, even if willing to take the time, which often is not available (Leonhardt 2006). Finally, there are also CDS utilities that are standalone. For example, there are systems that support infection control nurses to reduce incidence of hospital-acquired infections through quick assessments of data to which providers can respond rapidly with targeted treatment (Informa 2010). Still, overalerting is common and often results in all alerts being ignored.

The Agency for Healthcare Research and Quality commissioned a report on the state of CDS systems. The report cites that CDS is most effective when:

- CDS is matched to user intentions, noting that while on-demand reminders are less likely to be overridden, automatic alerts are often ignored
- Alerts are tiered so that those that prevent the most harmful results should be displayed for all users, whereas those with less impact may be displayed only for certain categories of clinicians

- CDS is integrated into work processes, as the system is more likely to be used in this configuration, although integration generally requires considerable customization (Berner 2009)

CDS systems must be kept current. There are many ways such systems can become obsolete or not function properly. If a rule directs a clinician to perform certain diagnostic examinations or studies are based on best practices and the best practices change, the rule needs to change as well. The medical literature is filled with examples of where new evidence has suggested that an old treatment is not as effective as a newer one or where a correlation once believed to have existed between certain factors no longer appears to be true.

In addition to keeping rules current, it is important to ensure that each rule has the correct information to process. For example, in an emergency situation where a patient presents with chest pain, there are several possible diagnoses, each based in a different body system, including cardiac, respiratory, digestive, and so forth. If a CDS system requires a specific set of data to be collected for every patient presenting with chest pain and all data requirements are met, the CDS will operate properly. However, if one data element is not entered, the rule either may not fire when it should or it may fire when unnecessary, causing an annoyance. If clinicians routinely override the rule and identify such inconsistencies in the rule firing, they will lose trust in all the CDS and the purpose of CDS is lost. Many organizations will not permit a required field to be overridden for this reason. Other organizations allow the override but have the EHR produce an alert that indicates that CDS has been negated due to lack of information, so that the users are advised that they are on their own for making the applicable decision.

However, even in cases where all necessary data are entered and a rule fires appropriately, physicians may need to override a CDS rule. For example, it may be that a patient is allergic to a medication, but having tried other medications and in consultation with the patient it is agreed to give a lower dose of the medication with heightened monitoring. This is a legitimate clinical reason for the override. Some organizations do not require explicit documentation of the rationale for overriding an alert, citing that such rationale was not previously required. However, because EHRs retain metadata indicating that a rule has fired, an attorney may question why attention was not paid to the alert in case of a lawsuit. Even if this never happens, the fired alert is likely to cause a nurse or pharmacist to double-check with the provider, and that ensuing telephone call and potential delay in getting medication to the patient could be eliminated by a simple acknowledgment that the alert was purposely overridden. The EHR should enable a pop-up for the rationale to be recorded by one simple click. Just the same, there are times when rules themselves need to be modified or turned off. In some cases, clinicians find certain rules highly repetitive and annoying. In evaluating whether a rule should be changed, a designated clinical committee should review the rule to determine whether its impact on the ultimate result warrants the change. It is also possible, however, to fire rules in accordance with classes of users. For example, when a house staff member logs on, he or she could have more CDS than when an attending physician logs on, or certain specialties may want more rules than others.

There are also concerns about overdependence on alerts where professional judgment may not be applied. For example, always assuming that a drug-allergy alert must be obeyed could lead to delayed or less effective treatment.

Both ignoring alerts and overdependence on alerts have caused vendors to introduce "hold harmless" clauses into their EHR contracts. Unintended consequences from either situation or other ineffective use of the EHR has also caused the Food and Drug Administration (FDA) to take notice and observe that it is within its power to regulate the EHR as a medical device, although such action has yet to be taken (Raths 2011).

Reporting and Analytics

While reporting and analysis of data have been performed even with paper-based health records, reporting and analytics are considered core clinical EHR applications because previously they required manual abstraction of data—even from electronic systems. A significant level of POC documentation (including CPOE and BCMAR) of structured data is necessary for the types of analytical reports clinicians and administrators need for clinical and business decisions. Analytics are also required to support accountable care organizations (ACOs) and patient-centered medical homes (PCMHs), which are reimbursement models and whose care coordination structures are designed to link patient outcomes more closely with risk and reward structures of reimbursement (Kelly 2011).

Reporting and analyzing data have been time-consuming and error-prone tasks. Data are often not required to conform to a standard vocabulary and are therefore virtually incomparable. While the Joint Commission and the Centers for Medicare and Medicaid Services (CMS) have required reporting of core measures and CMS posts the findings on its Hospital Compare website, there is little ability to use the data for real-time or even near-real-time analytics. In fact, it has been observed that healthcare primarily performs quality measurement and reporting, but the improvement aspect is limited and not required to be reported. Physician practices do not fare any better in their quality activities.

As a result of the increasing availability of patient data in the EHR, healthcare is now beginning to routinely use advanced analytics in clinical decision making (Dolan 2011). Clinical analytics is the process of gathering and examining data in order to help gain greater insight about patients (Dolan 2011). Health plans also are starting to use predictive modeling to evaluate what their future costs will look like in order to develop products accordingly, reduce cost, and ensure adequate resourcing.

Supporting Infrastructure for EHR

There are some important elements of the EHR that need special attention once the core clinical EHR components are acquired. These include the nature of the databases used in managing EHR data, storage management and e-discovery, special software to support application software, human–computer interfaces, and enhanced security controls.

Databases Databases are the means to hold data for processing. Every application has its own database. But the integration of data from multiple independent systems into a central database is generally considered an essential element for a comprehensive EHR. This not only provides access to data but also integrates them in a manner that makes them more readily processable in real time and for CDS. For example, the CPOE system is able to process drug-allergy and drug-drug contraindication alerts in its own database (although in this case it taps into a separate drug knowledge base to do so). The CPOE database, however, does retain lab results. To support drug-lab checking, such as whether a patient will tolerate a drug known to be contraindicated in patients with poor liver function, there must be the ability to use both drug and lab data. In order to collect and process data in this integrated manner, a special database is used that incorporates special indexing and management functions to capture, sort, process, and present information back to users—specific to a patient and in a split second of time. Such a database is called a data repository. To distinguish repositories that focus on clinical information (instead of financial or administrative data), the term *clinical data repository* (CDR) is used. The clinical data repository is a component of the EHR that captures data.

CDRs are relational databases that have been optimized to perform online transaction processing (OLTP). Each and every time a user enters data, retrieves data, views data, and is supplied an alert specific to a given patient, that action is considered a transaction.

A CDR is typically used for processing transactions, and even though they may be very complex, each transaction does not require processing an immense amount of data at one time. When complex reporting and analytics are to be performed on data, a clinical data warehouse (CDW) may be the more appropriate database structure to use. **Data warehouses** are often hierarchical or multidimensional and are designed to receive very large volumes of data (often as an extraction of data from a repository) and perform complex, analytical processes on the data. This processing is referred to as online analytical processing (OLAP).

Data can be mined and processed in many ways. For example, a data warehouse may be used for clinical quality improvement and best practice guideline development. It is not to suggest that reports cannot be generated from any individual application or from a CDR; however, complex, analytical processing will degrade the processing power of the CDR and frustrate users. Hence, small organizations that do not acquire a CDW tend to generate fewer complex reports, process them at night or on weekends when the CDR is less active, or rely on external CDWs to which they send data for processing.

Storage Management and e-Discovery Storage management is increasingly important in an EHR environment (Hardy 2010). The volume of data captured by information systems in general, and in particular by EHRs, is becoming immense. In addition, there is a growing expectation in the industry that data should be accessible in real time for very long periods of time. Finally, as clinicians become dependent on the computer for all their data needs, they will not tolerate downtime or delays for retrieving archived data. As a result, while storage media are becoming less expensive, managing data storage has become increasingly important. Many hospitals are creating specific storage management service units within IT departments. Storage management is the process of determining on what type of media to store data, deciding how rapidly data must be accessible, arranging for replication of storage for backup and disaster recovery, and determining where storage systems should be maintained. Storage management requires an understanding of the nature of the data to be maintained and its potential future use.

New technologies should aid storage management. Many healthcare organizations use storage area networks, which are networks whose sole purpose is the transfer of data between computers and storage elements (Tate et al. 2006). Some healthcare organizations are beginning to look at virtualization to reduce both processing and storage hardware costs. **Virtualization** is the emulation of one or more computers within a software platform that enables one physical computer to share resources across other computers (Blokdijk 2010). Even newer to healthcare is **cloud computing**, which is the application of virtualization to a variety of computing resources to enable rapid access to computing services via the Internet (Mell and Grance 2011). Cloud computing is not limited to storage management, as some EHR vendors are providing EHRs as **Software as a Service (SaaS)**— a subscription service to EHRs delivered over the cloud. Although more than storage, **redundancy** in servers, networking, and telecommunications capabilities such that there are at least two means of processing, moving, and exchanging data must also be part of contingency planning that includes backup, emergency mode operations, and disaster recovery. These are often new strategies for many care delivery organizations as they approach adopting the mission-critical systems that are EHR components.

The introduction of an EHR should trigger a review of the organization's retention schedule, with an eye toward potentially enabling a realistic retention schedule for electronic data. Another element of the retention schedule should be to understand the impact of e-discovery and address what will be retained for what period of time. E-discovery refers to the Amendments to Federal Rules of Civil Procedure and Uniform Rules Relating to Discovery of Electronically Stored Information. E-discovery makes audit trails, the source code of software used, **metadata** ("data about data"), and any other electronic information that is not typically considered the legal health record subject to a motion for compulsory discovery. Three examples serve to illustrate this.

- Nurses have long used a card system for annotating their care plans for their patients— written in pencil so they may be updated as needed. On discharge, these have been discarded and were not considered part of the legal health record. This has been the standard of practice, but in an EHR the care plans are recorded permanently. It may be feasible to delete these from the EHR. But it is yet another new step, which some nurses may always remember to do and others may not; and some nurses may choose to

delete or not, based on certain circumstances they perceive to be important. The inconsistency of the practice is very likely subject to question in a court, which may request this information through an e-discovery motion. Because the EHR will record this, it is probably best to retain the information in light of the potential for e-discovery.

- Documentation of system crashes in the IT department is actually a HIPAA requirement (under the Security Rule standard on information system activity review). There has been more than one incident of a lawsuit lost or large settlement made when an information system activity log could not be produced for the court as proof of the timing of a system crash in comparison to the timing of a specific data entry, dictation, transcription, or signature on a document.

- Documentation associated with CDS systems is increasingly important. This includes what changes are made to the EHR's data dictionary that may impact the firing of a CDS rule, changes made to the rules themselves, as well as documentation of overrides and their rationale. For instance, if a data element is required and users want to make it optional, a data analyst should study the potential impact of this change. If it is very likely to cause a CDS rule to misfire and there is a high risk for a negative result, the change probably should not be made. If a change is made, it should be made only with the approval of a clinical committee that has studied the impact and determined that the organization is willing to take whatever risk exists. This should be documented within the data dictionary as the change is made. Likewise, if a CDS rule is turned off or changed, the risk must be understood. Finally, if a clinician is provided with an alert and ignores it, it is possible that an attorney may request a motion to review both the software and an audit trail, asking why the alert was overridden. If not documented, the clinician may not be able to recall or may be found in noncompliance with standards of practice (Amatayakul 2013).

Support Software Special software to support application software is increasingly needed in an EHR environment. Such software includes interfaces and interface engines and their associated data exchange standards, as well as inference engines, registry systems, and knowledge bases previously described.

Because an EHR relies on exchanging data with multiple source (and destination) systems, communication across these systems is essential. But few of these systems are fully integrated. Integration in this context means that the systems exchange data seamlessly without the need for an interface, or special software to negotiate the exchange. In most cases, however, source systems are from different vendors, or from vendors who have acquired different products and "bolted" them together with a strong interface. The result is often that applications do not exchange data easily with one another, or with a CDR into which much of the data should be placed for ease of EHR use. In order for an interface to be written, however, the applications' software must be written to conform to a data exchange standard protocol. HL7 is the predominant standards development organization that creates standards for exchange of clinical data. Likewise, the Accredited Standards Committee X12 (ASC X12) develops standards for exchange of the HIPAA Transaction Code Sets (TCS). Digital Imaging and Communications in Medicine (DICOM) develops standards for exchange of clinical images, and the NCPDP develops standards for exchange of retail pharmacy financial and administrative data and for prescriptions. Where a hospital may have as many 200 to 500 different applications and an increasing number of medical devices that now must be connected to information systems (physician practices will have fewer applications, but still the potential exists to have at least 2 if not 20 or more), there are potentially even more interfaces needed, as an application may need to communicate with several other applications. Consider only the R-ADT application that must communicate with virtually every other clinical system. The result, then, could be that hospitals may have hundreds of interfaces. While many vendors do write their software to comply

with the protocols so that interfaces can be written, there are nuances in the standards that do not make them as "standard" as desirable and the interfaces must be kept up-to-date as changes are made to both the underlying applications and the standards themselves. Hence an interface engine is a tool to manage the multiplicity of interfaces and track changes.

Recall that data exchange standards only focus on syntax, or structure and format, of the data. Data exchange standards are often called message format standards for this reason. The interoperability achieved through application of message format standards is often referred to as technical interoperability. Technically, the data from one application can be exchanged with another application. Technical interoperability, however, does not address semantics, or the meaning of the data. Semantic interoperability requires use of a standard vocabulary to ensure that when data are exchanged the meaning of the data will be understood.

While data exchange standards are challenging today, there is the expectation that applications will ultimately be moved from a client/server architecture to a web services architecture (WSA) that can take advantage of Extensible Markup Language (XML) constructs. XML is a specification for creating custom markup languages that uses a set of annotations to text that gives instructions regarding how text is to be displayed. HL7 Version 3 messages are based on an XML encoding syntax. However, the message standard is not backward compatible with its Version 2.x protocols; until such time that care delivery organizations move from a client/server architecture to WSA, the value of the HL7 Version 3 messaging component is somewhat limited for use in structured data exchange. There are, however, some new uses that are being made of the Version 3 standard, and it is widely deployed in Europe and in countries that did not have the legacy infrastructure as the United States.

Data capture and retrieval technology must also be reassessed in light of the EHR and its clinical users. The term human–computer interface (HCI) is used to describe these technologies because they are the construct that enables exchange of data between the human and the computer. That interface is improving, but still challenging. HCIs must direct data capture in a clear and concise manner for both the novice and the power user. Data capture as well as visualization techniques, which were mentioned when describing clinical analytics (how data, alerts, reminders, and other elements of EHR use are displayed), have a significant impact on patient safety. Consideration must be given to screen size and effective use of screen "real estate," the nature of icons and the universality of their meaning; and even sound, animation, and color with respect to the healthcare environment, which has a lot of sounds and different types of lighting. It has been mentioned that clinicians are mobile and often work in teams that require viewing the same information simultaneously. Structured data entry is counterintuitive to most clinicians, so these tools must be easy to use. Especially for documentation of progress notes, clinicians prefer to be able to read narrative, so structured data entry must be able to be converted to a narrative output. Different techniques are available, each with its own benefits and risks. These include the computer wrapping narrative around structured data to produce sentences or paragraphs, DRT, or more sophisticated NLP, or through macros or copy and paste techniques that reuse standard phraseology.

Usability, or the overall ability of a user to capture and retrieve data efficiently and effectively, has been an increasingly recognized issue of importance. The Certification Commission for Health Information Technology (CCHIT 2009) was the original organization that certified EHR products and was one of several ONC-authorized testing and certifying bodies (ONC-ATCBs). It offered a comprehensive certification program—certifying beyond the basic MU criteria. For its comprehensive certification of ambulatory EHRs, CCHIT provided a usability rating it called PERUSE (from perceived usability). Meaningful Use Stage 2 required EHR vendors to adopt user-centered design principles and demonstrate they used them to test their products for patient safety.

Enhanced privacy and security controls may be both more available in an EHR and more needed in an EHR environment. This has been recognized by the proposed modifications to the HIPAA Privacy and Security Rules in HITECH. Although most of HIPAA's privacy requirements are accomplished through administrative and operational activities, EHR technology can assist in carrying out a number of the privacy standards. An EHR can provide highly effective access controls to meet the HIPAA Privacy Rule minimum necessary standard requirements. Role-based access controls (RBACs) are used where only specific classes of persons may access protected health information (PHI). Context-based access controls (CBACs) add the dimensions that control not only class of persons but specific categories of information and under specific conditions for which access is permitted. Because the minimum necessary requirement does not pertain to disclosures for healthcare treatment, some care delivery organizations have interpreted this so broadly as to include that any healthcare professional may have access to any patient, or at least any physician or nurse may have such access. (This form of access control is usually referred to as user-based access control [UBAC]). It must be observed, however, that not every clinician has a treatment relationship with every patient. In an emergency, the EHR should have emergency access procedures that can be invoked by a simple additional click on a pop-up window, for instance, indicating the nature of the emergency. This function is often called "break-the-glass," a term that is taken from the action one takes to break the glass to reach a fire alarm. This usually also generates a special audit log that can be reviewed later to ensure that the situation was truly an emergency. Having such a strong control has been a huge deterrent for the curious. In another example, when a patient requests confidential communication, there needs to be a way to notify providers that an alternate address or phone number must be used to contact the patient concerning certain information. Again, a note on the chart cover may be the only available solution in the paper environment, but a flag that pops up on a computer screen or that automatically routes calls or correspondence would provide much greater assurance that the patient's request is being carried out. Many technical measures are available to help protect patient privacy.

HIPAA's security requirements are generally more technical than the privacy requirements, but they also require establishing policies to direct how the technical tools will be applied. As noted under the privacy discussion, access controls used in healthcare organizations in the past have been quite weak. As a result of heightened concerns on the part of the public and because of an increasing rate of identity theft in general and medical identity theft in particular (Irby 2010), state governments and now the federal government under the HITECH data breach notification requirements (45 CFR Parts 160, 162, and 164 2013) are cracking down. As a result, many care delivery organizations are adopting more stringent security controls, sanctions, and other formal processes to aid in data protection. Because so many security incidents have occurred surrounding the use of laptops, other portable and mobile devices, remote storage services, and remote access capabilities, the federal government issued a HIPAA Security Guidance document in December 2006, providing specific cautions and recommendations for policy development, heightened training, and addressing incidents. It also strongly recommended possible risk management strategies including two-factor authentication, increased backup, password protection for all files, encryption for all portal devices, strong physical security protections for mobile devices, and prohibition against transmission of PHI via open networks,

such as the Internet. Yet again in 2009, the federal government issued guidance specifying the technologies and methodologies that render PHI unusable, unreadable, or indecipherable.

More attention is being paid to security, but apparently it is not considered enough. The MU incentive criteria added a requirement for a security risk analysis to be conducted to determine the appropriate level of security controls to put into place to ensure not only confidentiality of PHI within EHRs (so it is not wrongfully disclosed), but also data integrity (such as encryption and other security controls so data are not altered as they are stored on electronic media or transmitted) and data availability (through various forms of contingency planning—backup, emergency operations, and disaster recovery). A risk analysis, as illustrated in figure 12.4, is a systematic process of identifying security measures to afford protections given an organization's specific environment, including where the measures are located, what level of automation they have, how sensitive the information is that needs protection, what remediation will cost, and many other factors. A security risk analysis should lead to ongoing security (and privacy) compliance auditing (Amatayakul 2009).

Other heightened security controls are also being mandated, such as the use of **two-factor**

Figure 12.4. A security risk analysis

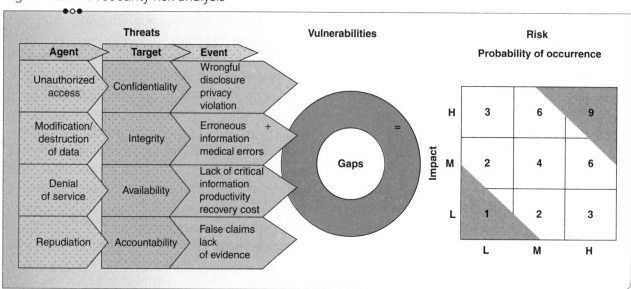

Source: Copyright © 2005, Margret\A Consulting, LLC.

authentication (that is, a password and token) for e-prescribing of controlled substances (21 CFR Parts 1300, 1304, 1306, and 1311 2010). Modifications to the HIPAA Privacy and Security Rules will make business associates directly accountable to the regulations and not just via a contractual obligation with the covered entity. Health breach notification from PHRs has also been mandated by the Federal Trade Commission (16 CFR Part 318 2009).

EHRs in Other Types of Healthcare Institutions

Hospitals and physician practices have generally been the early adopters of EHRs. They have been discussed together in this chapter because increasingly they are using the EHR systems from the same vendor, they are connecting on a much more regular and intensive basis, and hospitals depend on their physicians to adopt the technology in the hospital as well as in their own practices. Other types of healthcare providers, however, are adopting various forms of EHRs in increasing numbers.

Behavioral health facilities find the integration of data from multiple sources especially helpful in coordination of care. A number of behavioral health EHR products are on the market, and some were certified under the original EHR product certification program. At this time, however, behavioral health professionals who are not physicians do not qualify for MU incentives. Somewhat related to behavioral health are human services agencies. These often have a behavioral health component but also manage assisted living facilities, child care services, adult day care, and many other programs that have at least some need for EHR types of recordkeeping and are, in fact, moving to adopting automated systems to support their needs.

Long-term and post-acute care (LTPAC) has been a relatively early adopter of health IT components. Home health agencies have for some time adopted handheld devices to capture data in compliance with regulatory requirements. Nursing home facilities have a difficult time affording systems, but their highly structured data-reporting requirements also make them good candidates for simple EHR systems.

Finally, health plans collect a tremendous amount of data about individuals from claims, direct feeds from commercial labs, and claims attachments. Most health plans are creating databases that can be sorted by patients as their EHRs for disease management or data in aggregate can be used for analytics.

Check Your Understanding 12.6

Instructions: **Answer the following questions on a separate piece of paper.**

1. The standards related to archiving images is
    A. Accredited Standards Committee X12 (ASC X12)
    B. Health Level Seven (HL7)
    C. Radiological Society of North America (RSNA)
    D. Digital Imaging and Communications in Medicine (DICOM)

2. Which of the following is a form of clinical decision support (CDS)?
    A. Drug-allergy alert
    B. Presentation of a context-sensitive template
    C. Workflow support
    D. All of the above

3. Which of the following provides for the five rights of safe medication administration?
    A. Barcode medication administration record
    B. Computerized provider order entry
    C. Electronic medication administration record
    D. All of the above

4. A clinical data repository (CDR) is a relational database optimized to
    A. Archive data for real-time accessibility
    B. Conduct online transaction processing
    C. Perform online analytical processing
    D. Store documents and other digital information

Match the category of EHR system components to the specific functionality and technology:

5. _____ Storage area network

6. _____ E-prescribing

7. _____ Eligibility verification

8. _____ Nutrition and food services system

9. _____ Clinical analytics

10. _____ Usability

11. _____ Inference engine

12. _____ Practice management system

A. Financial and administrative system

B. Ancillary or clinical departmental system

C. Core clinical EHR applications

D. Data quality management

E. Supporting infrastructure

F. Systems to provide connectivity

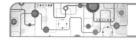

References

Amatayakul, M.K. 2013. Electronic Health Records: Conceptual Framework. Chapter 5 in *Health Information Management: Concepts Principles and Practice*, 4th ed. Edited by LaTour, K.M., S. Eichenwald Maki, and P. Oachs. Chicago: AHIMA

Amatayakul, M.K. 2009. *Guide to HIPAA Privacy and Security Auditing: Practical Tools and Tips to Ensure Compliance*, 2nd ed. Marblehead, MA: HCPro.

American Health Information Management Association. 2011a. CAC 2010-2011 Industry Outlook and Resources Report. http://library.ahima.org/xpedio/groups/public/documents/ahima/bok1_048947.pdf

American Health Information Management Association. 2011b. *Pocket Glossary of Health Information Management and Technology*. Chicago: AHIMA.

Ball, M.J. and S. Bierstock. 2007 (Summer). Clinician use of enabling technology. *Journal of Healthcare Information Management* 21(3):68–71.

Berner, E.S. 2009. Clinical decision support systems: State of the art. AHRQ Publication No. 09-0069-EF. Rockville, MD: Agency for Healthcare Research and Quality. http://healthit.ahrq.gov/images/jun09cdsreview/09_0069_ef.html

Blokdijk, G. 2010. *Virtualization—The Complete Cornerstone Guide to Virtualization Best Practices*, 2nd ed. Newstead, Australia: Emereo Pty Ltd.

Blumenthal, D. 2009 (Dec. 27). Presentation to the American Medical Informatics Association. http://www.informationweek.com/blog/healthcare/229204271?printer_friendly=this-page

Bufton, M. 1999. Electronic health records and implementation of clinical practice guidelines. In *Electronic Health Records: Changing the Vision*. Edited by Murphy G.F., M.A. Hanken, and K.A. Waters. Philadelphia: W.B. Saunders Company.

Cerrato, P. 2012 (Jan. 5). Is your clinical database up to speed? *InformationWeek*. http://www.informationweek.com/news/healthcare/clinical-systems/232301360

Certification Commission for Healthcare Information Technology. 2009. Usability Testing Guide. http://www.cchit.org/get_certified

Chi, N-C. and G. Demiris. 2015. A systematic review of telehealth tools and interventions to support family caregivers. *Journal of TelemCusacedicine and Telecare* 21(1):37–44.

Dolan, P.L. 2011 (May 2). Electronic Medical Records: What Your Data Can Tell You. amednews.com. http://www.ama-assn.org/amednews/2011/05/02/bisa0502.htm

Friedlin, J., P.R. Dexter, and J.M. Overhage. 2007. Details of a successful clinical decision support system. *AMIA Annual Symposium Proceedings* 2007:254–258.

Friedman, C.P. 2009. A "fundamental theorem" of biomedical informatics. *Journal of American Medical Informatics Association* 16:169–170.

Hardy, K. 2010 (May 19). Data storage of top concern to healthcare providers. *Healthcare IT News*. http://www.healthcareitnews.com/news/data-storage-top-concern-healthcare-providers

HIMSS Analytics™. 2010 (January 7). Clinical Analytics: Can Organizations Maximize Clinical Data? http://www.himssanalytics.org/docs/clinical_analytics.pdf

IEEE. 2015. IEEE 802.11™: Wireless LANs. http://standards.ieee.org/about/get/802/802.11.html

Informa. 2010(July 13). Clinical surveillance system documents interventions to help reduce catheter-related infections. *Infection Control Today*. http://www.infectioncontroltoday.com/news/2010/07/clinical-surveillance-system-documents-interventions-to-help-reduce-catheter-related-infections.aspx.

Institute of Medicine. 2003. Key capabilities of an electronic health record system. Letter Report. Washington, DC: IOM. http://www.nap.edu/books/NI000427/html

Institute of Medicine. 1991. *The Computer-Based Patient Record: An Essential Technology for Health Care.* Washington, DC: National Academies Press.

Irby, L. 2010 (March 23). Medical Identity Theft on the Rise—Statistics. http://www.spendonlife.com/blog/medical-identity-theft-statistics

Kelly, F. 2001. Implementing an Executive Information System (EIS). http://www.dssresources.com

Kelly, J. 2011 (April 18). Lack of EHR standards hampering healthcare data analytics. http://siliconangle.com/blog/2011/04/18/ehr-standards-healthcare-data-analytics/

Kohn, D. 2003. The technologies behind document management systems. *Advance Healthcare* 13(14):24

Kohn L., J. Corrigan, and M. Donaldson. 2001. *Crossing the Quality Chasm: A New Health System for the 21st Century*. Committee on Quality of Health Care in America, Institute of Medicine. Washington, DC: National Academies Press.

Kohn L., J. Corrigan, and M. Donaldson. 2000. *To Err Is Human: Building a Safer Health System*. Washington, DC: National Academies Press.

Leonhardt, D. 2006 (Feb. 22). Why doctors so often get it wrong. *The New York Times*. http://www.nytimes.com/2006/02/22/business/22leonhardt.html

Lundberg, C.B., J. Warren, J. Brokel, G. Bulechek, H. Butcher, J. McCloskey Dochterman, M. Johnson, M. Mass, K. Martin, S. Moorhead, C. Spisla,

E. Swanson, E. and S. Giarrizzo-Wilson. 2008 (June). Selecting a standardized terminology for the electronic health record that reveals the impact of nursing on patient care. *Online Journal of Nursing Informatics*. http://ojni.org/12_2/lundberg.pdf

Mell, P. and T. Grance. 2011 (Sept.). *The NIST Definition of Cloud Computing*. NIST Special Publication 800-145. Gaithersburg, MD: National Institute of Standards and Technology.

National Alliance for Health Information Technology. 2008 (April 28). Defining key health information technology terms. http://healthit.hhs.gov/portal/server.pt/...0...0.../10_2_hit_terms.pdf

Nuance Communications. 2008. Dragon Medical: Speech-enable the Practice's EMR for Faster, More Efficient and Profitable Clinical Documentation [Product sheet]. http://www.nuance.com/naturallyspeaking/pdf/ds_DNS10_Medical.pdf

Office for Civil Rights. 2011 (Dec. 31). Health Information Privacy Rule Enforcement Highlights. http://www.hhs.gov/ocr/privacy/hipaa/enforcement/highlights/index.html

Open Source Initiative. 2012. The Open Source Definition. http:// http://www.opensource.org/docs/osd

Pulley, J. 2010 (June 1). EHRs not so user-friendly. *Health IT Update*. http://healthitupdate.nextgov.com/2010/06/the_usability_or_lack_thereof.php

Raths, D. 2011 (April 8). Report from PharEHR Summit: Will FDA regulate EHRs? *Healthcare Informatics*. http://www.healthcare-informatics.com/article/report-pharmehr-summit-will-fda-regulate-ehrs

Resnik, P., M. Niv, M. Nossal, A. Kapit, and R. Toren. 2008 (Fall). Communication of clinically relevant information in electronic health records: A comparison between structured data and unrestricted physician language. *Perspectives in HIM, CAC Proceedings*. http://perspectives.ahima.org/index.php?option=com_content&view=article&id=136:communication-of-clinically-relevant-information-in-electronic-health-records-a-comparison-between-structured-data-and-unrestricted-physician-language&catid=58:conference-paper&Itemid=110

Schnitzer, G. 2000. Natural language processing: A coding professional's perspective. *Journal of AHIMA* 71(9):95–98.

Stead, W.W. and H.S. Lin, eds. 2009. *Computational Technology for Effective Health Care: Immediate Steps and Strategic Directions*, 2–5. National Research Council. National Academy of Sciences. Washington, DC: National Academies Press.

Stead, W. and M. Lorenzi. 1999. Health informatics: Linking investment to value. *Journal of the American Medical Informatics Association* 6(5):341–348.

Strong, K. 2008. Enterprise content and records management. *Journal of AHIMA* 80(2):38–42.

Tate, J., P. Beck, H. Hugo Ibarra, S. Kumaravel, and L. Miklas. 2006. *Introduction to Storage Area Networks*, 4th ed. IBM Redbooks. http://www.redbooks.ibm.com/redbooks/pdfs/sg245470.pdf

Tonelli, M. 2006 (Feb.). Evidence-based medicine and clinical expertise: Physicians should incorporate a balance of evidence-based medicine with expertise and experience in their clinical decision-making process. *AMA Journal of Ethics* 8(2):71–74. http://journalofethics.ama-assn.org/2006/02/ccas1-0602.html

TripleTree. 2006. Healthcare Revenue Cycle Management. Spotlight Report. http://www.connextions.com/files/TripleTreeRevenueCycle.pdf

Versel, N. 2011 (Dec. 19). 10 innovative clinical decision support programs. *Information Week*. http://www.informationweek.com/news/galleries/healthcare/clinical-systems/232300511

Warner, H. 2000. Can natural language processing aid outpatient coders? *Journal of AHIMA* 71(8):78–81.

Witry, M.J., W.R Doucette, J.M Daly, B.T Levy, and E.A Chrischilles. 2010 (Winter). Family physician perceptions of personal health records. *Perspectives in HIM* 7. http://www.ncbi.nlm.nih.gov/pmc/articles/PMC2805556/

Wright, A., D.F. Sittig, J.S. Ash, J. Feblowitz, S. Meltzer, C. McMullen, K. Guappone, J. Carpenter, J. Richardson, L. Simonaitis, R.S. Evans, W.P. Nichol, and B. Middleton. 2011 (May). Development and evaluation of a comprehensive clinical decision support taxonomy: Comparison of front-end tools in commercial and internally developed electronic health record systems. *Journal of the American Medical Informatics Association*. 18(3):232–242.

Wunderlich, G and P. Kohler, eds. 2001. *Improving the Quality of Long-Term Care*. Institute of Medicine Committee on Improving the Quality of Long Term Care. Washington, DC: National Academies Press.

16 CFR Part 318: Health Breach Notification Rule. 2009 (Jan. 1).

21 CFR Parts 1300, 1304, 1306, and 1311: Electronic Prescriptions for Controlled Substances. 2010 (June 27).

45 CFR Parts 160, 162, and 164: HIPAA Transactions and Code Sets, Security Rule, Privacy Rule, Breach Notification for Unsecured Protected Health Information. 2013 (Jan. 25).

13

Health Information Systems Strategic Planning

Margret K. Amatayakul, MBA, RHIA, CHPS, CPEHR, FHIMSS

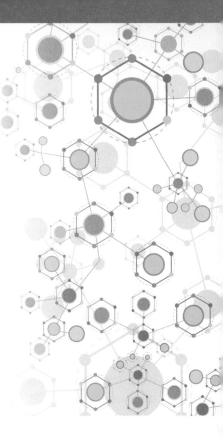

Learning Objectives

- Participate in strategic planning of the systems development life cycle for health information systems
- Facilitate the design, implementation, and ongoing maintenance of health information systems

- Examine health information systems from a utilization perspective to help optimize their use
- Analyze health information systems from an information and data governance perspective to help ensure their value

Key Terms

Accountable care organization (ACO)
Administrative data
Administrative metadata
Adoption
Application service provider (ASP)
Benefits realization
Best of breed
Best of fit
Change control
Chart conversion
Chief information officer (CIO)
Chief medical informatics officer (CMIO)
Chief technology officer (CTO)
Clinical data
Clinical data analyst
Clinical transformation

Cloud computing
Contract negotiation
Data administrator
Data conversion
Data governance
Data model
Data provenance
Data quality management
Data quality measurement
Database administrator
Decision support
Dependency
Descriptive metadata
Due diligence
e-discovery
End user
Environmental scan
Financial data

Go-live
Governance
Health data
Health informatics
Health information
Health information system
Health information technology
Health reform
Implementation
Implementation plan
Information governance
Installation
Interface
Interoperability
Legacy system
Metadata
Migration path
Optimization

Patient safety
Personal health data
Planning horizon
Policy
Population health data
Procedure
Project manager
Project plan
Public health data
Request for proposal (RFP)
Requirements analysis
Requirements specification

Research data
Return on investment (ROI)
Risk management
Scribe
SMART goals
Software as a service
   (SaaS)
Steering committee
Stewardship
Strategic plan
Structural metadata
Sunsetting

Super user
System
System configuration
System development
   life cycle
System integrator
Tactical plan
Thoughtflow
Usability
Value
Value-based purchasing
Workflow

Although many people use computers and other types of electronic systems on a daily basis almost without thought, automating health information is still relatively new to healthcare. There remain many users who do not take full advantage of a computer's benefits. Although the first computers were created in the 1940s and automation has been used in many healthcare settings since the 1970s for processing financial and administrative data, it was not until 2010, when federal incentives were offered for making meaningful use of electronic health records (EHRs), that healthcare became serious about implementing and using information systems. The healthcare industry remains very much in the process of fully acquiring, implementing, and adopting health information systems. Furthermore, as anyone with a smartphone knows, the life cycle of new technology moves so rapidly that what we buy today practically becomes obsolete tomorrow. Health information systems are much more expensive, complex, and time-consuming to implement than smartphones, so their life cycle is somewhat longer—but still necessitate upgrades, enhancements, and sometimes replacements. This chapter focuses on strategic planning for the life cycle of needs identification, requirements specification, acquisition, implementation, maintenance, and monitoring of results to ensure health information systems address desired needs.

A Systems View

In general, a **system** is a set of components that work together to achieve a common purpose. For example, the circulatory system includes the heart, arteries, veins, and blood that help nourish our bodies. A computer system is a set of devices that support the programing of electrical pulses to represent and process data. An information system is generally regarded as including humans and computers. Humans build the computer hardware, write software so that computers process data, connect various applications to one another, and also address the operational issues relating to people, policy, and process. Such operational components include, for example, training on use of the various information system applications, establishing policy for how applications will be used, and improving associated processes. Ideally, the result is information that has value and can improve the quality of care, patient safety, access to care, cost of care, efficiency of care processes, patient experience of care, and the health of the nation in general. Figure 13.1 summarizes the scope of a health information system.

Many people involved in design, implementation, or use of information systems often do not think about the components as part of an overall system and how all of the parts must work together to achieve the desired result. There is a need to take a systems view of looking at any major project or program to appreciate the interrelationships

Figure 13.1. Scope of a health information system

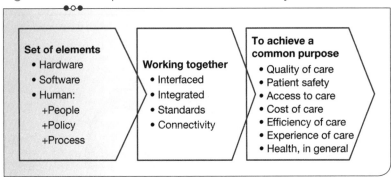

Copyright © 2015 Margret\A Consulting, LLC. Reprinted with permission.

between the components and how each component affects the whole (Haines Centre for Strategic Management 2013). Ultimately, a systems view should ensure that all needed components exist and are working together properly. Without a systems view, it is possible—and very likely—that components may not work together or there may be gaps that need filling so the result is not what was desired. For example, in implementing information systems in healthcare, it is often found that intended users do not want to take the time to learn how to use the systems or to have their processes redesigned. The result of these gaps frequently causes the information systems to be used poorly, or in some cases abandoned.

The healthcare industry sometimes uses the terms *health information system* and *health information technology* synonymously. This chapter distinguishes their meaning.

Health information system is used to refer to all the components—human and computer—that ensure health data are processed into useful health information. The human component will include everyone and their associated practices from the computer hardware designer and software engineer to the process improvement specialist and end user of the information being derived from the data being processed; and many others. The computer component includes hardware, software, cables, radio waves, and much more.

Health information technology is reserved to describe computer systems used to process health data into health information.

Figure 13.2 illustrates a health information system(s), comprised of many computer (software

applications and other health information technology) as well as human (people, policy, and process) components. A local health information system exists in each organization; and as a nation, the local health information systems collectively are a health information system, whether or not they share data directly.

Health data and health information are increasingly defined very broadly. **Health data** are the raw facts or figures that are processed into useful health information. **Health information** supplies value to the management of illness, injury, or maintenance of health and wellness. Health data include data created by an individual as well as data created by a healthcare organization or health plan.

The following example illustrates how all types of health data are processed into useful health information by the various components of a health information system.

An individual experiencing symptoms of contaminated food documents the symptoms and a food diary in a personal health record, and seeks treatment. A diagnosis is confirmed by a provider in a local emergency department with the aid of a laboratory test performed on a specimen from the individual. This information is available for the individual to view from a portal to the provider's information system and/or to the lab's information system. The provider writes a prescription that is electronically transmitted to a local pharmacy. Part of the cost of the drug may be covered by the individual's insurance and the individual keeps a record of the co-pay for income tax purposes. The provider should convey the potential for food contamination to the local public health department who will manage further contamination.

Figure 13.2.   Health information system

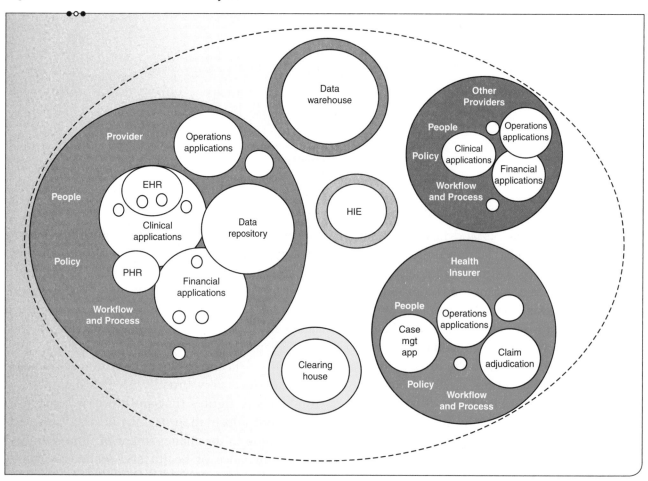

Copyright © 2015 Margret\A Consulting, LLC. Reprinted with permission.

If the food contamination can be spread, an entire region's population may be impacted.

Until very recently in healthcare, the lack of sharing of health information across disparate systems has not been valued. With a new focus on health reform and accountability for the quality of healthcare delivered, the ability to share information across the continuum of care has become essential.

System Development Life Cycle

As suggested by the fast pace at which health information technology changes and the many processes and components entailed in processing health data, it should be clear that health information systems have life cycles that, when fully understood, can be used to manage changes so the system continues to produce the desired results. The **system development life cycle** (SDLC) refers to the steps taken from an initial point of recognizing the need for a desired result, through the steps taken to ensure that all components needed for the system to achieve the desired result are addressed, to repeating this cycle whenever the result of the system fails to continue to produce the desired result (NIST 2009). Failure of a system to produce the desired result may be due to internal or external changes. For example, if a health information system was acquired a number of years ago and there is a new federal mandate for a change in a code system or the operating system software is no longer being supported, the healthcare organization must address needed changes in the system (or acquire a replacement) to continue to produce desired results. The general nature of an SDLC is illustrated in figure 13.3.

There may be variations in how the steps in the SDLC are described depending on the context in which it is used. For example, a hardware or software developer may go through an SDLC when creating a new product. The vendor may identify need for a new product; then determine the feasibility of creating the new product with specifications that would satisfy the new product needs, design the product, develop it for mass production, maintain the product as small changes in the environment

Figure 13.3. System development life cycle

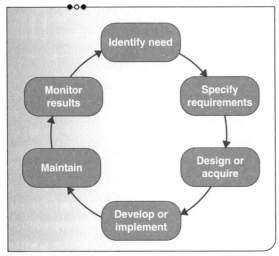

Copyright © 2015 Margret\A Consulting, LLC. Reprinted with permission.

may impact it, and monitor sales to justify continued maintenance or sunsetting (no longer selling or supporting) the product. As another example, when a provider identifies a need for health information systems support, the provider will specify the requirements needed, acquire the new system, implement the new system, maintain it, and monitor that it continues to meet needs over time. Sometimes a health information system may need to be fully replaced (for various reasons), in which case the SDLC of acquiring a new product is repeated.

Each of the major steps in the SDLC generally includes a number of smaller steps. For example, when an upgrade to a provider's health information system becomes available from the vendor, a provider may determine if it wishes to accept the upgrade (identify need); develop a plan for implementation (specify requirements such as when the upgrade should occur and who will perform the implementation); acquire the upgrade; implement it; and continue to use it for its operations (maintain it) until monitoring proves the need for another upgrade, replacement, staff retraining, or other action.

The SDLC is most often applied when information systems are being developed or acquired. However, the SDLC should also be applied as part of a continuous improvement process to assure that systems meet ongoing and any new needs. Taking a systems view and applying the SDLC can also be a useful process when planning any new program, expanding service offerings, and addressing other needs. The key value of the SDLC is to apply a formal, logical process to ensure that all components needed for a system to optimally achieve its value are in place.

Strategic Planning for Health Information Systems

The SDLC can be especially useful when developing a strategic plan, especially for health information systems. Generally a **strategic plan** is long term, covering a period of at least three to five years, and focused on the direction needed to accomplish the organization's mission.

Because computer systems have a short life cycle, many organizations develop plans for information systems that are often only one or two years. This is actually a **tactical plan** (short term, focused on one component or project) rather than a strategic plan. Tactical plans often do not fully address the SDLC. The result may be one where the short-term project focused on only one component does not work well with other components of the larger health information system.

Strategic Planning Purpose

Strategic planning is necessary to assure that all parts of a health information system are addressed, especially as new components continuously are developed and many systems are expanding beyond organizational boundaries to connect large systems with other large systems. Most providers find that the timeline for planning information systems is at least three to five years, and many have already exceeded 10 or even 20 years—especially when considering all of the components that must be addressed. For example, in order to implement an EHR, most providers need, at a minimum, a patient registration system to supply patient demographic data to the EHR. Hospitals need many additional systems, such as laboratory information systems, nursing documentation systems, release of information systems, food and nutrition systems, human resource systems, patient financial systems, and such. Most hospitals will have upwards of 100 systems, and very large healthcare delivery networks may have several hundred systems. The smallest physician office may have as many as 10 different types of health information systems. Even when most of the health information systems are acquired from the same vendor and look like they are only one system; they are actually many components, often installed separately over time.

If a health information system, as defined previously, includes human and computer components, then both human and computer components must be planned. Technology impacts people in different ways. In a physician's office, for example, the practice management system (PMS) is primarily used by practice administrators for patient demographic data and billing processes. They often have previous experience using these functions as standalone systems; and clinicians—physicians and nurses—rarely, if ever, use the PMS. But when an EHR that integrates the PMS with EHR functionality is acquired, practice administrators and clinicians are impacted. The practice administrator may need very little additional training and may

be excited by new functionality available from the new system. Alternatively, the EHR may be feared by the clinicians who often have little or no experience using information systems, at least in their working environment. Clinicians will need considerable training, time for workflow and process redesign, information on change management, and strong usage monitoring to determine if they should celebrate success or correct course. Taking a systems view when implementing the new, integrated system not only assures that the technology will be addressed, but that "people, policy, and process" factors will be addressed to ensure users achieve value from the new technology.

Another strategic planning consideration from a systems view is the need to sequence the implementation of the technical components within the health information system and the need to recognize the impact of the sequencing on people, policy, and process.

For example, many hospitals early in the process of implementing EHRs decided to implement barcode medication administration record (BCMAR) systems that nurses would use to ensure the right medication was given to the right patient at the right time. From a strategic planning view, these hospitals often thought that nurses would learn these systems very easily and then be able to assist physicians when it came time to implement computerized provider order entry (CPOE) systems. The result of not addressing the full SDLC, however, led to many hospitals finding that nurses did not like these systems and often did not use them properly. For example, when a barcode reader was tethered to a computer by cable, the cable often did not comfortably reach to the patient's barcoded wrist band. Those tasked with acquiring and implementing the technology must not have considered the component of how the barcode reader would be used in actual practice. Nurses also did not like the increase in medication "errors" that resulted from using the system—often because the default policy in BCMAR systems was set to record any delay of more than a few minutes in administering medication as an error, even if the patient was in surgery at the time the medication was originally programmed to be administered.

Without strategic planning from a systems view to identify the need to evaluate policy, many nurses created workarounds such as scanning copies of the patients' wrist bands at the nursing station and then actually administering the medications whenever the patient was available.

Interestingly, the plan to sequence the implementation of computerized provider order entry (CPOE) systems after the implementation of BC-MAR systems backfired when the federal incentive program for Meaningful Use (MU) of EHRs was adopted, requiring CPOE in Stage 1 and BC-MAR not until Stage 2.

The incentive program may also be an example of lack of a systems view and the need for more strategic planning at the national level. The incentive program timelines have slipped and the goals for each stage have had to be modified (see figure 13.4).

For example, many providers found it took longer than two years to fully implement Stage 1 requirements. In some cases, their vendors were not ready; in other cases implementation challenges such as those described in the previous examples precluded timely attestation to meaningful use of the EHR. There were also challenges in meeting Stage 2 requirements, especially for **interoperability** (ability to share data across separate systems). The federal government had not fully established electronic processes for collecting quality data to measure health system improvement, so that quality data were not being derived directly from the EHR but by intermediary processes. By the end of 2015, not only had the timelines slipped for both Stages 1 and 2, but there was uncertainty surrounding whether Stage 3 would be implemented or the MU incentive program shut down to be substituted with other strategies. It was also not until 2015 when the Office of the National Coordinator for Health Information Technology (ONC) released its first 10-year Nationwide Interoperability Roadmap with increasing focus on sharing health information and health IT beyond the EHR. Clearly health information systems are not only major investments, but complex systems that require extensive preparation, time to implement, and attention to human factors to get people to use them correctly and achieve results.

Preparing for Strategic Planning for Health Information Systems

Strategic planning for a health information system should adopt a systems view. The life cycle of strategic planning should begin with addressing its governance and planning horizon. Then, much like the SDLC for the health information system itself, strategic planning should:

- Describe needs to be met in the form of goals for the system.

- Identify challenges that must be addressed in specifying the system's design requirements. These challenges can often be identified through an environmental scan.

- Document the design of the health information system in a migration path that provides a reference point for acquiring and implementing the components of the health information system.

- Establish maintenance requirements for the system.

- Put forth a monitoring program that assures the goals for the system are being met; and if they are not, take steps to examine new

Figure 13.4. Goals and timeline for federal incentive program for Meaningful Use of EHR

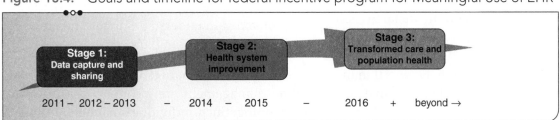

Source: Adapted from ONC 2013.

needs, specify requirements for addressing new needs, design and implement changes in the system, and keep those changes current and appropriate for continuous goal achievement.

The components of strategic planning mirror the components of the SDLC.

Governance

Governance of the strategic planning process should be established before strategic planning begins. **Governance** refers to the establishment of policies and the continual monitoring of their implementation for effectively and efficiently managing an organization's assets (Business Dictionary 2015). Effective governance results from interactions between key stakeholders to which the stakeholders are accountable and who follow a transparent, responsive, equitable, and inclusive process to make decisions about how an organization will use its assets to achieve a specific goal or set of goals (Good Governance Guide 2012). Governance for strategic planning of a health information system must reflect the components of the health information system (human and computer) and how the organization's information assets support the healthcare delivery process (Cole 2015).

The governance of the strategic planning process for a health information system, therefore, will be performed by representatives from senior management (financial, operational, and clinical) and the leadership of information technology and enterprise health information management.

Senior managers should be involved in health information system strategic planning. The following are the roles of senior managers involved in such planning:

- The chief financial officer (CFO), or a deputy, should participate in strategic planning both to impart knowledge about financial feasibility and financing for the system and to learn and appreciate opportunities for return on investment from the system. Financial managers need to get an overall perspective on how a health information system can impact

the total value of healthcare; **value** is defined as a combination of quality, cost, and patient experience of care. In addition, the patient financial manager in combination with the finance officer is increasingly involved in various strategies the nation is adopting for **health reform** (that is, major policy changes to improve the quality and manage the cost of healthcare). **Value-based purchasing** (VBP), a key health reform strategy, is a specific program of enhanced payment to deliver care that takes into consideration access, price, quality, efficiency, and alignment of incentives rather than volume alone, which has been the hallmark of fee-for-service payment mechanisms (NBCH 2011). Strategic planning for a health information system today needs to recognize the need for and how patient financial and cost information can integrate with clinical data.

- The chief operations officer (COO), or a deputy, should be responsible for ensuring that the health information system is used by all applicable persons within the healthcare delivery process. Input provided by this representative to the strategic planning for a health information system can help anticipate and prepare the organization for the myriad changes in processes and workflows that will occur as part of health information system adoption, and the broader context of health reform.

- Senior clinical officers, including the chief medical officer and chief nursing/patient care officer, represent the primary users of the clinical components of health information systems. As such, their contributions to strategic planning for a health information system are vital to getting grassroots adoption of the systems to be implemented. They provide input and gain understanding to generate trust in the systems from their peers.

Leaders of information technology and information management are also involved in strategic planning. Such individuals have the technical knowledge and skills to help direct the implementation of the health information system being planned:

- **Chief medical informatics officers** (CMIOs) are physicians who have special interest in health information systems and technology (McNickle 2012). They typically are practicing physicians who can put policy into practice. While the CMO represents the medical staff as a whole on all matters relating to their practice of healthcare, the CMIO is the bridge between the medical staff and administration of a healthcare organization implementing a health information system. They are enlightened advocates, but also strong proponents of system **usability**—the efficiency, effectiveness, and satisfaction with which users achieve results from health information systems (Pfister and Ingargiola 2014), and **patient safety**—preventing harm to patients, learning from errors, and building a culture of safety (Hughes 2008). The CMIO is focused how data and information may be analyzed, transformed, used in decision support, and disseminated within a learning health system (AMIA/AHIMA 2012).

- Other informatics professionals include those specific to nursing and other clinical disciplines. They are focused on individuals and patients. Public health informaticians focus on populations and society. Together these professionals are referred to as health informatics professionals (AMIA/AHIMA 2012) and may provide one or more representatives to the strategic planning process for a health information system depending on the size of the organization and the current status of building a robust health information system. **Health informatics** is a growing field focusing on the intersection of technology, clinical practice, and financial affairs (AHIMA 2014).

- The **chief information officer (CIO)** is responsible for the "management, implementation and usability of information and computer technologies" (Rouse 2015a) for an organization. The CIO should offer the strategic planning process; both current state of the art information regarding health information technology and level-setting for the planning timeline over which changes and new technology can realistically be implemented. The CIO also manages staff members who play important roles in incorporating health information technology into the organization's health information system strategic plan.

- A **chief technology officer (CTO)** is responsible for overseeing current technology and creating relevant policy for its use (Rouse 2015b.).

- **Clinical data analysts** contribute to configuring information systems specific to organizational needs, conduct training on use of technology and specific healthcare applications, and may be engaged in creating reports and monitoring data usage for specific clinical applications—especially those related to clinical research (Darling 2011).

- **Database administrators** are technical staff members within information technology departments who design and manage the technical implementation and maintenance of databases.

- **Data administrators** are persons who apply domain expertise to the logical design of a database, establish policies and standards governing creation and use of data, maintain data dictionaries, and manage the quality of data. Data administrators may have backgrounds in health information management and/or health informatics.

- The health information management (HIM) professional complements the perspectives provided by the CIO in planning health information system strategy. Where the CIO addresses the technical components of health information as processed by health information technology, the HIM professional provides information and data governance perspectives. These focus on managing the input (data) and output (information) of the health information system. They specifically address the components of data design (that is, data models) and capture, data security, data quality, information access and use, information retention and disposal, documentation requirements, legal and regulatory compliance, ethical use of information, and the intellectual property ownership of information (Kloss 2015, 40).

Planning Horizon

The **planning horizon** for the strategic planning of a health information system refers to both the scope of the system to be addressed and the number of years estimated for planning, acquiring, and implementing the components identified. The planning horizon helps anticipate the resources that will be needed and the feasibility for carrying out the plan. If there are insufficient resources, the planning horizon may need to be lengthened, the scope narrowed, or alternatives considered.

Components of Strategic Planning

Following a systems view, the components for strategic planning for a health information system include identifying needs for the organization that can be addressed through a health information system, recognizing challenges that may get in the way of assuring needs are met, designing a plan that ensures challenges can be overcome, and maintaining the plan via ongoing monitoring.

Describe Needs

Needs for the organization that a health information system can address are most commonly expressed as goals. Goals for what and how the health information system will achieve desired results reflect current and anticipated needs and should drive all subsequent elements of the planning process. **SMART goals** are statements that identify results that are:

- Specific
- Measurable
- Attainable
- Relevant
- Time-based

An example of a SMART goal for a hospital performing strategic planning for a health information system is to:

Improve the near-miss medication error rate (specific) by 80 percent (measurable) using a BCMAR system (relevant) that is implemented with adequate training and process improvement (attainable) over a period of one year (time-based).

Another goal for this same hospital planning its health information system may be:

By the time BCMAR is fully implement (time-based), nurses will spend 50 percent (measurable) less time on paperwork in order to spend at least a half hour more per patient on education (measurable) by using a single nurse assessment template (specific), tailored to the data identified by nurses as necessary for patient care (relevant) and for which nurses will receive help from a consultant successfully implementing such a process in several other hospitals (attainable).

Any given organization will have several SMART goals for its health information system. For example, a clinic may include the following goal in its planning:

Physicians will aid in reducing unnecessary diagnostic studies tests by 10 percent (measurable) over the next two years (time-based) through the interoperability capability of the system (relevant) making available (attainable), at the time an order is placed for a test, the results from previous tests performed across the enterprise within a time period specific to the type of test and schedule for the patient (specific).

SMART goals incorporated into a strategic plan should address all system components, including desired functionality, specific technology requirements to support the desired functions, and the expectations for people to adopt new policies and processes to ensure the goals' achievement and, therefore, provide value back to the organization for its investment (Amatayakul 2013, 139).

Identify Challenges

Challenges are those inevitable elements that pose barriers to achieving success with a health information system. Without recognizing them as early in the planning process as possible, it becomes very difficult to overcome them. An **environmental** scan is a process to formally identify challenges that considers both internal and external factors (SHRM 2012). (Challenges are often described as opportunities for improvement.) The following are a few of the many ways to collect information about these environments.

- Published data can help identify lessons learned from others. For example, determining how many hospitals already had an EHR prior to implementing the incentive program may have been the trigger for federal government to implement such a program. However, in its strategic planning for the incentive program's timeline, the federal government did not apply the fact that most hospitals took much longer to implement their systems than the timeline the federal government set forth. A hospital seeking to implement an EHR under the incentive program would recognize the opportunity for funding an EHR, but in its environmental scan may have identified as a challenge the average cost of EHRs and average timelines for implementation. Looking to overcome these barriers led some hospitals and a number of physicians to acquire EHRs that matched the incentive funding and timeline—only later to find that these vendors were struggling to implement Stage 2 requirements at low cost or had not earned sufficient money to stay in business.
- Surveys are another important way to understand the potential challenges to be addressed in strategic planning for a health information system. A simple survey of staff and members of the medical staff of a hospital might have identified that, on average, low numbers of potential users regularly use a computer. This is factual data. Perceptions are also important to understand. If a survey of potential users finds concerns about using an EHR, immediate work can begin on helping overcome this challenge.
- Anecdotal information from observations and interviews are also important in helping identify challenges. Prior to the

EHR incentive program, there were already articles published about unintended consequences of EHR use. These articles described issues with how the system was designed, lack of user training, and the like. All of these issues could be overcome by attention to people, policy, and process issues; but the headlines only added to distrust of EHRs by clinicians that to this day are challenging to address.

The sources of information gathered about the environment should be many and varied. This ensures a comprehensive understanding of the environment and reduces bias.

Document Design

Design refers to a picture or framework for how a health information system being planned is expected to look. It is a high level outline of all components the organization has identified as needed to achieve its goals. This high level view is much like a map at a 30,000 foot level. General statements of goals for each part of the timeline and the general nature of the applications (software), technology (computer systems), and operational elements (people, policy, and process) are documented. This documentation of the strategic plan may be referred to as a **migration path** (Amatayakul 2013, 170)

The migration path should reflect the IT architecture of hardware and software as well as the operational elements of people, policy, and process changes to address improvements in clinical quality, patient safety, evidence-based practices, cost of care, productivity, user satisfaction, patient experience of care, and more.

The migration path is then supported by additional documentation that more specifically provides the SMART goal statements; describes the detailed nature of the information technology infrastructure; and addresses the policies, procedures, training, workflow changes, and other operational elements that need to be put into place. Staffing, budgets, detailed requirements specifications, and other elements of more detailed planning follow from the migration path. Figure 13.5 provides an

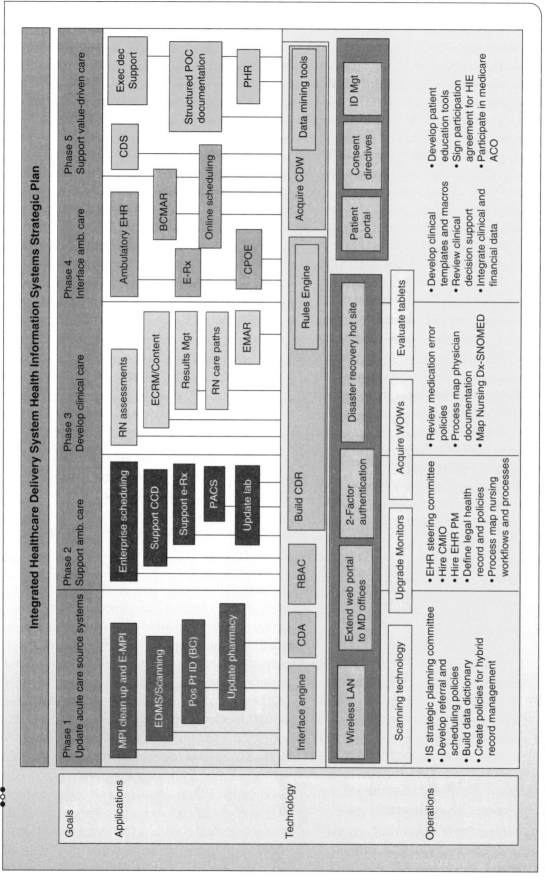

Figure 13.5. Example migration path

Copyright © 2015 MargretA Consulting, LLC. Reprinted with permission.

example of a migration path for an integrated healthcare delivery system. It is essentially a one page map illustrating where the organization is going with its health information system. Details are then spelled out in accompanying materials.

Some healthcare organizations question why they need a migration path when either their vendor heavily dictates the components to be implemented or the federal incentive program for meaningful use of the EHR directs required elements. While these circumstances do provide a framework for a strategic plan for health information systems, they do not afford a complete picture of all the major elements a healthcare organization may wish to include in its strategic plan.

For example, an EHR vendor may not supply all the software desired by an organization, such as that for integrating clinical and financial data needed to participate in a Medicare **accountable care organization (ACO)**, which is an organization of providers that work together collaboratively to improve the quality and cost of a population of patients (Council of Accountable Physician Practices of the American Medical Group Foundation 2015). In an ACO, providers are paid for the quality of care rendered, not the volume of care. In addition, most health information system vendors will acknowledge that the people, policy, and process issues associated with gaining adoption and optimizing system use are very important, but they are the responsibility of the healthcare organization. Organizations must determine when certain types of staff are needed, what policies are needed, and how processes need to change to ensure goal achievement.

There are also timelines and sequencing decisions that the healthcare organization should be making. Again, it is true that the federal incentive program dictated that there were three stages over which incentives would be paid. However, there is more to a health information system—and even more to an EHR—than what is included in the federal MU of EHR incentive program. Furthermore, the elements of what is included in each stage have shifted, as has the timeline. Finally, although implementation of CPOE

was specified for Stage 1, that does not mean that a hospital could not have implemented a full BCMAR system sometime prior to, or concurrent with, CPOE. The organization constructing its strategic plan for a health information system makes its own decisions about the timeline and sequencing, obviously considering all factors including any incentive programs and other factors identified from its environmental scan.

There are also dependencies between applications and across applications, technology, and operational elements. A **dependency** exists when one component cannot operate without another component. An example is that software cannot be used without hardware. Not all dependencies are quite so obvious. For example, a nurse acuity system that supports scheduling nurses for shift duty based on historical patient volumes and acuity levels requires administrative data from a human resource system to identify nurse credentials, a patient acuity classification system, clinical data to classify patients, and a scheduling system that tracks patient volumes by type of patient acuity. Another example that many experts are just coming to recognize is that it is advisable for EHR users to review the clinical decision support system (CDSS) rules prior to their implementation. This gives users the opportunity to learn how such CDSS is constructed, develop trust in the rules or modify them per local practices and policies, and as a result be more inclined to use the CDSS effectively.

It is important to note that a migration path is a high-level view of the strategic plan, not an implementation plan for each component. An **implementation plan** is used to manage the thousands of tasks in selecting, acquiring, and implementing the various hardware, software, and operational components of the health information system. Implementation plans are tactical, relatively short term, and often repeated with only slight variation for every component implemented.

Maintain Strategic Plan

Once the migration path is developed, it should be reviewed regularly and updated as needed.

It becomes the road map for all decisions relative to going forward with health information systems. Achieving consensus on the migration path keeps organizations from making reactive decisions. Except for unanticipated changes in current applications, technology, or operations or unexpected external mandates, the migration path should be relatively stable. Every organization has its own migration path and there is no one right or wrong path—only one that is most appropriate for a particular organization given its current situation and future goals.

 ## Check Your Understanding 13.1

Instructions: Answer the following questions on a separate piece of paper.

1. True or False: The focus of strategic planning for health information systems is implementation of health information technology.

2. True or False: The systems development life cycle encourages systematic thinking for many different types of contexts.

3. True or False: Governance of the strategic planning process should be led by the chief information officer.

4. True or False: A migration path is a tool to document potential challenges to implementing a health information system strategic plan.

5. Who is the primary advocate for usability of an EHR in heath information systems strategic planning?
   A. Chief medical officer
   B. Chief medical informatics officer
   C. Chief technology officer
   D. Chief nurse informaticist

6. The role of the health information manager in health information strategic planning is:
   A. Database administration
   B. Informatics governance
   C. Project management
   D. Technical security

7. Conducting an environmental scan as part of strategic planning may help identify:
   A. Barriers to using health information technology due to staff inexperience with computers
   B. Challenges with respect to organizational goals
   C. Operational elements needed to support application software and technology
   D. Which vendors sell products that meet the organization's requirements specifications

8. The systems development life cycle step in which it may be found that an information technology component is no longer of value is:
   A. Identify needs
   B. Specify requirements
   C. Design or acquire
   D. Monitor results

9. The purpose of an implementation plan is to:
   A. Create a budget
   B. Document the strategic plan
   C. Manage project tasks
   D. Select a vendor

Carrying Out the Strategic Plan

The strategic plan becomes a tool to identify the components that need to be acquired in addition to those that the organization already has in place. These are then implemented, often as one or more projects, each with a project manager and project plan. A project represents a specifically defined scope of work. This work includes specifying detailed requirements for each component, acquiring and putting in place the appropriate resources, implementing the components, monitoring the components' use, providing ongoing maintenance, and determining when it is appropriate to upgrade, enhance, or (in some cases replace) a component.

From a systems view, as each component is implemented and ongoing monitoring occurs, reference to the strategic plan assures that the components are still contributing to the strategic goals and that they will fit with the remaining components being acquired and implemented. As this assessment occurs, the strategic plan may need to be modified or enhanced, pushing forward into further planning horizons.

Project Management

Project management generally includes appointing a steering committee and project manager.

The **steering committee** is a representative group of key stakeholders who provide advice and guidance in the acquisition of the health information system components under consideration. The steering committee members are generally managers and representative users from the departments that will be most impacted by the given component or components of the health information system being acquired and implemented.

Although some organizations do not identify a project manager until implementation of a new health information system gets underway, many are finding that putting project planning in place earlier is needed. Planning for acquisition and implementation are significant project components. In addition, the project manager gets engaged sufficiently early in the process so that no learning curve needs to be experienced at the critical juncture of implementation readiness. As such, the organization typically appoints a project manager and, for large organizations or large projects, a project team.

The **project manager** is responsible for developing a detailed project plan and for ensuring that all tasks are successfully performed on time and on budget. The **project plan** for a health information system will very likely have hundreds, if not close to a thousand or more tasks. Details of each task's timeline, dependencies, and resources required are included on the project plan. For large organizations, some system components may be phased in over time. For example, CPOE may be implemented prior to BCMAR. Each system component itself may also have a turnover plan. For example, it was quite common to implement CPOE in the emergency department during Stage 1 of the MU program. The number of physicians using the CPOE in the emergency department generally met the initial use requirement. This allowed the organization to work very closely with these physicians and learn lessons for the remainder of the rollout. Similarly, a hospital with many nursing units might implement BCMAR on only one or two units at a time until all are implemented. A multispecialty clinic may decide that primary care physicians will be trained to use the EHR before specialists. This type of staging is often referred to as a turnover strategy.

The project manager is also responsible for the project budget; managing all contractors involved in the project as well as the internal project team; identifying and getting resolution for all issues that occur during the implementation; and performing risk management. Contractors would predominantly be the vendor's team, but might also include other contractors who assist with special activities, such as workflow and process redesign, coaching physicians, building special databases, or writing interfaces not supplied by the primary vendor, and others.

The project team consists of dedicated information technology staff from the organization (or contracted for the project specifically), super users, and operations staff who assist with workflow and process redesign, policy development, and other tasks. **Super users** are typically staff members who will ultimately be **end users** (those using the system for everyday tasks), but who have agreed to help with the implementation, testing, training, and post go-live troubleshooting. Super users may be trained and, in some cases, certified by the vendor to the specific product being implemented.

During any implementation there will be a number of risk factors that arise. Risk management is also a task at which the project manager must be skilled. **Risk management** is a process that identifies where there is the possibility that a key step or series of steps may not be performed on time, where a component of the system is not working properly and may potentially delay other aspects of the implementation or will cost more to fix, and other risks.

Although it should go without saying, communication is a vital role for the project manager and is essential throughout the entire project life cycle. Regular communication about the status of the project, invitations to contribute to requirements specifications, announcements about vendor selection, progress on implementation, and regular expressions of appreciation for support and celebration of accomplishments help reduce stress in the highly demanding experience of health information system adoption. Many project managers use a communication plan specifying the types of communications needed at various stages of the project, who should deliver the communications, the medium for the communications, and the communication that was undertaken, and any feedback or lessons learned from it. (See chapter 27 for more details on managing projects.)

Requirements Analysis

Requirements analysis is the step that identifies, in detail, the precise requirements needed for both health information technology (that is, hardware and software) and operational components (people, policy, and process) of the health information system to meet the goals specified in the strategic plan. It is not enough to say "we want an EHR" or even something expressed as a SMART goal, such as "we want to provide patients easy, electronic access to their health information within 24 hours of their encounter with the healthcare system." It is necessary to describe much more specifically what functionality the organization means by EHR or patient access to health information.

Functionality requirements include those relating to data entry, information retrieval, storage of data and information, analytics to be performed on data, management of the quality of the data, security and privacy protection of the data and information, data integrity, provision of access to information, sharing of data and information, and others.

Even though the federal government spells out the standards an EHR must have in order to be certified under federal government requirements (ONC 2015a) and for the organization to earn the federal MU program incentives (CMS 2015), buyers must be aware that not all certified EHRs are the same. The certification standards specify the minimum functionality for the minimum components comprising an EHR. From there, the possibilities are virtually endless.

For example, EHR certification does not include automation of every conceivable piece of health information that is captured in the course of caring for a patient. It does not address anesthesia records, nurses' notes, the patient's required diet, documentation of vital signs, a physical therapy plan, and other information that currently may be captured on paper or automated in standalone systems. EHR certification does not address document management, transcription of notes and reports, and incorporation of referral letters and consultations. Some healthcare organizations have not recognized these gaps in their haste to acquire an EHR and earn incentives. The result is a hybrid record of paper and electronic, or electronically scanned paper and electronic. In many cases, the vendor that offers an EHR for sale does not address these other components, leaving the organization to its own devices to attempt to integrate them.

The gaps identified previously only highlight gaps related to technology. There are also very likely to be gaps in operational elements. Some vendors supply extensive training on their system, including providing professional certification to "super users" who help implement and provide ongoing training on the system. Others vendors offer a website that intended users can go to for training as they wish.

As previously noted, many vendors acknowledge the importance of, but do not address changes in, workflow and processes. Few vendors will highlight the policy implications of implementing the technology. For example, if a physician uses a **scribe** (an individual who perform data entry functions at the point of care), what authority does the scribe have to document, sign a note, or override an alert?

Recognizing gaps is not to criticize any given vendor, but to assure that the strategic planning effort recognizes any gaps and that the organization addresses what it wants to do about them. For example, one organization may decide to scan all health information that is on paper and not really make plans for more than that. Another organization may prioritize automating all health information that is currently on paper so that ultimately scanning paper will be eliminated.

Gaps are not the only variations in EHRs or other health information system components. Looking "under the covers" is also important. What types of audit logging (that identifies who accessed what record, at what time, and what part of the record was viewed, added to, or changed) is performed by the system? For how long are these logs kept and is software supplied that will help analyze the logs (such as to help determine if access was to a record of a relative, done all at one time retrospectively of the care rendered, or concurrently at the point of care?) How are data about documentation retained and made visible to users as necessary? For example, most health information systems incorporate a process to correct a documentation error. But not all systems display that there was an error correction made, when, or by whom. Some of these errors could impact the patient. For example, an order for a wrong patient could have been entered, then recognized a few hours later and changed. While there should be failsafe policies and procedures for others to apply

professional judgment in carrying out all orders, it is possible that the incorrect order could have been carried out before the correction was made. Not only may this have had an immediate negative affect on the patient, but if not, it may later be missed by the person making the correction or another person that could compound the potential for negative impact.

Considering how a health information system will fit into the organization's workflow is also important. If workflows and processes are currently problematic and there is poor productivity that automation should improve, it is likely that not only some assistance with workflow and process redesign may be necessary, but also that the health information system may need to be flexible enough to accommodate some changes. An example is a physician who wanted an EHR that would support improvement in preventive service offerings for patients. The physician had in mind that some staff would address some of the preventive services at the point of registration (have you had your seasonal flu shot this year?), nurses would speak to patients about some other preventive services such as mammograms or prostate tests either before or after the patient's examination, and the physician would address more targeted preventive services with the patient at the conclusion of a patient visit. In the course of evaluating various vendor products, the physician found that not one met this requirement. One vendor, however, recognized that the physician was describing the ideal workflow for preventive services and offered to redesign the product. This vendor was then successful in selling this change to a number of other clients.

Once all the requirements that need to be acquired from a vendor are identified, they are put into a **requirements specification**, which is a formal document conveyed to vendors. Operational requirements should be treated similarly, though they are brought to senior management to assure they will be available as appropriate.

Acquisition

Acquisition of the health information system is a process that encompasses many considerations, including a vendor strategy that considers the type of vendors to be considered, issuing a request for proposal that includes the requirements specifications, and narrowing the field of vendors to the one with whom the organization negotiates a contract.

Vendor Strategy

Many organizations go through a process of considering whether they will select one or many vendors for the various components of its health information technology. Most healthcare organizations are currently leaning toward engaging a single vendor for most of the needed technology, but almost always find they need to fill in gaps with other vendors. The situation in which the goal is to minimize the number of vendors is referred to as a **best of fit** approach to acquisition. Alternatively, selecting a vendor for each type of technology throughout the migration path resulting in potentially a number of different vendors is referred to as **best of breed**. Generally it is believed that a best of fit approach will ensure that the technology components will work together, whereas the best of breed approach is used to acquire the very best any vendor has to offer. Unfortunately, this approach requires the organization to acquire software that works between two or more systems to enable the two systems to share data. This software is referred to as an **interface**.

Realistically, however, best of fit solutions do not necessarily work as smoothly as might be hoped. Sometimes a best of fit vendor is nothing more than a **system integrator**—a company that acquires products and develops permanent interfaces between them, selling them then as a single technology offering. This is not true of all best of fit vendors, but is important to determine how a given vendor compiles its technology offerings so that one can anticipate potential issues. For example, a system that has been integrated from multiple different vendors may actually exchange data well, but each component may have a different look and feel. This could be an issue for users having to learn various components. The tradeoff needs be considered before going to market.

Another consideration with respect to how health information technology may be acquired is to determine the organization's financing needs and preference for how products can be acquired. In the past, most healthcare organizations used client-server technology. The organization purchased computers that served as the location where software and data were stored and from which data and functionality were delivered to user's computers. Over time, this form of technology acquisition was replaced with an **application service provider (ASP)** strategy. In this case, the organization did not need to purchase servers. Instead, the ASP provided the servers, loaded the organization's software and data on these servers, and provided the organization's users with the data and functionality through a secure connection. In general, this was a somewhat less expensive acquisition strategy. More recently, **software as a service (SaaS)** has become popular. Much like the ASP housing the servers, the SaaS houses the servers and delivers data and functionality to the users via secure connection, but also provides the software. This strategy reduces cost to the organization further because the organization does not need to acquire the software. The disadvantage for some organizations, however, is that only minimal configuration can be made to the software to meet specific and different needs of the organization. Other organizations find this is an advantage in cost and helps standardize workflows and processes.

Many people equate SaaS with cloud computing. **Cloud computing** refers to servers that may be located anywhere in the world (where there is room on servers for a low price) and that supply data and functionality via the Internet, rather than a local place that provides data and functionality via virtual private network (VPN) or even direct cabling to a healthcare organization. The servers in the cloud can host software offered as SaaS, or can host an organization's own software, such as in an ASP strategy. Cloud computing has financial advantages, but there are risks regarding where data are actually stored and reliability and integrity of secure Internet connections. The healthcare industry is quite conservative and has only recently begun to adopt cloud computing, primarily as an offline storage option for (encrypted) data that are not routinely needed; and generally with contracts specifying that data must be stored on servers within the United States.

Request for Proposal

Once all requirements are determined for functionality, vendor strategy, and other elements being sought from a vendor, an organization typically compiles all of this information into a **request for proposal (RFP)**. This solicitation to vendors usually also includes basic information about the healthcare organization, such as how many users will be using the system, the timeline for implementation, and any special contractual issues that must be addressed. RFPs typically are sent to four to six vendors that the organization has prescreened during preliminary investigations such as at trade shows, through referrals from other organizations, and sometimes in a formal request for information (RFI) process. If a healthcare organization is early in the process of acquiring a health information system, the RFP may be lengthy and cover all or nearly all of the health information technology desired over the planning horizon. When a healthcare organization is in the middle of rolling out its strategic plan and finds it needs to fill a gap not covered by existing vendors, the RFP will be more focused. Even when the existing vendor could fill such gaps, some organizations will issue an abbreviated RFP to several vendors, especially to compare functionality. Such an RFP should include information about what other vendors are involved in the mix of components that already exist so that the vendor can determine what may be needed for system integration.

Evaluating Responses to the RFP

Evaluating responses to an RFP for a major health information system acquisition generally follows several steps.

1. An internal analysis of the proposal against the requirements specification and other components of the RFP should be conducted by the steering committee. The steering committee should also thoroughly analyze all components of the proposal, not just the price.

In fact, many organizations do not supply the steering committee with price information at the beginning of the RFP analysis. This can bias a steering committee for or against specific vendors, when in reality the price in the proposal is rarely the price after negotiation (Cohen 2005). Second, and perhaps more importantly, price may (though not always) reflect quality—not only of the health information technology itself, but the associated operational elements included such as timeliness of implementation completion, responsiveness of ongoing maintenance and upgrades, and other factors.

2. Once the internal review is complete, the steering committee should narrow the field of vendors where any vendors whose bids are deficient are dropped from consideration.

3. Remaining vendors (often this is three or four) who appear on internal review to meet the requirements specified in the RFP should then be invited to conduct a demonstration of their products. Ideally this should be an in-person demonstration so that not only can intended users see firsthand what the system can do, but the vendor also can get a better understanding of the organization. While the expectation is not that the vendor will attempt to upsell (that is, sell more than requested), there may be gaps the organization did not consider. There may also be other challenges that the vendors identify that may narrow or broaden their scope of response.

4. Following the demonstration, the vendor may be asked by the organization (or may ask the organization) to return a revised proposal. If this is not necessary, generally the next step is again narrowing the field so that any vendor whose product did not demonstrate well is dropped from consideration. Typically two or three viable vendors remain.

5. Remaining vendors from the second cut may be further analyzed by conducting various forms of **due diligence** (that is, steps taken to confirm various facts about the product). Due diligence for health information system

components acquisition almost always includes reference checks, frequent site visits to see how the products work in a real-life setting, and for very big acquisitions, corporate site visits and investigations. The extent to which an organization takes these steps is often determined by the scope of what is being acquired. Reference calls may be sufficient when acquiring a single component, such as a blood banking system, food and nutrition system, or respiratory therapy system.

6. Once all information is accumulated, the steering committee, potentially with the assistance of the finance department or procurement officer should consider all of the findings to date in light of the price and contract terms. At this point a contract issues checklist should be started. This can be a simple spreadsheet on which every issue is identified and then sent to the vendor to be addressed. An example of an issue might be that a desired (but not essential) function is missing and the healthcare organization wants to know if it will be provided in the next upgrade or, if not, what it would cost to include today. Another common issue with vendor contracts is that they can be fairly weak in their obligations to implement federally mandated changes. For example, many providers found vendors unwilling to implement and test ICD-10 changes immediately when the mandate first came out. Some vendors attempted to make the change contingent upon buying other components that were actually not necessary to have with ICD-10. Stronger contractual language may have made more organizations ready earlier. Price may also be an issue for negotiation, although asking for discounts or competitive bidding should wait until all other issues are addressed. Financing may be an exception, if not already included in the RFP. Most healthcare organizations have the contract issues checklist reviewed by their legal counsel prior to using it in contract negotiation. (Amatayakul 2013)

Contract Negotiation

Contract negotiation is the process of going back and forth with the vendor on the issues identified until all are resolved to the satisfaction of both parties. It is not advisable to start a negotiation discussing price, as the vendor typically will then address all other negotiable factors with price increases.

Once all factors other than price are addressed, the payment schedule, discounts, end-of-year concessions, and other price-cutting tactics should be discussed.

One very important issue related to price is the payment schedule. The payment schedule most vendors offer requires a breakdown such as the following: a down payment of 20 percent; then 50 percent upon installation; another 20 percent upon implementation; and the remainder on the first day users use the system in actual practice (that is, go-live day). This should not be considered an acceptable payment schedule. The organization should offer a small down payment of 10 percent; another 10 percent on installation; 40 percent on completion of implementation; 20 percent upon completion of training and go-live; and the remaining 20 percent 90 days after go-live to assure that there are no unforeseen issues from implementation (Stratis Health 2013).

One successful place to cut price is often on interfaces, which are software programs used to share data between different applications. For example, if the system being acquired is mainstream and the system that needs to be interfaced is also mainstream, chances are very high that the vendor has already written many such interfaces and should not charge for this, or should charge only a modest fee for minor adjustments and testing.

Another way to cut cost is for the healthcare organization to acquire its own hardware (especially user devices). Information technology vendors typically mark up the prices of hardware and most organizations have the ability to buy in quantity at a discount.

In general, organizations negotiating price should consider that expecting a vendor to deeply discount a price puts the vendor—and ultimately the organization—at risk. If a vendor loses too much money on deep discounts, the vendor may not be able to stay in business or may have to cut staff, and hence services. Unfortunately, this was an all-too-frequent occurrence during Stage 1 of the MU incentive program. Such vendors either found it very difficult to modify the systems for Stage 2 on a timely basis putting their clients at risk for not earning the next stage of incentives, or simply went out of business, leaving the health-care organization with no support or ongoing upgrades. Some small providers simply gave up. Others waited out the delays and were grateful for the federal extensions. Still other organizations sought to remove the old system and replace with a new system. The latter is a costly and time-consuming process; although some found that it resulted in acquiring a better system and users more willing to adopt the system.

Implementation

Implementation is the process in which the system is configured to meet a specific organization's needs. Implementation follows acquisition. Implementation includes a number of steps, including installation of hardware and software, system configuration, data conversion, chart conversion, workflow and process improvement, and policy and procedure development and documentation.

Installation

Installation is the process a vendor uses to load software onto the hardware being acquired. While technically it is part of implementation because it is not performed until after a contract has been negotiated, it is rarely a step that the implementing organization undertakes itself.

System Configuration

A significant part of implementation is system configuration (often referred to as system build). **System configuration** (or system build) includes loading data tables and master files (for example, files of all the names of staff members and their permissions for access to the system), adjusting decision support rules for transitioning, writing interfaces, customizing screens, and numerous other tasks that make the system work for the specific organization. For example, consider what is done when acquiring a word processing system where there are many options for how to display tools, proofing so EHR does not become HER, and customizing templates.

Data Conversion

Implementation may also include **data conversion** (that is, taking data already in one automated system and putting it into the new system). Many organizations evaluate the quality of their data, the cost of the conversion, and the extent of differences between the old and new system in deciding whether data conversion will be performed or if data will be re-entered into the new system. For example, many new practice management systems for physician offices have by far more revenue cycle management functions than old systems. Many old systems also do not have very good data quality (for example, duplicate patients, old account information). As a result, many clinics have decided to use the new system implementation as a means to enter all new patient information so there are fewer issues with data quality, and there are no issues regarding whether the data from the old system can accurately populate the various fields in the new system.

Chart Conversion

Another conversion issue, often referred to as **chart conversion**, refers to moving from paper to an electronic system; and it most often impacts physician offices and clinics moving from paper-based health records to EHRs. Chart conversion considers how much of the paper should be moved into the electronic system, and in what form (that is, scanned images or structured data entered manually from the paper files). Most find that physicians need much less of the old information on paper than they initially think. The clinics make the paper files available for the first one or two uses of the electronic system, at which time users enter only the data really needed for ongoing care, and then the paper file is provided only on request thereafter.

Workflow and Process Improvement

Implementation almost always entails considerable involvement by the organization. If workflow and process improvement steps were not started prior to implementation, during implementation is when it is essential to address the types of changes that can be made with the information technology in order to meet the organization's strategic goals for its health information system. A process is work performed; **workflow** is the sequence of steps in the process. Workflows and processes are often depicted in workflow diagrams, which are tools illustrating what process steps are performed by whom and when, often including information about the decision factors that play a role in the process. Health information technology can often help automate these decision factors. (See chapter 25 for examples of workflow diagrams.) Computers are tireless and once programmed correctly they follow the rules and do not forget. Hence reminders and alerts are a key distinguishing feature of automated processes in comparison to manual processes (Amatayakul 2012).

In healthcare, the concept of thoughtflow has also been introduced. **Thoughtflow** refers to a process and its sequence when the process is largely conducted mentally. This is true for most healthcare professional processes (Ball and Bierstock 2007). Thoughtflows are unique because they are not visible to others who might be tasked with helping identify workflow and process improvements. Thoughtflows are also very unique to the individual. This is the primary asset the health professional has. If thoughtflow needs to be changed without the individual internalizing and creating the change themselves, it can be extremely difficult to adjust. It is for this reason that many healthcare professionals have a difficult time adapting to EHRs and other health information systems.

Policies and Procedures

Policies and procedures about how to use the information technology are also important to address during implementation. **Policy** refers to the general direction in which action should be taken that reflects the organization's culture and mission. In some cases, existing policies can be improved upon because of the greater level of precision with which health information technology can capture and measure quality of care and other areas for

improvement. **Procedures** are step-by-step guides in how to carry out a process. Procedures that will be performed via the information technology almost always need updating. More detail on procedures, workflow, and process improvement can be found in chapter 25.

Testing

Testing the system to ensure it is working as intended should be performed as part of implementation and prior to training. Testing should be a formal process where test scripts or use cases (see chapter 25) are created and used by super users and others to verify that all processing can be performed as expected. As with any issues that arise during the project, any testing failures should be documented on an issues log and corrected by the vendor before the system is released for training.

Training

Training is the final step before go-live. All end users must be trained on the system. Two key issues with respect to training are pertinent to health information systems. First, training must be done after testing. It is not fair to new users to attempt to learn the system and have to also identify whatever may be wrong with it. Physicians may not tolerate this and some may be very resistant to use such a system. Second, everyone must be trained. Health information systems are complex tools configured to the specific organization in which they have been implemented. In fact, it is advisable to consider developing policy in advance of system acquisition relating to training compliance. See chapter 24 for details on training methodology.

Go-Live

Go-live is the final step in turning over the information system to the end users. Go-live should be planned as carefully as the entire project itself. The day of go-live can be stressful for everyone. Go-live is usually a time when all hands on deck are need. Usually no vacations are permitted in areas where go-live is occurring. In many cases, all available super users are brought to this area to support new users. "At the elbow" support, where someone is immediately available to help a new user having a problem, is essential for healthcare professionals starting to use a new information system. Many project managers set up a hotline for calls of concern, sometimes set up a command center for support staff to wait for issues, and also sponsor a break area where new users can relax, get a special treat, vent, or just relax and reflect—sometimes even celebrate that they made it through their first use with no problems. The project manager should also frequently check how things are going and be prepared to make any adjustments as needed. Many healthcare organizations find it helpful for senior management and executives also to have a visible presence, especially for implementation of major system components that impact patient safety, such as CPOE and BCMAR. It is not expected that these individuals can troubleshoot system issues, but their presence shows support for the system and the ability to mobilize staff or take other critical actions at any point. Finally, there should be at least a debriefing at the end of the first day, if not the first half of a shift and end of shift. The debriefing should celebrate success even where there may be some outstanding issues. Everyone should be thanked for their support, especially the new end users; even if it is a simple thing like giving gold stars to any user who logs on or at least views one thing on the system. It is amazing how such a minor thing can maintain the morale and motivation needed for a successful go-live.

Go-live activities will taper off after the first day of use. Generally by the end of the first week of use, most major issues are identified and hopefully resolved. Super users will be needed for a while, but the project manager should monitor ongoing use to determine if there are any areas or persons with special difficulties. The project manager should have the authority to require retraining, make workflow changes, or take other steps to ensure the system is both suitable for use and is being used. It is important to determine and address the root cause of any problems and not give in just because someone does not want to use the system.

Ongoing Monitoring, Benefits Realization, System Maintenance, Upgrades, Enhancements, and Replacements

Once the major aspects of implementation are generally completed, ongoing monitoring, benefits realization, system maintenance, upgrades, enhancements, and replacements are the components of the SDLC that follow.

Ongoing Monitoring

Ongoing monitoring refers to evaluating the level of usage and the value being achieved from the usage. This should be a routine task that begins immediately after go-live. If a user is not using the system, this should be investigated. If a report is produced that is not consistent with expectations, this should be evaluated. Formal complaints should be logged on to the issues log and addressed. The task of ongoing maintenance is often turned over from the project manager to a staff person at this time; as the project manager will likely move on to managing another new project. The staff person assigned to this function should have the ability to convene a task group to address any issues that are multidisciplinary or crosscutting throughout an organization.

Many organizations find it helpful to hold weekly, then monthly, and potentially even ongoing quarterly informal or social events that convey the notion of hospitality and equality among anyone interested. The chief medical information officer (CMIO), nurse informaticist, health informaticist, and/or other person involved in day-to-day operation of the health information system and who can bridge communications between users and information technology staff should attend, listen, and investigate. Many new ideas can come from such events. Persistent issues often can be resolved. An organization with many different locations might set up an electronic forum to accomplish something similar. Informal, in-person events at each location, however, should be encouraged. Issues with electronic systems can often persist if the only avenue for registering complaints is also electronic.

Benefits Realization

Benefits realization is a formal process of studying whether the value (for example, cost savings, productivity improvements, revenue enhancements, improved quality of care and patient safety, patient and provider experience of care satisfaction) was worth the investment of time, energy, and money. Benefits realization, however, can be a powerful motivator to keep pressing ahead and to value even small gains. It should start at the completion of the implementation. This is the point in time when all end users are trained, the system has gone live, and there has been some period of time to get acclimated and adopt as much of the process changes and functionality as possible.

Benefits realization begins with a review of the original SMART goals to determine whether the organization believes they have been met. Some goals may be in the form of financial rewards—where there is a specific return on investment to be achieved. Many goals for EHRs are related to patient safety and quality. These often are considered more qualitative than quantitative, yet still can be measured. Some goals depend on perception surveys, such as patient and provider experience of care satisfaction. Other goals may be recognized as achieved based on anecdotal evidence.

Goal achievement may be staged over time. For instance, in a physician office, the office may set a goal to reduce transcription by 50 percent within the first year of adoption, then to 85 percent within the second year. In a hospital, it may be that 75 percent of all medication orders and 30 percent of all other orders are entered on the CPOE system within three months of go-live, with full utilization by the end of the first year. If these milestones are not met, the organization then needs to determine why they were not met and take steps to correct course. Is it a system problem, user training issue, resistance to change, or technology issue? As an example, an organization may not have correctly anticipated the bandwidth necessary to support all the new users. System configuration may need changing or additional bandwidth acquired, even after careful system configuration tasks have been performed. In other cases, the goals may

have been unrealistic, in which case they should be modified.

A solid management theory that "you cannot manage what you cannot measure" is very true in a health information system project. If an organization cannot determine whether or not goals have been met, there is a management issue.

Some organizations include in their benefits realization a formal **return on investment (ROI)** analysis. ROI determines if the system has paid for itself, comparing the financial benefits to the total costs of the system. This is difficult in an information systems environment.

Health information systems are expensive, even as costs are decreasing. The cost of the EHR component for a hospital is very difficult to generalize because an EHR is a component of multiple components. Source systems and other applications also must be connected to these components. Costs also vary over time. However, estimates range from less than $1 million to $3 million for a critical access hospital; $5 to $15 million for a small community hospital with generally a single vendor; $10 to $25 million or more for a small to medium-sized community hospital with multiple vendors that require either extensive interfacing or complete replacement; to upwards of $100 million or more for a large integrated delivery network to acquire the hardware, software, and human resources to fully implement an EHR (Hoyt 2011). For physician practices, the cost is somewhat easier to estimate because the components being purchased are generally more integrated. For very small practices (one to three physicians), an EHR may cost around $5,000 to $15,000 per physician (Hoyt 2011). Costs increase as the practice grows in size because of the increase in complexity. Larger practices will generally have more source systems to interface, and often the practices want greater customization and more comprehensive functionality. Costs for such systems range from $25,000 to $50,000 or more per physician (also depending on whether a practice management system is acquired or replaced as part of the EHR acquisition) (Hoyt 2011). None of the costs described here include other direct and indirect costs of the organization necessary to implement the system, such as labor costs, contractors, consultants, training materials, staff time spent in training, and such.

In addition to the challenge of identifying the complete cost of a health information system, there are many other variables that may impact whether a system is returning its investment or not. Systems take a long time to implement and costs may have been spread out over a long period of time. Some costs may be shared between systems or with other types of expenditures. For example, medical devices are increasingly incorporating information system components—Are they costs of the process of care or information technology? Other factors may have caused expenditures or investment opportunities to be different than initially planned. Many CFOs have dropped formal return on investment analyses, but still do want to see changes that demonstrate achievement of other important goals.

System Maintenance

System maintenance refers to ongoing tasks that keep the system current with minor software fixes, new hardware requirements, security updates, and many other potential needs based on continuous monitoring. While system maintenance has been viewed more as a technology issue, applying a systems view should also recognize that maintenance of workflows, policy compliance, and other operational elements should be addressed. Technical system maintenance includes ensuring continuous system backups, installing updates to antivirus software, or adding new drug information to clinical systems. Workflow maintenance should look into whether there are workarounds to the use of a health information system. Even proactive investigation as to whether the clinical decision support rules reflect current, evidence-based medical knowledge should be a routine part of ongoing maintenance. Continuing maintenance, then, requires a variety of staff skills as well as a plan and checklist.

Upgrades

Upgrades to systems are more formal processes, generally supplied by the vendor when there is a major change. For example, the upgrade from ICD-9 to ICD-10 significantly impacted health information systems. It was estimated that the change impacted as many as 50 different components of a hospital's health information systems—from the obvious coding and billing system changes, to each system that contributed charge data to the billing system as well as others relying upon coded data for various quality reporting processes (ONC 2015b). Upgrades might also be released by vendors to fix system glitches that may have been identified by the vendor's clients or user groups; or there may be federal mandates such as ICD-10, MU incentives, new versions of HIPAA transaction standards, and others.

Enhancements

Enhancements to the health information system may be new functionality provided by the vendor to an existing system, or expansion of the health information system within the organization by adding an additional system component. New functionality provided by the vendor may be considered an upgrade and included in regular maintenance fees; or it may be considered a separate product that is optional and therefore is priced as a new product. It is very important to distinguish between what is an upgrade and what is optional. Vendors often require their clients to keep current with at least a certain level of upgrade. If this is not done, new upgrades, including those required by federal mandates, may be excluded from regular maintenance and a fee must be paid for their installation and implementation. This fee covers the cost of installing all previous upgrades so that the latest upgrade works properly. New system components continue to be common changes to an organization's health information systems. In fact, many of these may be included on the strategic plan as components specifically reserved for later implementation. Others may arise out of new demands in the industry. It is anticipated that health reform will require a number of new types of information technology support.

Replacements

The healthcare industry is at the point where many organizations have a significant amount of health information technology already in place. While this is good news, it also means that the time has come for replacements of older and out-of-date systems (sometimes referred to as **legacy systems**)—in some cases, recognition that poorly performing systems need replacement; and in yet other situations, the need to replace systems that have been sunsetted by the vendor. **Sunsetting** refers to the action taken by a vendor to no longer support ongoing maintenance or upgrades for a legacy system.

Replacement often means a reselection must be performed. Reselection is the process undertaken to acquire a replacement for an existing system. Reselection should reflect lessons learned from the primary selection, especially for replacement of poorly performing systems. For example, many

EHRs were selected in haste in order to help the organization meet the MU incentive program requirements. Such systems may have been acquired without any formal selection process. Many of these systems were implemented by information technology staff with minimal or no input from end users. Workflows and processes were not changed; components may not have been configured properly; and policy on use may have been haphazard. Contracts may not have been well-negotiated; upgrades not installed; or users not trained.

A reselection does not need to start with a totally clean slate. There are components of the strategic plan, requirements specifications, RFP, and other elements that should be reviewed and updated based on lessons learned.

 ## Check Your Understanding 13.2

Instructions: **On a separate piece of paper, match the activity to the process in which the activity is performed.**

1. _____ Return on investment analysis
2. _____ Steering committee formation
3. _____ Updating virus definitions
4. _____ Contract negotiation
5. _____ Goal setting
6. _____ Reselect a legacy system being sunset
7. _____ Functionality specification
8. _____ Evaluating system usage
9. _____ System configuration
10. _____ Add a new application

A. Health information system strategic planning
B. Project management
C. Requirements analysis
D. Acquisition
E. Implementation
F. Ongoing monitoring
G. Benefits realization
H. System maintenance
I. Upgrades/enhancements
J. Replacements

Strategic Planning for Health Information System Adoption and Optimization

Just as strategic planning addresses the full SDLC, distinguishing between implementation, adoption, and optimization of a system reflects very

important stages users need to move through in order to take full advantage of health information systems. While such stages occur for any system, they are particularly applicable to EHRs, where users have not been accustomed to using computers for their work, and especially not at the point of care (that is, concurrently with interviewing, examining, and treating the patient).

Implementation

Implementation, as previously described, is the process of putting a new system into place for an organization. At the conclusion of the implementation, users are trained to use the system. While it would be desirable for everyone to be sufficiently prepared to fully use the system immediately upon their training, this is rarely the case. Initial use is often slow. Sometimes organizations encourage new users of health information systems to perform only certain, limited functions on the computer initially, gradually over time increasing these functions. Some elements of training may need reinforcement. Workflows and processes that have been changed sometimes need to be changed again to better fit a personal style, while still producing the intended results. In some cases, not all components of the information system are fully implemented and the degree of use depends on their implementation status.

A key point to bear in mind from this distinction is that a system that has been implemented does not necessarily mean that all users are fully using the system.

Adoption

Adoption refers to the stage where every intended user is fully using the basic functionality of the system. Adoption requires a period of acclimation where users need time to work through how they are going to use the system, to identify what further configuration may be necessary, to acquire retraining and (further) redesign of workflows and processes, and to have changes reinforced. Clinicians who are new to health information systems often need time to see for themselves there has been improvement in quality of care, timeliness of treatment, and other benefits with use of the system.

There is currently debate in the industry about the use of scribes to achieve full utilization of basic functionality. The purpose of using a scribe is to reduce the data entry burden for physicians. The issues with use of a scribe revolve around verification and authentication of the entry, whether the scribe will identify and report to the physician a clinical decision support alert or reminder that occurs, and whether the scribe has authority to override alerts. There are also issues of who pays for the scribe's time. If most of the other documentation is also performed on the system, there can be a question of whether the provider will review such documentation online, or whether the scribe must read it to the provider—and when and where that will occur. Any organization in which providers wish to use a scribe should have a policy that addresses these and any other issues; as well as having a documentation auditing program in place to assure that policies are followed.

With or without scribes, some users may never reach the adoption stage, in which case counseling, workarounds, sanctions, terminating employment or medical staff privileges, or other strategies may be necessary to achieve the results needed by all.

Optimization

Optimization includes activities that extend use of information systems beyond the basic functionality. The term *power user* may be applied to users who know how to perform all or close to all of the available functions in the system. Optimization focuses on using a health information system to improve the clinical practice of medicine. Such profound changes often are referred to as **clinical transformation** (Pryor et al. 2006). For example, if a physician has always prescribed a certain medication for a given condition, the physician who has optimized use of CPOE will follow evidence-based medicine guidelines in selecting the appropriate medication. New knowledge coming from multiple sources, including the organization's own health information system can be made available at the point of care. Typically, optimization also includes the integration of clinical and financial data. For example, if there is a choice of medications but some are more expensive for the patient than others, provider and patient are given a more informed choice.

Optimization often leads to acquisition of additional technology, such as more sophisticated clinical decision support, different input devices, medical device integration, data analytics, or additional applications as they become available on the market. It could be said that optimization is a continuous state of quality improvement.

Strategic Planning for Ongoing Management of Health Information

In the context of strategic planning for the ongoing management of health information, management of health information refers to the process of ensuring the quality of data and information. While the health information management (HIM) professional should be engaged in strategic planning for the health information system and the acquisition and implementation of information system components; data governance and information governance are also key roles and responsibilities for HIM professionals.

Data governance is distinguished from information governance very precisely, with **data governance** being the "function of defining, implementing, and enforcing policies and standards for data," and **information governance** the "control and use of the actual documents, reports, and records created from data" (Johns 2015). (See also chapter 3.) Both data and information should be treated as strategic organizational assets (Troester and Haxholdt 2012). When viewed in this way, the importance of data and information is elevated to the same level as any other organizational assets, such as land, buildings, furnishing, and equipment. Some have suggested that data and information are the lifeblood of an organization—without data and information, it would be impossible to carry out the mission of the organization (Dravis 2013).

Unfortunately, health data and information are often not treated with the importance they deserve. There are several reasons for this. While clinicians value health information, they find the process of documenting health data to be cumbersome and time-consuming. Another reason for not treating data and information as strategic assets is that traditionally health data and information have been buried in mounds of paper that is very difficult and laborious to process. Privacy and security protections on health data and information often further contribute to not making health data and information as available for use as appropriate. Finally, some question the accuracy and completeness of health data and information. The purpose for which certain data (such as diagnoses and procedure data for claims) are collected may be inconsistent with other purposes for which that same data are needed (such as to determine the value of performing a given procedure for a specific diagnosis). To improve the value of healthcare, it is recognized that the industry must become a learning health system. This is a system that finds better ways to capture quality data, generate and apply best evidence for collaborative healthcare choices of each patient and provider, and unlock the power of health data and information safely and securely in order to ensure value in healthcare (IOM 2007). Refer to chapter 14 for more information on a learning health system. These considerations should be addressed in a health data and information governance plan that is part of the strategic plan for the health information system.

Health Data and Information Governance Plan

Strategic planning for ongoing management of health information must address the governance of all types of health data and information for which the organization is responsible and all processes performed on this data and information, such as their capture, use, storage, sharing, and disposal as applicable. It is essential for there to be governance and stewardship (that is, taking care of something you own or have been entrusted with) for the healthcare data life cycle. Such a data life cycle follows the SDLC (Kloss 2015, 38).

ARMA International has established Generally Accepted Recordkeeping Principles for information governance that include accountability for the governance program, integrity assurance so that data and information are not altered during the course of their being processed, protection of the data and information, compliance assurance for adherence to applicable laws and other requirements in collecting and using the data and information, assurance of the availability of the data and information for all authorized users and uses, appropriate retention and disposition of the health data and information, and transparency with respect to how the governance program operates (ARMA International 2005).

In addition to a focus on recordkeeping, data and information governance for healthcare must also assure that the data and information contained in records (of any type—EHR, accounting, personnel, and others) are accurate, comprehensive, consistent, current, used according to a standardized definition of the data, granular, precise, relevant, and timely (AHIMA 2015). The content of the record must also support effective patient care. Just as medication has five rights, EHR content also requires right actions. The right clinical data must be captured. The data must be presented in a usable manner. Right decisions must be able to be made from the data. Right work processes help support the right collection and use of the data. These "rights" should yield the desired outcomes for quality and cost-effective care.

Types of Health Data and Information

Health data and information are a healthcare organization's strategic assets over which governance is needed. The types of data and information over which governance is needed in healthcare delivery settings include:

- **Administrative data**—data associated with identifying patients, location of care, healthcare professionals, and more. These data are vital for organizational operations and to ensure accurate documentation about patients.

- **Clinical data**—data produced by healthcare providers in the process of diagnosing and treating patients. While the bulk of clinical data are processed within the EHR set of health information system components, there may be clinical data residing in standalone components. Some of this may be temporary data. Other clinical data should ultimately be incorporated into the EHR. These data require the same level of governance as all other data.

- **Financial data**—data associated with healthcare is produced by and often exchanged between healthcare providers and health plans, including eligibility and benefits information, healthcare claims, and the like. Increasingly, financial and clinical data are being merged to assess healthcare value. As a result, there is an increasing need to ensure common data definitions across what often are disparate financial and clinical components.

- **Research data**—data that may be the same as any of the previous data listed plus additional data associated with a specific research protocol. For example, a research protocol may require a patient to document and submit to the researcher diet, sleep, and other information not normally collected during a treatment episode in order to evaluate the pharmacodynamics of a new drug. Such research data are often housed in separate databases, but also must be governed in the same way as all other information assets of the organization.

- **Personal health data**—data maintained by an individual, often in a personal health record. Much of this data will come from the variety of healthcare organizations that treat the patient; but some of the data may be compiled by the patient directly, such as a diabetic blood sugar diary. Some healthcare organizations offer health information technology to support the compilation of personal health data by an individual. Whatever data is supplied to a patient or directly to a patient's personal health record should be governed with the same due diligence as data that may be maintained only by the healthcare organization itself. While it may seem obvious that data about a patient that goes to a patient from a healthcare organization should be the same data as retained by the patient, personal health records are fairly new and some of the data being contributed to personal health records do not have the same level of attention paid as that maintained by the healthcare organization.

- **Population health data**—data on the quality, cost, and risk associated with the health of a specific set of individuals (Esterhay et al. 2014). This set of data may be data about all of the patients seen by the healthcare organization, a subset of the patients seen, and (increasingly) a set of data about many more patients than being treated by a single healthcare organization. There are a variety of sources of data that contribute to the larger set of data. This data may be compiled by health plan, such as the Centers for Medicare and Medicaid Services (CMS). A number of Blue Cross Blue Shield (BCBS) plans in different states are starting to compile data for the entire population of a state, whether they are enrolled in BCBS or not. Health information exchange organizations (HIO) in a state or region may also compile population health data. The primary use of data for purposes of population health are to study trends in clinical (and often financial) data to determine best practices that can be fed back to the providers in the community to improve the quality and cost of care.

- **Public health data**—data used to prevent the spread of disease. Some public health data are generated by providers; and public health nurses, social workers, and others generate additional data. Any public health data generated by a healthcare organization should maintain the information in the applicable component(s) of the health information system. Public health departments have an obligation to their data following the same data governance principles.

While addressing virtually every possible form of health data and information, a formal governance program is key to ensuring the quality of such data and information.

Metadata

Metadata are a special type of data associated with all data and information in a health information system. Many define metadata as data about data. There are three types of metadata: descriptive, structural, and administrative (NISO 2004). Essentially any data about data in an information system is metadata. It is important to note that metadata is generally not considered part of the legal health record, but may be subject to compulsory discovery in a court of law under the Amendments to Federal Rules of Civil Procedure and Uniform Rules Relating to Discovery of Electronically Stored Information (referred to as **e-discovery**). It is very important to understand what metadata exist within the health information system, to establish policies for retention and about who may have access to the metadata, and to assure that these policies are being followed.

Descriptive Metadata

Descriptive metadata describes each data element to be captured and processed by information technology. A data dictionary is typically used for this purpose. For example, the term *principal diagnosis* would be something commonly collected in an EHR. The data put into the field called "principal diagnosis" should conform to the definition in the data dictionary. Data dictionaries are often maintained in databases. Table 13.1 provides an example of part of a data dictionary entry for the data element "principal diagnosis."

Structural Metadata

Structural metadata describes how the data for each data element are captured, processed, stored, and displayed. A form of data model is generally used to describe how data elements are used in processing data, including the various attributes and relationships between data. A data model ultimately contributes to the ability to write software to perform the processing of data described in the model. The data model is also used to troubleshoot issues with data entry, processing, or information generation after implementation of the software.

An example of a process that would be modeled for an EHR is the basic function "physician enters an order." *Physician* can be defined in a data dictionary; *order*, however, is a broader concept; and different types of orders will likely be processed differently in a health information system. For example, a medication order will be sent to a clinical pharmacy application in a hospital. An order for a laboratory test will be sent to a laboratory application. A series of data models, one for a drug order, another for a lab test order, and more are required. Even then, "drug order" would have a number of data elements, such as "drug name," "dose," and others. Each of these data elements would be defined in the data dictionary.

Figure 13.6 provides examples of the basic form of a data model (on top) and the more complete version of the same data model, with labels identifying the various features of the model. These data models are depicted in an entity relationship diagram type of data model. The model helps describe relationships between entities. For instance, the example here indicates that one physician must place an order, although the order may contain many attributes (such as several drugs, diet instructions, lab tests).

Administrative Metadata

The third type of metadata is administrative metadata. This type of metadata is programmed to be generated by the information technology. It provides information about how and when data were created and used. It also is a record of the instructions given to users about actions to be taken with the information technology and what the user response was.

Audit logs and information system activity review (ISAR) logs are examples of administrative metadata. Audit logs are records of actions taken on data within information technology. The content of audit logs range from basic—such as only identifying who accessed what component of the health information system, to complex—such as

Table 13.1. Example of part of a data dictionary entry

Data dictionary	Example
Name of data element	Principal diagnosis
Physical name in database	PCPL-DX
Synonyms	None
Definition	Condition, after study, which occasioned the admission to the hospital
Reference	Federal Official Guidelines for Coding and Reporting
Source of data	Physician
Derivations	None
Valid values	ICD-10-CM codes
Conditionality	None
Default	None
Lexicon	ICD-10-CM

Copyright © 2016 Margret\A Consulting, LLC Reprinted with permission.

Figure 13.6. Examples of basic and more complete version of a data model

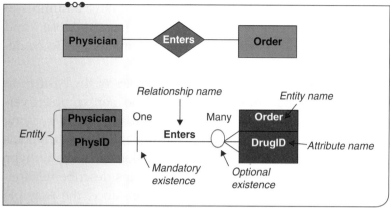

Copyright © 2015 Margret\A Consulting, LLC. Reprinted with permission.

recording who accessed what data when and what process (for example, view, copy, enter, delete) was performed on the data. Audit logs are often used as a security control, but may also help determine how a data entry error was made, when it was corrected, and who may have further accessed information about the error. Audit logs are sometimes used to evaluate the timeliness of actions performed, such as what time a drug was actually administered. Information system activity review logs (as required by the HIPAA Security Rule) documents the events that impact information technology, such as attempted hacks, system crashes, and other.

Another example of administrative metadata is decision support. **Decision support** rules are programmed into software to recognize various combinations of data that are being captured in information technology and to generate various types of actions by the technology according to the rule requirements. For instance, a data element is defined in the data dictionary as required to be entered. If a user does not enter data in this field, the software recognizes this as a result of the rule specifying this requirement and will display an alert to the user to enter data into this field. In health information systems there are many types of decision support and especially clinical decision support in an EHR.

Data provenance is another type of administrative data and refers to where data originated and where data may have moved between databases. This is becoming increasingly important as the healthcare industry shares data across many different stakeholders. For example, a physician may want to know if certain information it is acquiring into its EHR came from the patient's personal health record or another provider's EHR (Viola and Mookencherry 2012).

Data Quality Management

A last but not least element of strategic planning for ongoing management of health information is the assurance of the quality of the various types of data being used and the types of process performed on the data.

Data quality management is "the business processes that ensure the integrity of an organization's data during collection, application (including aggregation), warehousing, and analysis" (AHIMA 2015). AHIMA also distinguishes data quality management from **data quality measurement**, in which "a data quality measure is a mechanism to assign a quantity to quality of care by comparison to a criterion" (AHIMA 2015). Both data quality management and measurement are important, however the former assures good data and the later assures good care. It is believed that good care is not fully feasible without good data. AHIMA offers a data quality management model and characteristics of data quality (refer to chapter 6), including a checklist to assess data quality management efforts (AHIMA 2015).

With respect to strategic planning for health information systems, data and information governance must address how data quality issues can be discovered, how corrective action should be taken, and the necessary change controls that should reflect any changes made as a result of the corrective action.

Data Quality Discovery Process

Data quality issues can be discovered in a variety of ways—some of which are relatively easy, but others require resources for planning and carrying out. The four primary data quality discovery processes are listed in table 13.2.

Data entry errors can be easy to make, such as by clicking the wrong item, entering too many or too few digits in a number, copying narrative from one note to create another and not changing all the required variables, underusing structured data in favor of comments fields, or overriding CDS alerts and reminders. HIM professionals should assist their care delivery organizations in updating policies and procedures that describe the required documentation practices for the organization's health information system. These build on and refine documentation practices for paper-based records. The organization should also require checks and balances in the health information system to support data quality (such as valid values for a field, alerts to enter data for a required field, checks for internal consistency for right and left, and so on) and utilize regular data quality audits.

A special case of data quality concern centers on the common practice of data reuse in computer-based systems. Because it is easy to copy and paste, clinicians soon learn to use this capability where it exists. As mentioned earlier, such a practice often results in not fully addressing all the required

Table 13.2. Data quality discovery processes

Discovery process	Examples
Receiving complaints—frequent complaints about issues with specific data entry formats, or for specific data elements should be investigated	• Why do we have to enter these data? (May suggest that some of the data are not being entered) • I can't find the value for this field. (May reflect a training issue, or missing choices due to the choice either being out-of-date or very new) • This alert is always wrong. (May reflect a common data entry error or misinterpretation of guidance)
Observing use—particularly when a component of an information system is just implemented, a new user has difficulty using the system, or workarounds are suspected	• Are all users using the system at the point-of-care as intended? • Are data being documented on paper scraps (or a person's hand) and entered into the system later? • Are users skipping over data because workflow is an issue?
Auditing—a formal process to evaluate potential issues	*Auditing structured data entries* • Are data entered in comment fields where structured data choices exist? • Are data entered in comment fields because structured fields do not exist? • Are any choices never used, and why not? • Are certain data choices used too frequently, and why (for example, personal preference versus evidence-based guidelines)? *Auditing unstructured data entries (for example, comment fields, macros, copy and paste, short dictations)* • Are entries complete? • Are entries unique to the patient? • Could structured data entry generate sufficient narrative to reduce data entry burden and potential issues of repetition or other errors? *Auditing corrections, amendments, deletions* • Are corrections, amendments, deletions legitimately made, visible, date/time stamped and authenticated, linked to applicable entry?
Evaluating output—a process that evaluates the quality of the output of a process (for example, a report, graphic display of data) to identify issues that may reveal data entry problems	• Review a sampling of CDS overrides to determine if data entry errors are contributing to inaccurate alerts and reminders • Compare new, computer-generated reports to paper-based reports and reconcile differences as actual, more accurate due to better data, or less accurate due to data quality issues • Review contents of clinical summaries and other data generated automatically from the system for accuracy. (For example, this author found that her PHR identified her as a male.)

Source: Copyright © 2015 Margret\A Consulting, LLC. Reprinted with permission.

variables within the documentation. Even if the data element copied from one record to another does not contribute to a medical error, the inconsistency or incomplete documentation can result in the questioning of the entire record if the record is brought to court. Many organizations are disabling this capability where they can, or monitoring for it with applicable sanctions. Yet others have found that the practice is sufficiently useful so they put users on notice that they are individually at risk for errors that may result. Clearly, each organization should do a risk analysis to address such issues for itself.

Another factor to consider, that focuses on the EHR, is that many clinicians really do not appreciate that the EHR is more than an automated chart. They often are so grateful that they can access data they previously could not that they forget there are many other benefits that rely on structured data. However, if the findings of the audit reveal that the value placed in the comment field is one that is not on the drop-down menu and occurs frequently, there should be consideration for adding the choice or identifying it as a synonym, as applicable. Again, many new users will not think about how the system can be improved. They assume that what they are given is something with which they must work. The result can be some growing unhappiness that the EHR is not doing more than the paper chart is for the level of effort they put forth in learning to use it. Documentation audits within the EHR should look for completeness, timeliness, internal consistency, and other factors that have typically been evaluated in paper documentation. For example, when reviewing patients' data within the EHR, do all patients on a unit appear to have been given their morning meds only seconds apart? This is not feasible in walking from room to room, so it is possible that nurses have found a workaround where they are scanning all the meds at the nursing unit instead of at the point of care—defeating the medication five rights of ensuring right patient, right drug, right dose, right route, and right time.

In addition to reviewing the EHR content itself, it is important to do walkarounds to observe how systems are being used. This should be done periodically, and not just after go-live but also when upgrades or even slight modifications are applied.

For example, a desired fix may necessitate a slight change in the placement of a data entry field on an assessment form within the EHR, which then may cause an unexpected workflow and process change. While such a change (that is, a change in the placement of a data entry field) to the EHR should be communicated via pop-up at the time of login for affected users, choosing that same day to do a walkaround provides the extra emphasis on the commitment and support the organization is making in its EHR and to the clinical transformation initiative and provides an opportunity to observe any unexpected impact on workflow that may be revealed by the EHR users. Walking around also can demonstrate that those responsible for the technology and compliance are approachable. Just as in the paper world, documentation audits and walkarounds should not be punitive but serve to enhance the EHR's usefulness.

Finally, an increasing cause of data error is occurring as a result of heightened use of core clinical applications where source systems are either not connected or an audit of all changes in one application is not traced to potential impact on other applications. The Institute for Safe Medication Practices (ISMP) is an organization dedicated to medication error prevention and patient safety. ISMP (2007) describes where a hospital's pharmacy information system had recently been upgraded and new medication route codes implemented so they would be more descriptive and use more familiar abbreviations. However, when an order for "Humulin N 40 units" was entered into the computer, the pharmacist did not notice that the route of administration had defaulted to "IJ" on the BCMAR. Initially the nurse thought IJ was intrajugular, but the patient did not have a jugular line. After reviewing the original (handwritten) order, which did not include the route of administration, the nurse interpreted the "N" to be IV and administered the drug intravenously. However, Humulin N should never be administered IV and the patient became hypoglycemic. The changes made to the pharmacy information system were not evaluated to determine their impact on other systems. In addition, this is a case for CPOE that requires all components of the medication order to be entered. Finally, healthcare professionals must apply professional knowledge and judgment. If there is any uncertainty, the nurse should have accessed a drug knowledge database. If the hospital had a BCMAR component, the drug knowledge should have been available there as well.

When technology, software applications, and workflow processes throughout the organization are synchronized to support the work of the system's many end users, the organization has achieved process interoperability, a situation where all its subsystems are able to process data in like manner, with similar access controls and other policy and process constraints.

Corrective Action

For many of the examples used in this discussion, corrective action has been suggested. Discovering issues with data quality must lead to corrective actions, or the same errors will continue and users will continue their frustrations if they do not see their concerns addressed. Corrective actions generally entail making decisions about changes in data elements or pieces of software that generate CDS alerts and reminders, reports, and more. Such corrective actions should always be done in a formal manner. Some corrective actions simply entail retraining or revision of procedures to make them clearer. These should be documented that they were performed. If the data quality issues continue, other forms of corrective action may be needed.

Where corrective action entails a specific change in the information system, a work group of stakeholders to the issue should be convened to review corrective action needed, agree and formally approve the best approach to correction, ensure the corrections are carried out, and monitor that the corrections are effective.

Change Control

Change control is a formal process of documenting what change in an information system is needed, the rationale for the change, necessary approvals (for example, the stakeholder workgroup's approval to turn off a specific CDS alert), when the change was made, who made the change, that related documentation (for example, data model, data dictionary, policy, procedure) has been updated to reflect the change, and that monitoring for a period of time was performed. It is important to note that changes to information systems reflect metadata. Such a change could significantly impact patient care. For example, a CDS rule that is turned off or changed in some way should have a risk analysis performed: What is the likelihood that the change could result in significant harm? Is there evidence that clinicians apply sufficient professional judgment that such an event would be very unlikely? The answers to these and similar questions as applicable to the specific issue being studied should lead to appropriate action.

Health information systems can be powerful tools; but as with any tool, the tool must be properly built, the user of the tool must be properly trained, and the tool may need to be updated or replaced as the SDLC enfolds.

Check Your Understanding 13.3

Instructions: Answer the following questions on a separate piece of paper.

1. True or False: Data quality management uses specific measures to evaluate the quality of care.

2. True or False: Data quality management should follow the systems development life cycle of discovering an issue, implementing corrective action, and monitoring that corrections are followed.

3. True or False: In order to discover data quality issues, it is necessary to rely upon super users to report problems.

4. True or False: An example of a data entry error that can result in a patient safety issue is when an entry in a comment field is inconsistent with a structured data entry.

5. True or False: Change control is a process of not permitting changes to be made without necessary approvals.

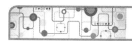 # References

American Health Information Management Association. 2015 (Oct.). Data Quality Management Model (Updated). *Journal of AHIMA* 86(10).

American Health Information Management Association. 2014 (Sept.). Defining the basics of health informatics for HIM professionals. *Journal of AHIMA* 85(9).

American Medical Informatics Association and American Health Information Management Association. 2012 (Jan. 16). Joint AMIA/AHIMA Summary of their Relationship and Links to the Informatics Field. https://www.amia.org/joint-amia-ahima-summary

Amatayakul, M.K. 2013 (Update). *Electronic Health Records: A Practical Guide for Professionals and Organizations.* Chicago: AHIMA.

Amatayakul, M. 2012. *Process Improvement with Electronic Health Records: A Stepwise Approach to Workflow and Process Management.* Boca Raton, FL: CRC Press.

ARMA International. 2005. Generally Accepted Recordkeeping Principles®. http://www.arma.org/r2/generally-accepted-br-recordkeeping-principles

Ball, M.J., and S. Bierstock. 2007 (Summer). Clinician use of enabling technology. *Journal of Healthcare Information Management* 21(3):68–71.

Business Dictionary. 2015. Governance. http://www.businessdictionary.com/definition/governance.html

Centers for Medicare and Medicaid Services (CMS). 2015. Electronic Health Records (EHR) Incentive Programs. https://www.cms.gov/Regulations-and-Guidance/Legislation/EHRIncentivePrograms/index.html?redirect=/EHRIncentivePrograms/

Cohen, M.R. 2005. Negotiating a Winning EHR Contract, TEPR 2005. http://www.mrccg.com/media/1643/tepr%20negotiating%20a%20winning%20contract.pdf

Cole, B. 2015 (May 19). Fresh Look at Governance Required to Maximize Information as an Asset. SearchCompliance. http://searchcompliance.techtarget.com/feature/Fresh-look-at-governance-required-to-maximize-information-as-an-asset

Council of Accountable Physician Practices of the American Medical Group Foundation. 2015. Accountable Care Facts, Top Questions About ACOs & Accountable Care. http://accountablecaredoctors.org/american-healthcare-whats-the-problem/

Darling, G. 2011 (Nov.). What Does a Clinical Informatics Data Analyst Do, Exactly? http://healthcareittoday.com/2011/11/08/clinical-informatics-data-analyst/

Dravis, F. 2013 (Jan. 3). Why Data is the Lifeblood of Your Business. http://www.utopiainc.com/insights/blog/417-data-lifeblood-of-business

Esterhay, R.J., L.S. Nesbitt, J.H. Taylor, and H.J. Bohn, Jr., eds. 2014. *Population Health: Management, Policy, and Technology.* Virginia Beach, VA: Convurgent Publishing.

Good Governance Guide. 2012. What Is Good Governance? http://www.goodgovernance.org.au/about-good-governance/what-is-good-governance/

Haines Centre for Strategic Management. 2013. A Systems View of the Organization. http://hainescentreasia.com/concepts/systems_view_of_organization.htm

Hoyt, B. 2011. Low Cost Electronic Health Records. Health Informatics in Developing Countries. http://www.healthinformaticsforum.com/forum/topics/low-cost-electronic-health.

Hughes, R.G., ed. 2008 (April). *Patient Safety and Quality: An Evidence-Based Handbook for Nurses.* Rockville, MD: Agency for Healthcare Research and Quality.

Institute of Medicine. 2007. *The Learning Healthcare System: Workshop Summary.* Washington, DC: National Academies Press. http://www.nap.edu/catalog/11903.html

ISMP. 2007 (July). Nurses' rights regarding safe medication administration. *ISMP Medication Safety Alert! Nurse Advise-ERR* 5(7). Horsham, PA: Institute for Safe Medication Practices.

Johns, M.L. 2015. *Enterprise Health Information Management and Data Governance.* Chicago: AHIMA

Kloss, L. 2015. *Implementing Health Information Governance: Lessons from the Field.* Chicago: AHIMA.

McNickle, M. 2012 (June 20). 5 Keys to Evolving Role of the CMIO. *Healthcare IT News.* http://www.healthcareitnews.com/news/5-keys-evolving-role-cmio

National Business Coalition on Health (NBCH). 2011. Value-Based Purchasing: A Definition. *Value-based Purchasing Guide.* http://www.nbch.org/Value-based-Purchasing-A-Definition

National Information Standards Organization (NISO). 2004. Understanding Metadata. http://www.niso.org/publications/press/UnderstandingMetadata.pdf

National Institute of Standards and Technology (NIST). 2009 (April). The System Development Life Cycle (SDLC) http://csrc.nist.gov/publications/nistbul/april2009_system-development-life-cycle.pdf

Office of the National Coordinator for Health Information Technology (ONC). 2015a (Jan. 30). Connecting Health and Care for the Nation: A Shared Nationwide Interoperability Roadmap, DRAFT Version 1.0. http://www.healthit.gov/policy-researchers-implementers/interoperability

Office of the National Coordinator for Health Information Technology (ONC). 2015b. About the ONC Health IT Certification Program. https://www.healthit.gov/policy-researchers-implementers/about-onc-health-it-certification-program

Office of the National Coordinator for Health Information Technology (ONC). 2013. EHR Incentives & Certification: How to Attain Meaningful Use. https://www.healthit.gov/providers-professionals/how-attain-meaningful-use

Pfister, H.R. and S.R. Ingargiola. 2014 (Feb. 20). ONC: Staying Focused on EHR Usability. iHealthBeat. http://www.ihealthbeat.org/insight/2014/onc-staying-focused-on-ehr-usability

Pryor, D.B., S.F. Tolchin, A. Hendrich, C.S. Thomas, and A.R. Tersigni. 2006. The clinical transformation of Ascension Health: Eliminating all preventable injuries and deaths. *Joint Commission Journal on Quality and Patient Safety* 32(6):299–308.

Rouse, M. 2015a. Chief Information Officer (CIO) Definition. TechTarget. http://searchcio.techtarget.com/definition/CIO

Rouse, M. 2015b. Chief Technology Officer (CTO) Definition. TechTarget. http://searchcio.techtarget.com/definition/CTO

SHRM (2012) Strategic Planning: What Are the Basics of Environmental Scanning? http://www.shrm.org/templatestools/hrqa/pages/cms_021670.aspx

Stratis Health. 2013. Vendor of Choice and Contract Negotiation for EHR and HIE. https://www.stratishealth.org/expertise/healthit/clinics/index.html

Troester, M. and M. Haxholdt. 2012. How to Manage Your Data as a Strategic Information Asset. SAS. http://www.sas.com/en_us/whitepapers/how-to-manage-your-data-as-strategic-information-asset-105843.html

Viola, A. and S. Mookencherry. 2012 (Feb.). Metadata and meaningful use. *Journal of AHIMA* 83(2). http://library.ahima.org/xpedio/groups/public/documents/ahima/bok1_049357.hcsp?dDocName=bok1_049357

14

Consumer Health Informatics

Ryan Sandefer, MA CPHIT

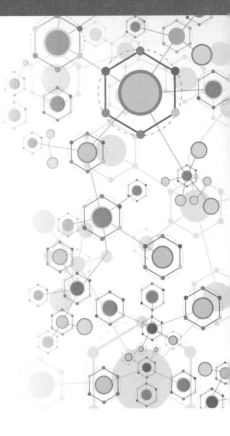

Learning Objectives

- Examine the topic of consumer health informatics
- Differentiate patient portals, personal health records, and personalized medicine
- Promote the importance of patient and family engagement
- Demonstrate knowledge of patient activation
- Analyze patient-centered care

Key Terms

Consumer health informatics
Continuity of care document (CCD)
Continuity of care record (CCR)
Health literacy
Internet forum
Learning health system
mHealth

Patient activation measure (PAM)
Patient-centered care
Patient-centered medical home (PCMH)
Patient engagement
Patient-generated health data

Patient portal
Personal health record (PHR)
Personalized medicine
Quantified self
Secure messaging
Social determinants of health
Telehealth

The personal use of technology and information is proliferating across nearly every dimension of modern life. Individuals bank, purchase books and music, and socialize using the Internet. Healthcare is not different in this respect. A growing number of individuals interact with some aspect of healthcare delivery through the use of technology. Individuals may seek information regarding their symptoms using the Internet, track their eating habits with a mobile application, access their clinical information through a secure web portal, or have a remote encounter with a healthcare provider through video technology. All of these examples are considered consumer health informatics. Consumer health informatics is largely focused on developing tools and processes to empower patients. By creating, using, and sharing health information, consumers are more engaged in their health and healthcare, which can lead to overall improvements in individual and population health outcomes.

To emphasize the importance of consumer engagement in the healthcare delivery process, the Office of the National Coordinator for Health Information Technology (ONC) produced a federal Health IT Strategic Plan that puts the consumer at the center of improving care quality, lowering costs, and improving population health (see figure 14.1). There are three major focus areas in the strategic plan (collect, share, and use), and the intent of the plan is to collect patient-generated data, share information more effectively with patients, and use technology and data to improve population health.

The model described in the strategic plan has been called the learning health system. The **learning health system** is

> an ecosystem where all stakeholders can securely, effectively, and efficiently contribute, share, and analyze data and create new knowledge that can be consumed by a wide variety of electronic health information systems to support effective decision making leading to improved health outcomes. A learning health system is characterized by continuous learning cycles at many levels of scale. (ONC 2015a)

Because the consumer is the central stakeholder in this care delivery model, it is essential that consumers can effectively contribute and use information for decision-making purposes. Figure 14.2 illustrates

Figure 14.1. Health IT strategic plan goals

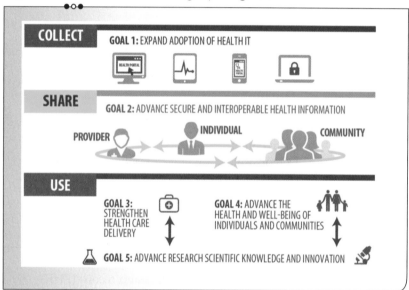

Source: ONC 2015a, 16.

Figure 14.2. The learning health system

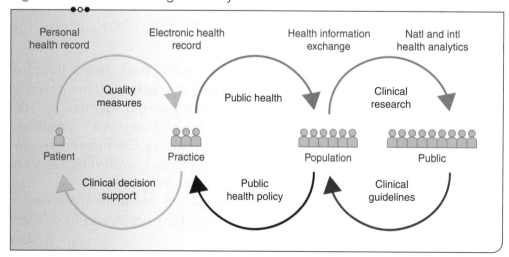

Source: ONC 2015a, 19.

how continuous learning cycles work across the healthcare continuum by showcasing how information collected throughout the care process can be used to inform care at each level.

This chapter examines the various aspects of consumer health informatics and discusses recent research that is shaping the future of the discipline. Ultimately, the goal of consumer health technology is for individuals to become more engaged in their health and healthcare, thereby improving the overall health experience and potentially health outcomes.

Consumer Health Informatics and Consumer Engagement

Consumer health informatics is the "field devoted to informatics from multiple consumer or patient views. These include patient-focused informatics, health literacy, and consumer education. The focus is on information structures and processes that empower consumers to manage their own health" (AMIA 2015). Where clinical or health informatics primarily focuses its attention on healthcare providers or organizations, the intent of consumer health informatics is to focus specifically on the needs of the consumer, whether the consumer is formally interacting with a healthcare provider or not. Consumer health informatics has also been described as the "branch of medical informatics that analyzes consumers' needs for information; studies and implements methods of making information accessible to consumers; and models and integrates consumers' preferences into medical information systems" (Eysenbach 2000, 1715). Because the needs of consumers are unique from those of other health informatics stakeholders (for example, clinicians), the design of products, services, and information displays need to be customized to ensure the greatest impact on engaging the patients in managing their health.

Consumer health informatics' focus on consumer needs and preferences speaks to its inherent link to consumer/patient engagement. The Center for Advancing Health defines **patient engagement** as

> actions individuals must take to obtain the greatest benefit from the healthcare services available to them. This definition focuses on behaviors of individuals relative to their healthcare that are critical and proximal to health outcomes, rather than the actions of professionals or policies of institutions (Chase 2013).

Patient engagement is related to more than healthcare and it is related to much more than informatics or technology. Patient engagement is patient centered as opposed to clinician or organization centered. It represents a shift in the way health and healthcare are viewed—it is focused on patient activities that support improved health and therefore health outcomes, rather than simply healthcare-related activities. As the former US Surgeon General, Dr. Regina Benjamin stated, patient engagement is "not just in the doctor's office. It's got to be where we live, we work, we play, we pray" (Brown 2011).

The application of consumer informatics to consumer engagement is not limited to the formal interactions between patients and clinicians, but rather encompasses a much wider view of how individuals work with technology and information to improve health understanding and health outcomes. The focus on consumer engagement is critical to the Institute for Healthcare Improvement's Triple Aim initiative that has a goal to optimize health system performance. The Triple Aim revolves around improving care outcomes, improving patient experience, and reducing healthcare costs. The aim focused on patient experience is intended to address patient experience from both the clinical quality and patient satisfaction perspectives (IHI 2015).

Models have been developed to illustrate consumer health informatics that places consumers at the center of a process that involves inputs, integrating processes, and outputs (see figure 14.3). The model depicts how the consumer is impacted by various factors, such as health status, culture, and

Figure 14.3. Model of consumer health informatics

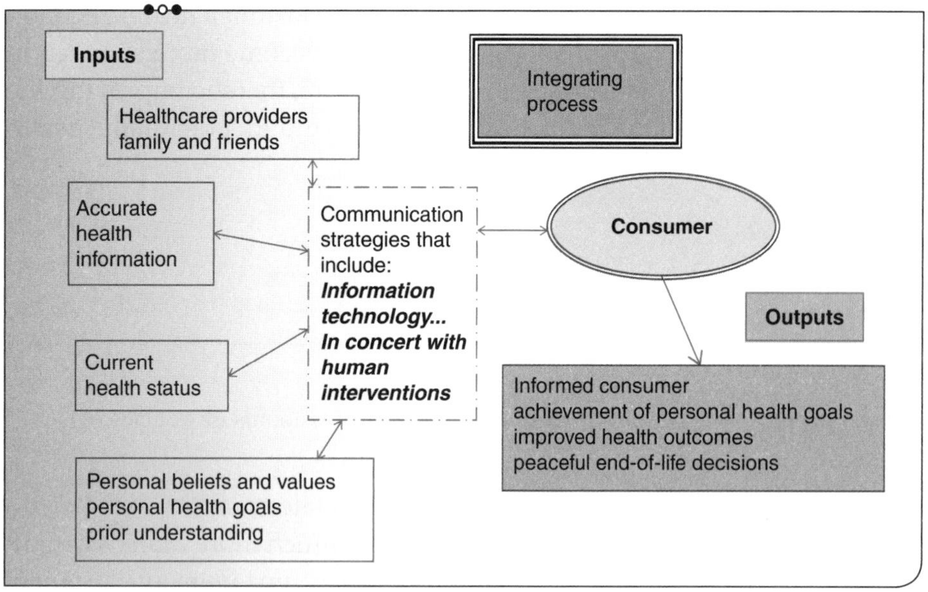

Source: Deborah Lewis, Betty L. Chang, Charles P. Friedman © 2005 Springer Science+Business Media, Inc. Reprinted with permission from Springer.

communication preferences, and how the method in which information is communicated to the patient (via technology or human–human interaction) impacts a variety of outcomes (Lewis et al. 2005).

The Evolution of Consumer Engagement in Healthcare

Historically, the US healthcare delivery system has focused on treating medical conditions by the encounter, not caring for the patient as an individual across the care continuum (Cassidy 2013; Lewis et al. 2005). The history of the patient encounter as been described as such:

> In the not-so-distant past, health information for patients was delivered from the perspective of the medical world. This model was understandable, as patients traditionally looked to their healthcare providers as the primary, and possibly only, source of information on health and disease. Although this approach may have been valuable in reducing access to misinformation, it also limited the range of information available to patients or consumers and placed the patient in a less engaged role. (Lewis et al. 2005, 1)

While this reliance on clinicians to be the sole source of health information was once the model, healthcare today is much more focused on team-based care where the patient is viewed as an integral member of the team.

Consumer Assessment of Healthcare Providers and Systems

An early attempt to evaluate consumer perception with health plans was launched in 1995 through a partnership between the Agency for Healthcare Research and Quality (AHRQ), Harvard Medical School, RAND Corporation, and the Research Triangle Institute. This partnership eventually led to the adoption of a standardized assessment of consumer perspectives regarding healthcare access and quality (CAHPS) by the Centers for Medicaid and Medicare Services (CMS). CMS has required certified organizations to evaluate the patient experience since the implementation of the Hospital Consumer Assessment of Healthcare Providers and Systems (HCAHPS) in 2002. Similarly, CMS has required clinicians and ambulatory care groups to survey patients on their experience since 2007 with the Clinician and Group CAHPS (CG-CAHPS) survey tool. There are also CAHPS surveys focused on the following healthcare settings: health plans, surgical care, dental plans, home health, hospice, nursing homes, and others (AHRQ n.d.). Despite this attention on patient experience of care through evaluation and monitoring, there has been little focus on widespread adoption of consumer tools and programs aimed at using health information for improved decision making. The rise of the Internet, patient-focused websites, information sharing portals, and other similar tools for tracking and sharing patient and organization-generated data has rapidly transformed this domain of informatics.

Numerous research studies have shown there is a clear link between patient engagement and improved clinical outcomes, including diabetes control, cancer screening, and depression follow-up care (Simon et al. 2011; Tenforde et al. 2012; Turvey et al. 2012). Patients who engage in using personal health information also have higher rates of patient satisfaction, health management, and patient loyalty to healthcare organizations (Finkelstein et al. 2012; Turley et al. 2012).

Patient-Centered Medical Home

With an increased focus on quality outcomes and patient satisfaction, as well as a changing healthcare reimbursement environment, there is increased attention to viewing patients and families as full members of the healthcare team and providing patient-centered care, which is defined as "relationship-based primary care that meets the individual patient and family's needs, preferences, and priorities" (AHRQ 2015). The patient-centered medical home (PCMH), for example, is a model that attempts to improve care outcomes and reduce care costs by reorganizing how primary care is delivered. There are five pillars to the PCMH model: a patient-centered orientation; comprehensive, team-based care; coordinated care; superb access to care; and a systems-based approach to quality and safety (AHRQ 2011).

EHR Incentive Program

The EHR (electronic health record) Incentive Program is another federal program that has attempted to improve consumer engagement in healthcare. The CMS EHR Incentive Program adopted the goals of the National Priorities Partnership and its National Quality Strategy when creating the goals and objectives for meaningful use of electronic health records. One of the goals is to "engage patient and families" by providing them with "timely access to data, knowledge, and tools to make informed decisions and to manage their care" (Tavenner and Sebelius 2012). Table 14.1 displays the EHR Incentive Program's objectives and measures for each of the three stages, and thus shows the program's emphasis on providing patients timely access to health information in an electronic format. Not only is the increased focus on providing access to health information in electronic format critically important in the evolution of the program, but also the significant increase in the proportion of patients who must engage in the use of these technologies to meet the threshold. For example, the proportion of patients who participate in secure messaging increases from 5 percent in Stage 2 to a proposed 35 percent in Stage 3 (CMS 2015).

The EHR Incentive Program included additional measures related to patient engagement apart from providing patients and families their health information. The program required changes in the way demographic information was collected, including preferred language, and it also required that demographic information be captured in structured format. The program also introduced measures related to sending patient reminders, using data analytics to create patient lists, utilizing the electronic health record (EHR) to identify patient-specific educational resources, and requiring patient family history to be recorded as structured data (CMS 2015).

The EHR Incentive Program is only one example of how patient engagement is being used to impact care outcomes, access, and cost.

Hospital Value-Based Purchasing Program

The CMS Hospital Value-Based Purchasing Program (HVBP) is another program that has placed significant value on patient experience. The HVBP provides financial incentives for hospitals that perform well. The total performance score that determines the incentive is based off of two domains—clinical processes and patient experience of care. The patient experience accounts for 30 percent of the total performance score. In other words, patient engagement as measure by nurse and physician communication with patients, discharge

Table 14.1.   EHR incentive program patient engagement objectives and measures

Objective	Stage 1	Stage 2	Stage 3 (proposed)
Provide patients their health information	More than 50 percent of all patients of the EP [eligible professional] who request an electronic copy of their health information are provided it within three business days.	Measure 1: More than 50 percent of all unique patients seen by the EP during the EHR reporting period are provided timely (available to the patient within four business days after the information is available to the EP) online access to their health information, with the ability to view, download, and transmit to a third party. Measure 2: More than five percent of all unique patients seen by the EP during the EHR reporting period (or their authorized representatives) view, download, or transmit to a third party their health information.	Proposed Measure 1: For more than 80 percent of all unique patients seen by the EP or discharged from the eligible hospital or CAH [Critical Access Hospital] inpatient or emergency department: (1) The patient (or patient-authorized representative) is provided access to view online, download, and transmit their health information within 24 hours of its availability to the provider; or (2) The patient (or the patient-authorized representative) is provided access to an ONC-certified API [Application Program Interface] that can be used by third-party applications or devices to provide patients (or patient authorized representatives) access to their health information, within 24 hours of its availability to the provider.
Use secure electronic messaging to communicate with patients on relevant health information.	Not applicable.	A secure message was sent using the electronic messaging function of CEHRT [Certified EHR Technology] by more than five percent of unique patients (or their authorized representatives) seen by the EP during the EHR reporting period.	Proposed Measure 2: For more than 35 percent of all unique patients seen by the EP or discharged from the eligible hospital or CAH inpatient or emergency department during the EHR reporting period, a secure message was sent using the electronic messaging function of CEHRT to the patient (or the patient's authorized representatives), or in response to a secure message sent by the patient (or the patient's authorized representative).
Provide clinical summaries for patients for each office visit.	Clinical summaries provided to patients for more than 50 percent of all office visits within three business days.	Clinical summaries provided to patients within one business day for more than 50 percent of office visits.	Proposed Measure 1: During the EHR reporting period, more than 25 percent of all unique patients seen by the EP or discharged from the eligible hospital or CAH inpatient or emergency department actively engage with the electronic health record made accessible by the provider. An EP, eligible hospital or CAH may meet the measure by either: (1) More than 25 percent of all unique patients (or patient-authorized representatives) seen by the EP or discharged from the eligible hospital or CAH inpatient or emergency department (POS [Place of Service] 21 or 23) during the EHR reporting period view, download or transmit to a third party their health information; or (2) More than 25 percent of all unique patients (or patient-authorized representatives) seen by the EP or discharged from the eligible hospital or CAH inpatient or emergency department during the EHR reporting period access their health information through the use of an ONC-certified API that can be used by third-party applications or devices.

Table 14.1. Continued

Objective	Stage 1	Stage 2	Stage 3 (proposed)
Incorporate patient-generated health data			Proposed Measure 3: Patient-generated health data or data from a nonclinical setting is incorporated into the certified EHR technology for more than 15 percent of all unique patients seen by the EP or discharged by the eligible hospital or CAH inpatient or emergency department during the EHR reporting period.

Source: CMS 2015.

information, and other patient-centered measures are critically important for those hospitals reimbursement (CMS 2011). Similarly, other programs related to healthcare reform, such as accountable care organizations that aim to improve how care is coordinated across the continuum of care, are not only required to engage in the care process, but patient engagement is seen by healthcare leaders as critical to the success of the delivery and payment model (Taylor et al. 2011).

Check Your Understanding 14.1

Instructions: **Answer the following questions on a separate piece of paper.**

1. Which of the following fields of informatics largely focuses on developing tools and processes to empower patients?
   A. Consumer
   B. Health
   C. Medical
   D. Nursing

2. What is "an ecosystem where all stakeholders can securely, effectively, and efficiently contribute, share, and analyze data and create new knowledge that can be consumed by a wide variety of electronic health information systems to support effective decision making leading to improved health outcomes"?
   A. Patient-centered medical home
   B. Meaningful Use
   C. Learning health system
   D. Consumer health informatics

3. Patient engagement is most characterized by:
   A. Actions and behaviors
   B. Technology
   C. Meaningful Use
   D. Healthcare teams

4. The patient-centered medical home model includes five pillars, including which of the following?
   A. EHR
   B. Coordinated care
   C. Teaching
   D. Informatics

5. Patient experience of care accounts for what percentage of the hospital value-based purchasing program?
   A. 10%
   B. 20%
   C. 30%
   D. 40%

Social Determinants of Health and Health Literacy

Consumer engagement in their healthcare has been noted in a number of Institute of Medicine (IOM) reports as key to addressing the issues of healthcare access, cost, and quality (Mills 2005; Page 2004; Knebel and Greiner 2003; IOM 2001; Kohn et al. 2000; Wunderlich and Kohler 2001). One of the central challenges facing the US healthcare system is the disparity in health outcomes based upon a variety of socioeconomic factors such as age, race, ethnicity, income level, education level, and healthcare access. These factors have been labeled by the World Health Organization (WHO) as the social determinants of health, defined as

> the conditions in which people are born, grow, work, live, and age, and the wider set of forces and systems shaping the conditions of daily life. These forces and systems include economic policies and systems, development agendas, social norms, social policies and political systems. (WHO 2015)

HealthyPeople 2020

HealthyPeople 2020, an initiative sponsored by the US Department of Health and Human Services (HHS), has organized the social determinants of health into five domains (see figure 14.4):

1. Economic stability,
2. Education,
3. Health and healthcare,
4. Neighborhood and built environment, and
5. Social and community context (HHS 2014a).

These domains reflect the social determinants of health (SDOH) that ultimately impact health outcomes. By developing this model, HHS goals and objectives can be developed within each domain.

The HealthyPeople initiative determines goals and objectives for each of the five domains, collects information to determine a baseline measure, and monitors this measure against the target. For example, one of the measures related to health and healthcare is the number of individuals with a "usual primary care provider." The rate in 2007 was 76.3

percent and the target is 83.9 percent (HHS 2014a). Figure 14.5 provides a snapshot of this measure by race and ethnicity in 2011 and illustrates that there is a clear divide between those who report having a usual primary care provider and those who do not. Overall, the percentage of individuals reporting a usual primary care provider decreased by 1.2 percent between 2000 and 2011. In 2011, nearly 69 percent of the Hispanic or Latino population reported having a usual primary care provider, as opposed to 84 percent of populations who reported two or more races (HHS 2014a). There are clear disparities in healthcare outcomes based upon social determinants. By better understanding the disparities and setting goals and objectives to address them, health disparities can be addressed.

Health Literacy

One of the social determinants of health outlined by HealthyPeople is health literacy. Health literacy is defined as

Figure 14.4. HealthyPeople 2020 model of social determinants of health

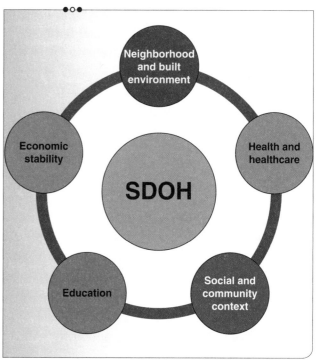

Source: HHS 2014a.

Figure 14.5. Usual primary care provider by race and ethnicity

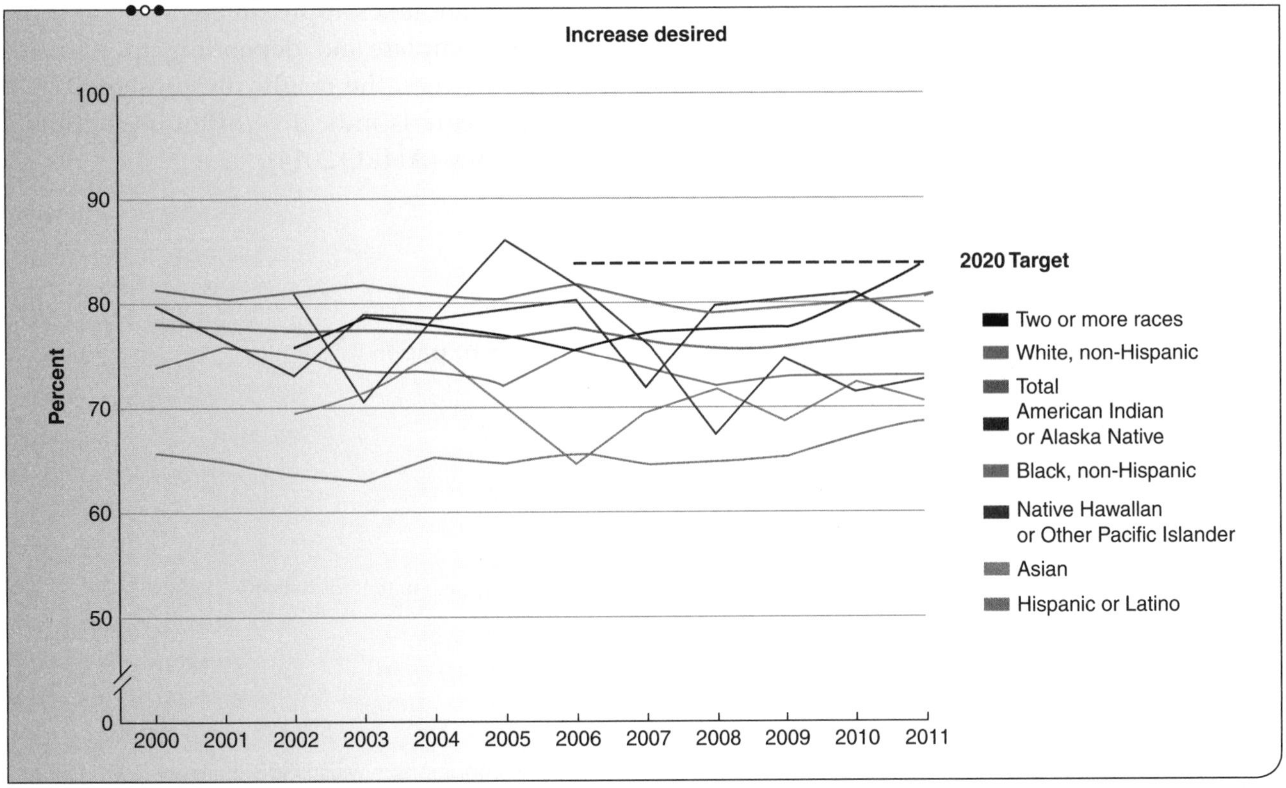

Source: HHS 2014b.

whether a person can obtain, process, and understand basic health information and services that are needed to make suitable health decisions. Health literacy includes the ability to understand instructions on prescription drug bottles, appointment cards, medical education brochures, doctor's directions, and consent forms. It also includes the ability to navigate complex healthcare systems. Health literacy is not simply the ability to read. It requires a complex group of reading, listening, analytical, and decision-making skills and the ability to apply these skills to health situations. (HHS 2014a)

Consumer informatics is focused on empowering patients by communicating effectively with them using a variety of methods, including health information in various formats. The communication of health information, whether in verbal or written format, relies on the ability of the individual to understand the information to achieve its desired purpose. However, the IOM reports that approximately half of the American adult population may "have difficulties acting on health information" (Sørensen et al. 2012, 3). While individuals may be searching for health information online or obtain-

ing their own health information from providers, they may not be able to fully understand the information or use the information for behavior change. Research has shown that individual health literacy level is a predictor of health outcomes, including medication adherence, self-management skills, and knowledge of disease (Sørensen et al. 2012). Every percentage increase in health literacy levels results in a two percentage increase in health status (Sentell et al. 2014). Because consumer health informatics largely involves developing technology for consumers to more effectively engage in healthcare, especially through the capture and use of health information, health literacy must be a key factor when developing tools and techniques to engage patients.

There are numerous valid and reliable measures of health literacy, including the Short Assessment of Health Literacy—Spanish and English (SAHL–S&E) and the Rapid Estimate of Adult Literacy in Medicine—Short Form. The Agency for Healthcare Research and Quality (AHRQ) produced a toolkit with access to validated tools that provide the ability to assess the health literacy of individuals. The tools can be used for research, clinical or programmatic purposes. For example, the SAHL–S&E instrument instructions and information regarding training are available for download. This measurement of health literacy includes 18 test terms that are meant to test an individual's vocabulary and comprehension. The assessment takes approximately two to three minutes to complete and, depending upon the individual answers, the results are presented as a score. The score is indicative of the individual's health literacy (AHRQ 2014).

Check Your Understanding 14.2

Instructions: **Answer the following questions on a separate piece of paper.**

1. Health literacy is focused on whether a person can do which of the following?
   A. Obtain basic health information and services
   B. Process basic health information and services
   C. Understand basic health information and services
   D. All of the above

2. Approximately what percentage of American adults have difficulty acting on health information?
   A. 30%
   B. 40%
   C. 50%
   D. 60%

3. True or False: Social determinants of health are only considered those conditions in which individuals are born.

4. True or False: According to HealthyPeople 2020, there are disparities in health outcomes based upon social determinants of health.

5. True or False: There are currently no valid and reliable measures of health literacy.

Health Information Online Resources

One of the most basic forms of consumer engagement is the use of the Internet for seeking health information online. An estimated 4.5 percent of all Internet searches are health related (Morahan-Martin 2004). According to research conducted by the Pew Research Center's Internet and American Life Project, 72 percent of American adults searched the Internet for information related to a health issue in the past twelve months, including 55 percent who searched for information regarding a specific medical diagnosis; 43 percent for a specific procedure or treatment; 27 percent for information regarding how to lose or manage weight; and 25 percent for information regarding health insurance. Interestingly, of those individuals who use the Internet for seeking health information, 60 percent reported that the information found online affected the decision regarding how to treat the illness or condition; 56 percent reported that it changed the approach to maintaining their health; and 53 percent reported that the information led them to ask a doctor new questions or seek a second opinion (Rainie 2013).

Healthcare-Focused Websites

There are many examples of health information maintained on the Internet and available for consumption. The Mayo Clinic has developed one of the most utilized patient education-focused websites. According to the Mayo Clinic (2014), its website receives over 50 million visitors per month (Plumbo 2015). The website allows users to access thousands of patient education materials, including content focused on symptoms, diseases and conditions, treatments and procedures, medications, research, and a variety of other topics and services. There are numerous other healthcare-focused websites where consumers seek information and guidance. The Medical Library Association's Consumer and Patient Health Information Section (CAPHIS) annually ranks the top 100 consumer-focused websites regarding their ability to provide information consumers can trust. The categories include general health, men's and women's health, and drug information resources, among others. The top rated websites include Aetna Intelihealth, Centers for Disease Control and Prevention, the Cleveland Clinic Health Information Center, Familydoctor. org, and Mayo Clinic (CAPHIS 2013).

Internet Forums

In addition to general health-related searches and healthcare-focused websites, another aspect of consumer health informatics is the rise of Internet-based forums. An **Internet forum** is a "web application for holding discussions and posting user-generated content, also commonly referred to as web forums, newsgroups, message boards, discussion boards, bulletin boards or simply a forum" (Ho 2009, 187). Internet forums are frequently used by individuals who share a common interest. One of the most popular healthcare Internet forums is PatientsLikeMe. PatientsLikeMe was created in 2004 and has a goal of connecting patients in a forum that allows them to better understand and manage their conditions by sharing their experiences and learning from others with similar conditions. Additionally, the website has a research mission. Members of PatientsLikeMe can provide data regarding their condition and experience to track and manage their health, and this data can be used in research studies. Currently, PatientsLikeMe.com has over 325,000 members, representing 2,400 conditions. The website boasts that over 60 research studies have been published using member data (there are currently over 27 million data points about disease) (PatientsLikeMe

2015). There are numerous Internet forums that are general (like PatientsLikeMe), but there are others that are more focused, such as IHadCancer.com (focused on cancer patients), CureDiva.com (focused on breast cancer patients), and ConnectedLiving. com (focused on seniors). Internet forums provide a venue for individuals to safely connect with each other to discuss health concerns. For individuals with rare conditions or who live in rural areas, for example, these forums allow them to pose questions, share stories, and generally connect with other individuals who have had similar health-related experiences. This ability to create communities through technology adds value to the individual in terms of addressing the isolation that oftentimes accompanies clinical diagnoses, and has resulted in improved healthcare outcomes.

Web 2.0 is considered the second generation of Internet-based services that emphasizes online collaboration and sharing among users. Some of these applications and technologies include blogs, social networks, content communities, wikis, and podcasts. Web 2.0 tools are characterized by being highly collaborative and participative, using multiple data sources and multimedia, and connecting communities through conversation and an open environment that is virtually available at any time. Although the first generation of Internet services was passive in nature, the Web 2.0 users are actively engaged through creating their own content, participating in discussions and communities, and sharing their own videos, photos, and information.

In the healthcare industry, Web 2.0 technologies and tools commonly are referred to as Health 2.0. Many consumers and providers are using Health 2.0 tools to better manage their health and that of their patients. Blogs are used to share clinical education information, wikis are used as healthcare reference tools, podcasting is used to provide continuing education for healthcare providers, and social networking is used by patients to develop condition-related communities.

Legal and ethical issues must be considered with the use of such technologies and tools. For example, the privacy of the patient and the confidentiality and transparency of the information must be addressed. Additionally, liability issues and the value of intellectual property come into play. Because the nature of Web 2.0/Health 2.0 is inherently open and collaborative, Web 2.0/Health 2.0 restrictions are few; and there is little control over data and information that is available for open distribution. Consequently, while the power of the Web 2.0/Health 2.0 technologies and tools is clear, also is the importance of harnessing its power for the greater good of the healthcare industry.

Technologists are beginning to discuss the concept of Web 3.0/Health 3.0. While the definitions vary widely, Web 3.0 will likely focus on expanding the participatory and collaborative nature of social networks that defined Web 2.0 to include more real-time video and three-dimensional elements. Other commentators argue that Web 3.0 will adopt semantic web standards, thereby allowing computers to read and generate content similar to humans.

Patient Activation Measure

Given the association between the level of health literacy and the overall level of engagement in healthcare and clinical outcomes (Sørensen et al. 2012), the **patient activation measure (PAM)** was developed as a way to be able to predict the patient's level of engagement in healthcare, including the knowledge, beliefs, skills, and behaviors that are necessary to manage one's health (Hibbard et al. 2004). The PAM is a 13-item Likert survey instrument (a Likert item is a statement that allows an individual to respond based upon their level of agreement with the statement) that scores patients on a scale of 1 to 100 and classifies patients as falling into one of four categories based upon their total score. The levels describe four progressive domains of activation—from passive health consumer to active health advocate. The PAM provides a useful tool for measuring one's level of engagement as it is a predictor of health outcomes:

> Those who are activated [based upon the results of the survey] believe patients have important roles to play in self-managing care, collaborating with providers, and maintaining their health. They know how to manage their condition and maintain functioning and prevent health declines; and they have the skills and behavioral repertoire to manage their condition, collaborate with their health providers, maintain their health functioning, and access appropriate and high-quality care. (Hibbard et al. 2004, 1010)

The four levels of the PAM are disengaged and overwhelmed; becoming aware, but still struggling; taking action; and maintaining behaviors and pushing further (Insignia 2015).

Research has shown that the PAM works to accurately predict a patient's level of activation (overall level of engagement in managing one's health), yet a patient's activation is minimally impacted by socioeconomic and demographic factors; thus the PAM score can be increased over time (Hibbard et al. 2013; 2005; 2001). Moreover, increasing PAM scores among patient populations has shown significant impact on improved healthcare outcomes and reductions in cost. For each percentage point increase in the PAM score, there is a two point reduction in hospital readmission rates and a two point increase in medication adherence rates (Insignia 2015). Organizations purchase the PAM, survey their respective patient populations, and can use the PAM scores as a tool for more effectively partnering with patients to meet their care goals.

Check Your Understanding 14.3

Instructions: **Answer the following questions on a separate piece of paper.**

1. Approximately what percentage of all Internet searches are health related?
   A. 1.5%
   B. 4.5%
   C. 10.5%
   D. 25.5%

2. What organization ranks consumer-focused healthcare websites?
   A. ONC
   B. CAPHIS
   C. CMS
   D. CAHPS

3. The patient activation measure (PAM) consists of how many levels?
   A. 2
   B. 4
   C. 6
   D. 8

4. True or False: There is no association between a patient's activation level and their health outcomes.

5. True or False: Web 2.0 emphasizes sharing of resources and collaboration.

Patient Portals, Personal Health Records, and Telehealth

The federally sanctioned definition of EHR includes the requirement for use of nationally recognized interoperability standards so data can be shared across more than one healthcare organization. The Meaningful Use (MU) incentive criteria require the ability to exchange key clinical information not only with providers but also with patients and includes the provision of electronic copies of discharge instructions, clinical summaries for office visits, and timely electronic access (CMS 2015). Coordinating care across the continuum and consumer empowerment are key principles of the federal government's focus on building a better health system. The consumer informatics tools that have been garnering significant attention in recent years are patient portals, personal health records, and telehealth encounters between patients and providers. The use of patient portals and personal health records has a significant impact on clinical outcomes, patient satisfaction, and professional and organizational efficiency (Dorr et al. 2007; Sequist et al. 2011; Simon et al. 2011).

Patient Portals

The ONC has defined a **patient portal** as a "secure online website that gives patients convenient 24-hour access to personal health information from anywhere with an Internet connection. Using a secure username and password, patients can view health information" (ONC 2014). Patient portals allow patients to view information from recent clinical visits, hospital discharge summaries, medications, immunizations, allergies, and lab results. Depending on the vendor or the organization, patient portals may allow patients to request prescription prefills, schedule appointments, make payments, and view educational materials.

Clinical messaging was an early form of connectivity, most commonly between providers. If any protected health information (PHI) was exchanged, encryption was sometimes deployed—although the lack of interoperability between encryption software products sometimes made that difficult to do. Web portals are more commonly used today to provide secure connectivity. This technology is a step up from clinical messaging because not only may messages be exchanged securely but also direct access to certain applications may be provided. For example, there may be a patient portal set up by a healthcare organization for use by patients. Patients may be able to exchange secure e-mail messages with their providers, such as to request an appointment, for access to lab results, to obtain access to a patient health summary, or for tailored instructions for taking medications, wound care, and so on. E-visits are online provider encounters, for which some health plans have started providing reimbursement and which can save patients an office visit and associated costs (Watson et al. 2010). The American Medical Association (Skoch and Taylor, 2010) and the American Academy of Family Practice (2008), among other specialty groups, have endorsed e-visits, providing guidelines for their use. Although the MU incentive program criteria do not require a portal for exchange of information, physician practices that are seeking recognition as a PCMH will find that a portal is encouraged by the National Committee for Quality Assurance (NCQA 2011).

Continuity of care record (CCR) or continuity of care document (CCD) standards are yet another form of connectivity, required in the MU incentive program. The CCR originally was conceived by the Massachusetts Medical Society as a means to standardize referral information and was ratified as a standard under ASTM International (2005) with assistance from HIMSS and other medical societies. The CCR is a specification of data that is most useful as a snapshot of a patient's health condition and the data that should be able to be produced in CCR (or CCD) format directly from the EHR. The CCR may be rendered as a PDF or as an XML file. The CCD is a combination of Health Level Seven's (HL7's) Version 3 clinical document architecture (CDA) and the CCR.

HL7's CDA is an XML-based markup standard that specifies the encoding, structure, and semantics of a healthcare document (not limited to the content of the CCR). It enables healthcare documents to be transported using HL7 Version 2.x, HL7 Version 3, DICOM, MIME attachments to e-mail, HTTP, or FTP. (When the HIPAA claims attachment standard was first proposed in 2005, the CDA was identified as one format for claims attachments. Today, the Affordable Care Act [ACA] requires adoption of a claims attachment standard—although its specification has not yet been finalized.) When the CDA and CCR are combined, the resultant CCD provides an XML-based markup standard to encode, structure, and identify the semantics of the CCR. Refer to chapter 5 for more information on standards.

Figure 14.6 provides an illustration of a patient portal offered by the US Department of Veterans Affairs. The application is called MyHealtheVet.

The web-based application allows a patient to access a variety of personal health information through one centralized repository, including information related to vital signs and readings, labs and tests, and health history. The figure also illustrates one of the key features of patient portals—secure messaging. Because of the requirements of the EHR Incentive Program, organizations or professionals are required to make patient portals available to patients, and the portals must allow for secure messaging between patients and providers. Secure messaging enables

> a user to electronically send messages to, and receive messages from, a patient in a manner that ensures: (1) Both the patient (or authorized representative) and EHR technology user are authenticated; and (2) the message content is encrypted and integrity-protected in accordance with the standard for encryption and hashing algorithms. (NIST 2013)

Personal Health Records

Personal health records (PHRs) are yet another form of connectivity that is becoming popular with some patients and the federal government, health plans, and employers who are promoting their use for value-driven healthcare. Personal health records are similar to patient portals. Whereas patient portals are typically tethered to and maintained by a healthcare organization on behalf of a patient, personal health records are created and maintained by the consumer. Personal health records have been defined as

> an electronic, lifelong resource of health information needed by individuals to make health decisions. Individuals own and manage the information in the PHR, which comes from healthcare providers and the individual. The PHR is maintained in a secure and private environment, with the individual determining rights of access. The PHR does not replace the legal record of any provider. (Wolter and Friedman 2005)

The detailed elements that are potentially available in a personal health record vary widely. Personal health records can include calendars and reminders, health record organizers, communication portals, cost management tools, wellness programs, and educational resources. The Mayo Clinic has developed

Figure 14.6. Example of web-based patient portal

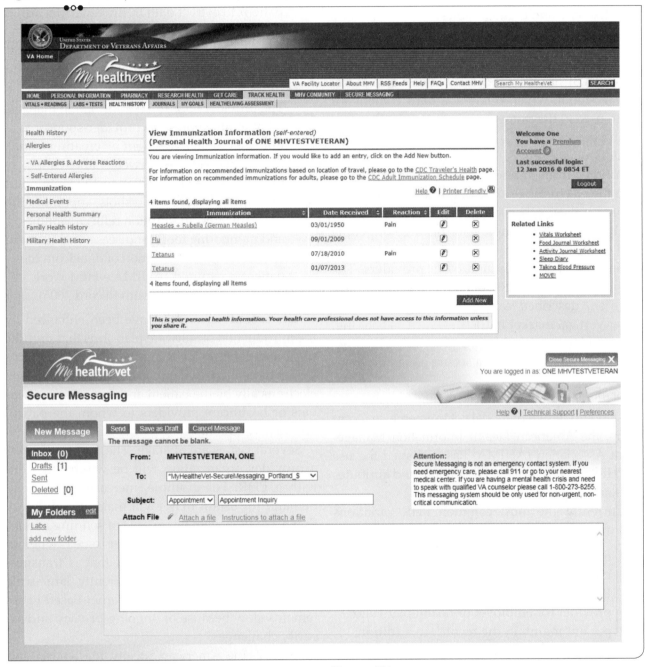

Used with permission from My HealtheVet (http://myhealth.va.gov) Department of Veterans Affairs.

the following list of elements that should be included in a personal health record as a means of assisting individuals to manage their health:

- Primary care doctor's name and phone number
- Allergies, including drug allergies
- Medications, including dosages

- Chronic health problems, such as high blood pressure
- Major surgeries, with dates
- Living will or advance directives
- Family history
- Immunization history
- Results of screening tests

- Cholesterol level and blood pressure
- Exercise and dietary habits
- Health goals, such as stopping smoking or losing weight (Mayo Clinic 2014)

HL7 (2008) has adopted the PHR-System Functional Model, which offers standard content for their use. PHRs come in many forms. Personal health records (PHRs) electronically populate elements or subsets of protected health information (PHI) from provider organization databases into the electronic records of authorized patients, their families, other providers, and sometimes health payers and employers. A range of people and groups maintain the records, including the patients, their families, and other providers. The development of PHRs parallels the consumer-centrism described earlier and long evident in other vertical market industries, such as banking, where consumers maintain and examine their activities 24 hours a day in a secure electronic environment.

PHRs come in a variety of forms and formats, with no standard design or model yet to emerge. In recent years, the American Health Information Management Association (AHIMA) has promoted the use of PHRs and has provided definitions and attributes for standardization.

Currently, the most common PHR variations and models include:

- *Shared data record:* The shared data record model consumes the largest number of PHRs and is the most effective. Here, both provider (or employer or health plan) and patient maintain the record. In addition, the provider (or employer or health plan) supports the record. As such, the patient receives and adds information over time. The focus of this model is to keep track of health events, medications, or specific physiological indicators, such as exercise and nutrition.

- *EHR extensions:* The EHR extensions model extends the EHR into cyberspace so that an authorized patient can access the provider's record and check on the record's content.

Often this model also allows an authorized patient to extract data from the healthcare provider's record. The record is still maintained by the provider but is available to the patient in an online format.

- *Provider-sponsored information management:* The provider-sponsored information management model represents provider-sponsored information management by creating communication vehicles between patient and provider. Such vehicles can include reminders for immunizations or flu shots, appointment scheduling or prescription refill capabilities, and monitoring tools for disease management in which regular collection of data from the patient is required (AHIMA e-HIM Work Group on the Legal Health Record 2005).

The preceding models have been enhanced by the introduction of software platforms that propose to store a patient's PHR in a health vault or bank. Under these models, data can be added and viewed electronically by the patient and any other individuals or healthcare providers to whom the patient allows permission.

Several issues are at stake. The first is whether a provider organization will be willing to work with a PHR. For example, increasing consumer demand for useful PHRs will make it mandatory that an EHR system be capable of sending and receiving data from a PHR. Another issue is whether a patient can trust the network that is transmitting his or her information. Currently, large-scale deployment and adoption of Internet-based PHRs remains slow because of ongoing privacy and security challenges.

In 2002, the American Society for Testing and Materials (ASTM) Committee E31 (Healthcare Informatics), Subcommittee 26 established a standard for PHRs on the Internet. Content for the standard was based on the e-health tenets developed by AHIMA in 2000. In 2007, Health Level Seven (HL7) announced the approval of the Personal Health Record System Functional Model (PHR-S FM) as a Draft Standard for Trial Use. The PHR-S FM defines the functions that may be present in PHR systems and provides guidelines that facilitate health information exchange (HIE) among different PHR systems and between PHR and EHR systems (HL7 2008).

Although fewer than expected, people are adopting PHRs (Lewis 2011). There are, however, an increasing number of EHRs that support a PHR, as well as commercial PHR vendors selling directly to consumers. In general, PHRs range from being fairly unsophisticated, where patients can direct providers to send an e-fax to a given website or they can upload documents or enter information themselves, to quite comprehensive, where direct feeds from a provider or health plan as well as structured templates for the individual to enter his or her own data are provided. Although many providers remain concerned that the volume of information they may have to review from a PHR is not reimbursable as well as being skeptical about the accuracy of patient-reported data, there is a small but growing interest in having patients more engaged in their healthcare through keeping a PHR.

Health plans are particularly interested in populating PHRs they support with problem lists and medication lists from claims data. While there are some concerns about how clinically relevant diagnosis information may be from claims data, the fact that the health plan can provide this information across all providers is attractive. The health plan can then provide direct disease management support to patients.

Similarly, PHRs that are linked, or tethered, to EHRs enable the provider to direct specific information to the patient's PHR as well as retrieve information from the patient's PHR (Connecting for Health 2006). In more comprehensive forms of PHRs, the source of the data is identifiable and the data entered by any given source is only able to be altered by that source—maintaining the integrity of all data. Although these tethered forms of PHR may only contain the information from the one provider that supports the PHR, the ability for the patient to enter his or her own data can be an aid to the provider. The patient can logon in advance of a visit or at a kiosk in the waiting room and enter his or her own medical history, family history, and history of present illness and respond to structured questions that provide a review of systems.

Some patient monitoring devices may also be connected to the PHR. These functions save considerable documentation time during the visit, where this information only needs to be reviewed and validated. The time savings can then be spent on more thorough examination, treatment planning, and education (Bachman 2007).

Patients and caregivers want access to personal health information (Fricton and Davies 2008; Markle Foundation 2003). The features that were rated the most important by patients were accessing an up-to-date health history, summaries for clinical encounters, current medication lists, and receiving email reminders regarding preventive care. The highest rated feature by patients was the ability to email providers, yet emailing providers was one of the lowest rated features by providers themselves. The lowest rated feature by patients was the frequency of using online resources for health information in the past year, yet this was highly rated by providers. Accessing health history was the highest overall rated feature by all stakeholders (Fricton and Davies 2008).

Telehealth

Unlike patient portals and personal health records, telehealth is not a web-based application to provide timely access to health-related information. Telehealth is "the use of electronic information and telecommunications technologies to support long-distance clinical healthcare, patient and professional health-related education, public health, and health administration. Technologies include videoconferencing, the Internet, store-and-forward imaging, streaming media, and terrestrial and wireless communications" (HRSA n.d.). Telehealth may be considered a form of connectivity. Telehealth includes a set of technology and processes that enables delivery of healthcare services (and information) via telecommunications technologies. Telehealth is not new and does not require an EHR. Telehealth supplements a healthcare organization's capabilities such as for remote intensive care unit monitoring (Wright 2005), although there are also questions as to whether critical care outcomes are actually improved (Kahn 2011) or are only supplements to staffing. Telehealth can be used to provide emergency care, offer consultations across great distances (or in limited access areas, even including inner-city areas), monitor local patients with chronic disease, track progress in recovery of certain types of illnesses or injuries (Melville 2012), and bring sign language to the hearing impaired during a local healthcare encounter (Hirsch and Marano 2007).

Telehealth is critical for patient engagement because it provides patients an alternative method for engaging with providers and receiving care. While telehealth involves, for example, the provision of psychiatry via high-definition video conferencing, it also involves the use of smart technologies to monitor patients in their homes. These smart technologies include devices for collecting vitals, tracking medication adherence, tracking movement and dietary habits, or glucometers.

Data Display

One of the critical questions facing the use of patient portals, personal health records, and telehealth involves information sharing and data visualization (see chapter 18 for more detail on data visualization). Data visualization is simply the display of data in pictorial or graphical format. Data visualization can aid with the interpretation of data (Sas n.d.). Not only do graphical displays have potential for effectively presenting data to health professionals, but patients may also benefit. Research has explored the efficacy of graphical displays of quantitative information targeted to patients and found that charts offer advantages over sharing or displaying numbers in comparing risks of various treatments (Feldman-Stewart et al. 2007). Because healthcare is moving toward a patient-centered health system (Clancy and Collins 2010), the patient will inevitably become a more active participant in decisions pertaining to treatment and continuity of care. A graphical depiction of data has been shown to assist patients in determining the relative risks of various treatments, and therefore holds promise as a tool for promoting patient-centered healthcare (Feldman-Stewart et al. 2007). A graphical display reduces the cognitive burden of patients for interpreting data, allowing them to make decisions more quickly and accurately (Feldman-Stewart et al. 2007; 2000).

With the expanding use of the electronic health record, patients will have more access to their health information, and therefore will be seeking ways to interpret this information. By depicting healthcare results graphically, a patient may be able to easily understand the results, decreasing the need for the physician or other caregivers to educate the patient on such matters. Also, with expanding development of patient portals via the World Wide Web, health information may be easily accessible and systems will be developed with the sole purpose of educating patients. When such portals are designed, a graphical display of healthcare data with accompanied interpretive text could improve a patient's understanding of their health status.

Check Your Understanding 14.4

Instructions: **Answer the following questions on a separate piece of paper.**

1. A patient portal includes which of the following elements?
   A. Security
   B. Accessibility 24 hours a day
   C. Contains personal health information
   D. All of the above

2. Secure messaging includes the use of which of the following standard documents?
   A. CDA
   B. HL7
   C. ONC
   D. HIPAA

3. Personal health records may include which of the following features?

   A. Allergies

   B. Immunizations

   C. Health goals

   D. All of the above

4. True or False: Personal health records must be tethered to a healthcare organization.

5. True or False: Telehealth is not considered a form of connectivity.

Patient-Generated Health Data

The Office of the National Coordinator for Health Information Technology defines **patient-generated health data (PGHD)** as "health-related data created, recorded, or gathered by or from patients (or family members or other caregivers) to help address a health concern" (ONC 2015b). PGHD can include "health history, symptoms, biometric data, treatment history, lifestyle choices, and other information" (Deering 2013). PGHD can improve the efficiency of organizations by reducing the frequency of office visits, improving the overall understanding of health condition among patients, the treatment of chronic conditions, patient–provider relationships, and generally improving the patient experience of care (Deering 2013). As opposed to other types of clinical data generated by clinical organizations, patients (or their caregivers) are responsible for recording this information and for determining who gets access to the generated information and when they are provided access to the information. Because of the value that PGHD can provide to individual patients and healthcare organizations, the ONC's Health Information Technology Policy Committee has adopted recommendations for including PGHD into future versions of the EHR Incentive Program. The proposed Stage 3 Meaningful Use requirement states that "patient-generated health data or data from a nonclinical setting is incorporated into the certified EHR technology for more than 15 percent of all unique patients seen by the EP during the EHR reporting period" (CMS 2015). Regardless of what happens with the Final Rule for Stage 3, it is clear that patient-generated health data is converging with the traditional medical record in new and innovative ways.

Figure 14.7 illustrates the process of recording PGHD and how the information could be used in the clinical process. First, the person (patient/consumer) either enters data into an electronic device or the information is captured by a remote monitoring device. Second, the person grants access to the information to a third party and transfers the data to them, in this case to a provider organization and a particular physician and staff member. The third step in the process is for the provider and staff to review the information and document the information (potentially within the EHR but not necessarily) and, depending on the type of information provided, they could provide feedback to the person. Examples of patient-generated health data are cardiac monitoring or blood pressure tracking.

In addition to the recording and collecting of data that can be used for routine engagements with healthcare providers, there is a global movement that promotes and supports the collection and use of large amounts of information regarding personal activity—diet, physical activity, psychological states and traits, mental and cognitive traits, environmental variables, and social variables (Swan 2013). This movement has been labeled the "Quantified Self"

Figure 14.7. Patient-generated health data flow

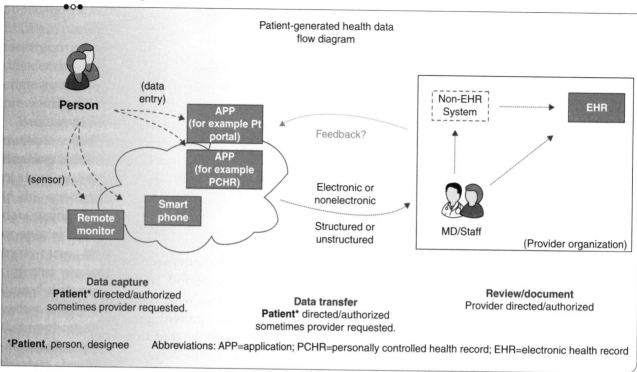

Source: Shapiro et al. 2012.

and is defined as any individual engaged "in the self-tracking of any kind of biological, physical, behavioral, or environmental information. There is a proactive stance on obtaining information and acting on it" (Swan 2013). The explosion of mobile cellular devices and other wireless personal devices focused on health and fitness monitoring has facilitated the growth of this movement. The use of these devices for health-related purposes has been labeled **mHealth** and has been defined by the Health Information Management and Systems Society (HIMSS) as the "the generation, aggregation, and dissemination of health information via mobile and wireless devices" (HIMSS 2015). For example, mobile phones have the capability to serve as a pedom-eter, connect with other wearable devices, and track weight, heart rate, respiration, sleeping activity, calories burned, and much more. There are also a variety of additional wearable devices that have made quantifying daily activity extremely easy—both for data collection and data analysis. The adoption and use of mobile device fitness applications is growing 87 percent faster than the entire mobile industry (Rhodes 2014). This growth in mobile devices has implications for consumer informatics. Individuals are engaging with health-related information at unparalleled rates. This engagement is altering expectations regarding the types of information that can be collected, how it is displayed, and how it can be used.

Personalized Medicine

Personalized medicine has been defined by the US Food and Drug Administration (FDA) as "the tailoring of medical treatment to the individual characteristics, needs, and preferences of a patient during all stages of care, including prevention, diagnosis, treatment, and follow-up" (FDA 2013). Personalized medicine focuses on utilizing very specific attributes of patients as a basis of providing treatment. One of the driving forces of personalized medicine is the collection and use of genetic information. For example, the FDA has approved a drug that treats cystic fibrosis caused by a specific gene mutation (the G551D mutation). The drug restores function to a specific protein that is affected by the gene mutation (FDA 2013). The ability to sequence or partially sequence patient genomes has the potential to revolutionize healthcare delivery by providing treatments that are tailored to these specific genetic markers. The Human Genome Project, which involved the sequencing of the 3 billion base pairs of the human genome,

took 13 years to complete and approximately $3 billion dollars (NIH 2010). This project has opened the door to using genetics to predict risks of future illnesses. Today, the cost for a complete genome sequencing costs approximately $5,000 (NIH 2015) (see figure 14.8 for a detailed breakdown of sequencing costs over time). As it becomes less expensive to learn more about our genes and how they influence our health, consumers will be able to engage with this information (and their providers) to create customized care plans that will potentially influence major decisions regarding healthcare interventions.

Consumer Informatics and Next Steps

The transition from the organization-focused system characterized by silos of care to a patient-centered system has been challenging. The patient-centered system that has teams of care delivery

using informatics, research, and evidence-based guidelines, including patients as key members of the team, has been called the learning health system. Consumer informatics plays a critical role in the learning health system. Consumers who access

Figure 14.8. Cost per genome from 2001 to 2015

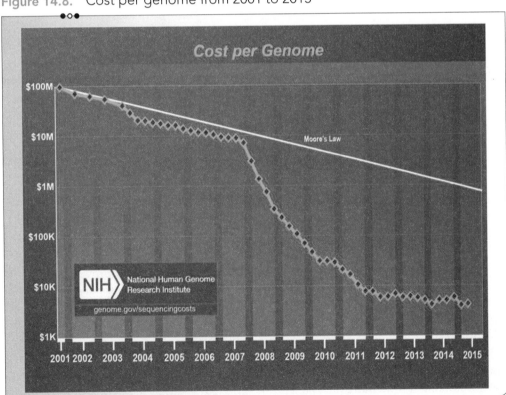

Source: NIH 2015.

and use health information report improved health outcomes and patient satisfaction levels, yet there are wide disparities in terms of the populations who use the tools that offer access to health information. Consumer informatics will be responsible for not only designing tools and resources to provide access to health information, collect and report data, and engage with providers and caregivers, but designing these tools in such a way that the consumer needs and preferences are integrated into the design of these resources to address the disparities that have impacted the adoption of tools in the past.

Check Your Understanding 14.5

Instructions: **Answer the following questions on a separate piece of paper.**

1. Patient-generated health data can include which of the following: Health Records may include which of the following features?
   A. Lab values
   B. CT Scan
   C. Symptoms
   D. CCR

2. True or False: mHealth has the potential to facilitate the adoption of PGHD practices.

3. True or False: Personalized medicine uses broad clinical guidelines for tailoring of medical treatment to the individuals.

4. True or False: The Quantified Self movement relies solely on obtaining information from healthcare providers to track personal health.

5. True or False: Meaningful Use promoted patient-generated health information.

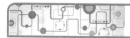

References

Agency for Healthcare Research and Quality. n.d. Clinician & Group. https://cahps.ahrq.gov/Surveys-Guidance/CG/index.html

Agency for Healthcare Research and Quality. 2015. Patient-Centered Care. http://www.pcmh.ahrq.gov/page/patient-centered-care

Agency for Healthcare Researcha and Quality. 2014. Health Literacy Measurement Tools (Revised). http:// www.ahrq.gov/professionals/quality-patient-safety/quality-resources/tools/literacy/index.html

Agency for Healthcare Research and Quality. 2011. The Patient-Centered Medical Home: Strategies to Put Patients at the Center of Primary Care. http://www.pcmh.ahrq.gov/sites/default/files/attachments/Strategies%20to%20Put%20Patients%20at%20the%20Center%20of%20Primary%20Care.pdf

AHIMA e-HIM Work Group on the Legal Health Record. 2005 (Sept.) Update: Guidelines for defining the legal health record for disclosure purposes. *Journal of AHIMA* 76(8):64A–G.

American Academy of Family Practice. 2008. E-visits. http://www.aafp.org/online/en/home/policy/policies/e/evists.printerview.html

American Medical Informatics Association. 2015. Consumer Health Informatics. https://www.amia.org/applications-informatics/consumer-health-informatics

ASTM International. 2005. ASTM E2369-05 Standard Specification for Continuity of Care Record (CCR). http://www.astm.org/Standards/E2369.htm

Bachman, J. 2007 (July/August). Improving care with an automated patient history. *Family Practice Management* 14(7):39–43.

Brown, E. 2011. Surgeon General Discusses Health and Community. *Los Angeles Times.* http://articles.latimes.com/2011/mar/13/health/la-he-surgeon-general-20110313

Cassidy, B. 2013. Envisioning the Future of the Health Information Management Profession. Chapter 30 in *Health Information Management: Concepts, Principles and*

Practice, 4th ed. Edited by LaTour, K.M., S. Eichenwald Maki, and P. Oachs. Chicago: AHIMA.

Centers for Medicaid and Medicare Services. 2015. Medicare and Medicaid Programs; Electronic Health Record Incentive Program-Stage 3. *Federal Register*. https://www.federalregister.gov/articles/2015/03/30/2015-06685/medicare-and-medicaid-programs-electronic-health-record-incentive-program-stage-3

Centers for Medicaid and Medicare Services. 2011. Open door forum: Hospital Value Based Purchasing. Fiscal Year 2013 overview for beneficiaries, providers and stakeholders. https://www.cms.gov/Medicare/Quality-Initiatives-Patient-Assessment-Instruments/hospital-value-based-purchasing/downloads/HospVBP_ODF_072711.pdf

Chase, D. 2013. The 7 Habits of Highly Patient Centric Providers. *Forbes*. http://www.forbes.com/sites/davechase/2013/02/18/the-7-habits-of-highly-patient-centric-providers/

Clancy, C. and F.S. Collins. 2010. Patient-Centered Outcomes Research Institute: The intersection of science and health care. *Science Translational Medicine* 2(37):37cm18.

Connecting for Health, Markle Foundation. 2006. Connecting Americans to Their Health Care: A Common Framework for Networked Personal Health Information. http://www.markle.org/sites/default/files/CF-Consumers-Full.pdf

Consumer and Patient Health Information Section (CAPHIS). 2013. Top 100 List: Health Websites You Can Trust. http://caphis.mlanet.org/consumer/index.html

Deering, M.J. 2013. Issue Brief: Patient-Generated Health Data and Health IT. http://wanghaisheng.github.io/images/pghd_brief_final122013.pdf

Dorr, D., L.M. Bonner, A.N. Cohen, R.S. Shoai, R. Perrin, E. Chaney, and A.S. Young. 2007. Informatics systems to promote improved care for chronic illness: A literature review. *Journal of the American Medical Informatics Association* 14(2):156–163.

Eysenbach, G. 2000. Recent advances: Consumer health informatics. *British Medical Journal* 320(7251):1713.

Feldman-Stewart, D., M.D. Brundage, and V. Zotov. 2007. Further insight into the perception of quantitative information: Judgments of gist in treatment decisions. *Medical Decision Making* 27(1):34–43.

Feldman-Stewart, D., N. Kocovski, B. A. McConnell, M. D. Brundage, and W.J. Mackillop. 2000. Perception of quantitative information for treatment decisions. *Medical Decision Making* 20(2):228-238.

Finkelstein J., A. Knight, S. Marinopoulos, M.C. Gibbons, Z. Berger, H. Aboumatar, R.F. Wilson, B.D. Lau, R. Sharma, and E.B. Bass. 2012 (June). Enabling Patient-Centered Care Through Health Information Technology. Rockville (MD): Agency for Healthcare Research and Quality (US); (Evidence Reports/Technology Assessments, No. 206.) Available from: http://www.ncbi.nlm.nih.gov/books/NBK99854/

Fricton, J.R. and D. Davies. Personal Health Records to Improve Health Information Exchange and Patient Safety. In *Advances in Patient Safety: New Directions and Alternative Approaches* (Vol. 4: Technology and Medication Safety). Edited by Henriksen, K., J.B. Battles, M.A. Keyes, et al. Rockville, MD: Agency for Healthcare Research and Quality (US); 2008 Aug. Available from: http://www.ncbi.nlm.nih.gov/books/NBK43760/

Health Information Management and Systems Society. 2015. mHealth. http://www.himss.org/library/mhealth

Health Resources and Services Administration. n.d. Telehealth. http://www.hrsa.gov/ruralhealth/about/telehealth/

Health Level Seven. 2008. *PHR-System Functional Model, Release 1 DSTU*. Ann Arbor, MI: Health Level Seven.

Hibbard, J.H., J. Greene, and V. Overton. 2013. Patients with lower activation associated with higher costs; Delivery systems should know their patients' "scores." *Health Affairs* 32(2):216–222..

Hibbard, J.H., E.R. Mahoney, J. Stockard, and M. Tusler. 2005. Development and testing of a short form of the patient activation measure. *Health Services Research* 40(6 Pt 1):1918–1930.

Hibbard, J.H., J. Stockard, E.R. Mahoney, and M. Tusler. 2004. Development of the patient activation measure (PAM): Conceptualizing and measuring activation in patients and consumers. *Health Services Research* 39(4 Pt 1):1005–1026.

Hibbard, J.H., M. Geenlick, H. Jimison, J. Capizzi, and L. Kunkel. 2001. The impact of a community-wide self-care information project on self-care and medical care utilization. *Evaluation and the Health Professions* 24(4):404.

Hirsch, J. and F. Marano. 2007. Better patient care through video interpretation. http://www.healthmgttech.com/index.php/solutions/hospitals/better-patient-care-through-video-interpretation/Print.html

Ho, J. 2009. Consumer health informatics. *Studies in Health Technology and Informatics* 151:185–194.

Insignia. 2015. Patient Activation Measure. http://www.insigniahealth.com/products/pam-survey

Institute for Healthcare Improvement. 2015. The IHI Triple Aim. http://www.ihi.org/Engage/Initiatives/TripleAim/pages/default.aspx

Institute of Medicine. 2001. *Crossing the Quality Chasm: A New Health System for the 21st Century*. Committee on Quality of Health Care in America. Washington, DC: National Academies Press.

Kahn, J.M. 2011 (January 1). The use and misuse of ICU telemedicine. *Journal of the American Medical Association* 305(21):2227–2228.

Knebel, E. and A.C. Greiner. 2003. *Health Professions Education: A Bridge to Quality*. Washington, DC: National Academies Press.

Kohn, L.T, J.M Corrigan, and M.S Donaldson. 2000. *To Err Is Human: Building a Safer Health System*. Washington, DC: National Academies Press.

Lewis, N. 2011 (April 8). Consumers slow to adopt electronic personal health records. *InformationWeek*. http://www.informationweek.com/news/healthcare/EMR/229401249

Lewis, D., B.L. Chang, and C.P. Friedman. 2005. Consumer health informatics. In *Consumer Health Informatics: Informing Consumers and Improving Health Care*. New York: Springer. 1–7.

Markle Foundation. 2003. Connecting for Health: A Public-Private Collaborative. The personal health working group final report. Washington, DC: http://www.providersedge.com/ehdocs/ehr_articles/The_Personal_Health_Working_Group_Final_Report.pdf

Mayo Clinic. 2014. Personal Health Record: A Tool for Managing Your Health. http://www.mayoclinic.org/healthy-lifestyle/consumer-health/in-depth/personal-health-record/art-20047273

Melville, N.A. 2012 (January 18). Teledermatology sessions improve diagnoses, outcomes. *Medscape Medical News*. http://www.medscape.com/viewarticel/757108

Mills, T.L. 2005. Insuring America's health: Principles and recommendations. *Journal of the National Medical Association* 97(8):1185.

Morahan-Martin, J. M. 2004. How Internet Users Find, Evaluate, and Use Online Health Information: A Cross-Cultural Review. *CyberPsychology & Behavior* 7(5):497–510.

National Committee for Quality Assurance. 2011 (February 1). *PCMH 2011 Standards*. Washington, DC: National Committee for Quality Assurance.

National Institutes of Health. 2015. DNA Sequencing Costs: Data from the NHGRI Genome Sequencing Program (GSP). http://www.genome.gov/sequencingcosts/

National Institutes of Health. 2010. The Human Genome Project Completion: Frequently Asked Questions. https://www.genome.gov/11006943

National Institute for Standards and Technology. 2013. Test Procedure for §170.314(e)(3) Secure Messaging—Ambulatory Setting Only. http://healthit.gov/sites/default/files/170.314e3securemessaging_2014_tp_approvedv1.3.pdf

Office of the National Coordinator for Health Information Technology. 2015a. Connecting Health and Care for the Nation: A Shared Nationwide Interoperability Roadmap. https://www.healthit.gov/sites/default/files/nationwide-interoperability-roadmap-draft-version-1.0.pdf

Office of the National Coordinator for Health Information Technology. 2015b. "Patient-Generated Health Data." Office of the National Coordinator for Health Information Technology Accessed June 29. http://www.healthit.gov/policy-researchers-implementers/patient-generated-health-data.

Office of the National Coordinator for Health Information Technology. 2014. What Is a Patient Portal? http://www.healthit.gov/providers-professionals/faqs/what-patient-portal

Page, A. 2004. *Keeping Patients Safe: Transforming the Work Environment of Nurses*. Washington, DC: National Academies Press.

PatientsLikeMe. 2015. PatientsLikeMe: Live Better, Together. https://www.patientslikeme.com

Plumbo, G. 2015. Mayo Clinic Announces Next Evolution of Web Presence. http://newsnetwork.mayoclinic.org/discussion/mayo-clinic-announces-next-evolution-of-web-presence/

Rainie, L. 2013. E-patients and Social Media. Pew Research Center. http://www.pewinternet.org/files/old-media/Files/Presentations/2013/2013%20-%2010.10.13%20-%20E-patients%20and%20social%20media_PDF.pdf

Rhodes, H. 2014. Accessing and using data from wearable fitness devices. *Journal of AHIMA* 85(9):48.

Sas. n.d. Data Visualization: What It Is and Why It Is Important. http://www.sas.com/en_us/insights/big-data/data-visualization.html

Sentell, T., W. Zhang, J. Davis, K.K. Baker, and K.L. Braun. 2014. The influence of community and individual health literacy on self-reported health status. *Journal of General Internal Medicine* 29(2):298–304.

Sequist, T.D., A.M. Zaslavsky, G.A. Colditz, and J.Z. Ayanian. 2011. Electronic patient messages to promote colorectal cancer screening: A randomized controlled trial. *Archives of Internal Medicine* 171(7):636–641.

Shapiro, M., D. Johnston, J. Wald, and D. Mon. 2012. Patient-Generated Health Data: White Paper. Office of the National Coordinator for Health Information Technology. http://www.healthit.gov/sites/default/files/rti_pghd_whitepaper_april_2012.pdf

Simon, G.E., J.D. Ralston, J. Savarino, C. Pabiniak, C. Wentzel, and B.H. Operskalski. 2011. Randomized trial of depression follow-up care by online messaging. *Journal of General Internal Medicine* 26(7):698–704.

Skoch, E. and T.B. Taylor. 2010 (February 4). AMA/TransforMed Webinar: Engaging patients in using technology to manage their personal health care.

Sørensen, K., S. Van den Broucke, J. Fullam, G. Doyle, J. Pelikan, Z. Slonska, and H. Brand. 2012. Health literacy and public health: A systematic review and integration of definitions and models. *BMC Public Health* 12(1):80.

Swan, M. 2013. The quantified self: Fundamental disruption in big data science and biological discovery. *Big Data* 1(2):85–99.

Tavenner, M. and K. Sebelius. 2012. Medicare and Medicaid programs; Electronic health record incentive program–Stage 2. *Federal Register* 77(171):53968–54162.

Taylor, E.F., T. Lake, J. Nysenbaum, G. Peterson, and D. Meyers. 2011. Coordinating care in the medical neighborhood: Critical components and available mechanisms. Mathematica Policy Research.

Tenforde, M., A. Nowacki, A. Jain, and J. Hickner. 2012. The association between personal health record use and diabetes quality measures. *Journal of General Internal Medicine* 27(4):420–424.

Turley, M., T. Garrido, A. Lowenthal, and Z.Y. Yvonne. 2012. Association between personal health record enrollment and patient loyalty. *American Journal of Managed Care* 18(7):e248–e253.

Turvey, C.L, D.M. Zulman, K.M Nazi, B.J Wakefield, S.S. Woods, T.P. Hogan, F.M. Weaver, and K. McInnes. 2012. Transfer of information from personal health records: A survey of veterans using My HealtheVet. *Telemedicine and e-Health* 18(2):109–114.

US Department of Health and Human Services. 2014a. Social Determinants of Health. http://www.healthypeople.gov/2020/topics-objectives/topic/social-determinants-health

US Department of Health and Human Services. 2014b. Access to Health Services. http://www.healthypeople.gov/2020/topics-objectives/topic/Access-to-Health-Services/national-snapshot

US Department of Veterans Affairs. n.d. MyhealtheVet. US Department of Veteran's Affairs Accessed June 29. https://www.myhealth.va.gov/mhv-portal-web/anonymous.portal?_nfpb=true&_nfto=false&_pageLabel=mhvHome

US Food and Drug Administration. 2013. Paving the Way for Personalized Medicine: FDA's Role in a New Era of Medical Product Development. http://www.fda.gov/downloads/ScienceResearch/SpecialTopics/PersonalizedMedicine/UCM372421.pdf)

Watson, A.J., H. Bergman, C.M. Williams, and J.C. Kvedar. 2010 (April). A randomized trial to evaluate the efficacy of online follow-up visits in the management of acne. *Archives of Dermatology* 146(4):406–411.

Wolter, J. and B. Friedman. 2005. Health records for the people touting the benefits of the consumer-based personal health record. *Journal of AHIMA* 76(10):28.

World Health Organization. 2015. Social Determinants of Health. http://www.who.int/social_determinants/en/

Wright, A., D.F. Sittig, J.S. Ash, J. Feblowitz, S. Meltzer, C. McMullen, K. Guappone, J. Carpenter, J. Richardson, L. Simonaitis, R.S. Evans, W.P. Nichol, and B. Middleton. 2011 (May). Development and evaluation of a comprehensive clinical decision support taxonomy: Comparison of front-end tools in commercial and internally developed electronic health record systems. *Journal of the American Medical Informatics Association*. 18(3):232–242.

Wunderlich, G.S. and P.O. Kohler. 2001. Improving the Quality of Long-Term Care (Institute of Medicine Committee on Improving the Quality of Long Term Care)." Division of Health Care Services, Washington, DC. https://iom.nationalacademies.org/~/media/Files/Report%20Files/2003/Improving-the-Quality-of-Long-Term-Care/LTC8pagerFINAL.pdf

15

Health Information Exchange

Phillip McCann, MSC, MS, RHIA, CISSP

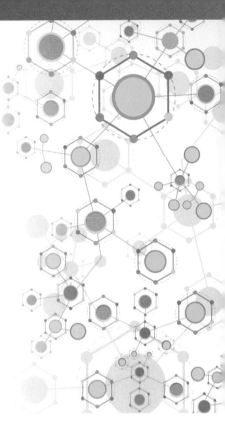

Learning Objectives

- Discover how health information exchange can transform healthcare delivery
- Determine the broad impact information technology has had on other industries and its potential to transform healthcare delivery
- Identify the challenges of standards in a highly fragmented and customized industry
- Differentiate between the pros and cons of different models of health information exchange
- Distinguish the importance of HIE in the context of healthcare quality improvement

- Identify the stages of a health information exchange implementation
- Explain the challenges of interoperability
- Explain the eHealth HealtheWay and its origins in the Nationwide Health Information Network
- Collaborate in the development of operational policies and procedures for health information exchange
- Conduct system testing to ensure data integrity and quality of health information exchange

Key Terms

Admit-discharge-transfer (ADT) message
Centralized model
Clinical Document Architecture (CDA)
Consumer-mediated exchange
Continuity of care document (CCD)
Data use and reciprocal service agreement (DURSA)
DIRECT exchange

eHealth Exchange
Federated model
Health information exchange (HIE)
Health Information Technology for Economic and Clinical Health (HITECH) Act
Health record banking model
Certified electronic health records technology (CEHRT)

Hybrid model
Interoperability
Master patient index (MPI)
Nationwide Health Information Network (NHIN)
Query-based exchange
Record locator service (RLS)
Trust community

Health information exchange (HIE) is defined as "the electronic movement of health-related information among organizations according to nationally recognized standards. The goal of health information exchange is to facilitate access to and retrieval of clinical data to provide safer, timelier, efficient, effective, equitable, patient-centered care" (HRSA 2013). Health information exchange is culture, process, and technology directed to deliver added value to patients, providers, healthcare organizations, and the public. It is the natural outcome of over 50 years of advances in biomedical knowledge, and the digitization of data to enable information to be accessible at the time and location it is most needed. Health information exchange also holds the promise of creating new knowledge and transforming care delivery and the care experience as dramatically as digitized information has transformed the consumer experience in industries like retail, music, and telecommunications. Digitized information has recreated the science of supply chain management, business knowledge, consumer insights, and production. Stakeholders in healthcare reason that it is possible to achieve similar advances in healthcare delivery through better management of the vast amounts of information that are generated during a healthcare event. Greater management and accessibility of health information are assumed to hold the key to better population health insights and higher quality of care. By making a patient's information available when needed and through data aggregation of best outcomes, a foundation for fact-based diagnosis and treatments is provided. It is assumed by many policy makers and diverse professionals in the healthcare industry that the aggregation of diagnostic and therapeutic processes will lead to a reduction of practice and diagnostic variability providing more consistent treatment based on best practices mined from large amounts of collected data.

Currently, a great deal of knowledge is not shared among practitioners and systems that could provide benefits for patients, healthcare providers, payers, and other stakeholders in the healthcare information continuum. Analysis of information and data points on best practices in surgeries and treatments across a wide range of ailments can be aggregated into new knowledge that is available to the industry, making many treatments safer and more efficient. Data mining of healthcare information by researchers may also lead to new human health insights and treatment discoveries. Health information exchange can enable health information to become accessible and shared healthcare knowledge.

Care Quality and Efficiency through an Infrastructure of Health Information Technology

In 2009, the **Health Information Technology for Economic and Clinical Health (HITECH) Act** was passed to promote the use of health IT. The objective of the legislation was to explore innovations in reimbursement; provide guidance on health IT standards, certification, and interoperability; and to provide incentives to healthcare providers to adopt electronic health record systems (HealthIT. gov 2015a). The goal of this legislation was to launch a number of initiatives that would potentially prove the benefits of information technology in relation to better healthcare delivery and coordination of services to the patient. Individually, electronic health records (EHRs) promised to provide a longitudinal patient record that could be used to better inform a patient's providers. In aggregate, electronic health records could be used to create new knowledge for population health and individual treatment. A shareable health record can also reduce treatment variability and minimize redundant testing. The overarching goal was to provide better and current information at the point of care delivery to inform diagnostic decision making.

In 2009, the Congressional Budget Office estimated that the HITECH Act would cost a total of $32.7 billion over the decade of 2009 to 2019 (ONC 2015a). Prior to the HITECH Act, adoption of EHRs among physicians and hospitals was quite low. Approximately only 22 percent of physicians had an EHR system that had even basic functionality when reviewed against the requirements of the Office of the National Coordinator for Health IT (ONC) **Certified Electronic Health Record Technology standards (CEHRT)** program (ONC 2015a). The CEHRT standards are used to inform technology vendors and providers about the functionality required to receive incentive payments for the implementation of EHR technology in the Centers for Medicare and Medicaid Services (CMS) EHR incentive program. Only 12 percent of hospitals had adopted a basic EHR system (ONC 2015a). Results from a 2013 survey of office-based physicians indicate that 48 percent have a system that conforms to CEHRT criteria, and hospitals' usage of EHR systems had increased to about 59 percent (ONC 2015a). These numbers indicate an accelerating rate of adoption of health information technology in the healthcare delivery marketplace incentivized by federal dollars but controlled by regional and local providers. This rapid diffusion of technology is creating a digital infrastructure upon which healthcare providers and business innovators can imagine new ways to improve care quality, efficiency, and consumer engagement in their wellness.

The adoption of health information technology (HIT) in the full range of healthcare provider organizations is a foundational step in the creation of the value chain that health information exchange represents. HIT infrastructure has the potential of managing the complexity that has become a part of the healthcare delivery system. Computer applications, processing power, networked workstations, and storage can facilitate the management of the abundance of information that is now available for every patient that is being treated.

Check Your Understanding 15.1

Instructions: **Answer the following questions on a separate piece of paper.**

1. What are some of the benefits that the health information exchange is expected to deliver to the healthcare industry?

2. What were the objectives of the Health Information Technology for Economic and Clinical Health Act?

3. What are the Certified Electronic Health Record Technology standards and why are they important?

4. Why did policy makers assume that information technology would improve quality and efficiency of healthcare delivery?

5. How is care quality intended to improve through the implementation of health information technology?

Interoperability and Its Challenges

HIMSS defines **interoperability** as "the ability of different information technology systems and software applications to communicate, exchange data, and use the information that has been exchanged" (HIMSS 2015). Watching entertainment content on television is a common example of this. It would be very difficult if every television and movie studio insisted upon releasing their entertainment content in proprietary file or signal formats that were not compatible with or only compatible with a few of the manufacturers of the video screens available in the market place. Interoperable technical standards for electronic signals and file formats in entertainment content distribution developed over decades have led to a level of interoperability between technology and content developers that has transformed the consumer experience, expanded the market reach of the industry, and enriched investors. In healthcare the variability of services, products and systems, and the lack of motivation to share information to achieve a common purpose continues to confound healthcare's efforts for interoperability. Some challenges to interoperability include the diversity of healthcare services, the wide range of information systems, and the numerous clinical domains with high levels of information complexity.

A single medication has a clinical, branded, generic, and chemical name. That same medication has multiple forms in which it can be administered. Add to this the different strengths the medication is available in as well as the combination of names, forms, and strengths that are available. The same medication can also be described using ingredient names and strengths, and via multiple ingredient names either clinical, branded, or generic. For example, acetaminophen has seven different forms; eight different strengths; eleven different clinical, branded, generic and clinical names; and six different combination names/forms/strengths (Shrestha and Gudivada 2015), and this is only a small sampling of the level of variability in descriptors for this common pharmaceutical.

Another area of information complexity is the document structure used to share patient information at transitions of care between providers. The organizations behind the ASTM Continuity of Care Record (CCR) and the Health Level 7 International Clinical Document Architecture (CDA) collaborated to create the **Continuity of Care Document (CCD)** to bring together the benefits of two complementary but incompatible XML document formats to better serve the purpose of health information exchange. The CCD is a more interoperable version of the two formats providing flexibility between systems while maintaining message context and accuracy (Corepoint Health 2009). The formatting flexibility that makes the CCD a valuable standard is also an attribute that can contribute to a lack of interoperability when

seeking to send messages to organizations outside of the originating organizations network.

Additional elements challenging interoperability include EHR vendor's implementations of protocols for information transmission, messaging and document frameworks such as Extensible Markup Language (XML), External Data Representation (XDR), Transmission Control Protocol (TCP), Health Level 7 International Admit Discharge Transfer message (HL7 ADT), Health Level 7 International Consolidated Continuity of Care Document (HL7 C-CCD), Health Level 7 International Fast Healthcare Interoperability Resources (HL7 FHIR), to name just a very few document formats, metadata descriptors, and transmission protocols. The numerous technology vendors in healthcare may also have slightly unique ways of implementing a standard within their systems. They may also provide system frameworks that are easily customized by their customers that can lead to nonstandard implementations of industry standards. This can interfere with interoperability with systems outside of a single enterprise technology implementation.

Healthcare delivery is highly fragmented in its knowledge base and consequently in its analysis and treatment of various diagnoses. It is challenging and expensive to integrate older computer hardware and software with newer technology for interoperability. Individual healthcare systems frequently customize their technology to better serve their internal constituents. Customizations can occur even with terminology standards such as Logical Observation Identifiers Names and Codes (LOINC) used for medical laboratory observations and the Systematized Nomenclature of Medicine–Clinical Terms (SNOMED-CT) used for general medical terminology in EHR systems, which are deployed within individual institutions information systems. (Refer to chapter 5 for more information on terminologies and standards.) Any customization of a standard renders it a nonstandard deployment and not interoperable with others using the standard.

Achieving interoperability with another facility or organization requires a cultural commitment and a strong trust relationship. Before the IT departments ever get involved there must be committed governance of the standards for classifications, terminologies, vocabularies, and other such structures that are used. Building a governance structure and agreeing upon the standards and how they are to be implemented for successful mapping between systems is the most difficult work to be accomplished in any health information exchange implementation. In spite of the funding provided by the American Recovery and Reinvestment Act (ARRA) of 2009 to incentivize the digitization of health records, the federal government only provides guidance and some incentives to motivate progress toward its regional, state, and national goals of interoperability in support of health information exchange. The ONC relies upon the industry and individual users to work out the details and make interoperability work for the benefit of healthcare delivery organizations and the consumer.

The American Health Information Community

In 2005, the American Health Information Community (AHIC) was chartered as an advisory committee to the US Department of Health and Human Services (HHS). This body was created to help the nation transition to electronic health records through common standards in support of interoperability through a process of advisory committee guidance and competition between technology companies within the industry. It was to initiate a common, open, transparent, collaborative framework, with just enough chaos to spark innovation efforts, for achieving interoperability between technology vendors. The Secretary of the Department of Health and Human Services at that time, Michael O. Leavitt, noted that

> a second challenge is achieving interoperability and minimizing the limitations of proprietary data that cannot be exchanged between different systems. The US health care system is complex, fragmented, and uses multiple standards for the use of technology. It is analogous to the railroad system that existed in America in the 1850s. Several railroad companies began laying tracks and competing for business, but the rail gauges (or, width of the tracks) varied, so that most trains couldn't switch from one network to another. The continent had multiple, incompatible networks instead of one interoperable network. We solved our rail problem long ago, but now we face a similar hurdle with health IT. (Leavitt 2005)

The community was chartered for two years, and the scope of its mission was:

- Security and privacy: Make recommendations on appropriate privacy and security protections
- Nationwide Health Information Network (NHIN) architecture: Make recommendations for a nationwide architecture using the Internet to share health information in a secure and timely fashion
- EHR standards certification: Prioritize health information technology achievements that will provide immediate benefits to consumers
- Standards harmonization: Make recommendations on standards harmonization for interoperable communications between EHRs
- Succession: Make recommendations on how the AHIC can transition within five years to a private sector health information community (Leavitt 2005)

The AHIC was successful as an incubator for the collaborations, standards, and technology development necessary to accelerate the improvements in the quality and value of healthcare delivery in the United States. The efforts of these committees established the foundations on which future innovations and progress could be built. In 2008, the National eHealth Collaborative (NeHC) was established as a public–private partnership to continue the work of the AHIC (Leavitt 2005). The NeHC was established through a grant from the ONC. Its mission was to promote the successful deployment of health IT and health information exchange nationwide (National eHealth Collaborative 2015).

Check Your Understanding 15.2

Instructions: Answer the following questions on a separate piece of paper.

1. What is interoperability?

2. What environmental factors make interoperability between health information technology providers so difficult to achieve?

3. What is the stated purpose of the Nationwide Health Information Network?

4. For what purpose was the American Health Information Community launched?

5. Provide some examples of information complexity that can cause problems with interoperability?

Models for Health Information Exchange

There are several conceptual models for health information exchange. The basic models are the centralized model, the federated or decentralized model, the hybrid model, and the health record banking model (HIMSS 2009). Participants, or members, in an HIE have the responsibility of making the HIE economically viable and governing the numerous details that define the relationships that comprise a health information exchange organization. Each model has pros and cons of sustainability, privacy and security, liability, interoperability, and development that must be considered in the early stages of planning. All of the models described have the potential to provide labs, imaging, medication lists, notes, and demographic information at the point of care delivery.

The Centralized HIE Architecture

In the centralized model, all data are stored in a shared data repository. Figure 15.1 illustrates at a high level how data is pushed to the centralized database and is received through queries to the database. The governance policies between the participants in the data warehouse dictate the scope of data usage, patient consent for data sharing, and the specific standards and information that are exchanged. Some of the advantages of this architecture are uniformity of data, quick response times to queries, and consistency in data accessibility. Disadvantages include increased chances of data duplication, information not being current due to scheduling of data transfers from participants, and increased costs for the development of a data warehouse and the supporting software.

The Decentralized HIE Architecture

The decentralized or federated model is an architecture most individuals are familiar with because it is the fundamental way that the Internet works. Figure 15.2 illustrates the decentralized model, indicating that the record locator service is the focal point for a query on a patient. Data and information remain on the servers of the participant hospitals until called for through a query. The HIE's record locator service (RLS) manages the pointers to the information on the servers of the HIE participants. The pointers in a RLS can include a person identification number (person ID) and metadata. The RLS does not provide information about the record, it merely points to where it might be found (HL7 2015a). Data are not stored in a centralized database and records are only provided when queried. Some advantages of the federated model include data remaining under the control of the HIE participant until needed, redundancy in the event of a disaster because multiple systems mitigate the risks caused by a single point of failure, and data is potentially more current. Disadvantages include data potentially not being available when needed due to technical challenges with a participant, a

Figure 15.1. The centralized HIE model

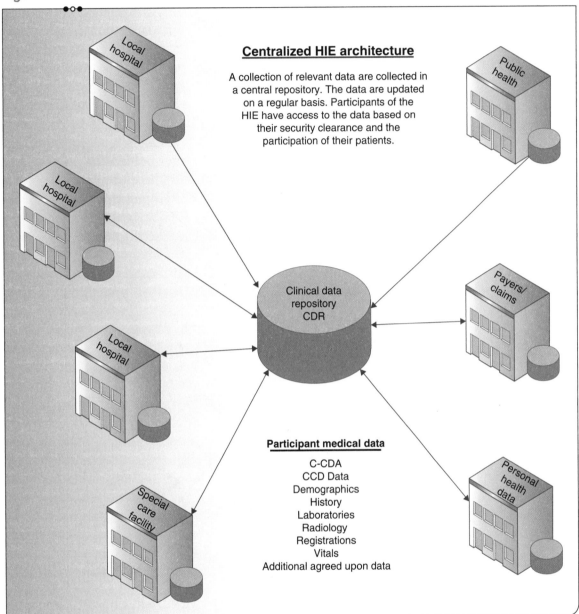

Centralized HIE architecture

A collection of relevant data are collected in a central repository. The data are updated on a regular basis. Participants of the HIE have access to the data based on their security clearance and the participation of their patients.

Local hospital

Public health

Local hospital

Clinical data repository CDR

Payers/ claims

Local hospital

Participant medical data

C-CDA
CCD Data
Demographics
History
Laboratories
Radiology
Registrations
Vitals
Additional agreed upon data

Personal health data

Special care facility

potential lack of data sharing for purposes or research, and incomplete data because a patient has records across several participants.

The Hybrid HIE Architecture

The **hybrid model** is a cross between the centralized and the decentralized models. Figure 15.3 illustrates the hybrid model, which combines the functionality of a record locator service and a centralized data repository. In a hybrid model, some data are stored in a centralized database and some

remain on the servers of the HIE participants until queried. In many respects the hybrid provides the best of two models. A centralized database enables the data for research queries from HIE participants and entities that have contracted for deidentified data for research purposes. A centralized warehouse makes the data available faster and potentially more available to patients through a common patient portal tethered to the HIE instead of one hospital. The decentralized aspects of the model provide more current data resident

Figure 15.2.   The decentralized HIE model

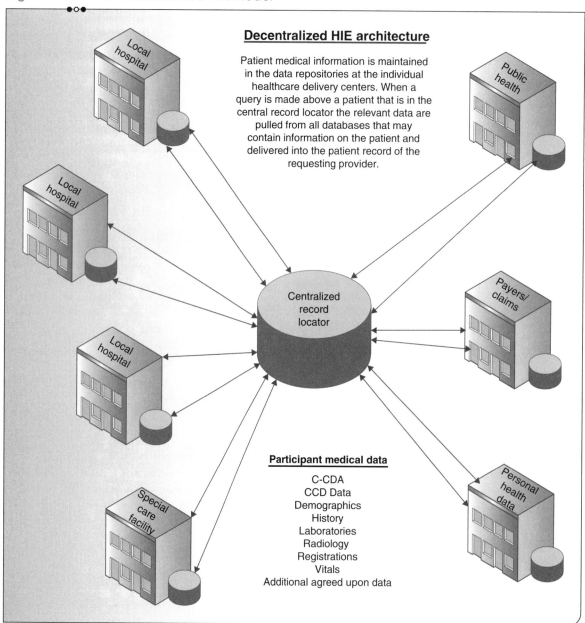

Decentralized HIE architecture

Patient medical information is maintained in the data repositories at the individual healthcare delivery centers. When a query is made above a patient that is in the central record locator the relevant data are pulled from all databases that may contain information on the patient and delivered into the patient record of the requesting provider.

Local hospital

Public health

Local hospital

Centralized record locator

Payers/ claims

Local hospital

Special care facility

Personal health data

Participant medical data

C-CDA
CCD Data
Demographics
History
Laboratories
Radiology
Registrations
Vitals
Additional agreed upon data

in each participants EHR, and enhanced security for patient records that remain within the systems of the most recent participant. Information also remains tied to the individual participants, creating a redundant data element that enhances data availability and integrity.

The Health Record Banking HIE Architecture

The **health record banking model** is an organization with information sharing agreements between a group of healthcare providers that enables the aggregation and delivery of patient information to the patient under the control of the patient. A health record bank utilizes a centralized data repository that receives patient information from participant organizations. Instead of the patient information being owned and controlled by the participant, individual patient information is controlled by the patient/consumer. Participant organizations push patient information out to the patient portal as they

Figure 15.3. The hybrid HIE model

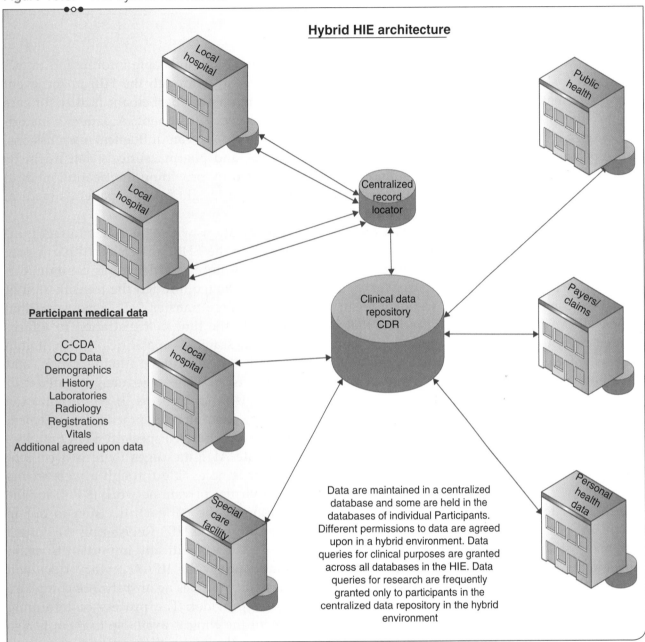

Hybrid HIE architecture

Local hospital

Public health

Centralized record locator

Local hospital

Participant medical data

C-CDA
CCD Data
Demographics
History
Laboratories
Radiology
Registrations
Vitals
Additional agreed upon data

Local hospital

Clinical data repository CDR

Payers/ claims

Special care facility

Personal health data

Data are maintained in a centralized database and some are held in the databases of individual Participants. Different permissions to data are agreed upon in a hybrid environment. Data queries for clinical purposes are granted across all databases in the HIE. Data queries for research are frequently granted only to participants in the centralized data repository in the hybrid environment

encounter the patient. The patient is delivered a standardized set of information that they can deliver to care providers on an as-needed basis, negating issues of patient privacy and ownership of the patient record. A health record bank (HRB) creates a record that stores a consumer's longitudinal health record. The HRB's focus is on collecting all of the necessary patient data instead of select data sets (Health Record Banking Alliance 2013).

The architectural models for HIE mask the issues that a lack of interoperability create below the surface of every discussion of health information exchange between technology vendors and healthcare organizations. Health information exchange can exist with minimum technology if there is an agreement between organizations that is beneficial to all involved. Technological interoperability can be developed between participants in stages once a shared vision and trust relationship is established.

Legal Issues in the Exchange of Electronic Protected Health Information

Health information exchange relies upon the patient to either opt in and agree to participate in the HIE, or opt out by choosing not to participate in the HIE. A patient's decision not to share health information is protected by the Health Insurance Portability and Accountability Act (HIPAA) and can have critical consequences for the healthcare provider if the decision is not respected. Fines to the provider can be significant if a complaint is filed with the Office of Civil Rights (OCR) and the OCR finds that the provider has been negligent or cavalier in their compliance with HIPAA privacy regulations. HIPAA (45 CFR 164.522) mandates that a covered entity that has agreed to restrict access to patients' information—except for emergency and other authorized purposes—must maintain that restriction or they will be in violation of HIPAA privacy laws. It is because of the HIPAA privacy regulations that significant resources and time are committed to the coordination of the accurate documentation of a patient's choice to participate or to not participate in health information exchange. Refer to chapter 11 for more information on HIPAA.

In many states, there is legislation that determines if the default decision for being part of an HIE is default-in or default-out. If a state is a default-in decision state, when a patient visits a healthcare provider that is a member of an HIE the provider will be required to provide the patient with meaningful disclosure of the right not to participate in the HIE and must ask the patient if there is a preference not to participate. If a state is a default-out decision state, the healthcare provider who is a participant in an HIE will provide the patient with the opportunity to join the HIE. Choosing to join the HIE makes the patient's information available to other participants in the HIE on an as-needed basis to be used in good faith for the benefit of the patient. Opting into

the HIE makes all available information immediately available through the HIE in the event of a visit to another participant facility for care or an emergency treatment. A patient's historical health record can influence readmissions, treatments, and pharmaceuticals that might be administered by providing the treating medical team through insight into the patient's medical history.

In organizations where the HIE interface is integrated into the EHR, a decision to participate in the HIE or not to participate is communicated to the exchange through the transmission of admit- discharge-transfer (ADT) messages that are coded at the time of registration to a facility. ADT messaging capabilities are built into many patient registration, administration, and EHR systems. ADT messages are generated during the registration process. If an organization is not using computerized practice management systems or has chosen a specialty EHR that does not generate ADT messages there is a consent portal that is accessible through a web browser and a virtual private network (VPN) for the registration of the patient's decision to opt in or to opt out of the HIE. Registering the correct patient decision is critically important to avoid noncompliance with HIPAA privacy rules and the possibility of fines against the noncompliant healthcare provider. The process of informing patients of the choices available to them is also important to the final outcome. Registration staff have scripts they must read to patients informing them of their choices to either not participate or participate in the HIE depending on state regulations.

Whether patients have chosen to opt in or opt out of an HIE sharing agreement, they can always reverse their decision the next time they present at an HIE participant facility. Because of the high stakes involved and the threat of legal sanctions, significant resources are allocated to testing, implementation, and training of personnel regardless of the participant's technology solution for documenting consent. ADT feeds are tested over an extended time period to ensure that the feed and the transmitted data conform to the agreed upon specifications.

The public has mixed feelings about the privacy of their personal health information and some will change their consent to share status frequently. Participant organizations in an HIE go to great lengths to ensure that they document their consumers' preference correctly.

Early HIE Initiatives

Innovation projects and programs, private and public, begin with an assumption of an end goal and then proceed to test various ways of attaining that objective. The innovation process will typically initiate numerous projects (prototypes) to test their viability and to attain the quick wins and failures that will inform the knowledge base and decisions in later stages of their initiative. The Beacon Community Cooperative Agreement was one of the innovation incubators that was funded in 17 communities throughout the United States. The purpose was to test the potential for building and strengthening HIT infrastructure, to streamline and modify workflows, and to adjust organizational culture sufficiently to leverage HIT tools to improve population health and improve the quality of care while reducing costs. The Beacon Communities initiated some of the early projects that addressed the issues of building trust communities and working with data standards to exchange basic health information for tracking patient movements (Commonwealth Fund 2012).

The **Nationwide Health Information Network (NHIN)**, established by the ONC in 2004 was initiated to create a governance, standards, and policy structure that could be easily adopted and scaled to enable health information exchange across organizational, regional and state boundaries. The NHIN is not a set of servers in the basement of the offices of ONC. Instead NHIN is a set of guidelines, recommended technology standards, and data use and service-level agreements that can facilitate data exchange. It is a public–private endeavor that encompasses a diverse group of entities from across the country. The standards and guidelines it established led to many initiatives such as DIRECT Protocols for secure messaging and CONNECT,

which initially served as a gateway for the processing of disability claims for the Social Security Administration (SSA) NHIN (HealthIT.gov 2015b).

The **eHealth Exchange** is the next iteration of the NHIN and most recently, under the umbrella of the Sequoia Project, no longer requires ONC funding. It started out as a public–private consortium utilizing the standards, governance, and legal agreements of the NHIN as a foundation for an exchange network that now spans across 50 states, 13,000 medical groups, 4 federal agencies, and 40 percent of US hospitals (eHealth Exchange 2015a). Membership in the eHealth Exchange provides the participant with a tested legal framework for their trust community, which is discussed later in the chapter, providing efficiencies in standards testing and exchange connectivity with governmental providers. A participant in the eHealth Exchange is able to exchange information with any other participant across the nation (eHealth Exchange 2015b).

The ONC has also been instrumental in providing funding to nurture health information exchange within the states. The state HIE program launched in 2010 with the goal of enabling statewide exchange using DIRECT and query-based exchange methods. Fifty states and eligible territories and state designated entities received awards. The goal was to rapidly build capacity for exchanging health information within and between the states. By accepting the funding, the participating bodies were required to:

- Create and implement up-to-date privacy and security requirements for HIE
- Coordinate with Medicaid and state public health programs to establish an integrated approach

- Monitor and track meaningful use HIE capabilities in their state
- Set strategy to meet gaps in HIE capabilities
- Ensure consistency with national standards (HealthIT.gov 2014)

Metrics to measure progress toward a goal are a significant part of program and project management processes. In the interest of transparency, and to gauge the progress toward its goals, a 2014 study funded by the ONC documented mixed results for success within the state HIE programs based on a six state review. The study found that the state HIE programs raised awareness for HIE within the state among potential participants. The challenges of interoperability remain a constant barrier as technology vendors and healthcare organizations grapple with a deeply ingrained culture of technology customizations to meet individual organizational needs making technology migrations for interoperability more costly. Sustainability of state HIE organizations continues to be a challenge as short-term value is difficult to demonstrate; healthcare organizations wait for the next wave of technology to resolve issues prevalent in solutions that are available today (Dullabh et al. 2015a).

Exchange Methodologies

A health information exchange does not contain the legal health record. The legal health record of participant patients is maintained by each participant organization in the HIE. Many exchanges are merely conduits of data facilitating the transmission, translation, and mapping of electronic protected health information (ePHI) between participant EHRs in the HIE. The medical information acquired through an HIE will be a collection of the information that is available on the patient. It is reliant upon the organization requesting the patient information to format the information so it is meaningful and easily readable to the requesting provider.

In order for exchange to be meaningful, a minimum required data set must be agreed upon between the participants in the HIE. If the HIE aspires to be able to connect to the NHIN or eHealthExchange, they will be required to conform to that network's minimum data set requirements. Additionally there are multiple transmission protocols to be considered. Health Level Seven (HL7) International is an organization that has focused on creating comprehensive frameworks and standards for integrating, sharing, exchanging, and retrieving ePHI. Many of its frameworks provide a structure for sharing and exchanging information like demographics, race, problems, allergies, medications, immunizations, labs, documents, radiology images, procedures, and language.

One of the main issues between providers can be the request for or the sending of too much information about a patient. Too much information can have the same effect as having no information because of the continuous time constraints everyone works under. It is for this reason that participants in an HIE must agree upon what information is valuable in specific situations and what the minimum set of information is that should be collected and shared in the course of ordinary operations. For example, the information needs of an emergency department encounter can be vastly different than the information needs of a cardiologist seeing a patient for a maintenance visit. In larger organizations, it is not the doctors that will typically be using the exchange technologies. Health information management staff or care coordinators will acquire the needed information on a patient based on the doctor's and organization's predetermined requirements for the unique circumstances of the patient visit.

The exchange methodologies that are currently available provide access to health information exchange across the economic spectrum of providers. DIRECT messaging exchange can be available to any provider that has access to an Internet connection. Query-based and consumer mediated exchange require a more sophisticated technology infrastructure. It is important to remember that all health information exchange relies on documenting the correct patient decision for participation or nonparticipation in the health information exchange.

DIRECT Exchange

DIRECT messaging exchange is an encrypted email platform. DIRECT messaging is used by a provider to push information to another provider. It does not ask a question of a database, it merely pushes a message in a secure format so it can be viewed by the intended recepient. A DIRECT healthcare Internet service provider (HISP) only enables an exchange between members who either have membership in that HISP or with a provider in a different HISP that is a member of the same trust community like DIRECT TRUST. Launched in March 2010 as a part of the Nationwide Health Information Network, the DIRECT Project was created to specify a simple, secure, scalable, standards-based way for participants to send (push) authenticated, encrypted health information directly to known, trusted recipients over the Internet (DIRECT Project 2015). This is referred to as **DIRECT Exchange**. A direct message is viewed as an email in an HTML format, and attachments (labs, CCD, images) are frequently sent as portable document format documents (PDFs). DIRECT exchange is currently used for referrals, discharge summaries sent to primary care physicians, transmission of lab reports to ordering physicians, and the transmission of continuity of care documents of various kinds.

This form of information exchange enables coordinated care, benefitting both providers and patients. DIRECT exchange is also being used for sending immunization data to public health organizations or to report quality measures to the CMS (HealthIT.gov 2014). DIRECT exchange is important because it is accessible to providers large and small. Service providers that have not been included in the EHR incentive programs, like medical specialists and long-term care and skilled nursing facilities, can utilize DIRECT messaging to exchange patient information and referrals. DI-RECT exchange is the entry-level information exchange that is available to the broadest healthcare delivery audience and requires membership in a Health Information Service Providers (HISP) network, Internet access, and a browser.

Query-Based Exchange

Query-based exchange is "used by providers to search and discover accessible clinical sources on a patient. A query on a database asks a question of the database and pulls information based on the keywords that are used in the query. This type of exchange is often used when delivering unplanned care such as ED visits" (HealthIT.gov 2014). Query-based exchange, depending on the technology vendor, uses Boolean search queries to locate patient information in either a centralized data repository or across a federated network of providers. In a Boolean search engine, the application combines the keywords used in the search string to retrieve an index of possible solutions from the queried database based on the keyword and the hierarchy in which those keywords appear in the search string. Participant organizations with the proper patient permission can pre-prepare a patient's health record before a patient visit to monitor if they have received treatment from another provider in a different facility that they should be aware of. This type of use can have positive implications for care coordination and quality of care. A query-based search can be used in emergency situations where the query might be carried out by staff seeking medication, allergies, and medical problems on a patient that presents at the emergency department. Health information exchange is a significant cultural and process re-engineering project. Use cases and their workflows must be worked out in advance and shared with the internal staff that will be expected to use the new technological capabilities effectively. Query-based capabilities are frequently integrated into an organization's EHR system making it easier to add queried information to the patient record that is searched. Standardizing data field specifications (data normalization) between the participants in the HIE enables queried data to be easily shared and used by all participant providers.

Consumer-Mediated Exchange

Consumer-mediated exchange provides patients with access to their health information allowing them to manage their healthcare online in a similar fashion to how they might manage their finances through online banking (HealthIT.gov 2014). An example of consumer-mediated exchange is the Blue Button initiative. Blue Button is a public–private partnership based within the ONC in close partnership with the White House and the Office of Veterans Affairs, CMS, and the Department of Defense (DOD). "Its objective is to engage and empower consumers and patients through electronic access to their individual health information, which they can use to manage and improve their health and health care" (Ricciardi and Dole 2014). Consumer-mediated exchange provides the ultimate solution to patient privacy by giving consumers control of who has access to their protected health information and when they have access to it.

HIE Implementation Considerations

Health information exchange implementations, whether internal or between competing organizations, are large technology implementations. Large technology implementations are programs comprised of multiple projects. Project programs are closely tied to strategic business strategy and require complicated governance processes to ensure that diverse stakeholder concerns and needs are always considered before decisions are implemented and changes made. Programs have long time horizons and in many cases are ongoing because they are the infrastructure on which the business operates. The projects that the program is comprised of will have shorter time horizons, less governance issues, and more restricted budgets. It is the projects within the program that the organization will reference for indications of success in the early stages of the program. Successful project completion adds momentum to the overall progress of the program to satisfy the strategy goals it was designed to fulfill. The completed project's resources can then be repurposed to the fulfillment of the objectives of the next project in the program project portfolio.

There is no prescriptive formula for the successful implementation of health information exchange practices. A 2014 study found that 74 percent of surveyed HIEs have issues with financial sustainability. There are interoperability issues between HIE technology vendors and only 30 percent of surveyed hospitals and 10 percent of ambulatory practices are connected to an HIE

(JASON, the MITRE 2014). These numbers indicate that there is no burning market demand for HIE capabilities and a large percentage of healthcare providers are waiting until the technology issues are resolved through their EHR vendors or interface engine providers, and the economies of scale bring the costs of the remaining software venders down to a more reasonable level. Vision is essential for organizations that choose to pursue cross-organizational information exchange now to have a strategic head start on the new payment and care frameworks that are coming from payers in the near future. Planning is essential, and the plan must develop a view of the future that guides current and future decision making. The business goals and strategic plans of all of the HIE participants must be in alignment for the services and products they will collaborate on through the implementation of the HIE.

Identification of a Trust Community

A **trust community** is a group of organizations that have identified a set of mutual goals and dependencies that through collaborative effort lead to mutual benefit. HIE is dependent upon the formation of a trust community. Many times these trust communities are formed between members of an integrated delivery network (IDN) to facilitate sharing of resources and to formalize the network connections they have for referrals and transitions of care. In the context of health information exchange outside of a single enterprise or IDN, a group of regional healthcare organizations can choose to collaborate to facilitate cross-organizational exchange of patient information in support of better patient care, quality of healthcare delivery, and population health. A trust community has common interest and goals and opportunities for collaboration that provide benefits for all involved.

Development of Governance Committees

Once the trust community has been identified, governance must be considered. There will be numerous committees to provide the many stakeholders across all participants with input into the decision making. Committees and workgroups may have titles like executive/advisory committee, technology and planning, data normalization, privacy and security, human resources, patient registration managers, health information managers, and so on. Like any large infrastructure investment, it will be important to identify and engage as many stakeholders as possible and involve them actively in the planning and decision making to minimize objections once the program is initiated. HIE implementations tend to be dominated by a company's IT department, similar to the implementation of EHRs in the early stages of meaningful use. Considering that health information exchange is a trust agreement between competing organizations, identifying return on investment and other organizational benefits can be challenging. Early involvement of the organizational and HIM teams may make the transition to HIE practices a smoother migration for all participants.

Identification of the Technology Platform

Once governance is in place, the selected committees should do the research necessary to determine what technology features are most important to their HIE operational needs. Teams should read about and benchmark the experiences of other HIEs and interview organizations that are operational to better understand the potential barriers to success and determine the best paths to consider. After the research and interviews are conducted, a request for proposal (RFP) will be issued to vendors that provide the required technology and service capabilities. Selection of the final vendor will be a function of the governing committees and a rigorous search in the HIE platform technology market through the RFP process. Preparing an RFP involves researching all of the specifications that are desired in a technology purchase and putting those specifications into a structured document so the applicants are forced to provide answers to questions designed for easy analysis. Once the RFP responses are reviewed by the committee, the answers are scored, and the candidates to be interviewed are chosen. Committee interviews with candidate executives and technologists lead to the final selection of a vendor.

Contracts and Participant Agreements

The eHealth Exchange has the **Data Use and Reciprocal Support Agreement (DURSA)**. The DURSA is a legally binding contract that draws from federal and local laws and defines the requirements for participation in the eHealth Exchange national network (HealtheWay 2015). The participants in an HIE should develop a legally binding agreement, similar to the DURSA, between all members. The participant agreement will provide very granular details of all obligations and responsibilities of all members. The agreement will also address the sanctions for violations of the contract. Once a technology platform is chosen, the participants should also create an equally binding contract between their HIE entity and the vendor.

Operational Policies

The agreements that are reached in the participant agreement and vendor contract should be developed into operational policies and procedures. Once created, they are distributed to all participants as a reference for the staff that will handle integrating technology and workflows into member organizations.

Development of Vendor and Participant Project Teams

The various governance committees that the trust community has created will initiate the planning cycle for the project. Project managers will be designated and plans developed. Technology implementations, as well as organizational change management projects, are deployed in stages. For the IT team, the initial step to be accomplished is to coordinate the communications from the participants' HL7 ADT feeds from their EHR interfaces to the HIE interface engine.

Data Governance

Data governance and normalization should be ongoing throughout the technology implementation. One of the initial projects requiring collaboration and governance will be the HL7 **Admit-discharge-transfer (ADT) message**. Data governance is important when sharing ADT messages between organizations to ensure that the exchanged data is interoperable between information technology systems created by different manufacturers. The HL7 ADT represents a flexible standard that can be modified to create greater efficiencies within a closed organizational system. Once that system is opened to sharing information, the affiliated organizations must work to standardize how they are using the standard so information can be shared. The ADT is a patient tracking mechanism that is transmitted from numerous systems within a healthcare facility as a patient moves through the system. An ADT message contains demographic information and other information. Payer systems, registration systems, and EHRs all have the capability to send an ADT message. HL7 provides the following description of the ADT message:

> Patient Administration, also known as admit-discharge-transfer (ADT), supports many of the core administrative functions in healthcare such as person and patient registration and encounter management. Information is entered into a patient or person registry or into a patient administration system, and then passed to other systems (for example, other registries, clinical, ancillary, and financial systems). The ADT provides the standards for bi-directionally transmitting administrative data for patients, persons, service delivery locations, and patient encounters. (HL7 2015c)

Accurately tracking administrative details and patient encounters is essential for billing and scheduling.

There are 51 different segments in an ADT message. Many of the segments are not used in most messages. A quick sampling of ADT segments looks like this

- A01   Admit/visit notification
- A02   Transfer a patient
- A03   Discharge/end visit
- A04   Register a patient
- A05   Pre-admit a patient
- A06   Change an outpatient into an inpatient
- A07   Change an inpatient to an outpatient
- A08   Update patient information
- A09   Patient departing—tracking
- A10   Patient arriving—tracking (HL7 2015c)

The messages are created and transmitted through trigger events that are programmed into the communications or administration systems. The interpretation of a standard is relevant because each healthcare facility will populate different segments in the ADT message, and they will use different structure standards within the segments. Data governance and data normalization are critical functions in the preplanning stages before the ADT feeds go-live into the HIE's interface engines. The HIM professional, in conjunction with the IT project manager of the organization and the technology vendor, can have a significant impact on the ease with which the initial stages of implementation progress.

The Creation of the Sandbox for System Testing

A sandbox is an isolated environment that simulates the production environment that will be used once testing is completed. Connecting to the sandbox and thoroughly testing and adjusting systems and applications to discover flaws in development and execution is a necessary step in the implementation cycle. Nothing leaves the sandbox before it is completely tested and proven to be 10 percent compatible with the live production environment. Once ADT feeds are proven reliable in the sandbox, the project managers schedule a date for go-live in the production environment.

Stages of HIE Implementation

There are three stages of implementation in a health information exchange project. They include ensuring proper connectivity and the aggregation of data, the exchange of clinical data, and finally making the exchange available to participants.

Stage 1 of Implementation

Once a participant is transmitting messages and data to the HIE's interface, the aggregation of data that will enable the creation of the registry that allows the system to identify patients within its system begins. Depending upon the HIE system, there are locator systems and structures that allow the retrieval of information on individual patients.

Master Patient Index (MPI)

AHIMA defines the **master patient index (MPI)** as "a list or database created and maintained by a healthcare system to record the name and identification number of every patient who has been admitted or treated in the facility" (AHIMA 2013). In the context of an HIE, the MPI will rely on algorithms that match elements of patient demographic information to determine relationships in patient identity. During the testing stages of the implementation, these algorithms and criteria will be adjusted until a designated performance metric for accuracy is met (AHIMA 2013).

Record Locator Service (RLS)

The **record locator service (RLS)** provides the ability to identify where records are located based upon criteria such as a person ID and record data type, as well as provides functionality for the ongoing maintenance of this location information (HL7 2015a).

The RLS handles the bookkeeping and allows the identification of the server instances that contain categories of registered information about a person. The locator service maintains the following knowledge:

- At a minimum, given an identity, the RLS shall retrieve all appropriate locations with information associated with that identity.

- Provides for context-sensitive information location based upon matching metadata requirements. It is also desirable to allow for labeling technology like extensible metadata that can be embedded within the file.

- Retains what categories or registered patterns of information (HL7 Templates) a given location knows about.

- Recognizes what categories of information (topics) a given location wants to receive messages.

- Identifies individuals for which is information stored (HL7 2015a).

In many HIE environments, it is desirable to measure how many patients move between facilities within the participant trust community. ADT messages are monitored (deidentified) to build reports on the movements of patients between facilities. ADT messages can also capture the information needed to track patient opt-in or opt-out status either initiating or terminating participation in the HIE. The patient consent profile is updated every time the patient presents at an HIE participant organization depending upon relevant local legislation. Stage one is also when connectivity to public health and disease registries will occur; and DIRECT messaging will be implemented.

Stage 2 of Implementation

Stage 1 operations will run long enough for the technology and project management teams to mitigate any challenges that arose with any participant or the vendor before moving to Stage 2. Stage 2 of implementation will initiate the exchange of clinical data (labs, radiology reports, medications, CCDs, discharge summaries, physician notes, and others). HL7 **Clinical Document Architecture (CDA)** is used as the standard for document exchange. HL7 defines the CDA as "a document markup standard that specifies the structure and semantics of 'clinical documents' for the purpose of exchange between healthcare providers and patients" (HL7 2015b). The CDA framework is both human and machine readable. A CDA document can include text, images, and even multimedia content. It is this level of flexibility that enables its ability to contain any type of clinical content. A common use for the CDA document is as a discharge summary, imaging report, admission and physical, pathology report, and more (HL7 2015b). The CDA framework has enabled several additional document standards and architectures that have improved and stabilized some elements of interoperability across multiple technology vendors.

All of the governance, normalization, and testing activities conducted in Stage 1 implementation will be repeated for Stage 2 because the information exchange and standards conformity must be exact to enable interoperability between EHR and information location systems. Issues that can arise include nonconformance of usage of coding systems like LOINC, SNOMED-CT, and medication nomenclatures and vocabularies.

Stage 3 of Implementation

In the third stage of an implementation, the HIE is made available to the ambulatory care facilities and providers that refer patients to the acute-care facilities. It is in this phase that the HIE is considered a community.

The Value-Added Enterprise

The adoption of information technology in other industries has enabled a rapid restructuring of the internal and external business environment. This adds value to the enterprises that have embraced the technology adoption, and to the consumer whose expectations of products and services has been transformed. Adding value to the enterprise and to the consumer experience is what differentiates a great business from the rest of the competitors in its marketplace. In the healthcare delivery market HIMSS identifies five categories of value that HIT provides:

1. Improved communications with all stakeholders.
2. Improved patient safety through a reduction in medical errors and readmissions.
3. Increased use of evidence-based medical guidelines through clinical decision support (CDS).
4. Improved population health and quality measure reporting.
5. Greater support for preventative medicine through wellness initiatives and supply chain and patient scheduling efficiencies. (HIMSS 2009)

The value in health information exchange mirrors the HIMSS value-added processes. An HIE's value is in assisting participants in meeting meaningful use stages, patient engagement, monitoring hospital 7- and 30-day readmissions, and patient movements between medical facilities and providers. The HIE will be beneficial in referral management, payer engagement, and in documenting patient outcomes to specific treatments. Information and knowledge derived from data are the foundation of value and will lead the HIE to create services for the community that will enhance revenue and build participation.

 Check Your Understanding 15.3

Instructions: **Answer the following questions on a separate piece of paper.**

1. What are the five categories of value that are identified by the Health Information Management and Systems Society?

2. Name the three methods for health information exchange and explain their differences.

3. What role has the ONC played in the development of health information exchanges across the country?

4. Why is trust important in health information exchange?

5. What role does governance play in the successful deployment of a health information exchange?

Meaningful Use for HIE

In 2009, the American Recovery and Reinvestment Act (ARRA) authorized CMS to provide incentive payments to eligible professionals and hospitals who adopt, implement, upgrade, or demonstrate meaningful use of certified electronic health record technology. Through incentives paid directly to providers, or the organizations that hire providers, CMS was creating the digital infrastructure that, once completed, would create the pathway for information transmission. Key parts of this information could then be used for a number of quality healthcare delivery monitoring and population health purposes (CMS 2014). Stage 1 Meaningful Use had very basic requirements for health information exchange that could be met by merely attempting an exchange of information with another organization. DIRECT exchange was very instrumental in enabling healthcare providers and organizations to meet the simple requirements of Stage 1 Meaningful Use.

Meaningful Use has progressed from its Stage 1 implementation (the broad adoption of certified electronic health record systems) into Stage 2, which is intended to advance clinical processes and require greater use of health information exchange between EHR systems from different vendors. Interoperability between technology companies has always been a fundamental objective of the CMS EHR incentive program. The federal government's goal of only providing guidance on interoperability standards enabled the industry to maintain the status quo in standards-based information exchange. Interoperability in other technology sectors has usually been driven by a single dominant manufacturer who has imposed standards that were quickly adopted by consumers and consequently by suppliers and smaller manufacturers. The fragmented nature of healthcare delivery and the lack of a dominant technology provider left the marketplace with numerous technology solutions competing and not cooperating with the development and use of interoperability standards. This understanding of the power of the marketplace is one of the reasons why the government has provided funding to programs like the state HIEs, the Beacon Communities, NHIN, CONNECT, and DIRECT Project to test and advance interoperability standards. Stage 3 will be implemented in 2016 and 2017 and will focus on improved outcomes and interoperability between EHR systems with essential communications and access to health information for patients (CMS 2014). Success of the Meaningful Use programs means that the technologies that were promoted will fall into the background and become invisible, like good infrastructure should. It is uncommon in this era for individuals to engage in discussions about national electrification, a nationwide telecommunications network, the national highway system, or banking ATMs. All of the mentioned technologies redefined their industries, modern culture, and lifestyles. Health information exchange, once successfully embedded, will become invisible while radically changing the ways individuals consume and perceive healthcare delivery.

Additional Health Information Exchange Initiatives

The American Health Information Coalition was commissioned with the intent of creating a public–private coalition to develop the conceptual foundations and organizational structures for changing the healthcare delivery paradigm in the United States from one that was event and provider focused to one that was more systematic (holistic) in its approach to public and individual wellness and healthcare delivery. The NHIN was one of the conceptual spin-offs from this early coalition. The NHIN has evolved into the eHealth corporation chartered to advance the implementation of secure, interoperable nationwide health information exchange (HealtheWay 2015). One recent evolution of this public–private initiative is the Sequoia Project.

The eHealth Exchange Sequoia Project is "a group of federal agencies and non-federal organizations that came together under a common mission and purpose to improve patient care, streamline disability benefit claims, and improve public health reporting through secure, trusted and interoperable health information exchange" (eHealth Exchange 2015b). ONC transitioned management of its eHealth Exchange to Sequoia Project for maintenance in 2012. Since 2012 eHealth Exchange has grown to become the largest health information exchange network in the country (The Sequoia Project 2015).

The eHealth Exchange represents a trust community that is creating a system of networks across the nation allowing electronically captured protected health information to be pushed to and queried wherever it is needed. DIRECT messages can already be transmitted across the nation. As more health information exchanges are onboarded, the value of the system of networks will increase exponentially. eHealth Exchange has a very rigorous onboarding process that includes extensive testing of interoperability, transmission standards, codes, and vocabularies.

The CommonWell Health Alliance is a coalition of mid- to small-sized EHR manufacturers that have organized to accelerate interoperability between different technology organizations using standards promoted by the eHealth Exchange and HL7. This coalition is a marketplace response to maintain relevance for smaller technology groups who want to remain competitive in the health information exchange environment (CommonWell Health Alliance 2015).

Adherence to the processes of change management is enabling the ONC to lead the market to where the market should be focused. Initiatives like the Beacon Communities, state HIE programs, and the health information technology regional extension center (HITREC) programs are changing the culture of healthcare delivery in small stages. The ONC remains focused on driving quality improvement and greater efficiency by providing a strong and evolving vision, maintaining diverse stakeholders in the vision's creation, and in providing incentives for reaching goals and disincentives for not reaching goals.

The Nationwide Interoperability Roadmap

Connecting Health and Care for the Nation Draft Version One is the latest evolution in ongoing communications that support the ONC vision of "supporting the adoption of health IT and promoting nationwide health information exchange to improve health and care" (ONC 2015b). Figure 15.4 is a high-level timeline of how ONC anticipates interoperability progressing from 2015 through 2020. The emphasis in the interoperability roadmap is on the 10-year vision for health information exchange. It contains detailed descriptions of the needed collaborations, standards, governance, regulatory environment, cultural changes, monitoring, and flexibility in processes that will be required to meet ONC's deadlines. The interoperability roadmap describes the actions and roles of a variety of health IT stakeholders needed to achieve ONC's 10-year interoperability vision.

Consistent with the ONC's operating procedures, the interoperability roadmap was open for comment from stakeholders and the public and then moved to a completed version that was published toward the end of 2015. A final document will be released in 2016 and will be subject to ongoing updates, based on progress toward its goals and the political climate of the time.

The guiding principles of nationwide interoperability are intended to focus collective efforts to make practical and valuable progress and encourage innovation. Figure 15.5 illustrates the principles as metaphorical building blocks. The 10 principles that provide guidance follow:

Figure 15.4. Initial interoperability timeline

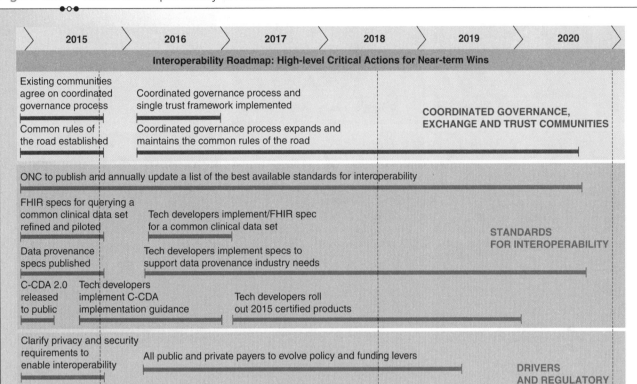

Source: ONC 2015b, 15.

1. Build upon existing health IT infrastructure, (existing healthcare organizations have significant investments in existing technology [sunk costs] and newer technologies will need to integrate with the existing ones to add value to an institution's IT infrastructure).

2. One size does not fit all—healthcare organizations have unique needs based on its location, the demographics of its patient base, its internal specialties. and its integration into the surrounding community. They remained viable by customizing technologies to meet a unique set of circumstances.

3. Empower individuals—silos of knowledge and information suppress creativity and innovation. The benefits of information in motion are better realized when cross-disciplinary teams within organizations work together to maximize the potential that is available within new information technology capabilities.

4. Leverage the market—competition between technology competitors should create better products and lower costs as marketplace competitors work to enhance their product and service offerings to capture a larger share of customers.

5. Simplify—collaboration and governance provide a faster path to a return on investment than technology ever can. Lead HIE initiatives

Figure 15.5. Interoperability principals

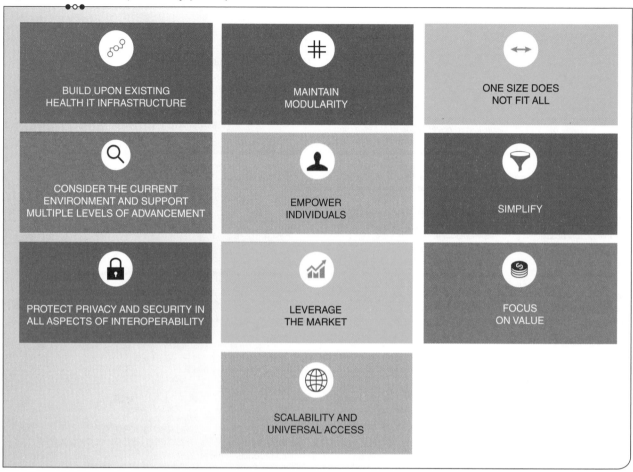

Source: ONC 2015b, 9.

with trust and cooperation and simplify the requirements for everything that follows.

6. Maintain modularity—customization is expensive. For every dollar spent customizing something it requires six to make modifications to the customization. Modular components in a network facilitate common standards and plug and play simplicity.

7. Consider the current environment and support multiple levels of advancement—engagement from all users and structured feedback processes within an organization ensures responsiveness to a dynamic environment and adjustment to processes that ensure ongoing progress toward stated goals.

8. Focus on value—marketplace competition and common standards between technology competitors leads to greater buyer choice

and increased value for the buyer as the marketplace products move toward Commoditization over time.

9. Protect privacy and security in all aspects of interoperability—HIE is reliant on the ability to provide total compliance with all applicable privacy and security requirements for the patient. Trust is the currency of the HIE.

10. Ensure scalability and universal access— piloting technology and processes that provide significant benefit can be scaled to a size that will share the benefits to a broad audience and make sure that innovations funded by public money remain accessible to the public without burdensome licensing fees (ONC 2015b, 20).

Consistent standards and governance policies will enable successful HIE practices to be scaled from organizations to regions and across states providing greater access to the benefits HIE can provide to a wide range of stakeholders.

The stated building blocks of the interoperability roadmap include the following.

1. **Core technical standards and functions:** The technical standards and functions are outcomes of good governance and successful collaboration in the interest of interoperability. At the organizational level it is important to minimize or eliminate customizations in core applications and technology to please a few internal clinicians.

2. **Certification and testing to support adoption and optimization of health IT products and services:** Guidelines for technology performance created by ONC and industry contributors is another element of trust that can be relied upon. Standards for information capture and transmission have been created in a collaborative fashion by ONC and the industry. Vendor conformance to the established standards through testing and certification provides a guarantee of quality in the products and services they are delivering to care practitioners.

3. **Privacy and security protections for health information:** The security of information at rest and in transmission is essential to developing trust with the consumer. Protected health information is an essential component of the goal to provide better care outcomes and greater cost and time efficiency in treating chronic and acute illnesses. The value of being able to use deidentified big data in the pursuit of best practices and better control of illness within populations is dependent upon the public having trust that their information will not be used for fraudulent purposes. It is also essential that consumers have the ability to control the use of their information and to have the trust in the methods and technology that is used to enforce their wishes.

4. **Supportive business, clinical, cultural, and regulatory environments:** Healthcare is an old industry and there is a significant amount of old clinical practices, cultural artifacts, and technology (sunk costs) that must be overcome to make progress toward transforming healthcare delivery to a consumer and wellness-centric activity. Regulations must be harmonized across 50 states to provide a framework for information exchange that is conducive for standardized information sets. The numerous suppliers of clinical technology and materials must coordinate around the vision for delivering better quality and efficiency to the consumer of healthcare. In addition to the needed changes within competitive organizations, individuals providing care must embrace the benefits that technology can provide and make fact-based decision making an essential element of their diagnostic workflows.

5. **Rules of engagement and governance:** There is a diverse field of stakeholders involved in healthcare delivery and in the exchange of information supporting healthcare payments, care, care coordination, care quality, material supply, and the like. It is important to engage stakeholders in the decision making that supports the ONC guidelines for interoperability. Industry and consumer participation in the vision and goals of interoperability ensure that the benefits derived from the transformation in care delivery are mutually shared (ONC 2015a, 31).

These five items are identified by ONC as the foundations of interoperability. It is important to remember that health information exchange is a small component of an overall plan to transform healthcare delivery in the United States. The past years have been spent incentivizing the digitization of medical recordkeeping. Now the emphasis is on making sure the information is mobile and exchangeable between providers of all types and accessible by the consumer when and where it is needed.

Governance

HIE governance is concerned with the establishment of a shared set of behaviors and standards that enable trusted electronic health information exchange among participants (ONC 2015b, 27). Participants must agree on controls such as ID validation, access, cryptography, and standards for data transmission, normalization, and minimum data sets. The goal is to increase trust among all participants so that they incur no additional liabilities through information exchange because they all share a particular set of values, processes, and standards. Since its inception, the ONC has supported the creation of public–private collaborations to address the issues of governance in HIE. DIRECT Trust, the New York eHealth Collaborative (NYeC), the National eHealth Collaborative (which has recently merged with the Health Information and Management Systems Society), HealtheWay's Care Quality Principles of Trust, and the Sequoia Project's eHealth Exchange DURSA are examples of organizations involved in governance that have received support and provided insights to ONC's HIE governance initiatives.

The ONC's interoperability roadmap is a vision statement that provides a 10-year high-level plan of what needs to occur to achieve health information technology interoperability and the learning healthcare system within the scope of its timeline. This vision provides an overview of its governance principles aggregated from the numerous forums and body of work that it has initiated from public–private collaborations. The ONC's rules of the road are guidance statements of principle meant to overcome market place entropy among technology vendors and healthcare corporate cultures around the practices of information exchange and responsiveness to customer requests for patient information. The rules of the road are broad principles understood to add or create value for diverse stakeholders through the use of mobile information.

Levers to Drive Interoperability

In spite of the ONC's targeted marketplace incentives and policy guidance EHR interoperability and health information exchange have remained an elusive goal to achieve. Market forces, a fear of competition, and structural impediments across an extremely fragmented healthcare delivery environment has inhibited the adoption of interoperability standards. The ONC, with the support of CMS, is now focused on providing additional incentives and local regulatory oversight to further modify the behaviors of reluctant technology vendors and healthcare delivery organizations to drive support needed to accelerate interoperable standards and practices across all levels of the health IT marketplace.

Value-based payment is the conceptual replacement for fee-for-service. Value-based payment pays for an episode of care and incentivizes a system-based methodology of delivering care instead of paying for each service delivered in an episode-of-care delivery. A value-based payment establishes a fee for an episode of care and requires providers for that episode to work as a team in support of the care delivery. Efficient work practices can result in profit for the team. Inefficient work practices or poor quality care delivery (redundant, unnecessary tests, readmissions within 7 or 30 days) result in a loss of profit. The interoperability roadmap calls for 30 percent of Medicare payments to be paid to providers through alternative payment models by 2017 and 90 percent between 2018 and 2020 (ONC 2015d, 10). Health information exchange and its many governance structures, trust networks, and technology interface engines, are the infrastructure upon which ONC is relying to make value-based payments a successful reality. Care coordination in support of a patient's episode of care relies upon efficient communications about a patient's treatment status within a medical home or managed care network environment. As EHRs become more interoperable, health information exchange will become more efficient. HIE is expected to greatly reduce redundant testing, treatment variability, and wasteful practices within any given episode of treatment.

To support value-based payment, the federal government will exert its guidance on technical standards through new grants and contracts that fund health IT adoption. CMS will emphasize the medical home model through its Medicaid managed care programs along with its quality and performance metrics. There will be a call to action to state HIEs to adopt interoperability standards recommended by ONC. Medical homes and new health care delivery models will drive the adoption of health information exchange through their focus on care coordination. ONC and CMS will work to influence private payers and purchasers of healthcare services to insist upon technologies and practices that support health information exchange and new payer models.

The ONC's interoperability roadmap calls for empowering broad-based action, generating short-term wins, consolidating gains, while building on past successes and anchoring the new approach in the culture. The roadmap calls for federal, state, business, and individual involvement to change the delivery paradigm from one that is focused on the treatment of singular incidents of illness to a learning health system that takes a holistic approach to the wellness of its constituents. These data driven delivery networks are anticipated to deliver the triple aim of improving patient quality and satisfaction, improving population health, and reducing the per capita cost of healthcare (Institute for Healthcare Improvement 2015).

The Nationwide Privacy and Security Framework

Trust is the currency that makes everything in health information exchange possible. Being able to guarantee privacy and security of patient health information at rest and in transit is a primary concern of all stakeholders. Figure 15.6 is illustrating the privacy and security framework that ONC is promoting within its interoperability roadmap guidance document. In spite of the significant regulations around privacy and security that exists within HIPAA, there remains significant variability within implementation across the industry. The nationwide privacy and security framework is designed as guidance to industry participants on the consistent adoption and implementation of standards that address cyber security, encryption, ID validation, and permissions to collect, share, and use PHI. Addressing the issues of trust for the exchange and use of regular and sensitive information across regional, state, and national boundaries remains one of the more challenging issues facing the adoption of health information exchange.

Core Technical Standards and Functions

The Interoperability Standards Advisory is published by the ONC to support its earlier nationwide interoperability roadmap. The ONC's guidance on interoperability is fundamental to achieving its learning health system framework through public–private alliances. The 2016 iteration of the standards advisory reflects the ONC's decision to pursue a straightforward approach to advising the industry on interoperability standards and implementation (ONC 2015c). The ONC expects to annually update the advisory based on feedback it receives from the HIT Standards Committee and the public at large. The ONC will collaborate, facilitate, and provide the mechanisms to create the dialog with all stakeholders and will annually publish a new Advisory each December. The ONC's 10 principles of interoperability will be maintained and future advisories will seek to minimize the potential for unnecessary sunk costs while enabling and promoting the entry of new innovative standards. Because of the rapidly changing technological environment and the ever-evolving healthcare delivery system, each advisory reflects the best available standards, practices, and characteristics at a given point in time (ONC 2015c).

The ONC does not expect all stakeholders to agree with its interpretation of "best available" but welcomes feedback and the opportunity for

Figure 15.6.　The privacy and security framework

Nationwide Privacy and Security Framework (based on the FIPPs)

1. **INDIVIDUAL ACCESS:** Individuals should be provided with a simple and timely means to access and obtain their individually identifiable health information in a readable form and format.

2. **CORRECTION:** Individuals should be provided with a timely means to dispute the accuracy or integrity of their individually identifiable health information and to have erroneous information corrected or to have a dispute documented if their requests are denied.

3. **OPENNESS AND TRANSPARENCY:** There should be openness and transparency about policies, procedures and technologies that directly affect individuals and/or their individually identifiable health information.

4. **INDIVIDUAL CHOICE:** Individuals should be provided a reasonable opportunity and capability to make informed decisions about the collection, use and disclosure of their individually identifiable health information.

5. **COLLECTION, USE, AND DISCLOSURE LIMITATION:** Individually identifiable health information should be collected, used, and/or disclosed only to the extent necessary to accomplish a specified purpose(s) and never to discriminate inappropriately.

6. **DATA QUALITY AND INTEGRITY:** Persons and entities should take reasonable steps to ensure that individually identifiable health information is complete, accurate and up-to-date to the extent necessary for the person's or entity's intended purposes and has not been altered or destroyed in an unauthorized manner.

7. **SAFEGUARDS:** Individually identifiable health information should be protected with reasonable administrative, technical and physical safeguards to ensure its confidentiality, integrity and availability and to prevent unauthorized or inappropriate access, use, or disclosure.

8. **ACCOUNTABILITY:** These principles should be implemented and adherence assured, through appropriate monitoring and other means and methods should be in place to report and mitigate non-adherence and breaches.

Source: ONC 2015b, 65.

dialog on criteria that will apply to the widest possible audience. More guidance on the advisory process can be found at HealthIT.gov. The interoperability standards are subject to continuous review. A link to the 2016 Interoperability Standards Advisory can be found at https://www.healthit.gov/standards-advisory.

The Consumer as the Driver of Change in Healthcare Delivery Cultures

The importance of consumers moving from being passive to active healthcare consumers has been well recognized. Patients and their families can bring useful and often critically important knowledge if they are empowered to do so. The wellness programs instituted by payers and supported by employers are tools for educating the consumer about the importance of maintaining their health and being aware of changes in their health status before conditions escalate. Initiatives like the Blue Button provide the public using their services with the ability to access and download their personal health information to a file. The Blue Button provides the user with control over their health information, and it makes it easy to share with anyone they choose without issues of consent management.

Healthcare delivery is not currently consumer centered like the retail, entertainment, and electronics industries; however, patient-centered care is gaining traction as more initiatives for care coordination, new payer models, and patient-directed consent for uses of their health information take hold. Health information exchange is a convergence of standards, trust, and security controls that will provide patients with the information access and usefulness and value that they experience from other business sectors.

HIM in HIE

The creation of a health information exchange is traditionally viewed, inside of a health organization, as just another large-scale information technology implementation. Because of the scarcity of resources that many provider organizations experience, there is frequently the desire to minimize the involvement of employees not directly related to the IT department. The extreme compartmentalization that occurs within healthcare has also made information about health information exchange invisible because of a lack of proximity or access to relevant information. Many who might become involved do not become involved because they may not have knowledge of an internal implementation, they may not want to increase their workloads unnecessarily, or they may think they do not have the necessary knowledge to add value to the project. HIM professionals have a great deal of information to share with the organization. Involvement in a data governance or data normalization committee or workgroup is clearly within the scope of the HIM professional. The HIM professional can add great value in user groups when information of the benefits of HIE workflows should be distributed to multiple departments within the healthcare organization. The HIM professional can serve as a project manager working with clinical units, registration, and IT to create functional workflows for the correct processing of patient opt-in and opt-out decisions. The HIM professional can also add great value as the organizational bridge between the IT team and the clinical teams that will ultimately determine the value of the HIE to the organization by facilitating the integration of the HIE's capabilities into the daily routines of the different clinical domains.

It is important for the professional who wants to become involved to ask for the opportunity to be involved. Like the implementation of EHRs and other business information systems, HIE implementation requires the involvement of many organizational disciplines. Asking to participate is a good place to start. The HIM professionals' knowledge of informatics, codes, business practices, and vocabularies makes them a valuable asset to any project management team.

Check Your Understanding 15.4

Instructions: **Answer the following questions on a separate piece of paper.**

1. What is the purpose of the Meaningful Use program?

2. What is the purpose of the eHealth Exchange?

3. Why has the Office of the National Coordinator published the interoperability roadmap? What purpose does it serve for the healthcare industry?

4. What are some of the levers that can drive the adoption of interoperability standards within a healthcare delivery organization?

5. What role does the consumer have in the future of healthcare delivery?

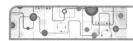 # References

American Health Information Management Association. 2013. *Health Information Management: Concepts, Principles, and Practice*, 4th ed. Chicago: AHIMA.

Centers for Medicare and Medicaid Services. 2014 (Oct. 06). 2013 Definition Stage 1 of Meaningful Use. https://www.cms.gov/Regulations-and-Guidance/Legislation/EHRIncentivePrograms/2013Definition_Stage1_MeaningfulUse.html

Commonwealth Fund. 2012 (Jan.). Early Findings from the Beacon Community Program Evaluation Teams. http://www.commonwealthfund.org/~/media/Files/Publications/Issue%20Brief/2012/Jan/1576_Rein_beacon_communities_phase_1_evaluation_ib_v2.pdf

CommonWell Health Alliance. 2015 (May 22). http://www.commonwellalliance.org/

Corepoint Health. 2009. The Continuity of Care Document. http://www.corepointhealth.com/sites/default/files/whitepapers/continuity-of-care-document-ccd.pdfs

DIRECT Project. 2015 (May 15). Interoperability Portofolio (Archive). http://www.healthit.gov/policy-researchers-implementers/direct-project

Dullabh, P., L. Hovey, and P. Ubri. 2015a (June). Provider Experiences with HIE: Key Findings from a Six-State Review. https://www.healthit.gov/sites/default/files/reports/provider_experiences_with_hie_june_2015.pdf

eHealth Exchange. 2015a (June). The Sequoia Project. file:///C:/Users/PGM/Documents/AHIMA%20Textbook/eHealth-Exchange-Overview-7-23-15.pdf

eHealth Exchange. 2015b. (May 15). What Is eHealth Exchange. http://healthewayinc.org/ehealth-exchange/

Health Level International. 2015a (April). Record Locator Service. https://www.hl7.org/documentcenter/public/wg/servicesbof/Record%20Locator%20Integrated%20Description%20v0.9.doc

Health Level Seven International. 2015b (May 17). CDA Release 2. http://www.hl7.org/implement/standards/product_brief.cfm?product_id=7

Health Level Seven International. 2015c (May 17). HL7 Version 3 Standard: Patient Administration. http://www.hl7.org/implement/standards/product_brief.cfm?product_id=92

Health Record Banking Alliance. 2013 (Jan. 4). A Proposed National Infrastructure for HIE Using

Personally Controlled Records. http://www.healthbanking.org/docs/HRBA%20Architecture%20White%20Paper%20Jan%202013.pdf

Healthcare Information and Management Systems Society. 2015 (April). What is Interoperability. http://www.himss.org/library/interoperability-standards/what-is-interoperability

Healthcare Information and Management Systems Society. 2009 (Nov.). HIE Technical Models. https://www.himss.org/files/HIMSSorg/content/files/2009HIETechnicalModels.pdf

HealtheWay. 2015 (April 22). About HealtheWay. http://healthewayinc.org/

HealthIT.gov. 2015a (May 3). Select Portions of the HITECH Act and Relationship to ONC Work. http://healthit.gov/policy-researchers-implementers/select-portions-hitech-act-and-relationship-onc-work

HealthIT.gov. 2015b (April). Interoperability Portfolio Archive. https://www.healthit.gov/policy-researchers-implementers/interoperability-portfolio

HealthIT.gov. 2014 (May 12). Health Information Exchange (HIE). http://www.healthit.gov/providers-professionals/health-information-exchange/what-hie

Health Resources and Services Administration (HRSA). 2013 (March 3). What is Health Information Exchange? http://www.hrsa.gov/healthit/toolbox/RuralHealthITtoolbox/Collaboration/whatishie.html

Institute for Healthcare Improvement. 2015 (May 22). IHI Triple Aim Initiative. http://www.ihi.org/Engage/Initiatives/TripleAim/Pages/default.aspx

JASON, The MITRE Corporation. 2014. *A Robust Health Data Infrastructure*. Washington DC: AHRQ.

Leavitt, M.O. 2005 (July 20). Secretary, Department of Health and Human Services. http://www.hhs.gov/asl/testify/t050720.html

National eHealth Collaborative. 2015 (Oct. 21). Healthcare IT Index. http://www.healthcareitnews.com/directory/national-ehealth-collaborative-nehc

Office of the National Coordinator for Health Information Technology. 2015a (May 3). 2014 Report to Congress on Health IT Adoption and HIE. http://www.healthit.gov/sites/default/files/rtc_adoption_and_exchange9302014.pdf

Office of the National Coordinator for Health Information Technology. 2015b (March 10). Connecting

Health and Care for the Nation. http://www.healthit.gov/sites/default/files/nationwide-interoperability-roadmap-draft-version-1.0.pdf

Office of the National Coordinator for Health Information Technology. 2015c (May 22). 2015 Interoperability Standards Advisory. http://www.healthit.gov/standards-advisory

Office of the National Coordinator for Health Information Technology. 2015d (Feb. 10). *Federal Health IT Strategic Plan: 2015–2020*. http://www.healthit.gov: http://www.healthit.gov/sites/default/files/federal-healthIT-strategic-plan-2014.pdf

Ricciardi, L. and A. Dole. 2014 (Feb. 24). HealthIT Buzz. http://www.healthit.gov/buzz-blog/consumer/introducing-blue-button-connector/

Shrestha R. and R.C. Gudivada. 2015 (April 16). Beyond the Hype: Achieving True Semantic Interoperability in Healthcare. Seminar Presentation. Chicago, IL: HIMSS Annual Conference.

The Sequoia Project. 2015 (Oct. 22). About The Sequoia Project. http://sequoiaproject.org/about-us/

45 CFR 164.522: Rights to request privacy protection for protected health information. 2011 (Oct. 1).

PART IV
Analytics and Data Use

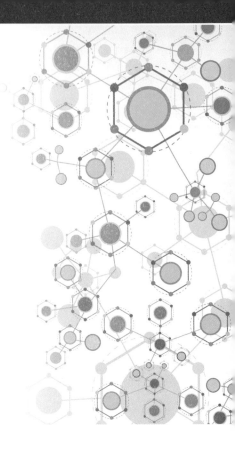

16
Healthcare Statistics

Cindy Glewwe Edgerton, MHA, MEd, RHIA

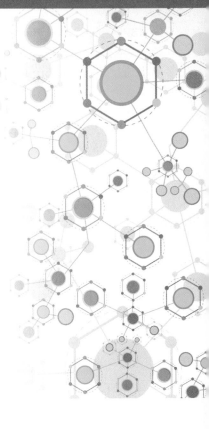

All healthcare organizations depend on accurate, reliable, and robust data to report outcomes and make important decisions. Many of the data used in the decision-making process are presented as statistics in tables, spreadsheets, reports, or graphs. This data should be readily available and usable by healthcare managers and other staff who use data in their job.

Health information management (HIM) professionals are often at the heart of the data collection process that provides data to other departments and administrators who gather that data and organize it into valuable information. Because much of the data collected in the healthcare environment is abstracted from the patient health record, the HIM department plays an important role in the process. HIM professionals ensure that patient data is complete and accurate so that statistics and information used throughout the organization will be reliable.

Statistics can be intimidating. This chapter intends to make healthcare statistics less scary and show how they can be easily calculated to assist with organizational decision making.

Introduction to Healthcare Statistics

Statistics can be defined as "a branch of mathematics concerned with collecting, organizing, summarizing, and analyzing data" (Horton 2012, 2). In the healthcare environment, statistics are usually referring to clinical data, but can also involve data that assists with the operations of a healthcare facility. The US Library of Medicine (2012) describes health statistics as "providing information for understanding, monitoring, improving, and planning the use of resources to improve the lives of people, provide services, and promote their well-being." Healthcare statistics are an important source of information for daily operations and decision making by administrators and supervisors. Even staff use statistics in their daily work at times, to report information and make decisions.

Use of Statistics

In many ways, health statistics help to improve healthcare quality and improve business operations. Statistical data is used by a wide variety of healthcare professionals from administrators, to providers and caregivers, to ancillary departments, department managers, researchers, and many others. With such a wide variety of users come a wide variety of uses and needs for healthcare statistics.

Healthcare administrators and department managers use healthcare statistics to make operations and business decisions on a day-to-day basis. Budgets, capital expenditures, staffing, and strategic plans all involve complex decisions that are supported by data and statistical analysis. Clinical care statistics are also used to report on quality of care issues and patient care outcomes.

An example of using data and healthcare statistics for operational decision-making follows. A hospital chief financial officer (CFO) has been closely monitoring the budget because the hourly wage expense has spiked over the last couple of months. However, admissions and revenue has increased at the same pace. The CFO has been speaking with the departments affected to determine if the increased hourly wage expense is because of a need for more staffing due to increased admissions. For three months, he graphed the three sets of data (hourly wage, admissions, and revenue) to illustrate the relationship between the data in each month as seen in figure 16.1.

This graph in figure 16.1 shows that as admissions increased, so did hourly wage and revenue, at about the same pace. For example, in January as admissions increased 15 percent over budget, revenue increased 21 percent and hourly wages increased 11 percent. February and March also show

Figure 16.1.   Analysis of hourly wages in relation to admissions and revenue

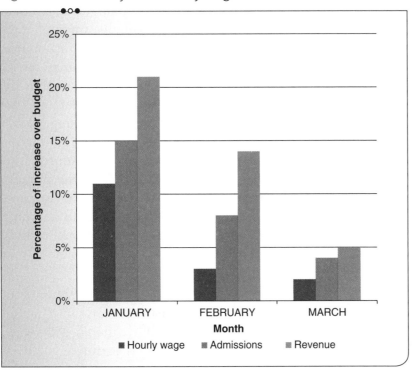

corresponding increases over budget between the three variables that provides evidence that the variables are related. The CFO will continue to monitor this to be sure that a decrease in admissions and revenue is matched with a decrease is hourly wage.

In another example, clinical analysis can be used to make decisions that may impact quality of care. The nursing manager collects infection data each week and monitors hospital-acquired infections by computing statistics that show daily, weekly, monthly, quarterly, and then yearly numbers of these infections. If the statistical information indicates an infection rate higher than the standard, the nursing manager will work to find trends and issues and put processes into place to improve the infection rates. She graphs the data to report to the nurses at their monthly staff meeting and provides the infection control committee with this data that they need for their quarterly meetings.

Ancillary departments such as lab, radiology, and pathology use similar statistical data to make the same types of decisions. They use the data to make decisions about budget and staffing, and they use statistics to monitor quality within their department. All departments have goals and standards, and the statistical data is needed to measure if those standards are met. For instance, if the lab has a process standard that all hematology lab results are placed on the patient's chart within three hours of the blood draw, then statistical data regarding turnaround time must be collected and monitored to determine if the department is meeting that standard.

Researchers use existing data to compute statistics for their research studies or they collect their own data for statistical analysis. These statistics help them determine if their hypothesis is supported by the data or if the results are not what they were hoping for. An immense amount of statistics are used in pharmaceutical studies and studies that are done to find treatments or cures for diseases. Researchers must be experts in data collection and analysis. Public health agencies, such as the Centers for Disease Control (CDC), rely on statistics to inform them of disease trends, survival rates, and other public health concerns. This data is used to direct public health education initiatives and make decisions about which areas will receive the most financial support.

Another example of how statistics are used to improve patient health comes from the CDC's Morbidity and Mortality Weekly Report. It focuses on the value of electronic quality data to public health reporting. "With greater EHR use, more health data are linked with available patient demographic information in a format that is easily retrievable and collected at the point of care" (CDC 2015a). One example provided in the report was on the use of electronic clinical quality measures (eCQM). There were 63,000 healthcare providers who submitted data to the Medicare Electronic Health Records Incentive Program so that the data could be analyzed with the goal of improving blood pressure control for hypertension patients. In a three-year reporting period, it was found that 62 percent of the patients achieved controlled blood pressure. This statistical data is being used to evaluate nationwide progress toward public health improvement goals (CDC 2015a). It is through public health agencies that the nightly news reports how many people had a heart attack last year, for example and how many people were diagnosed with lung cancer.

Sources of Data

In any study of statistics, it is important to consider the sources of the data that are used for statistical analysis. As mentioned earlier, the patient record tends to be the most commonly used source for statistical information in a healthcare organization. The health record is usually a primary data source. This means that it is a "record that was developed by healthcare professionals in the process of providing care" (Horton 2012, 3). It is the first place the data was recorded. Therefore, secondary data sources are created using the information from a primary data source. Some examples of secondary data sources are indices, registries, and reports created within the healthcare organization to manage data and assist with operations and decision making. To create secondary data sources, data and information is abstracted from the primary data source. This means that the data is pulled from the primary data source and placed in a database or in a special form used to collect data. Refer to chapter 6 for more detail on using secondary data for indices and registries.

Descriptive vs. Inferential Statistics

When conducting statistical analysis, it is important to understand the difference between the two classifications of descriptive statistics and inferential statistics. Descriptive statistics are meant to *describe* a large amount of data by illustrating the data with charts, graphs, and tables in a way that the data is summarized and organized. Descriptive statistics are not used to draw conclusions about the population that the data is describing. On the other hand, inferential statistics are used to test a hypothesis and draw conclusions about the population. The conclusions are used to *infer* that the conclusions about the sample are reflective of the whole population from which the sample was taken. Refer to chapters 17 and 19 for more detail on descriptive and inferential statistics.

Review of Basic Mathematical Calculations

Before anyone can begin to learn to use statistical formulas or understand statistical analysis, knowledge and review of some basic mathematical calculations is important. Mathematical calculations are the basis for many statistical formulas.

Ratio

A ratio is a comparison of two numbers of the same type of data. The ratio is spoken as "a to b" but is usually written as a:b. For instance, an analysis of adult to pediatric patients at a local clinic finds that the ratio is five adult patients for every two pediatric patients. The ratio would be spoken as "five to two" and would be written as 5:2.

For small numbers in a population or set of data, the ratio can be seen without any mathematical calculation, but for large numbers there is a simple division equation, shown in the following formula, to ensure the ratio is stated in the lowest numbers possible. For example, a clinic has 5,000 adult patients and 2,000 pediatric patients. One way to show the ratio would be 5,000:2,000, however that is cumbersome. In this case, both numbers are divisible by 1,000 as shown in the formula:

$$\text{Ratio} = \frac{x}{y} = \frac{5000}{2000} = \frac{5000/1000 = 5}{2000/1000 = 2}$$

The ratio is $5 : 2$

Rate

A **rate** is a type of ratio where the two numbers are representing different things. For example, a rate may compare the number of patients and the number of days in a time period, or the number of patients and the number of patients who have a certain disease. Rates are usually expressed as a percentage. For this reason, most rates should include the percent (%) sign after the value.

To calculate a rate, there is a formula that is important to remember. Once this formula is known, any type of rate can be easily calculated. The general rate formula is

$$\frac{\text{The number of times something happened}}{\text{The number of times it could have happened}} \times 100$$

Multiplying the rate by 100 puts the decimal point in the right place for a percentage. It means the difference between 0.305 percent (forgetting to multiply by 100) and 30.5 percent. This is a critical difference so it is a step that must not be skipped.

Most often the smaller number will be divided by the larger number. For example, a health information manager wants to know the productivity rate of the coders in the HIM department this week. There were 239 discharges this week, so potentially, the coders could have coded all 239 discharged charts.

However, in reality they coded 192 of the charts. To calculate the rate, the HIM manager divides 192 (the number of times something happened) by 239 (the number of times something could have happened) and multiplies it by 100, for a rate of 80.33 percent:

$$\frac{192 \text{ (Number of discharges coded this week)}}{239 \text{ (Total number of discharges this week)}} \times 100 = 80.33\%$$

When reporting rates in healthcare, it is important not to round to less than two decimal places. In reporting healthcare statistics, it is often meaningful to show more detail than less. In quality or disease reporting, 5.09, 5.37, and 5.49 can signify important differences even though they could all be rounded down to 5. For instance, if these were lab results, the small differences could mean the difference between a normal and abnormal level.

Average

The next important calculation to understand is the average. This is also referred to as the arithmetic average, or the arithmetic mean. Arithmetic mean is the most common type of average. To calculate the **arithmetic mean**, the sum of all of the numbers in a group of data is divided by the number of items in that group of data. For example, there may be a need to know the average age of the patients who attended a small diabetes seminar at the clinic. Ten patients attended:

- *Step 1*: Add all of the ages of the attendees. 49 + 62 + 68 + 54 + 42 + 31 + 62 + 48 + 38 + 36 = 490
- *Step 2*: Divide the total by the number of items in the data. 490/10 = 49

The average age of attendees at the diabetes seminar is 49.

Although the arithmetic mean is the most commonly reported type of average (Salkind 2011), there are two other types of average—median and mode. The **median** is the middle number in a set of scores, or the midpoint in a list of numbers or data. Values are listed in order and then the middle number is located and that is the median. It is used instead of the mean when there is an extreme low or high score (outliers) that would skew the results in a way that they would not be valid or realistic (Salkind 2011). To calculate median in the previous example:

1. Place the list of numbers in the set of data into numerical order.

   The set of data: 49, 62, 68, 54, 42, 31, 62, 48, 38, 36

   Listed in numerical order: 31, 36, 38, 42, 48, 49, 54, 62, 62, 68

2. Choose the number in the middle of the list:

   31, 36, 38, 42, **48**, 49, 54, 62, 62, 68

3. The median in this set of data is 48. If there is an even number of values in the data then two numbers will be in the middle. If this is the case, the mean of those two numbers will need to be calculated and that will be the median.

The **mode** is calculated by finding which number in a set of data occurs most often. To calculate the mode:

1. List the numbers in the set of data into numerical order.

The set of data: 5, 7, 9, 8, 9, 5, 6, 4, 2, 2, 3, 2, 5, 9, 8, 5, 5, 7, 5, 6, 5

Listed in numerical order: 2, 2, 2, 3, 4, 5, 5, 5, 5, 5, 5, 5, 6, 6, 7, 7, 8, 8, 9, 9, 9

2. Count how many times each number occurs in the list:

   2–3

   3–1

   4–1

   5–**6**

   6–2

   7–2

   8–2

   9–3

3. The value of 5 occurs more times than any other of the values so 5 is the mode.

The mode is used to find the most common or frequent value. For example, the mode may be used to find the most frequent MS-DRG for patients admitted in the month of December.

Check Your Understanding 16.1

Instructions: **Answer the following questions on a separate piece of paper.**

1. If there are 10 family practice physicians at Center Clinic and two pediatricians, what is the ratio of family practice physicians to pediatricians?

2. Midwest Hospital admitted 780 patients for cancer diagnosis procedures in 2015. Of those patients, 430 were diagnosed with cancer. What is the rate of cancer diagnosis for this group of admissions?

3. What is the average (mean) age for the following group of OB/GYN patients?

Admission	Discharge	Department	Patient age
6/15/15	6/16/15	OB/GYN	26
6/15/15	6/17/15	OB/GYN	32
6/15/15	6/17/15	OB/GYN	29
6/16/15	6/20/15	OB/GYN	36
6/17/15	6/18/15	OB/GYN	28
6/17/15	6/20/15	OB/GYN	40
6/18/15	6/20/15	OB/GYN	32

4. For the same group of patients in this table, what is the median of the patient ages?

5. For the same group of patients in this table, what is the mode of the patient ages?

Terminology Related to Healthcare Statistics

Studying any topic requires commitment to learning the terminology that is common to the topic. The study of statistics is no different. There are many statistical terms that are important for health information management professionals to be familiar with in the study of healthcare statistics. HIM professionals may assist with the calculations of these types of statistics or the collection and reporting of the data. These are also important statistical terms that affect coding accuracy and the understanding of reimbursement issues.

- **Hospital inpatient**: A patient who is "provided with room, board, and continuous general nursing service in an area of an acute-care facility where patients generally stay at least overnight" (HHS HIS n.d.).
- **Hospital outpatient**: A hospital patient who receives services in one or more of the hospital's facilities when he or she is not currently an inpatient or home care patient. An outpatient may be classified as either an emergency outpatient or a clinic outpatient.
  - An emergency outpatient is admitted to the emergency department of a hospital for diagnosis and treatment of a condition that requires immediate medical, dental, or other emergency services.
  - A clinic outpatient is admitted to a clinical service of the clinic or hospital for diagnosis and treatment on an ambulatory basis.
- **Hospital newborn inpatient**: A patient born in the hospital at the beginning of the current patient hospitalization.
  - Newborns are usually counted separately because their care is so different from that of other inpatients.
  - Infants born on the way to the hospital or at home are considered hospital inpatients, not hospital newborn patients.
- **Inpatient admission**: An acute-care facility's formal acceptance of a patient who is to be provided with room, board, and continuous nursing service in an area of the facility where patients generally stay overnight.
- **Inpatient discharge**: The termination of hospitalization through the formal release of an inpatient by the hospital.
  - The term includes patients who are discharged alive (by physician's order), who are discharged against medical advice (AMA), or who died while hospitalized.
  - Unless otherwise indicated, inpatient discharges include deaths.
- **Inpatient service day**: The unit of measure denoting the services received by one inpatient in one 24-hour period. It is often referred to in the shortened version of patient day.
- **Inpatient census**: Indicates the number of patients present in the healthcare facility at a particular point in time (AHIMA 2012).

Statistics Related to Volume of Service and Utilization

An important factor in managing healthcare services is monitoring the volume of service, regardless of the type of facility. In other words, monitoring how many patients are served in a specific period of time and the type of services each patient receives. It is important for administrators to keep a constant watch on numbers of patients, numbers and types of services provided, and utilization of resources. The data collected that is related to volume of service is critical to making daily operational decisions that affect staffing and budgeting, inventory of supplies, space needs, and technology needs.

Inpatient Census

Inpatient census is an important volume measure tracked in the hospital environment. The inpatient census indicates the number of patients present in the healthcare facility at a particular point in time. Before hospitals had robust automated systems that can track the status of inpatients, the census reporting was a manual process. Today, it is an automated process due to the fact that the movement of patients from nursing unit to nursing unit, or from inpatient status to discharged, is entered into the computer and the software can be used to pull census data at any given time.

Because there is continuous activity during the course of any given day, with patients being discharged, new patients being admitted, and patients transferring to a different unit within the hospital, the census data can be different throughout the day. For instance, at 9:00 a.m. six patients are discharged; but at the same time two patients are admitted. Between 9:15 and 10:00 a.m. three more patients are admitted. This would make the census at 9:00 a.m. different than census data at 10:00 a.m., and this will change throughout the day. For this reason, each hospital must decide on a consistent time to take the census and use that time every day. This ensures consistent and valid data. Midnight is a common census taking time.

Daily Inpatient Census

The daily inpatient census is the technical name for the census data reported at midnight or other official census taking time. The daily inpatient census will include all patients present as inpatients at 12:00 midnight, plus any patients admitted and discharged during the same day. These patients are referred to as **A&D**, which symbolizes patients admitted and discharged on the same day. These patients are not present at midnight for the census taking time, but they must still be counted because they were classified as an inpatient at some point during that day. For example, a patient is admitted through the emergency room at 6:49 p.m. on June

15 but the patient dies at 9:22 p.m. on the same day. Because this patient was an inpatient and received inpatient services, they must be counted in the daily inpatient census. Forgetting to include the A&D patients in the census would not accurately reflect service volume. The daily inpatient census should reflect all of the patients treated as inpatients during the 24-hour period. In table 16.1, a daily census report is illustrated. Notice that there is a separate column for newborn (NB) reporting as well as a column labeled **A&C**. A&C stands for adults and children. In a daily census, newborns are reported separately because they require a different type and volume of service and care compared to inpatient adults and children.

Also note that the daily census indicates numbers transferred in and transferred out. When case managers and physicians talk about transferring a patient at discharge, they are usually discussing a transfer to another facility; in the case of the daily census, transfers are simply patients transferring from one nursing unit in the hospital to another, or intrahospital transfers. For instance, an 89-year-old patient was admitted to the intensive care unit after suffering a heart attack, but three days later was moved out of the ICU to the cardiac care unit. This patient has been transferred out of the ICU and transferred in to the cardiac care unit. In this 24-hour period this would count as one transfer out and one transfer in. In the daily census, the totals for transferred in and transferred out should be equal. Any transfer to another facility would

Table 16.1. Daily census

LINE #		Newborns	A&C
1	Remaining last report	11	159
2	Admitted	5	42
3	Transferred in	0	8
4	**Total (sum of lines 1, 2, 3)**	16	209
5	Transferred out	0	8
6	Discharged	8	49
7	Died	0	2
8	**Total (sum of lines 5, 6, 7)**	8	59
9	**Remaining midnight (Line 4 – Line 8 =)**	8	**150**

be a discharge and recorded in the daily census as such.

Inpatient Service Days

A unit of measure that reflects the services received by one inpatient during a 24-hour period is called an inpatient service day (IPSD) (Horton 2012). An IPSD can be thought of as one for each patient treated. Therefore, the daily inpatient census will be equal to the number of inpatient service days for that day. Inpatient service days is an important measure of volume of services provided by the facility. IPSDs will be reported on a daily, weekly, monthly, quarterly, and annual basis to track volume of service that has a direct correlation to amount of revenue. Chief financial officers will be very interested in inpatient service day reports as the reports will be one reflection of the facility's financial condition because IPSDs are included in calculations determining cost per patient and revenue totals per patient.

Census Calculation

As seen in table 16.1, calculating the daily census consists of counting the patients who remained at the previous midnight, adding the admissions for the next 24-hour period, and subtracting the discharges in that same period. This is typically automated, and a report similar to table 16.1 could be generated daily if needed. Another important calculation in daily census reporting is the average daily census. The **average daily census** is the average number of inpatients treated during a given period of time (Horton 2012). The formula for calculating the average daily census is:

$$\text{Average daily census} = \frac{\text{Total number of inpatient service days for a given period}}{\text{Total number of days in the period}}$$

Just as newborns (NBs) and adults and children (A&C) are reported separately on the daily census report, they can be reported separately for the average daily census as well. This helps managers and administrators with planning for the different

levels of services and budgeting for the newborn unit separately from other nursing units. The formula for calculating the average daily census for adults and children is:

$$\text{Average daily census for A \& Cs} = \frac{\text{Total number of inpatient service days for A \& Cs for a given period}}{\text{Total number of days in the period}}$$

The formula for calculating the average daily census for newborns is:

$$\text{Average daily census for NBs} = \frac{\text{Total number of inpatient service days for NBs for a given period}}{\text{Total number of days in the period}}$$

Using Census Reports

In addition to the daily census report shown in table 16.1, other census reports such as monthly, quarterly, and annual census reports are created to give managers and administrators a bigger picture of the census activity. While daily and monthly census reports are used to react to current budget needs, quarterly and annual reports are used for future staffing and budgeting considerations. The census data is also used in strategic planning when deciding on areas for expansion or development. The following examples illustrate real-life scenarios where census data is used on a daily basis.

Hospital Census in Practice Liz Taylor, MS, RHIT, from Sharon Hospital in Sharon, CT, explains that

> As part of the daily organizational safety huddle, we review the patient census statistics to determine our patient volume for the day, what departments may be overburdened or at full capacity as well as address any immediate or urgent staffing and/or resource needs. This discussion also provides an opportunity for other departments and ancillary services to know and be prepared

for downstream effects of an overburdened or full capacity unit. Quick discussions and requests for assistance are held, opportunities to address or elicit assistance for other resources or needs for a particular service or assessments/resources can be noted and more detailed discussions held as appropriate outside of the huddle.

The patient statistics discussion at the huddle alerts other departments and services of volume, resources, critical patients, needs for staffing and/or opportunities for service and/or service recovery. Patient engagement and patient satisfaction is known to be an outgrowth (at times) of patient census (high volume, staffing shortages, resources) and helps the organization to recognize such trends and take appropriate action. Patient census statistics and patient engagement (satisfaction) is crucial to the future of value based purchasing initiatives for healthcare organizations. First and foremost, the patient census statistics discussion at the daily morning huddle is a safety first initiative and brings patient safety to the forefront of every discussion every day. (Taylor 2015)

This is an example of how the census is used on a daily basis by various departments in a hospital. It shows how the census data is used to make both operational and patient care decisions. This hospital's daily census huddle equips staff with data and knowledge from which decisions can be made throughout the day.

The Important Use of a Daily Census Report   Jen Hoefs, registration–scheduling and communications supervisor at Burnett Medical Center, a Critical Access Hospital in Grantsburg, WI, explains how a daily census report is used in various areas of the hospital:

The utilization of the daily census report is a vital component of patient case management by key staff members in the healthcare setting. It serves as an overall snapshot of how many patients are in the hospital at a given

moment in time and under what type they have been registered (inpatient, observation, swing bed).

The census report is generated by a designated registration staff member each morning after ensuring that any and all overnight registrations to an inpatient and/or observation status have been completed. This report is verified against a hard copy of the current patients on the acute floor that was created by the acute station health unit coordinator. This report is then distributed to key staff members involved in the patients' care/management.

Listed are a few examples of how some of these key staff members utilize and rely on this report.

Utilization review (UR) coordinator: This staff member utilizes the report to keep track of the number of days patients have been in the hospital, to which doctor they have been admitted and what type of patient status they fall under; for example, inpatient medical, inpatient respite, inpatient hospice, inpatient surgery, observation, or OB observation. The UR coordinator also uses this to prep for the daily patient planning meeting to ensure that the length of stay is correct and in line with the patient's insurance guidelines for that specific diagnosis and treatment currently taking place.

Dietitian/dietary department: The dietary department uses this report to determine how many meals they will need to prepare while working closely with the dietitian on staff to ensure the patients' specific diet requirements are being met. The dietitian uses this report to review the patients' charts in regard to their diets that are ordered by the providers; for example, a diabetic diet, gluten-free diet, low sodium diet, cardiac diet, or a liquid diet.

Business office manager: This staff member uses this report to track who is placed in a bed currently and under what patient type class they fall; for example, inpatient, observation, or swing bed. They use this report to prepare for the daily patient care planning meeting looking at it from the facility's financial perspective to ensure that the proper steps are being completed to bill the patients' insurance appropriately, accurately, and promptly. This staff member works closely with the UR coordinator.

Social services: These staff members utilize this report to visit with the patients and determine and assist the patient in arranging and discussing any services that may be needed upon discharge; for example, a nursing home placement, in-house assistance once returning to home, questions related to living wills and advanced directives for healthcare, and medical power of attorney.

Infection control: This staff member uses this report to review patient charts to determine if appropriate infection control precautions are in place, being followed, and if there are any cases of infection that need to be reported.

Ancillary department (Radiology, Pharmacy, and Physical/Occupational Therapy): These departments use this report as a case management tool in determining the patient's name, room number, patient class status, and to verify if any of the current orders are for procedures, therapies, or medications for patients who are currently in-house. (Hoefs 2015)

This is another example of how patient census is used by various departments to make crucial decisions throughout the day. It is clear that census data is much more than numbers that are posted in the system daily. This data is tracked, analyzed, used, and discussed within healthcare teams on a daily basis and is a very important statistic.

Occupancy Data

Along with inpatient census, another important measure of volume of service and utilization is inpatient bed occupancy. Bed occupancy is monitored and occupancy rates are used for decisions about staffing, materials, and other budget items. Occupancy rate, or percentage of occupancy, is an important indicator of the hospital's financial picture. The **inpatient bed occupancy rate** is the percentage of official beds occupied by hospital inpatients for a given period of time. Hospitals strive for a high occupancy rate because that usually equates with higher revenues.

Bed Count

In order to calculate occupancy rate, the bed count must also be known; that is, "for a bed to be included in the official count, it must be set up, staffed, equipped, and available for patient care" (Horton 2012, 44). Bed count is one of the ways a hospital is classified. For example, it is likely that bed count will be indicated in the overview of the hospital on a hospital website. For instance:

> *Valley Hospital is a 129-bed acute-care hospital with a 72-bed skilled care nursing home, and a 156-bed assisted living facility. Valley Hospital also operates three outpatient multispecialty clinics within the Valley community.*

There are also times when a hospital may need to set up temporary beds, especially at the time of a disaster or an epidemic when the need for care in the community is greater than the normal number of beds that exist. The hospital is allowed by their licensing body to set up beds as needed. In these unusual cases, the temporary beds do not count as part of the official bed count.

Calculating Inpatient Bed Occupancy Rate

When calculating inpatient bed occupancy rate, the numerator is the total number of inpatient service days for the given period and the denominator is the total possible inpatient service days for the given period. The maximum number of inpatient service days indicates that every available bed in the hospital is occupied every single day (Horton 2012, 46). The occupancy rate compares the number of patients treated daily to the number of patients who could have been treated. The formula for calculating the inpatient bed occupancy rate is:

$$
\begin{aligned}
&\text{Inpatient bed occupancy} = \\
&\frac{\text{Total number of inpatient}}{\text{Total number of inpatient bed}} \times 100 \\
&\text{count for the same period}
\end{aligned}
$$

For example, if 325 patients occupied 370 beds on July 25, the inpatient bed occupancy rate would be 87.8 percent (325/370 × 100). If the rate were for more than one day, the number of days would have to be factored in, so the number of beds would be multiplied by the number of days in the given time period. For instance, if the occupancy rate was being calculated for a week, the number of beds would be multiplied by seven for the seven days in the week. If the same hospital wanted to measure occupancy rate for the week of July 25, 370 (number of beds) would be multiplied by 7 (number of days in the week). Therefore, there are a possible 2,590 inpatient service days in a week at this hospital. In this given week, there were 2,190 inpatient service days. To calculate the occupancy rate, the equation would look like this: ([2,190/{370 × 7}] × 100). The occupancy rate at this hospital for the week of July 25 would be 84.55 percent.

It is possible that a hospital could report an occupancy rate of greater than 100 percent. When a hospital is full and uses temporary beds, the temporary beds are not added to the denominator when calculating occupancy rate. If the inpatient bed count at the hospital is 290 and 5 temporary beds are used for a certain time period, the total number of inpatient bed count is still 290. For example, on October 2, Community Hospital has 279 patients occupying their 290 inpatient beds. But a tragic train derailment occurs in the afternoon and 16 patients are rushed to the hospital and temporary beds are set up to serve all of the patients. The inpatient service days for October 2 is 295 (279 + 16). The occupancy rate for the day would be calculated as 295/290 × 100, which equals 101 percent. If an occupancy rate is greater than 100 percent, it can be concluded that all of the hospital beds are occupied with the addition of temporary beds.

Hospital Bed Turnover

Another important measure of volume of service and utilization at a hospital is the bed turnover rate. This measure indicates how many times each bed was occupied in a given period. This information is a statistic that helps administrators make decisions about budgeting and staffing, as well as strategic planning. For instance, if the hospital has a high turnover rate, this means that it experiences many short stays. Administrators know that every time a patient leaves, the room and bed must be cleaned and sterilized at a higher level than the daily cleaning that happens when a patient remains in the room. This means that high turnover requires a higher level of cleaning staff and this will increase the budget for housekeeping. High turnover also increases the workload for case managers, nurses, and many other staff throughout the hospital. The formula for the bed turnover rate is:

$$
\begin{aligned}
&\text{Bed turnover rate} = \\
&\frac{\text{Number of discharges for the time period}}{\text{The bed count for the time period}}
\end{aligned}
$$

For example, City Hospital had 1,899 discharges and deaths for the month of July. The bed count is 420. Therefore, the bed turnover rate is 4.5 percent (1,899/420). This illustrates that, on average, each bed had 4.5 patients occupying the bed during the month of July.

Length of Stay

Length of stay (LOS) is an important measure of utilization and volume of service at any hospital. When a patient is discharged, the length of stay is indicated. Length of stay is the number of days a patient occupied a hospital bed. An important thing to remember when counting length of stay is that the day of discharge is not counted. If patient A was admitted on August 4 and discharged on August 7, his or her length of stay is three days. To calculate this using a mathematical equation, the day of admission is subtracted from the day of discharge. For patient A, this would be calculated as (7 − 4 = 3). There is an extra step if the patient is discharged in a different month than the admission. "One way to calculate the LOS in this case is to subtract the date the patient was admitted and then add the total number of hospitalized days for the month in which the patient was discharged" (Horton 2012, 58). For example, the LOS for a patient admitted on July 28 and discharged on August 4 is seven days: ([July 31 – July 28 = 3 days] + [August 1 – August 4 = 4 days]), 3+4 = 7.

In today's healthcare environment, it is common for a patient to be admitted and discharged on the same day. In this case, regardless of how many hours they were an inpatient, the LOS is one day. Remember, the day of discharge is not counted when figuring length of stay, so a patient who is admitted one day and discharged the next is also counted as a LOS of one day. The LOS for a patient who is admitted on November 5 at 6:30 a.m. and discharged on November 5 at 4:50 p.m. is one day. The LOS for a patient who is admitted on November 5 at 6:30 a.m. and discharged on November 6 at 11:00 a.m. is also one day.

In a given period of time, the LOS for all of the patients is added up for a total length of stay. For example, if the chief of staff would like to know the total length of stay for the intensive care unit (ICU) for July 15. Table 16.2 may be assembled as an illustration of this total length of stay.

This total length of stay indicates the number of days care was provided to these patients who were either discharged or died. It is typical that LOS will be calculated for each department or nursing unit, and then for the hospital as a whole.

Administration may also want to know the average length of stay (ALOS) for each day,

Table 16.2.   Total length of stay

Patient	LOS
1	2
2	7
3	5
4	9
5	6
6	3
Total LOS	32

each week, each month, each quarter, and then the annual LOS (ALOS). ALOS is calculated from the total LOS data collected each day. The total LOS is divided by the number of patients discharged in the same time period. Using table 16.2, the average length of stay for the six patients discharged from the ICU on July 15 is 5.33 (32/6). The general formula for calculating ALOS is:

$$\text{Average length of stay} = \frac{\text{Total length of stay for a given period}}{\text{Total number of discharges, including deaths, for the same period}}$$

Along with the measures discussed earlier, the ALOS for adults and children (A&C) would be reported separately from the newborn ALOS.

Table 16.3 is an example of a summary report that illustrates all of the statistics discussed in this section. The HIM department may be responsible for compiling this type of report periodically for meetings and planning sessions.

Table 16.3.   Statistical summary, Community Hospital, period ending July 20XX

Admissions	July 20XX		Year-to-Date 20XX	
	Actual	Budget	Actual	Budget
Medical	728	769	5,075	5,082
Surgical	578	583	3,964	3,964
OB/GYN	402	440	2,839	3,027
Psychiatry	113	99	818	711
Physical medicine and rehab	48	57	380	384
Other adult	191	178	1,209	1,212

Table 16.3.   *Continued.*

Admissions	July 20XX		Year-to-Date 20XX	
	Actual	**Budget**	**Actual**	**Budget**
Total adult	2,060	2,126	14,285	14,380
Newborn	294	312	2,143	2,195
Total admissions	2,354	2,438	16,428	16,575

Average length of stay	July 20XX		Year-to-Date 20XX	
	Actual	**Budget**	**Actual**	**Budget**
Medical	6.1	6.4	6.0	6.1
Surgical	7.0	7.2	7.7	7.7
OB/GYN	2.9	3.2	3.5	3.1
Psychiatry	10.8	11.6	10.4	11.6
Physical medicine and rehab	27.5	23.0	28.1	24.3
Other adult	3.6	3.9	4.0	4.1
Total adult	6.3	6.4	6.7	6.5
Newborn	5.6	5.0	5.6	5.0
Total ALOS	6.2	6.3	6.5	6.3

Patient days	July 20XX		Year-to-Date 20XX	
	Actual	**Budget**	**Actual**	**Budget**
Medical	4,436	4,915	30,654	30,762
Surgical	4,036	4,215	30,381	30,331
OB/GYN	1,170	1,417	10,051	9,442
Psychiatry	1,223	1,144	8,524	8,242
Physical medicine and rehab	1,318	1,310	10,672	9,338
Other adult	688	699	4,858	4,921
Total adult	12,871	13,700	95,140	93,036
Newborn	1,633	1,552	12,015	10,963
Total patient days	14,504	15,252	107,155	103,999

Other key statistics	July 20XX		Year-to-Date 20XX	
	Actual	**Budget**	**Actual**	**Budget**
Average daily census	485	492	498	486
Average beds available	677	660	677	660
Clinic visits	21,621	18,975	144,271	136,513
Emergency visits	3,822	3,688	26,262	25,604
Inpatient surgery patients	657	583	4,546	4,093
Outpatient surgery patients	603	554	4,457	3,987

Source: Horton 2013, 291.

Check Your Understanding 16.2

Instructions: **Answer the following questions on a separate piece of paper.**

1. Match the term to the correct definition:

_____ A patient who is provided with room, board, and continuous general nursing service in an area of an acute-care facility where patients generally stay at least overnight

    A. Inpatient service day

    B. Hospital newborn inpatient

    C. Hospital inpatient

_____ A hospital patient who receives services in one or more of the hospital's facilities when he or she is not currently an inpatient or home care patient.

_____ A patient born in the hospital at the beginning of the current patient hospitalization

_____ An acute-care facility's formal acceptance of a patient who is to be provided with room, board, and continuous nursing service in an area of the facility where patients generally stay overnight

_____ The termination of hospitalization through the formal release of an inpatient by the hospital

_____ The unit of measure denoting the services received by one inpatient in one 24-hour period; it is often referred to in the shortened version of patient day

_____ Indicates the number of patients present in the healthcare facility at a particular point in time

D. Inpatient census

E. Hospital outpatient

F. Inpatient admission

G. Inpatient discharge

2. What is the average daily census for A&C for January if the total inpatient service days was 4,792?

3. What is the daily census for July 16 if the census at midnight for July 15 was 239, there were 59 discharges, 67 admissions, and 24 A&Ds?

4. For the following table, calculate length of stay for each patient.

	Admission	Discharge	Length of stay
Patient A	June 5	June 8	
Patient B	June 6	June 6	
Patient C	June 11	June 16	
Patient D	June 29	July 3	
Patient E	June 15	June 15	
Patient F	June 21	June 28	
Patient G	June 26	July 2	

5. For the following table of patient data, calculate the average length of stay statistics.

Date	Number of patients discharged	Discharge days	Average length of stay
June 2	16	89	
June 3	22	119	
June 4	12	54	
June 5	19	105	
June 6	15	45	
June 7	24	118	
June 8	18	68	

Statistics Related to Clinical Services and Patient Care

Along with the many calculations this chapter has introduced to measure utilization and volume of service, there are many other important statistical calculations in the healthcare environment that indicate levels of clinical services and patient care. These statistics often relate to quality of patient care, or the severity of illness of each facility's patient demographics. Each hospital reports morbidity and mortality rates for all patients discharged within a certain time period. The New York Department of Health defines *morbidity* as another word for illness and *mortality* as another word for death (New York State Department of Health 1999). This data helps to identify opportunities for improvement, trends, and any issues that may need immediate attention. These types of statistics can be reported as a whole for the hospital, but can also be broken down by department, nursing unit, or individual physician to determine if any cases of excellence or any issues are isolated to just one certain area, or if they are hospitalwide.

Death Rates

An important measure of quality of care and patient demographic for each hospital is the **hospital death rate**. This is calculated using the number of patients discharged from the hospital (both alive and dead) during a specific time period. As discussed earlier, deaths are always counted as discharges because it is one way to end a patient's hospitalization. Following are the types of death rates that may be calculated for each hospital.

Gross Death Rate

The **gross death rate** is the number of all hospital discharges compared to the number of deaths from that same group of patients. It indicates the proportion of deaths, or mortality, that the hospital experiences in a given time period. The gross death rate is calculated by dividing the total number of

deaths occurring in a given time period by the total number of discharges, including deaths, for the same time period. The formula for calculating the gross death rate is:

$$\text{Gross death rate} = \frac{\substack{\text{Total number of inpatient deaths} \\ \text{(including NBs) for a given period}}}{\substack{\text{Total number of discharges, including} \\ \text{A \& C and NB deaths, for the same} \\ \text{time period}}} \times 100$$

For example, Midwest Hospital reported 19 deaths (both A&C and NB) during the month of August. There were 689 total discharges, including deaths. The gross death rate is 2.75 percent ([19/689] × 100).

Net Death Rate

The **net death rate** is a death rate that is adjusted so that certain deaths are not counted against the hospital. The net death rate does not include any deaths that occurred within 48 hours of the patient's admission to the hospital. This is an important measure because 48 hours is not usually enough time to improve the patient's health. Especially if the patient was admitted to the hospital gravely ill and died within 48 hours, it is assumed that the care providers did all that they could but the patient was too ill upon admission. There was just not enough time to treat the patient to result in a positive outcome. The formula for calculating the net death rate is:

$$\text{Net death rate} = \frac{\substack{\text{Total number of inpatient deaths} \\ \text{(including NBs) minus deaths} \\ < 48 \text{ hours of admission for a} \\ \text{given period of time}}}{\substack{\text{Total number of discharges} \\ \text{(including NBs) minus deaths} \\ < 48 \text{ hours for the same period}}} \times 100$$

Using the data from the previous example of gross death rate, Midwest Hospital reported 19 deaths (both A&C and NB) during the month of August. Six of those were within 48 hours of admission. There were 689 total discharges. Therefore, the net death rate is 1.9 percent ([{19 − 6} / {689 − 6}] × 100). It is important to report the net death rate because it will usually be a lower death rate and may be a more accurate indicator of quality care.

Newborn Death Rate

Although newborn deaths are included in a hospital's gross death rate and net death rate calculations, it can also be valuable to calculate a newborn death rate separately. This measure can give important information about mortality and morbidity of newborns at each individual hospital. The number of newborns at a hospital include only those born alive at the hospital. The **newborn death rate** is the number of newborns who died in comparison to the total number of newborns discharged, alive and dead. In order to be counted as a newborn death, the newborn must have been delivered alive (Horton 2012). A stillborn infant is not counted in any death rate statistics, because by definition of a stillborn, the infant was not born alive. The formula for calculating the newborn death rate is:

$$\text{Newborn death rate} = \frac{\substack{\text{Total number of NB deaths for} \\ \text{a given period}}}{\substack{\text{Total number of NB discharges} \\ \text{(including deaths) for the same period}}} \times 100$$

For example, Midwest Hospital reported three newborn deaths during the month of August. There were 69 newborn discharges (including these three deaths). The newborn death rate is 4.34 percent ([3/69] × 100).

Fetal Death Rate

A fetal death is the healthcare terminology for what is better known as a stillborn infant. A **fetal death** is the death of an infant while still a fetus, before the mother gives birth, regardless of the length of the pregnancy. Stillborn infants are not considered to be either admitted or discharged from the hospital because they were never a live infant. A fetal death is reported when the physician determines that the fetus no longer has a heartbeat or shows any other evidence of life.

The World Health Organization (WHO) recommends that fetal deaths be classified as early, intermediate, and late (Barfield 2011). Statistics are calculated using this classification system. (See table 16.4.) This is also important information during the coding process because the code choices are based on the same classification system. Hospitals and public health agencies calculate fetal death rates for reporting purposes. To calculate the **fetal death rate**, divide the total number of intermediate and late fetal deaths for the period by the total number of live births and intermediate and late fetal deaths for the same period. Early fetal deaths are not included in the fetal death rate. The formula for calculating the fetal death rate is:

$$\text{Fetal death rate} = \frac{\substack{\text{Total number of intermediate and late} \\ \text{fetal deaths for a given period}}}{\substack{\text{Total number of live births plus total} \\ \text{number of intermediate and late fetal} \\ \text{deaths for the same period}}} \times 100$$

For example, Midwest Hospital reported 329 live births and 8 intermediate and 2 late fetal deaths during the month of August. The fetal death rate is 2.94 percent ([8 + 2/{329 + 8 + 2}] × 100).

Table 16.4. Classification of fetal deaths

Term classification	Gestation	Group classification
Early fetal deaths	Less than 20 completed weeks of gestation	Group I
Intermediate fetal deaths	20 completed weeks of gestations but less than 28	Group II
Late fetal deaths	28 completed weeks of gestation and over	Group III
Fetal deaths with gestation not stated	Presumed 20 weeks or more	Group IV

Source: CDC n.d.

Maternal Death Rate

Another specific area of death rates that hospital administrators and managers find important to track is the maternal death rate. A **maternal death** is the death of any woman from any cause related to, or aggravated by, pregnancy or its management, regardless of the duration of the pregnancy or the site of the death. Maternal deaths that are not related to the pregnancy, such as a car accident, are not counted in the maternal death rate.

Maternal deaths are referred to as either direct or indirect. A direct maternal death is the death of a woman resulting from obstetrical (OB) complications of the pregnancy state, labor, or puerperium (the period including the six weeks after delivery). Direct maternal deaths are included in the maternal death rate. Some examples of direct maternal causes of death would be infection, hemorrhage, obstructed labor, and hypertensive disorders such as eclampsia. An indirect maternal death is the death of a woman from a previously existing disease or a disease that developed during pregnancy, labor, or the puerperium that was not due to obstetric causes, although the physiologic effects of pregnancy were partially responsible. Maternal death rates are tracked as an indicator of quality of care but they can also help researchers and public health agencies understand trends in prenatal care and conditions that may be increasing in prevalence. The statistics can identify prenatal care needs in certain communities that will lead to public health initiatives.

The formula for calculating the maternal death rate is:

$$\text{Maternal death rate} = \frac{\substack{\text{Total number of direct maternal deaths} \\ \text{For a given period}}}{\substack{\text{Total number of maternal (OB)} \\ \text{discharges, including deaths, for} \\ \text{the same period}}} \times 100$$

As an example, in August, Midwest Hospital reported 330 maternal discharges. Two of these patients died. The maternal death rate for August is 0.60 percent ([2/330] × 100).

Autopsy Rates

An **autopsy**, also known as a postmortem examination, is the examination and study of a dead body to determine the cause of death. Although autopsies are not performed for every death, they are very helpful in the education and training of medical and other clinical care students. They are also valuable for continued research of the human body and cause of disease. Family members also find autopsy results very useful in identifying diseases that are hereditary so that family members can be proactive in disease prevention and treatment. Autopsies in the hospital are usually conducted by pathologists or some other physician who has been trained in this area. When the autopsy is complete, the autopsy report is created and documented in the patient's health record. The next sections discuss the different types of autopsies that are commonly conducted in a hospital.

Gross Autopsy Rate

The **gross autopsy rate** includes all of the deaths that occurred with inpatients, and it indicates the proportion of those on which an autopsy was performed. The formula for calculating the gross autopsy rate is:

$$\text{Gross autopsy rate} = \frac{\substack{\text{Total number of autopsies on inpatient} \\ \text{deaths for a given period}}}{\substack{\text{Total number of inpatient} \\ \text{deaths for the same period}}} \times 100$$

For example, at Midwest Hospital during the month of September, the hospital reported 18 deaths. Autopsies were performed on five of those patients. The gross autopsy rate is 27.7 percent ([5/18] × 100).

Net Autopsy Rate

The **net autopsy rate** is calculated in the same way, but the bodies of patients who were not available for autopsy are removed from the denominator. The reason some bodies may not be available for autopsy is that there are times that the coroner or medical examiner may remove the body from the premises. This is usually done for legal reasons, such as a patient who was involved in a crime that led to their death. Using the same example for the gross death rate, where there were 18 deaths and 5 autopsies, in calculating the net autopsy rate the numerator will still be 5 because 5 autopsies were performed at the hospital. However, one body was removed from the city by the medical examiner. Therefore, that person would be removed from the denominator. The net autopsy rate would be 29.4 percent ($[5/18 - 1] \times 100$). The formula for calculating the net autopsy rate is:

$$\text{Net autopsy rate} = \frac{\begin{array}{c}\text{Total number of autopsies on}\\ \text{inpatient deaths for a given period}\end{array}}{\begin{array}{c}\text{Total number of inpatient deaths}\\ \text{minus unautopsied coroner or medical}\\ \text{examiner cases for the same period}\end{array}} \times 100$$

Hospital Autopsy Rates

Another type of autopsy rate is the hospital autopsy rate. This autopsy rate includes anyone who had an autopsy at the hospital. While the gross autopsy rate and net autopsy rate only include those patients who died while an inpatient at the hospital, the hospital autopsy rate includes any former patients who died anywhere other than as a hospital inpatient. Upon death, if an autopsy is needed, these former patients are brought to the hospital for the autopsy.

Newborn Autopsy Rate and Fetal Autopsy Rate

The newborn autopsy rate and the fetal autopsy rate would be calculated in the same way as the gross autopsy rate.

The formula for the newborn autopsy rate is:

$$\text{Newborn autopsy rate} = \frac{\begin{array}{c}\text{Total number of autopsies on NB}\\ \text{deaths for a given period}\end{array}}{\begin{array}{c}\text{Total number of NB deaths}\\ \text{for the same period}\end{array}} \times 100$$

The formula for the fetal autopsy rate is:

$$\text{Fetal autopsy rate} = \frac{\begin{array}{c}\text{Total number of autopsies on}\\ \text{intermediate and late fetal deaths for}\\ \text{a given period}\end{array}}{\begin{array}{c}\text{Total number of intermediate and late}\\ \text{fetal deaths for the same period}\end{array}} \times 100$$

Hospital Infection Rates

Although hospital infection rates have been calculated for a very long time, in today's healthcare environment where patient care outcomes are emphasized more than ever, infection rates are a focus of healthcare facilities, such as the Joint Commission, CMS, and public health agencies. Infections are a major focus because they can lead to other complications, longer inpatient stays, and even death. A low infection rate can be an indicator of quality care.

Hospital-Acquired Infection Rates

Hospital-acquired infection rates, or nosocomial infection rates, indicate the rate of infections that were acquired during the hospital stay. These rates are calculated for the entire hospital, but will also be calculated for each unit to monitor any issue that may be affecting only a certain unit. Hospitals want to have a hospital-acquired infection rate of 0.0 percent, but it is common to have a very low infection rate. A spike in the infection rate will warrant immediate attention of administrators, medical staff, and nurses who will work to determine a reason for the sudden increase.

The formula for calculating hospital-acquired infection rates is:

$$\text{Hospital-acquired infection rates} = \frac{\begin{array}{c}\text{Total number of hospital - acquired}\\ \text{infections for a given period}\end{array}}{\begin{array}{c}\text{Total number of discharges, including}\\ \text{deaths for the same period}\end{array}} \times 100$$

For example, if there were 196 discharges last week and 2 hospital-acquired infections were reported, the hospital-acquired infection rate would be $(2/196) \times 100 = 1.02$ percent.

Postoperative Infection Rates

Another important indicator of quality care is the postoperative infection rate. A postoperative infection is one that occurs after a clean surgical case, meaning that there was no infection before the surgery. A postoperative infection could indicate poor wound care or some type of surgical contamination.

The formula for calculating postoperative infection rate is:

$$\text{Postoperative infection rates} = \frac{\substack{\text{Number of infections in clean surgical} \\ \text{cases for a given period}}}{\substack{\text{Total number surgical operations} \\ \text{for the same period}}} \times 100$$

For example, if there were 582 surgical operations performed in March, and 3 postoperative infections were reported for March, the postoperative infection rate would be calculated as $(3/582) \times 100 = 0.515$ percent.

Check Your Understanding 16.3

Instructions: **Answer the following questions on a separate piece of paper.**

1. Calculate the death rate in the following cases:

	Gross death rate	Net death rate
City Hospital reported 49 deaths in June. There were 489 discharges. Eight of those deaths occurred within 48 hours of admission.		
County Hospital reported 62 deaths in May. There were 524 discharges. Seventeen of those deaths occurred within 48 hours of admission.		

2. Calculate the autopsy rate in the following cases:

	Gross autopsy rate	Net autopsy rate
City Hospital reported 49 deaths in June. Twelve of those bodies were autopsied. Four of the 49 bodies were removed from the hospital for examination by the medical examiner.		
County Hospital reported 62 deaths in May. Sixteen of those bodies were autopsied. Nine of the 62 bodies were removed from the hospital for examination by the medical examiner.		

Ambulatory Care Statistics

Although the statistics discussed so far have focused on hospital inpatients, all healthcare environments have statistics that they monitor on a regular basis. Ambulatory care, or outpatient care, must track number of patients, volume of service, quality of care, and many related rates. For example, while hospitals calculate and report census, ambulatory facilities track number of daily visits or encounters. While hospitals track length of stay and average length of stay, physician clinics track length of appointments and average length of appointments. Administrators in ambulatory settings use this data for decision making, staffing and budgeting, just as hospital administrators do. Regardless of the setting, statistical reporting is crucial to the success of healthcare service and financial stability. Monitoring a variety of statistical data lends valuable information for strategic planning.

Statistics in Reimbursement Management

As discussed throughout this chapter, statistics are used for decision making and budgeting in all healthcare environments. Statistics are also used in reimbursement management, which is directly related to the budget and the financial success of a healthcare organization. Some important areas administrators monitor in relation to reimbursement are:

- Coding and billing errors
- Accounts receivable
- Level of care and resources used per case
- Claims turn-around time

Case-Mix Analysis

The **case-mix index (CMI)** at each hospital informs administrators about resources consumed for patients with similar diagnoses and treatments. Case-mix index is "a weighted average of the sum of the relative weights of all patients treated during a specified time period" (Casto and Forrestal 2015, 115). Relative weights can also be stated as comparable values. Case mix gives details about how complex the patient cases are at each hospital, or a picture of the severity of illness typical at each hospital. This information is important because the complexity of the hospital's patients reflects on the cost of treating those patients.

Along with CMI, diagnosis-related groups (DRGs) are used "for hospital reimbursement because it measure the resources consumed for clinically similar patients" (Casto and Forrestal 2015, 115). The DRG method assigns a numeric value to an acute-care inpatient hospital episode of care, which serves as a relative weighting factor intended to represent the resource intensity of hospital care of the clinical group that is classified to that specific DRG. As a reimbursement system, the DRG assignment determines the payment level the hospital will receive (AHIMA 2010).

Case-mix index is calculated by adding the DRG weights for all Medicare discharges and dividing by the number of discharges. Using the data in table 16.5, if the total of the MS-DRG weights for the top 10 MS-DRGs at Community Hospital Neurology Center is 2,726.269, this total would be divided by the number of discharges. If the number of discharges were 2,439, the calculation would be 2,726.269 divided by 2,439 for a CMI of 1.1177. The MS-DRG system is the newest Medicare DRG system that went into effect October 1, 2007. The MS stands for Medicare severity.

Example One of Usage

The State of California gives the following example of how case-mix index might be used:

> The case-mix index (CMI) can be used to adjust the average cost per patient (or day) for a given hospital relative to the adjusted average cost for other hospitals by dividing the average cost per patient (or day) by the hospital's calculated CMI. The adjusted average cost per patient would reflect the charges reported for the types of cases treated in that year.
>
> For example, if Hospital A has an average cost per patient of $1,000 and a CMI of 0.80 for a given year, their adjusted cost per patient is $1,000/0.80 = $1,250. Likewise, if Hospital B has an average cost per patient of $1,500 and a CMI of 1.25, their adjusted cost per patient is $1,500/1.25 = $1,200.
>
> Therefore, if a hospital has a CMI greater than 1.00, their adjusted cost per patient or per day will be lowered and conversely if a hospital has a CMI less than 1.00, their adjusted cost will be higher (OSHPD 2014).

Table 16.5.   Calculation of case-mix index for the top 10 MS-DRGs at Community Hospital Neurology Center

MS-DRG	Number (N)	MS-DRG weight	N x MS-DRG weight
056	223	1.7368	387.3064
058	560	1.6027	897.512
059	419	1.0399	435.7181
060	166	0.7899	131.1234
073	129	1.3014	167.8806
074	242	0.0786	19.0212
053	319	0.8746	278.9974
054	83	1.3195	109.5185
055	229	1.0100	231.29
089	69	0.9406	64.9014
TOTAL	2,439		2726.269
CMI			1.1177

Example Two of Usage

The State of California also provides the following example of how their Office of Statewide Health Planning and Development uses case-mix and MS-DRG data:

> To calculate the CMI, the Office of Statewide Health Planning and Development (OSHPD) uses MS-DRG weights assigned by CMS. Patients are assigned to one of over 700 MS-DRGs (based on the principal and secondary diagnoses, age, procedures performed, the presence of co-morbidity and/or complications, discharge status, and gender).
>
> Each MS-DRG has a numeric weight reflecting the national "average hospital resource consumption" by patients for that MS-DRG, relative to the national "average hospital resource consumption" of all patients. CMS implements revisions to the MS-DRG weights on October 1, the beginning of the federal fiscal year. These are published annually in Table 5 of the *Federal Register*. OSHPD uses the version released October 1 on their data for the following calendar year.
>
> Although the MS-DRG weights are based on resource consumption by Medicare patients, OSHPD applies them to all patient discharge data reported by hospitals in California during the course of a calendar year. The OSHPD case-mix index is then calculated by averaging the MS-DRG weight of patients discharged within the calendar year, namely, the sum of the MS-DRG weights divided by the number of patients (OSHPD 2014).

Public Health and Epidemiology Data

Vital statistics are based on the reporting of the vital events of births, deaths, marriages, divorces, and fetal deaths. All 50 states are required to register all births, deaths, marriages, divorces, and fetal deaths; and this information is shared between various governmental organizations. Each state's government is responsible for keeping a registry of vital events and for issuing birth, death, marriage, and divorce certifications (CDC 2015c).

The **National Vital Statistics System (NVSS)** is used to collect the nation's vital statistic information. It is the data-sharing organization to which each state disseminates their vital statistic registry data. Traditionally, all vital event information is registered with the NVSS using standardized forms. However, electronic reporting will certainly become the norm as work continues on developing secure electronic reporting systems (CDC 2015c).

The following is a description of the eVitals Standards Initiatives the CDC is implementing to work toward these secure reporting systems.

> The CDC/NCHS' Division of Vital Statistics (DVS), in conjunction with the Classifications and Public Health Data Standards Staff (CPHDSS), is working with the National Association for Public Health Statistics and Information Systems (NAPHSIS), state representatives, and other vital records stakeholders to develop vital records standards to enable interoperable electronic data exchanges among electronic health record systems, US vital records systems, and potentially other public information systems for birth, death, and fetal death events. (CDC 2015c)

This will be important for access to real-time data rather than having to wait until an annual report is published. As-needed data will help public health agencies, government entities, and researchers move forward with reporting and studies without delaying their work until the data is available.

Epidemiology Statistics

Epidemiology statistics are based on large populations through public health agencies. According to the CDC,

> epidemiology is the study of the distribution and determinants of health problems in specified populations and the application of this study to control health problems. Epidemiology is the scientific method used by 'disease detectives'—epidemiologists—to get to the root of a public health problem or emerging public health event affecting a specific population (CDC 2015d).

Populations may include a city, a county, a neighborhood, a healthcare facility, a school, or any other entity to be studied (CDC 2015d). These studies assist health researchers in assessing current health issues that should be further studied. The data collected in the studies lead to public health education initiatives.

Epidemiologists conduct research studies on a public health issue for a certain population and collect large amounts of data. This data is analyzed with statistical formulas used by researchers to determine if the data and information they have gathered in their research has significance. Any significant findings may be researched further, and results are used to create initiatives to impact the issues that were identified. For instance, if research and statistics show that one city has a significantly higher prevalence of skin cancer, public health agencies may wish to launch an education campaign about the use of sunscreen and other skin protections. These statistics are referred to as **population-based statistics** because they track the mortality and morbidity of a population.

Some typical population-based statistics reported are birth rates, infant mortality rates, general death rates, and cause-specific death rates. Disease-specific data is also collected and rates are reported regarding the frequency, or **incidence rate**, of disease, along with reports of specific diseases along with prevalence rates. **Prevalence rates** report the proportion of persons with a certain disease to the number of persons in a population. Prevalence rates are used to track severity of diseases and can indicate whether a disease may be at an epidemic proportion. These statistics help public health professionals plan where research dollars will be allocated, where community education is needed, and what initiatives should be a focus in future public health initiatives. Figure 16.2 is a graph of the prevalence of cancer in males from 1999 to 2012 to illustrate an example of the use of public health statistics. This type of public health data can inform decisions about cancer treatment and research.

Community-Based Disease Tracking

Another important mechanism for tracking disease incidence and prevalence is the National Notifiable Diseases Surveillance System (NVDSS).

Figure 16.2. Prevalence in cancer from 1999 to 2012

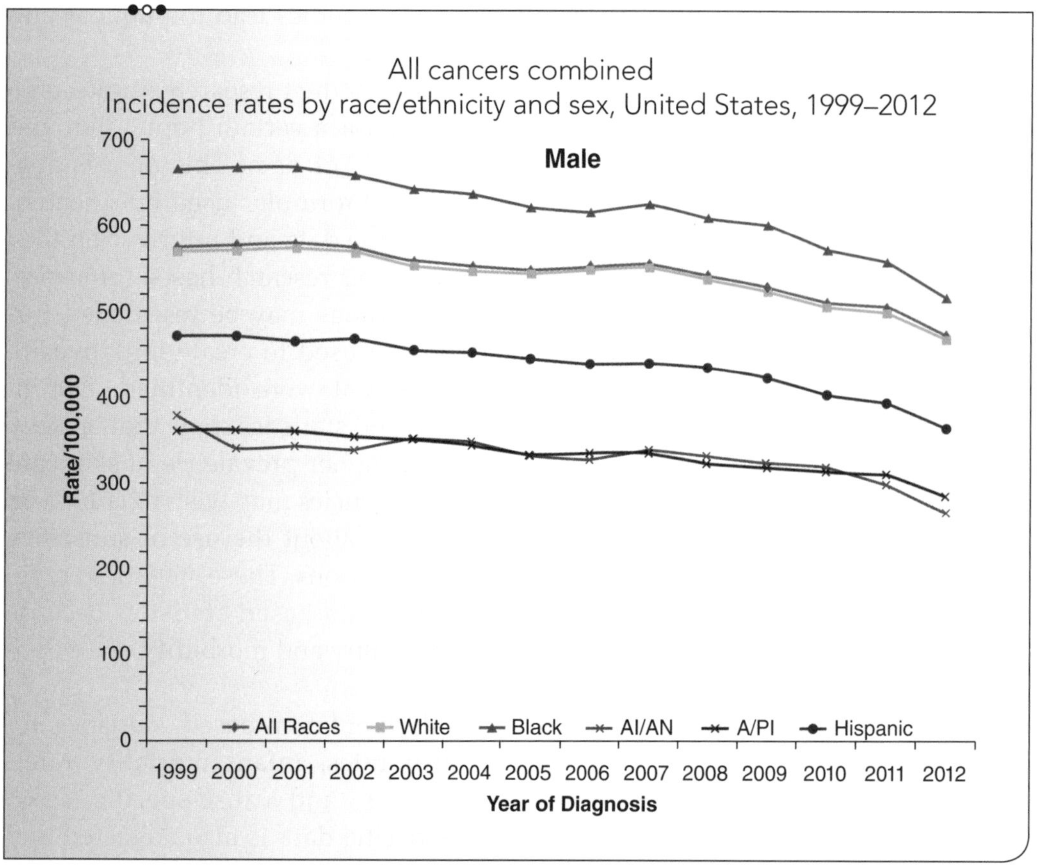
All cancers combined
Incidence rates by race/ethnicity and sex, United States, 1999–2012
Male
Rate/100,000
700
600
500
400
300
200
100
0
All Races
White
Black
AI/AN
A/PI
Hispanic
1999 2000 2001 2002 2003 2004 2005 2006 2007 2008 2009 2010 2011 2012
Year of Diagnosis

U.S. Cancer Statistics Working Group. United States Cancer Statistics: 1999-2012 Incidence and Mortality Web-based Report. Atlanta: U.S. Department of Health and Human Services, Centers for Disease Control and Prevention and National Cancer Institute; 2015. Available at: http://www.cdc.gov/cancer/dcpc/data/index.htm

Like the National Vital Statistics System, it is managed by the CDC. The system tracks notifiable diseases. **Notifiable diseases** are those that a state must report to the CDC when the diseases are identified by hospitals or other healthcare facilities. The list of notifiable diseases changes over time and can vary by state. The information that is reported is specific to the disease and demographics of the patient, but patient identifiers are not reported.

National morbidity data is reported each week. This timely data is used by public health administrators to act quickly on any data that may signify an epidemic or a crisis situation. The data is analyzed on a regular basis to find trends, changes, and patterns that should be monitored and investigated. Each annual list of notifiable disease can be found on the website for the CDC. If needed, past years' lists can also be downloaded on the site.

Using Healthcare Statistics

Healthcare statistics are widely used in the healthcare environment. Health information management professionals are often involved in the data collection process but they also must know how to calculate various statistics to use in their day-to-day decision making and reporting. Health information management professionals may be responsible for calculating or finding statistical information for administrators who need the information for strategic planning, budgeting, and staffing decisions.

Finding and Using Existing Statistics

Researchers know that they do not always have to do their own data collection studies because a wealth of databases and statistics already exist. Healthcare managers may also use existing data for reports, presentations, decision making, justifications, and benchmarking. Online search engines have made it possible to find valuable statistics fairly easily. It is also important for health information management professionals and other healthcare administrators to be able to locate existing statistics and use them in projects, studies, decision making, and benchmarking. There is a wealth of valuable healthcare data available and becoming a practiced researcher is an important skill to have. Figure 16.3 illustrates helpful steps to take in a search for statistics. Following these steps, the researcher would first need to establish goals for the research project, then search publications and the Internet for existing research and data found in publications. Next, the researcher should go to the original sources and analyze the information and collect the data. If they find they need more information or different types of data, they would need to reassess their needs, and go back to the beginning of the process to find even more data. As shown, searching publications and the Internet can help the researcher find valuable information. However, time must be taken to evaluate the data found to assess its value and validity and determine if the source can be used or if more sources should be sought.

As an example of the value of existing statistics, a health information manager has volunteered to be part of a team at a clinic that is focusing on the adolescent population in their community. The goal is to increase the adolescent visits at the clinic,

with a focus on well visits for health maintenance. The project manager asks for a volunteer to find some national data of how many adolescents typically have well visits in any given year. This information will be used as a benchmark that your clinic will try to exceed. The HIM manager has volunteered for this task and finds some excellent data through the Healthy People 2020 initiative (HealthyPeople.gov). Since one of the goals of Healthy People 2020 is to increase the proportion of adolescents who have had a wellness visit in the past 12 months, the HIM manager is able to find national data on this topic for the past seven years. A printout of this data can be taken to the next project meeting. The project manager may decide that the team can use this data as the benchmark.

Figure 16.3. Steps in searching for existing health statistics

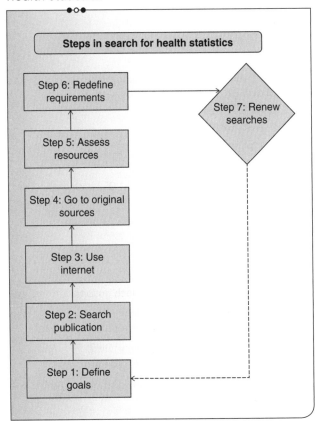

Source: US Library of Medicine 2008.

Check Your Understanding 16.4

Instructions: **Answer the following questions on a separate piece of paper.**

1. The arithmetic average is the:
   A. Middle
   B. Mode
   C. Mean
   D. Median

2. Data and statistical analysis is valuable in which of the following HIM tasks?
   A. Budgeting
   B. Staffing
   C. Strategic planning
   D. All of the above

3. The middle number in a set of scores is the:
   A. Average
   B. Mode
   C. Mean
   D. Median

4. Which of the following terms indicates the number of patients present in the healthcare facility at a particular point in time?
   A. Inpatient service day
   B. Hospital newborn inpatient
   C. Hospital inpatient
   D. Inpatient census

5. The termination of hospitalization through the formal release of an inpatient by the hospital is known as which of the following?
   A. Inpatient census
   B. Hospital outpatient
   C. Inpatient admission
   D. Inpatient discharge

6. Community Hospital admitted 1,052 patients for orthopedic procedures in 2015. Sixteen of those patients developed a postoperative infection. What is the postoperative infection rate for this group of admissions?
   A. 65.75%
   B. 1.52%
   C. 0.015%
   D. 34.25%

7. The case-mix index (CMI) at each hospital informs administrators about which of the following?
   A. Resources consumed for patients with similar diagnoses and treatments
   B. How many DRGs are reported for the hospital
   C. Statistical significance of each diagnosis code
   D. Total MS-DRGs reported for the year

8. How often is national morbidity data reported?
   A. Annually
   B. Quarterly
   C. Monthly
   D. Weekly

9. A unit of measure that reflects the services received by one inpatient during a 24-hour period is called a(n):
   A. Daily census
   B. Admission
   C. Transfer in and transfer out
   D. Inpatient service day

10. A&C on a census report is referring to which of the following?
   A. Admissions and consults
   B. Appendicitis and colitis
   C. Adults and children
   D. A.M. and clock

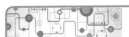

References

American Health Information Management Association. 2012. *Pocket Glossary of Health Information Management.* Chicago: AHIMA.

American Health Information Management Association. 2010 (April). Evolution of DRGs (updated). *Journal of AHIMA* web exclusive. http://library.ahima.org/xpedio/groups/public/documents/ahima/bok1_047260.hcsp?dDocName=bok1_047260

Barfield, W. 2011. Standard terminology for fetal, infant, and perinatal deaths. *Pediatrics* 128(1): 177–181.

Casto, A. and E. Forrestal. 2015. *Principles of Healthcare Reimbursement*, 5th ed. Chicago: AHIMA.

Centers for Disease Control and Prevention. Morbidity and Mortality Weekly Report. 2015a. Using Electronic Clinical Quality Measure Reporting for Public Health Surveillance. http://www.cdc.gov/mmwr/preview/mmwrhtml/mm6416a3.htm

Centers for Disease Control and Prevention. 2015b. Cancer Rates by Race/Ethnicity and Sex. http://www.cdc.gov/cancer/dcpc/data/race.htm

Centers for Disease Control and Prevention. 2015c. About the National Vital Statistics System. http://www.cdc.gov/nchs/nvss/about_nvss.htm

Centers for Disease Control and Prevention. 2015d. What Is Epidemiology? http://www.cdc.gov/EXCITE/epidemiology.html

Centers for Disease Control and Prevention. n.d. Technical Appendix—Fetal Death. ftp://ftp.cdc.gov/pub/health_statistics/nchs/Datasets/mmb/i_Fetappd.pdf

HealthyPeople.gov. 2015. Healthy People 2020. http://www.healthypeople.gov/

Hoefs, J. 2015 (May). Personal communication with author.

Horton, L. 2012. *Calculating and Reporting Healthcare Statistics*, 4th ed. Chicago: AHIMA.

Horton, L. 2013. Healthcare Statistics. Chapter 18 in *Health Information Management: Concepts, Principles and Practice*, 4th ed. Edited by LaTour, K.M., S. Eichenwald Maki, and P. Oachs. Chicago: AHIMA.

New York State Department of Health. 1999. Basic Statistics: About Incidence, Prevalence, Morbidity, and Mortality—Statistics Teaching Tools. https://www.health.ny.gov/diseases/chronic/basicstat.htm

Office of Statewide Health Planning and Development. 2014 (July 8). Healthcare Information Division: Case Mix Index. http://www.oshpd.ca.gov/HID/Products/PatDischargeData/CaseMixIndex/

Salkind, N. 2011. *Statistics for People Who (Think They) Hate Statistics*, 4th ed. Thousand Oaks, CA: SAGE Publications, Inc.

Taylor, L. 2015 (May). Personal communication with author.

US Department of Health and Human Services. Indian Health Service. n.d. Indian Health Manual. https://www.ihs.gov/ihm/index.cfm?module=dsp_ihm_pc_p3c3

US Library of Medicine. 2012. Finding and Using Health Statistics. http://www.nlm.nih.gov/nichsr/usestats/index.html

US Library of Medicine. 2008. National Information Center on Health Services Research and Health Care Technology (NICHSR). http://www.nlm.nih.gov/nichsr/usestats/steps_in_successful_search_diagram.html

17

Healthcare Data Analytics

Susan White, PhD, RHIA, CHDA

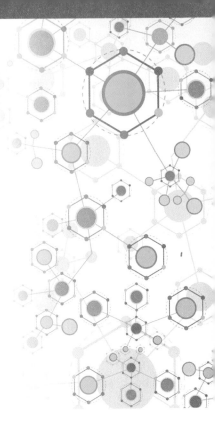

Learning Objectives

- Examine the role of data analytics in healthcare operations
- Apply statistical techniques to healthcare data
- Apply statistical inference
- Calculate hypothesis tests and confidence intervals
- Evaluate the role of HIM professionals in healthcare data analytics

Key Terms

Accountable care organizations
Alternative hypothesis
Cluster sampling
Coefficient of determination
Confidence interval
Continuous data
Continuous variables
Correlation
Data analytics
Data mining
Dependent variable
Descriptive statistics
Discrete data
Healthcare data analytics
Hypothesis test

Independent variable
Indirect standardization
Inferential statistics
Interval data
Mean
Median
Mode
Nominal data
Normal distribution
Null hypothesis
One sample t-test
Ordinal data
Pay for performance
Predictive modeling
P-value

QualityNet
Range
Rate
Ratio data
RAT-STATS
Simple linear regression (SLR)
Simple random sample
Standard deviation
Stratified random sample
Structured data
Systematic random sampling
Type I error
Type II error
Unstructured data
Variance

The term **data analytics** is used to describe a variety of approaches to using data to make business decisions. **Healthcare data analytics** is, therefore, the practice of using data to make business decisions in healthcare. More specifically, healthcare data analytics is the application of statistical techniques to allow informed decisions to be made based on the data. A variety of descriptive statistics are used in healthcare including rates and proportions as well as measures of central tendency such as the mean, median, and mode. Inferential statistics include techniques such as confidence intervals and hypothesis testing, and are used to determine if a provider's performance is significantly better or worse than national norms. In this chapter, both sets of statistical techniques will be applied in the healthcare operations and business context.

The business of healthcare requires the management of both clinical and financial decisions. Healthcare is rich with a wide variety of data sources that may be analyzed to drive those decisions. Professionals working in the field of analytics do not typically collect data for the purpose of a research study (perform primary research) and design experiments to prove or disprove theories. The field of analytics often leverages the use of secondary data already collected by others for various purposes (to help improve business decisions going forward). Sampling and experimental design may be used to collect primary data to answer specific business analysis needs, but that is often a time-consuming and expensive task. The healthcare industry produces a tremendous amount of clinical and operational data. The secondary use of that data is often used in analytic projects to measure and improve the performance of healthcare entities.

Healthcare Initiatives and the Impact on Data Analytics

Electronic health records (EHRs) bring a flood of data into the already data-rich healthcare environment. The true value of that data may only be realized through applying analytic techniques to distill the raw data into information that can support decision making. The results of data analytics can have a significant impact on both the clinical and financial outcomes of the healthcare system.

The SAS Institute is an industry leader in the area of business analytics and distributes a statistical software program that is used by many business and government entities called statistical analysis software, more commonly called SAS. The SAS Institute listed the following concepts to support the effective use of EHR data:

- A centralized data repository that synthesizes data from currently incompatible data silos on any platform and format
- Sophisticated data extract, transform, and load (ETL) processes that maintain data

quality, so that one can have faith in the accuracy of research based on that data

- Healthcare-specific analytics that enable nonstatisticians to reveal meaningful intelligence from vast amounts of information about patients, populations, providers, procedures, and risks
- Predictive analytics to deliver more accurate research forecasts, evidence-based treatment protocols, and improved patient outcomes
- Query, reporting, and visualization tools that give various types of users the highest quality of information, where and when needed, via multiple platforms and channels (SAS Institute 2006)

Many recent federal initiatives have put the spotlight on the importance of data analytics in healthcare. A few samples of these initiatives are discussed here.

Pay for performance (P4P) programs are based on data-driven metrics to measure both the quality and efficiency of a healthcare provider.

Bonus payments may be awarded or penalties imposed on providers depending on their level of performance. The Centers for Medicare and Medicaid Services (CMS) implemented the first stages of their P4P program in July 2003 with the National Voluntary Hospital Reporting Initiative (CMS 2009). In their 2009 report "Roadmap for Implementing Value Driven Healthcare in the Traditional Medicare Fee-for-Service Program," CMS staff identified key factors for consideration in the implementation of P4P:

1. Identification and promotion of the use of quality measures through pay for reporting
2. Payment for quality performance
3. Measures of physician and provider resource use
4. Payment for value—promote efficiency in resource use while providing high quality care
5. Alignment of financial incentives among providers
6. Transparency and public reporting (CMS 2009)

Each of these factors is related to the use of healthcare data and analytic techniques. CMS is in various stages of the implementation of these components throughout the Medicare system. In the hospital setting, both the inpatient prospective payment system (IPPS) and the outpatient prospective payment system (OPPS) include a penalty for providers that do not report the required quality indicators.

In the area of financial analytics, the Healthcare Financial Management Association (HFMA) developed a set of indicators to measure revenue cycle performance. These so-called MAP (measure, apply, perform) indicators include financial metrics that may be derived from healthcare data. They provide a framework for benchmarking the ability of a healthcare provider to collect the money owed for the treatment of patients. The MAP indicators measure performance in four key areas—patient access, revenue integrity, claims adjudication, and management (HFMA 2015). Refer to chapter 8 for more detail about these indicators.

The arrival of the **accountable care organization** (ACO) begins to tie together the use of clinical and financial analytics throughout the healthcare delivery system (White et al. 2011). The ACO is an integrated delivery system that includes physicians, hospitals, and other providers all focused on the delivery of care to a particular geographic segment of the Medicare population. The ACO receives incentive payments for delivering care in an efficient manner and providing a level of preventive care and education that may avoid subsequent treatment for chronic diseases. The intent of the ACO program is to improve the efficiency of care delivered to Medicare beneficiaries. In order to do so effectively, the ACO must have a robust database regarding the care delivered to the beneficiaries they are to serve as well as a broad spectrum of analytics to understand the patterns of care and chronic diseases present in the population.

All of the examples presented in this section highlight the growth of analytics in the healthcare setting. The demand for professionals with solid analytic skills and the ability to interpret the results of analysis to non-analytics staff is outpacing availability at this time. HIM professionals that can demonstrate these skills will become an invaluable resource in their organization.

Types of Data

Data can be characterized in a number of ways. The most broad categorization is structured versus unstructured. **Structured data** are data that are comprised of values that can be stored as either numbers or a finite number of categories. Healthcare data such as height, weight, age, gender, and MS-DRG are all examples of structured data. Conversely, **unstructured data** cannot be expressed as numbers or categories. The classic example of unstructured data in healthcare are the clinician notes that are recorded in an EHR. The notes often contain valuable data regarding treatment protocols and documentation of comorbid conditions (the presence of one or more additional disorders along with a primary disorder) (Krajniak et al. 2016), but they are recorded as freeform text and are therefore difficult to use in analyses. Analytic tools such as natural language processing (NLP) or other methods of characterizing key words or concepts may be used to analyze unstructured data. For example, NLP engines are used in computer-assisted coding programs to identify key medical terms found in clinical documentation such as nursing notes.

Structured data may further be broken down into levels of measurement. Care should be taken to understand the level of measurement of each data element that may be analyzed so that the proper statistical method is applied. The four basic levels of measurement are displayed in table 17.1. Ordinal and nominal data are both **discrete data** types. They take on categorical values and cannot be added together or divided. **Nominal data** is expressed as categories that represent names of items, but do not have a natural order. Examples of data with a nominal measurement level include gender, color, MS-DRG,

CPT codes, and ICD codes. **Ordinal data** is also expressed as categories, but in this case the categories do have a natural order. Patient severity level, trauma center level, and trimester of gestation are all examples of ordinal data found in healthcare.

Ratio and interval data are both considered **continuous data**. They can take on a continuum of values as opposed to discrete categories. Their values may be added and subtracted for comparison. **Ratio data** examples include length of stay, charges, hemoglobin levels, and such. **Interval data** is also continuous, but does not have a true zero value. An example of interval data is temperature. The temperature may be zero, but that does not represent the absence of temperature. Only that it is very cold. Another distinction between ratio and interval data is that the concepts of "half of" or "twice" has meaning. For instance, if the average length of stay at one unit is five days and the average length of stay in another unit is half as long, the value is 2.5 days. The concept of twice as cold does not have a practical interpretation. The interval between two temperature values does have an interpretation. This is where the term *interval* was derived. If the difference or interval between two data values has meaning, then the measurement level is interval. If the ratio or multiplication of two data values has meaning, then the measurement level is ratio.

Table 17.1. Basic levels of measurement

Data type	Examples	Appropriate descriptive statistics
Nominal—categorical data where the categories are mutually exclusive, but do not have a natural order	Gender, HCPCS codes, department or unit	Frequency counts, proportions, mode
Ordinal—categorical data where the categories are mutually exclusive and they do have a natural order	Patient satisfaction scores, severity scores, trauma center level, surveys measured on a Likert scale	Frequency counts, proportions, mode, range
Interval—naturally numeric data where the distance between two values has meaning, but multiplying values and zero value has no interpretation	Temperature, pH level, dates	Mean, median, standard deviation, range
Ratio—naturally numeric data where zero has an interpretation and the values may be doubled or multiplied by a constant and still have meaning	Charges, length of stay, age	Mean, median, standard deviation, range, geometric mean, coefficient of variation

Descriptive versus Inferential Statistics

The science of statistics is segmented into two broad categories—descriptive and inferential. **Descriptive statistics** are used to describe the distribution of the variable of interest. **Inferential statistics** are used to test hypotheses or make decisions. These hypotheses have a probability or risk of making an error based on the data collected. This probability is referred to as the Type I error or p-value. Inferential statistics help analysts trend and summarize the data to determine whether or not they are seeing significant results in the sample or simply observing an event that occurred due to chance.

The appropriate descriptive statistic is determined by the type of data analyzed. If the intent is to describe how often an event of interest occurs, then rates and proportions are often used. For instance, a mortality rate is used to measure how many subjects died compared to the total number of subjects. A proportion is the appropriate statistic to use when describing the breakout of MS-DRG cases with no complication or co-morbidities (CC), complications or co-morbidities (CC), and major complications or co-morbidities (MCC). If the intent is to analyze a variable that is interval or ratio in nature, then the appropriate descriptive statistic is likely the mean, median, or mode. For instance, length of stay for inpatient services is described using mean (average) or median. Table 17.1 lists types of data and the appropriate descriptive statistics.

The appropriate inferential statistic method is determined by the hypothesis to be tested or the question to be answered. An analyst may be asked to compare their facility's length of stay or mortality rate to a state standard or to determine if the MS-DRG change rate is different from the value typically observed at the facility. These questions may be answered using inferential techniques. The appropriate statistical method is dependent on the question and the type of data available for the analysis.

Basic healthcare operations questions may often be analyzed using confidence intervals or hypothesis tests. A **confidence interval** is a range of values, such that the probability of that range covering the true value of a parameter is a set probability or confidence. A **hypothesis test** allows the analyst to determine the likelihood that a hypothesis is true given the data present in the sample with a predetermined acceptable level of making an error.

For instance, suppose the goal of a study is to determine the typical wait time in a hospital's emergency department (ED). A random sample of patients is selected from the population of patients visiting the ED during the previous month. The average wait time, 53.5 minutes, is a statistic that describes the typical wait time, but that statistic alone does not give any information about the precision of the estimate or how certain it is that the true population ED wait time is a range of around 53.5 minutes.

A confidence interval may be used to provide that additional information. A 95 percent confidence interval for the ED wait time was calculated and found to be: (50.1, 56.9). The value 95 percent is the confidence level or the probability that the confidence interval contains the true population average. In this case, there is a probability of 95 percent that the interval (50.1, 56.9) includes the true population average ED wait time. Recall that these figures are based on a sample and we do not know the entire population value. The sample is used to make inferences or conclusions about the population. The width of the confidence interval is a measure of the precision of the estimate. A narrower interval is more precise.

Continuing with this same ED wait time example, suppose the goal was to test to determine if the average wait time was meeting a facility standard of 60 minutes. In this case, a hypothesis test is the correct statistical method. Hypothesis testing requires the definitions of the null hypothesis to be tested versus an alternative hypothesis.

The **null hypothesis** is typically the status quo (White 2015). The **alternative hypothesis** is sometimes called the research hypothesis and is a conclusion that typically requires some action to be taken (White 2015). The null hypothesis is that the ED wait time is less than or equal 60 minutes; the alternative hypothesis is that the ED wait time is greater than 60 minutes. In hypothesis testing, an acceptable Type I error level should be selected prior to calculating the result. **Type I error** is the probability of incorrectly rejecting the null hypothesis given the values present in the sample. In this example, Type I error is making the conclusion that the wait time is longer than 60 minutes when it is truly less than or equal to 60 minutes. Analysts must also be aware of Type II error in hypothesis testing. **Type II error** occurs when the null hypothesis is not rejected when it is actually false (White 2015). Type II error may be controlled by adjusting the sample size used for the study; a larger sample will decrease the likelihood of committing a Type II error.

The practical implications of making a Type I error in this situation is the expense that may be incurred to study the root cause of the long wait times and make operational corrections. For this example the Type I error is set to be 5 percent or 0.05. The probability of making a Type I error may be calculated using the sample data and the appropriate test statistic. The probability of making a Type I error based on a particular set of data is called the **p-value**. If the p-value or probability of making a Type I error is less than the Type I error level set prior to testing, then the null hypothesis may be rejected. After calculating the test statistic and determining the p-value is 0.03, the null hypothesis is rejected and the conclusion is made that the ED wait time is longer than the standard.

The first step in any study is to identify the research question (discussed further in chapter 19). Many data analysis projects start without a clear idea of the exact question to be answered. The analyst becomes so concerned with summarizing the data and producing reports that they forget their efforts may be wasted if the question is not well defined at the outset. Examples of some of the research questions that may be of interest include:

- What is the typical ED wait time?
- Does our ED wait time meet our facility standard?
- What is the percent of lab orders that are not signed by a physician?
- What is the coding accuracy rate for secondary diagnosis codes?

Once the research question is defined, the unit of analysis must also be determined. For example, to determine the percentage of lab orders that are not signed by a physician, the unit of analysis is the entire set of lab orders for the time period of interest. This set of lab orders serves as the population of interest. It is practically impossible to collect the entire population of lab orders to definitively answer the questions posed. The data required is often selected via a sampling plan and then analyzed to make inferences or conclusions about the percentage of lab orders unsigned in the population.

In practice, it is sometimes difficult to determine the unit of analysis. For instance, in determining the coding accuracy rate for secondary diagnosis codes, should the unit of analysis be each code or the claim on which the code appears? There is a critical difference between the two units of analysis. If the unit of analysis is the code, then the resulting rate would be the proportion of correct codes and not the proportion of correct claims. If the research question is to estimate the number of claims correctly coded, then the claim should be the unit of analysis.

Impact of Sampling

If the entire population of units of analysis were available for a study, then there would be no reason to use inferential statistics. Consider the previous lab order example. If the entire population of lab orders submitted at the facility during the time period of interest could be profiled, then the signature rate could be calculated exactly and compared to a standard. Unfortunately, the availability of the population or the time required to review the population is often not practical.

Figure 17.1. AMI measure set sample size requirements

Quarterly sample size
Based on initial patient population size for the AMI measure set
Hospital's measure

Average quarterly initial patient population size "N"	Minimum required sample size "n"
≥1551	311
391–1550	20% of initial patient population size
78–390	78
6–77	No sampling; 100% initial patient population required
0–5	Submission of patient level data is encouraged but not required: • CMS: if submission occurs, one to five cases of the initial patient population may be submitted • Joint Commission: if submission occurs, 100% initial patient population required

The most common types of random sampling are simple, stratified, systematic, and cluster sampling. These are discussed further in chapter 19. In **simple random sampling**, every member of the population has an equal probability of inclusion in the sample. A **stratified random sample** is selected by first dividing the population into subsets or strata. A simple random sample is then selected from each strata from the sample. **Cluster sampling** is similar to stratified sampling in that the population is divided into subsets, called clusters here. The clusters are then randomly selected. All units within the randomly selected clusters are included in the sample. **Systematic random sampling** is a method used to determine a simple random sample. In systematic random sampling every N/nth record is selected from the population. N is the number of units in the population and n is the sample size (White 2015).

The particular statistical method used is dependent on the sampling method used to collect the data. Stratified and cluster sampling require a more complex set of statistical methods than simple random sampling.

Sampling techniques are used frequently in the healthcare setting. For instance, CMS allows hospitals to report many of the required quality indicators based on a sample of claims and not the full population. Figure 17.1 is an example of the sample size requirements outlined in the **QualityNet** Hospital Inpatient Measures Specification Manual (QualityNet 2015). QualityNet is a Centers for Medicare and Medicaid Services (CMS) website that provides information about quality measurement and serves as the basis for communication between CMS, their contractors, and healthcare providers regarding quality data and metrics.

CMS reports the sample size and rate for measures that are based on samples rather than full population statistics. In table 17.2 the values for University Hospital are based on a sample. This table demonstrates the types of comparisons that are made using a sample of the patients treated by a provider. Notice that University Hospital's statistics are all based on a sample, but the sample of n = 16 submitted for the measure Heart Attack Patients Given PCI within 90 Minutes of Arrival is deemed too small to be sure how they are performing.

CMS (2016) also includes guidance on how to calculate a confidence interval for rates based on samples. These instructions may be found in table 17.3.

Using the guidance in table 17.3 and the data presented in table 17.2, confidence intervals may be formed for the example quality indicators.

Table 17.2.   Example hospital comparison based on sample

Hospital process of care measures tables	Average for all reporting hospitals in the United States	Average for all reporting hospitals in the state	General hospital	University hospital	Data collected	
					From	To
Heart attack patients given aspirin at arrival	99%	99%	99% of 747 patients	100% of 173 patients[1]	1/1/2010	12/31/2010
Heart attack patients given ACE inhibitor or ARB for left ventricular systolic dysfunction (LVSD)	96%	97%	100% of 116 patients	97% of 71 patients[1]	1/1/2010	12/31/2010
Heart attack patients given PCI within 90 minutes of arrival	91%	93%	96% of 154 patients	88% of 16 patients[1,2]	1/1/2010	12/31/2010

[1] The hospital indicated that the data submitted for this measure were based on a sample of cases.
[2] The number of cases is too small to be sure how well a hospital is performing.
Source: CMS 2015.

Table 17.3.   Guide to calculating confidence intervals for rates based on samples

Estimating confidence intervals for the process of care measures: estimated values for proportion data

Sample size	Observed rate								
	10%	20%	30%	40%	50%	60%	70%	80%	90%
<25	–	–	24.9%	26.6%	27.2%	26.6%	24.9%	–	–
25–75	8.3%	11.1%	12.7%	13.6%	13.9%	13.6%	12.7%	11.1%	8.3%
76–125	5.9%	7.8%	9.0%	9.6%	9.8%	9.6%	9.0%	7.8%	5.9%
126–175	4.8%	6.4%	7.3%	7.8%	8.0%	7.8%	7.3%	6.4%	4.8%
176–225	4.2%	5.5%	6.4%	6.8%	6.9%	6.8%	6.4%	5.5%	4.2%
226–275	3.75%	5.0%	5.7%	6.1%	6.2%	6.1%	5.7%	5.0%	3.7%
276+	2.9%	3.9%	4.5%	4.8%	4.9%	4.8%	4.5%	3.9%	2.9%

Source: CMS/OCSQ/QIG: The values in the table are the approximate amount to add and subtract from the observed rate to estimate a 95 percent confidence interval for the given sample size. (Interpolation between the values in the table is appropriate.) Estimates of an interval in these cells exceed the natural limits for proportions.
Source: CMS 2016.

For example, a 95 percent confidence interval for the proportion of Heart Attack Patients Given ACE Inhibitor or ARB for Left Ventricular Systolic Dysfunction (LVSD) for University Hospital is 97 percent +/– 8.3 percent. The 8.3 percent comes from table 17.3 looking up the value for the row with a sample size of 71 or 25–75 and the column for the observed rate of 90 percent (highest available in the table). Based on the sample selected, one can be 95 percent sure that the population compliance with this quality indicator is between 88.7 percent and 100 percent at University Hospital. Notice that the upper bound, or limit, on the confidence interval should be 97 percent + 8.3 percent, but in practical terms the percentage cannot be more than 100 percent and therefore that is the reported upper limit.

Notice the pattern of the values presented in table 17.3. The values in the table represent the half-widths of the confidence interval or the amount to be added and subtracted from the observed rate to formulate the 95 percent confidence interval. For a fixed value of the observed rate (column in the figure), the half-width values decrease as the sample size increases. This makes intuitive sense. As the sample size increases, the analyst knows more about the population and therefore may formulate narrower or more precise intervals for the rate. For a fixed sample size (row in the figure), the half-width values increase until the observed rate is 50 percent and then decreases across the row as the observed rate decreases. This pattern is due to the fact that the standard deviation of the rate statistic is equal to the rate multiplied by one minus the rate, which is maximized at 50 percent. This also makes intuitive sense. If an event has an equal chance of occurring or not, like flipping a coin, then it is difficult to make precise estimates; and therefore, the confidence interval must be wider or less precise for a fixed sample size.

Tools for Sampling and Design

The sample size for a study is determined by the amount of precision desired for the study. There are a number of tools available to assist analysts in calculating the required sample size. Traditional statistical software packages such as SAS offers a module for sample size calculation. G-Power is a public domain software application that may be used to calculate sample size for a number of statistical methods (Buchner et al. 2007). The Office of the Inspector General (OIG) offers a statistical package called **RAT-STATS** (OIG 2007) that is free to download. RAT-STATS can be used for both sample size determination and the generation of the random numbers required for sampling.

The OIG developed RAT-STATS to help providers select samples for audits required for those under corporate integrity agreements to resolve compliance issues. The OIG also requires random sample audits to support the estimation of amounts subject to repayment under self-disclosure agreements. The claim error rate and overpayment per claim is estimated from the sample and then extrapolated to determine the repayment amount. CMS Medicare Integrity Contractors use a similar methodology to determine amounts of over- or underpayments during their audits (CMS 2010). See chapters 9 and 10 for more information on coding and organizational compliance.

Using RAT-STATS to Determine Appropriate Sample Size

Suppose a health data analyst at a recovery audit contractor (RAC) is asked to select a sample of medical records to determine if a provider is accurately coding the CC and MCCs for their congestive heart failure (CHF) cases for discharges from 10/1/2009 to 9/30/2010. The analyst knows that CHF groups to MS-DRGs 291, 292, and 293. It is also known that the provider of interest submitted 953 claims for these MS-DRGs during the time period. The RAC's medical record reviewers will make a correct or incorrect coding determination for each claim and then estimate the total amount of payment error for this MS-DRG set. The Program Integrity Manual (CMS 2010) suggests that contractors use a one-sided lower 90 percent confidence interval to determine the amount of the payment error (CMS 2010). They claim this is a conservative estimate of overpayment since there is a 90 percent probability that the true overpayment amount is more than the one-sided lower 90 percent confidence bound.

The unit of analysis in this study is the claim. The population to be sampled is the 953 claims that the provider submitted during the study period for the MS-DRGs of interest. The research question is to determine the average amount of payment error for claims assigned to an incorrect MS-DRG. In RAT-STATS this is referred to as a variable study since the goal is to measure a continuous variable such as currency or time for each sampling unit (OIG 2007).

To determine the sample size required for this audit, the analyst must set a precision range and confidence level. Suppose he or she wishes to draw a simple random sample, with a precision range of +/−5 percent and a confidence level of 80 percent. This level is selected since an 80 percent confidence level in RAT-STATS is equivalent to the one-sided 90 percent confidence interval suggested for RAC use in the CMS Program Integrity Manual (CMS 2010). The sample size calculation also requires a prior estimate of the overpayment amount average and standard deviation. These statistics are typically determined via a probe sample or pilot study, which is a version of the study performed using a small sample. From previous studies the analyst knows that the typical provider audit yields an average overpayment of $500 with a standard deviation of $150.

To determine the required sample size within RAT-STATS:

1. Open RAT-STATS
2. Click Sample Size Determination
3. Click Variable Sample Size Determination
4. Click Unrestricted
5. Click Using a Probe Sample
6. Select the No Probe Sample radio button since the mean and standard deviation from the probe sample are known and do not need to be calculated
7. Enter the Universe Size and select all confidence and precision levels (figure 17.2)
8. Click OK
9. The mean ($500) and standard deviation ($150) from the probe sample should be entered when requested
10. The required sample sizes are then presented (See figure 17.3.)

Figure 17.2. RAT-STATS variable sample size determination screen

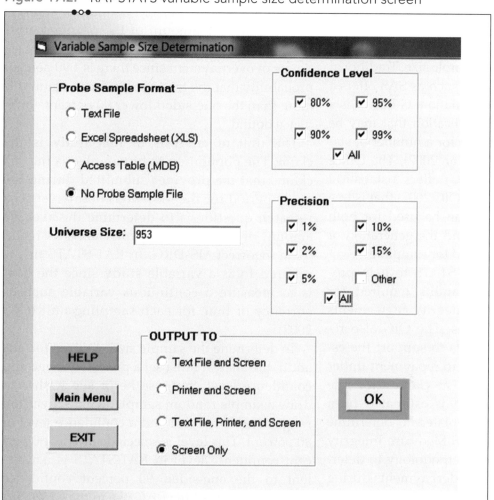

Source: OIG 2007.

Figure 17.3. RAT-STATS variable sample size output

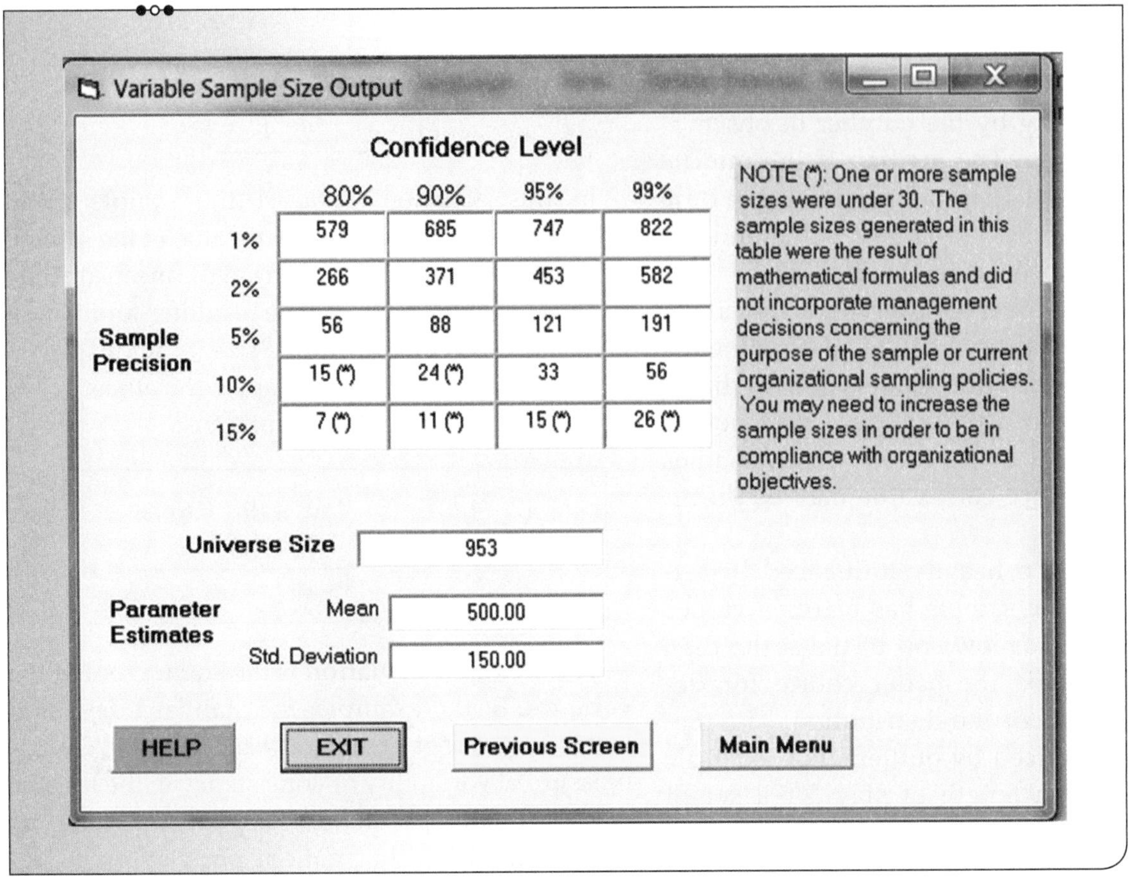

Source: OIG 2007.

The sample size required for the audit to result in the desired confidence level of 80 percent and the desired precision of 5 percent is 56. Notice that the required sample size increases as the confidence level increases and as the desired precision decreases. Decreasing precision levels are equivalent to narrower or more precise confidence intervals. This is the same pattern noted in the CMS confidence interval guidance presented in table 17.3.

Analyzing Continuous Variables

Interval and ratio scales of measurement are also referred to as **continuous variables**. Examples of continuous variables in healthcare include length of stay, charges, reimbursement, wait time, patient body mass index (BMI), and minutes to code a medical record. Descriptive statistics such as the arithmetic mean, geometric mean, median, standard deviation, and standard error may all be used to describe the distribution of a continuous variable.

Measures of Central Tendency

The center of the distribution of a continuous variable is typically described by the **mean** (arithmetic average), median, or mode. Each of these statistics has properties that make them the correct choice in a particular situation. The mean is the most common statistic used in practice. The mean is found by adding up all of the values and dividing by the number of observations in the sample. The **median** is the middle value in the sample. To find the median, the data is sorted from smallest to largest value and the center value is chosen as the median. If the sample has an even number of observations, then the two middle values are averaged to determine the median. The **mode** is the value with the highest frequency of occurrence. There may not be a unique mode for some continuous variables such as charges since each value may be different in the sample.

The mean can be heavily influenced by extreme values. If the sample has extreme values on either the high or low end of the scale, then the median may be the better choice for describing the center of the distribution. The median is less influenced by outliers. For example consider the mean length of stay for a set of patients with the following values: 2, 5, 9, 1, 6 days. The mean length of stay is 4.6 days and the median length of stay is 5 days. If the patient who stayed 9 days is replaced by a patient with a 20-day stay, the mean length of stay becomes 6.8 days while the median is still 5 days. The outlier value of 20 pulls the mean higher, but the median is unchanged by the extreme value. The mode is most often used when summarizing categorical data, since the values in continuous variables may not repeat. For instance, multiple patients are not likely to have the same charge for an admission or the same blood pressure measure. Since the number of possible values for categorical variables is typically limited to a relatively small set, repeating values are more likely and the mode is a more meaningful statistic.

Measures of Spread

The most common measures of spread of a continuous variable are the variance, standard deviation, and range. The sample **variance**, or measure of variability, is calculated as the average squared deviation from the mean. The formula for the sample variance is:

$$s^2 = \frac{\sum (y - \overline{y})^2}{n-1}$$

In this equation, subtract the sample mean (y with a bar over it) from each value in the sample (y). Each of these differences from the mean are then squared and summed up. The resulting summation is then divided by the sample size (n) minus 1.

In the length of stay example with values: 2, 5, 9, 1, 6 days, the variance calculation is:

$$s^2 = \frac{\begin{array}{c}(2-4.6)^2 + (5-4.6)^2 + (9-4.6)^2 + \\ (1-4.6)^2 + (6-4.6)^2\end{array}}{5-1} = 10.3$$

The **standard deviation** is the square root of the variance. In the example, the standard deviation is the square root of 10.3 or 3.2. The value 3.2 is a measure of variability or consistency in the lengths of stay for this population of patients. This may be compared to other patient populations to determine if the lengths of stay are more or less variable. The variance and standard deviation are both influenced by outliers. The median absolute deviation is occasionally used as an alternative measure of spread if the data includes extreme outliers, but the variance and standard deviation are the most common measures of spread used in practice.

The **range** is the difference between the minimum and maximum values. The range is very sensitive to outliers, since by definition it is calculated as the difference between the two most extreme values. The range in our example data is the maximum value (9) minus the minimum value (1) or $9 - 1 = 8$.

Inferential Statistics for Continuous Data

The presentation of the full spectrum of inferential techniques used with continuous variables is beyond the scope of this text. However, the following sections present two common methods that demonstrate the utility of statistical inference in the healthcare setting.

Inference Example: One Sample t-Test

Hypothesis tests are a common technique used to determine if the results for the sample are truly significant or if they are simply due to random chance. The **one sample t-test** is used to compare a population to a standard value. The example regarding the wait times in an ED is an application of the one sample t-test.

The first step in performing any hypothesis test is to determine the null and alternative hypotheses. Suppose in the ED wait time example, the ED director is concerned that the wait times exceed the standard of 60 minutes. The marketing director would like to run a new campaign that touts ED wait times that are significantly shorter than the standard of 60 minutes. In this case, the research question is to determine if the ED wait times are significantly shorter or longer than 60 minutes and a two-sided alternative hypothesis will be used. The null and alternative hypotheses are:

$$H_0: \mu = 60$$
$$H_1: \mu \neq 60$$

The lower case Greek letter μ (mu) represents the true population mean. This is a two-sided hypothesis test since the alternative is not equal. The next step is to determine the acceptable level of Type I error. Recall that Type I error is the probability of rejecting the null hypothesis when it is actually true. In this example, the Type I error level is set to be 5 percent. Since Type I error or rejecting the null hypothesis when it is true may cause the analyst to come to a conclusion that may cause some change in process or patient care, the level of Type I error or alpha-level for a statistical test should be selected based on the context of the test. If an error would be costly, then the Type I error should be set to a very small value. Many researchers use 5 percent or 0.05 as the acceptable level of Type I error.

A sample of 20 patients is selected and the sample mean ED wait time is 53.5 minutes with a standard deviation of 7.23 minutes. The null hypothesis may be tested using the following formula:

$$t = \frac{(\bar{x} - \mu_0)}{s / \sqrt{n}}$$
$$t = \frac{(53.5 - 60)}{7.23 / \sqrt{20}}$$

Studying the anatomy of the t-test can help formulate the intuition regarding hypothesis tests in general. In general, the null hypothesis is rejected when the test statistic, t in this case, is an extremely large positive value or extremely small negative value. The numerator of the t statistic is the difference between the sample mean (μ_0) and the null hypothesis (H_0) value. If that difference is large (positive or negative), then the t statistic is large. The denominator of the t statistic is the standard error or the standard deviation (s) divided by the square root of the sample size (n). This value is directly proportional to the standard deviation and indirectly proportional to the sample size. In other words, the standard error increases if the standard deviation is larger and decreases as the sample size grows. The t statistic increases as the standard error decreases. The t statistic is comparing the difference between the sample mean and the null hypothesis value relative to the spread in distribution and the sample size.

The determination of the value of the t statistic that is extreme enough to reject the null hypothesis is dependent on the t distribution and the acceptable level of Type I error. The t statistic is compared to the t distribution, which is similar in shape to the standard normal distribution. Using the t distribution, a cut-off or critical value can be determined so that the probability of observing a value that large by chance is the Type I error level. The critical value is determined by the Type I error level and the degrees of freedom or the sample size minus one ($n - 1$). The degrees of freedom for a statistical test is the number of observations (n) minus the number of parameters estimated when calculating the test statistic. In this case, the sample mean is estimated and then used to calculate the t test value. Therefore, the degrees of freedom for the one-sample t-test is $n - 1$. In this example, the degrees of

Figure 17.4. T distribution with 19 degrees of freedom

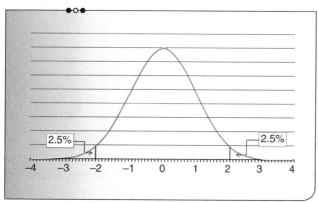

freedom are 20 − 1 = 19 and the error level is 0.05. The test statistic must be greater than 2.09 or less than −2.09 to reject the null hypothesis. This value may be derived from a table of the *t* distribution found in most statistical tests or from Microsoft Excel by using the TINV function: =TINV(0.05,19). TINV is a function in Microsoft Excel that returns the inverse of the *t* distribution given the alpha or Type I error level and degrees of freedom for a two-sided t-test. Figure 17.4 shows the shape of the *t* distribution and the probability represented by the 2.09 and −2.09 critical values. The probability of observing a value outside of −2.09 and 2.09 on the *t* distribution with 19 degrees of freedom is 2.5 percent + 2.5 percent = 5 percent.

Based on the sample the *t* statistic is:

$$t = \frac{(53.5 - 60)}{7.23/\sqrt{20}} = \frac{-6.5}{1.62} = -4.02$$

Since −4.02 is less than −2.09, the null hypothesis is rejected and the conclusion is that the ED wait time is less than the 60 minute standard. [Note: In hypothesis testing, the null hypothesis is either rejected or not rejected. The null hypothesis is never accepted.]

Inference Example: Confidence Interval for Mean

Since the null hypothesis was rejected in favor of the alternative that the ED wait times are significantly lower than the standard, the marketing director is interested in finding out how far below the standard the ED wait times might be. She is interested in publishing a figure in the new campaign, but needs to be sure the value is defensible. A confidence interval will result in a range of values with an associated level of confidence that the interval contains the population average ED wait time. The confidence level is designated to be 95 percent. The formula for the 95 percent confidence interval for the mean is:

$$\left(\bar{x} - t_{\alpha/2, n-1} \times \frac{s}{\sqrt{n}}, \; \bar{x} + t_{\alpha/2, n-1} \times \frac{s}{\sqrt{n}} \right)$$

Where $\bar{x}$ is the sample mean, $t_{\alpha/2, n-1}$ is the critical value from the *t* distribution at $\alpha/2$ with $n - 1$ degrees of freedom, s is the sample standard deviation and n is the sample size.

The confidence interval is centered at the sample mean. The width of the confidence interval is a function of the *t* distribution (confidence level), the sample standard deviation and the sample size. To calculate a 95 percent confidence interval, we set $\alpha = 0.05$ to determine the critical value of $t_{\alpha/2, n-1}$. Notice that a larger standard deviation results in a wider interval. A larger sample size results in a narrower or more precise interval. Recall that the earlier discussion about sample size selection was dependent on the sample standard deviation, the desired precision, and the confidence level. The concept of sample size selection is directly related to the width or precision of the desired confidence interval. $t_{\alpha/2, n-1}$ is the value from the *t* distribution with $n - 1$ degrees of freedom where there is an $\alpha/2$ chance of observing a value that extreme by chance. A 95 percent confidence interval may also be expressed as a $(1 - \alpha)$ percent confidence interval. In this case α is 0.05 and the degrees of freedom are 20 − 1 = 19.

$$t_{\alpha/2, n-1} = 2.09$$
$$\frac{(53.5 - 2.09 \times 7.23)}{\sqrt{20}}, \; \frac{(53.5 + 2.09 \times 7.23)}{\sqrt{20}}$$
$$(53.5 - 3.4, 53.5 + 3.4)$$
$$(50.1, 56.9)$$

The result of this analysis is that the marketing director can be 95 percent sure that the true population average ED wait time is between 50.1 and 56.9 minutes.

Two-sided hypothesis test and confidence interval for the population mean are related. The formulas contain the same sample statistics and if the confidence level is one minus the Type I error rate then the null hypothesis will be rejected for any value outside of the confidence intervals. For the ED wait time example, notice that the 95 percent confidence interval does not contain 60 minutes. The null hypothesis that the ED wait time was equal to 60 minutes was rejected at the 5 percent level. The confidence interval end points tell us that any null hypothesis greater than 56.9 minutes or less than 50.1 minutes would be rejected at the 5 percent level since those values are outside of the upper and lower bounds of the 95 percent confidence interval.

Normal Distribution

The distribution of data values may be described with statistics. The **normal distribution** is the formal name of the distribution known as the bell-shaped curve. The shape of the normal distribution is uniquely defined by its mean and standard deviation. Figure 17.5 shows the standard normal distribution, which is a special case where the mean is zero and the standard deviation is equal to one. All normally distributed variables may be transformed to the standard normal distribution

Figure 17.5. Standard normal distribution function

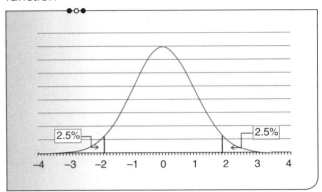

by subtracting the mean and dividing by the standard deviation.

The normal distribution is often used to describe the approximate distribution of variables. It is used in quality control charts and other tools because the percentage of the distribution within multiples of the standard deviation is easily defined. For instance, 66 percent of the distribution is concentrated between one standard deviation below to one standard deviation above the mean; 95 percent of the distribution is concentrated between two standard deviations below to two standard deviations above the mean; and over 99 percent of the distribution is concentrated between three standard deviations below the mean to three standard deviations above the mean.

Check Your Understanding 17.1

Instructions: **Answer the following questions on a separate piece of paper.**

1. Which of the following is a measure of central tendency?
   A. Variance
   B. Median
   C. Standard deviation
   D. Range

2. When describing the typical length of stay for patients admitted for congestive heart failure, which is the most appropriate measure of central tendency when there are a number of long stay outliers?
   A. Minimum
   B. Mean
   C. Median
   D. Mode

3. The one sample t-test may be used to:
   A. Determine if a distribution is highly variable
   B. Determine if a population mean is likely to be different from a standard value
   C. Determine the most likely value of the population mean
   D. Define a range of likely values for the population mean

4. Type I error in an hypothesis test is:
   A. The probability of rejecting the null hypothesis when it is false
   B. The probability of rejecting the null hypothesis when it is true
   C. The probability of not rejecting the null hypothesis when it is true
   D. The probability of not rejecting the null hypothesis with it is false

5. If the average length of stay for a sample of 15 patients is 2.3 days and the standard deviation is 1.5 days, which of the following statements is true?
   A. A 95 percent confidence interval will be wider than a 90 percent confidence interval.
   B. A 95 percent confidence interval and 90 percent confidence interval will be the same.
   C. A 95 percent confidence interval will be narrower than a 90 percent confidence interval width.
   D. Not enough information is provided to answer.

Analyzing Rates and Proportions

Rates and proportions are actually summary statistics based on either a sample or population. A **rate** is the number of times an event of interest occurs divided by the number of times that event could have occurred. The event and the number eligible must be carefully defined so that the calculations of rates are valid and reproducible.

Descriptive Statistics for Rates and Proportions

Rates may be reported as percentages, counts per 1,000, or as a fraction as in x out of y. When calculating a rate, the numerator (top number in a fraction) is the number of subjects with the trait of interest. The denominator (bottom number in a fraction) is the number of subjects that could have had the trait of interest.

Consider the example of measuring the mortality rate at a facility. The mortality rate may be interpreted as the probability of any one of the 100 patients dying. In other words, in the context of this analysis each patient has two outcomes—living or dying. The mortality rate calculated from a sample is an estimate of the population probability of dying or p.

It is always good practice to not only estimate the probability or p of an event, but to also estimate the variance or spread around the sample proportion estimate. If our sample of size n produces a proportion estimate of p, denoted as $\hat{p}$, then standard error of a proportion estimate is:

$$SE_p = \sqrt{\frac{\hat{p} \times (1 - \hat{p})}{n}}$$

The standard error of the sample proportion is the standard deviation divided by the square root of the sample size. In this formula, $\hat{p}$ is the estimated proportion based on the random sample. Therefore, both the mean and the standard error of the sample proportion depends on the estimated value. Notice that the standard error decreases and the sample size increases. The value of SE_p is maximized when the sample proportion is 0.5 or 50 percent. Recall from the discussion of the CMS quality indicators that the confidence intervals using their guidance were the widest when the observed rate was 50 percent.

Inferential Statistics for Rates and Proportions

The most common types of inferential statistical techniques used with rates and proportions are hypothesis tests to compare rates to a standard or confidence intervals. If an analyst is trying to determine if a rate is higher or lower than a standard, then a hypothesis is the correct statistical technique. In hypothesis testing, the first step is to define the null hypothesis (status quo)(H_0) and the alternative or research hypothesis (H_1).

$$H_0 : p = p_0$$
$$H_1 : p \neq p_0$$

The test is performed to determine if the analyst should reject the null hypothesis at a given error level. This is called the Type I error level. The error level should be set low (0.01 or 0.05) as the action to be taken is costly in terms of money, time, or patient lives. If the question is less critical, then the error level may be set higher. The test statistic used in this situation is a z test. A z test should be used to test hypotheses regarding proportions:

$$z = \frac{(\hat{p} - p_0)}{\sqrt{p_0 \times (1 - p_0)/n}}$$

In this formula, n is the sample size, p_0 is the null hypothesis value and $\hat{p}$ is the estimated proportion based on the random sample. If the test statistic z is greater than $z_{\alpha/2}$ or less than $-z_{\alpha/2}$ where α is the predefined Type I error level. For this test, the standard normal distribution is used to determine a critical value beyond which the null hypothesis should be rejected. If the error level of the test is 0.05 or 5 percent, then the critical value or $z_{\alpha/2}$ is 1.96. This may be derived from the standard normal table found in most statistics text books or from using the following formula in Excel: =NORMSINV(0.025). NORMSINV(0.025) will return a z score that represents the point for which 2.5 percent of the curve is outside +/− that point. The argument 0.025 is used because the Type I error level was set to 0.05 and this is a two-sided test (0.05/2 = 0.025). Figure 17.5 shows the critical values on the probability curve of the standard normal distribution. As with the t-test, one half of the Type I error is allocated to each side of the curve. Notice that the critical value for the standard normal distribution is slightly smaller than that from the t distribution

with 19 degrees of freedom. As the degrees of freedom for the t distribution increases, it becomes closer to the standard normal distribution.

One of the CMS quality indicators measures the proportion of Pneumonia Patients Assessed and Given Influenza Vaccination. A facility may wish to compare their rate to the national vaccination rate. If 80 percent of the patients out of a sample of 74 eligible patients received a flu vaccine at University Hospital can we conclude that their vaccination rate is significantly different from the national rate of 91 percent?

The hypothesis to be tested here is:

$$H_0 : p = 0.91$$
$$H_1 : p \neq 0.91$$

The test statistic is:

$$z = \frac{(0.80 - 0.91)}{\sqrt{0.91 \times (1 - 0.91)/74}} = \frac{-0.110}{0.033} = -3.33$$

Since the test statistic, $z = -3.33$, is less than the critical value, -1.96, the null hypothesis is rejected. The conclusion is that University Hospital's flu vaccine rate for pneumonia patients is significantly lower than the national rate.

The $z_{\alpha/2}$ is the same critical value identified for the two-sided hypothesis test presented. A 95 percent confidence interval for the flu vaccine rate at University Hospital is:

$$\left(\hat{p} - z_{\alpha/2} \times \sqrt{\frac{\hat{p} \times (1 - \hat{p})}{n}}, \hat{p} + z_{\alpha/2} \times \sqrt{\frac{\hat{p} \times (1 - \hat{p})}{n}} \right)$$

$$\left(0.80 - 1.96 \times \sqrt{\frac{0.80 \times (1 - 0.80)}{74}}, \right.$$
$$\left. 0.80 + 1.96 \times \sqrt{\frac{0.80 \times (1 - 0.80)}{74}} \right)$$

$$\left(0.80 - 1.96 \times \sqrt{\frac{0.80 \times (1 - 0.80)}{74}}, \right.$$
$$\left. 0.80 + 1.96 \times \sqrt{\frac{0.80 \times (1 - 0.80)}{74}} \right)$$

$$(0.80 - 0.09, 0.80 + 0.09) \; or \; (0.71, 0.89)$$

The 95 percent confidence interval for the population pneumonia patient flu vaccine rate is from 71 percent to 89 percent. This precision for this interval is +/− 9 percent. If a more precise interval is desired, then a large sample size should be collected for the next measurement period.

Check Your Understanding 17.2

Instructions: **Answer the following questions on a separate piece of paper.**

1. The sample mean and standard error of a proportion is dependent on:
   A. The estimated proportion
   B. The sample size
   C. Both of these values
   D. Neither of these values

2. Which distribution is used to test a hypothesis regarding proportions?
   A. Normal distribution
   B. T-distribution
   C. Uniform distribution
   D. F-distribution

3. If we wish to test the hypothesis that a facility's mortality rate is significantly different than the state average of 5 percent, which of the following null and alternative hypotheses are appropriate?
   A. H_o: p ≤ 5%; H_1: p≥5%
   B. H_o: p = 5%; H_1: p≠5%
   C. H_o: p > 5%; H_1: p≤5%
   D. H_o: p≠ 5%; H_1: p=5%

4. If a 95 percent confidence interval for the proportion of postoperative infections is (0.9 percent, 1.5 percent), what is the precision of that interval?
   A. ±1.5%
   B. ±0.6%
   C. ±0.9%
   D. ±0.3%

5. If the test statistic for testing the hypothesis that the readmission rate at General Hospital is different from zero is $z = 3.45$, what would the conclusion of the test be at the 0.05 level?
   A. Accept H_o
   B. Reject H_1
   C. Reject H_o
   D. Do not reject H_o

Analyzing Relationships between Two Variables

A data analyst may need to explore the relationship between two variables. Examples include the relationship between length of stay and charges, patient age, and mortality, or number of coding staff members and number of records coded per shift.

Correlation

Correlation is the statistic that is used to describe the association or relationship between two variables.

In the healthcare setting, we may note that length of stay and charges are highly related or correlated. Since charges increase as length of stay increases, it is said that the two variables are positively correlated. An example of two variables that are negatively correlated may be years of coder experience and time to code a medical record. If the more experienced coders have shorter review times, then the two variables are negatively correlated.

Pearson's Correlation Coefficient

Pearson's correlation coefficient or r measures the strength of the linear relationship between two variables. The statistic can range from -1 to $+1$. Negative one is perfect negative correlation while positive one is perfect positive correlation. The formula for calculating Pearson's correlation coefficient is:

$$r = \frac{\sum_{i=1}^{n}(X_i - \bar{X}) \times (Y_i - \bar{Y})}{\sqrt{\sum_{i=1}^{n}(X_i - \bar{X})^2} \times \sqrt{\sum_{i=1}^{n}(Y_i - \bar{Y})^2}}$$

Where $\bar{X}$ and $\bar{Y}$ are the mean of the variables X and Y respectively and n is the number of data points.

Notice that the numerator of the statistic will determine the sign of the correlation. Confidence intervals and hypothesis tests may be performed to make inference about the strength of association between two variables. Pearson's r is a measure of correlation and not causation. Causation is far more difficult to prove via data and really requires a carefully designed and controlled experiment to prove.

Suppose an analyst wishes to study the relationship between number of years of coding experience and time required to code an outpatient medical record. The analyst selects a random sample of seven coders and collects the data presented in table 17.4 (answers are rounded to two decimal places).

The Pearson's r for experience and time is:

$$r = \frac{\sum_{i=1}^{n}(X_i - 3.0) \times (Y_i - 41.6)}{\sqrt{\sum_{i=1}^{n}(X_i - 3.0)^2} \times \sqrt{\sum_{i=1}^{n}(Y_i - 41.6)^2}}$$

$$r = \frac{-56.93}{\sqrt{21.50} \times \sqrt{286.00}} = -0.83$$

The interpretation of the negative value of the correlation coefficient is that time to code records decreases as experience increases. A scatter plot of two variables is a useful tool for exploring the relationship. Figure 17.6 shows the decreasing trend in coding time as the years of experience increase for each subject in the sample.

Pearson's r may be converted to the **coefficient of determination** or r^2. The r^2 measures how much of the variation in one variable is explained by the second variable. In this example, $r^2 = (-0.83)^2 = 0.68$. Therefore 68 percent of the variance in coding time may be explained by the years of experience.

Simple Linear Regression

Simple linear regression (SLR) is another type of statistical inference that not only measures the strength of the relationship between two variables, but also estimates a functional relationship

Table 17.4. Example calculation Pearson's correlation coefficient

Subject	X: Experience (yr)	Y: Time (min)	$(X_i - \bar{X}) \times (Y_i - \bar{Y})$	$(X_i - \bar{X})^2$	$(Y_i - \bar{Y})^2$
1	5.00	30.00	(20.94)	3.72	117.88
2	1.00	55.00	(29.30)	4.29	200.02
3	2.50	45.00	(2.37)	0.33	17.16
4	4.50	35.00	(8.37)	2.04	34.31
5	3.50	45.00	1.78	0.18	17.16
6	2.00	39.00	1.99	1.15	3.45
7	3.00	37.00	0.28	0.01	14.88
Total	**21.50**	**286.00**	**(56.93)**	**11.71**	**404.86**

Figure 17.6. Example of relationship between two continuous variables

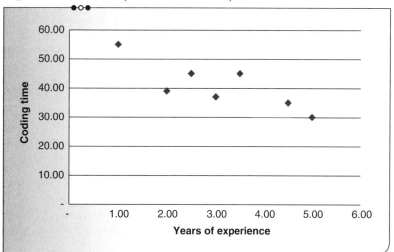

between them. SLR may be used when one of the two variables of interest is dependent on the other. For instance, the total charge incurred during an inpatient stay is often dependent on the length of time spent in the hospital. Regression may also be used to describe the relationship between coder experience and time per record beyond simply stating they have a negative correlation or inverse relationship. In general the variable that is used to predict is called the **independent variable**. The outcome or variable to be predicted is called the **dependent variable** (White 2015).

SLR is typically performed by fitting a line via a least squares algorithm. Basically, the least squares method selects the line that minimizes the vertical (Y) distance between all points and the selected line. The result is a line that may not actually go through any points, but comes as close as possible to all points. The least squares line for this example is displayed in figure 17.7.

The slope of the least squares line is always the same sign as the correlation between the two variables. The formula for the least squares line for this data is:

$$[Coding\ time] = -4.86 \times [Experience] + 55.78$$

The SLR line represents the predicted or expected values of the dependent variable given various values of the independent variable. The interpretation of this relationship is that the predicted coding time for a coder with no experience is 55.78 minutes. This value, 55.78, is referred to as the y-intercept of the line. Each year of experience reduces the predicted time to code records by 4.86 minutes. This value, –4.86, is referred to as the slope of the line. The slope is an estimate of the change in the dependent variable, y, which is expected for each one unit change in the independent variable, x. The line displayed in figure 17.7 states that the expected coding time for a coder with four years of experience is y = –4.86 × 4 + 55.78 = 36.34 minutes. The coefficient of determination is used to measure the explanatory power of the linear regression line. As previously calculated, the $r^2 = 0.68$. The years of experience of a coder explains 68 percent of the variance in coding time. One application of this regression line is to create personalized workload expectations for each coder based on experience. A performance ratio could then be calculated as the observed coding time divided by the expected coding time for each coder to monitor performance and provide feedback for improvement. A performance ratio greater than one would indicate better than expected performance and a performance ratio less than one would indicate a performance that requires improvement.

Figure 17.7.   Example of least squares line

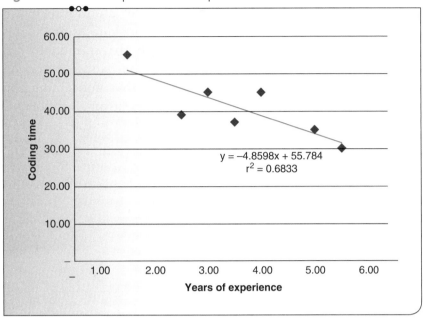

Figure 17.8.   Relationship between length of stay and total charge for CHF inpatient stays

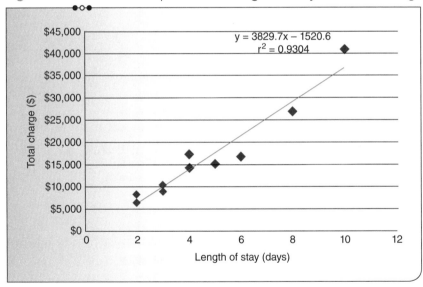

Another interesting application of SLR is studying the relationship between charge per inpatient visit and length of stay for inpatient stays. The least squares line may be used to break out the fixed and variable portions of the charges.

Figure 17.8 displays the relationship between patient length of stay and total charges for congestive heart failure. The relationship between length of stay and total charge is very strong with an r^2 of 0.93. In other words, length of stay explains 93 percent of the variance in total charge. This strong relationship between total charge and length of stay is true for many medical inpatient stays. The relationship between these two variables may be less strong for surgical inpatient stays if the charge for the surgery is a large proportion of the total charge.

The model in figure 17.8 states that the predicted total charge equals $1,521 + $3,830 × LOS. The intercept of the line, $1,521, represents the fixed charge of a CHF inpatient stay. Fixed charge items are registration, administration, initial laboratory, or radiology work ups that are not dependent on how long the patient stays. The slope of the line represents the variable component of the charge. Variable charge items are nursing care, dietary, maintenance medications, and other resources that are used each day of the stay. Breaking the charges into the fixed and variable components facilitates root cause analysis studies into the variation in resources used to treat various types of patients. For instance, the charges for CHF patients are clearly driven more by the variable component than the fixed component. CHF treatment protocols that concentrate on length of stay reduction may be an effective way to ensure proper resources are used to treat these patients. For a joint replacement or other surgical case with significant medical supply costs, it is unlikely that a length of stay study would be very effective.

Check Your Understanding 17.3

Instructions: Answer the following questions on a separate piece of paper.

1. If the correlation between patient lung volume level and BMI is 0.6, which of the following conclusions is correct?
   A. Patients with low BMI have large lung volume
   B. Patients with high BMI have large lung volume
   C. High BMI causes large lung volume
   D. Large lung volume causes high BMI

2. Which statistic measures the strength of the linear relationship between two variables?
   A. Slope of the linear regression line
   B. t-test
   C. Correlation
   D. Intercept of the linear regression line

3. If the coefficient of determination for this SLR model: Cost = 1,500 + 300 × LOS is 0.8, then which of the following statements is correct?
   A. 80 percent of the variance in length of stay is explained by cost
   B. 20 percent of the variance in cost is explained by length of stay
   C. 80 percent of the variance in cost is explained by length of stay
   D. 20 percent of the variance in length of stay is explained by cost

4. Using the model in questions 3: Cost = 1,500 + 300 × LOS, what is the interpretation of the slope of the line?
   A. The typical cost of care is $1,500
   B. For every one day increase in length of stay, the cost will decrease by $300
   C. For every one day increase in length of stay, the cost will increase by $300
   D. The cost of care and length of stay are not related

5. Using the model in question 3: Cost = 1,500 + 300 × LOS, what is the interpretation of the intercept of the line?
   A. For every one day increase in length of stay, the cost will increase by $1,500
   B. The fixed cost of admitting a patient is $1,500
   C. For every one day increase in length of stay, the cost will decrease by $1,500
   D. The fixed cost of admitting a patient is $300

Analytics in Practice

There are numerous practical applications of data analytics in healthcare. Just a few examples include data mining, predictive modeling, analysis of risk adjusted quality indicators, and real-time analytics.

Data Mining

The techniques of data analytics may be used to perform data mining. In **data mining**, the analyst performs exploratory data analysis to determine trends and identify patterns in the data set. Data mining is sometimes referred to as knowledge discovery.

In healthcare, data mining may be used to determine if it is cost effective to expand facilities. An analysis of appointment wait times for patients to see a certain type of specialist or to receive a particular diagnostic test might indicate a need to expand that service. Data mining may also be used to analyze referral patterns of physicians within a particular network.

In traditional data analytics, data is collected for a specific purpose to answer a business or research question. In data mining, data is often used for secondary analysis. That is, the data is used for a purpose that was not the primary reason for collection. Claims data is an excellent data source for mining and finding patterns, but the primary purpose of claims data is for submission to ask for payment and not data mining (White 2015).

In data mining, historical data is analyzed to find trends and patterns. Those trends and patterns are then used in business planning or process improvement. This historical technique may be extended to predict future behavior based on the data via predictive modeling techniques.

Predictive Modeling

Predictive modeling is another application of data analytics in healthcare. Predictive modeling is actually a special application of data mining. CMS is using predictive modeling to identify potential fraudulent Medicare claims (White 2011).

The pattern of claims submitted by a provider is analyzed to identify trends that are unlikely given the claims history of the provider or the patient. For instance, predictive modeling may be used to identify a provider that submits a claim for a service that is unrelated to their specialty or a high cost service for which they have not submitted a previous claim. The goal of this technique is to target claims that are unlikely to be valid and select them for further review.

Predictive modeling applies statistical techniques to determine the likelihood of certain events occurring together (White 2011). Statistical methods are applied to historical data to learn the patterns in the data. These patterns are used to create models of what is most likely to occur. Predictive modeling is used by credit card issuers to determine if transactions are likely fraudulent. Customers who receive a phone call from their credit card company verifying that they authorized a transaction were the subjects of a predictive model.

For example, a customer's typical credit card transaction is $100. The credit card issuer notices that the customer submitted three $5,000 transactions in one day. Given the customer's history and the credit card issuer's historical data regarding fraudulent transactions, those transactions look suspicious. The credit card company may then put a hold on the card and call to verify that the customer really did authorize the suspect transactions. The triggers that tell the credit card company when to suspect a fraud issue are created via predictive modeling techniques.

Predictive modeling techniques use multiple data sources. Data such as the provider's claim history, the patient's demographics and health status, the services included on the claim, and the attributes associated with previously identified fraudulent claims may all be used to develop a statistical model. Statistical techniques used to create the model may include logistic regression, cluster analysis, or decision trees. All of these statistical techniques allow the user to combine multivariate (more than one outcome variable) historical data into a model that may be used to assess the probability or likelihood that current claims are fraudulent.

In logistical regression, the likelihood that a claim is fraudulent is estimated based on a series of historical data. In cluster analysis, historical data are used to build a model that will measure the distance of a claim from the typical claims submitted by that provider or for that type of service. Decision trees use a series of screens or yes or no questions to determine the probability that a claim is valid. The output of each of these methods is the probability of a claim's validity that is expressed as a claim score.

The claim score is typically structured so that it is directly related to the probability that a claim is in error. A high score may indicate a high probability that a claim is not legitimate. If the score meets a criteria (either above or below a cutoff value), then it is identified as a potential error. The criteria or cutoff value may be used to tune the model to control the sensitivity and specificity of the model. If the cutoff is too extreme, then the model may not be sensitive enough and will allow fraudulent claims to be paid. If the cutoff is not extreme enough, then the model may not be specific enough and identify a large number of false positives.

In the healthcare setting the cost of paying fraudulent claims must be weighed against the cost of withholding payment and reviewing the claim prior to payment. For high-cost/low-volume claims, the cutoff may be set lower to ensure that no questionable claims are paid. The cost of paying an invalid claim outweighs the cost of reviewing a few false positive claims. The model may be adapted and adjusted as more claims history is aggregated.

Many commercial payers currently use predictive modeling as one of their fraud prevention techniques. The UnitedHealth Group (UnitedHealth Group 2009) estimated that the use of predictive modeling in the Medicare and Medicaid programs could save the programs $113 billion over the first 10 years of use. A study from the Lewin Group (Lewin Group 2009) validated the UnitedHealth Group's estimates and further estimated savings of $128.6 billion over the same first 10 years of use.

Risk-Adjusted Quality Indicators

The values for some quality and outcomes indicators in healthcare are dependent on the mix of patients treated at that facility. For example, the 30-day mortality rate at a major academic medical center cannot be directly compared to the 30-day mortality rate at a rural community hospital without some sort of adjustment for the difference in acuity of the patients. CMS uses a hierarchical regression model to adjust for both individual patient characteristics as well as hospital characteristics. The model calculates an expected 30-day mortality rate for each hospital and then compares the expected rate to the observed rate when reporting statistics on their Hospital Compare website. The method is similar to the observed versus expected productivity ratio presented in the simple linear regression portion of this chapter. The model used to calculate the expected mortality is far more complex, but the interpretation is the same. CMS calculates a risk standardized mortality rate (RSMR) based on the expected mortality rate and the observed mortality rate for each condition and hospital profiled (CMS 2011). Lower RSMR implies a hospital has better quality as measured by these rates.

Although the details involved in hierarchical regression are beyond the scope of this text, the concept that an observed rate is compared to an expected rate to determine relative performance makes intuitive sense. The exact methodology to derive the expected rate may vary depending on the research question and the data available for modeling.

A more straightforward method for calculating a RSMR is to use **indirect standardization** (Osborn 2005) to derive the expected rate for an outcome variable. Indirect standardization is appropriate to use for risk adjustment when the risk variables are categorical and the rate or proportion for the variable of interest is available for the standard or reference group at the level of the risk categories. The expected outcome rate for each risk category is calculated based on the reference group and then weighted by the volume in each risk group at the population to be compared to the standard.

Table 17.5. MS-DRG 308, 309, 310 mortality rates

MS-DRG and name		Estimated US in-hospital mortality rate	The Hospital statistics			
			The hospital discharges	Observed in-hospital deaths	Observed mortality rate	Expected deaths
308	Cardiac arrhythmia and conduction disorders w mcc	4.9%	152	6	3.9%	7.39
309	Cardiac arrhythmia and conduction disorders w cc	0.8%	158	2	1.3%	1.31
310	Cardiac arrhythmia and conduction disorders w/o cc/mcc	0.2%	191	0	0.0%	0.46
Totals		1.3%	501	8	1.6%	9.16

Source: HHS 2009.

Indirect standardization is not useful when trying to compare the outcomes at two facilities, but is useful when comparing a facility to a standard.

The example data presented in table 17.5 presents the in-hospital mortality rate for the family of cardiac arrhythmia and conduction disorder MS-DRGs for the United States as well as The Hospital. The observed overall in-hospital mortality rate for The Hospital, 1.6 percent, is higher than the national rate, 1.3 percent. The Hospital actually recorded lower mortality rates for patients assigned to two of the three individual MS-DRGs. The Hospital actually had lower mortality in MS-DRG 308, which includes patients with major complications and co-morbidities. The proportion of the patients in each MS-DRG is not available for the national statistics, it is not known if The Hospital's mix is more concentrated in the MS-DRGs with major complications or co-morbidities. The national rates for each MS-DRG may be used to estimate the expected mortality rate for The Hospital using indirect standardization.

The first step in indirect standardization is to use the hospital's volume and the national in-hospital mortality rate for each risk category to calculate the expected number of deaths. In this example, the MS-DRGs represent the risk categories. Based on the data in table 17.5 the expected number of deaths for each of the MS-DRGs is:

- MS-DRG 308: $0.049 \times 152 = 7.39$
- MS-DRG 309: $0.008 \times 158 = 1.31$
- MS-DRG 310: $0.002 \times 191 = 0.46$

The three MS-DRG expected deaths are then added together to yield the expected number of deaths at the hospital: $7.39 + 1.31 + 0.46 = 9.16$. The expected in-house mortality rate for the hospital is then $9.16/501 = 1.8$ percent. The observed and expected mortalities may then be used to calculate a standardized mortality ratio (SMR).

$$SMR = \frac{Observed\ Mortality\ Rate}{Expected\ Mortality\ Rate}$$

The SMR for the hospital is 1.6 percent / 1.8 percent or 0.89. An SMR value less than one means the observed mortality rate is lower than expected and an SMR greater than one means the observed mortality rate is higher than expected. The SMR for the hospital is 0.89 indicating that the observed in-hospital mortality rate is lower than expected. Note that the unadjusted observed mortality rate for the hospital was actually higher than the national rate. Indirect standardization gave the hospital credit for the lower mortality rate in the most resource intense cases and therefore allowed an apples-to-apples comparison to the national rate.

Real-Time Analytics

As data analysis tools mature and the granularity of the data available in a healthcare entity increases, real-time analytics and performance dashboards based on key performance indicators (KPI) are becoming the norm. Once a set of KPIs is identified, data elements to drive those indicators are created in real-time and not based on static historical databases. For example, a KPI for a HIM manager at a hospital may be the level of charges in the set of discharged and not final billed (DNFB) charts. If the level of charges goes above a predefined threshold, then an e-mail is sent to the manager to notify him of that fact so that action may be taken quickly. Without real-time analytics producing the KPI and alert, the manager may not have been alerted of the high level of DNFB until a weekly or monthly report was produced.

Some of the KPIs that may be included in real-time dashboards include both financial and clinical indicators, such as:

- Days in accounts receivable
- Charges in DNFB
- Patient census by unit
- Number of patients in ED waiting for inpatient bed
- ED wait time

- Number of patients waiting for discharge
- Time for housekeeping to return a bed to service

KPI dashboards are now used throughout healthcare organizations. Many healthcare IT vendors now include at least some level of KPI dashboard functionality in their systems. The difficulty in implementing such systems effectively is setting thresholds for the various KPIs that are meaningful and do not identify false positives. Many hospital performance indicators such as volume, length of stay, and emergency department wait times have a certain amount of typical variability. Setting thresholds that are too sensitive could result in management investigating issues that are not unusual. Combining KPIs with the concepts of analytics such as confidence intervals and other statistical inference tools can produce a system of real-time alerts that are both sensitive enough to identify performance issue yet specific enough to avoid false positives.

Opportunities for Health Information Management Professionals in Healthcare Data Analytics

Health information management (HIM) professionals are uniquely positioned to take on a variety of roles related to healthcare data analytics. Combining the following skills transforms the traditional HIM role into one of a business analyst:

- Understand data structures and coding systems
- Understand available data and methods for integration
- Communicate with both finance and IT staff
- Act as a business analyst—far more valuable than a pure data analyst

For instance, in revenue cycle management, the identification of missed charges is challeng-

ing. The traditional approach to identifying missed charges is to perform a charge description master (CDM) review and interview unit staff to ensure charge codes are utilized as designed. The staff may also review departmental order sheets to ensure they include complete and accurate listings of the services available in the department. A HIM professional with strong analytic skills may take a data-driven approach to study this issue. Credentials such as AHIMA Certified Health Data Analyst (CHDA) allow HIM professionals to demonstrate their expertise in this area.

The charge codes that occur together often may be identified through profiling of the historical claims data. Claims with only one of those codes may be selected for focused review. A chart review on that set of records that are most likely to include missed charges may then be completed to understand the root cause of the missing charges. The use of analytics on the historical claims may save a significant amount of time in the identification of particular codes that are problematic. Corrective action may be designed and implemented in a much more efficient manner.

Opportunities to apply analytics to common operational issues are present throughout the healthcare business setting. AHIMA's Healthcare Data Analysis Toolkit lists a number of responsibilities that may be required of HIM professionals to perform analysis-based jobs in healthcare (Bronnert et al. 2011).

An entry-level health data analyst position may include the following analytic responsibilities:

- Identify, analyze, and interpret trends or patterns in complex data sets
- In collaboration with others, interpret data and develop recommendations on the basis of findings
- Develop graphs, reports, and presentations of project results, trends, data mining
- Perform basic statistical analyses for projects and reports
- Create and present quality dashboards
- Generate routine and/or ad hoc reports

A mid-level health data analyst position may include the following additional analytic responsibilities:

- Work collaboratively with data, reporting, and the database administrator to help produce effective production management and utilization management reports in support of performance management related to utilization, cost, and risk with the various health plan data; monitor data integrity and quality of reports on a monthly basis
- Work collaboratively with data and reporting in monitoring financial performance in each health plan
- Develop and maintain claims audit reporting and processes
- Develop and maintain contract models in support of contract negotiations with health plans

- Develop, implement, and enhance evaluation and measurement models for the quality, data and reporting, and data warehouse department programs, projects, and initiatives for maximum effectiveness
- Recommend improvements to processes, programs, and initiatives by using analytical skills and a variety of reporting tools
- Determine the most appropriate approach for internal and external report design, production, and distribution, specific to the relevant audience

A senior-level health data analyst position may include the following additional analytic responsibilities:

- Understand and address the information needs of governance, leadership, and staff to support continuous improvement of patient care processes and outcomes
- Lead and manage efforts to enhance the strategic use of data and analytic tools to improve clinical care processes and outcomes continuously
- Work to ensure the dissemination of accurate, reliable, timely, accessible, actionable information (data analysis) to help leaders and staff actively identify and address opportunities to improve patient care and related processes
- Work actively with information technology to select and develop tools to enable facility governance and leadership to monitor the progress of quality, patient safety, service, and related metrics continuously throughout the system
- Engage and collaborate with information technology and senior leadership to create and maintain a succinct report (for example, dashboard), as well as a balanced set of system assessment measures, that convey status and direction of key systemwide quality and patient safety initiatives for the trustee quality and safety committee and senior management; present this information regularly to the quality and safety

committee of the board to ensure understanding of information contained therein

- Actively support the efforts of divisions, departments, programs, and clinical units to identify, obtain, and actively use quantitative information needed to support clinical quality monitoring and improvement activities
- Function as an advisor and technical resource regarding the use of data in clinical quality improvement activities
- Lead analysis of outcomes and resource utilization for specific patient populations as necessary
- Lead efforts to implement state-of-the-art quality improvement analytical tools (that is, statistical process control)

- Play an active role, including leadership, where appropriate, on teams addressing systemwide clinical quality improvement opportunities

The level of understanding of the relationship between variables analyzed and the complexity of the analytic techniques increase as an HIM professional advances from the entry to senior level. The common thread through all of these job responsibilities is strong basic analytic skills and understanding of the healthcare application of those techniques. HIM professionals that have a solid grasp of statistical techniques can combine those skills with their knowledge of the clinical application of data to assist with the interpretation and application of the results of analysis projects.

 ## Check Your Understanding 17.4

Instructions: Answer the following questions on a separate piece of paper.

1. Analysis of data to find trends and patterns is called:
   A. Data warehousing
   B. Data governance
   C. Data mining
   D. Data transfer

2. What type of data is used for a purpose that was not the primary reason for collection?
   A. Secondary data
   B. Primary data
   C. Statistical data
   D. All of the above

3. What application of data mining is used to identify potential fraudulent Medicare claims?
   A. Database modeling
   B. Knowledge management
   C. Total quality management
   D. Predictive modeling

4. Which of the following statistical techniques can be used to create a model to assess the probability that current Medicare claims are fraudulent?
   A. Logistic regression
   B. Cluster analysis
   C. Decision trees
   D. All of the above

5. Credentials that demonstrate expertise in data analytics are:
   A. CHDA
   B. CHPS
   C. CHDI
   D. CPHQ

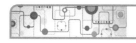

References

Bronnert, J., J. Clark, L. Hyde, J. Solberg, S. White, and M. Wolin. 2011. *Health Data Analysis Toolkit*. Chicago: AHIMA.

Buchner, A., E. Erdfelder, F. Faul, and A.G. Lang. 2007. G*Power: Statistical Power Analyses for Windows and Mac. http://www.psycho.uni-duesseldorf.de/abteilungen/aap/gpower3

Centers for Medicare and Medicaid Services. 2016. Confidence Interval. https://www.medicare.gov/HomeHealthCompare/Data/Confidence-Interval.html

Centers for Medicare and Medicaid Services. 2015. Hospital Compare. http://www.hospitalcompare.hhs.gov

Centers for Medicare and Medicaid Services. 2011. Statistical Methods Used to Calculate Rates. https://www.medicare.gov/homehealthcompare/Data/Statistical-Methods.html

Centers for Medicare and Medicaid Services. 2010. Program Integrity Manual. 2010. https://www.cms.gov/Regulations-and-Guidance/Guidance/Manuals/Internet-Only-Manuals-IOMs-Items/CMS019033.html

Centers for Medicare and Medicaid Services. 2009. Roadmap for Implementing Value-Driven Healthcare in the Traditional Medicare Fee-for-Service Program. Technical Report. Baltimore, MD: CMS. http://www.cms.gov/Medicare/Quality-Initiatives-Patient-Assessment-Instruments/QualityInitiativesGenInfo/Downloads/VBPRoadmap_OEA_1-16_508.pdf

Healthcare Financial Management Association. 2015. HFMA's MAP. http://www.hfma.org/map

Krajniak, M.I., K. Anderson, and A.R. Eisen. 2016. Separation Anxiety. In *Encyclopedia of Mental Health*, 2nd ed. Edited by Friedman, H.S. Waltham, MA: Elsevier.

Office of the Inspector General. 2007. RAT-STATS Statistical Software. http://oig.hhs.gov/compliance/rat-stats/index.asp

Osborn, C. 2005. *Statistical Applications for Health Information Management*, 2nd ed. Sudbury, MA: Jones and Bartlett.

QualityNet. 2015. Specifications Manual for National Hospital Inpatient Quality Measures, Version 5.0b. https://www.qualitynet.org/dcs/ContentServer?c=Page&pagename=QnetPublic%2FPage%2FQnetTier4&cid=1228774725171

SAS Institute. 2006. *White Paper: Analytics in Healthcare*. Cary, NC: SAS.

UnitedHealth Group. 2009 (June). Health Care Cost Containment—How Technology Can Cut Red Tape and Simplify Health Care Administration. http://www.unitedhealthgroup.com/~/media/UHG/PDF/2009/UNH-Working-Paper-2.ashx

US Department of Health and Human Services. 2009. Welcome to HCUPnet. http://hcupnet.ahrq.gov/HCUPnet.jsp

White, S. 2015. *A Practical Approach to Analyzing Healthcare Data*, 3rd ed. Chicago: AHIMA.

White, S. 2011 (Sept.). Predictive modeling 101. *Journal of AHIMA* 82(9): 46–47.

White, S., C. Kallem, A. Viola, and J. Bronnert. 2011 (June). An ACO primer. *Journal of AHIMA* 6(82):48–49.

18

Data Visualization

David Marc, MBS, CHDA

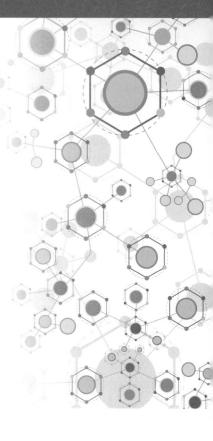

In medicine, practitioners and other professionals are faced with almost insurmountable amounts of data pertaining to clinical symptoms, laboratory results, medications, quality reporting, reimbursement and cost data, survey data, and such. This information is ultimately utilized for decision making.

However, given the volume, variety, and complexity of the data, there is the potential for errors in decision making. As such, methods are continually being developed to aid in the decision-making process by presenting information using charts. Charts can help supplement human information processes to maximize the efficiency of interpreting data while minimizing interpretation errors.

The purpose of a chart is to display information, and when the chart is viewed by a person, the information is interpreted by the viewer's visual system. **Graphical perception** is the term referring to the visual interpretation process and was originally described as the ability to unconsciously extract information from graphics (Cleveland and McGill 1984). Presenting data with charts has vast implications in healthcare related to presenting information in an abbreviated and easily understood manner. Since the volume of data that health information management (HIM) professionals are held accountable for is vast and continuing to grow with technological advancements, including the electronic health record and improved data storage capabilities, there is a need to examine more efficient ways to present information. In addition, new data is constantly being collected in healthcare, which ultimately increases the data complexity, thereby offering further considerations for presenting data graphically.

With increasing data complexity, there is an increased likelihood for failures in recognizing important findings to guide decision making. The capacity for a human being to process large amounts of information is limited; therefore, new strategies are being explored to improve the presentation of data in order to enhance efficiency and effectiveness of an interpretation. Not all charts are created equal. Exploration of the theoretical foundation of graphical presentations allows for a better understanding of the charts that lead to the most effective visualization of data by overcoming human limitations of processing data and making decisions.

Graphical perception research is about human graphical perception and how the interpretation of data is time- and task-dependent. That is, the time of accurately extracting information from visual displays is dependent on the position, length, angle, area, and volume of the chart. Table 18.1 ranks various graphical techniques based on the most accurate presentation methods (Cleveland and McGill 1985; 1984).

When data is presented as a position along a common scale, the information can be extracted faster and with greater accuracy than other methods. By choosing a graphical method that ranks higher on table 18.1 than other methods, one can enhance the accuracy and efficiency of interpreting the data. There are various types of charts that can be used to present data across the various graphical techniques.

- A **bar plot** is used for presenting data as a position along a common scale.
- A line chart can also be used for presenting data as a position along a common scale.
- A stacked bar plot is used for presenting data using length.
- A scatterplot is used to depict direction.
- A pie chart is used to present data by comparing area.
- A 3D bar plot is used for comparing volume.
- A heat map is used to present data using shading and color saturation.

There are many different types of charts that can be applied along the continuum of the ranked techniques. Notably, the purpose of any type of graphic is to display information to facilitate rapid and accurate interpretation to ultimately guide decisions. Therefore, when designing a chart, it is important to consider using a method that offers greater interpretation efficiency and accuracy.

Table 18.1 Ranking of graphical techniques from most to least accurate

Rank	Graphical technique
1	Position along a common scale
2	Position along nonaligned scales
3	Length, direction, angle
4	Area
5	Volume, curvature
6	Shading, color saturation

Source: Adapted from Cleveland and McGill 1984.

Check Your Understanding 18.1

Instructions: **Answer the following questions on a separate piece of paper.**

1. Provide an example of a graphical technique that uses area to present data.

2. Provide two examples of graphical techniques that present data along a common scale.

3. True or False: A graphical technique that uses length, direction, or angle is the most accurate.

4. Which of the following terms refer to the visual decoding (interpretation) process and was originally described as the ability to unconsciously extract information from graphics?
   A. Charts
   B. Graphical perception
   C. Data visualization
   D. Decision making

Effects of Graphical Presentation on Decision Making

Early research in behavioral decision making has observed that when individuals make decisions, they trade off the effort required to make a decision versus the accuracy of the outcome (Beach and Mitchell 1978). The use of decision aids, such as charts, have been found to be used only to reduce effort and not to improve accuracy; however, depending on the task, the use of charts does not extensively compromise the accuracy of the outcome (Speier 2006).

When considering the implications of presenting and visualizing data, one must consider how humans trade accuracy for effort. One example may be when physicians compare changes in laboratory data over time. Rather than taking an approach where the physician must calculate the exact difference in values over time, the physician most likely examines the dimensional differences in the data over time (that is, determines if the value decreases or increases since the previous test). Given this scenario, a graphical display of the laboratory data may be better suited for a dimensional interpretation without compromising on accuracy when compared to the standard approach of presenting laboratory data in a table with only the numbers presented.

Charts Versus Tables

The most common type of data that is displayed graphically is quantitative data. For example, the weight of a child can be tracked over their lifetime. Weight is a quantitative data element. When presenting the weight of a child over the period of their childhood, the data can be presented in a table where the numeric values for weight are displayed. Alternatively, a chart can be generated, such as a line chart, that displays how weight trends over a period of time. An example on how this data can be presented using a table or a line chart is shown in figure 18.1. If a user was tasked with identifying the exact weight at four years old, the simplest way to complete this task is by referring to the table. To extract the exact weight at four years old from the chart would require more complex perceptual tasks. However, if the task was to identify the trend in weight over time, the simplest way to complete this task is by referring to the chart. The line plot quickly reveals an upward trend in weight for each year. The table would require a user to examine the relationship between the discrete, or specific, numbers for each year to interpret a trend. This example highlights the importance of displaying information with a method that accommodates the desired task.

Charts employ spatial arrangement of information, whereas tables utilize a symbolic arrangement (Speier 2006). Charts emphasize a spatially-related relationship in data but typically do not present discrete data values. Tables, however, are symbolic since they emphasize discrete data values, but do not present the relationship between the data. **Spatial representations** allow information to be viewed at a glance utilizing perceptual processes without needing to address the individual elements of the information separately or analytically. **Symbolic representations** require analytical processes where information is extracted from specific data values. When considering the advantages and disadvantages of each arrangement, spatial data supports more of a dimensional interpretation, which may decrease effort yet limits the consideration of discrete data points, which may decrease accuracy. Symbolic representations, however, support more of a holistic interpretation where discrete data points may be determined, allowing for increased accuracy yet requiring increased effort. Simply put, a chart offers the advantage of seeing the general trend of data and comparing differences in data between groups or over time. However, the precise numeric values are more easily discerned when reading a table. Each method has advantages depending on the context of the situation and therefore each can be thought of as task-dependent.

The effectiveness of charts to support decision making can be dependent on the task environment. The task content, task complexity, and task structure can influence the accuracy and efficiency of an interpretation. Charts do not have total superiority over tables and the benefit of charts is task-dependent (Dickson et al. 1986; Hartley and Cabanac 2014; Speier 2006). In tasks where an accurate interpretation of values is important, especially when a user has experience with tables or tabular presentations, tables are better suited than charts. For tasks that involve viewing the time dependency of large amounts of data, charts are better suited than tables. When the task involves conveying a message from several sets of data on a common subject, presenting subsets of data using both charts and tables is best. Finally, when the task involves large amounts of data and the goal is to recall fairly specific details after the presentation, charts offer better performance than tables. In medicine, data is often presented as both discrete data and time-dependent data depending on the type of data and the context of the situation.

Figure 18.1 Displaying quantitative data in a table versus a chart

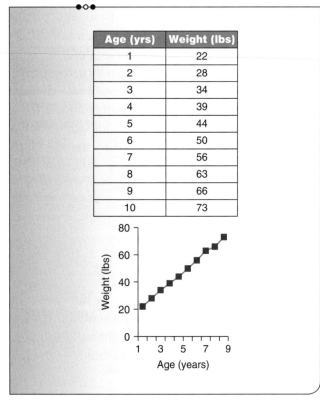

Age (yrs)	Weight (lbs)
1	22
2	28
3	34
4	39
5	44
6	50
7	56
8	63
9	66
10	73

Therefore, both tables and charts may be applicable for presenting data depending on the situation.

To expand on the previous explanation, the most suitable situations to provide a chart versus a table depends on the intended use of the information. The presentation method, whether using charts or tables, needs to be considered in context to the task at hand knowing that each presentation method has advantages in different situations. However, there are factors other than the context of the task that can influence the utility of charts versus tables, such as the experience of the user and the complexity of the data, which will be explored further in this chapter.

Check Your Understanding 18.2

Instructions: **Answer the following questions on a separate piece of paper.**

1. If you were asked to create a method for presenting data to help a patient identify their latest cholesterol level, would a table or chart be preferred?

2. If you were asked to create a method for presenting data to help a patient identify the trend in their last five cholesterol levels, would a table or chart be preferred?

3. _____ allow information to be viewed at a glance utilizing perceptual processes without needing to address the individual elements of the information separately or analytically.
   A. Spatial representations
   B. Symbolic representations
   C. Charts
   D. Tables

4. _____ require analytical processes where information is extracted from specific data values.
   A. Spatial representations
   B. Symbolic representations
   C. Charts
   D. Tables

5. True or False: Charts represent a spatial representation of data.

Considerations for Adopting Visualization Techniques

Several factors can have an impact on the effectiveness of a visual display, including the

- Context of the situation,
- Experience of the user,
- Type of chart, and
- Complexity of the data.

Research has just begun exploring the impact these factors have on interpreting visual displays of healthcare data. For example, a prior study in radiology proposed four potential measures to consider recording when designing a visual display: accuracy, which is the measure of correctness; latency, which describes the amount of time it takes to answer a question; compactness of the display; and user preference (Starren and Johnson 2000). Although, it may not be necessary to explore each of these measures each time a visual display is being designed, the accuracy and latency of interpreting a visual display tend to be the most common measures to consider.

The remainder of the chapter explores how situations with users of varying experience, using different types of charts, and displaying data of varying complexity can influence the adoption and use of visual displays of data.

Context of the Situation

As described previously, there are certain situations where it may be necessary to present data using numerical values and other situations where a graphical display is ideal. Research has been conducted to compare whether numbers, charts, or a combination of both are best for presenting quantitative data (Feldman-Stewart et al. 2000). One study compared six different display methods including pie charts, vertical bar plots, horizontal bar plots, numbers, systematic ovals, and random ovals. The patients were presented information pertaining to the probabilities of treatment risks and benefits using a combination of methods (figure 18.2). **Systematic ovals** are a graphical technique that displays stacked ovals with the height of the stack corresponding to the maximum of the scale. The ovals are separated into discrete units with each oval corresponding to a specific unit of measurement. The value for the result is summarized by the ovals that are filled in. Figure 18.2 displays an example of systematic ovals where each oval corresponds to one unit. Since the value is 45, there are 45 ovals filled in. A **random oval** display is similar to systematic ovals but it is not as uniform; the ovals are randomly filled in.

The ability to interpret the data presented in figure 18.2 can vary depending on the type of task. If the task required choosing a larger or smaller object, the symbolic representation using vertical bars results in the most accurate and rapid processing, followed by systematic ovals. When the task required an estimate of the value, which requires greater precision, numbers resulted in the most accurate estimates, followed by systematic ovals (Feldman-Stewart et al. 2000). These results suggest that quantitative information be presented in one of two ways—either by presenting both vertical bars and numbers or only presenting systematic ovals. Studies such as this demonstrate that the performance of charts to convey quantitative information is highly dependent on the type and complexity of the task at hand, and in some cases the display of both numbers and charts is best.

There are certain characteristics of healthcare data that can be used for determining whether a chart or table is the best method for displaying data. For example, the presentation of a specific number, or set of numbers, is necessary to carry out a task of revealing the last known value for a patient's HbA1c (glycated hemoglobin). The reason the number is the best method is because the task requires an accurate interpretation of a discrete value. Yet when the purpose is to view trends over a period of time, such as monitoring HbA1c in a diabetic patient over the period of several months, a graphical presentation is more appropriate. The reason is that a rapid comparison of several values over time is required for this task.

Figure 18.2.   A comparison of six different graphical presentations of numeric information

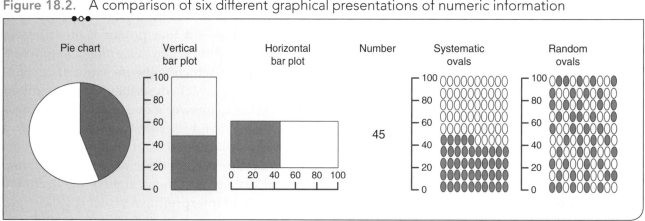

Source: Adapted from Feldman-Stewart et al. 2000.

However, to facilitate an accurate and rapid interpretation, one may consider presenting both the specific numbers and a corresponding chart.

Experience of the User

The ability to interpret data using visual displays is largely dependent on the experience of the person interpreting that display. This is especially relevant in the healthcare setting where health professionals make decisions subconsciously or implicitly and where many tasks are routine and nonreflective when they are in familiar situations such as in interpreting commonly seen data (Eva 2005). The degree of implicit, nonreflective cognitive processing may be directly related to the experience of the physician (Eva 2005). When considering the impact of charts, more experienced health professionals who are trained to look at tabular data (tables) may find a graphical presentation to be a hindrance in effort and accuracy. However, charts can improve the accuracy of interpreting data with less experienced health professionals. Experience must be considered when designing a visual display of data. It is often best to discuss and evaluate the impact that a visual display has on users that vary in terms of experience. That is, assess whether a visual display improves or hinders the performance of users with varying levels of professional experience.

Presentation Method

Health professionals often find themselves immersed in data, which can lead to **information overload**, defined as a difficulty in making decisions due to the presence of excessive amounts of information. Presentation methods should maximize information retrieval while not causing information overload (Caban and Gots 2015). The advantage of a chart, if done correctly, is to present the task information externally thereby limiting cognitive processing. A graphical display should use tasks as high in the ordering of processing as possible (see table 18.1). If information could be presented in more than one way, the one that proves to be the most accurate should be favored. For example, if the average time to code an inpatient chart was assessed across six months in three different coders, values could be displayed using a stacked bar plot or a side-by-side bar plot (figure 18.3). If the task was to identify the month that had the lowest average time to code an inpatient chart for each coder, the side-by-side bar plot offers an advantage because it only requires judgments regarding the position along a common scale, rather than judgments regarding position on identical but nonaligned scales (figure 18.3). The side-by-side bar plot reveals that the lowest average time to code an inpatient chart for coder 1 is in April, for coder 2 is in May, and for coder

Figure 18.3. Stacked bar plot versus side-by-side bar plot comparing the average time for three coders to code an inpatient chart over six months

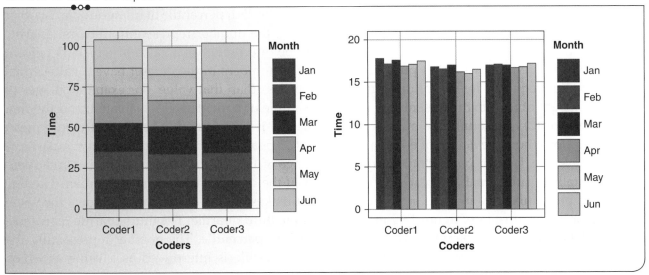

3 is in April. If this task were completed with the stacked bar plot, it would be very difficult to ascertain which month has the lowest average time to code an inpatient chart for each coder.

A **histogram** displays a frequency or density distribution of a single numeric variable. Categorizing or sorting these numeric variables together is called binning. The numeric variable is broken down into groups based on specific ranges of values to establish the widths of each bar in a histogram. The height of each bar represents the frequency or density of each of the binned groups. The distribution can be described as normally distributed when the pattern follows a bell-shaped pattern. If the histogram has the highest point to the left side of the graph and a right trailing tail, it is referred to as right skewed or positively skewed. If the histogram has the highest point to the right side of the graph and a left leading tail, it is referred to as left skewed or negatively skewed. A bimodal distribution occurs when there is more than one peak in the data. Figure 18.4 displays an example of each of these distribution categories.

The speed and accuracy of interpreting various medical parameters has been researched in depth (Baur et al. 2010; Lesselroth and Pieczkiewicz 2011; Thomas and Powsner 2005; Tufte 2006; West et al. 2015). In these studies, there were numerous graphical methods that were emphasized as effective ways for presenting data. The methods are largely dependent on the type of data that is available (namely, frequency, mean, median). Figure 18.5 displays some of the most common graphical methods along with an explanation regarding the most appropriate data to use with each method.

A bar plot is used for two main purposes: (1) for plotting the frequency for one or more groups where the height of each bar represents the count or frequency, or (2) for plotting the mean for one or more groups where the height of each bar represents the average. The bars can be drawn vertically or horizontally. A horizontal bar plot is typically used when presenting data in an ascending or descending order. For instance, figure 18.5 presents a horizontal bar plot to compare the average total performance score by the type of hospital in de-

scending order. When a bar plot is used for plotting the mean for one or more groups, the standard deviation or standard error for each level of a group may be added to the plot to show the range of data. When a large number of groups are compared in descending or ascending order on a bar plot, an alternative method for presenting the data is the use of a dot plot.

A **dot plot** presents the frequency or means to compare many groups using dots. The dot plot offers a less cluttered view of the data when there are many groups to compare. An example of a dot plot is shown in figure 18.5.

A **pie chart** is used to present the count or proportion of subgroups to the whole. The component parts of a pie chart represent the subgroups of a single factor. If each proportion that is presented in a pie chart is summed, the total should always equal 100 percent.

A **line plot** is used for two main purposes: (1) to present trends or patterns in the number of occurrences between groups, or (2) to present trends or patterns in the mean of a variable between groups. Typically, the change of a variable over time is compared. When more than one group is compared in a line plot, a separate line is drawn for each group.

A **boxplot** displays the descriptive statistics of a continuous variable including the minimum, first quartile, medium, third quartile, maximum, and potential outlier values. The line that makes the bottom of the box represents the value for the first quartile; the first quartile of a dataset is used to represent the 25th percentile of numeric data. In other words, the number representing the first quartile can be interpreted as a value at which 25 percent of the numbers in the dataset have a value equal to or less than that value. For example, if ages of a sample of patients were evaluated, and the first quartile is determined to be 15, that would mean that 25 percent of the patients in your sample have an age of 15 years or less. The bold line in the center of the boxplot represents the median. The line that makes the top of the box represents the value for the third quartile. The third quartile represents the 75th percentile. The number representing the third quartile is interpreted as a value at which

75 percent of the numbers in the dataset have a value equal to or less than that value. If there are dots above and below the boxes, these dots represent potential outliers. An outlier is a value that is distant from other values. For example, if the age of 250 years were present in the dataset, this would represent an outlier. Potential outliers are determined on a boxplot when there are values in the dataset that are lower than the first quartile value minus 1.5*IQR and above the third quartile plus 1.5*IQR. IQR stands for interquartile range and is calculated as the value of the third quartile minus

Figure 18.4. Histogram distribution categories

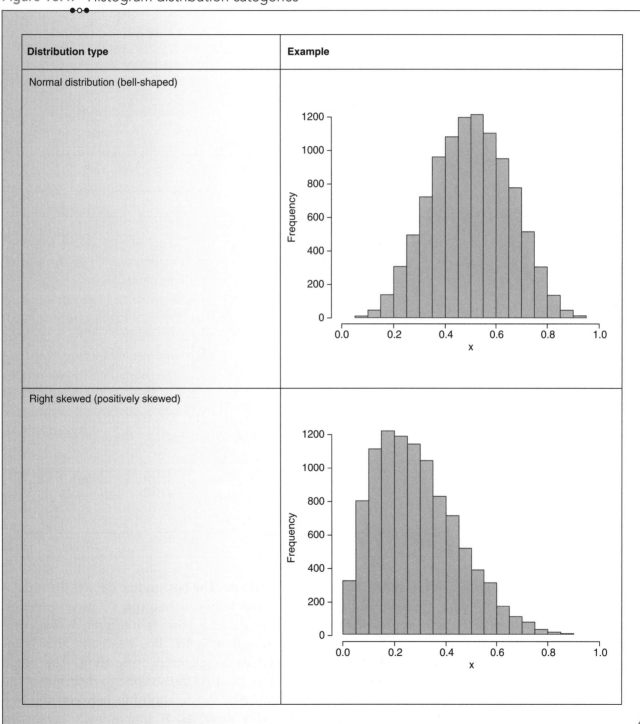

Figure 18.4   *(Continued)*

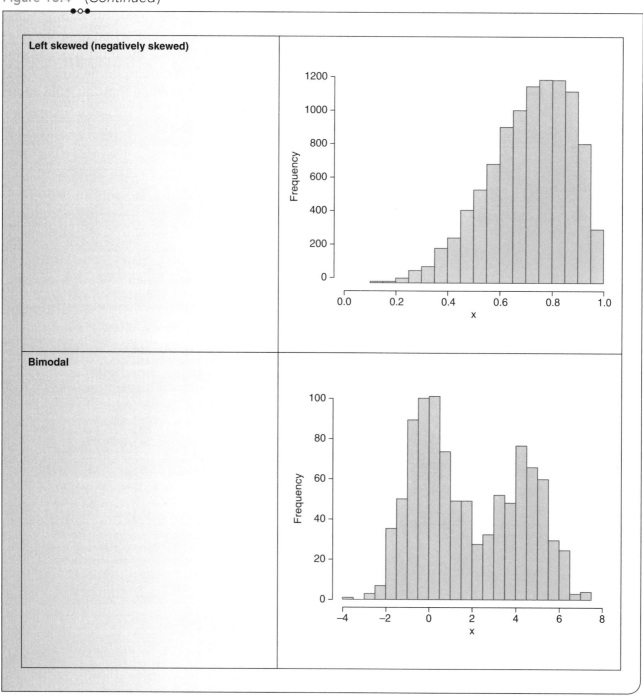

the value of the first quartile. When outliers are not present, the whiskers—the lines protruding from the top and bottom of the box—represent the minimum and maximum values.

A **scatterplot** displays the relationship between two quantitative variables. A line is typically drawn through the middle of the points and represents the trend of the data, which is known as

the best-fit line. The best-fit line depicts the type of relationship between two quantitative variables. If the line ascends, this is interpreted as a positive association; if the line descends, this is interpreted as a negative association. The slope of the line (that is, the steepness) determines the significance of the relationship between the two quantitative variables. A simple linear regression

Figure 18.5.   Explanation of the most common graphical methods

Plotting frequencies

Graph type	Definition	Example
Bar plot	Displays the frequencies for one or more groups. The bars can be drawn vertically or horizontally.	The count of females and males in the selected patient population 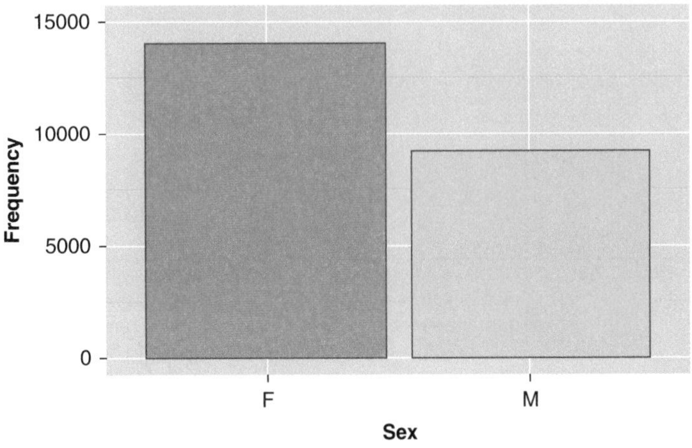
Pie chart	The count or proportion of subgroups. The component parts of a pie chart represent the subgroups of a single variable.	The count and percentage of females and males in the selected patient population 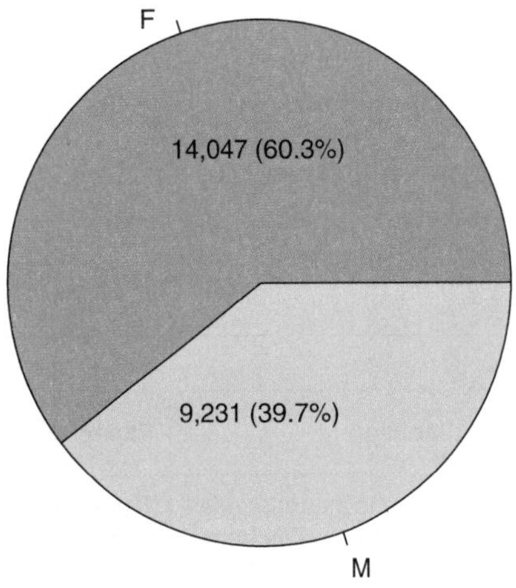
Line plot	Displays trends or patterns in the number of occurrences between groups. Typically, the change of a variable over time is compared.	The number of patient visits for males and females for the years 2009 through 2012

Figure 18.5   (*Continued*)

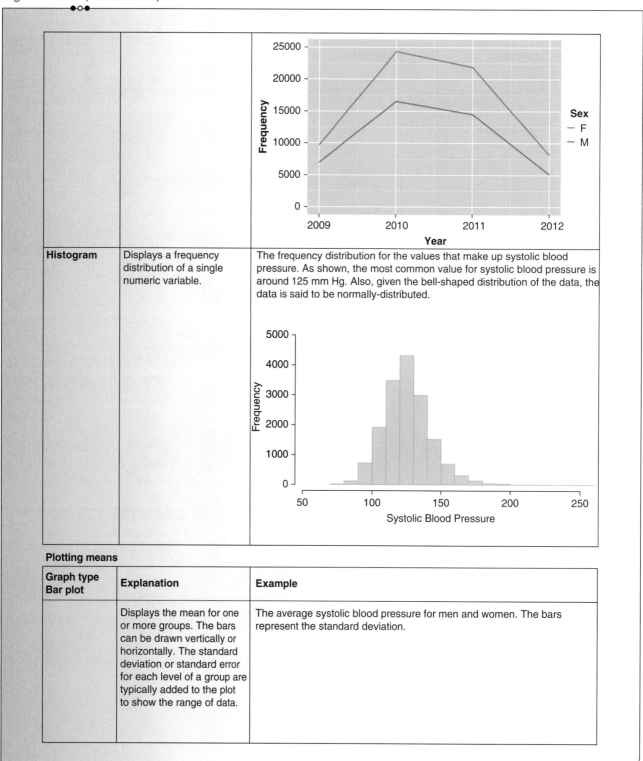

| Histogram | Displays a frequency distribution of a single numeric variable. | The frequency distribution for the values that make up systolic blood pressure. As shown, the most common value for systolic blood pressure is around 125 mm Hg. Also, given the bell-shaped distribution of the data, the data is said to be normally-distributed. |

Plotting means

Graph type Bar plot	Explanation	Example
	Displays the mean for one or more groups. The bars can be drawn vertically or horizontally. The standard deviation or standard error for each level of a group are typically added to the plot to show the range of data.	The average systolic blood pressure for men and women. The bars represent the standard deviation.

Figure 18.5 (*Continued*)

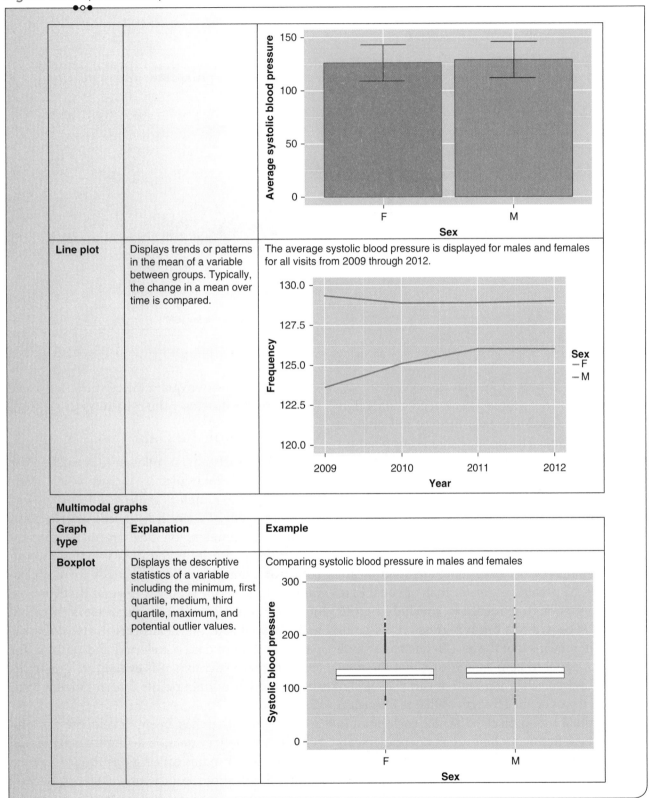

Line plot	Displays trends or patterns in the mean of a variable between groups. Typically, the change in a mean over time is compared.	The average systolic blood pressure is displayed for males and females for all visits from 2009 through 2012.

Multimodal graphs

Graph type	Explanation	Example
Boxplot	Displays the descriptive statistics of a variable including the minimum, first quartile, medium, third quartile, maximum, and potential outlier values.	Comparing systolic blood pressure in males and females

Figure 18.5 *(Continued)*

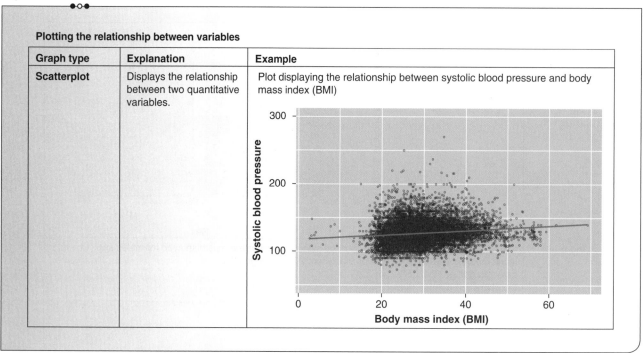

Plotting the relationship between variables

Graph type	Explanation	Example
Scatterplot	Displays the relationship between two quantitative variables.	Plot displaying the relationship between systolic blood pressure and body mass index (BMI)

is the statistical procedure that is associated with a scatterplot. The simple linear regression offers information related to the significance and strength of an association. The p-value that is supplied for a simple linear regression establishes whether the best-fit line has a slope that is significantly different from zero. A p-value is used for determining significance of a statistical test. The p-value should be compared to a predefined significance level, known as α. If the p-value is less than α, there is enough evidence to conclude a significant finding. If the p-value is greater than or equal to α, there is not enough evidence to conclude significance. With regard to a linear regression, a significant finding means that the best-fit line has a slope that is not equal to zero, suggesting that the relationship between the quantitative variables is significant. However, the strength of that relationship is determined based on the distance each point is from the best-fit line. If there are many points scattered far from the best-fit line, the association between the quantitative variables is said to be weak. If the points are close to the best-fit line, the relationship is stronger. The statistic that represents the strength of the relationship is the r^2 value, which can range from 0 to 1. The strength of the relation-ship between the two quantitative variables is said to be stronger the closer the r^2 value is to 1.

Complexity of the Data

Data complexity, as it relates to visualization of healthcare data, usually arises when there are multiple parameters that need to be viewed simultaneously. When it is necessary to view multiple parameters on one graphical display, difficulties can arise if the data is not standardized (for example, different ranges for each parameter), does not follow a normal distribution, or a relationship between parameters is meant to be visualized. As healthcare technology expands and more data is collected and utilized, the level of complexity expands even more due to the sheer number of data points that are meant to be displayed.

A method that has been developed for presenting a variety of data on a single display in an easy-to-read format is called a **dashboard**. For example, the dashboard in your vehicle presents a variety of data that is important for operating the vehicle. In healthcare, dashboards are used for different purposes including viewing organization performance data, financial data, and clinical data.

The dashboards may use various graphics including bar plots, pie charts, numbers, textual summaries, and other methods. A dashboard is meant to support a high-level understanding of the data. If additional information is necessary to drill down into more specific findings, a process called slicing and dicing can be adopted. **Slicing and dicing** refers to the process of taking what is known at the highest level of understanding and working downward to identify the underlying causes for the high-level observation. A dashboard helps facilitate a greater understanding of financial, operational, and clinical processes to identify problems and successes.

An example of a dashboard is shown in figure 18.6. This dashboard was created by Dundas

Figure 18.6. Example of a dashboard for hospital management

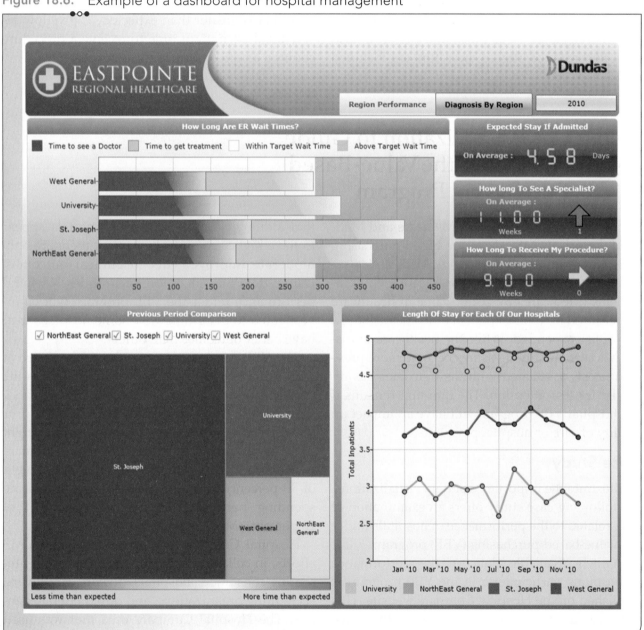

Source: Used with permission from Dundas Data Visualization, Inc. ©2015 - www.dundas.com

Data Visualizations, Inc., and displays key performance indicators (KPIs) for hospitals within a fictitious hospital system named Eastpointe. The regional performance dashboard, which is the tab that is selected in figure 18.6, displays KPIs such as time to see a doctor, time to get treatment, expected stay if admitted, and length of stay (per hospital), among other measures. Users can examine numerous date ranges such as today, the current week, the current year, and other configurable ranges. Interactive tooltips display the values shown via the interactive charts, which consist of line charts, stacked bar plots, and digital indicators. For instance, digital indicators are included as arrows for some measures. A user can quickly determine if the length of time to see a specialist or to receive a procedure is greater than expected, as expected, or less than expected by viewing the direction of an arrow and the color. If the arrow points up and is red, this indicates a time that is greater than expected. If the arrow points to the side and colored yellow, this indicates a time as expected. If the arrow points down and is green, this indicates a time less than expected. The red arrow for the length of time to see a specialist indicates a time that is greater than expected. The yellow arrow for the length of time to receive a procedure shows a length of time that is as expected.

Using Data Visualization to Guide Decisions Under the Value-Based Purchasing Program

According to the Centers for Medicare and Medicaid Services (CMS), the value-based purchasing (VBP) program is an effort to link Medicare's payment system to the quality of care provided to inpatients (Medicare.gov 2015). Value in healthcare is measured in terms of patient outcomes achieved per dollar expended. While the healthcare industry has seen quality measures become more prevalent, costs associated with the outcomes has received far less attention. The question remains if the hospital VBP program will have an impact on quality of care or hospital payments.

Case Study

To illustrate the importance of data visualizations, the following case study offers an examination of data related to the performance of hospitals under the value-based purchasing (VBP) program.

Publicly available data on the performance of hospitals participating in the VBP program is published on the Hospital Compare website. This data was used to examine if hospitals that have reported greater VBP program total performance actually present with better clinical outcomes. From the analysis that follows, it was discovered that although high performing hospitals appear to have higher patient satisfaction, there are only moderate improvements in clinical outcomes. Using data visualization techniques, hospital performance under the VBP program will be investigated to determine why some hospitals may have better outcomes than others.

The VBP program presents the performance of each hospital using a rating system known as the total performance score. The total performance score is calculated based on the following four domains: clinical process of care domain (weight of 20 percent), patient experience of care domain (weight of 30 percent), outcome domain (weight of 30 percent), and efficiency domain—Medicare spending per beneficiary measure (weight of 20 percent) (Medicare.gov 2015).

Hospital Compare was created through CMS efforts, in collaboration with organizations representing consumers, hospitals, doctors, employers, accrediting organizations, and other federal agencies. The Hospital Compare data that was used in the following analysis was based on hospital VBP performance data from the January 1, 2013 through December 31, 2013 reporting period. VBP performance data was compared based on the hospital ownership status and the state where the hospitals were located.

The charts in this case study were created using the R Statistical Software package with the ggplot2 package. R is open source software (available as a free download) that uses a command line language.

When comparing the total performance score by the hospital ownership status using a horizontal bar plot, those hospitals that are physician-owned had the highest total performance score. The lowest total performance score occurred in the state government-owned hospitals (figure 18.7).

The observed differences may be partly related to the perceptions of patients regarding hospital quality. Some research demonstrates that patient surveys may not be a reliable measure of hospital quality based on the observation that patients' views can be swayed by the type of hospital. That is, hospitals treating the very sickest patients often received low patient satisfaction evaluations while physician-owned hospitals, with just a few specialties, tended to have higher satisfaction rates (Rau 2013). Therefore, the lower total performance score in some hospital types may be in part due to lower patient satisfaction. In addition, patient experience in safety-net hospitals had an overall lower performance than non–safety-net hospitals (SNHs) on patient experience metrics (Chatterjee et al. 2012). SNHs care for vulnerable and poor populations. However, even if a hospital demonstrated improvements they may lose money under the VBP program if those improvements were not as great as peer hospitals (Rau 2013). Under the VBP program, hospitals are expected to meet certain quality standards but are also expected to show improvement compared to prior years. Therefore, if a hospital shows improvements in quality from prior years, but not

Figure 18.7. Comparing the average total performance score by hospital ownership status

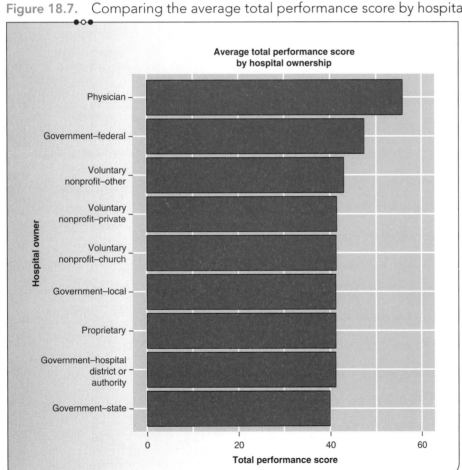

to the extent of peer hospitals, they may still lose money.

Total Performance Score by Hospital Location

When comparing the total performance score of each state using a dot plot, Hawaii, South Dakota, Alaska, and Minnesota have the highest scores, while District of Columbia, Nevada, New Jersey, and Connecticut have the lowest scores (figure 18.8).

The patient experience of care domain score is calculated based upon patient satisfaction surveys and represents 30 percent of the total performance score. Therefore, if patients report dissatisfaction with a hospital, this can negatively impact the total performance score. To get a sense of which states are performing best with regard to patient satisfaction, the average patient experience of care domain score was compared across each state using a dot plot. South Dakota, Louisiana, Wisconsin,

Figure 18.8.   Average total performance scores by each state

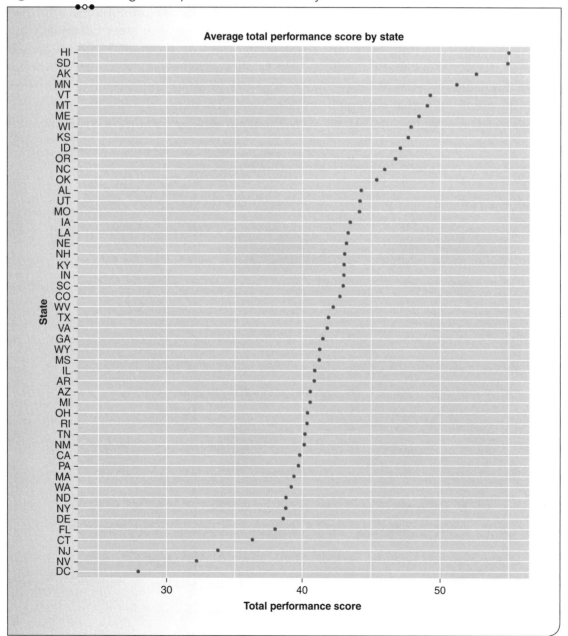

and Maine are the states that have the highest patient experience of care domain score, while District of Columbia, New York, Nevada, and New Mexico have the lowest score (figure 18.9). Many of the same states that fell within the higher and lower quartiles of the total performance score remained higher or lower when compared to the overall patient experience scores.

When looking at a clinical outcome, such as acute myocardial infarction (AMI) readmission rates, New Jersey, Connecticut, Massachusetts, and New York had the highest AMI readmission rate while Wyoming, New Mexico, Utah, Kansas, and Oklahoma had the lowest (figure 18.10). AMI readmission rates are worthwhile to compare since this outcome is one of the primary causes of Medicare penalties for hospitals participating in the VBP program (Rau 2013).

It is interesting to note that there are some inconsistencies in the readmission rates relative

Figure 18.9.   Average patient experience of care domain score by each state

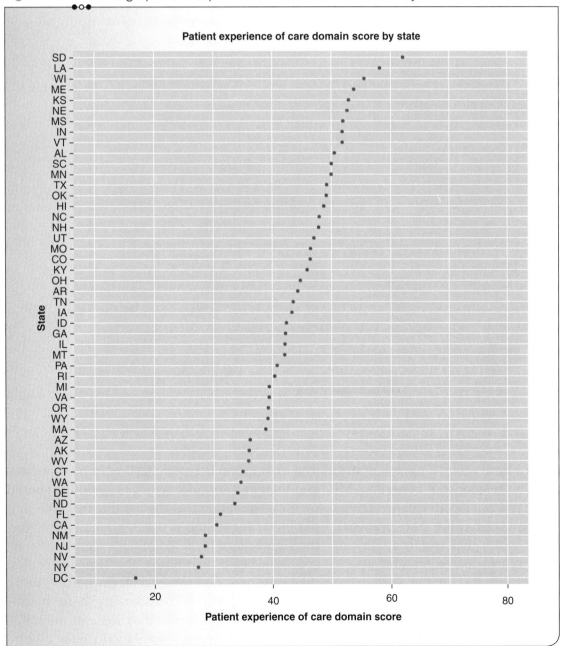

Figure 18.10.   Average AMI readmission rates by state

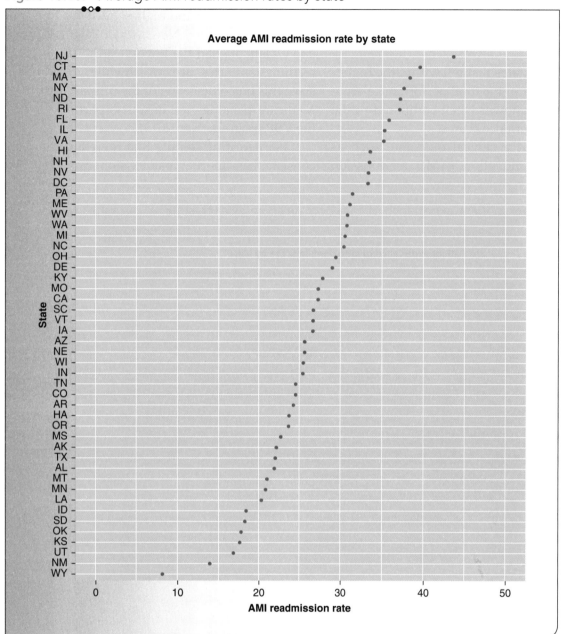

to the total performance score for some states. When examining the relationship between AMI readmission rates and total performance scores for each state using a scatterplot, there is a weak correlation (figure 18.11). For instance, Hawaii has a high total performance score and also a high AMI readmission rate in the scatterplot shown in figure 18.10. New Mexico has one of the lowest AMI readmission rates but only a moderately high total performance score. The association between AMI readmission rates and total performance scores is significant based on the observation that the p-value from the simple linear regression is 0.003, which is less than the significance level (α) of 0.05. Despite the association being significant, the strength of that relationship is said to be weak since the r^2 value is only 0.17, which is considerably lower than 1. Overall, the trend shows that some of the states with a higher average total performance score

Figure 18.11. Association between AMI readmission rates and total performance score for each state

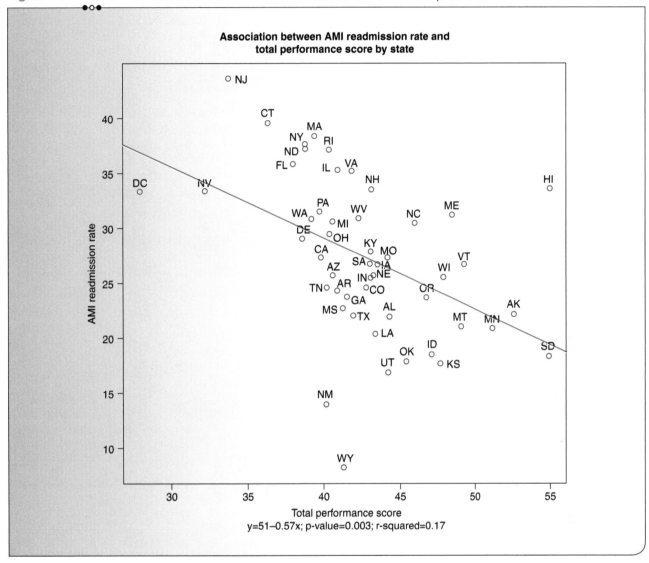

also have a lower average AMI readmission rate. However, this finding is not consistent for all hospitals. From the analysis described, it was discovered that states with high performing hospitals appear to have only small improvements in clinical outcomes.

The use of data visualization techniques offered a method for examining if VBP is associated with improved outcomes. Based on the analysis, VBP does not appear to strongly correlate with improvement in health outcomes, as evident by AMI readmission rates. Possible causes for this observation may be that either the total performance score does not measure what it should, or the outcome measurement does not reflect the quality of the total performance scores measure. That is, there is uncertainty as to how the total performance score equates to quality of care. Based on the findings from this analysis, further studies can be conducted to identify the impact of the weighted measures on the total performance score and to identify if there is one measure that affects the total performance score more adversely when a hospital is not performing well.

Check Your Understanding 18.3

Instructions: **Answer the following questions on a separate piece of paper.**

1. If you were tasked with presenting the changes in revenue over the last five years, what would be the best graph to adopt?
   A. Bar plot
   B. Line plot
   C. Histogram
   D. Boxplot

2. True or False: A chart is always preferred over a table of data.

3. What is the highest ranked method for presenting data?
   A. Length, direction, angle
   B. Position along nonaligned scales
   C. Position along a common scale
   D. Volume, curvature

4. What does a scatterplot reveal?
   A. The average differences between two groups
   B. The relationship between two variables
   C. The distribution of data
   D. The frequency of data

5. Which of the following should be considered when designing a chart?
   A. The context of the situation
   B. The type of graph
   C. The experience of the user
   D. All of the above

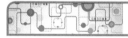

References

Beach, L.R. and T.R. Mitchell. 1978. A contingency model for the selection of decision strategies. *Academy of Management Review* 3:439–449.

Caban, J.J. and D. Gotz. 2015. Visual analytics in healthcare: Opportunities and research challenges. *Journal of the American Medical Informatics Association* 22:260–262.

Chatterjee, P., K. Joynt, E. Orav, and J. Ashish. 2012. Patient experience in safety-net hospitals: Implications for improving care and value-based purchasing. *Archives of Internal Medicine* 172(16):1204–1210.

Cleveland, W.S. and R. McGill. 1985. Graphical perception and graphical methods for analyzing scientific data. *Science* 229:828–833.

Cleveland, W.S. and R. McGill. 1984. Graphical perception: Theory, experimentation, and application to the development of graphical methods. *Journal of the American Statistical Association* 79:531–554.

Dickson, G.W., G. DeSanctis, and D.J. McBride. 1986. Understanding the effectiveness of computer graphics for decision support: A cumulative experimental approach. *Communications of the ACM* 29:40–47.

Dundas Data Visualization, Inc. 2015. Dundas Dashboard. http://www.dundas.com/

Eva, K.W. 2005. What every teacher needs to know about clinical reasoning. *Medical Education* 39:98–106.

Feldman-Stewart, D., N. Kocovski, B.A. McConnell, M.D. Brundage, and W.J. Mackillop. 2000. Perception of quantitative information for treatment decisions. *Medical Decision Making* 20: 228–238.

Hartley, J. and G. Cabanac. 2014. Do men and women differ in their use of tables and graphs in academic publications? *Scientometrics* 98(2):1161–1172.

Lesselroth, B.J. and D.S. Pieczkiewicz. 2011. *Data Visualization Strategies for the Electronic Health Record.* Nova Science Publishers.

Medicare.gov 2015. The Total Performance Score Information. https://www.medicare.gov/hospitalcompare/data/total-performance-scores.html

Rau, J. 2013. Nearly 1,500 Hospitals Penalized Under Medicare Program Rating Quality. Haiser Health News. http://kaiserhealthnews.org/news/value-based-purchasing-medicare/

Speier, C. 2006. The influence of information presentation formats on complex task decision-making performance. *International Journal of Human-Computer Studies* 64(11):1115–1131.

Starren, J. and S.B. Johnson. 2000. An object-oriented taxonomy of medical data presentations. *Journal of the American Medical Informatics Association*. 7:1–20.

Thomas, P. and S. Powsner. 2005. Data presentation for quality improvement. *AMIA Annual Symposium Proceedings* 2005:1134.

Tufte, E.R. 2006. *Beautiful Evidence*. Cheshire, CT: Graphics Press.

West, V.L., D. Borland, and W.E. Hammond. 2015. Innovative information visualization of electronic health record data: A systematic review. *Journal of the American Medical Informatics Association* 22(2):330–339.

19

Research Methods

Elizabeth Forrestal, PhD, RHIA, CCS, FAHIMA

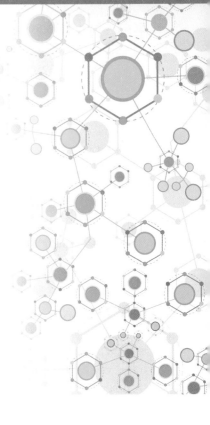

Nonparticipant observation
Nonrandom (nonprobability) sampling
Observational research
Outcome evaluation
Outcomes research
Participant observation
Pilot study
Policy analysis
Primary analysis
Primary source
Problem statement
Process evaluation
Prospective

Protocol
Qualitative approach
Quantitative approach
Quasi-experimental method
Questionnaire survey
Random sampling
Randomization
Randomized controlled trial (RCT)
Reliability
Research
Research design
Research frame
Research method
Research methodology

Research question
Retrospective
Sample
Scale
Secondary analysis
Secondary source
Simulation observation
Survey
Systematic review
Theory
Treatment
Triangulation
Validity
Variable

Research is a systematic process of inquiry aimed at discovering or creating new knowledge about a topic; confirming or evaluating existing knowledge; or revising outdated knowledge. Knowledge of research and research methods supports health informatics and health information management (HIM) professionals in their use of evidence to answer a question or to make a decision. This chapter discusses research theories and models, describes research designs and methods, and provides a step-by-step process of conducting research. Examples of HIM research studies are given and the linkage between research and the HIM practitioner is shown.

Research Frame

A **research frame** comprises the theory underpinning the study and the model illustrating the factors and relationships that the study is investigating. The frame also includes the assumptions of the researcher's field and the field's typical methods and analytical tools. A research frame provides an overarching structure for a research project.

Theories and Models

HIM is at the intersection of many different fields of study. As a result, HIM researchers draw on theories and models not only from healthcare, but also from computer science and business. Many theories and models exist from these fields. Researchers select the theory or model that best suits their purpose and addresses their question or problem.

A **theory** is the systematic organization of knowledge that explains or predicts phenomena, such as behavior or events. "Theories explain phenomena by interrelating concepts in a logical, testable way" (Karnick 2013, 29). Theories provide definitions, relationships, and boundaries. The best theories simplify the situation, explain the most facts in the broadest range of circumstances, and most accurately predict behavior (Singleton and Straits 2005, 20). For example, the theory of diffusion of innovations is a commonly used theory in studies related to health information technologies. The theory explains how new ideas and products—innovations—spread. The theory includes definitions of innovation and communication and elements (concepts) of the process of diffusion (Rogers 2003, xvii–xviii, 11). Researchers used the theory in their study to understand the factors affecting patients' acceptance and use of consumer e-health innovations (Zhang et al. 2015, 1).

A **model** visually depicts a theory. Models can portray theories with objects, can be smaller-scaled versions, or can be graphic representations. A model includes all of a theory's known properties. For example, figure 19.1 is a model showing factors critical to successfully implementing barcoding in hospital pharmacies. The researchers identified three factors as potential barriers to successful implementations (Alharthi et al. 2015, 1). In their study, the researchers found that pharmacists perceived resistance and particularly its category, fear of change, as the most critical success factor of the three factors.

Figure 19.1. Hierarchy model of critical success factors (CSFs) for pharmacy barcode implementation

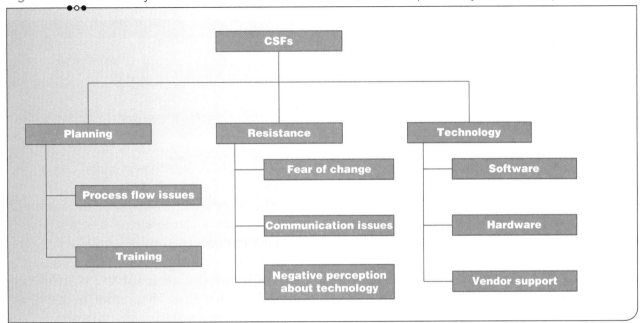

Source: Alharthi et al. 2015, 11.

Research Methodology

Research methodology is the study and analysis of research methods and theories. Generally, there are two types of research: basic research and applied research and these two types are ends of a continuum, not separate entities. Therefore, the distinction between them is sometimes unclear, however, they can be differentiated as follows.

- **Basic research** answers the question "Why?" and focuses on the development of theories and their refinement. Basic research is sometimes called bench science because it often occurs in laboratories.

- **Applied research** answers the questions "What?" and "How?" and focuses on the implementation of theories into practice. Applied research, particularly clinical applied research, may occur in healthcare settings, such as at the bedside.

Research methodologists also describe two overarching approaches to research: the quantitative approach and the qualitative approach.

- **Quantitative approach** is the explanation of phenomena by making predictions, collecting and analyzing evidence, testing alternative theories, and choosing the best theory. Objective knowledge that is **generalizable**, applicable to other similar situations and people, is the desired end result. As the word *quantitative* implies, the data often can be quantified and lead to statistical or numerical results. In HIM, an example would be a study that calculates the percentage of a healthcare organization's patients that use its patient portal.

- **Qualitative approach** is the interpretation of nonnumerical observations. These nonnumerical observations include words, gestures, activities, time, space, images, and perceptions. These observations are placed in context which means the specifics of the situation. Context includes time, space, emotional attitude, social situation, and culture. In HIM, an example would be an exploration of the reasons why patients are uncomfortable using a healthcare organization's patient portal.

The purpose of the research determines the approach. Research that investigates numerically measurable observations is quantitative; while research that explores reasons or interprets actions is qualitative. Within both approaches, researchers make certain basic assumptions. (See table 19.1.)

Table 19.1.   Comparison of assumptions in quantitative and qualitative research approaches

Quantitative	Qualitative
Single truth exists	Multiple truths exist simultaneously
Single truth applies across time and place	Truths are bound to place and time (contextual)
Researchers can adopt neutral, unbiased stances	Neutrality is impossible because researchers choose their topics of investigation
Chronological sequence of causes can be identified	Influences interact with one another to color researchers' views of the past, present, and future

Mixed methods research is a third approach that combines quantitative and qualitative techniques within a single study or across multiple, complementary studies. Mixed methods research is suited to investigations of large topics or complex phenomena, such as in healthcare.

In a series of studies, HIM researchers can use all three approaches. For example, in a quantitative study, researchers might investigate the effectiveness of a community health center's program to educate elders with low incomes on the reliability of health websites. In a qualitative study, researchers may explore the impact of the educational program on elders' application of information from the websites. In a mixed methods study, researchers could investigate factors associated with the implementation of the program, such as the health director's selection of the educational materials and the director's views on barriers and facilitators of the program's implementation.

Researchers use inductive reasoning or deductive reasoning to justify their decisions and conclusions about phenomena.

- **Inductive reasoning**, or induction, involves drawing conclusions based on a limited number of observations. Inductive reasoning is "bottom up." Researchers employing inductive reasoning begin with observations, detect patterns or clusters of relationships, form and explore tentative hypotheses, and generate provisional conclusions or theories. For example, during his professional practice experience, a student might observe that all coders in the coding department at XYZ hospital had the RHIT credential. Thus, he might conclude that all coders have the RHIT credential.

- **Deductive reasoning**, or deduction, involves drawing conclusions based on generalizations, rules, or principles. Deductive reasoning is "top down." Researchers using deductive reasoning begin with a theory, develop hypotheses to test the theory, observe phenomena related to the hypotheses, and validate or invalidate the theory. For example, the same student might use the generalization that all coders have the RHIT credential. He sees that Jane Doe is a coder in the department. Therefore, he concludes that Jane Doe must have the RHIT credential.

As the examples demonstrate, neither induction nor deduction alone is completely satisfactory. Early, exploratory research often takes an inductive approach. Once researchers have generated a theory, they use the deductive approach to test the theory.

Check Your Understanding 19.1

Instructions: On a separate piece of paper, indicate whether the following statements are true or false (T or F).

1. Research is the study and analysis of research methods and theories.

2. An aspect of a theory is that it predicts behavior.

3. A model is the systematic organization of knowledge that explains or predicts behavior or events.

4. Research conducted by HIM professionals that answers the question "how?" is considered applied research.

5. A researcher using inferential statistics to analyze data is taking a quantitative approach.

Research Process

The research process is orderly problem solving using the following basic components:

- Defining the research question (problem)
- Performing a literature review
- Determining a research design and method
- Gathering data
- Analyzing the data
- Presenting results

These components are the basis of a step-by-step process to collect accurate and reliable data, to conduct appropriate analyses, and to provide sound information.

Knowing the purpose of the research is critical. The researchers' purpose should be to answer a significant question, to solve a meaningful problem, or to contribute to the body of knowledge. Purpose drives decisions in each of the components of the research process.

Defining the Research Question (Problem)

Research begins with defining the research question or the problem within a topic. (Refer to figure 19.2 for examples of topics.) A **research question** is a clear statement in the form of a question of the specific issue within a topic that a researcher wishes to study. An example of a research question related to the first topic in figure 19.2 would be: What is the effect of competitive market forces on the exchange of information among healthcare organizations?

Process of Development Purpose assists researchers in developing their research question. Quantitative researchers with the purpose of generating objective information develop clearly defined research questions. They follow a linear process focusing the question to a researchable issue. Qualitative researchers with the purpose of interpreting nonnumerical observations develop initial, preliminary research questions. They follow an iterative or cyclical process refining the questions as their research study progresses. Investing time and effort in developing the research question is crucial. Criteria for a well-developed research question include (Aveyard 2010, 23–37):

- The question is clearly and exactly stated.
- The question has theoretical significance, practical worth, or both.
- The question has obvious and explicit links to a larger body of knowledge, such as a theory or a research model.
- The research results advance knowledge in a definable way.
- The answer to the question or the solution to the problem is worthwhile.

Developing the research question begins with identifying a question or problem. Sources of research questions include research models, recommendations of previous researchers, and gaps in the body of knowledge.

- *Research models:* Research models show the factors and relationships in a theory. Researchers can select one or two factors that other researchers have raised questions about or have found problematic.
- *Recommendations of previous researchers:* In journal articles, theses, and dissertations, researchers specifically make recommendations

Figure 19.2. Examples of topics in health informatics and information management

- Interoperability and exchange of information among healthcare organizations, accrediting bodies, regulatory agencies, and other authorized entities
- Findings of evaluation studies of health information systems and technology
- Information technology and improvement of clinicians' performance, clinical care, and health outcomes
- Factors in the adoption and use of health information technologies and systems
- Standards for reporting on studies in health informatics and information management
- Access, use, quality, and types of consumer e-health initiatives
- Classifications, terminologies, coded data, and structured reports

for additional research based on the results of their own research. For example, researchers may identify unintentional flaws in their own study that future researchers could correct in a replication study.

- *Gaps in the body of knowledge:* Published as journal articles, comprehensive reviews of the literature on a problem or question identify gaps or problematic areas. (See the section on performing a literature review.) These review articles can be examined for research questions.

Next, researchers narrow the focus of the question to a manageable and researchable issue. Researchers begin with a broad, general question and then gradually pinpoint the topic into a problem statement. For example, the researcher might begin the description of the problem as a general societal concern. Supporting citations would come from popular magazines and opinion articles. Then, he or she would focus the discussion by explaining how this problem or question affects the field of health informatics and information management. Supporting citations here would come from scholarly journal articles, technical government reports, or other credible, scientific papers. Finally, the researcher writes the problem statement.

Problem Statement

A **problem statement** is a single sentence with an action verb, such as explore or compare, that specifically and succinctly states what the researcher will be doing to investigate the problem or question (Colling 2003, 226). An example of a problem statement related to the first topic in figure 19.2 would be: This exploratory study compares the effects of competitive market forces on the exchange of information between healthcare organizations in states with managed care penetration greater than the national percentage of penetration with states with managed care penetration less than the national percentage of penetration. The action verb *compare* tells the reader that the researchers will be comparing effects.

Quantitative researchers operationalize their problem statement, which means that they formulate the problem statement using operational definitions obtained during their literature review. Operational definitions are measurable terms that are capable of generating data and that satisfactorily capture the issues of the question or problem. On the other hand, in qualitative research the problem statement is a tentative supposition. As a working possibility, the problem statement guides initial data collection and is revised during the study based on the data obtained. For both quantitative and qualitative researchers, the problem statement also limits the study's scope by setting its boundaries—aspects of the problem or question that the researcher will *not* be investigating. Finally, the action verb in the problem statement indicates the study's research design.

Check Your Understanding 19.2

Instructions: On a separate piece of paper, indicate whether the following statements are true or false (T or F).

1. The first component in the research process is to select a research method.

2. Purpose drives decisions in each of the components of the research process.

3. A research question is a single sentence with an action verb that directly states what the researcher will be doing to investigate an issue.

4. A criterion for a well-developed research question is that it explicitly links to a larger body of knowledge.

5. Using a research model as the source of a research question is a poor practice because a research model is a visual depiction and a research question is a written format.

Performing a Literature Review

A literature review is a systematic and organized compilation of the important information about a topic. Literature review has three meanings defined as follows:

- Meaning 1: *Process* of identifying, reading, summarizing, analyzing, and synthesizing the writings of recognized scholars and experts.

- Meaning 2: *Product* that is the introduction to a manuscript or an article in which researchers explain how they arrived at their research question.

- Meaning 3: *Product* in which the introduction of meaning 2 is expanded and refined into an entirely separate, independent, and peer-reviewed article or book chapter. Known as a systematic review or meta-analysis, this literature review is a specialized type of research and is discussed in greater detail in a later section on secondary analysis.

Purposes of the Literature Review Literature reviews have three purposes: (1) to orient readers to the issue and to persuade them of the necessity of the research study; (2) to assure the reader that the researcher has conducted a thorough review of all aspects of the topic; and (3) to build the researcher's knowledge in the topic.

The literature review should guide the reader to conclude that the logical and necessary next step is the research proposed by the researchers. The thoroughness of the literature review lends credibility to the study. Researchers, as a result of their literature review, come to a complete understanding of the topic and can demonstrate the competencies in figure 19.3. Researchers who can apply these competencies are able to clearly explain their research topic and are more likely to conduct a research study that yields valuable evidence for practice.

Process of the Literature Review A literature review is a systematic process consisting of four steps:

1. Identify sources of the literature.
2. Seek and retrieve the literature.
3. Collect and record information underlying the competencies (see figure 19.3).
4. Analyze and synthesize the information obtained in the previous step.

Sources of Information In the first step, the researcher identifies the sources of literature for the review. Many sources of information exist, such as printed works, audiovisual media, and electronic media. (See figure 19.4.)

Figure 19.3. Competencies resulting from a strong knowledge base

- Outline a historical overview of a topic including turning points, trends, and controversies
- Describe research frames and approaches in the topic
- Explain the evolution of major theories being able to differentiate between accepted theories and those outside the mainstream
- Relate leading theorists and researchers with their ideas and findings
- Determine applicable models, appropriate research designs and methods, interventions, and pertinent and confounding factors
- Clarify concepts, identify relevant variables and main outcome measures with their operational definitions, and describe expected results
- State advantages and disadvantages of various research methods
- Identify sources of data, populations, and sampling techniques
- Cite the strengths and weaknesses of commonly used instruments
- Select appropriate analytical techniques
- Assess the thoroughness of literature reviews in published studies
- Identify competently conducted research and inadequately conducted research
- Detect unexplored issues, gaps, or discrepancies in the body of knowledge that his or her research can investigate, fill, or resolve

Figure 19.4. Sources of information

Periodicals
Abstract
Annual review
Cartoon
Journal
Magazine
Monograph
Newsletter
Newspaper
Press release

Books, brochures, and book chapters
Book
Book chapter
Brochure
Dictionary
Encyclopedia
Legal citation
Manual
Map or chart
Pamphlet
Product insert
Published or archived letter

Technical and research reports
Government bulletin
Government report
Industry report
Issue brief
Monograph

Nongovernment agency report
Position paper
Reference report
University report
White paper
Working paper

Proceedings of meetings
Conference
Meeting
Poster session
Symposium
Unpublished proceeding paper

**Doctoral dissertations
and Master's theses**
Abstract of dissertation
Abstract of thesis
Dissertation
Thesis

Unpublished works
Submitted manuscript
Unpublished letter
Unpublished manuscript
Unpublished raw data

Reviews
Book
Film
Video

Audiovisual media
Address
Audiotape
Chart
Film
Lecture
Music recording
Performance
Published interview
Recorded interview
Slide
Speech
Television broadcast and
    transcript
Television series and
    transcript
Unpublished interview
Work of art

Electronic media
Computer program
Computer software
Electronic database
Internet website
Online abstract
Online book
Online journal
Social media
Software manual

Many of these sources of information are available to HIM researchers through educational institutions' libraries or through reciprocal agreements between the researchers' employers and educational institutions. Libraries' extensive holdings, also called collections, include paper and online journals, books and electronic books, reference manuals, maps, videotapes, and audiotapes. Libraries typically list their holdings on webpages. Many of these holdings can be accessed through the library's catalogs, bibliographic databases, and other databases.

Usually, the majority of a literature review is based on published literature. However, for some research methods, other information sources may be important such as audiovisual media for the qualitative approach. Therefore, consideration should be given to identifying all the potential information sources for the literature review.

The published literature comprises primary and secondary sources. **Primary sources** are the original works of the researchers who conducted the research study. Research-based articles in *Educational Perspectives in Health Informatics and Information Management, Journal of Medical Internet Research,* or *International Journal of Medical Informatics* are examples of primary sources. **Secondary sources** are summaries of the original works. Encyclopedias and textbooks are familiar secondary sources. For literature reviews, primary sources are preferable to secondary sources.

Additionally, peer-reviewed (refereed) journals, also called research or academic journals, are preferable to popular (trade) magazines. Peer-reviewed journals are a type of professional or scientific journal for which content experts evaluate articles for quality and relevance prior to publication. This evaluation, namely peer review, ensures that the information reported in the journal is of the highest quality (Dine et al. 2015, 8). Examples of peer-reviewed journals are *Perspectives in Health Information Management, Journal of the American Medical Informatics Association, Journal of the American Medical Association, New England Journal of Medicine,* and *Science.* Popular magazines, for example, are not peer-reviewed.

For HIM researchers, an important information source is the grey literature (British spelling because the term originated in the United Kingdom). The grey literature is the body of publications that is available in print, electronically, or both, but that is not published in easily accessible journals (Eden et al. 2011, 98–99). It is produced by government agencies (such as the Institute of Medicine), academic institutions, or companies in business and industry, such as Deloitte LLP and RAND Corporation. Examples include technical reports, technology assessments, pamphlets, and product inserts.

Search and Retrieval of Information Sources

In the second step, researchers search and retrieve information sources from knowledge bases, such as bibliographic databases and digital collections. **Bibliographic databases** are databases of published literature such as journals, magazines, newspaper articles, books, book chapters, and other information sources. The databases' scopes vary by type of information source indexed and by academic disciplines covered. For example, some databases only index peer-reviewed journals while others also index conference proceedings and book chapters. Also, in terms of scope, some databases focus on indexing publications from certain academic disciplines, such as health sciences or computer science, while others are multidisciplinary. Finally, many databases have evolved beyond mere indices into digital libraries, providing the full texts of their indexed contents.

HIM researchers need to search a variety of databases because HIM is multidisciplinary. Moreover, some of the grey literature is also available through digital collections, such as the resources of the Centers for Medicare and Medicaid Services and the Agency for Healthcare Research and Quality. Table 19.2 provides a list of selected databases and digital collections covering business and management, computer science and engineering, health services administration, and medicine and allied health sciences.

To organize and manage information sources, researchers use reference management software, such as Reference Manager, EndNote, RefWorks, BiblioExpress, Zotero, and others. These software packages allow researchers to:

- Create personal bibliographic databases
- Utilize the packages' search engines that directly download citations and full-text articles into the researchers' personal bibliographic databases
- Import the contents of databases into word-processing software
- Transform bibliographic entries into the required style of the journal (styles editor)

The following methods describe ways to search for and retrieve peer-reviewed journal articles.

1. Generate a list of key terms, known as medical subject headings (MeSH) in the health and medical databases, and synonyms.

2. Generate a list of target databases such as JSTOR and PubMed. JSTOR, PubMed, and many other databases provide online tutorials on how to query them. University libraries also provide online tutorials on how to search many of the databases.

3. Enter queries using the key terms and synonyms and focus your queries using limits, such as publication type (refereed journal), language (English), and time periods.

4. Scan the abstracts of the retrieved articles to determine their relevance and to identify pivotal articles. Abstracts briefly summarize the major parts of a research study.

5. Save the articles that are available electronically; photocopy the articles that are unavailable electronically. Note that although it may be convenient to only use online articles, the resulting literature review will be incomplete and biased.

6. Run new queries on the databases or retrieve additional articles based on information obtained while scanning abstracts and articles initially retrieved, such as previously unretrieved articles written by leading theorists or researchers, references cited at the end of the pivotal articles, and new terms based on the MeSH headings of the pivotal articles.

Table 19.2.   Selected bibliographic databases and other digital collections

Bibliographic database or digital collection	Description
ABI/INFORM Complete	Journals, dissertations, working papers, business newspapers, trade publications, business and economics magazines, and country- and industry-focused reports in business, health services and information management, accounting, and finance
ACM Digital Library (Association for Computing Machinery)	Journals, magazines, and conference proceedings in computer science and engineering
Agency for Healthcare Research and Quality ("Effective Health Care Program Library of Resources" and "Research Tools and Data")	PowerPoint presentations, full research reports, summaries of evidence-based research, educational materials, and other resources on healthcare interventions and treatment options for a variety of health conditions
	Statistical data on healthcare delivery and summaries and full reports of research findings and technology assessments
AHIMA Body of Knowledge (BoK)	Articles from the *Journal of the American Health Information Management Association* and *AHIMA Advantage*; proceedings from AHIMA's Annual Convention and Exhibit; AHIMA practice briefs, toolkits, leadership models, position statements, reports, guidelines, and white papers; and government publications, such as the *Federal Register* and documents from the US Department of Health and Human Services
Business Source Complete	Journals and books covering business, management, economics, banking, finance, accounting, and others
Centers for Medicare and Medicaid Services' Research, Statistics, Data and Systems	Broad range of quantitative resources, summary information, and research reports on Medicare and Medicaid programs, demonstration projects, health expenditures, and key statistics
CINAHL (Cumulative Index of Nursing and Allied Health Literature)	Journals and publications in nursing, biomedicine, health sciences librarianship, consumer health, and allied health disciplines
Federation of American Scientists' Office of Technology Assessment Archive	US Office of Technology Assessment's reports, background papers, and contractor papers analyzing scientific and technical policy issues of the 1970s–1990s
Google Scholar	Journals, dissertations, books, abstracts, and court opinions covering multiple fields from academic publishers, professional societies, online repositories, universities, and other websites
IEEE Xplore (Institute of Electrical and Electronics Engineers)	Transactions, journals, magazines, and conference proceedings in computer science and engineering
JSTOR (Journal Storage)	Journals in the humanities, social sciences, and sciences
LexisNexis Academic	Foreign and domestic newspapers, magazines and trade journals, federal and state cases and statutes, law reviews, company financial information, medical news, and state and country profiles in accounting, marketing, business, and law.
MEDLINE	Medicine, nursing, allied health, dentistry, veterinary medicine, healthcare system, and preclinical sciences
National Information Center on Health Services Research and Health Care Technology (NICHSR)	Publications and web materials such as data, funding announcements, reports, and links to websites, produced by the National Library of Medicine and other organizations that are of interest to the health services research community
New York Academy of Medicine Library's Grey Literature Report	Medical and public health topics not indexed in academic databases
PubMed	Service of the US National Library of Medicine covering MEDLINE, life science journals, and online books in biomedicine and health, behavioral sciences, chemical sciences, and bioengineering

Collection and Recording of Information from Sources   The third step is to collect and record information from the sources. Be sure to capture complete citation data (see figure 19.5). Collect and record all the information that forms a strong knowledge base (information in competencies in figure 19.4). Researchers write a recap of the research of previous scholars and researchers and record key information from this recap in a summary table (see table 19.3). A summary table identifies key information from previous research studies by listing each study in a row, with columns displaying

Figure 19.5. Citation data required for various style guides

- Full name of the author, including first name and middle initial or name (be aware that some entries in websites have authors)
- Full title of the journal, book, video, or website
- Complete information about dates of publication, including the year, month, and season (be aware that some entries in websites are dated)
- Complete name and address of the publisher (for books and videos)
- Inclusive page numbers
- Volume number and issue number (sometimes these data are only on the front of the publication)
- Accurate URL and access date (for Internet sources)
- Accurate DOI (Digital Object Identifier) for all articles that have them. The DOI is a unique, stable identifier for articles in an online environment. The DOI is alphanumeric, beginning with the number 10, then a prefix (four or more digits representing the publisher), a forward slash, and a suffix (numbers assigned to the article by the publisher)

Table 19.3. Summary table of the information from peer-reviewed journal articles

Author	Year	Approach, design, and method	Time frame	Sample and response rate	Analytical techniques	Key findings, limitations, and recommendations
X	2012	• Mixed methods • Descriptive • Interview survey	Not stated	• Convenience sample of 209 patients • Participation rate not stated	• Percentages • Thematic analysis of participants' comments	• Goal of after-visit summary as a communication tool to engage and support patients is often unmet • Limitation of convenience sample at two primary care clinics • Recommends survey sent to larger group of participants and studies on physicians' perceptions about using after-visit summaries random sample
A, B, and C	2015	• Quantitative • Correlation • Data mining	2 years	• 18 physicians • 100%	Bivariate correlation	• Physicians' use of specialized software showing integrated information from four sources was strongly positively correlated with patients' disease control • Limitation of already high values impeded study's ability to demonstrate improved patient satisfaction ("ceiling effect") • Recommends development of new platform so software can be used with other computer systems and subsequent follow-up studies on these other systems
L, M, and N	2015	• Quantitative • Quasi-experimental • Cohort study	3 years	• 565 physicians in year 1, 678 physicians in year 2, and 626 physicians in year 3 • 48%, 62%, and 61%, respectively	Multivariate linear regression	• Use of the tool improved clinical outcomes for patients with diabetes and team cohesion was a significant positive moderator of the effect • Limitation of study's setting in primary care in one integrated delivery system • Recommends additional study of the effects of team cohesion

its features, such as publication year or approach, design, and method. Capturing data and recording information initially during the first reading of the information source help to reduce rework during the manuscript's composition.

Analysis, Evaluation, and Synthesis of Information from Sources In the fourth step, researchers analyze, evaluate, and synthesize the information that they have captured and recorded in the third step. The summary table, created in the third step, can act as an analytical and evaluative tool by identifying and emphasizing features, common characteristics, trends, and gaps in the published literature or other information sources (table 19.3). Merely chronicling a long series of descriptions of previous studies is inadequate.

Instead, in synthesis, researchers compare similarities and contrast differences among the previous studies, critically evaluate the previous studies' methods and analytical tools, interpret the findings, and draw conclusions about the information that the previous studies present. Synthesis makes sense of all the information that has been captured.

Development of Literature Review After completing the literature review process, researchers develop the introduction to their paper or their article. These two documents—the introduction or the article—are the literature review products. The characteristics of a well-developed literature review include:

- Comprehensiveness that is also relevant and focused
- Conciseness in stating what is known and unknown about a topic
- Logical and succinct summary comprised mainly of primary sources
- Critical analysis and evaluation that includes strengths, weaknesses, limitations, and gaps
- Synthesis

Common conventions guide the development of literature reviews. These conventions include:

- Brief descriptions of the scope of the literature review. For example: "The topic of health information systems is broad. This literature review focused on research articles related to mental health."
- Statement of the strategies used to identify literature. For example: "To identify relevant articles, we used the following inclusion and exclusion criteria."
- Use of an organizing function to create a coherent and logical order to the literature review. Examples of organizing functions include the research model and chronology.
- Inclusion of pertinent research studies. Pertinent studies include turning points in the development of knowledge about a topic, such as research studies that moved the topic forward or added new factors to the topic. Researchers provide enough information about these studies, such as the features listed in the summary

table (table 19.3) that their quality can be assessed. These key studies are described in greater detail than replication or duplicative studies. Research studies that have the same findings with the same factors are bundled. For example: "Research (citation one, citation two, citation three, and so on) has shown that cost is an obstacle to the implementation of electronic health records in small primary care practices." The pertinence of tangentially related studies, if included, is explicitly stated. The studies most-related to the researchers' proposed study are discussed last.

- Inclusion of important studies with contradictory findings. Readers could interpret their absence as evidence of the researchers' bias. Evidence of bias detracts from the credibility of the literature review. Explanations of the contradictory findings based on evaluation and analysis are suggested.
- Inclusion of research studies that either were conducted inadequately or resulted in gaps or conflicting results, especially if the researcher is rectifying the errors. The researcher specifically points out the inadequacies, gaps, or conflicting results.
- Verb tenses that traditionally situate the event or idea in time. Present tense is used to express truths, accepted theories, and facts and to explain recent, valid studies. The past tense, with the relevant date, is used to describe past studies with continued historical significance. Examples are:
  - *Accepted theory*: Specific goals motivate employees more than vague goals.
  - *Recent study*: Johnson's results illustrate the importance of specific goals.
  - *Study of historical importance*: In 1972, the study of Smith et al. showed the importance of expectancy in motivation.

Finally, the literature review concludes with a sentence that specifically links the previous research to the researchers' study. In quantitative studies, the literature review concludes with a clear and explicit **hypothesis**, a statement that describes a research question in measurable terms.

Check Your Understanding 19.3

Instructions: On a separate piece of paper, indicate whether the following statements are true or false (T or F).

1. The term *literature review* can refer to both a process and a product.

2. The literature review is important because it guides readers to conclude that the researcher's project is necessary.

3. Information sources should always be printed publications.

4. An example of a primary source is an entry in an encyclopedia.

5. Peer-reviewed (refereed) journals are a type of professional or scientific journal for which content experts evaluate articles for quality and relevance prior to publication.

6. For HIM researchers, technical reports from government agencies may be an important information source.

7. Searching bibliographic databases with different scopes, such as business and medicine, retrieves differing sets of journal articles.

8. In the literature review, researchers orient readers to recognized scholars' research related to the research question.

9. Synthesis means compiling a long, comprehensive paragraph detailing every research study described in the retrieved journal articles.

10. Studies with contradictory results should be excluded from the literature review because they confuse the reader and interrupt the logical flow of information.

Determining a Research Design and Method

The **research design** is the infrastructure of a study. A **research method** is a set of specific procedures used to gather and analyze data. Researchers can investigate the same broad question or problem using different research designs and research methods. (See table 19.4.) The selection of the appropriate research design and method increases the likelihood that the data (evidence) collected are relevant, high quality, and directly related to the research question or problem.

Research Design A research design is a plan to achieve the researchers' purpose: answering a question, solving a problem, or generating new information. There are six common research designs: historical, descriptive, correlational, evaluation, experimental, and causal-comparative. Which design is appropriate depends on the researchers' purpose and statement of the problem.

Preliminary, exploratory investigations are often descriptive or correlational. As researchers refine these investigations, they conduct causal-comparative and experimental studies. Researchers also combine designs to address their particular research questions or problems. For instance, studies may include both descriptive and correlational findings.

Historical Research Historical research investigates the past. Researchers examine primary and secondary sources. Primary sources include wills, charters, reports, minutes, eyewitness accounts, letters, and e-mail records. Secondary sources are derived from primary sources; secondary sources summarize, critique, or analyze the primary sources. Primary sources are superior to secondary sources. Examining both primary and secondary sources, HIM researchers could explore the origin of standards organizations, the development of transaction standards, and the history of code sets.

Descriptive Research Descriptive research determines and reports the current status of topics and

Table 19.4.   Designs of research, their applications, their associated methods, and examples of HIM studies

Design	Application	Method	Example of HIM study
Historical	Understand past events	Case study Bibliography	The factors leading to the creation and development of clinical decision support systems in the 1960s and 1970s
Descriptive	Describe current status	Survey Observation	A survey of clinicians to determine how and to what degree they use clinical decision support systems
Correlational	Determine existence and degree of relationship	Survey Secondary analysis	A study to determine the relationship among individual clinicians' attributes, the health team's characteristics, the setting, and use of clinical decision support systems
Evaluation	Evaluate effectiveness	Survey Case study Observation Randomized, double-blind, controlled trial	A study to evaluate the efficacy of the implementation of a clinical decision support system in a specialty clinic in an academic health center
Causal-Comparative (Quasi-Experimental)	Detect causal relationship	Cohort study Case-control (retrospective) study	A study to compare the antibiotic prescribing practices for acute respiratory infections of primary care clinician teams using a clinical decision support system versus primary care clinician teams not using a clinical decision support system
Experimental	Establish cause and effect	Parallel group trial Cluster trial Randomized, double-blind, controlled trial	A study to evaluate the influence of a clinical decision support system on clinicians' antibiotic prescribing practices for acute respiratory infections with clinicians randomized into an intervention group and a control group

subjects. The shortcomings of descriptive research include the lack of standardized questions, trained observers, and high-response rates. HIM researchers have conducted many descriptive studies, such as the status of the HIM workforce, coding accuracy, the extent of electronic health record (EHR) implementation, and levels of agreement on terms in clinical terminologies.

Correlational Research   Correlational research detects the existence, the direction, and the degree of relationships among factors. The factors in correlational research and other research designs are called **variables**.

In correlational research, there are at least two measured variables. For example, correlational researchers conducted a study investigating the association between stress and anxiety. They found that the scores for the two variables, stress and anxiety, both moved in the *same* direction—

as one increased so did the other. This association is a positive relationship because the variables' scores are moving in the same direction. The researchers also investigated the participants' feelings of personal accomplishment. In this case, the researchers found that the scores for the variables, stress and feelings of personal accomplish, moved in *opposite* directions—as stress increased the feelings of personal accomplishment decreased and vice versa. This association is a negative (inverse) relationship because the variables' scores are moving in opposite directions. However, the design of the researchers' study—correlational—did *not* permit them to state that stress caused anxiety (or vice versa) or that stress decreased feelings of personal accomplishment (or vice versa). Many other factors, such as financial problems, poor coping skills, or low self-confidence could have been associated with stress, anxiety, and feelings of personal accomplishment.

The degree or strength of the relationship among variables can range from 0.00 to +1.00 (or –1.00), detailed as follows:

- Strength of 0.00 means absolutely no relationship
- Strength between 0.00 and +1.00 or between 0.00 and –1.00 means that the variables sometimes, but not always, move together
- Strength of 1.00 or –1.00 means a perfect relationship, with the variables moving exactly in tandem

The value of correlational research is that it indicates the existence of associations that can be examined and possibly explained using experimental research studies.

HIM researchers have conducted studies on factors related to the adoption of health information technologies, rates of social media usage and opinions about healthcare laws, rankings of adverse drug effects and their mortality rates, healthcare professionals' security practices and their personal characteristics, use of electronic mobile applications and maintenance of health regimens, and many more.

Evaluation Research Evaluation research is the systematic application of criteria to assess value (Øvretveit, 2014, 6–13). Researchers can assess the value of programs, projects, organizations, interventions, policies, technologies, products, and other activities or objects. Criteria to assess these activities or objects can be related to many of their aspects, such as conceptualization, design, components, implementation, effectiveness, efficiency, impact, scalability, and generalizability.

Common types of evaluation studies are needs assessments, process evaluations, outcome evaluations, and policy analyses (Shi 2008, 213).

- **Needs assessment:** Collecting and analyzing data about proposed programs, projects, and other activities or objects to determine what is required, lacking, or desired by an employee, group, or an organization. The HIM professional could survey patients to determine their preferences and priorities for various features in the healthcare organization's patient portal.

- **Process evaluation:** Monitoring programs, projects, and other activities or objects to check whether their development or implementation is proceeding as planned (also known as formative evaluation) (Robson 2010, 253). A research team could assess whether the roll-out of the new features in the organization's patient portal is occurring per the project's milestones and within budget. Adjustments can be made as needed.

- **Outcome evaluation:** Collecting and analyzing data at the end of an implementation or operating cycle to determine whether the program, project, or other activity or object has achieved its expected or intended impact, product, or other outcome (also known as summative evaluation) (Robson 2010, 253). Researchers could conduct a study comparing the level of patients' interaction with their organization's patient portal to the level of interaction reported by their industry peers. Organizational leaders can use the findings to help decide whether the vendor's contract should be renewed or revised.

- **Policy analysis:** Identifying options to meet goals and estimating the costs and consequences of each option prior to the implementation of any option (Shi 2008, 219–220). For a federal agency, a research team could identify various ways to increase patient self-management and engagement using health information technologies and, for each way, analyze its benefits and costs, and predict its consequences.

Other terms are used for the large umbrella of evaluation research depending upon the focus of the research, the researchers' educational background, and the research's funding source. These terms include outcomes research, health services research, health technology assessment, and comparative effectiveness research.

- **Outcomes research** is defined as research that seeks to improve the delivery of patient care by studying the end results of health services, such as quality of life, functional status, patient satisfaction, costs, cost-effectiveness, and other specified outcomes (In and Rosen 2014, 489). An example of outcomes research is a study investigating whether a clinical decision support system that links the EHR to treatment protocols, drug information, alerts, and community resources for the care of patients with HIV infection improves a patient's quality of life.

- **Health services research** is multidisciplinary research that studies how social factors, financing systems, organizational structures and processes, health technologies, and personal behaviors affect access to healthcare, its quality and cost, and overall health and well-being (AcademyHealth 2015). The research is usually concerned with relationships among need, demand, supply, use, and outcome of health services. An example of health services research is a study that investigates whether the degree of adoption of health information technologies affects patient safety.

- **Health technology assessment (HTA)** is the evaluation of the usefulness (utility) of a health technology in relation to cost, efficacy, utilization, and other factors in terms of its impact on social, ethical, and legal systems. The purpose of HTA is to provide individual patients, clinicians, funding bodies, and policymakers with high quality information on the benefits and cost effectiveness of health interventions (Ware and Hicks 2011, 64S). Technology, in this context, is broadly defined as the application of scientific knowledge to practical purposes and includes methods, techniques, and instrumentation. Health technologies promote or maintain health; prevent, diagnose, or treat acute or chronic conditions; or support rehabilitation (INAHTA 2015). They include pharmaceuticals, medical devices, medical equipment, medical diagnostic and therapeutic procedures, organizational systems, and health information technologies. For example, the Technology Assessment Program at the Agency for Healthcare Research and Quality (AHRQ) conducts technology assessments based on primary research, systematic reviews of the literature, meta-analyses, and appropriate qualitative methods of synthesizing data from multiple studies. The Centers for Medicare and Medicaid Services (CMS), one consumer of the AHRQ's HTAs, uses them to make its national coverage decisions for the Medicare program (AHRQ 2015).

- **Comparative effectiveness research (CER)** is research that generates and synthesizes "evidence that compares the benefits and harms of alternative methods to prevent, diagnose, treat, and monitor a clinical condition, or to improve the delivery of care. The purpose of CER is to assist consumers, clinicians, purchasers, and policy makers to make informed decisions that will improve healthcare at both the individual and population levels" (IOM 2009, 13). Specifically, CER can help determine which intervention, such as a drug or a surgery, may be most effective or beneficial for a given patient. For example, under the Affordable Care Act (ACA) of 2010, the AHRQ is charged to disseminate information gained by federally funded CER. Recent CER information that the AHRQ has disseminated includes stroke prevention in atrial fibrillation and treatment of tinnitus (GAO 2015, 31).

Experimental Research   **Experimental research** is a design in which the researcher directly manipulates factors in carefully controlled interventions and according to strict **protocols** (detailed sets of rules and procedures). The purpose of the control in the interventions and protocols is to maintain uniform conditions during the research so that no extraneous factors, known as **confounding variables**, affect the study's outcome. The researchers' end goal is to be able to pinpoint the cause of the intervention's effect without any possible, alternative explanations. Thereby, experimental research establishes **causal relationships**—relationships that show cause and effect. For example, smoking (the cause) results in lung cancer (the effect).

Researchers conducting experimental research work with two types of variables. **Independent variables** are antecedent or prior factors that researchers manipulate directly; they are also called treatments or interventions. **Dependent variables** are the measured variables; they depend on the independent variables. The dependent variables reflect the results that the researcher theorizes. They occur subsequently or after the independent variables. Therefore, the independent variable causes an effect in the dependent variable.

Experimental researchers design their studies to maximize the likelihood of establishing causal relationships and to minimize any potential effects of confounding variables. To achieve these aims, experimental researchers design into their studies the following four key features (Campbell and Stanley 1963, 13).

- *Randomization*: The process begins with random sampling— the unbiased selection of subjects from the population of interest. (Random sampling is discussed in greater detail in the section on gathering data.) Then **randomization**, or the arbitrary allocation of subjects between comparison groups, occurs. Of the comparison groups, the **experimental (study) group** comprises the research subjects who receive the study's intervention.

- *Observation*: Measurement of the dependent variable *before* and *after* the treatment. Observation is used generically and could be a pretest and a posttest.

- *Presence of a control group*: Another group, the **control group**, comprises the control subjects who do not receive the intervention.

- *Treatment (intervention)*: Process in which the researcher manipulates the independent variables. In this context, **treatment**, also known as intervention, is defined generically or broadly, beyond its usual meaning of therapy. Treatment could mean a physical conditioning program, a computer training program, a particular laboratory medium, or the timing of prophylactic medications.

As an example of an experimental study, HIM researchers could investigate the effects of an Internet-based health promotion program. Adult participants could be randomized between an experimental group and a control group. All participants' base-line data on their consumption of fruits and vegetables could be collected via an online survey prior to the start of the intervention. The intervention could be a multimedia online module containing information and guidance on the benefits of eating fruits and vegetables. Members of the experimental group could be given a link to the program; members of the control group could be told that they were on the wait list and that their access was delayed. Members of the experimental group could access the module via the link from their homes. After three months, all participants could be sent online questionnaires about their consumption of fruits and vegetables. Subsequently, the two groups' data could be analyzed and compared in terms of their initial consumption patterns and their post-intervention patterns.

Causal-Comparative Research **Causal-comparative research** is a type of quasi-experimental design. *Quasi* means resembling or having some of the characteristics. Therefore, causal-comparative research resembles experimental research by having many, but not all, of its characteristics. Causal-comparative research lacks two characteristics of experimental research: manipulation of treatment and random assignment to a group. Causal-comparative research is also called *ex post facto*, meaning retrospective, because some past variable or phenomenon has already occurred.

Three situations, logistically and ethically, require the causal-comparative design:

- The variables cannot be manipulated (gender, age, race, birthplace).
- The variables should not be manipulated (accidental death or injury, child abuse).
- The variables represent different conditions that have already occurred (medication error, heart catheterization performed, smoking, environmental exposure).

These situations prevent people from being assigned randomly into groups. However, by relinquishing manipulation of treatment and randomization, causal-comparative (quasi-experimental) research can only determine the *possibility* of causal relationships.

In an example of a causal-comparative study, HIM researchers may look back in time (retrospective) to investigate the factors associated with inpatient medication errors when a computerized alert system was in place. Identifying inpatient admissions with and without medication errors in the database, researchers could look for patterns in the records associated with errors, such as the patients' diseases, location of care (intensive care unit versus regular nursing floor), providers' characteristics, organizational features, and other factors.

A schema, based on the previously described four features (randomization, observation, control group, treatment), can be used to differentiate experimental research designs and causal-comparative (quasi-experimental) research designs (Campbell and Stanley 1963). Studies having all four key features are classified as experimental (one acceptable omission is the prior observation). Studies totally missing any feature are classified as quasi-experimental.

Time Frame as an Element of Research Design

The element of time frame cuts across all six types of designs. There are two pairs of time frames—retrospective versus prospective and cross-sectional versus longitudinal.

- **Retrospective** time frame involves looking back in time. For example, leadership studies in which the researcher asks the leader to list factors that led to his or her success are examples of a retrospective time frame. For some types of questions, such as those related to historic events, a retrospective design is the only possible design.

- **Prospective** time frame follows subjects into the future to examine relationships between variables and later occurrences. For example, researchers identify individuals or subjects with certain variables and then follow these individuals or subjects into the future to see what occurs.

- **Cross-sectional** time frame involves collecting or reviewing data at one point in time. As snapshots, these studies face the potential danger of collecting or reviewing data during an unrepresentative time period. For example, researchers could conduct a study for a professional association on the characteristics of its members, such as age, gender, job titles, educational attainment, and opinions of the associations' web page.

- **Longitudinal** time frame requires collecting data at multiple points in time. Examples include studies of breast cancer and cardiovascular disease, such as the Nurses' Health Study that has followed the health of more than 238,000 nurses since 1976 (Nurses' Health Study 2015).

Check Your Understanding 19.4

Instructions: On a separate piece of paper, indicate whether the following statements are true or false (T or F).

1. A researcher's choice of a research design depends upon the researcher's purpose and statement of the problem.

2. To examine the effect of legislation on the number of hospitals in rural areas in the 1950s and 1960s, a researcher would use a historical design.

3. A positive relationship is described when a supervisor's feelings of personal efficacy decrease as her number of subordinates increases.

4. Health technology assessment is considered applied research.

5. The variable that reflects the outcome of the research's intervention is the independent variable.

Research Methods A research method is the particular strategy that a researcher uses to collect and analyze data. Certain research methods are more closely associated with one design than another (table 19.4). However, considerable overlap exists among methods and designs. For example, researchers can use the survey research method in both descriptive and correlational research designs.

Survey **Surveys** systematically collect data about a population (entire group) to determine its current status with regard to certain factors. Surveys are a form of self-report research in which the individuals themselves are the source of data. Two formats of surveys are interviews (oral) and questionnaires (written or electronic). Census surveys collect data from all the members of the population. Sample surveys collect data from representative members of the population.

Census surveys are conducted when the population is fairly small. For example, the Health Information Management Association of Australia (HIMAA) conducted a census survey. HIMAA surveyed all of its members, approximately 800, to obtain feedback on its members' views of current challenges facing the profession, challenges facing the profession in the next five to ten years, and other issues (Wissmann 2015, 4). On the other hand, when data about a large population is needed, researchers conduct a sample survey. Researchers collected data from a random sample to examine the readiness of baby boomers (about 75 million people age 46 to 64 years) to adopt consumer health technologies (Colby and Ortman 2014, 2; LeRouge et al. 2014, e200).

In **interview surveys**, researchers orally question the members of the population. Examples of interview surveys are telephone surveys and focused studies. Researchers can question members of the population as individuals or as a group. Additionally, they can conduct a structured interview controlling the questions and responses or they can conduct an unstructured interview allowing a free-flowing conversation. In the structured interview, researchers use a written list of questions called an interview guide. Using an interview guide ensures that all individuals or focus groups are asked the same questions. The structured interview has the advantages of being easier to quantify, tabulate, and analyze than the unstructured interview. However, the unstructured interview is often chosen when the topic is unexplored, poorly understood, or ill-defined. Typically, both types of interviews are recorded and transcribed for later analyses.

For example, using telephone interviews, researchers explored the public's attitudes concerning the potential of health information technologies, particularly EHRs, to improve healthcare (Gaylin et al. 2011, 920–928). The researchers interviewed a random sample of 1,015 US households with telephones or cell phones. The interviewers had in-depth training and followed a strict protocol. The researchers found that the respondents believed EHRs could improve healthcare and reduce its costs and that positive attitudes toward health information technologies and EHRs were related to higher incomes and an affinity for technology.

Investigating physicians' adoption of patient portals, researchers conducted interviews during a focused study as a phase of a larger study (Vydra et al. 2015, 1). In a **focused study**, researchers and a small number of participants, known as the **focus group**, have a group interview on the researchers' topic to uncover information through the participants' discussion of their thoughts and experiences. The researchers orally question the focus group and moderate the resulting discussion. In this HIM research, the researchers questioned four physicians who had responded to an earlier phase of the study—an electronic survey. The purpose of the focused study was to gain additional clarity on the physicians' integration of the organization's patient portal into their work flow, their actual use of the portal, and their perception of their use of it. This discussion was audio-recorded and the transcription analyzed. The researchers' findings concluded that while the physicians perceived portals positively as a means to increase patients' engagement and satisfaction, their own utilization with the technology was limited because of the lack of reimbursement for the time spent (Vydra et al. 2015, 1).

Questionnaire surveys query members of a population by providing participants a means to record and submit their responses electronically or in print form. Questionnaire studies are efficient because they require less time and money than interview studies do and because they allow the researchers to collect data from many more members of the population.

For example, in the previously discussed investigation on physicians' adoption of patient portals, an earlier phase of the study was an electronic survey (Vydra et al. 2015, 1). Electronic surveys were sent to all 89 primary care physicians affiliated with a university medical center and subject to the departmental patient portal policy. Among the items on the surveys were questions asking the respondents to estimate average amounts of time that they spent on various activities associated with the organizational patient portal. Fifty-four physicians (60.6 percent) responded. The results showed that the respondents overestimated the average time that they spent on the patient portal's activities (12.5 hours per week) as compared to the institutional log-in records (8.2 hours per week) by approximately 34 percent (Vydra et al. 2015, 14).

Observational Research   In **observational research**, researchers observe, record, and analyze behaviors and events. Typically, researchers spend prolonged periods in the setting or events under research; however, some research topics, such as behaviors in natural disasters, prevent this prolonged engagement. Observational research is used in multiple research designs, but is often classified with the qualitative approach. Highly detailed, observational research provides insight about what subjects do, how they do it, and why they do it. Three common types of observational research discussed in this chapter are nonparticipant observation, participant observation, and ethnography.

In **nonparticipant observation**, researchers act as neutral observers who neither intentionally interact with nor affect the actions of the population being observed. The researchers record and analyze the observed behaviors and also the content of modes of communication, such as documentation, speech, body language, music, television shows, commercials, and movies. Three common types of nonparticipant observation include:

- **Naturalistic observation**: Researchers record observations that are unprompted and unaffected by their actions. It is difficult to remain unobtrusive in naturalistic observation because the researchers' mere presence can affect people's behavior and other activities. In one naturalistic study, researchers examined the effects of a tailored, web-based chronic pain management program on participants' subjective assessment of their pain and other aspects of their lives (Nevedal et al. 2013, e201). Making the study naturalistic, the program was fully automated via its tailoring algorithms to relevant participant variables and included no telephone, e-mail, nor face-to-face contacts with another person. The 645 participants were either employed by a company or were a member of a healthcare plan. The participants accessed the online management program and completed assessments at baseline, one month, and six months. The researchers' results showed that after the intervention, the participants assessed their pain as significantly decreased in terms of its intensity, unpleasantness, and interference in their lives. The researchers concluded that further research in a randomized controlled trial is warranted to determine the magnitude of the intervention's effects (Nevedal et al. 2013, e201).

- **Simulation observation**: Researchers stage events rather than allowing them to occur naturally. Researchers can invent their own simulations or use standardized vignettes to stage the events. HIM researchers often have a model of a system or computer application and, in a simulation study, are attempting to imitate its function to analyze and improve its performance. For example, HIM researchers had designed an information system with decision support tools for medication administration (Moss and Berner 2015, 308). The researchers conducted a simulation study to evaluate the tools' use, content, and format. A simulation laboratory had been built to resemble an actual intensive care unit (ICU) and to allow the screens of its three computers (nursing station, medication cart, and patient bedside) to project on its walls so that everyone present could see the screens. Five simulation sessions were held (one for each ICU specialty group) with a total of 17 ICU nurse participants. Each session lasted about seven hours, during which each nurse individually received information ("report") on a patient and was asked to give medications to the simulated patient. While administering the medications, the nurses could use any or none of the decision support tools or available printed references. During the simulation, the nurses were interrupted at least twice by typical interruptions, such as telephone calls and clinical team member questions. The researchers observed and recorded the process as each nurse administered medications. Among the study's results, the researchers reported that nurses underestimated their need for support and that nurses preferred decision support tools that were short, color-coded, and easily accessed. The researchers cautioned that their study's results could not be generalized to other hospitals; however, their method to design and test the clinical decision support tools could be transferred to other settings (Moss and Berner 2015, 308).

- **Case study**: Researchers conduct an in-depth investigation of one or more examples of a phenomenon, such as a trend, occurrence, or incident. The case is a person, event, group, organization, or a set of similar institutions. The researchers identify characteristics of the case with the purpose of shedding light on similar cases. Case studies are intensive, and researchers amass rich data. Rich data are layers of extensive details from multiple sources including administrative records, financial records, policy and procedure manuals, legal documents, government documents, surveys, interviews, and other sources.

In one case study, healthcare management researchers mined a single year's data of a large, urban healthcare system "to quantify its market opportunities for medical tourism" (patients traveling domestically or internationally for health services) (Fottler et al. 2014, 49). The healthcare system comprises a full-service medical–surgical acute-care hospital (with emergency department), women's and babies' hospital, trauma hospital, cancer center, children's hospital, and three smaller regional hospitals. The system annually treats 2 million patients, 2,000 of whom are international patients (Fottler et al. 2014, 49). The data source was the system's electronic health records from which medical and sociodemographic data were collected and analyzed through frequency distributions. The researchers' findings could be used by the systems' executives to focus its marketing initiatives on specific areas of the United States and foreign countries and on health services attractive to medical tourists.

Case studies are common in evaluation research on health information technologies and systems. HIM researchers conducted a case study in two hospitals that had used a commercially available computerized physician order entry (CPOE) system or a clinical decision support (CDS) system for at least two years (Cresswell et al. 2014, e194). These two hospitals were categorized as "early adopters" of technology. The purpose of the case study was to understand the midterm consequences of implementing the systems for early adopters. At both hospitals, the data collected included:

- Forty-three audio-recorded and transcribed interviews (interviews were about 30 minutes each and were partially structured using an interview guide)
- Twenty one and a half hours of non-participant observations of various healthcare professionals during morning work rounds and meetings as recorded on a recording sheet and in field notes that included the setting, participants, interactions, medication and computer-related activities, and sequences of events
- Eleven documents of the hospital plans for the systems' implementations (Cresswell et al. 2014, e194)

The researchers used both inductive and deductive reasoning to identify themes in their data. The researchers also analyzed the data from the two hospitals separately. This separation allowed the researchers to subsequently use triangulation to assess the consistency of their evidence. **Triangulation** is the use of multiple sources or perspectives to investigate the same phenomenon. Theses multiple sources or perspectives include data (multiple times, sites, or respondents), investigators (researchers), theories, and methods (Carter et al. 2014, 545). The results or conclusions are validated if the multiple sources or perspectives arrive at the same results or conclusions. The three overarching themes that the researchers found were (1) impact on individual healthcare professionals, such as greater legibility of prescriptions and, for some, increased workloads; (2) introduction of perceived new safety risks related to accessibility and usability of the systems' hardware and software; and (3) realization of organizational benefits through secondary uses of the hospitals' data, such as reports on adherence to clinical guidelines (Cresswell et al. 2014, e194).

In **participant observation**, researchers are participants in the observed actions, activities, or processes. They can participate overtly (openly) or covertly (secretly). The researchers not only record their observations of other people's daily lives and the contexts of actions, but also record their own experiences and thoughts. Participant observation research is used to investigate groups, processes, cultures, and other phenomena.

A research team used overt participant observation in one phase of its research studying personal health records (PHRs) and their effects on communications among healthcare practitioners, pediatric patients with diabetes, and their caregivers (Piras and Zanutto 2014, 421–422). Members of the research team came from a hospital's pediatrics department and an HIT research institute. Their joint project was a PHR that integrated a logbook application for patients' smartphones and a dashboard for visualizing data to be used by physicians, patients, and caregivers. Prior to the introduction of the PHR, the HIT members of the team conducted the participant observation phase to investigate the doctor–patient relationship. This phase's

"purpose was to understand the practices, places, and artifacts [items that people create, such as diaries, tools, buildings, and many more items] related to the management of clinical data by doctors and patients before the technology came into use" (Piras and Zanutto 2014, 426). Five sessions of participant observation occurred during patients' appointments in which patients' laboratory tests were reviewed, their paper-based diabetic management logbooks analyzed, and their therapies adjusted, as necessary. The preliminary analysis of the materials collected during the observations was shared with the doctors and the resulting discussion was audio-recorded and transcribed. The comments and observations made during the discussion became an integral part of the next phase of the research.

Ethnography is the investigation of a culture by collecting data and making observations while being in the field (naturalistic setting). Ethnographers amass great volumes of detailed data while living or working with the population that they are studying. Coming from anthropology to healthcare, this observational method includes both qualitative and quantitative approaches and both participant and nonparticipant observation.

HIM researchers used an ethnographic study to reveal workarounds that clinicians used to evade security as they accessed the healthcare organization's computer systems in their care of patients (Koppel et al. 2015, 215). To obtain perceptions of computer security rules, the researchers conducted interviews and observations with hundreds of medical personnel (nurses, doctors, line workers, and managers) and with 19 cybersecurity experts, chief information officers, chief medical informatics officers, chief technology officers, and IT personnel. They collected reports from online medical discussion lists and the literature. The researchers also shadowed many clinicians as they worked to understand the clinicians' motivations and tradeoffs for circumvention. The researchers found that to accomplish their essential task of caring for patients clinicians had invented dozens of ingenious ways to circumvent what they viewed as onerous and irrational computer security rules. For example, the researchers found that "clever clinicians at one hospital defeated proximity-sensor-based timeouts [computer session terminations] by putting Styrofoam cups over the detectors" (Koppel et al. 2015, 217). The researchers pointed out that auditing and analyzing computer access logs would fail to catch these clever circumventions of cybersecurity rules. The researchers concluded that "in the inevitable conflict between even well-intended people vs. the machines and the machine rule makers, it's the people who are more creative and motivated," especially for healthcare "professionals who carry the responsibility for patient care" (Koppel et al. 2015, 219).

Experimental Method In **experimental methods**, researchers randomly assign participants into an experimental group or into a control group. In these methods, researchers actively intervene to test a hypothesis. They manipulate an independent variable (treatment or intervention) in order to assess its effect on the dependent variable (the outcome). The procedures of these methods attempt to make the dependent variable—the outcome variable—the only difference between the two groups and, thereby, establish a causal relationship between the treatment and the outcome. Experimental research methods demonstrate the key features of randomization, observation, a control group or groups, and a treatment as previously discussed in the section on experimental research design.

A **randomized controlled trial (RCT)** is an example of the experimental methods. The word *controlled* refers to the control group. Alternate terms for RCTs are clinical trials and randomized clinical trials. The word *clinical* refers to *at the bedside*, meaning the experiment involves investigations of diagnostic and therapeutic procedures, drugs and devices, and other biomedical and health interventions. Terms associated with RCTs include *arm*, *usual care*, and *blinding*.

- *Arm*: Another term for group, such as an experimental arm and a control arm. Studies that have more than one intervention or more than one version of the intervention have multiple experimental arms. For example, a three-armed study would have an arm for the participants who receive a web-based

intervention and a monthly e-mail from the researchers; a second arm for the participants who only receive the web-based intervention; and a third arm for the control group.

- *Usual care*: Typical therapy for a condition. In some experiments, the subjects in the control arm receive usual care rather than no treatment. Examples of these experiments include studies of investigational devices and studies that compare the outcomes of an experimental treatment and the typical therapy.

- *Blinding*: Process of preventing the parties involved in an RCT (subjects, researchers, and study managers or analysts) from knowing to which group, experimental or control, a participant belongs (also known as masking). Its purpose is to minimize the risk of subjective bias stemming from expectations and perceptions. In a single-blind study, only the subjects are blinded to knowing whether they are receiving the intervention or not. In a **double-blind study**, both researchers and subjects are blinded. In a triple-blind study, the staff members managing the study's operations and analyzing the data are blinded, as well as the researchers and subjects.

Researchers can use multiple types of RCTs. The most common type of RCT is the parallel-group (independent-group) trial, described previously in this section, in which the experimental group and the control group are concurrently compared. Two other types of RCTs that readers might encounter in the literature are the crossover trial and the cluster trial. In the crossover trial, each arm receives a consecutive sequence of two or more treatments. At the end of their sequence, the participants crossover and repeat the other arm's sequence. In cluster trials, groups such as clinics, families, and geographical areas are randomly assigned to different arms rather than individuals themselves.

For example, researchers conducted a parallel-group trial to examine the impact of PHRs on medication-use safety among older adults (Chrischilles et al. 2014, 679). The researchers randomized participants between an experimental PHR-user group and a usual-care control group. After the six-month trial, the PHR-user group was significantly less likely to use multiple nonsteroidal anti-inflammatory drugs (a medication-use risk) than the control group. However, there was no difference between groups in use of inappropriate medications or adherence measures. The researchers concluded that while PHRs could engage older adults to self-manage their medications, longer-termed studies were needed to evaluate the effect of this behavior change on health outcomes (Chrischilles et al. 2014, 685).

Quasi-experimental Method In **quasi-experimental methods**, researchers cannot randomly assign participants into two groups. Instead, the researchers observe the effect of an intervention that has already occurred. These interventions could be diagnostic or therapeutic procedures, risk factors, exposures, or other events. The researchers cannot fully control for potentially confounding variables and, as a result, cannot establish causal relationships. Types of quasi-experimental methods include the cohort study and the case-control retrospective study.

- **Cohort study**: A cohort is a defined group of people who share some characteristic (CMS 2006). After an intervention (such as exposure to a factor of interest), researchers observe what happens to the cohort. The cohort's outcomes are then compared to the outcomes of a similar group that has not received the intervention.

- **Case-control (retrospective) study**: *Cases* are people with a specific disease or outcome of interest and *controls* are people from the same population as the cases, but who do not have the disease or outcome. By comparing the cases to the controls, the researchers look for associations between the outcome and an intervention, such as a prior exposure to a particular risk factor. Epidemiological studies of disease outbreaks may use this type of study because the outcome is rare and the past exposure can be reliably measured.

For example, using a retrospective cohort study, researchers investigated the association between use of a community-wide health information exchange (HIE) system and 30-day same-cause hospital readmissions during a six-month period in a metropolitan area (Vest et al. 2015, 435). The researchers obtained claims files from two health plans that insure 60 percent of the area's population. The HIE's portal automatically recorded users' access. The researchers found that providers' access of patient information from the HIE system post-discharge was associated with a 57 percent lower odds of 30-day same-cause readmission, controlling for patient, utilization, and hospital factors. The researchers estimated that the annual savings from avoided readmissions totaled about $605,000 (Vest et al. 2015, 437).

Secondary Analysis Researchers distinguish between primary analysis and secondary analysis. **Primary analysis** refers to analysis of original research data by the researchers who collected them. **Secondary analysis** is the reanalysis of the original data of another organization or researcher to answer new questions or by using different statistical techniques (Cheng and Phillips 2014, 371–372). Secondary analysis includes data mining and systematic reviews.

Data mining is use of various analytical tools to discover new facts, valid patterns, and relevant relationships in large databases (Naidu and Tiwari 2014, 109). Data mining is considered secondary data analysis because data miners use databases created by others, often for purposes unrelated to research and data mining. Data mining is covered in more detail in chapter 17.

A **systematic review** is a comprehensive review of the evidence on a clearly formulated question that uses systematic and explicit methods to identify, select, and critically appraise relevant published and unpublished research studies; to extract and analyze data from the studies that are included in the review; and to present integrated and synthesized information (Green et al. 2011, 1.2.2). Systematic reviews must meet strict standards to avoid bias.

Systematic reviews are characterized by the following:

- Focusing on a well-defined question
- Using explicit search criteria to identify literature and, if appropriate, grey literature

- Employing inclusion and exclusion criteria to select articles and information sources
- Evaluating evidence in literature against consistent methodological standards
- Including relatively homogeneous (similar) studies with common underlying features

Also known as qualitative (narrative) systematic reviews, these reviews may take from 6 to 24 months to complete.

Three other types of systematic reviews exist based on their purpose and on analytical techniques:

- Scoping systematic reviews are exploratory reviews that map the range, extent, and breadth of relevant evidence and literature and other available information resources on a topic.
- Rapid reviews are simplified, less-comprehensive reviews that generally conceptualize questions and are conducted when decision makers or policymakers need information within one to six months.
- **Meta-analyses** are a specialized type of systematic review that introduces statistical techniques to combine summary-level information from at least two studies. Meta-analyses estimate the overall, combined effect of several studies' outcomes (effects) for an intervention. This estimate of effect is expressed as an effect size, such as an odds ratio or a Pearson r correlation coefficient (see chapters 16 and 17 for details on statistics). Meta-analyses may also be called an overview or a quantitative systematic review.

The advantages of systematic reviews are that they integrate and weigh findings from many studies, some of which are contradictory. Researchers synthesize the results from multiple studies in order to reach overall conclusions.

For example, researchers conducted a systematic review to assess the effectiveness of Internet-based interventions in decreasing nonprofessional caregivers' stress (Hu et al. 2015, e194). The researchers listed all the terms related to caregiver and Internet-based interventions that they used to search four identified databases. The researchers' criteria specified that the studies be open-label (not blinded to either researcher or participant) or RCTs published in peer-reviewed English language journals. The researchers then documented their search and their results are typical of systematic reviews:

- Identification of 1,485 articles in which initial database searches retrieved 1,474 articles and the authors identified 11 more articles through other sources
- Exclusion of 162 of the 1,485 articles as duplicates
- Exclusion of 1,014 articles by screening the articles' titles and abstracts and finding that the studies did not meet inclusion criteria
- Exclusion of 285 articles by reading their full text and finding that the studies did not meet inclusion criteria
- Inclusion of 24 studies of which 8 were open-label studies and 16 were RCTs (Hu et al. 2015, e194)

In analyzing the features of the 24 studies, though the outcomes in 18 of the studies were either positive or partially positive, the researchers identified no clear patterns such as duration of study or the complexity of the intervention. The researchers concluded that Internet-based interventions are mostly effective in reducing caregivers' stress and that future research is warranted. They also recommended that future studies investigate outcomes for recipients' health and for different technologies and the cost of the interventions (Hu et al. 2015, e207).

Selection of a Research Design and a Research Method In selecting a research design and method, the most important factor that researchers should consider is their purpose as reflected in their problem statement. Additionally, researchers consider the following factors:

- *Skills:* Can the researcher conduct the laboratory experiments, moderate the discussions, or perform the analytical techniques necessary for the research?

- *Time:* Does the researcher have the time to devote to conducting the research, such as in the case of a longitudinal study over a period of 10 years?

- *Money and resources:* Can the researcher afford the equipment and other costs of the research, such as setting up the simulation laboratory described earlier in the section on nonparticipant observation?

- *Potential subjects:* Are sufficient numbers of subjects available and are they willing to participate, given their busy schedules? Will people who volunteer to be subjects in the research differ from those who do not volunteer?

Researchers should establish a match among the research design and method, their purpose, and the other factors.

Check Your Understanding 19.5

Instructions: On a separate piece of paper, indicate whether the following statements are true or false (T or F).

1. Census surveys collect data from representative members of a population.

2. Focus groups allow researchers to uncover information about a topic through participants' discussion of their thoughts and experiences.

3. A potential complication of naturalistic studies is that the researcher's mere presence could affect their participants' reactions.

4. Rich data are amassed in case studies.

5. An RCT can establish causation.

Gathering Data

High-quality research depends on a carefully conceived plan and flawless execution. Prior to beginning their research study, researchers must write a step-by-step plan that considers every logistical detail from the start of their study to its completion. It is important to document the procedures of and adherence to the plan because the methods section of the study reports the plan's execution in such detail so that other researchers can replicate the study.

Validity and Reliability   Researchers who fail to plan their study's logistics may violate principles associated with the validity and reliability. Researchers whose study procedures violate principles of validity and reliability contaminate their data and may also compromise their ability to analyze their data.

Validity   There are three types of validity—internal validity, external validity, and validity.

Internal validity and external validity involve the integrity of the research plan. Validity without a modifier refers to an attribute of instruments (tools or devices that measure or record observations).

Internal validity is an attribute of a study's design that contributes to the accuracy of its findings. Threats to internal validity come from factors outside the study (confounding variables) and are potential sources of error that could contaminate a study's results (Campbell and Stanley 1963, 5). Figure 19.6 lists and defines eight common threats to internal validity that researchers attempt to avoid in the design of their research study. If internal validity is breached, researchers cannot state for certain that the independent variable caused the effect.

External validity involves the generalizability of the study's findings to other people or groups, such as patients, hospitals, and countries. Internal validity represents the bare minimum; internal validity combined with external validity is the ideal.

Figure 19.6. Threats to internal validity

History	Unplanned events occur during the research and affect the results
Maturation	Subjects grow or mature during the period of the study
Testing	Taking the first test affects subsequent tests; "practice effect"
Instrumentation	There is a lack of consistency in data collection
Statistical Regression	Subjects are selected because of their extreme scores
Differential Selection	Control group and experimental group differ, and the difference could affect the study's findings
Experimental Mortality	Loss of subjects occurs during the study
Diffusion of Treatment	Members of the control group learn about the treatment of the experimental group

For example, researchers within the Department of Veterans Affairs (VA) evaluated the use of automated encoders in the VA system (Lloyd and Layman 1997, 73–74). Eight VA medical centers tested encoding software programs from three vendors. During the course of the study, an earthquake badly damaged one of the VA medical centers, which never reopened. Therefore, no final data on the software program were available from that center. This event represents the threat to internal validity of mortality (attrition), meaning the loss of subjects. In addition, the VA centers were not covered by Medicare's inpatient prospective payment system (PPS). This uniqueness represents a threat to external validity because most hospitals are covered by the PPS. Thus, the findings lacked generalizability.

An instrument's **validity** is the extent to which the tool (questionnaire) or device (counter) measures what it is intended to measure. Two important aspects of an instrument's validity are content validity and construct validity, described follows:

- Content validity concerns whether the instrument's items (content) relate to the topic. For example, a coding test with content validity would have items related to key aspects of coding, such as uses of codes, the appropriate code set to use for healthcare services in various healthcare settings, and sources of guidelines for coding.

- Construct validity is the instrument's ability to measure hypothetical, nonobservable traits called constructs. Classic examples of constructs are psychological concepts, such as intelligence, motivation, and anxiety. Although intelligence itself is not visible, its effects are. Therefore, if an instrument is intended to measure patient satisfaction, it should include issues associated with patient satisfaction.

Reliability **Reliability** involves the consistency and stability of an instrument's measurements. Over time, a test or observation dependably measures whatever it was intended to measure. Repeated administrations of the instrument will result in reasonably similar findings. Two aspects of reliability are intrarater reliability and interrater reliability:

- **Intrarater reliability** means that the same person repeating the test will have reasonably similar findings.

- **Interrater reliability** means that different persons completing the test will have reasonably similar findings.

Instruments' validity and reliability are often stated in journal articles. Electronic databases of instruments also provide the validity of instruments.

Selecting an Instrument An **instrument** is a standardized, uniform way to collect data. Examples of instruments include not only the previously discussed interview guides and questionnaires, but also checklists, rating scales, scenarios, and vignettes, among others.

Using a well-designed instrument minimizes bias and maximizes certainty of the variable's (treatment's) effect on the dependent variable (outcome). Researchers can find standardized instruments in electronic databases. These databases provide descriptions of instruments, often with their validity and reliability. Examples of electronic databases related to HIM research that researchers could use to begin their search for an appropriate instrument include:

- Health IT Survey Compendium (AHRQ 2014)
- HF (Human Factors) Tools (FAA 2015)
- HaPI (Health and Psychosocial Instruments) (Behavioral Measurement Database Services 2015)
- Mental Measurements Yearbook with Tests in Print (Buros Center for Testing 2015).

Researchers can also find standardized instruments during their literature review as they read articles. Examples of instruments used in HIM research include the System Usability Score (SUS) (Brooke 1986); the Software Usability Measurement Inventory (SUMI) (Kirukowski and Corbett 1993); and the Questionnaire for User Interaction Satisfaction (QUIS™) (University of Maryland 2015).

Factors in Selection The most important factor in selecting an instrument is the purpose of the research so that the data collected are relevant to the research question. Other factors to consider include:

- Satisfactory ratings for validity and reliability
- Clarity of language
- Brevity and attractiveness
- Match between the theories underpinning the instrument and the researcher's investigation
- Match between the level of measurement (nominal, ordinal, interval, or ratio scales of data—see chapter 17) and the proposed statistical analyses
- Features (see next section)
- Public domain (used for free and can be copied, often with citation) or proprietary (must be purchased and cannot be copied without permission)
- Cost

Researchers should obtain a sample of the instrument (often for free or at a nominal cost) and read it in its entirety to be sure that it collects what they want to collect and that it operationalizes terms the same way they do. For example, researchers studying workplace social support would want to ensure that the instrument collects data about social support in the workplace from colleagues rather than social support in the home from family members.

Selecting an existing instrument with established validity and reliability is easier than developing one's own instrument. For example, to conduct a statewide assessment of HIT workforce needs, HIM researchers developed a quantitative employer needs assessment survey (Fenton et al. 2013, 1–2). First, the researchers conducted 12 focus groups with employers to obtain qualitative data from which to develop the survey. The researchers then constructed the survey through multiple cycles during which they analyzed transcripts of the focus groups' discussions and content of facilitators' whiteboards, reviewed the survey, checked its validity, and tested it. Drafting the written survey consumed five to six weeks of intensive work of a research team. After the paper version of the survey was completed, it was loaded into an online survey tool for which additional testing was required. For the online survey, the research team also spent time considering web design features, such as a progress completion bar and navigational buttons (Fenton et al. 2013, 3).

Features of Instruments Researchers consider the following features of instruments in terms of the type of data that they are collecting:

- Structure of questions
  - Structured (closed-ended) questions list all the possible responses.
  - Unstructured (open-ended) questions allow free-form responses.
  - Semistructured questions begin with structured questions and then follow with open-ended questions to clarify.

The advantages of structured questions are that they are easier for the participant to complete and for the researcher to tabulate and analyze than unstructured questions. The advantages of unstructured questions are that they allow in-depth questions and may uncover aspects of a problem unknown to the researcher. Semistructured questions have the advantages of obtaining comparable data for analysis and potentially providing insights.

- Numeric or categorical data
  - Numeric items request the respondent to enter a number in terms of specific unit of measure, such as day, week, or year.
  - Categorical items classify respondents into groupings. The categories must be *all-inclusive* (all respondents fit into a category, even if it is "other"), *mutually exclusive* (no overlapping among categories), *forming meaningful clusters* (logical and understandably different), and *sufficiently narrow or broad* (number of categories may range from two to eight, but respondents should be able to see substantive shades of meaning among the categories).
  - Numeric items are preferable to categorical items when feasible (Alreck and Settle 2004, 113).

- Scaled categorical items. **Scales** are progressive categories such as size, amount, importance, rank, or agreement. (See table 19.5.) Each category is also called a point; a scale

with five categories is a five-point scale. A commonly used scale is the **Likert scale**, which allows respondents to record their level of agreement or disagreement along a range (see table 19.5). HIM researchers used a scale on a survey that allowed respondents to categorize their competence, from very weak to very strong, in educational subdomains related to health information management (Sandefer and Karl 2015, 26). (See figure 19.7.) To ascertain perspectives or public relations images, researchers use semantic differential scales that allow respondents to rate products, healthcare organizations, or other services. (See figure 19.8.) The scale places adjectives that are polar opposites on the ends of the continua. Up to 20 adjective pairs may be used with half the items beginning with the positive adjective of the pair and the other half beginning with the negative adjective.

- Availability of various formats, such as paper-based, Internet, and multiple languages (English, Spanish, Korean, and others). Prior to using an instrument, researchers should confirm that its validity and reliability have been established for the format they intend to use and in the setting (patient's home, academic health center, and such) of their study.

Table 19.5. Common scales

Scale	Purpose	Example
Two-Point	Dichotomous question	Yes, no Favor, oppose True, false
Three-Point	Importance, interest, or satisfaction	Very, fairly, not at all
	Satisfaction with amounts	Too much (many), just (about) right, not enough (too few)
Four-Point	Generic	Excellent, good, fair, poor
	Measurement of amounts	Very much, quite a bit, some, very little
Likert (Five-Point)	Indication of agreement or disagreement	Strongly agree, agree, neutral, disagree, strongly disagree
Verbal Frequency (Five-Point)	Frequency	Always, often, sometimes, rarely (seldom), never
Expanded Likert (Seven-Point)	Extra discrimination desirable	Very strongly agree, strongly agree, agree, neutral, disagree, strongly disagree, very strongly disagree

Figure 19.7.   Excerpt from survey

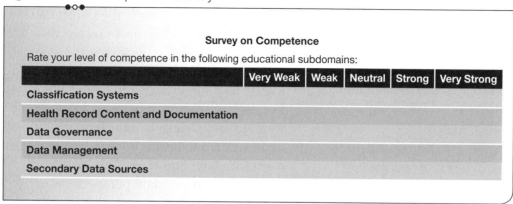

Source: Content derived from Sandefer and Karl 2015.

Figure 19.8.   Example of a semantic differential scale

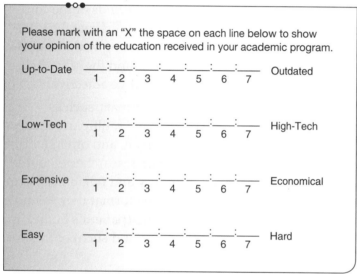

Target Population and Sample   A target population is the large group that is the focus of the research study. Target populations can be health information professionals, physicians, US patients, households, hospitals, schools, university students, US citizens, voters, people with diabetes, and websites. A **sample** is a portion of a target population; it is a set of units. Researchers often use samples because studies involving entire populations can be impractical or unfeasible.

Data Sampling Methods and Types of Samples   Sampling is the process of selecting the units to represent the target population. The sample frame is the list of subjects from which the sample is drawn (Dillman et al. 2014, 3). Researchers should ensure that the list is representative of all the elements of the target population. A coverage error occurs when elements of the population are missing from the sample frame, creating a systematic (nonrandom) discrepancy between the target population and the sample frame (Dillman et al. 2014, 3). For example, a coverage error could occur if researchers used web access to determine the sample frame for a study of Medicare beneficiaries' opinion of using an electronic personal health record. Not all people have access to the Internet.

Two major methods of sampling are random sampling and nonrandom sampling as follows:

- **Random sampling** is a method of selecting a sample from a target population in which all its members have an equal and independent chance of being selected for the research study. This method underpins many statistical analytical techniques that HIM professionals encounter. To generate random samples, researchers can use either a feature of spreadsheet applications called the random number generator, an option of statistical packages called select cases, or a table of random numbers from a basic statistics textbook. Four common types of random sampling are simple random sampling, stratified random sampling, systematic sampling, and cluster sampling. (See table 19.6.) Researchers using these methods attempt to make the random sample as representative of the population as possible.

- **Nonrandom (nonprobability) sampling** does not use statistical methods of probability to select samples and all members of the target population do *not* have an equal and independent chance of being selected for the research study. Three common types

of nonrandom sampling are convenience sampling, purposive sampling, and snowball sampling.

Sample Size   Sample size is the number of subjects the researcher determines should be included in the study in order to represent the population. The sample size must be large enough to support the planned statistical analyses and to detect statistical significance (Farrokhyar et al. 2013, 207, 209)(see chapter 17 about statistics and statistical significance). Other considerations include the population's heterogeneity and its typical response and attrition rates (Brink et al. 2006, 137). **Heterogeneity** means variation or diversity. The more heterogeneous a population, the larger the sample needs to be to ensure that it includes all the diverse units in the population. Similarly, the sample size increases as the response rate declines or the attrition rate rises. Finally, the size of the sample should be economical, providing the level of detail needed to answer the question, but not wasting time, money, and resources through excessive numbers of participants (Brink et al. 2006, 137; Noordzij et al. 2010, 1388).

Statistical formulae are used to calculate adequate sample sizes (Osborn 2006, 145–149).

Table 19.6.   Methods and types of sampling

Type of sampling	Description
Random sampling	
Simple	The selection of units from a population so that every unit has exactly the same chance of being included in the sample. When a unit has been selected, it is returned to the population so that the other units' chances remain identical.
Stratified	Some populations have characteristics that divide them. For example, the human population is male and female. The male and female subgroups are called strata (singular, stratum). The percentage of the stratum in the population should equal the percentage of the stratum in the sample. Therefore, the sample should be 50 percent male and 50 percent female. Other percentages would cast doubt on the results.
Systematic	Units of the sample are selected from a list by drawing every *n*th unit. For example, health information professionals could choose every fourth surgery on the surgical schedule for surgical case review.
Cluster	The sample is clusters of units. The population is first divided into clusters of units, such as family, school, or community.
Nonrandom sampling	
Convenience	Opportunistic use of any unit that is handy. Also known as an accidental sample, its use diminishes the generalizability and credibility of the research.
Purposive	Qualitative researchers use their expertise to select both representative units and unrepresentative units of the population.
Snowball	Initial contacts (units) suggest additional contacts who also could be informative.

Formulae depend on the sampling method used, such as simple random sampling or stratified random sample, and on the amount of information the researcher has about the population.

One commonly used formula for determining optimal sample size requires the researcher to know or to decide on the size of the population, the proportion of subjects needed, and an acceptable amount of error. The formula results in the number of responses needed from the sample. This number must be adjusted by the target audience's typical response rate to arrive at the number of instruments to be distributed. The following example walks through the formula for arriving at the sample size. (See figure 19.9.) Suppose a research team at a health center wanted to determine the sample size for a study on clinicians' opinions of a feature of the center's clinical decision support system. In this instance, the team knows that the number of clinicians is 800 but has little other information. Having no other specific data, the general convention is to select $p = 0.5$ and $\beta = 0.05$. Using the basic formula, the team members calculate that in this situation a sample of 267

Figure 19.9.   Basic example of sample size calculation

Sample size = n Proportion of subjects needed = p

Size of the population = N Acceptable amount of error = β

Formula

Data from the case

$$n = \frac{Np(1-p)}{(N-1)\frac{(B^2)}{4}+(p)(1-p)}$$

$N = 800$

$p = 0.5$

Calculations

$\beta = 0.05$

$$n = \frac{(800)(0.5)(1-5)}{(800-1)\frac{(0.05^2)}{4}+(0.5)(1-5)}$$

$$\frac{200}{(799)(0.000625)+25}$$

$$n = \frac{200}{0.75}$$

$n = 267$

is needed if they are willing to accept 5 percent error due to variability in the sampling. Finally, the team determines the number of surveys to distribute by multiplying the sample size by the typical response rate. Thus, if half of the clinicians typically respond to surveys, the team must double the sample and distribute 534 surveys for the opinion study.

Data Collection Procedures   Data collection procedures differ between quantitative and qualitative studies. Quantitative researchers conduct their studies in a linear fashion. They plan their study, collect data, analyze their data, and present their findings. Qualitative researchers conduct their studies in a cyclical, iterative fashion. They plan their study, collect data, analyze the data, revisit and revise their initial questions, create new questions, and collect more data. In collecting more data, they may seek other sources of data and participants and may add alternate techniques for data collection.

Depending upon the method, issues related to data collection include:

- Obtaining approvals of oversight committees
- Listing each data element required to perform the appropriate statistical techniques
- Training for data collection procedures
- Conducting a pilot study
- Considering the response rate
- Assembling and preparing the data for analysis

Prior to conducting studies, researchers must obtain written approvals from the institutional review board (IRB) and other oversight entities of their organizations. To obtain approvals, researchers complete the organization's documentation, providing descriptions of their research plan and copies of their informed consent forms. (See chapter 20 for a complete discussion of IRBs.) Of note for this chapter on research methods is that researchers must allow sufficient time in their plan for the IRB to review the research, meet, and respond.

Researchers should list each data element required for each statistical analysis that they plan to conduct and determine whether their data collection strategies will obtain all these data elements. Therefore, it is advisable to conduct mock statistical analyses on fabricated data and to create tables and figures for the manuscript early in the planning of the research. Running mock statistical analyses also assists researchers in determining their sample size.

Researchers and those they employ to assist them may require special training. For example, publishers of some psychological tests require verification of training to administer the tests. The researchers must obtain this verification (or select another instrument). To effectively conduct interviews or to observe vignettes, researchers and their assistants also need training.

Conducting a **pilot study** is a trial run that allows researchers to work out the logistical details of their research plan and enhances the likelihood of the research's successful completion. Pilot studies obtain valuable information for researchers as follows:

- Confirmation of details: Volumes of materials or numbers of study assistants needed, costs, and likely response rates.

- Detection of potential problems: Biases in sample selection; flawed performance of equipment, hardware, software, or the website; poorly worded instructions, unclear questionnaire items, and leading questions in interviews; log jams (gridlock) in the distribution method; errors in the scoring key; and discrepancies between the order of items on the data collection instrument and the order on the data entry screen.

Ensuring an adequate response rate is of particular concern for surveys. Low response rates jeopardize a study's internal validity. Researchers should carefully review the literature for the response rates of their intended audience, factors affecting response rates, and successful strategies. Experts recommend a mixed-mode approach that contacts participants in multiple ways and also allows them to respond in the mode of their choice (Dillman et al. 2014, 14). The mixed-modes approach combines postal paper questionnaires, telephone interviews, web-based surveys, and other contact mechanisms. Using an approach for a survey that combined postal letters and e-mails, paper and web-based questionnaires, and offered a $2.00 incentive, researchers were able to achieve a 63 percent response rate within 10 days and a 77 percent response rate within 2 months when data collection ended (Dillman et al. 2014, 22–23).

Researchers also must be on guard for bias in response. Participants may differ from nonparticipants. Responders to the survey may differ from nonresponders. Researchers must establish the similarity of the participants, nonparticipants, responders, and nonresponders to the population.

Finally, researchers must include a mechanism in the plan for assembling their data and preparing them for analysis. Depending upon the research method, procedures should be in place for transcribing interviews, data entry, scoring, and quality checks on data entry. In data preparation, missing values and data cleansing must be addressed. Missing values are variables that do not contain values for some cases. Missing values must be resolved before statistical techniques can be applied. Two common rudimentary techniques to resolve missing values are case deletion in which all cases with a missing value are deleted and single imputation in which the missing value is replaced with the average of the available values. The disadvantages of both techniques are the loss of cases and the potential for bias because the missing data may not be random. Multiple imputation avoids these disadvantages by substituting missing values that have been predicted based on producing multiple data sets using existing values, performing statistical analyses on each of them, and combining the results. Data cleansing (data cleaning, data scrubbing) is the "process of detecting, diagnosing, and editing faulty data" (Van den Broeck et al. 2005, 0966). Data cleansing includes finding duplications (such as the return of two questionnaires by the same participant), checking internal consistency (mismatch between city and zipcode), and identifying outliers (values outside the expected range, such as 42 years in study on infant mortality). The process requires many hours of detailed work for which researchers should allow time in their plan.

Check Your Understanding 19.6

Instructions: On a separate piece of paper, indicate whether the following statements are true or false (T or F).

1. Internal validity involves being able to apply a study's results to another type of healthcare organization.

2. Interrater reliability is consistency in results across different test takers or data collectors.

3. Researchers should develop their own instruments because they are the content experts.

4. A seven-point scale has seven categories.

5. A coverage error occurs when the sample frame systematically excludes some members of a population.

6. A simple random sample is appropriate when the population has characteristics that divide it into strata.

7. Purposive sampling has occurred when, in setting up a focused study, a qualitative researcher selected some participants who were representative and some who were unrepresentative of the group.

8. An adequate sample size for a homogeneous population is typically smaller than an adequate sample size for a heterogeneous population.

9. A pilot study is an unnecessary waste of time and resources when the researcher is experienced.

10. Internet-delivered surveys are better than ground-mail-delivered surveys because they can guarantee a higher response rate.

Analyzing the Data

In this analytical phase of the research process, researchers try to determine what they have found or what the data reveal. In their plan for the study, the researchers decided which analytical techniques they would use. These techniques are described in the methods section of the manuscript with sufficient detail and clarity so that other researchers can duplicate them.

Techniques for quantitative data analysis and the statistical packages for these techniques are discussed in chapter 17. This chapter on research methods adds complementary information on analytical techniques and software analytical packages for qualitative studies.

Techniques for Qualitative Data Analysis
Qualitative data analysis is a systematic process of working with data to create coherent descriptions and explanations of phenomena (Miles et al. 2014, 10). Qualitative researchers interpret their data, seeking patterns and connections, to make sense and understandings (Merriam 2009, 175–176). Analysis of qualitative data is a cyclical and iterative process with data collection, data analysis, and generation

of hypotheses and theories as concurrent, intertwined activities. Although there are many techniques to analyze qualitative data, generally the process is described as having three major activities: data condensation, data display, and conclusion drawing and verification (Miles et al. 2014, 10). Two common qualitative analytical techniques are grounded theory and content analysis.

Grounded Theory
Grounded theory refers both to the theories generated using the analytical technique and the technique itself. Researchers, using grounded theory, code (attach meaningful labels), categorize, and compare their data. The term evolved because its early users spoke of their work being "grounded in data." Thus, the term emphasizes that the data generate the theories.

Grounded theory is an iterative or cyclical process. During data collection, researchers using grounded theory record and code their observations (called incidents). However, analysis begins during data collection. From the analysis, the researchers begin creating conceptual categories to fit their data. Both data collection and analysis may uncover gaps or discrepancies that require additional data collection or participants. The grounded theory technique has four stages:

1. Comparing incidents applicable to each category (includes comparing categories' relationships)
2. Integrating categories and their properties (cyclical process)
3. Delimiting theory (reducing and integrating core categories, tying theory to core categories, and achieving higher level conceptualizations)
4. Writing theory (validating theory by pinpointing data behind it) (Glaser 1965, 439–443)

Development of grounded theory consists of intertwined and concurrent data collection, data coding, categorization, and analysis. Because of the constant analysis and comparisons of categories, the theory and technique are sometimes called *constant comparative method*.

This process results in complex theories that fit the data closely. In grounded theory, researchers seek to develop theories that are unique to groups or settings, unlike quantitative researchers who seek to develop theories that are generalizable.

Content Analysis   Content analysis is the systematic and objective analysis of communication to describe and to make inferences about behaviors. Most often, researchers analyze written documentation. However, they may analyze other modes of communication, such as speech, body language, music, television shows, commercials, and movies. Both qualitative and quantitative researchers use content analysis to analyze data.

Content analysis is "essentially a coding operation" (Babbie 2016, 328). Researchers iteratively cycle through a process of coding and categorizing their data until all the meanings of their data have been categorized. Researchers code the text, image, or other means of communication. Coding is the labeling of words or word groups (segments) or images with annotations or scales. These labels are characteristics of the segments. To assess reliability, the agreement between and among coders may be checked. From the coding, researchers identify key terms, characteristics, or other attributes. The coded text (or communication) becomes the data. The data are then categorized into overarching themes. In a quantitative aspect of content analysis, some researchers also tabulate the frequency of coded data. Generally, content analysis is an iterative process characterized by progressively reducing the units of analysis into fewer and fewer categories and, eventually, into themes.

Qualitative Analytical Software   Qualitative researchers conduct data analysis; qualitative analytical software does *not* conduct analysis. Known as CAQDAS (computer-aided qualitative data analysis software) programs, the software assists researchers in analyzing their data. For example, the programs facilitate manual tasks, such as organizing data and retrieving specific coded excerpts from transcripts of interviews. However, the researchers perform the actual analysis and interpretation of their data (Humble 2012, 125). Experts advise though that researchers carefully explore the program's features to ensure a fit between the program's features and the researchers' question, design, and methods (Cope 2014, 323; Humble 2012, 129).

Several qualitative analytic software programs exist to aid investigators in their organization, management, collection, coding, and analysis of data. Some software is freeware; some is proprietary. Table 19.7 describes features of some of the common CAQDAS programs.

Presenting Results

Researchers provide other HIM professionals with techniques to answer questions and to solve problems in the workplace and with new knowledge. Without presentation and interpretation, the techniques and knowledge would be unavailable to practitioners.

Process   Researchers follow a two-step process when presenting their results. In the first step, they report their research findings with no commentary, explanation, or interpretation. This section of a manuscript is called *research findings*. In the second step, the researchers comment on, explain, and interpret their findings. This section of the manuscript is called *discussion*. Also included in the discussion are conclusions and recommendations for future research.

In research findings, the researchers describe their results in the past tense; general truths are stated in the

Table 19.7. Free and proprietary qualitative analytical software

Qualitative analytical software	Description
ATLAS.ti	Codes and analyzes text-based data from open-ended surveys, transcriptions of focus groups, or other sources. ATLAS.ti can be used to code other types of qualitative data, such as photographs. ATLAS.ti allows the retrieval of specific information based on search criteria. ATLAS.ti also has the ability to export data as an SPSS dataset (ATLAS.ti 2015).
CDC EZ-Text	Free software program from the US Centers for Disease Control and Prevention assists investigators to create, manage, and analyze semi-structured qualitative databases. Investigators can use the software to enter data, create online codebooks, apply codes to specific response passages, develop case studies, conduct database searches to identify text passages, and export data in a wide array of formats for further analysis with other analytic software programs (CDC EZ-Text 2015).
Code-A-Text Integrated System for the Analysis of Interviews and Dialogues (C-I-SAID)	Codes and analyzes documents, transcripts, and sound files. Coding is labeling words or word groups (segments) with annotations or scales. These labels are characteristics of the segments. This software allows investigators to specify labels and easily insert them into the document or sound file. Once the investigator has coded what the subjects said, the investigator can analyze the content of the document or sound file using this software. C-I-SAID produces descriptive statistics and tables and charts that support analysis. The software also assists investigators to categorize the segments into themes, known as content analysis. C-I-SAID can be applied to field notes, open-ended questionnaires, and interviews. A multimedia version codes video and pictures (LingTranSoft 2015).
HyperRESEARCH and HyperTRANSCRIBE	HyperRESEARCH is a cross-platform software for qualitative analysis that assists in coding and retrieving data, in building theories, and in conducting analyses of data. The software has multimedia capabilities that allow work with text, graphics, audio, and video sources. HyperTRANSCRIBE assists the transcription of audio or video data from its source to a text file by giving keyboard control over the looping and playback of audio or video files (Researchware, Inc. 2015).
NVivo	Analyzes unstructured data. It is used to code and analyze text-based data from open-ended surveys, transcriptions of focus groups, or other sources. NVivo allows investigators to retrieve specific quotes based on search criteria. The software also can create tabular data representing the counts of specific codes. The data can be exported to quantitative statistical packages (QSR International 2015).

present tense. The style of writing for scientific manuscripts is objective, precise, and factual. Maintaining a neutral tone, the researchers are merely recording their findings in narrative form. They describe the results for each hypothesis (quantitative study) or research question (qualitative study). Researchers state whether or not the results support the hypotheses. They also record characteristics about the sample and, depending upon the approach, describe the results of the analyses that investigate whether the sample is similar to or different from the population. Supplemental statistical analyses also are described. Researchers are careful to correctly use the terms *statistical significance* (see chapter 17) and *significance* (practical or making a difference).

For research findings, researchers generate tables, graphs, and figures to support their narrative reporting of their findings. (See chapter 18 on data visualization for detailed descriptions of tables and graphs and their use.) One rule of thumb is that data should be presented in only one mode (Day and Gastel 2011, 92). Researchers present the data in the mode of communication, narrative text, table, or figure, which is most effective for that particular data element.

In the discussion section, researchers create new knowledge and put their findings in the context of the existing knowledge. The section is not a superficial repetition of the findings section. Researchers compare their findings to the findings in the literature, describing similarities and discrepancies and providing some rationale to explain why their findings were the same or different. In writing this section, researchers answer the following questions:

- How do their findings answer their research question or address their problem statement?
- What theoretical significance do their findings have?
- What practical significance do their findings have?
- How do their findings explicitly link to the larger body of knowledge?
- How have their findings improved the field's research model?

- How have their findings expanded the body of knowledge?
- What new definitions have they added to the field's area of practice?
- How do their findings support practitioners in the workplace?
- What valid conclusions can the researchers and the readers draw?

In closing their discussion of the findings, researchers state the limitations of their research. A researcher describing a questionnaire survey might state that one limitation is that the data are self-reported. Researchers also make recommendations for future research. In conducting their study, researchers could have seen ways to improve the study or uncovered layers of other questions. These potential improvements and additional questions become the recommendations for further research.

Dissemination of Research Dissemination makes knowledge public. Knowledge is disseminated and examined through poster sessions, presentations at professional meetings, and journal articles. For the researchers' information to be useful, it must be available and accessible to practitioners and other researchers.

Poster sessions and presentations occur at professional meetings, conferences, and symposia. Up to 12 months before a professional meeting, professional associations will issue a call for session proposals. In response to the call, researchers send brief descriptions of their proposed session. The meeting planners determine which proposals to accept based on the submission's quality, the number of submissions, and relevance of the submission's topic to the theme of the conference.

Poster Session Researchers must conform to the conference's poster guidelines when participating in a poster session. Prior to the event, meeting planners send out the requirements for the poster, such as its size and other requirements. Meeting planners will also state the session's time slot on the meeting agenda. During the time slot, the researcher stands near the poster and answers questions about the research study. Often, researchers have available their research paper that expands upon the poster's content and give it to interested people.

Institutional printing departments offer services that enhance posters. Commercial printing companies with staffs of commercial artists and graphic designers also will print the posters. The departments and companies have submission guidelines. Websites that offer printing of posters may be a cost-effective alternative. These websites may have templates that researchers can use. Posters typically include:

- Banner (header) with title of study, names of researchers, and institutional affiliation
- Abstract
- Purpose
- Method
- Results
- Discussion and conclusions

Posters should be colorful and readable at a distance. Charts and graphics are particularly striking.

Presentation Professional presentations occur during sessions of regional, state, national, and international meetings. As described previously, researchers submit proposals in response to a call and, if accepted, receive a notice of their time slot. Presenters should be prepared to talk about their research to the audience. Recommendations for effective presentations advise that presenters:

- Know the background(s) of the audience, such as being members of the general public or technical experts
- Focus on their "take-home message," such as their actual findings or implications for practice
- Keep it simple
- Allow one minute per slide
- Use a logical flow that tells a story
- Practice their presentation (Reumann 2012, 7)

Publication Research that is published can be examined and critically analyzed by practitioners and other researchers. Scientific manuscripts commonly are organized in a prescribed structure. An unpublished paper is known as a manuscript. A manuscript or paper that has been published in a journal is known as an article.

Editors and researchers have agreed upon reporting guidelines for the content of many types of scientific papers. Using these preexisting guidelines assists authors in producing quality manuscripts. One general guideline for scientific papers is called *IMRAD* (introduction, methods, results, and discussion) (Cooper 2015, 67). The website of EQUATOR: **E**nhancing the **QUA**lity and **T**ransparency **O**f Health **R**esearch (2015) is a source of many reporting guidelines for health research. Examples of specific guidelines include:

- Consolidated Standards of Reporting Trials (CONSORT 2010) (Schulz et al. 2010)
- Consolidated criteria for reporting qualitative research (COREQ) (Tong et al. 2007)
- Preferred Reporting Items for Systematic Reviews and Meta-analyses (PRISMA) (Moher et al. 2009)

These preexisting guidelines help authors include all key data and information. Table 19.8 serves as a final checklist for the composition and revision of the manuscript.

Table 19.8. Organization of research publications

Section	Contents
Title page	Concise and descriptive title, author, author's affiliation, grant information, disclaimer, corresponding author's address, telephone, fax, and e-mail
Abstract	Background, purpose, methods, results, conclusions Context; objective; design, setting, and participants; interventions; main outcome measures; results, conclusions 45 to 250 words dependent upon call for papers or journal instructions 3 to 10 key words using medical subject headings (MeSH)
Introduction	Background; pertinent literature review that provides rationale for research; brief statement of research plan; purpose, objectives, or research question
Methods	Protocol with detail for replication Design, setting, and participants Definition of variables Reference to established methods Sampling strategy Collection of data Statement about approval of IRB or other oversight entity Analytical strategy
Results	Core Important results followed by less important results Neutral reporting
Discussion	Relationship between results and purpose, objectives, or research question Evidence of relationship Similarities to and differences from previous research New knowledge in terms of theoretical framework Limitations Conclusions as related to purpose, objectives, or research question Implications for future research Recommendations as warranted Summary
Acknowledgment	Contributors whose level of involvement does not justify authorship
References	Citations per format in instructions
Tables	Consistent with narrative Expand abbreviations Format per instructions
Figures	Consistent with narrative Expand abbreviations Legend Format per instructions

Check Your Understanding 19.7

Instructions: On a separate piece of paper, indicate whether the following statements are true or false (T or F).

1. Data analysis of qualitative data is a cyclical process.

2. In grounded theory, once data analysis has started, known as "grounding," no additional data collection may occur.

3. Qualitative analytical softwares conduct the analyses for researchers.

4. As a general rule, data elements should be presented in tables or graphs to save space.

5. For an audience of practitioners, presenters should, to establish their credibility, focus on the theoretical bases and models upon which their research study was founded rather than providing their actual findings.

Data Access

Access to data is critical for researchers who conduct secondary analyses or combine their primary research with public databases. Access to data depends on obtaining approval or permission, the type of data, and their location. In addition, researchers must arrange a secured way to collect their data, in accordance with Health Insurance Portability and Accountability Act (HIPAA) of 1996, other applicable rules and regulations, and the organization's policies.

Approval or Permission

Researchers need to obtain approvals or permissions from relevant oversight entities and, in the case of individually identifiable data, additional approvals may be required. Data can range from totally uncontrolled to highly protected. For example, data on the Internet are easily accessed whereas healthcare organizations' proprietary financial data are much more difficult to obtain. Researchers need to allow sufficient time to obtain the approvals or permissions.

Public or Proprietary Data

Public data are often accessible under the Freedom of Information Act; some have been posted on the Internet. State registry data also are often accessible. Proprietary data require permission of the owner of the database.

Individual or Aggregate Data

Data that identify one individual are less accessible than aggregate data. Protections exist for identifiable data. To use identifiable data, researchers must obtain approvals from all involved IRBs. For example, researchers may need to obtain the approval of the IRB of the university where they work and from the IRB of the healthcare organization from which they received the identifiable data. (See chapter 20 for additional information on the IRB.) Some organizations may require informed consents to review data. In addition, access to personally identifiable data has become more complex with the implementation of the provisions of HIPAA, the Health Information Technology for Economic and Clinical Health (HITECH) Act of 2009, and the federal Common Rule. (See chapter 11 for additional information on HIPAA.)

Location of Data

The ease of access varies widely by the location of data. As an example of easy access, anonymized data in public databases can be transferred in files over the Internet. As an example of difficult access, historical paper records can only be accessed by physically going to the site of storage within the organization's hours of operation and in accordance with its security rules.

Check Your Understanding 19.8

Instructions: On a separate piece of paper, indicate whether the following statements are true or false (T or F).

1. Analysts of secondary data need *not* concern themselves with HIPAA because the researchers who conducted the original (primary) research have already established compliance with HIPAA.

2. Healthcare organizations' proprietary data are obtainable under the Freedom of Information Act.

3. Researchers who are using *only* publicly available databases for their research must still obtain IRB approvals.

4. As a consequence of federal laws, researchers no longer have access to any individually identifiable data.

5. States and the federal government have digitized all paper records making historical research much more logistically feasible than in the past.

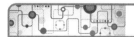 # References

AcademyHealth. 2015. What Is HSR. http://www.academyhealth.org/About/content.cfm?ItemNumber=831

Agency for Healthcare Research and Quality. 2014 (July). Health IT Survey Compendium. http://healthit.ahrq.gov/health-it-tools-and-resources/health-it-survey-compendium

Agency for Healthcare Research and Quality. 2015. Technology Assessment Program. http://www.ahrq.gov/research/findings/ta/index.html

Alharthi, H., N. Sultana, A. Al-amoudi, and A. Basudan. 2015 (Winter). An analytic hierarchy process–based method to rank the critical success factors of implementing a pharmacy barcode system. *Perspectives in Health Information Management.* http://perspectives.ahima.org/wp-content/uploads/2015/12/AnalyticHierarchyProcessbasedMethod.pdf

Alreck, P.L. and R.B. Settle. 2004. *The Survey Research Handbook,* 3rd ed. New York: McGraw-Hill/Irwin.

Aveyard, H. 2010. *Doing a Literature Review in Health and Social Care.* Maidenhead, England: McGraw-Hill Education.

Babbie, E. 2016. *The Practice of Social Research,* 14th ed. Boston, MA: Cengage Learning.

Behavioral Measurement Database Services. 2015. HaPI. http://bmdshapi.com/

Brink, H., C. van der Walt, and G.van Rensburg. 2006. *Fundamentals of Research Methodology for Health Care Professionals,* 2nd ed. Cape Town, South Africa: Juta Press.

Brooke, J. 1986. SUS [System Usability Scale]; A Quick and Dirty Usability Scale. http://www.usability.gov/how-to-and-tools/methods/system-usability-scale.html

Buros Center for Testing. 2015. Test Reviews and Information. http://buros.org/

Campbell, D.T. and J.C. Stanley. 1963. *Experimental and Quasi-Experimental Designs for Research.* Chicago: Rand McNally.

Carter, N., D. Bryant-Lukosius, A. DiCenso, J. Blythe, and A.J. Neville. 2014 (Sept.). The use of triangulation in qualitative research. *Oncology Nursing Forum* 41(5):545–547.

CDC EZ-Text. 2015. http://www.cdc-eztext.com/

Centers for Medicare and Medicaid Services. 2006 (May 14). Glossary. https://www.cms.gov/apps/glossary/default.asp?Letter=C&Language=English

Cheng, H.G. and M.R. Phillips. 2014 (Dec.). Secondary analysis of existing data. Opportunities and implementation. *Shanghai Archives of Psychiatry* 26(6):371–375.

Chrischilles, E.A., J.P. Hourcade, W. Doucette, D. Eichmann, B. Gryzlak, R. Lorentzen, K. Wright, E. Letuchy, M. Mueller, K. Farris, and B. Levy. 2014. Personal health records: A randomized trial of effects on elder medication safety. *Journal of the American Medical Informatics Association* 21(4):679–686.

Colby, S.L. and J.M. Ortman. 2014. The Baby Boom Cohort in the United States: 2012 to 2060. Population Estimates and Projections—Current Population Reports. https://www.census.gov/prod/2014pubs/p25-1141.pdf

Colling, J. 2003. Demystifying nursing research: Defining the problem to be studied. *Urologic Nursing* 23(3):225–226.

Cooper, I.D. 2015 (April). How to write an original research paper (and get it published). *Journal of the Medical Library Association* 103(2):67–68.

Cope, D.G. 2014 (May). Computer-assisted qualitative data analysis software. *Oncology Nursing Forum* 41(3):322–323.

Cresswell, K.M., D.W. Bates, R. Williams, Z. Morrison, A. Slee, J. Coleman, A. Robertson, and A. Sheikh. 2014. Evaluation of medium-term consequences of implementing commercial computerized physician order entry and clinical decision support prescribing systems in two "early adopter" hospitals. *Journal of the American Medical Informatics Association* 21(e2):e194–e202.

Day, R.A. and B. Gastel. 2011. *How to Write and Publish a Scientific Paper,* 7th ed. Santa Barbara, CA: Greenwood Press.

Dillman, D.A., J.D. Smyth, and L.M. Christian. 2014. *Internet, Phone, Mail, and Mixed-Mode Surveys: The Tailored Design Method,* 4th ed. Hoboken, NJ: John Wiley & Sons.

Dine, C.J., A.S. Caelleigh, and J.A. Shea. 2015 (Aug.). Selection and Qualities of Reviewers. Chapter 2 in *Review Criteria for Research Manuscripts,* 2nd ed. Edited by Durning, S.J. and J.D. Carline. Washington, DC: Association of American Medical Colleges.

Eden, J., L. Levit, A. Berg, and S. Morton, eds. 2011. *Finding What Works in Health Care: Standards for Systematic Reviews.* Washington, DC: The National Academies Press.

EQUATOR: Enhancing the QUAlity and Transparency Of Health Research. 2015. http://www.equator-network.org/

Farrokhyar, F., D. Reddy, R.W. Poolman, and M.Bhandari. 2013 (June). Why perform a priori sample size calculation? *Canadian Journal of Surgery* 56(3):207–213.

Federal Aviation Administration. 2015. HF [Human Factors] Tools. http://www.hf.faa.gov/workbenchtools/default.aspx

Fenton, S.H., E. Joost, J. Gongora, D.G. Patterson, C.H.A. Andrilla, and S.M. Skillman. 2013. Health information technology employer needs survey: An assessment instrument for hit workforce planning. *Educational Perspectives in Health Informatics and Information Management* Winter:1–36.

Fottler, M.D., D. Malvey, Y. Asi, S. Kirchner, and N.A. Warren. 2014. Can inbound and domestic medical tourism improve your bottom line? Identifying the potential of a US tourism market. *Journal of Healthcare Management* 59(1):49–63.

Gaylin, D.S., A. Moiduddin, S. Mohamoud, K. Lundeen, and J.A. Kelly. 2011 (June). Public attitudes about health information technology and its relationship to health care quality, costs, and privacy. *Health Services Research* 46(3):920–938.

Glaser, B.G. 1965 (Spring). The constant comparative method of qualitative analysis. *Social Problems* 12(4):436–445.

Government Accountability Office. 2015. Comparative Effectiveness Research: HHS Needs to Strengthen Dissemination and Data-Capacity-Building Efforts. Report No. GAO 15-280. http://www.gao.gov/assets/670/668804.pdf

Green, S., J.P.T. Higgins, P. Alderson, M. Clarke, C.D. Mulrow, and A.D. Oxman. 2011 (March).What is a systematic review (1.2.2.)? In: *Cochrane Handbook for Systematic Reviews of Interventions Version 5.1.0* [Updated March 2011]. Edited by J.P.T. Higgins J.P.T. and S. Green. http://handbook.cochrane.org/

Hu, C., S. Kung, T.A. Rummans, M.M. Clark, and M.I. Lapid. 2015. Reducing caregiver stress with Internet-based interventions: A systematic review of open-label and randomized controlled trials. *Journal of the American Medical Informatics Association* 22(e1): e194–e209.

Humble, A.M. 2012 (June). Qualitative data analysis software: A call for understanding, detail, intentionality, and thoughtfulness. *Journal of Family Theory and Review* 4(2):122–137.

In, H. and J.E. Rosen. 2014 (Oct.). Primer on outcomes research. *Journal of Surgical Oncology* 110(5):489–493.

Institute of Medicine. 2009. *Initial National Priorities for Comparative Effectiveness Research.* Washington, DC: The National Academies Press.

International Network of Agencies for Health Technology Assessment. 2015. HTA Glossary. http://htaglossary.net/HomePage

Karnick, P.M. 2013 (Jan.). The importance of defining theory in nursing: Is there a common denominator? *Nursing Science Quarterly* 26(1):29–30.

Koppel, R., S. Smith, J. Blythe, and V. Kothari. 2015. Workarounds to computer access in healthcare organizations: You want my password or a dead patient? *Studies in Health Technology & Informatics* 208:215–220.

Kirukowski, J. and M. Corbett. 1993. SUMI: The Software Usability Measurement Inventory. *British Journal of Educational Technology* 24(3):210–212.

LeRouge, C., C. Van Slyke, D. Seale, and K. Wright. 2014. Baby boomers' adoption of consumer health technologies: Survey on readiness and barriers. *Journal of Medical Internet Research* 16(9):e200.

LingTranSoft. 2015. C-I-Said. http://lingtransoft.info/apps/c-i-said

Lloyd, S.C. and E. Layman. 1997. The effects of automated encoders on coding accuracy and coding speed. *Topics in Health Information Management* 17(3):72–79.

Merriam, S.B. 2009. *Qualitative Research: A Guide to Design and Implementation.* San Francisco, CA: Jossey-Bass.

Miles, M.B., A.M. Huberman, and J. Saldaña. 2014. *Qualitative Data Analysis: A Methods Sourcebook*. 3rd ed. Thousand Oaks, CA: Sage.

Moher, D., A. Liberati, J. Tetzlaff, D.G. Altman, and the PRISMA Group. 2009 (July 21). Preferred reporting items for systematic reviews and meta-analyses: The PRISMA statement. *PLoS Medicine/Public Library of Science* 6(7):e1000097.

Moss, J. and E.S. Berner. 2015. Evaluating clinical decision support tools for medication administration safety in a simulated environment. *International Journal of Medical Informatics* 84(5):308–318.

Naidu, H. and A. Tiwari. 2014 (Nov.). Data mining and data warehousing. *International Journal of Engineering Sciences and Research Technology* 3(11):109–111.

Nevedal, D.C., C. Wang, L. Oberleitner, S. Schwartz, and A.M. Williams. 2013. Effects of an individually tailored web-based chronic pain management program on pain severity, psychological health, and functioning. *Journal of Medical Internet Research* 15(9):e201.

Noordzij, M., G. Tripepi, F.W. Dekker, C. Zoccali, M.W. Tanck, and K.J. Jager. 2010 (Oct.). Sample size calculations: Basic principles and common pitfalls. *Nephrology Dialysis Transplantation* 25(5):1388–1393.

Nurses' Health Study. 2015. http://www.channing.harvard.edu/nhs/

Osborn, C.E. 2006. *Statistical Applications for Health Information Management*, 2nd ed. Sudbury, MA: Jones and Bartlett.

Øvretveit, J. 2014. *Evaluating Improvement and Implementation for Health*. Maidenhead, England: McGraw-Hill Education.

Piras, E.M. and A. Zanutto. 2014. "One day it will be you who tells us doctors what to do!" Exploring the "personal" of PHR in pediatric diabetes management. *Information Technology & People* 27(4):421–439.

QSR International. 2015. NVivo. http://www.qsrinternational.com/product

Researchware, Inc. 2015. HyperRESEARCH: What It Is. http://www.researchware.com/

Reumann, M. 2012 (May–June). Preparing for conferences—basic presentation skills. *IEEE Pulse* 3(3):6–7, 12.

Robson, C. 2010. Evaluation Research. Chapter 21 in Gerrish, K. and A. Lacey. *Research Process in Nursing*, 6th ed. Chichester, United Kingdom: Blackwell Publishing, 248–256.

Rogers, E.M. 2003. *Diffusion of Innovations*, 5th ed. New York: Free Press.

Sandefer, R. and E.S. Karl. 2015. Ready or not: HIM is changing—results of the new HIM competencies survey show skill gaps between education levels, students, and working professionals. *Journal of the American Health Information Management Association* 86(3):24–27.

Schulz, K.F., D.G. Altman, D. Moher, and the Consort Group. 2010. CONSORT 2010 statement: Updated guidelines for reporting parallel group randomized trials. *Annals of Internal Medicine* 152(11):726–732.

Shi, L. 2008. *Health Services Research Methods*, 2nd ed. Albany, NY: Delmar.

Singleton, R.A., Jr. and B.C. Straits. 2005. *Approaches to Social Research*, 4th ed. New York: Oxford University Press.

Tong, A., K. Flemming, E. McInnes, S. Olive, and J. Craig. 2012. Enhancing transparency in reporting the synthesis of qualitative research: ENTREQ. *BMC Medical Research Methodology* 12:181.

University of Maryland. 2015. Questionnaire for User Interaction Satisfaction (QUIS™). http://www.lap.umd.edu/QUIS/index.html

Van den Broeck, J., S.A. Cunningham, R. Eeckels, and K. Herbst. 2005(October). Data cleaning: Detecting, diagnosing, and editing data abnormalities. *PLoS Medicine* 2(10):0966-0970.

Vest, J.R., L.M. Kern, M.D. Silver, R. Kaushal, and the HITEC Investigators. 2015. The potential for community-based health information exchange systems to reduce hospital readmissions. *Journal of the American Medical Informatics Association* 22(2):435–442.

Vydra, T.P., E. Cuaresma, M. Kretovics, and S. Bose-Brill. Diffusion and use of tethered personal health records in primary care. 2015. *Perspectives in Health Information Management* (Spring):1–16.

Ware, R.E. and R.J. Hicks. 2011 (Dec.). Doing more harm than good? Do systematic reviews of PET by health technology assessment agencies provide an appraisal of the evidence that is closer to the truth than the primary data supporting its use? *Journal of Nuclear Medicine* 52(12, Suppl 2):64S–73S.

Wissmann, S. 2015. Addressing challenges to the health information management profession: An Australian perspective. *Perspectives in Health Information Management* International issue:1–10.

Zhang, X., P. Yu, J. Yan, and I. Ton A M Spil. 2015. Using diffusion of innovation theory to understand the factors impacting patient acceptance and use of consumer e-health innovations: A case study in a primary care clinic. *BMC Health Services Research* 15:71.

Resources

Agency for Healthcare Research and Quality. Effective Health Care Program Library of Resources. http://www.ahrq.gov/professionals/clinicians-providers/ehclibrary/

Agency for Healthcare Research and Quality. Research Tools & Data. http://www.ahrq.gov/research/index.html

Agency for Healthcare Research and Quality. Results of ARRA-funded CER Dissemination Activities. http://www.ahrq.gov/cpi/about/mission/arra/index.html#s1

Agency for Healthcare Research and Quality. Technology Assessment Program. http://www.ahrq.gov/research/findings/ta/index.html

Federation of American Scientists. 2015. Office of Technology Assessment Archive, Technology Assessment and Congress. http://ota.fas.org/technology_assessment_and_congress/

Garrard, J. 2013. *Health Sciences Literature Review Made Easy: The Matrix Method*, 4th ed. Sudbury, MA: Jones and Bartlett.

National Information Center on Health Services Research and Health Care Technology (NICHSR) of the National Library of Medicine. http://www.nlm.nih.gov/hsrinfo/cer.html

Strunk, W., Jr. and E.B. White. 2000. *The Elements of Style*, 4th ed. New York: Longman.

20

Biomedical and Research Support

Valerie J.M. Watzlaf, PhD, RHIA, FAHIMA

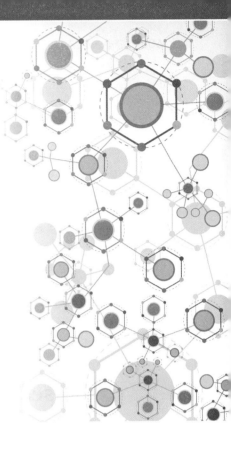

Learning Objectives

- Interpret inferential statistics that are part of research studies
- Analyze statistical data for decision making in research support
- Apply principles of research and clinical literature evaluation to improve outcomes
- Plan adherence to Institutional Review Board (IRB) processes and policies
- Comply with ethical standards of practice when conducting research or providing research support
- Identify laws and regulations applicable to biomedical research

- Analyze legal concepts and principles to the practice of HIM in research support
- Protect electronic health information through confidentiality and security measures, policies and procedures when used in biomedical research
- Examine the role of the health information management (HIM) professional both as a researcher and in a supportive role to research conducted in healthcare facilities
- Analyze the various research designs for conducting biomedical research

Key Terms

Attributable risk (AR)
Beneficence
Biomedical research
Case-control study
Clinical trial
Cohort study
Cross-sectional study
Double-blind study
Epidemiological study
Experimental study

Health Research Extension Act
Health services research
Human subjects
Incidence
Informed consent
Institutional Review Board (IRB)
Justice
Morality
National Committee for Quality Assurance (NCQA)

Observational study
Odds ratio
Office for Human Research Protections (OHRP)
Office of Research Integrity (ORI)
Prevalence
Principal investigator
Privacy Rule
Prospective study

Protected health information (PHI)
Protocol
Randomized clinical trial (RCT)

Relative risk (RR)
Research
Respect for persons

Retrospective study
Single-blind study
Vulnerable subjects

Biomedical research is a search for knowledge that often leads to advances in medicine. It determines what new drugs and other types of treatments, as well as new technology, are safe and effective for patients. When new treatments and technologies ultimately reach the consumers of healthcare, long-term studies of outcomes and effectiveness begin.

This chapter explores the various methods by which biomedical research is conducted. It also examines methods of assessing outcomes and effectiveness, including programs initiated by the Agency for Healthcare Research and Quality (AHRQ), Joint Commission, National Committee for Quality Assurance (NCQA), and the Patient-Centered Outcomes Research Institute (PCORI).

Clinical and Biomedical Research

Clinical and biomedical research studies are conducted to evaluate disease processes and interventions and the safety, effectiveness, and usefulness of drugs, diagnostic procedures, and preventive measures such as vaccines, mammography, and diets. The broad objective of these studies is to establish reproducible facts and theory that help solve human problems. The most common examples of these research studies are called **clinical trials**, in which a specific type of clinical or biomedical intervention is tested to determine its effectiveness. **Health services research** examines the quality, access, cost, staffing, utilization, and safety of healthcare services in order to improve the overall quality of care provided to patients. For example, *Health Services Research* is

a journal that publishes studies that focus on quality and outcomes of care, healthcare organizations and their use of technology, cost and utilization of care, the impact of health policy, and research methods used in health services research. Much of the research published by this journal focuses on health information management issues. Some examples include examining health information technologies, such as the use of the electronic health record (EHR) to investigate improvements in patient safety; public attitudes on health information technology (HIT) and HIT's relationship to quality, cost, and privacy; or the examination of hospital report cards, readmission rates, or the use of patient-centered medical homes and the impact on emergency room visits (Research and Educational Trust 2015)

Ethical Treatment of Human Subjects

Human subjects are often used in biomedical research studies. Because human subjects are involved, researchers are required to follow certain ethical principles that guide their behavior, morality, and decisions. **Morality** includes two separate requirements related to research: the requirement to acknowledge autonomy (being capable of making decisions) and the requirement to protect those

with decreased autonomy (due to changes in their health capacity) (NIH 1979).

Research ethics provide a structure for analysis and decision making, supporting and reminding researchers to protect human subjects, and providing workable definitions of benefits and risks.

Risk versus benefit is critical in weighing the advantages of biomedical research. A benefit is a positive value of being part of the clinical research study. A benefit may be specific to the individual subject in that it provides a good therapeutic outcome, or it may be a direct advantage to society as a whole rather than to the individual subject.

Risks are concerned with the probability or magnitude of harm to the research subject. Stating that 1 in 100 patients may experience a certain risk suggests probability of harm. A rash as a minor effect of the treatment or liver failure as a major effect of the treatment suggests magnitude of harm.

The challenge for the researcher is to weigh risks to the subject against potential benefits. This is difficult because not all potential benefits and risks are known in advance and, as stated earlier, the benefit may be for society at large rather than for the individual subjects who assumed the risks. However, there are many clinical and biomedical research studies in which the benefits far outweigh the risks to the individual. For example, an individual with stage IV pancreatic cancer may only see how the benefits outweigh the risks to enroll in a clinical trial that examines the effectiveness of a medication to stop the advancement of this devastating illness.

The Nuremberg Code and the Declaration of Helsinki

International guidelines also govern the ethical conduct of human research. The Nuremberg Code outlines research ethics that were developed during the trials of Nazi war criminals following World War II. These trials addressed charges that medical experiments were conducted on concentration camp prisoners without their consent. The code was widely adopted as a standard for protecting human subjects in the 1950s and 1960s. The basic tenet of the Nuremberg Code is that "voluntary consent of the human subject is absolutely essential" (Nuremberg Code 1949, 181). It is the duty and responsibility of the individual initiating, directing, or conducting the experiment to ensure the quality of the informed consent. Additionally, the Nuremberg Code requires that research be based on knowledge from previous animal work, the risks be justified by the anticipated benefits, only qualified scientists conduct the research, and physical and mental suffering be avoided. Research in which death is expected should not be conducted.

The Declaration of Helsinki is a code of ethics for clinical research which was approved by the World Medical Association in 1964. It was a reinterpretation of the Nuremberg Code directed toward medical research with a therapeutic intent. It is a statement of ethical principles that provides guidance to physicians and other participants in medical research involving human subjects, including research on identifiable human material or identifiable data. The document has been revised a number of times, most recently at the 64th World Medical Association General Assembly in Fortaleza, Brazil, October 2013 (WMA 2015).

Despite the Nuremberg Code and the Declaration of Helsinki, controversial ethical practices in biomedical research continued to be a problem. In 1966, Dr. Henry K. Beecher, an anesthesiologist, described several examples of research studies with controversial ethics that had been published by prominent researchers in major journals (Beecher 1966). Beecher's article increased public awareness of the ethical problems related to biomedical research, including:

- Lack of informed consent
- Coercion of, or undue pressure on, volunteers
- Use of a vulnerable population
- Information being withheld
- Available treatment being withheld
- Information about risks being withheld
- Subjects put at risk
- Risks to subjects that outweigh the benefits
- Deception
- Violation of rights

The work of Beecher enabled others who are doing research or working with researchers to pay attention to these ethical issues and work toward preventing them from occurring during biomedical research studies.

The US Public Health Services Syphilis Study

A study conducted in the United States that brought ethical issues in research to the forefront

Figure 20.1. Tuskegee syphilis study

The Tuskegee Syphilis Study is a notorious chapter in medical research in the United States. From 1932 to 1972, the US Public Health Service conducted research that had the stated purpose of obtaining more information about the clinical course of syphilis. The medical researchers from the US Public Health Service experimented on 399 African American males in Macon County, Alabama. The medical researchers told the men that they were being treated for "bad blood." In fact, the researchers were deceiving the men and were denying them treatment for syphilis. Many of the men's wives were infected, and their children were subsequently born with congenital syphilis. The US Public Health Service continued the study despite the advent of penicillin in 1947. The Tuskegee Syphilis Study is a symbol of unethical research.

Source: CDC 2013.

was the US Public Health Services Syphilis Study. This study was designed to study the natural history of syphilis in African-American men (see figure 20.1). At the time the study began, there was no treatment for syphilis. However, by the 1940s penicillin had proved to be safe and effective. The men enrolled in the study were denied treatment. They continued to be followed until 1972, when the first public accounts began to appear in the national press. The study resulted in 28 deaths, 100 cases of disability, and 19 cases of congenital syphilis (CDC 2013).

After the press blew the whistle, Congress formed an ad hoc panel that determined the study should be stopped immediately and that oversight of human research was inadequate. It was recommended that federal regulations be implemented to protect human research in the future. In 1974, Congress authorized formation of the National Commission for the Protection of Human Subjects in Biomedical and Behavioral Research. The Commission was charged with identifying the basic ethical principles that underlie the conduct of human research.

In 1979, the Commission published the *Belmont Report: Ethical Principles and Guidelines for the Protection of Human Subjects of Research* (HHS 1979). This report identifies the following three basic ethical principles that underlie all human subject research:

Respect for persons requires that individuals be treated as autonomous human beings and not used as a means to an end. Elements of autonomy include the ability to understand and process information and the freedom to volunteer for research without coercion or undue influence from others. Respect for persons requires informed consent and respecting the privacy of research subjects.

Beneficence is minimizing harms and maximizing benefits. Beneficence requires the best possible research design to achieve its goals. It also requires that researchers be able to perform the research and handle the risks.

Justice requires that people be treated fairly and that benefits and risks be shared equitably among the population. Justice requires that subjects be selected equitably and that vulnerable populations or populations of convenience not be exploited. (HHS 1979)

In 1981, the Department of Health and Human Services (HHS) revised its regulations on the protection of human subjects and made them available within the Code of Federal Regulations (45 CFR part 46). In 1991, subpart A of those regulations, was broadened to include 15 other federal departments, creating the Common Rule. Technical amendments, which are amendments that are not substantial, were made to the Common Rule in 2005. Also, the Office of Management and Budget (OMB) developed a workgroup to examine possible revisions to the Common Rule. Its draft, Advance Notice of Proposed Rulemaking (ANPRM), was circulated for comment, and the ANPRM entitled *Human Subjects Research Protections: Enhancing Protections for Research Subjects and Reducing Burden, Delay and Ambiguity for Investigators* was developed (HHS 2011a). On September 8, 2015, proposed revisions to the Common Rule were made in a Notice of Proposed Rulemaking (NPRM) published in the Federal Register (HHS 2015a). Just like the ANPRM, the NPRM seeks comments on this proposed rule. A summary of the changes include: broadening protections for research subjects, such as more focused informed consent documents that are shorter and clearer;

and a focus on more oversight for those studies that hold more risk for the research subject and less oversight on those that pose less risk. Public comments will be used in the process of developing proposed revisions to the Common Rule (Emanuel and Menikof 2011; HHS 2015b).

The Office for Human Research Protections (OHRP) of the HHS monitors compliance with the federal regulations that govern the conduct of research conducted or supported by HHS (HHS 2009). OHRP is a federal agency that provides leadership and oversight on all matters related to the protection of human subjects participating in research conducted or supported by HHS, as outlined in the regulations. OHRP provides clarification and guidance, develops educational programs, maintains regulatory oversight, and provides advice on ethical and regulatory issues in biomedical and behavioral research. The federal regulations for the protection of human subjects include Title 45 of CFR 46. The Food and Drug Administration (FDA) has a separate set of regulations governing human subjects research (21 CFR Part 56 IRBs and 21 CFR Part 50 Protection of Human Subjects). The basic requirements for IRBs and protection of human subjects are similar between the HHS and FDA regulations.

Check Your Understanding 20.1

Instructions: **Answer the following questions on a separate piece of paper.**

1. What is the origin of the Nuremberg Code? What are its basic tenets?

2. Which study brought ethical issues in research to the forefront and why did this occur?

3. A researcher fails to inform a study participant of the reasonable risks in a study on the effectiveness of a new chemotherapy agent. What ethical principle was violated?

4. List five ethical issues in the conduct of biomedical research in the United States cited by Beecher.

5. What were the major changes to the Common Rule proposed in 2015?

Protection of Human Subjects

The HHS regulations contain three basic provisions for the protection of human subjects (45 CFR 46):

- Institutional assurances of compliance
- Institutional review board review and approval
- Informed consent

Institutional Assurances of Compliance

An institutional assurance of compliance is a commitment of an institution to comply with HHS regulations for the protection of human subjects by documenting this commitment. HHS will support nonexempt research (research that receives a more extensive review by the IRB such as clinical trials or expedited research) covered by the regulations only if the organization has an OHRP-approved assurance on file; the research has been reviewed and approved by the organization's IRB; and the IRB will continue to review the research, as necessary (HHS 2009).

Protection of human subjects is required under the HHS Code of Federal Regulations. OHRP has formal agreements with more than 10,000 federally funded universities, hospitals, and other medical and behavioral research institutions in the United States and abroad (45 CFR 46). These organizations must agree to abide by the human subject protection regulations found in the Code of Federal Regulations. The OHRP's duties include:

- Establishing criteria for, and approving assurance of, compliance for the protection of human subjects with institutions engaged in HHS-conducted or HHS-supported human subject research
- Providing clarification and guidance on involving humans in research
- Developing and implementing educational programs and resource materials
- Promoting the development of approaches to enhance human subject protections

The OHRP also evaluates substantive allegations or indications of noncompliance with HHS regulations regarding the conduct of research involving human subjects (45 CFR 46.103). It also provides education and development on the complex ethical and regulatory issues relating to human subjects protection in medical and behavioral research. The OHRP helps institutions assess and improve their own procedures for protecting human subjects through a quality improvement program.

Institutional Review Board

The **Institutional Review Board (IRB)** is a committee established to protect the rights and welfare of human research subjects involved in research activities. The IRB members are appointed by the specific organization conducting the research.

The IRB determines whether research that is conducted is appropriate and that it protects human subjects as they participate in this research. The primary focus of the IRB is not on whether the type of research is appropriate for the organization to conduct but upon whether or not human subjects are adequately protected (45 CFR 46.111).

The purpose and responsibility of the IRB is to protect the rights and welfare of human subjects as they engage in research activities. The IRB must abide by the regulations as listed in 45 CFR 46.111 and 21 CFR 56.111. The IRB must first determine if research is being conducted and then determine if human subjects are being protected. **Research** is defined by the regulations as "a systematic investigation, including research development, testing and evaluation, designed to develop or contribute

to generalizable knowledge" (45 CFR 46.102). **Human subjects** are defined by the regulations as "living individual(s) about whom an investigator (whether professional or student) conducting research obtains (1) data through intervention or interaction with the individual, or (2) identifiable private information" (45 CFR 46.102).

An IRB must review all research activities covered by the HHS regulations and either (1) approve, (2) require changes to obtain approval, or (3) disapprove any research activity. An IRB must perform continuing reviews of ongoing research as often as necessary per degree of risk, but not less than one year. The IRB has the authority to suspend or terminate approved research that is not being conducted in accordance with IRB requirements or that has caused unexpected or serious harm to the subject. If a suspension or termination occurs, the IRB must include a documented statement for the reason and must report this immediately to the investigator, appropriate institutional officials, and HHS.

The protection of human subjects is a shared responsibility between the institutional officials, the IRB, and the investigator. It should not rest solely with the IRB. The institutional official is responsible for choosing one or more IRBs to review research; providing enough space, staff, and other resources to support the IRB's review and record-keeping responsibilities; providing education and training for the IRB staff and investigators; providing effective communication and guidance on human subject research; ensuring that investigators carry out their research responsibilities with the utmost respect for human subjects; and serving as the point of contact for OHRP or designating another individual to undertake this responsibility.

The IRB is made up of at least five members with diversified backgrounds per federal regulation, such as including at least one member with a scientific background and at least one member in a nonscientific area. However, most organizations have more than that number. For example, many large universities are composed of 10 IRB members, each functioning as a separate IRB under a central administration and support from the main IRB office. An IRB vice chairperson and several members with expertise in many diversified areas comprise the IRB committee. Also, the IRB office includes additional staff that reviews exempt or expedited research proposals (University of Pittsburgh 2015a).

Conflict of Interest

No IRB member may participate in the review of a research project in which he or she has a conflict of interest. A conflict of interest may include serving as an IRB committee member to review a research study protocol (a plan or proposal for the study) in which one has a definite interest in the outcome of the specific medical device or medication. If this situation arises, the IRB committee member should remove himself or herself from the composition of the committee (University of Pittsburgh 2015b).

Before IRB submissions are reviewed, investigators may be required or recommended to complete different educational modules. These modules may include education on research integrity, conflict of interest, use of lab animals in research and education, human embryonic and stem cell research, Health Insurance Portability and Accountability Act (HIPAA) researchers' privacy requirements, blood borne pathogens, chemical hygiene, responsible literature searching, IRB member education, research with children, and Good Clinical Practices module (recommended for those investigators involved in FDA-regulated research)(University of Pittsburgh 2015c). Some universities will require students, faculty, and staff to complete CITI training for all individuals involved in research. CITI is the Collaborative Institutional Training Institute, and some universities will draw on resources provided by them as well as those from the university in order to provide research training modules for all individuals involved in research (University of Pittsburgh 2015d).

Procedures for IRB submission

Exempt, expedited, and full board approval are the three major categories of IRB review for research study proposals. OHRP recommends that clear procedures be developed by organizations so that IRBs can determine whether research is exempt.

Exempt research activities include the involvement of human subjects in one or more of the listed categories according to the HHS Federal Policy regulations (45 CFR 46.101(b)(1–6)). Research that is exempt does not mean that the researchers have no ethical obligations to the participants, but that the regulatory requirements such as informed consent and yearly renewal from IRB do not apply to this type of research. The IRB still reviews research protocols to determine their exempt status.

Exempt research activities may include the involvement of human subjects in one or more of the following categories:

- Educational settings (45 CFR 46.101(b)(1)): Research conducted in educational settings involving normal educational practices such as testing different instructional methods (for example, differences in learning outcomes between distance education and traditional classroom)
- Use of educational tests, surveys, interviews, or observation (45 CFR 46.101(b)(2)): Research conducted in any setting in which educational tests such as aptitude or achievement tests are conducted unless participants are identified in any way when data are collected
- Use of educational tests, surveys, interviews, or observation (45 CFR 46.101(b)(3)): Research conducted that is not exempt under paragraph (b)(2) if (i) the human subjects are elected or appointed public officials or candidates for public office; or (ii) federal statute(s) require(s) without exception that the confidentiality of the personally identifiable information be maintained throughout the research and thereafter
- Research involving the collection or study of existing data, documents, records, pathological specimens, or diagnostic specimens (45 CFR 46.101(b)(4)): If these sources are publicly available or if the information is recorded by the investigator in such a manner that subjects cannot be identified, directly or through identifiers linked to the subjects

- Research and demonstration projects that are conducted by or subject to the approval of department or agency heads, and are designed to study, evaluate, or otherwise examine (45 CFR 46.101(b)(5)): (i) Public benefit or service programs; (ii) procedures for obtaining benefits or services under those programs; (iii) possible changes in or alternatives to those programs or procedures; or (iv) possible changes in methods or levels of payment for benefits or services under those programs

- Taste and food quality evaluation and consumer acceptance studies (45 CFR 46.101 (b)(6)): (i) If wholesome foods without additives are consumed; or (ii) if a food is consumed that contains a food ingredient at or below the level and for a use found to be safe, or agricultural chemical or environmental contaminant at or below the level found to be safe, by the Food and Drug Administration or approved by the Environmental Protection Agency or the Food Safety and Inspection Service of the US Department of Agriculture

Expedited research includes those activities that (1) present no more than minimal risk to human subjects, and (2) involve only procedures listed in one or more of the following categories as authorized by 45 CFR 46.110 and 21 CFR 56.110. The categories for expedited IRB review include:

1. Clinical studies of drugs and medical devices only when an investigational new drug application or medical device application is not required or when the medical device is cleared or approved for marketing and the medical device is being used in accordance with its cleared or approved labeling.
2. Collection of blood samples by finger stick, heel stick, ear stick, or venipuncture.
3. Prospective collection of biological specimens for research purposes by noninvasive means. Examples include hair and nail clipping or placenta removed at delivery.

4. Collection of data through noninvasive procedures (not involving general anesthesia or sedation) routinely employed in clinical practice, excluding procedures involving x-rays or microwaves. Examples include magnetic resonance imaging, electrocardiography, exercise testing, muscle strength testing, and so forth.
5. Research involving materials (data, documents, records, or specimens) that have been collected, or will be collected solely for nonresearch purposes (such as medical treatment or diagnosis). (*Note*: Some research in this category may be exempt from the HHS regulations for the protection of human subjects [45 CFR 46.101(b)(4)]. This listing refers only to research that is not exempt.)
6. Collection of data from voice, video, digital, or image recordings made for research purposes.
7. Research on individual or group characteristics or behavior (including, but not limited to, research on perception, cognition, motivation, identity, language, communication, cultural beliefs or practices, and social behavior) or research employing survey, interview, oral history, focus group, program evaluation, human factors evaluation, or quality assurance methodologies. (*Note*: Some research in this category may be exempt from the HHS regulations for the protection of human subjects [45 CFR 46.101(b)(2) and (b)(3)]. This listing refers only to research that is not exempt.)
8. Continuing review of research previously approved by the convened IRB as follows:
   - Where (i) the research is permanently closed to the enrollment of new subjects; (ii) all subjects have completed all research-related interventions; and (iii) the research remains active only for long-term follow-up of subjects; or
   - Where no subjects have been enrolled and no additional risks have been identified; or
   - Where the remaining research activities are limited to data analysis.

9. Continuing review of research, not conducted under an investigational new drug application or investigational device exemption where categories two (2) through eight (8) do not apply but the IRB has determined and documented at a convened meeting that the research involves no greater than minimal risk and no additional risks have been identified.

10. An expedited review procedure consists of a review of research involving human subjects by the IRB chairperson or by one or more experienced reviewers designated by the chairperson from among members of the IRB in accordance with the requirements set forth in 45 CFR 46.110.

All other research projects that do not qualify under exempt or expedited review must be reviewed and approved at the full board level.

Once the category of submission is determined, the investigator must complete the proper forms for submission to the IRB. The types of forms that must be completed depend upon the level of review. Most IRBs require that research protocols be submitted electronically. An IRB protocol checklist is usually provided so that the investigator can determine what types of documents need to be completed and submitted. See appendix E for a copy of the IRB checklist used at the University of Pittsburgh IRB office.

Once the appropriate forms are submitted to the IRB, the investigator awaits a decision from the IRB committee. The decisions from the IRB can include one of the following four categories:

- Full approval
- Approval subject to modifications—protocol is recommended for approval pending inclusion of changes
- Reconsideration—when there are a number of questions and concerns regarding the protocol and full board review and approval may be necessary once all questions and concerns are addressed
- Disapproval—when major scientific or ethical problems cannot be resolved (University of Pittsburgh 2015c)

Management of Handling Problems Related to Risk to Human Subjects

Sometimes during the course of the research study protocol reportable events occur. When this happens the investigator must notify the IRB and complete an unanticipated problem involving risk to human subjects report. The reportable event report should include the following (University of Pittsburgh 2015e):

- Principal investigator's (PI) name
- Title of the study
- IRB study number
- Funding source
- Brief description of the problem
- Severity of the event
- Causality of the event (Was it due to the study protocol or procedure?)
  - Corrective action plan, if necessary
- Whether protocol modification is necessary and, if so, a revised protocol and informed consent must be submitted
- Signature of the PI and date

It is important to document any reportable event that may occur while conducting research. The information listed is critical in order to protect the safety of future subjects that may participate in the study and also for IRB reporting purposes.

Recordkeeping and Retention

The IRB should prepare and maintain adequate documentation of all IRB activities. This documentation may include the following (45 CFR 46.115).

- Copies of all research study protocols reviewed, sample consent forms, progress reports, and reports of injuries to subjects or adverse event reports
- Minutes of IRB committee meetings
- Records of continuing review activities
- Listing of IRB members and their responsibilities
- All written procedures for the IRB
- Statements of significant new findings provided to subjects

The records related to this policy should be retained for at least three years, and records relating to research conducted should be retained for at least three years after completion of the research. All records shall be accessible for inspection and copying by authorized representatives of the department or agency at reasonable times and in a reasonable manner.

Informed Consent

Informed consent is more than just completing a form. It is a thoughtful and respectful explanation of information so that a person can decide whether to participate in a research study. The process that encompasses informed consent should not just regurgitate research study information but educate possible participants in terms they can understand. Informed consent should contain three fundamentals: information, comprehension, and voluntariness. The written presentation of information should document the basis for consent and for the participant's future reference. The consent document should also be revised when necessary to include changes to improve the consent procedure (45 CFR 46.116).

In most cases, biomedical research requires that subjects be given informed consent. **Informed consent** is a person's voluntary agreement to participate in research or to undergo a diagnostic, therapeutic, or preventive procedure. It is based on adequate knowledge and an understanding of relevant information provided by the investigators. In giving informed consent, subjects do not waive any of their legal rights nor do they release the investigator, sponsor, or institution from liability for negligence. Federal regulations require that certain information be provided to each human subject. This information includes the following:

- A statement that the study involves research, the purpose of the research, the expected duration of subject participation, a description of the procedures to be followed, and the identification of procedures that are experimental.

- A description of reasonably foreseeable risks or discomforts. The description must be accurate and reasonable, and subjects must be informed of previously reported adverse events.

- A description of the benefits to the subject or others who may reasonably benefit from the research.

- A disclosure of the appropriate alternative procedures or courses of treatment, if any, that might be advantageous to the subject. When appropriate, a statement that supportive care with no additional disease-specific treatment is an alternative.

- A statement describing the extent to which confidentiality of records identifying the subject will be maintained. The statement should include full disclosure and description of approved agencies such as the FDA that may have access to the records.

- For research involving more than minimal risk, an explanation as to whether any compensation or medical treatments are available if injury occurs and, if so, what they consist of or where further information may be obtained. Injury is not limited to physical injury. Research-related injury may include physical, psychological, social, financial, or otherwise.

- An explanation of who to contact for answers to pertinent questions about the research and research subjects' rights and who to contact in the event of a research-related injury to the subject.

- A statement that participation is voluntary and that the subject may discontinue participation at any time without penalty or loss of benefits to which he or she is otherwise entitled (45 CFR.116).

The federal regulations further require that additional consent information be provided when appropriate (45 CFR 46.116), including:

- A statement that the treatment or procedure may involve risks to the subject (or embryo or fetus if the subject is pregnant) that are unforeseeable
- Anticipated circumstances under which the subject's participation may be terminated by the investigator without regard to the subject's consent
- Any additional costs that a subject may incur as a result of participating in the research
- The consequences of a subject's decision to withdraw from the research and procedures for orderly termination of participation by the subject
- A statement that significant new findings developed during the course of the research that may relate to the subject's willingness to continue participation will be provided to the subject
- The approximate number of subjects involved in the study

Federal regulations also require that informed consent be presented in a language that is un-derstandable to the subject. If it is not, the consent form must be translated into the appropriate language. Subjects who are illiterate must have an interpreter present to explain the study and translate questions and answers between subject and investigator. A model consent form appears in appendix F. In institutions where biomedical research is conducted, consent forms are usually maintained in storage facilities monitored by the **principal investigator**. The principal investigator is the director of the research project and has full responsibility for all parts of the research conducted. Copies of the consent may or may not be kept in the medical record depending upon organizational policy. Consent forms often contain sensitive information such as that related to genetic testing. Results of tests related to genetic testing are not to be provided to insurers or other parties, and sometimes not to the subject. To help ensure that this information is not released inadvertently in the regular course of business related to the release of information process, some organizations choose to maintain these important documents separately. Examples of documents that are kept in the study center files are listed in figure 20.2.

Figure 20.2. Study center file contents

- Investigator's brochure
- Signed protocol
- Revised protocols (if applicable)
- Protocol amendments (if applicable)
- Continuing review documents
- Informed consent form (blank)
- HIPAA consent form (blank)
- Copies of signed consent forms
- Curriculum vitae (resumes) of principal investigator and coinvestigators
- Documentation of IRB or ethical review board (ERB) compliance
- All correspondence between the investigator, IRB or ERB, and study sponsor or contract research organization relating to study conduct
- Copies of safety reports sent to the FDA
- Lab certifications
- Normal laboratory value ranges for tests required by the protocol
- The FDA's Clinical Investigator Information Sheet
- Clinical research associate monitoring log
- Drug invoices
- Study site signature log
- Financial disclosure statement

Source: 45 CFR 46.115.

Vulnerable Subjects

HHS regulations include additional protections for vulnerable or special subject populations as subparts of 45 CFR Part 46. Federal regulations require that "when some or all of the subjects are likely to be vulnerable to coercion or undue influence, additional safeguards have been included in the study to protect the rights and welfare of these subjects." (45 CFR 46.111(b); 21 CFR 56.111(b)). When a subject has limited mental capacity or is unable to freely volunteer, the subject is considered a **vulnerable subject**. Examples of vulnerable subjects include the following:

- *Children* may be vulnerable depending on age, maturity, and psychological state. There is potential for control, coercion, undue influence, or manipulation by parents, guardians, or investigators. The risk is greater for particularly young children.

- *Pregnant women, human fetuses, and neonates* may be vulnerable because of the increased potential risk to them. There is potential for interventions or procedures to cause greater risk for both the pregnant woman and the fetus or neonate.

- *Mentally disabled individuals* have problems with capacity. They may not have freedom to volunteer because they may be institutionalized or hospitalized, are economically and educationally disadvantaged, and suffer from chronic diseases.

- *Educationally disadvantaged subjects* may have limitations on understanding the study they will be participating in; some may be illiterate. There is potential for undue influence and manipulation.

- *Economically disadvantaged subjects* may volunteer only because they will benefit economically. That is, because they will receive payment for participating in the research, they may volunteer. They may enroll in research only to receive monetary compensation or medical care they cannot otherwise afford.

- *Individuals with incurable or fatal diseases* may volunteer to participate out of desperation. In many cases, these individuals have failed many treatments and view volunteering in biomedical research as their last chance at surviving their illness. Also, because of disease progression or effects of medications, they may not have the mental capacity necessary to make an informed decision. These individuals may accept high risk because they are desperate for a cure, even when there is little or no prospect of direct benefit.

- *Prisoners* have limited autonomy and may not be able to exercise free choice. They may believe that they will receive adverse treatment or be denied certain privileges if they refuse to participate in the research study. In addition, cash payments may be an inducement to participate in research; thus, it could be said that they are not truly volunteering but only participating for the cash benefit. Prisoners represent a population of convenience; that is, they are readily accessible and available. Studies on a contained population can be done more quickly and more cheaply. Lastly, prisoners may not realize benefits from their participation in research because of their incarceration and social and economic status.

Check Your Understanding 20.2

Instructions: Answer the following questions on a separate piece of paper.

1. What is exempt research?

2. What is nonexempt research? Provide examples.

3. True or False: In signing an informed consent, a subject releases the research sponsor from any liability or negligence.

4. True or False: Individuals who may be subject to undue influence to enroll in biomedical research are considered vulnerable.

5. True or False: A subject may withdraw from a research study at any time.

6. True or False: A patient agrees to be a subject in a clinical trial assessing the effectiveness of the combination of two cancer agents. Because the patient is part of this research, all medical expenses are covered by the sponsoring organization. True or false?

Role of HIM Professionals in Research

The role of the health information management (HIM) professional in the research they do can take on two different functions. First, the HIM professional may serve as the PI for a particular research project. In this capacity, it is the responsibility of HIM professionals to submit their research study to the appropriate level of IRB review and approval. HIM professionals should follow the IRB checklist (refer to appendix E). They should also complete any appropriate consent forms (appendix F) so that the forms meet all of the essential rules and regulations that govern the IRB. As the PI of a research project, HIM professionals must follow all of the procedures just as they are written in their research study protocol. Since this is the original protocol that was approved by the IRB, any changes to this protocol should be submitted to the IRB again for review and approval. Second, HIM professionals can serve in a supportive role to investigators conducting research in healthcare facilities. In this capacity, they can provide education and information regarding the necessary policies and procedures that an investigator must follow when conducting research. They can inform the PI about the proper procedures to follow when undergoing IRB review and approval and provide consultation on the development of the research study protocol and consent forms. They can also serve as a patient advocate by educating patients about their rights when involved in research. Finally, HIM professionals may be asked to serve as members of or consultants to the IRB as subject matter experts in data and information handling as well as the protection of patient privacy and confidentiality.

Privacy Considerations in Clinical and Biomedical Research

In response to a congressional mandate in HIPAA, HHS issued regulations entitled Standards for Privacy of Individually Identifiable Health Information. Known as the **Privacy Rule**, the regulations protect medical records and other individually identifiable health information from being used or disclosed in any form (HHS 2013).

The Privacy Rule establishes a category of **protected health information (PHI)**, which may be used or disclosed only in certain circumstances or under certain conditions. PHI is a subset of what is called individually identifiable health information. It includes information in the patient's medical records as well as billing information for services rendered. PHI also includes identifiable health information about subjects of clinical research. Patient information considered protected is listed in chapter 11. Deidentification is important in protecting patient privacy and includes removing identifying information from patient records and can include patient name, zip code, and so forth.

The Privacy Rule defines the means by which human research subjects are informed of how their protected medical information will be used or disclosed. It also outlines their rights to access the information. The Privacy Rule protects the privacy of individually identifiable information while ensuring that researchers continue to have access to the medical information they need to conduct their research. Investigators are permitted to use and disclose PHI for research with individual authorization or without individual authorization under limited circumstances (HHS 2013).

A valid Privacy Rule authorization is an individual's signed permission that allows a covered entity to use or disclose the patient's PHI for the purpose(s) and to the recipient(s) stated in the authorization (HHS 2004a). When an authorization is obtained for biomedical research purposes, the Privacy Rule requires that it pertain only to a specific research study, not to future unspecified projects. See chapter 11 for information regarding elements of the Privacy Rule authorization.

For some types of research, it is impracticable for researchers to obtain written authorization from research participants. Therefore, the Privacy Rule contains criteria for waiver or alteration of the authorization requirement by an IRB or a privacy board. Under the Privacy Rule, either board may waive or alter, in whole or in part, the Privacy Rule's authorization requirements for the use and disclosure of PHI in connection with a particular research project. For example, an IRB may partially waive the authorization requirement so that the covered entity can provide contact information to investigators so that they can contact and recruit subjects into their research study (HHS 2004b; 2013).

It is believed that the Privacy Rule will promote participation in clinical trials. Reasons for lack of participation in clinical trials cited most often are concern about health insurance discrimination and loss of privacy should the information be released.

Oversight of Biomedical Research

Because of past abuses of human subjects in the conduct of biomedical research in the United States, Congress began hearings in 1981 to investigate scientific misconduct. Twelve cases of scientific misconduct were reported in the country between 1974 and 1981 (HHS 2011b). Representative Albert Gore Jr, chairman of the Investigations and Oversight Subcommittee of the House Science and Technology Committee, held the first hearing. Continued abuses were reported throughout the 1980s, which resulted in the creation of the Office of Research Integrity to provide oversight of biomedical research. Examples of scientific misconduct include researchers falsifying research data, enrolling study subjects who did not qualify for the protocol, disregarding the well-being of vulnerable human subjects, and falsifying personal information in grant applications (HHS 2011b).

In response to the public outcry over scientific misconduct in biomedical research, Congress passed the **Health Research Extension Act** in 1985 (Public Health Service regulation 42 CFR 493). The act requires the secretary of HHS to issue a regulation requiring applicant or awardee institutions to establish "an administrative process to review reports of scientific fraud" and "report to the Secretary any investigation of scientific fraud which appears substantial" (42 CFR 493).

Before 1986, reports of scientific misconduct were received by funding institutes within the Public Health Service (PHS). In 1986, the National Institutes of Health (NIH) assigned responsibility for receiving and responding to complaints of scientific misconduct to its Institutional Liaison Office. This was the first step in creating a central locus of responsibility for scientific misconduct within HHS. In March 1989, the PHS created the Office of Scientific Integrity (OSI) and the Office of Scientific Review (OSIR) in the Office of the Assistant Secretary for Health (OASH). In 1992, the OSI and the OSIR were consolidated to form the **Office of Research Integrity (ORI)** in the OASH. The creation of these groups removed responsibility for reviewing complaints of scientific misconduct from the funding agencies.

In 1993, the NIH Revitalization Act established the ORI as an independent agency within HHS. The role, mission, and structure of the ORI are focused on preventing misconduct and promoting research integrity principally through oversight, education, and review of institutional findings and recommendations (HHS 2011b). Responsibilities of the ORI include:

- Developing policies, procedures, and regulations related to the detection, investigation, and prevention of research misconduct and the responsible conduct of research
- Reviewing and monitoring research misconduct investigations conducted by applicant and awardee institutions
- Implementing activities and programs to teach the responsible conduct of research, promote research integrity, prevent research misconduct, and improve the handling of allegations of research misconduct
- Providing technical assistance to institutions that respond to allegations of research misconduct
- Conducting policy analyses, evaluations, and research to build the knowledge base in research misconduct and research integrity (HHS 2011c)

The ORI within HHS conducted a study that examined scientists' reports on suspected research misconduct. From this study, it found that investigators believe that the best way to detect and prevent research misconduct is to have the PI supervise research work closely by reviewing data and applying quality control procedures or audits on the data. The ORI also found that more open communication is necessary to detect research misconduct and that anonymity is necessary for the person reporting the possible misconduct. Policies and an effective training guide with a system for reporting were also found to be important (HHS 2011d).

Types of Biomedical Research Designs

The more common types of designs for research involving human subjects include:

- Epidemiological studies
- Cross-sectional study
- Case-control studies
- Cohort studies
- Clinical trials

Epidemiological Studies

Epidemiology is the study of health and disease in populations rather than individuals. It examines epidemics as well as chronic diseases. The purpose of an epidemiological study is to compare two groups or populations of individuals, one group with the risk factor of interest and one without it. In such studies, the investigator attempts to identify risk factors for diseases, conditions, behaviors, or risks that result from particular causes, such as environmental factors and industrial agents.

The goals are to quantify the association between exposures and outcomes and to test hypotheses about causal relationships. Epidemiological research has several objectives:

- Identify the cause of disease and its associated risk factors
- Determine the extent of disease in a given community
- Study the natural history and prognosis of disease
- Evaluate new preventive and therapeutic measures and new modes of healthcare delivery
- Provide the foundation for public policy and regulatory decisions relating to environmental problems

Epidemiological studies may be observational or experimental. In an observational study, the exposure and outcome for each individual in the study is studied (observed). In an experimental study, the exposure status for each individual in the study is determined and the individuals are then followed to determine the effects of the exposure.

Observational studies are used to generate hypotheses for later experimental studies. They may consist of clinical observations at a patient's bedside. For example, Alton Ochsner observed that every patient he operated on for lung cancer had a history of cigarette smoking (Gordis 1996). If he had wanted to explore the relationship further, he would have compared the smoking histories of a group of his lung cancer patients with a group of his patients without lung cancer. This would be a case-control study. Research designs that are considered observational are cross-sectional studies, prospective cohort studies, retrospective cohort studies, and case-control studies.

In biomedical research, experimental studies consist primarily of randomized clinical trials. In randomized clinical trials, individuals are randomly assigned to experimental and control groups in order to study the effect of an intervention, such as an experimental drug.

A major purpose of epidemiological studies is to determine risk. In prospective studies, a 2 × 2 table is a tool that is used to evaluate the association between exposure and disease. (See table 20.1.) The table is a cross-classification of exposure status and disease status. The total number of individuals with the disease is $a + c$, and the total number without disease is $b + d$. The total number exposed is $a + b$, and the total number not exposed is $c + d$.

The number of individuals who had both exposure and the disease is recorded in cell a; the number who had exposure, but no disease, is recorded in cell b; the number who had the disease, but no

exposure, is recorded in cell c; and the number who had neither the disease nor exposure is recorded in cell d.

Cross-Sectional Studies

In a cross-sectional study, both the exposure and the disease outcome are determined at the same time in each subject. A cross-sectional study may also be referred to as a prevalence study because it describes characteristics and health outcomes at a particular point in time. It provides quantitative estimates of the magnitude of a problem. After the population has been defined, the presence or absence of exposure and of disease can be established for each individual in the study. Each subject is then categorized into one of four subgroups that correspond to the 2 × 2 table that appears in table 20.2. An example of a cross-sectional study is determining the prevalence rate of individuals who receive yearly eye exams with type 2 diabetes mellitus.

The prevalence of disease in persons with exposure ($a/a + b$) is compared with persons without exposure ($c/c + d$). Alternatively, the prevalence of exposure in persons with the disease ($a/a + c$) is compared to the prevalence of exposure to persons without the disease ($b/b + d$).

A major advantage of the cross-sectional study is that it is relatively easy to conduct and may produce results in a short period of time. The disadvantage is that because exposure and disease are determined at the same time in each subject, the time relationship between exposure and onset of the disease cannot be established. It describes only what exists at the time of the study.

Table 20.1. 2 × 2 table for classifying disease status and exposure status

		Disease status		
		Yes	No	Total
Exposure status	Yes	a	b	$a + b$
	No	c	d	$c + d$
		$a + c$	$b + d$	$a + b + c + d$

Table 20.2. 2 × 2 table for cross-sectional studies

	Disease	No disease	Totals	Prevalence of disease for exposed/not exposed
Exposed	a	b	$a + b$	$a/a + b$
Not exposed	c	d	$c + d$	$c/c + d$
Totals	$a + c$	$b + d$	$a + b + c + d$	$a + b + c + d$
Prevalence of exposure for disease/no disease	$a/a + c$	$b/b + d$		

Group a: Persons exposed with the disease
Group b: Persons exposed without the disease
Group c: Persons with the disease, but not exposed
Group d: Persons without disease and without exposure

Case-Control Studies

Case-control studies are a major component of epidemiological research. In them, persons with a certain condition (cases) and persons without the condition (controls) are studied by looking back in time. The objective is to determine the frequency of the risk factor among the cases and the frequency of the risk factor among the controls in order to determine possible causes of the disease. In a case-control study, if there is an association between exposure and disease, the prevalence of history of exposure will be higher in persons with the disease (cases) than in those without it (controls). For a case-control study, see the 2 × 2 table in table 20.3. The proportion of cases exposed is $a/a + c$, and the proportion of controls exposed is $b/b + d$. For example, a researcher may be interested in examining the relationship between cell phone use and brain cancer. The researcher selects the cases as those individuals with brain cancer and the controls as those individuals without brain cancer but very much like the cases in all other characteristics. So, when selecting the controls, the researcher may choose a sibling or friend of the cases, as long as he or she does not have brain cancer. Then, the researcher may review cell phone records or conduct a person-to-person interview asking them questions about their past cell phone use. Odds ratios will be determined. The odds ratio is the probability that a certain outcome will occur if an individual is exposed to a certain variable or risk factor. This finding is then compared to the odds that a certain outcome will occur for those individuals not exposed to that variable or risk factor. For example, if the odds ratio is 5, the researcher can conclude that those individuals who use cell phones are five times more likely to develop brain cancer than those individuals who do not use cell phones (see Risk Assessment later in the chapter).

The advantages of case-control studies are that they are easy to conduct and cost-effective, with minimal risk to the subjects. Also, existing records may be used to conduct the studies. Case-control studies also allow the researcher to study multiple causes of disease. Although the use of existing health records is advantageous, there are problems associated with using them for retrospective research. One major problem is that the cases are based on hospital admissions. Admissions are based on patient characteristics, severity of illness and associated conditions, and admission policies. All of these vary from hospital to hospital, making standardization of the study difficult. In addition, there are problems related to poor documentation, illegibility, and missing records. Lack of consistency in diagnostic and clinical services between hospitals also makes comparability difficult. Further, validation of the information can be difficult. An important aspect of epidemiological studies is the identification of risk. In studies using medical records, the population at risk is generally not defined.

Cohort Studies

A cohort study is a prospective study in which the investigator selects a group of exposed individuals and unexposed individuals who are followed for a period of time to compare the incidence of disease in the two groups. The length of time for follow-up varies from a few days for acute diseases to several decades for cancer and cardiac diseases. For a cohort study, see the 2 × 2 table in table 20.4. If there is an association between exposure and disease,

Table 20.3. 2 × 2 table for case-control studies

	Cases (with disease)	Controls (without disease)
Exposed	a	b
Not exposed	c	d
Total	a + c	b + d
Proportions exposed	a/a + c	b/b + d

Group a: Persons exposed with the disease
Group b: Persons exposed without the disease
Group c: Persons with the disease, but not exposed
Group d: Persons without disease and without exposure

Table 20.4. 2 × 2 table for cohort studies

	Disease develops	Disease does not develop	Totals	Incidence rates of disease
Exposed	a	b	a + b	a/a + b
Not exposed	c	d	c + d	c/c + d

Group a: Persons exposed with the disease
Group b: Persons exposed without the disease
Group c: Persons with the disease, but not exposed
Group d: Persons without disease and without exposure

the incidence of disease is greater in the exposed group (a/$a + b$) than in the unexposed group (c/$c + d$). New cases of the disease are identified as they occur so that it can be determined whether a time relationship exists between exposure to disease and development of disease. The time relationship must be established if the exposure is to be considered the cause of the disease.

One of the most famous cohort studies is the Framingham Study, which began in the 1950s (Framingham Heart Study 2015). The research project was designed to monitor the incidence of coronary artery disease in more than 5,000 residents who were examined every two years for a period of 20 years. This study has provided important data demonstrating the relationship between the development of heart disease and risk factors such as smoking, obesity, diet, and high blood pressure.

Cohort studies offer several advantages. First, the researcher can control the data collection process throughout the study. Also, outcome events can be checked as they occur; many outcomes can be studied, including those that were not anticipated at the start of the study. The disadvantages of cohort studies are that they are costly and there is a long wait for the study results. Also, subjects may be lost to death, withdrawal, or lack of follow-up.

One difference between case-control and cohort studies is that the former is a retrospective study and the latter is a prospective study. A **retrospective study** is conducted by reviewing records from the past; a **prospective study** is designed to observe events that occur after the subjects have been identified. The advantages and disadvantages of retrospective and prospective studies are outlined in tables 20.5 and 20.6.

Another difference is that in a cohort study the subjects are individuals with or without the disease and the focus is disease status; in the case-control study, the subjects are individuals who have been exposed or not exposed to the disease and the focus is exposure status.

Clinical Trials

Clinical (medical) research is a specialized area of research that primarily investigates the efficacy

Table 20.5. Advantages and disadvantages of retrospective studies

Advantages	Disadvantages
Short study time	Control group subject to bias in selection
Relatively inexpensive	Biased recall possible
Suitable for rare diseases	Cannot determine incidence rate
Ethical problems minimal	Relative risk is approximate
Hospital medical record may be used	
Small number of subjects	
No attrition problems	

Table 20.6. Advantages and disadvantages of prospective studies

Advantages	Disadvantages
Control group less susceptible to bias	Requires more time
No recall necessary	Costly
Incidence rate can be determined	Relatively common diseases only
Relative risk is accurate	Ethical problems may be considerable and influence study design
	Volunteers needed
	Results may not be generalizable to a larger population
	Requires a large number of subjects
	Problems with attrition

of preventive, diagnostic, and therapeutic procedures. Efficacy involves both safety and effectiveness.

Clinical trials are the specific, individual studies within the field of clinical research. They offer a systematic way to introduce, evaluate, and monitor new drugs, treatments, and devices prior to their dissemination throughout the healthcare system. As a result, they have proved to be effective means of advancing knowledge about medicine and health and, thus, improving the quality of healthcare in the United States. Because clinical trials involve patients, they can begin only after the researcher has shown promising results in the laboratory or the results have been well documented in the literature. Clinicaltrials.gov from the National Institutes of Health is a database of clinical trials that have been and are currently being conducted around the globe. Examples of certain types of clinical trials can be searched in this database to determine if a specific topic or disease has been researched. It is required by the FDA that the researcher post a description of the clinical trial on the database and make the subject aware of this through the informed consent (NIH 2015).

The NIH supports thousands of clinical trials (NIH 2015). Private organizations such as drug companies and health maintenance organizations (HMOs) also support them. Trial sites are teaching and community hospitals, physician group practices, or health departments. Many clinical trials are multicentered; that is, a number of research institutions cooperate in conducting the study. In **randomized clinical trials (RCTs)**, participants are assigned to a treatment or a control group. They may be **single-blind studies** in which case the subject does not know the treatment or **double-blind studies**, in which case the investigator and the subjects do not know who is in the treatment or control group until the end of the study.

Researchers conduct clinical trials using protocols. **Protocols** are sets of strict procedures that specify the language of informed consent, the types of subjects, the timing of treatments, the period of participation, and the evaluation of efficacy. For example, in RCTs, researchers must follow strict rules in assigning patients to groups. The rules ensure that both known and unknown risk factors will occur in approximately equal numbers between the group of patients receiving the treatment and the group of patients not receiving it.

Most clinical trials consist of three phases. For example, in a phase 1 drug trial, studies are performed on 20 to 80 healthy volunteers who are closely monitored (NIH 2015). The objectives of phase 1 drug trials are to determine the metabolic and pharmacological actions of the drug in humans, to determine the side effects associated with increasing dosages and to gain early evidence of effectiveness. Historically, phase 1 trials are considered the safest and usually involve administering a single dose to healthy volunteers (NIH 2015). But they also can pose a high level of unknown risk because this is the first administration of a drug to a human. When the drug is highly toxic, such as cancer chemotherapies, cancer patients are usually the subjects for phase 1 trials.

In a phase 2 drug trial, the number of participants is usually increased to between 100 and 200 (NIH 2015). The purposes of this trial are to evaluate the drug's effectiveness for a certain indication in patients with the condition under study and to determine the short-term side effects and risks associated with the drug. Subjects included in phase 2 studies are usually those with the condition the drug is intended to treat. Phase 2 studies are randomized, well controlled, and closely monitored. They may include randomization to treatment and control groups and be double-blinded. Treatment and control groups allow for comparison between subjects who received the drug and those who did not.

Phase 3 drug trials involve the administration of a new drug to a larger number of patients in different clinical settings to determine its safety, effectiveness, and appropriate dosage. The number of subjects involved may range from several hundred to several thousand. Phase 3 trials are conducted only after evidence of effectiveness has been obtained. Phase 3 studies are designed to collect more information on drug effectiveness and safety for evaluating the drug's overall risk benefit.

The FDA, in collaboration with the research study sponsor, may decide to conduct a phase 4 postmarketing study to obtain more information about the drug's risks, benefits, and optimal use. Phase 4 studies may include studying different doses or schedules of administration than what was used in phase 2 studies, the use of the drug in other patient populations or other stages of the disease, or the use of the drug over a longer period of time. See table 20.7.

Risk Assessment

As stated earlier, one objective of epidemiological studies is to assess risk. Risk is the probability that an individual will develop a disease over a specified period of time, provided that he or she did not die as a result of some other disease process during the same time period. It is usually expressed as **relative risk (RR)**. Before risk can be assessed

Table 20.7. Phases of clinical trials

Phase	1	2	3	4
Number of subjects	20–80	100–300	1,000–3,000	Multitudes postmarketing
Purpose	Evaluate safety Determine dosage Identify side effects	Evaluate safety Determine effectiveness	Collect more information about safe usage Confirm effectiveness Monitor side effects Compare to alternatives	Collect data on effect on specific groups (population) Monitor long-term side effects

Source: NIH 2015.

properly, prevalence and incidence should be defined. Prevalence refers to the number of existing cases of a particular disease. Incidence refers to the number of new cases of a disease. The prevalence rate is therefore the number of existing cases of disease in a particular region during a specific time period divided by the number of individuals in the specific region for a specific time period. The incidence rate is the number of new cases of disease in a particular region during a specific time period divided by the number of individuals in the specific region for a specific time period. RR is calculated from cohort studies and compares the risk of some disease in two groups differentiated by some demographic variable such as sex or race. The group of interest is referred to as the exposed group and the comparison group is the unexposed group. The risk ratio is calculated as:

$$\frac{\text{Risk for exposed group or the incidence rate of the exposed group}}{\text{Risk for unexposed group or the incidence rate of the unexposed group}}$$

A relative risk of 1.0 indicates that there is identical risk in both groups. A RR that is greater than 1.0 indicates an increased risk for the exposed group; a RR of less than 1.0 indicates a decreased risk for the exposed group.

Odds Ratio

In a case-control study, the objective is to identify differences in exposure frequency associated with one group having the disease under study and the other group not having it. The incidence of disease in the exposed and unexposed populations is not known because persons with the disease (cases) and without the disease (controls) are identified at the onset of the study. Thus, RR cannot be calculated directly. So the question becomes: what are the odds that an exposed person will develop the disease? Or, put another way, what are the odds that a nonexposed person will develop the disease?

In a case-control study, the odds ratio compares the odds that the cases were exposed to the disease with the odds that the controls were exposed. Using the 2 × 2 table in table 20.1 as a reference, the odds ratio is calculated as:

$$\frac{(a/a+c)}{(b/b+d)}$$
$$\text{or}$$
$$\frac{(ad)}{(bc)}$$

The odds ratio measures the odds of exposure of a given disease. For example, an odds ratio of 1.0 indicates that the incidence of disease is equal in each group; thus, the exposure may not be a risk factor for the disease of interest. An odds ratio of 2.0 indicates that the cases were twice as likely to be exposed as the controls. This implies that the exposure is associated with twice the risk of disease.

Attributable Risk

The attributable risk (AR) is a measure of the public health impact of a causative factor on a population. In this measure, the assumption is that the occurrence of a disease in an unexposed group is the baseline or expected risk for that disease. Any risk above that level in the exposed group is attributed to exposure to the risk factor. It is assumed that some individuals will acquire a disease, such as lung cancer, whether or not they were exposed to a risk factor such as smoking. The AR measures the additional risk of illness as a result of an individual's exposure to a risk factor. The AR is calculated as risk for the exposed group minus the risk for the unexposed group. AR percent is calculated as follows:

$$\frac{(\text{Risk for exposed group}) - AR =}{(\text{Risk for unexposed group})} \times 100$$
$$\frac{}{\text{Risk for exposed group}}$$

Check Your Understanding 20.3

Instructions: **Answer the following questions on a separate piece of paper.**

1. Describe the relationship of the HIPAA Privacy Rule to clinical research.

2. What is an odds ratio?

3. What are some of the common types of research designs used in studies of human subjects?

4. What is the difference between incidence and prevalence?

5. What are the characteristics of a case-control study?

6. What are the characteristics of randomized clinical trials?

7. What is relative risk?

8. What is attributable risk?

Use of Comparative Data in Outcomes Research

Healthcare organizations such as the **National Committee for Quality Assurance (NCQA)** and the Joint Commission have developed measures for evaluating the effectiveness of healthcare providers. The purpose of the measures developed by the NCQA is to provide purchasers of healthcare, primarily employers, with information about the cost and effectiveness of organizations with which they contract for services. The Joint Commission measures also are designed primarily to encourage organizations to improve their own performance and to provide a comprehensive picture of the care provided within the organization. A full discussion of performance measures used in healthcare and by healthcare providers, is presented in chapter 21.

The Patient Protection and Affordable Care Act (ACA) established the Patient-Centered Outcomes Research Institute (PCORI) (ACA 2010). PCORI was established to provide evidence that will assist patients and healthcare providers about prevention and treatment care options and the research or comparative evidence that supports these decisions. The major difference in this type of research is that patients will play a major role in the types of research that are conducted as well as receiving information and research results that are clear and easy to understand. These studies will compare medications, medical devices, assistive technologies, surgeries, and such to determine the best ways to provide healthcare to patients. The National Strategy for Quality Improvement of Healthcare (2011) was developed by HHS as part of the ACA. It sets priorities and a strategic plan for quality improvement of healthcare in the United States. The Hospital Consumer Assessment of Healthcare Providers and Systems (HCAHPS), under Medicare, now requires all hospitals to publicly report standardized information on the perspectives of all patients to include the patient experience and patient satisfaction in the quality reporting. The Agency for Healthcare Research and Quality (AHRQ) has established a patient-centered care improvement guide. It provides best practices to assist hospitals in moving toward patient-centered care. It also provides evidence behind these best practices and examines barriers to establishing patient-centered care.

A major part of patient-centered research is developing questions that are important to patients and providers of care. Such questions include the following:

- Given my personal characteristics, conditions, and preferences, what should I expect will happen to me?
- What are my options, and what are the benefits and harms of those options?
- What can I do to improve the outcomes that are most important to me?
- How can the healthcare system improve my chances of achieving the outcomes I prefer?

To answer these questions, PCORI will

1. Assess benefits and harms to inform decision making, highlighting comparisons that matter to people.
2. Focus on outcomes that people notice and care about, and
3. Incorporate a wide variety of settings and diversity of participants (PCORI 2015)

A patient-centered research question should include the following elements:

1. Population of patients and research participants
2. Intervention(s) relevant to patients in target population
3. Comparator(s) (usual care or no specific intervention) relevant to patients in target population

4. Outcomes meaningful to patients in target population
5. Timing: outcomes and length of follow-up
6. Setting and providers (PCORI 2015)

PCORI explains that people sometimes care about outcomes that are different than the outcomes of interest to investigators (PCORI 2015). They care about things they notice such as pain and fatigue levels even though these elements may be more difficult to measure. For example, when measuring the outcomes related to a new drug for cancer, investigators may measure the difference in blood markers, while patients will focus on an end result of nausea.

The role and goal of PCORI is to redirect research investigations so that they include patient-centered outcomes such as nausea, pain, and functional status as well as the other scientific elements that may be important. PCORI strives to engage the end users to help shape the research so that the outcomes are going to matter to them—survival, function, symptoms, health-related quality of life, versus biomarkers, chemistry panels, and cost of end-of-life care.

A priority of the National Quality Strategy in Person and Family-Centered Care is to increase the use of EHRs that capture the voice of the patient by integrating patient-generated data in EHRs and routinely measuring patient engagement, self-management, shared decision making, and patient-reported outcomes. One of its indicators for doing this is to collect the percentage of patients asked for feedback. This is an example of how the EHR will be used to demonstrate at what rate the patient is involved in his or her care, and patient-centered outcomes research will be a major component in this data analysis.

Therefore, the HIM professional will play a vital role in making effective decisions about how to incorporate patient- and family-centered data within the EHR so that research in this area can be continued and needed outcomes generated.

Check Your Understanding 20.4

Instructions: **Answer the following questions on a separate piece of paper.**

1. Differentiate between the purpose of NCQA measures and Joint Commission measures?

2. What is required of the Hospital Consumer Assessment of Healthcare Providers and Systems (HCAHPS)?

3. How does the National Quality Strategy in Person and Family-Centered Care plan to increase the use of the EHR in patient-centered care?

4. What is the major focus of PCORI?

5. How is patient-centered outcomes research different than research historically performed by investigators?

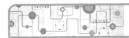 # References

Beecher, H.K. 1966 (Jan.). Consent in clinical experimentation: Myth and reality. *Journal of the American Medical Association* 195(1):34–5. http://www.ncbi.nlm.nih.gov/pubmed/5951827

Centers for Disease Control and Prevention. 2013. US Public Health Service Syphilis Study at Tuskegee—The Tuskegee Timeline. http://www.cdc.gov/tuskegee/timeline.htm

Emanuel, E. and J. Menikoff. 2011. Reforming the regulations governing research and human subjects. *New England Journal of Medicine* 365:1145–1150.

Framingham Heart Study. 2015. https://www.framinghamheartstudy.org

Gordis, L. 1996. *Epidemiology.* Philadelphia: W.B. Saunders.

National Institutes of Health. 2015. Clinicaltrials.gov. http://clinicaltrials.gov

National Institutes of Health, Office of Human Subjects Research. 1979. *The Belmont Report: Ethical Principles and Guidelines for the Protection of Human Subjects of Research.* The National Commission for the Protection of Human Subjects of Biomedical and Behavioral Research. http://ohsr.od.nih.gov/guidelines/belmont.html

National Strategy for Quality Improvement in Healthcare. 2011. Healthcare.gov. http://www.healthcare.gov/law/resources/reports/quality03212011a.html

Nuremberg Code. 1949. Reprinted in *Trials of War Criminals before the Nuremberg Military Tribunals under Control Council Law* 2(10):188–182. Washington, DC: US Government Printing Office. https://www.loc.gov/rr/frd/Military_Law/pdf/NT_war-criminals_Vol-II.pdf

Patient-Centered Outcomes Research Institute (PCORI). 2015. http://www.pcori.org/about/

Patient Protection and Affordable Care Act (ACA). 2010. http://housedocs.house.gov/energycommerce/ppacacon.pdf

Research and Educational Trust. 2015. Health Services Research. http://www.hsr.org/hsr/index.jsp

University of Pittsburgh. 2015a. Chapter 6: IRB Committees. Human Research Protection Office, Policies and Procedures. http://www.irb.pitt.edu/content/chapter-6-irb-committees

University of Pittsburgh. 2015b. Chapter 18: Conflict of Interest. Human Research Protection Office, Policies and Procedures. http://www.irb.pitt.edu/content/chapter-18-conflict-interest

University of Pittsburgh. 2015c. Training Requirements. Human Research Protection Office, Policies and Procedures. http://www.irb.pitt.edu/content/training-requirements

University of Pittsburgh. 2015d. Welcome to CITI. http://irb.pitt.edu/sites/default/files/corpus/files/citi/Welcome_to_CITI.pdf

University of Pittsburgh. 2015e. Chapter 17: Reportable Events. Human Research Protection Office, Policies and Procedures, http://www.irb.pitt.edu/content/chapter-17-reportable-events

US Department of Health and Human Services. 2015a (Sept. 8). Protection of Human Subjects (Common Rule). *Federal Register* 80(173).

US Department of Health and Human Services. 2015b. Regulations. Office of Human Research Protections. http://www.hhs.gov/ohrp/humansubjects/index.html

US Department of Health and Human Services. 2013. Research. Office for Civil Rights, Health Information Privacy. http://www.hhs.gov/ocr/privacy/hipaa/understanding/special/research/index.html

US Department of Health and Humans Services. 2011a (July 26). Human Subjects Research Protections: Enhancing Protections for Research Subjects and Reducing Burden, Delay and Ambiguity for Investigators. *Federal Register* 76(143). http://www.gpo.gov/fdsys/pkg/FR-2011-07-26/pdf/2011-18792.pdf

US Department of Health and Human Services. 2011b. The Office of Research Integrity Historical Background. http://ori.hhs.gov/historical-background

US Department of Health and Human Services. 2011c. The Office of Research Integrity About ORI. http://ori.hhs.gov/about-ori

US Department of Health and Human Services. 2011d. The Office of Research Integrity https://ori.hhs.gov/sites/default/files/gallup_finalreport.pdf

US Department of Health and Human Services. 2009. OHRP Fact Sheet. Office of Human Research Protections. http://www.hhs.gov/ohrp/about/facts/ohrpfactsheetdec09.pdf

US Department of Health and Human Services. 2004a. HIPAA Authorization for Research. NIH Pub. No. 04-5529. http://privacyruleandresearch.nih.gov/authorization.asp

US Department of Health and Human Services 2004b. Institutional Review Boards and the HIPAA Privacy Rule. NIH Pub. No. 03-5428. http://privacyruleandresearch.nih.gov/irbandprivacyrule.asp

US Department of Health and Human Services. 1979. *The Belmont Report: Ethical Principles and Guidelines for the Protection of Human Subjects of Research.* http://www.hhs.gov/ohrp/policy/belmont.html

World Medical Association (WMA). 2015. Declaration of Helsinki Ethical Principles for Medical Research Involving Human Subjects. http://www.wma.net/en/30publications/10policies/b3/

21 CFR 56: IRBs. 2015.

21 CFR 50: Protection of Human Subjects. 2015.

21 CFR 56.101: Scope. 2015 (April 1).

21 CFR 56.110: Expedited review procedures for certain kinds of research involving no more than minimal risk, and for minor changes in approved research. 2015 (April 1).

21 CFR 56.111(b): IRB. 2015 (April 1).

42 CFR 493: Public Health Service Act laboratory requirements. 1990 (March 14).

45 CFR 46: Protection of human subjects. 2009 (July 14).

45 CFR 46.101(b)(1-6): To what does this policy apply? 2009 (July 14).

45 CFR 46.102: Definitions. 2009 (July 14).

45 CFR 46.103: Assuring compliance with this policy–research conducted or supported by any Federal Department or Agency. 2009 (July 14).

45 CFR 46.110: Expedited Review Procedures for certain kinds of research involving no more than minimal risk and for minor changes in approved research. 2009 (July 14).

45 CFR 46.111: Criteria for IRB approval of research. 2009 (July 14)

45 CFR 46.111(b): Criteria for IRB approval of research. 2009 (July 14)

45 CFR 46.115: IRB records. 2009 (July 14)

45 CFR 46.116: General requirements for informed consent. 2009 (July 14).

21

Clinical Quality Management

Rosann M. O'Dell, DHSc, MS, RHIA, CDIP

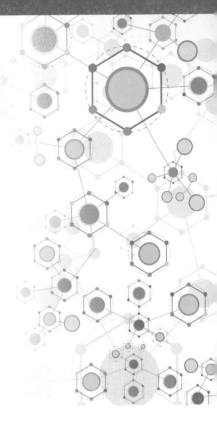

Patient Protection and Affordable
   Care Act (ACA)
Performance
Performance improvement
Plan-do-check-act (PDCA)
Quality

Quality indicators
Quality management
Quality professional
Tacit knowledge
Telehealth

Total quality management
Tracer methodology
Triple Aim
Value-based payments
Vision statement

Quality management and performance improvement are important concepts in the delivery of healthcare services. In healthcare literature, a definition of **quality** is "the degree to which health services for individuals and populations increase the likelihood of desired health outcomes and are consistent with current professional knowledge" (IOM 2001). Achieving quality is influenced by a variety of factors including effective and knowledgeable clinicians and staff, processes and systems that support care, engaged leaders, as well as the ongoing evaluation of clinical care to identify opportunities for improvement.

Quality management refers to processes utilized within healthcare organizations to assess, measure, and evaluate the quality of care provided to patients. Quality management efforts are interprofessional and multidisciplinary in nature, and no single health profession is solely responsible for quality management. Instead, quality management is the responsibility of all health professionals. Emerging healthcare professionals should appreciate that upon entering the healthcare workforce, their daily work is influenced by organizational efforts, initiatives, and requirements centered on quality management. **Total quality management** is "a management philosophy that includes all activities in which the needs of the customer and the organization are satisfied in the most efficient manner by using employee potentials and continuous improvement." (AHIMA 2014a). Quality management efforts are valuable because they produce data and information to assist an organization and its units of operation with understanding how well it performs any given task or function, as well as provides an objective mechanism to identify opportunities for

improvement. An effective quality management program instills a complimentary focus on performance improvement in all that surrounds quality management efforts.

Defined in a basic sense, **performance** is "the action or process of carrying out or accomplishing an action, task, or function" (Oxford Dictionaries 2015). In the context of clinical care, a complex myriad of actions, tasks, and functions occur involving a multidisciplinary and interprofessional team of health professionals. The complex nature of patient care is precisely why quality is managed and opportunities to improve performance are identified. Without concerted efforts on quality and performance, little would be known about outcomes of care or patient satisfaction. **Performance improvement** is processes and steps involved in taking identified areas needing improvement and using actionable efforts to improve performance.

Today's healthcare environment is increasingly driven by stakeholder expectations for safe and effective care. All the while, numerous policy changes, regulations, and the need to reduce costs influence day-to-day operations in healthcare. Health information professionals must possess an understanding of quality management and performance improvement, as well as the context of their professional contributions and roles in these areas. This chapter examines historical and current trends related to quality, and considers the role of organizational influence and uses of tools and processes to affect quality and performance. An overview of professional certifications and roles related to healthcare quality are described. Emerging topics influencing health services provision and quality are also discussed.

Historical Perspectives in Clinical Quality

Clinical care should be provided with a focus on quality. In the context of the entire history of medicine and healthcare, quality management is a more recent development. A lack of focus on quality was not because of a historical disregard for patients. Instead, the evolution of science and technology brought forth an understanding that certain protocols and evidence-based approaches could reduce the risk of death, injury, and unfavorable outcomes among patients.

Patient Safety Concerns Emerge

Some of the most significant threats to quality of care have stemmed from infections and the lack of infection control processes. For example, surgical procedures were noted as occurring hundreds of years before risks of infection were understood and even before anesthesia was available (Alexander 1985). It was not until the mid-18th century that pioneers in medicine and nursing began to identify infections as primary culprits to unfavorable patient care outcomes.

One such pioneer was Joseph Lister, a physician who is often referred to as the father of modern day surgery. Lister was an 18th century physician who devoted his career to not only being a surgeon, but also as a researcher who identified that microorganisms such as bacterium were dangerous when not mitigated in surgical settings (Alexander 1985). His work included the earliest uses of infection control measures in operating rooms such as placing anti-infective agents inside wounds as well as on dressings applied to surgical sites and instrument sterilization.

Another physician who devoted his career to patient safety research was Ignaz Semmelweis. Semmelweis is also credited in healthcare quality literature with enhancing patient safety and reducing infections in clinical settings by being one of the earliest and most steadfast champions of handwashing (Best and Neuhauser 2004). Another noteworthy early pioneer on patient safety was

nurse Florence Nightingale. Nightingale began her nursing career in Germany and then went on to manage nursing services in British hospitals. Her years of nursing experience led to her role in investigating the sanitation, mortality rates, and provider training in military hospitals, where she identified woefully unsanitary and unsafe conditions leading to negative patient outcomes. Nightingale was a nurse who conducted extensive research and applied statistical analyses to her findings to identify that unfavorable sanitation increased mortality (UK National Archives n.d.). Her findings spurred policy changes to public health programs including those related to the role and use of nurses in healthcare, nurse training, and government's role in healthcare facility sanitation (Monteiro 1985).

As an increasing body of knowledge emerged about opportunities to reduce mortality in healthcare settings in the early 1900s; the American College of Surgeons began advocating for sweeping changes in United States. By the 1920s, the American College of Surgeons championed a variety of opportunities to improve healthcare. These included the recommendation that complete health records be created and maintained for all patients and peer-review processes as well as uniform approaches to medical education in the training of physicians be developed (Fahrenholz 2013).

By 1928, the American College of Surgeons established the American Association of Medical Record Librarians, which is today known as the American Health Information Management Association. The creation of a professional association related to health records helped ensure that health records in patient care settings remained a high priority and support for those working with health records was available. It was around this time that hospitals and other care settings in the United States increasingly began creating and maintaining health records on patients to document care provided.

Legal Implications Related to Quality of Care

By the time World War II ended and American soldiers were returning home, healthcare services in the United States became more expansive to support a growing population. As the American healthcare infrastructure grew, it developed initially with limited regulatory influences or standards. Legal issues and liability related to clinical care were among the earliest indicators that an increased focus on quality would inform the future of American healthcare.

One case discussed in educational, healthcare, and legal venues is *Darling v. Charleston Community Memorial Hospital,* for which a final decision was rendered in appellate court in 1965 (Wiet 2005). In *Darling,* a young man was injured while playing football and broke his leg. Upon receiving emergency services and being admitted to Charleston Community Memorial Hospital, a series of clinical errors and miscommunication among Darling's care team ensued. The young man who entered the hospital with a broken leg was later transferred to another hospital because a series of errors, including unidentified infection of the broken leg inside a cast and inadequate oversight in care processes—such as improperly trained clinicians directing care decisions—resulted in the leg having extensive necrosis and damage requiring specialty care at an academic medical center. After a series of procedures performed at the receiving hospital, the leg could not be restored and required amputation (*Darling v. Charleston* 1965).

Darling was a landmark case in health law because the final legal judgment found both the treating physician as well as Charleston Community Memorial Hospital liable for the harm caused to Darling. Prior to *Darling,* it had never occurred in the history of medical malpractice liability that a healthcare organization was held legally responsible for clinical errors occurring in the care of a patient. **Medical malpractice liability** refers to instances where a civil claim for damages against a healthcare provider successfully proves that the provider was negligent in their care of the patient leading to injury or death. From this point forward, a legal precedent was set that healthcare organizations possessed a shared responsibility for patient care and safety, and healthcare organizations were no longer immune to liability for medical errors occurring within the walls of a healthcare facility (Wiet 2005). Drivers of quality and safety in patient care began to emerge, such as federal requirements and regulations, accreditation standards, and quality and safety advocacy groups.

Toward Systematic Quality and Performance Initiatives

As the *Darling* case was underway in 1965, another significant change was occurring in the US healthcare system. Title XIX of the Social Security Amendments of 1965 (Public Law 89-97) created the Medicare and Medicaid programs—the former providing health insurance coverage to Americans aged 65 and older as well as those with disabilities and certain medical conditions, and the latter providing insurance coverage to low income individuals and families. As the Medicare and Medicaid programs became operational and began providing insurance coverage to populations with unique vulnerabilities, a variety of standards and requirements were set forth by the federal government to promote safe care environments for Medicare and Medicaid beneficiaries. While providers and healthcare entities providing services to beneficiaries must adhere to numerous regulations, the baseline requirements stem from the **Conditions for Coverage** and **Conditions of Participation**. These conditions are those that "healthcare organizations must meet in order to begin and continue participating in the Medicare and Medicaid programs" (CMS 2013).

The Conditions for Coverage and Conditions of Participation are health and safety standards and are developed for each provider setting. The following types of healthcare organizations are subject to Conditions for Coverage and Conditions of Participation created specifically for the respective settings:

- Ambulatory surgical centers
- Community mental health centers
- Comprehensive outpatient rehabilitation facilities

- Critical access hospitals
- End-stage renal disease facilities
- Federally qualified health centers
- Home health agencies
- Hospices
- Hospitals
- Hospital swing beds
- Intermediate care facilities for individuals with intellectual disabilities
- Organ procurement organizations
- Portable x-ray suppliers
- Programs for all-inclusive care for the elderly organizations
- Clinics, rehabilitation agencies, and public health agencies as providers of outpatient physical therapy and speech-language pathology services
- Psychiatric hospitals
- Religious nonmedical health care institutions
- Rural health clinics
- Long-term care facilities
- Transplant centers (CMS 2013).

Today, manuals are available on the Centers for Medicare and Medicaid Services (CMS) website that define all standards applicable to various healthcare settings (CMS 2013). These standards address a multitude of topics ranging from environment of care standards to health record requirements. The standards required by healthcare organizations accepting Medicare and Medicaid patients help ensure that all aspects of an organization focus its efforts on quality management as a means to promote a safe care environment for patients as well as promote clinical documentation as a mechanism to capture factual details about care provided.

Another driving influence on quality management in healthcare includes the patient advocacy movement that has roots dating to the 1970s. While the education of clinical health professionals today instills the notion that clinical professionals have a role not only in patient care but also in patient advocacy, patient advocacy efforts stemming from

patients and consumers have also influenced the focus on quality in healthcare.

The patient advocacy movement arose because of the recognition that patients are due certain rights in their pursuit of health services. In 1973, the American Hospital Association published *A Patient's Bill of Rights*, which indicated what a patient should expect and is entitled to while receiving hospital-based care and treatment (Carroll College 1992). A new iteration of the bill of rights is known as the *Patient Care Partnership* (AHA n.d.). Because the intent of the *Patient Care Partnership* is to demonstrate the rights and responsibilities of patients in their pursuit of quality healthcare services, many hospitals share the *Patient Care Partnership* brochure with patients.

One of the earliest patient-established organizations in the patient advocacy movement was Consumers for Medical Quality in 1983. Consumers for Medical Quality was a nonprofit organization promoting safety in patient care and was founded by a cancer patient. It focused its resources on information sharing and support for patients who had experienced medical harm (Haskell 2014). As patients became increasingly interested in voicing their concerns about medical harm, third party payers for health services also became increasingly vocal about quality in patient care.

The 1980s are sometimes referred to as the era of managed care in textbooks and health policy literature. This decade is predated by the passage of the Health Maintenance Organization Act of 1973. This legislation allowed for federal funding in the exploratory implementation of health maintenance organizations. The government believed that health maintenance organizations had the ability to influence healthcare delivery by lowering costs and increasing quality. Among the basic requirements of the organizations receiving funding was that they focused on quality control. Each health maintenance organization was required to have a quality assurance program that "must emphasize health outcomes and provide for physician review and for review by other health professionals" (Social Security Administration 1974).

By the 1990s and 2000s, patient safety once again became a forefront topic in American healthcare. An increasing body of evidence suggested that healthcare delivery was suboptimal at best (IOM 2003; 2001). A slew of challenges existed within healthcare such as high rates of patient safety issues, lacking mechanisms for coordinated care, increasingly high healthcare expenditures, and inequity in access to health services.

During the 1990s, the Institute of Medicine (IOM) collaborated with healthcare quality and patient safety experts to conduct an exhaustive analysis of the United States healthcare system (IOM 2001). At the time, much had been published about medical errors but little was occurring systematically to improve safety in healthcare. The first groundbreaking publication related to the IOM's work was titled *To Err is Human: Building a Safer Health System*. This publication was an eye opening analysis of the staggering numbers of lives lost and billions of dollars wasted due to ineffective care and processes ultimately causing harm to patients. It became increasingly evident that until safety improved, quality of care would remain lackluster (Kohn et al. 2000).

The healthcare industry took note and the IOM continued their advocacy efforts for improved patient safety as a mechanism to enhance clinical quality. By 2001, IOM followed up its previous work with a publication titled, *Crossing the Quality Chasm: A New Health System for the 21st Century* (IOM 2001). This publication served as a formal call for complete redesign of the American healthcare system. Redesign in this context was not a roadmap for healthcare organizations. Instead, their recommendations centered on approaching healthcare from a "new perspective on the purpose and aims of the healthcare system, how patients and clinicians should relate, and how care processes can be designed to optimize responsiveness to patient needs" (IOM 2001). The findings from the IOM were timely because healthcare industry stakeholders, legislators, and health policy specialists were increasingly concerned that the current infrastructure of American healthcare delivery was not sustainable and left room for improvement. The IOM offered evidence about the shortcomings suspected by most stakeholder groups and their findings provided a basis for informed dialogue about necessary improvements and opportunities.

Crossing the Quality Chasm: A New Health System for the 21st Century outlined that healthcare ought to be safe, effective, patient-centered, timely, efficient, and equitable (IOM 2001). Ten redesign components were believed to be necessary for improvements in patient safety and clinical quality to occur. These redesign essentials included:

1. Care should be based on continuous healing relationships;
2. Care should be customized to align with individual patient preferences and values;
3. The patient should serve as the central source of control on the care team;
4. Information should flow freely to bolster knowledge and communication;
5. Decision making ought to be evidence based;
6. The healthcare system should focus on safety as a hallmark priority;
7. Increased transparency is needed;
8. Needs of patients should be anticipated versus addressed reactively;
9. Waste should be consistently and continuously decreased; and
10. Collaboration and cooperation among clinicians is essential (IOM 2001).

Another organization that has continuously influenced healthcare quality is the Institute for Healthcare Improvement. The Institute for Healthcare Improvement has worked on a variety of issues in healthcare all with a focus on applying scientific methods in quality management to improve healthcare's most challenging issues, such as the capability for improvement in healthcare delivery; person- and family-centered care; patient safety; and achieving quality, cost, and value (Institute for Healthcare Improvement 2015a). The Institute for Healthcare Improvement is recognized as a leader for work on creating the concept of the Triple Aim. The **Triple Aim** identifies that vast and systematic improvements are needed in order to improve experiences for patients in their pursuit of healthcare, enhance health among the population, and lower per capita costs (Institute for Healthcare Improvement 2015b).

Today's Drivers of Clinical Quality

Healthcare today is delivered with a keen focus on quality. Rarely does a new regulation or policy occur at the national level without significant quality elements embedded deeply within. While many concepts, initiatives, and groups drive quality management efforts such as those previously described, a few key drivers are introduced as particularly noteworthy at the present such as accreditation standards, regulatory requirements, advocacy groups focused on safe and effective care, quality indicator reporting and transparency, value-based payment efforts, and consumer engagement from patients.

Accreditation Standards

Accreditation refers to a voluntary process of organizational review in which an independent body created for this purpose periodically evaluates the quality of the entity's work against pre-established written criteria (AHIMA 2014a). Achieving accreditation is one way to demonstrate a commitment to quality and continuous improvement to patients, communities, and other stakeholders. Accreditation is also a pathway for ongoing participation in the Medicare and Medicaid programs. Regardless of the accrediting body, standards must be met by the healthcare organization that illustrates compliance with a wide array of requirements related to patient safety, the environment of care, information management and governance, medical staff obligations, staffing, and others.

In today's environment, a healthcare organization cannot sit on the sidelines and avoid the undertaking of accreditation. One reason why accreditation is an undertaking worth its investment is that it helps portray a healthcare organization as committed to meeting high standards, and accreditation status can be used in marketing strategies to attract patients. In addition, as previously noted, accreditation is a pathway for healthcare organizations to maintain their participation in the Medicare and Medicaid programs. It is noteworthy that the federal government is the largest single payer for health services. Because many patients are covered with insurance through programs such as Medicare and Medicaid, it makes strategic and business sense for a healthcare organization to accept patients with these types of insurance coverage or else they would lose out on a large market share of patients. Stakeholder groups that expect organizations to be accredited include third party payers, professional liability insurance providers, healthcare professionals, and patients to name a few. It should be understood, however, that being an accredited healthcare organization does not automatically indicate that excellence is achieved in patient care without quality issues arising. Instead, it illustrates a commitment of striving to meet standards that promote quality and safety in patient care. See table 21.1 for examples of accreditation organizations for a variety of facility types.

Regulatory Requirements

There are a variety of federal regulations that influence healthcare. All federal regulations of healthcare stem from federal law. Examples of legislation include:

- **Emergency Medical Treatment and Active Labor Act (EMTALA)**, which was enacted to "ensure public access to emergency services regardless of ability to pay" (CMS 2012).

- **Clinical Laboratory Improvement Amendments (CLIA)**, where "the objective of the CLIA program is to ensure quality laboratory testing" (CMS 2015a).

- **Medicare Prescription Drug, Improvement, and Modernization Act** was enacted to "amend title XVIII of the Social Security Act to provide for a voluntary program for prescription drug coverage under the Medicare Program, to modernize the Medicare Program, to amend the Internal Revenue Code of 1986 to allow a deduction to individuals for amounts contributed to health savings security accounts and health savings accounts, to provide for the disposition

Table 21.1. Examples of accreditation organizations

Name of accreditation organization	Description
Joint Commission	Accredits a variety of healthcare organizations including hospitals. It focuses on continuously improving "healthcare for the public, in collaboration with other stakeholders, by evaluating healthcare organizations and inspiring them to excel in providing safe and effective care of the highest quality and value" (Joint Commission 2015).
Accreditation Association for Ambulatory Health Care	Accredits a variety of ambulatory healthcare organizations including ambulatory surgery centers and community health centers. It exists to "encourage and assist ambulatory health-care organizations to provide the highest achievable level of care for recipients in the most efficient and economically sound manner . . . accomplishes this by the operation of a peer-based assessment, consultation, education, and accreditation program" (AAAHC 2015).
American College of Radiology	Accredits radiology facilities and "offers accreditation programs in CT, MRI, breast MRI, nuclear medicine, and PET as mandated under the Medicare Improvements for Patients and Providers Act as well as for modalities mandated under the Mammography Quality Standards Act" (American College of Radiology n.d.).
Commission on Accreditation of Rehabilitation Facilities	Accredits healthcare organizations providing services focused on "addiction and substance abuse, rehabilitation of a disability, home and community services, retirement living, and other health and human services" (CARF 2015).

of unused health benefits in cafeteria plans and flexible spending arrangements, and for other purposes" (Medicare Prescription Drug, Improvement, and Modernization Act 2003).

- **Health Information Technology for Economic and Clinical Health (HITECH) Act** was "enacted as part of the American Recovery and Reinvestment Act of 2009 . . . to promote the adoption and meaningful use of information technology . . . addresses privacy and security concerns associated with the electronic transmission of health information" (HHS n.d.).

- **Patient Protection and Affordable Care Act (ACA)** is a federal law reforming healthcare. The focus of the law includes quality, affordable healthcare for all Americans; the role of public programs; improving the quality and efficiency of healthcare; prevention of chronic disease and improving public health; healthcare workforce issues; transparency and program integrity; improving access to innovative medical therapies; community living assistance services and supports; and revenue provisions pertaining to premiums and taxation (ACA 2010).

When considering each of these, two things are noticeable. The first is that the major issue addressed in each one is unique from the others. The second thing to appreciate about each of these laws is that each includes requirements pertaining to quality and safety, which in turn influences the quality management undertakings of healthcare organizations. Those working in healthcare should continue to expect quality-related requirements embedded into forthcoming laws and related regulations.

Various stakeholders such as patients and their families as well as payers, advocacy groups, regulators, and accreditation organizations expect that safe and effective care is achieved and continues to improve.

The costs of healthcare continue to soar, room for improvement exists throughout the healthcare system, advocates and researchers illustrate the risks to human life when quality does not improve, and patients expect more from healthcare providers (Bowling et al. 2012; Lateef 2011). There are also growing expectations from advocacy groups and government agencies that science and technology support improved quality when used intelligently and in accordance with established evidence-based guidelines (AHRQ n.d.(a)).

Quality Indicator Reporting and Transparency

In healthcare today, quality indicators are reported from healthcare providers and organizations to a host of government agencies, nonprofit organizations, accreditation bodies, and payers to illustrate performance of meeting quality measures. Quality indicators identify performance or nonperformance of established quality measurements. When healthcare organizations collect quality indicator data, the data is used internally for performance improvement benchmarking. When the data is reported to external bodies, it is also used by external stakeholders to evaluate and compare healthcare providers and organizations.

A significant amount of quality data is available online for public viewing. Some of this data is offered from CMS through their Compare websites (CMS 2015b). These searchable websites provide data from Medicare-certified providers such as hospitals, nursing homes, and physicians among others. The Leapfrog Group is another organization offering transparent healthcare quality data that has been voluntarily reported to their organization (Leapfrog Group 2015). The Joint Commission Quality Check website allows the public to search in geographic locations for quality indicator results of various healthcare organizations. The Joint Commission Quality Check tool allows data to be represented based on type of clinical service or provider setting (Joint Commission Quality Check 2015). See table 21.2 for a list of sources of publicly available quality indicator data.

Transparency in sharing quality data is increasingly important. Historically in healthcare when quality was not achieved and performance was unfavorable, there was a tendency to keep these facts concealed from the public. It is recognized by healthcare professionals, patients, and policy makers alike that in today's environment the public has the right to transparent data about healthcare providers and organizations so they are most informed in their roles as patients and consumers. Nearly all health professions are increasingly engaged in empowering patients toward more informed engagement in healthcare. Within the profession of health information management (HIM), for example, AHIMA has led efforts to inspire HIM professionals to engage in new professional endeavors related to assisting patients with access to and use of their own health information (AHIMA 2014b).

Value-Based Payment Reforms

Payment for healthcare services by third party payers has been based more on the quantity of services provided instead of the quality of care rendered. This model offers little incentive for improved quality and is an ineffective use of limited financial resources available to pay for health services. A variety of value-based payment models are currently being implemented or piloted.

Table 21.2. Sources of publicly available quality indicator data

Organization name	Organization website	Overview of quality indicator data provided
Centers for Medicare and Medicaid Services	www.medicare.gov/hospitalcompare www.medicare.gov/nursinghomecompare www.medicare.gov/homehealthcompare www.medicare.gov/physiciancompare	Quality data reported from a variety of healthcare settings to the Medicare program as required by law. Examples of quality data available for consumers to review includes readmission rates, infection rates, staff-to-patient ratios, and patient satisfaction scores.
The Leapfrog Group	www.leapfroggroup.org	Quality data submitted voluntarily from hospitals to the Leapfrog Group. Examples of data available includes details on the use of computerized medication ordering, presence of specialty trained ICU physicians, use of processes to avoid harm, managing errors when they occur, maternity care, high-risk surgeries, and hospital-acquired conditions.
Joint Commission	www.qualitycheck.org	Quality data collected by the Joint Commission from organizations accredited by them. Data include accreditation status and links to reports for each organization that illustrate their performance with accreditation standards.

Value-based payment methods intend to direct the basis for reimbursement toward methodologies focused on paying for quality in clinical care versus quantity. **Value-based payments** can be thought of as any method of healthcare reimbursement that either financially incentivizes providers for good quality and outcomes or those that penalize providers for inadequate quality and unfavorable outcomes. This new paradigm of reimbursement methods will continue to influence quality management efforts throughout healthcare. In an environment where payment is increasingly linked to the quality of care and not the quantity of care provided, healthcare organizations and providers must increasingly focus their efforts on enhanced quality and performance or else significant losses in revenue will occur. This paradigm shift in payment also challenges the current healthcare system to move toward an environment focused more on continuous follow-up and engagement with patients after they complete an episode of care to ensure their needs are met and their health is positively progressing.

The Patient as a Consumer

Patients today are increasingly more savvy consumers of healthcare. The Internet provides unfiltered access for a patient to compare providers and insurance plans, as well as research any healthcare topic for which they have an interest. As patients become more savvy consumers, the stakes are higher for healthcare providers and organizations to attract and retain patients. One way that healthcare providers and organizations can attract patients is to be known for excellence in clinical quality and patient safety. While accreditation was previously described as one way to become known for quality and safety, healthcare providers and organizations can also increase their community engagement activities and patient outreach efforts to maintain a good reputation. The patient of today is an important driver of why quality is managed in healthcare. Because the multitude of drivers and influences of clinical quality are growing, healthcare organizations must continually focus on quality management.

Check Your Understanding 21.1

Instructions: **Answer the following questions on a separate piece of paper.**

1. Which of the following is the term for "processes and steps involved in taking identified areas needing improvement and using actionable efforts to improve performance"?
   A. Quality
   B. Quality management
   C. Performance
   D. Performance improvement

2. The court case *Darling v. Charleston Community Memorial Hospital* is best known for which of the following in healthcare settings?
   A. Hospitals are legally liable when patients are injured by care processes during hospitalizations.
   B. Physicians are the only legally liable party when patients are injured by care processes during hospitalizations.
   C. Nursing staff are the only legally liable party when patients are injured by care processes during hospitalizations.
   D. None of the above are true about *Darling*.

3. The Conditions for Coverage and Conditions of Participation relate to which programs?
   A. Medicare
   B. Medicaid
   C. Military health services
   D. Both A and B are correct

4. Which of the following is true about the Leapfrog Group?
   A. They are affiliated with CMS
   B. Submitting data to the Leapfrog Group is voluntary
   C. Submitting data to the Leapfrog Group is mandatory
   D. Data submitted to the Leapfrog Group is not visible to the public

5. Value-based payments may be structured to do which of the following?
   A. Incentivize good performance
   B. Reimburse providers in full
   C. Penalize poor performance
   D. Both A and C are correct

Organizational Influence on Clinical Quality

Organizations are organic in that everything within an organization is interrelated; the sum of all its parts influences an organization as a whole, to include its successes or failures. One way to consider this is to imagine a hospital in which every employee might indicate on a survey that they are committed to safe and effective care. However, if all these employees work for an organization that does not truly embrace within its culture a commitment to quality, clinical quality will be difficult to achieve and quality management efforts will appear futile. An organization and all its members must wholeheartedly embrace quality and performance improvement throughout the enterprise for either to be meaningful undertakings. Organizational mission and vision, leadership, organizational culture, interprofessional education and practice, and change management, play a role in influencing quality and performance improvement.

Organizational Mission and Vision

The mission and vision of an organization represent more than words printed on a brochure or published on a website. The purpose of an organization and how it hopes to exist in the future are necessary areas of understanding for employees and providers within an organization. In the example of healthcare organizations, it is common that mission and vision statements indicate quality as a tenet to the organization's mission and vision. What is sometimes overlooked about mission and vision statements is that for them to have any meaning, what is stated in the mission and vision must be carried out daily within the organization and embraced by staff and providers in all levels and departments of the organization.

A **mission statement** is a written statement that defines an organization's general purpose for existing, whereas a **vision statement** refers to what an organization sees as its ideal future state. In essence, the mission describes the current existence of an organization while the vision articulates goals for the future existence of an organization.

An example of a mission and vision statement includes:

- *Mission*: Above all else, we are committed to the care and improvement of human life.
- *Vision*: Together, we will be the premier healthcare destination for all we serve. (Overland Park Regional Medical Center 2015)

Organizational mission and vision relate to quality in that they go beyond being statements advertised to the public. Instead, mission and vision are created based on the organizational goals, strategic initiatives, and organizational culture. In the previous example statements, the mission succinctly articulates that the organization commits itself to the care and improvement of human life and the vision articulates that the organization hopes to become a premier destination for patients to seek health services. If the mission and vision are carried out and pursued daily in all areas of a healthcare organization, quality is a much more tangible and achievable goal. While everyone within an organization must share in the commitment to quality, those in formal and informal leadership positions play essential roles in inspiring organizational commitment to quality.

Influence of Leadership

Leadership often occurs within organizations through two primary groups of leaders. These groups include those in formal management roles who are expected to provide leadership as well as everyday personnel who naturally exhibit leadership qualities and are regarded as leaders by their peers. For managers who are expected to provide leadership by virtue of their jobs, there are three sources of managerial influence in healthcare organizations. These three sources include those formally responsible for the overall governance of a healthcare organization (such as a board of directors), chief level officers and senior managers, and appointed leaders of medical staff or other licensed independent providers (Schyve 2009).

Managers in healthcare organizations have the authority and obligation to influence an organizational culture of quality and safety, plan for the needs of patients, make available necessary resources for patient care, staff the organization according to needs, and commit to ongoing performance improvement (Schyve 2009). Because the management infrastructure of hospitals and other types of healthcare organizations is uniquely complex, those individuals assigned to perform management functions are most effective when they possess leadership skills. Without effective leadership skills, managers likely find themselves unable to influence staff and provider commitment to quality.

As previously mentioned, there are also leaders who arise within organizations without a formal job title placing them in a leadership role. **Leadership** can be thought of as roles or functions that advance an organization toward meetings its goals. Anyone within an organization who enhances its effectiveness is playing a leadership role (Scholl 2003). Considering the aims of quality management and related performance improvement, it is evident why leadership from within a healthcare organization is also embraced. Healthcare professionals often relate well to their peers. Leadership among peers provides a respected avenue and basis to improve collaboration and efforts focused on improved clinical quality. See chapter 22 for more discussion regarding organizational leadership.

Organizational Culture

An organization's mission and vision, leadership influence, and human resources work in concert to inform the organizational culture. The culture of an organization may have many attributes and culture can change over time. **Organizational culture** is what is felt by staff on any given day that is intangible but greatly influences how an employee feels about their job and the environment in which they perform it. In relationship to quality in clinical care, the ability for staff to perform clinical duties with a focus on quality is in part dependent on working in an environment that is positive, supports goals of excellence, and promotes teamwork.

Interprofessional Education and Practice

Historically when healthcare professionals provided their services to patients in patient care settings, the various health professions worked in silos, meaning they worked in isolation from each other. While these types of challenges remain, there are efforts underway to reshape the ways by which health professionals work together and view each other's contributions to patient care. The Institute of Medicine was one of the first organizations to vocalize that having silos in place, which prevent connecting all the moving parts of clinical care, is unacceptable. Released in 2003, the report *Health Professions Education: A Bridge to Quality* called for changes to education in the health professions (IOM 2003). The premise of this publication centered on the need for enhanced opportunities for health professions students to receive education alongside their peers in other specializations as a means to promote teamwork; this approach to education also allows for those entering the healthcare workforce to better understand the various professions versus only possessing an understanding of one's own professional role (IOM 2003).

Collaboration and teamwork among the various health professions can positively influence clinical quality. For this reason, many accreditation bodies responsible for accrediting academic programs in the health professions now incorporate standards requiring interprofessional education into the curriculum. For example, standard 11 from the Accreditation Council for Pharmacy Education standards is titled "Interprofessional Education." It requires curriculum in pharmacy academic programs to prepare students "to provide entry-level, patient-centered care in a variety of practice settings as a contributing member of an interprofessional team. In the aggregate, team exposure includes prescribers as well as other healthcare professionals" (Accreditation Council for Pharmacy Education 2015). **Interprofessional education** occurs when two or more professions learn about, from, and with each other to enable effective collaboration to improve health outcomes" (WHO 2010).

A benefit to introducing interprofessional education to students is that students can in turn enter the workforce and influence it by implementing interprofessional practice into daily work. Without interprofessional teamwork, clinical quality is compromised in a variety of ways. If those working for the care of a patient do not understand how all the needs of the patient are met, this diminishes the ability to provide optimal care. Lacking teamwork also negatively influences communication among the variety of professionals who support and provide patient care. Organizations that promote teamwork and interprofessional practice are often noted to experience less staff turnover. More consistency among staff and reduced turnover leads to a team of professionals more comfortable with each other and familiar with internal processes in the care of patients. It was noted earlier that not all healthcare organizations have broken down professional silos to achieve interprofessionalism. These silos can be broken down and change management techniques offer approaches to do so.

Change Management

Change management is the formal process of introducing change, getting it adopted, and diffusing it throughout the organization (AHIMA 2014a). Effectively instituting change can be challenging, and some aspects of change management relate to psychology and behavior. Change presents potential challenges among staff because even if change is needed, moving forward with change can initiate feelings of insecurity, and performance among staff may decline (Naghibi and Baban 2011). In addition, discussing patient safety and quality versus moving the needle in terms of improving quality in patient care sometimes stalls in healthcare. However, evidence is mounting that this way of working must change. Increased expectations for the healthcare industry to improve quality, safety, and value exist from various influential stakeholders including state and federal governments, accreditation organizations, and third party payers. If an organization cannot improve quality and patient care, meeting the varied expectations previously noted leaves an organization at risk to lose funding or experience reduced reimbursement, as well as potentially lose its accredited status. See chapter 22 for techniques for managing change.

In some organizations, a culture embracing quality comes naturally. Other organizations may experience challenges in achieving a culture with a deeply embedded appreciation for quality due to limitations in leadership and staff morale. Regardless of the organization, to maintain an existing culture or initiate a new culture focused on quality, ongoing change management techniques may be useful.

Clinical Quality Management Tools and Processes

While an organization itself has influence on clinical quality, it is also important to appreciate the ongoing processes and mechanisms that support operational oversight of quality.

Ongoing Quality Measure Reviews

Within a healthcare organization, a variety of reviews occur daily to evaluate the quality of care provided to patients. Reviews of clinical care are often performed by reviewing a patient's health record and extracting necessary data to identify performance or nonperformance of established quality measures. Table 21.3 provides examples of data abstracted from patient records to identify clinical quality.

Data collected during reviews to measure quality are often based on the needs of the organization, the type of organization, as well as requirements from accreditation standards, regulatory requirements, or payer guidelines. For example, in table 21.3 the CMS quality measurement for catheter associated urinary tract infections was noted. If a patient has a catheter associated urinary tract infection (CAUTI), CMS will not reimburse a hospital for care and resources used to treat the infection because if the infection is catheter associated this suggests that care processes and catheter management were suboptima, leading to the infection.

Stakeholders to clinical quality such as the Agency for Healthcare Research and Quality, National Quality Forum, and Joint Commission support the use of "valid and reliable measures of quality and patient safety to improve healthcare" (Hughes 2008). As previously noted, a variety of factors indicate which quality measures will be evaluated by a healthcare organization. It is also important to understand that the widespread support from stakeholders regarding quality measures stems from the fact that these measures are established because they have been scientifically validated and are considered to be evidence-based approaches to quality.

Data collected for quality reviews are used by providers and organizations to conduct internal and external benchmarking. **Benchmarking** is "the systematic comparison of the products, services, and outcomes of one organization with those of a similar organization, or the systematic comparison of one organization's outcomes with regional or national standards" (AHIMA 2014a). There are two types of benchmarking—internal and external. **Internal benchmarking** is used "to identify best practices within an organization, to compare best practices within an organization, and to compare current practice over time" (Hughes 2008). An example of internal benchmarking would be to compare rates of hospital-acquired pressure ulcers per nursing unit within the same hospital. This type of comparison may yield valuable information for understanding which units are experiencing the fewest pressure ulcers as well as why their rates are low. From this, best practices to reduce instances of pressure ulcers can be identified and implemented throughout the hospital.

External benchmarking occurs when an organization uses "comparative data between organizations to judge performance and identify improvements

Table 21.3.   Examples of data abstracted from patient health records to identify clinical quality

Description of quality measure	Data abstracted from the health record to identify compliance
One CMS quality measure evaluates the rate at which heart attack patients are prescribed a statin at discharge.	Analysts may review documentation in the record such as the discharge medication reconciliation form, prescriptions, and discharge instructions.
One CMS quality measure evaluates if patients with urinary tract infections acquired the infection via a catheter during the hospitalization.	Analysts may review documentation in the health record such as consultation notes, discharge summaries, physician progress notes, or nursing progress notes to identify if the urinary tract infection was catheter associated

that have proven to be successful in other organizations" (Hughes 2008). Data available for external benchmarking are readily available in today's transparent healthcare environment through a variety of online dashboards. For example, hospitals must report data during billing to CMS to identify if patient diagnoses are hospital acquired. Hospitals might choose to compare their rates of hospital-acquired conditions with those from similar hospitals to identify how they are performing in comparison. These resources are often searchable and provide mechanisms for comparing performance among providers and organizations.

Quality Measure Review Findings

Quality management efforts require time, money, and human resources; and are comprehensive and ongoing. It is important that data attained through quality management activities are used in meaningful ways. If vast amounts of data are collected within an organization but nothing meaningful occurs related to the data, then the efforts seem fruitless. However, if the data can be used to better inform an organization on their performance, aid in the identification of areas for improvement, as well as provide a basis for action and improvement, more people within the organization will appreciate the efforts and buy in to the rationale for quality management activities.

One might consider the potential value of quality measure data through the lens of the hierarchical relationship between data, information, knowledge, and wisdom. Without data and information, knowledge cannot be generated within an organization to understand the current state of quality nor the wisdom to recognize necessary future efforts to improve it. Knowledge exists in two forms—explicit and tacit. **Explicit knowledge** includes "documents, databases, and other types of recorded and documented information"; and **tacit knowledge** is "the actions, experiences, ideals, values, and emotions of an individual that tend to be highly personal and difficult to communicate" (AHIMA 2014a). This hierarchy indicates the following:

- Data in crude format has little meaning (for example, raw facts stored as characters, symbols, measures, statistics)

- Information is the convergence of data with relevant and meaningful details (for example, processed data)

- Knowledge depicts that which is known based on available information (for example, information combined with experience and context)

- Wisdom is the ability to translate knowledge into informed actions, behaviors, and changes (for example, actionable and long-term application of knowledge) (Rowley 2007)

As healthcare organizations enhance their knowledge about internal successes and opportunities in the context of quality, long-term efforts to improve in necessary areas will occur from an informed perspective. The hierarchy from data to wisdom illustrated in figure 21.1 shows that the vast amounts of data collected and reported during quality measure review processes holds potential value that can transform a healthcare organization and improve quality and safety in patient care.

Plan-Do-Check-Act Cycle

A commonly used process in clinical quality management is the **plan-do-check-act (PDCA)** cycle. PDCA is also referred to as the plan-do-study-act (PDSA) cycle, the Deming Wheel, or the Deming Cycle. PDCA is an ongoing process entailing "a systematic series of steps for gaining valuable learning and knowledge for the continual improvement of a product or process" (W. Edwards Deming Institute 2015). Healthcare organizations frequently use the PDCA cycle within quality and performance improvement activities.

This four-step process is cyclical in nature and intended to be never-ending. See figure 21.2 for an illustration of this cyclical process. The basis for the PDCA cycle is that constant evaluation of activities and processes should occur to ensure quality and identify when change is necessary. The W. Edwards Deming Institute describes the PDCA cycle as follows:

> The cycle begins with the Plan step. This involves identifying a goal or purpose, formulating a theory, defining success metrics and putting a

Figure 21.1.   Hierarchy of data, information, knowledge, and wisdom

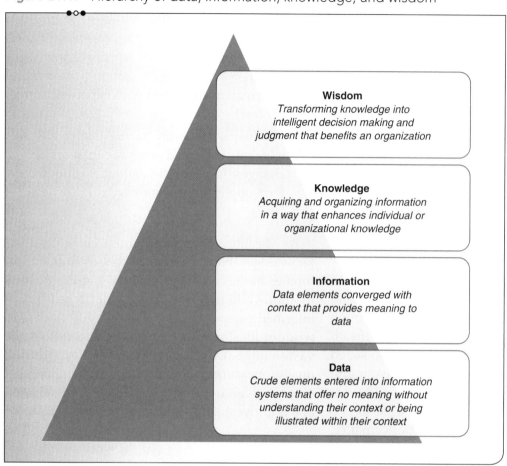

Wisdom
Transforming knowledge into intelligent decision making and judgment that benefits an organization

Knowledge
Acquiring and organizing information in a way that enhances individual or organizational knowledge

Information
Data elements converged with context that provides meaning to data

Data
Crude elements entered into information systems that offer no meaning without understanding their context or being illustrated within their context

Source: Rowley 2007.

Figure 21.2.   PDCA cycle

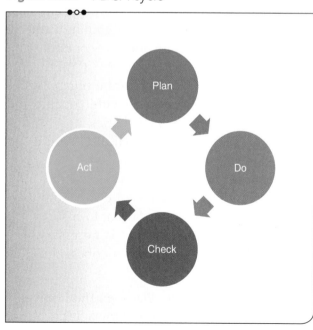

plan into action. These activities are followed by the Do step, in which the components of the plan are implemented, such as making a product. Next comes the Study step, where outcomes are monitored to test the validity of the plan for signs of progress and success, or problems and areas for improvement. The Act step closes the cycle, integrating the learning generated by the entire process, which can be used to adjust the goal, change methods, or even reformulate a theory altogether. These four steps are repeated over and over as part of a never-ending cycle of continual improvement. (2015)

An example is to use the PDCA cycle to reduce errors in clinical documentation. Assume a healthcare organization becomes concerned about the quality of its clinical documentation within the electronic health record (EHR). One particular area of concern is that documentation about the stage of pressure ulcers is often not sufficient, even if the documentation indicates the presence of a pressure ulcer on a patient. An interprofessional committee forms and determines that documentation must improve about pressure ulcer stages. To improve this documentation, the committee develops an educational activity that will be required of all nursing staff. The committee members provide the training session to all nursing staff. Two weeks after all nursing staff undergo the training, HIM analysts conduct retrospective chart reviews of records on patients with pressure ulcers. The chart review identifies that all but two nursing units have improved pressure ulcer staging documentation. The next step of action is to retrain the two nursing units still struggling with documentation. The PDCA cycle is:

- Plan—identify pressure ulcer documentation issues, form an interprofessional committee to evaluate the problem, and create a training program comprise the plan.
- Do—offer the required training session for all nursing staff
- Check—perform retrospective chart review to gauge documentation quality after training was provided
- Act—retrain two deficient nursing units

The PDCA cycle is used to comprehensively identify an issue, create and implement a plan of action, check to ensure the plan is working, and continue to improve.

Peer Review

While many quality management efforts, techniques, and tools focus on evaluating systematic processes, there are instances in which the actions and behaviors of clinical staff are evaluated. One example of a method to evaluate clinical staff is peer review. The first professional group in healthcare to grapple with the concept of peer review was physicians (Vyas and Hozain 2014). Medical peer review is

the process by which a professional review body considers whether a practitioner's clinical

privileges or membership in a professional society will be adversely affected by a physician's competence or professional conduct. The foremost objective of the medical peer review process is the promotion of the highest quality of medical care as well as patient safety. (AMA n.d.)

The Healthcare Quality Improvement Act of 1986 was the first federal legislation to address peer review. Medical malpractice lawsuits occurred at high rates during the 1970s and over time a growing concern emerged that physicians could move freely around the country and reestablish their practice with little question after having been found liable for injury, death, or other harm experienced by patients under their care. There were also concerns during this time that without legal protections in place for healthcare providers to participate in peer-review activities, physicians may be reluctant to evaluate their peers when doing so was necessary. The Healthcare Quality Improvement Act of 1986 is a federal law that established standards and requirements related to peer review among physicians. In the legislation, peer review is also referred to as professional review. When an incident has occurred and it is believed that peer review should occur, healthcare organizations must follow standards to ensure that any actions taken against the physician are appropriate and justifiable. This includes that the review is occurring to advance quality, includes reasonable efforts to obtain all relevant facts pertaining to the incident, the physician under review is given advance notice and is afforded a fair hearing, and that any actions taken are justified based on facts (Healthcare Quality Improvement Act 1986). An example of when peer review may be used is when a patient dies from a surgical complication. In this example, it may be determined by hospital policy that a team of peer physicians review the performance of the surgeon to ensure that standards of care were met.

The Healthcare Quality Improvement Act of 1986 also provides legal immunity to other physicians who participate in peer review activities; this helps ensure that competent physicians will willingly participate in review of their peers without the threat of legal implications when the review occurs in accordance with the law. This legislation also describes a variety of reporting requirements when malpractice occurs, other reportable actions occur, and/or payments are made related to malpractice. (Healthcare Quality Improvement Act 1986).

The **National Practitioner Data Bank (NPDB)** is "an information clearinghouse . . . to collect and release certain information related to the professional competence and conduct of physicians, dentists, and, in some cases, other healthcare practitioners" (HHS 2015). The NPDB was created due to requirements for its establishment per the Healthcare Quality Improvement Act of 1986. The NPDB is also now influenced by other federal laws such as the Medicare and Medicaid Patient and Program Protection Act of 1987 and the Health Insurance Portability and Accountability Act of 1996. Data reported to and stored in the NPDB includes provider-specific instances of medical malpractice and adverse events. For example, it is required that providers report the following events to the NPDB:

- Medical malpractice payments
- Federal and state licensure and certification actions
- Adverse clinical privileges actions
- Adverse professional society membership actions
- Negative actions or findings by private accreditation organizations and peer-review organizations
- Healthcare-related criminal convictions and civil judgments
- Exclusions from participation in a federal or state healthcare program
- Other adjudicated actions or decisions (HRSA n.d.(a))

The NPDB allows for eligible entities to report and query such information. Information about providers housed within the database is provided by or viewed by eligible entities including "medical malpractice payers, hospitals and other healthcare entities, professional societies, health plans, peer review organizations, private accreditation organizations, quality improvement organizations, and certain federal and state agencies . . . healthcare practitioners, entities, providers, and suppliers are authorized to query on themselves for information reported to the NPDB" (HHS 2015).

In settings such as hospitals, physicians undergo rigorous screenings before they are allowed to become members of the medical staff. **Medical staff** refers to physicians and other approved practitioners granted rights and responsibilities to admit patients into a healthcare facility for medical care. CMS provides required specifications that the medical staff must include members who are doctors of medicine and osteopathy, and may also include doctors of dental medicine or surgery, podiatric medicine, optometry, and chiropractic. Further, CMS indicates that if states grant certain privileges to other practitioners such as nurse practitioners or physicians, these professionals may be included in the medical staff infrastructure (CMS 2008).

If a physician or other practitioner hopes to join a hospital medical staff and are eligible to do so, they must undergo the credentialing process. **Credentialing** is a screening process to evaluate and validate a physician's qualifications for staff membership (AHIMA 2014a). One tool utilized extensively in the credentialing process is the NPDB. As described earlier, details included in the NPDB relate to a provider's historical performance related to quality of care, adverse issues, and medical malpractice, among other details. As hospitals and other healthcare facilities strive for a talented medical staff to provide the best possible care, the NPDB is an important tool in the credentialing process and medical staff management.

Tracer Methodology

Healthcare organizations often replicate accreditation surveyor processes to conduct internal evaluations of daily operations and clinical care to identify compliance with accreditation standards that by and large focus on quality and patient safety. Tracer methodology is one such example of a process used by surveyors who conduct on-site accreditation surveys for the Joint Commission that is replicated within a healthcare organization to evaluate performance. **Tracer methodology** is

> a process the Joint Commission surveyors use during the on-site survey to analyze an organization's systems, with particular attention to identified priority focus areas, by following individual patients through the organization's healthcare process in the sequence experienced by the patients; an evaluation that follows (traces) the hospital experiences of specific

patients to assess the quality of patient care; part of the new Joint Commission survey processes (Joint Commission 2014).

Healthcare organizations using tracer methodology, or as it is sometimes referred to as *tracers*, allow for peers within the organization to assess care processes, evaluate the environment of care, and conduct benchmarking with accreditation standards. The participation of staff from all units within an organization is particularly useful when conducting tracers. This type of interprofessional involvement best ensures that various professionals of differing expertise in healthcare can thoroughly evaluate the who, what, where, when, why, and how of clinical care, with the understanding that each professional provides a unique and valuable point of view.

Check Your Understanding 21.2

Instructions: **Answer the following questions on a separate piece of paper.**

1. Which of the following may be members of a medical staff?
   A. Registered nurses
   B. Physicians
   C. Chiropractors
   D. Both B and C are correct

2. Which of the following legislation was the first to address peer review?
   A. Emergency Medical Treatment and Active Labor Act
   B. Healthcare Quality Improvement Act
   C. Patient Protection and Affordable Care Act
   D. Health Information Technology for Economic and Clinical Health Act

3. Which of the following is used to evaluate and validate a physician's qualifications for staff membership?
   A. Credentialing process
   B. NPDB query
   C. Peer review
   D. PDCA cycle

4. Databases and records stored within an organization are examples of which of the following?
   A. Tacit knowledge
   B. Data, information, knowledge, wisdom hierarchy
   C. Explicit knowledge
   D. Knowledge management

5. Which of the following is reported to the National Practitioner Data Bank?

   A. Unfavorable patient satisfaction scores

   B. Medical malpractice incidents

   C. Adverse effects

   D. Both B and C are correct

Outcomes and Effectiveness Research in Healthcare

The major objective of **outcomes and effectiveness research (OER)** is to understand the end results (outcomes) of particular healthcare practices and interventions. Examples of patient outcomes include the ability to function, quality of life, satisfaction, and mortality. By linking the care that patients receive to the outcomes they experience, OER has helped to develop better ways to monitor and improve the quality of care.

Outcomes and Effectiveness Research Strategies

OER may be conducted at the community, system, institutional, or patient level. At the community level, outcomes research focuses on the population as a whole or on specific communities. For example, the *Dartmouth Atlas Report: Improving Patient Decision Making in Health Care* (2011) has found that the rate for mastectomy for early stage breast cancer in women over 65 in Victoria, Texas, was more than seven times higher than for women living in Muncie, Indiana.

OER at the system level refers to the healthcare system as a whole. It may include the entire country or a specific region. Examples of geographic variations in medical care at the national level cited by the *Dartmouth Atlas of Health Care* include the following:

- In Casper, Wyoming, the rate for back surgeries is 10.0 for every 1,000 Medicare recipients, more than six times higher than in Honolulu, Hawaii, where there are 1.7 surgeries for every 1,000 Medicare recipients.

- Heart patients in Albuquerque, New Mexico, receive carotid endarterectomies at a rate four times higher than in Roswell, New Mexico; a difference of about 200 miles away.

- Men in Wilmington, North Carolina, receive prostate-specific antigen (PSA) at a rate more than ten times higher than do men in Minot, North Dakota (Dartmouth Atlas 2011).

OER at the institutional level refers to the sites in which healthcare is delivered: hospitals, clinics, or health maintenance organizations (HMOs). An example outcome study performed at the institutional level is a review of health records and clinical data of patients with a principal diagnosis of acute myocardial infarction who expire during hospitalization. At the patient level, interest is on the interaction between one provider and one patient. An example is the ongoing assessment of patient satisfaction.

There is no standard method for conducting outcomes research at the institutional level or any level. Avedis Donabedian (1966) proposed the first model for evaluating patient outcomes. His model focused on measuring the structure, process, and outcomes of medical care. Structure is the setting in which the healthcare is provided and the resources available to provide it. Process is the extent to which professionals perform according to accepted standards. Process also is a set of activities that take place between providers. Outcomes include changes in the patient's condition, quality of life, and level of satisfaction. Other models used for the study of outcomes include the disease model and the health and wellness model. Epidemiological approaches are often used to study outcomes.

In the hospital setting, the health record often serves as the data source for outcomes studies.

Outcomes and Effectiveness Measures

Several types of measures are used in OER. Examples include clinical performance measures, patient perceptions of care and services, health status measures, and administrative and financial performance measures.

- *Clinical performance* measures are designed to evaluate the processes or outcomes of care associated with the delivery of clinical services. They allow for intra-organizational and interorganizational comparisons to be used to improve patient health outcomes. Clinical measures should be condition specific or procedure specific or should address important functions of patient care, such as medication use and infection control.

- *Patient perceptions of care and services* focus on the delivery of clinical services from a patient's perspective. Aspects of care that may be addressed are patient education, wait times, medication use, pain management, practitioner bedside manner, communication regarding current care and future plans for care, and improvement in health status.

- *Health status* measures address the functional well-being of specific populations, both in general and in relation to specific conditions. They indicate changes that have occurred in physical functioning, bodily pain, social functioning, and mental health over time.

- *Administrative and financial performance* measures address the organizational structure for coordinating and integrating service, functions, or activities across organizational components. Examples of administrative and financial measures are those related to financial stability, utilization, length of stay (LOS), and credentialing.

These types of measures range from the quality of care delivery to patient outcomes, including clinical, administrative, and financial performance.

Current Outcomes Movement

The current outcomes movement gained momentum in the 1980s when the prospective payment system (PPS) for Medicare inpatient care was implemented. The public and policymakers were concerned that Medicare patients were being forced out of hospitals. The fear was that patients were being discharged based on their LOS rather than when they were clinically ready for discharge. Medicare databases were promoted and used to monitor the quality of care through measurement of mortality rates, readmission rates, and other adverse outcomes.

Simultaneously, others were advancing the outcomes movement, which contained elements of research, measurement, and management. Other research efforts on geographic variations in medical practice, appropriateness of care, and the poor quality of medical evidence to support various interventions and treatments resulted in establishment of the Agency for Health Care Policy and Research (AHCPR) in 1989. The Healthcare Research and Quality Act of 1999 changed the agency's name to the **Agency for Healthcare Research and Quality (AHRQ)**. The mission of AHRQ is to support health services research designed to improve the outcomes and quality of healthcare, reduce its costs, address patient safety and medical errors, and broaden access to effective services. The research sponsored by AHRQ provides information that helps people make better decisions about healthcare. The goals and research priorities of AHRQ include

- Supporting improvement in health outcomes
- Strengthening quality measurement and improvement
- Identifying strategies to improve access, foster appropriate use, and reduce unnecessary expenditures (AHRQ 2015a)

A component of AHRQ is the AHRQ quality indicators (QIs) (AHRQ 2015a) QIs are measures that address various aspects of quality. The various types of QIs include the following:

- *Prevention QIs* identify hospital admissions that could have been avoided, at least in part, through high-quality outpatient care

- *Inpatient QIs* reflect quality of care inside hospitals, including inpatient mortality for medical conditions and surgical procedures. Four dimensions are used to assess inpatient quality: volume, mortality for inpatient procedures, mortality for inpatient conditions, and utilization indicators

- *Patient safety indicators* also reflect quality of care inside hospitals but focus on potentially avoidable complications and iatrogenic (caused by treatment) events. Patient safety indicators screen for problems that patients experience as a result of exposure to the healthcare system and that can be prevented by changes at the provider level or the area level. Provider-level indicators include only those cases where a secondary ICD diagnosis code flags a potentially preventable complication. Area-level indicators capture all cases of potentially preventable complications in a given area either during a hospitalization or resulting in subsequent hospitalization. Area-level indicators are identified by both principal and secondary ICD diagnosis codes

- *Pediatric quality indicators* use one or more of the other indicators listed previously and adapt them for use with children and neonates to reflect quality of care inside hospitals in different geographic areas across the United States to identify potentially avoidable hospitalizations (AHRQ 2015a)

Examples of AHRQ quality indicators appear in tables 21.4 through 21.6.

Table 21.4. AHRQ inpatient quality indicators

Type of indicator	Definition	Indicators
Volume	Indirect measure of quality based on evidence suggesting that hospitals performing more of certain intensive, high-technology, or highly complex procedures may have better outcomes for these procedures.	Esophageal resection volume Pancreatic resection volume Abdominal aortic aneurysm (AAA) repair volume Coronary artery bypass graft (CABG) volume Percutaneous transluminal coronary angioplasty (PTCA) volume Carotid endarterectomy (CEA) volume
Mortality Indicators for Inpatient Conditions	Conditions where mortality has been shown to vary substantially across institutions and where evidence suggests that high mortality may be associated with deficiencies in the quality of care.	Acute myocardial infarction (AMI) mortality rate Congestive heart failure mortality rate Acute stroke mortality rate Gastrointestinal hemorrhage mortality rate Hip fracture mortality rate Pneumonia mortality rate
Mortality Indicators for Inpatient Procedures	Procedures where mortality has been shown to vary substantially across institutions and where evidence suggests that high mortality may be associated with deficiencies in the quality of care.	Esophageal resection mortality rate Pancreatic resection mortality rate AAA repair mortality rate CABG mortality rate PTCA mortality rate CEA mortality rate Craniotomy mortality rate Hip replacement mortality rate
Utilization	Procedures whose use varies significantly across hospitals and for which questions have been raised about overuse, underuse, or misuse. High or low rates are likely to represent inappropriate or inefficient delivery of care.	Cesarean delivery rate Primary cesarean delivery rate Vaginal birth after cesarean (VBAC) rate VBAC rate, uncomplicated Laparoscopic cholecystectomy rate Incidental appendectomy in the elderly rate Bilateral cardiac catheterization rate

Source: AHRQ 2015b.

Table 21.5. AHRQ patient safety indicators

Indicator name
Death rate in low-mortality diagnosis-related groups (DRGs)
Pressure ulcer rate
Death rate among surgical inpatients with serious treatable complications
Foreign body left during procedure
Iatrogenic pneumothorax
Selected infections due to medical care
Postoperative hip fracture
Postoperative infection or hematoma
Postoperative physiologic and metabolic derangements
Postoperative respiratory failure
Postoperative pulmonary embolism or deep vein thrombosis
Postoperative sepsis
Postoperative wound dehiscence
Accidental puncture or laceration
Transfusion reaction
Birth trauma—injury to neonate
Obstetric trauma—vaginal with instrument
Obstetric trauma—vaginal without instrument
Obstetric trauma—cesarean delivery
Obstetric trauma with 3rd-degree lacerations—vaginal with instrument
Obstetric trauma with 3rd-degree lacerations—vaginal without instrument
Obstetric trauma with 3rd-degree lacerations—cesarean delivery

Source: AHRQ 2015c.

Table 21.6. AHRQ prevention quality indicators

Indicator name
Diabetes short-term and long-term complication admission rate
Perforated appendix admission rate
Chronic obstructive pulmonary disease (COPD) or Asthma in Older Adults admission rate
Hypertension admission rate
Congestive heart failure (CHF) admission rate
Dehydration admission rate
Bacterial pneumonia admission rate
Urinary tract infection admission rate
Angina without procedure admission rate
Uncontrolled diabetes admission rate
Asthma in younger adult admission rate
Rate of lower-extremity amputation among patients with diabetes

Source: AHRQ 2015d.

An analytical tool that AHRQ supports is the **Healthcare Cost and Utilization Project (HCUP)**. The HCUP database, called HCUPnet, is an online query system that gives instant access to the largest set of all payer healthcare databases that are publicly available (AHRQ 2012). It contains web-based tools that can be used to identify, track, analyze, and compare trends in hospital care at the national, regional, and state levels. HCUP data are used for research on hospital utilization, access, charges, quality, and outcomes. This database can be queried for information when doing internal assessments related to the AHRQ QIs.

Check Your Understanding 21.3

1. What are some examples of patient outcomes?
2. What is the mission of the Agency for Healthcare Research and Quality (AHRQ)?
3. Who sponsors the Health Care Utilization Project (HCUP)? What is the purpose of its database?
4. What types of performance measures were part of the first model for evaluating patient outcomes?
5. Describe four types of AHRQ quality indicators.

Systematic and Process-Driven Focus to Improve Performance

While it is important to appreciate quality management approaches and techniques, it is equally as valuable to examine concepts related to supporting improved performance in patient care. The IOM report, *To Err is Human*, was groundbreaking in many ways. Among the ways this publication reshaped thinking about safe patient care was that it was the first time that an acknowledgment was made that lackluster processes compromise clinical quality as much if not more so than individual errors. The following sections describe approaches and processes used in healthcare to support quality and improve performance.

Evidence-Based Care and Treatment

The expansive growth in clinical research and scientific discovery in the health sciences has benefited patient care in a number of ways. Among the ways that healthcare has benefited from information garnered through the application of the scientific method in clinical endeavors is the acquired appreciation that certain approaches, methods, protocols, and treatments have been proven to produce the best results for patients. The care and treatment of patients based on proven approaches is considered evidence-based practice.

Evidence-based practice is the application of "the best available research results (evidence) when making decisions about healthcare" (AHRQ n.d.(a)). The ability of healthcare professionals to locate and apply evidence in patient care requires them to possess knowledge and skills related to information appraisal and research. Because of early concerns that evidence-based medicine thwarted physician autonomy, some providers opposed the concept and suggested it was an unfavorable approach because it negated the role of physician judgment in patient care (Gerber and Lauterbach 2005). However, increased knowledge and understanding has led to widespread support for evidence-based practice because it not only provides a more proven basis for

clinical judgments among providers, but also relies on provider expertise and patient engagement in care decisions. Some evidence-based practice protocols are illustrated in CMS quality measures. The following are a few examples of evidence-based care that are also CMS quality measures:

- Patients should undergo percutaneous coronary intervention (PCI) within 90 minutes of arriving to a hospital when they have had a heart attack
- Patients with pneumonia should be given oxygenation assessment
- Patients undergoing surgery should receive appropriate antibiotics within one hour before surgery to prevent infection (CMS 2009)

Clinical Pathways

Clinical pathways, also sometimes referred to as critical pathways, are "structured multidisciplinary care plans, which detail essential steps in the care of patients with a specific clinical problem" (Rotter et al. 2010). Evidence-based practice relates to clinical pathways in that clinical pathways are informed by evidence-based approaches in the care and treatment of patients. For example, colorectal cancer screening is largely informed by evidence-based practice guidelines and clinical pathways have been published to address care processes related to colorectal screenings. One step of the clinical pathways for colorectal cancer screening is to identify if a patient meets the screening criteria based on evidence-based guidelines. From there, the clinical pathway includes two steps:

1. Provide documentation of the evidence-based guidelines for colorectal cancer screening to the patient and provide information about assessing colorectal cancer risk; and

2. Consider performing a health literacy screening on the patient to ensure that they understand the material provided and the implications of their decision to undergo the screening (HRSA n.d.(b)).

The use of clinical pathways in patients has been shown to reduce readmissions, improve outcomes, as well as support consistency in clinical care (Haddad 2010).

Clinical pathways expand the concept of a care plan because the pathway is established with the intent that the care plan accounts for the needs of the patient as well as promotes the interdependent nature of the health professions to achieve more cohesive patient care. Clinical pathways and their relationship to evidence-based practice illustrate the changing landscape in healthcare in which efforts to facilitate patient care are enhanced by scientific discovery, collaboration, and communication.

Case Management

Another example of a process-driven concept in healthcare that benefits patients and improves performance in clinical care is case management. Case management refers to the "collaborative process of assessment, planning, facilitation, care coordination, evaluation, and advocacy for options and services to meet an individual's and family's comprehensive health needs through communication and available resources to promote quality, cost-effective outcomes" (Case Management Society of America n.d.). The unique needs of each individual patient must be accounted for to maximize outcomes—both during an episode of care as well as afterward. The complex nature of the US healthcare system poses significant challenges to patients and families when they are faced with navigating it after a complex acute illness. For example, research has shown in recent years that patients with chronic health conditions less frequently see a primary care provider, even though research has also suggested that primary care management of chronic conditions optimizes continuity of care for patients with chronic conditions (Ladapo and Chokshi 2014). However, seeking primary care services and maintaining a patient–provider relationship in a primary care setting can be complicated by a variety of factors such as inadequate access to care in rural or underserved locations, lack of health insurance coverage, or changes to health insurance plans. Fragmentation in American healthcare is not necessarily decreasing. New opportunities offering convenience to patients such as immediate care services via clinics at pharmacies and other retail locations, as well as virtual e-visits via apps and websites are increasingly utilized and offer many benefits. Considering how these new models of care fit into care continuity is a worthy consideration (Ladapo and Chokshi 2014). Because the system itself is not intuitive to navigate, patients discharged from healthcare facilities find themselves at risk when follow-up care, ongoing services, and medication management are necessary.

Case management offers a solution to help ensure that the needs of patients are met during a hospitalization or other care episode as well as after they are discharged from a healthcare setting. Often healthcare organizations, such as hospitals, psychiatric hospitals, and long-term care facilities, staff a team of case managers. The case managers are assigned to a patient during their stay, remain with the patient during their care to ensure their medical and psychosocial needs are more appropriately being met, and assist in facilitation of ongoing needs after discharge. Without these types of coordinated efforts, patients are more likely at risk for readmission, poor medication management, or not receiving necessary ongoing care. It is also noteworthy that case management is becoming more common in ambulatory healthcare settings as primary care settings begin to embrace patient-centered medical home models of care, where a significant number of patients are managed for chronic conditions on a continuous basis (AHRQ n.d.(c)).

Care Coordination

Care coordination is reflected in clinical pathways as well as case management. In addition, healthcare providers engage in care coordination in the scope of ongoing management of a patient. Care coordination is the act of "organizing patient care activities and sharing information among all of the participants concerned with a patient's care to achieve safer and more effective care" (AHRQ 2015e).

Care coordination is necessary to ensure that a patient is provided care at the appropriate level, as well as to ensure that care is coordinated in thoughtful and proactive ways. Care coordination reflects an opportunity to provide healthcare services in a way that is proactive versus reactive in nature, for example care coordination relies on better communication among health professionals as well as early identification of a patient's current and future healthcare needs. If care is coordinated more effectively, this reduces oversights that could pose risks to the patient.

Effective Deployment and Use of Information Technology

Effective implementation and use of electronic health records (EHRs) and other health information systems provide mechanisms embedded within the systems to support improved patient care. Some functionalities in EHRs and other health information systems include visual and audio alerts when a patient has a known drug allergy, visual and audio alerts when a patient has a do-not-resuscitate order, as well as mechanisms to identify when ordered medications may be contraindicated by existing medications taken by a patient. Varieties of evidence-based guidelines are available as references as well as

set up to produce reminders and alerts within EHRs and health information systems. The ability for healthcare providers to have these resources available at their fingertips while they are already documenting in and reviewing a patient's health record is beneficial. Immediate and easy access to current evidence in the care and treatment of patients assists in creating a more appropriate plan of care.

Health information technology systems also support clinical pathways, case management, and care coordination. Clinical pathways rely on interprofessional and multidisciplinary collaboration based on evidence to maximize patient outcomes. Case management requires the appreciation for social and cultural needs of a patient, as well as a comprehensive understanding of their emotional and physical health status and future needs. Care coordination occurs when decisions related to ongoing or next levels of care are made proactively and timely. When functionalities of EHRs and other clinical information systems are continually optimized and used to their fullest potential with a focus on thorough documentation and effective information sharing, there is a potential for care coordination to improve because decisions regarding care can be based on meaningful real-time information.

Professional Designations and Roles in Healthcare Quality

It is important for emerging professionals to familiarize themselves with credentials and roles related to all areas of professional specialization within healthcare, including those related to quality management. Upon entering the workforce, many in HIM perform work that overlaps with organizational quality management efforts, serve on organizational quality-related committees, and sometimes even choose to work in a quality management role. Therefore, understanding credentials, roles, and functions of quality management are important for effective workforce preparation. Appreciating the variety of designations related to quality management is important for navigating one's career as well as working in the interprofessional environment of healthcare.

Certifications Related to Quality Management

Some professionals who work in quality management roles may choose to or are required to obtain certifications related to their work.

Certified Professional in Healthcare Quality (CPHQ)

The Certified Professional in Healthcare Quality (CPHQ) is a common designation obtained by those with experience in healthcare quality. The CPHQ is a certification exam offered by the National Association for Healthcare Quality. A **quality professional** is one who possesses a variety of knowledge and skills including those related to data analytics and information management, quality and performance improvement, leadership, and patient safety and risk management (NAHQ n.d.(a)). Any healthcare professional is eligible to take the CPHQ, although the National Association for Healthcare Quality indicates that possessing at least two years of experience in healthcare quality is a general rule of thumb for identifying readiness to take the CPHQ and also notes that the CPHQ is not an entry-level certification exam (NAHQ 2015b).

Certification in Health Care Quality and Management

The certification in Health Care Quality and Management (HCQM) is another certification option for health professionals working in roles related to quality. The HCQM is offered by the American Board of Quality Assurance and Utilization Review Physicians. This certification option focuses on the typical tenants of quality management; it also allows for those obtaining the certification to optionally complete subspecialty certifications in categories such as physician advisor, transitions of care, managed care, patient safety and risk management, case management, or workers' compensation (American Board of Quality Assurance and Utilization Review Physicians n.d.).

Certified Professional in Healthcare Risk Management

Those employed in risk management roles in healthcare work with issues related to healthcare quality each day. Among the duties of risk managers are evaluating instances of potential or actual medical errors and other patient safety issues that produce risk to a healthcare organization. Those working in risk management may also be certified as a Certified Professional in Healthcare

Risk Management (CPHRM). The CPHRM is administered by the American Hospital Association's Certification Center. Two eligibility pathways to the CPHRM certification exam exist. One is based on education and healthcare experience with the other solely based on risk management experience.

Health Information Managers

Health information managers credentialed as Registered Health Information Administrators (RHIAs) or Registered Health Information Technicians (RHITs) who are working in quality management and related roles find value in adding the CPHQ, HCQM, and/or CPHRM credentials to their resume. Because so many functions and roles related to quality management rely on professionals understanding healthcare data, care processes, and data science, health information managers are uniquely equipped to work in roles related to quality management.

The Health Information Manager Role in Clinical Quality

The ability to effectively evaluate the quality of care provided to patients and measure performance related to quality indicators hinges on documentation in health records as well as astutely skilled professionals who understand healthcare data and information science. The health record and documentation therein is considered the keeper of truth in recording care provided to patients. Health information managers possess a unique understanding and insight into diminished quality in documentation and how that relates to various uses of data. For these reasons, many health information professionals pursue careers in and around quality management.

Some with health information backgrounds fill positions in departments of healthcare organizations in positions ranging from a data analyst to a manager in departments such as quality management or quality improvement, performance improvement, or risk management. Others with health information expertise may choose to apply their understanding of quality management to roles related to the quality assurance of functions performed in health information management and information technology departments. Regardless of the way a health information manager applies their knowledge and skills to quality functions, they possess several underlying areas of expertise that are highly valued in healthcare and applicable to quality management.

Data Stewardship and Information Governance

As electronic health records emerge, data stewardship and information governance are increasingly important. Data stewardship and information governance are strategic concepts in the management of health information. **Health data stewardship** pertains to responsibilities that best ensure appropriate use of health data (NCVHS 2009). The concept of data stewardship in healthcare relates to information governance. **Information governance** is an "organizational-wide framework for managing information throughout its life cycle and supporting the organization's strategy, operations, regulatory, legal, risk, and environmental requirements" (AHIMA 2014c). See chapter 3 for more detail.

In the electronic data environment of healthcare today, governance of all information generated is necessary to improve the quality and safety of patient care, enhance population health, increase efficiencies in operations, as well as to reduce and mitigate risk and loss to the enterprise (AHIMA 2014c). Effective data stewardship and information governance are necessary to maximize the value of health information available in health records used to evaluate and measure quality of care. Without a robust framework focused on the quality, usability, and availability of healthcare data and information, evaluation of clinical care through data analysis is challenging and limits the potential for knowledge generation.

Data Analytics

The increasing volume of data created each day in healthcare provides opportunities to better understand quality of care, clinical outcomes, and performance related to meeting quality standards and metrics. As end users grapple with technologies such as electronic health records and other information systems, there are growing expectations that meaningful data can be garnered from these systems.

While health information managers working in quality management roles historically have focused much of their efforts extracting data from health records to help identify performance in meeting quality measures, health information managers today and in the future will also assume roles performing data analytics. In relationship to measuring quality and evaluating performance in clinical care, data analytics affords opportunities to statistically examine large amounts of data to identify trends, opportunities, and probabilities in the care of patients.

Application of data analytics to measure quality and performance offers great potential to strategically assess and improve all aspects of care delivery. Effective data analytics only occurs when those performing the analysis fully comprehend the complexity, limitations, meaning, and uses of healthcare data. To this end, the health information manager has the necessarily skills and knowledge to lead in the era of big data. See chapter 17 for more details.

Regulatory Compliance

Another area in which health information managers provide expertise to quality management relates to providing leadership in regulatory compliance efforts. Within a healthcare organization, there is a need for professionals who can understand sources of regulation, interpret regulation, and operationalize compliance with regulations.

This chapter described the regulatory environment in healthcare by which all regulations fully or partially focus on improving quality, which in turn influences quality management efforts. Often these types of regulations require that specific measurements of quality are conducted or that new quality management efforts are initiated in healthcare settings. Health information management professionals possess knowledge and skills related to health information and its regulated uses, and also have backgrounds in quality management; these complimentary domains afford health information professionals many opportunities to provide leadership in quality programs and processes to best ensure regulatory compliance.

Emerging Trends Impacting Industry Conversations about Clinical Quality

There are many emerging trends in healthcare and noting them in their entirety is not possible. However, several emerging concepts in health service delivery are increasingly relevant to the topics of clinical quality, quality management, and performance improvement.

Reputation, Brand Image, and Social Media

Social media is revolutionizing all aspects of society. The influence of social media on healthcare organizations is evidenced by information sharing in these mediums by patients about their experiences, to include providing ratings about satisfaction with health services, and healthcare is not immune from the transparent and accessible nature of immediate information that becomes viral by virtue of a "share" or "tweet." An initial hurdle that healthcare organizations faced at the advent of social media was deciding when to create accounts on social networking sites to engage patients and consumers. The challenge primarily existed because of concerns about how to compliantly interact with patients and consumers through a medium that was considered uncharted territory and do so in a way that avoided non-compliance with laws such as HIPAA.

Today, many healthcare organizations and providers are active on social media. Even if a healthcare organization or provider chooses to not have a social media presence, the reality is that the general public is very active on social media. Social media provides immediate information sharing to include instances in which patients are either satisfied or dissatisfied with care they have received. To this end, continually improving quality and safety in patient care is not only an ethical imperative, it is also necessary to maintain good relations and ratings among patients and consumers. Because

patients and consumers have immediate access via social networks to rate an organization, comment on an organization, or recommend an organization, healthcare organizations and providers are given yet another reason to enhance quality and performance improvement efforts to become a first-choice destination for patient care.

Increased Utilization of Telehealth Services

The Internet, apps, and smart devices are also revolutionizing patient care. **Telehealth** is the use of electronic information and telecommunications technologies to support long-distance clinical healthcare, patient and professional health-related education, public health, and health administration. Technologies include videoconferencing, the Internet, store-and-forward imaging, streaming media, and terrestrial and wireless communications (Health Resources and Services Administration n.d.). Not only are healthcare organizations and providers offering increased services through virtual consultations via telehealth mediums, a variety of medical startup organizations are also providing primary care consultations via app-based solutions.

Telehealth provides convenience to patients and expands access to health services. An emerging concern about telehealth pertains to how quality management will apply to virtually provided healthcare, particularly in instances when the care is ad hoc and offered as a one-time patient–provider exchange via an app and webcam. As telehealth emerges as an approach to expanding access to care, organizations offering these services must consider a variety of factors related to quality management such as:

- What processes are used to identify appropriate physician partners from remote locations to offer clinical services via telehealth?

- Are health services beyond traditional medical care of use to patients such as consultations from physical, occupational, and audiology therapists?
- How are telehealth services documented and how are health records managed?
- Will patient satisfaction be measured for patients seen in telehealth settings?
- How does telehealth affect care continuity?

Reimbursement for telehealth services is expanding, which is another indicator that telehealth consumption will increase. The future of measuring clinical quality in this environment provides opportunities and challenges, and emerging leaders in healthcare must consider how they will contribute to advancing goals of safe and effective care in these settings. Refer to chapters 12 and 14 for more information regarding telehealth.

The Learning Health System

The concept of embracing and initiating a learning health system in the United States is a popular topic with widespread support by healthcare stakeholders. Achieving quality in patient care remains a struggle in American healthcare, despite what is known about quality and safety and its implications (IOM 2013; 2003; 2001). Published in 2013, the Institute of Medicine brought a new focus to how increased quality and lowered costs could be achieved by sharing their findings after examining this topic in a publication titled *Best Care at Lower Cost: The Path to Continuously Learning Health Care in America.*

In today's healthcare system, the very best care actually is possible and it is attainable at a lower cost (IOM 2013). Despite the fact these things are possible, they too often remain unachieved. It is noted that "the foundation for a learning healthcare system is continuous knowledge development, improvement, and application . . . although unprecedented levels of information are available, patients and clinicians often lack access to guidance that is relevant, timely, and useful for the circumstances at hand" (IOM 2013). Relevant to the practice of HIM, it is noteworthy that the concept of the learning health system relies in large part on smart and effective use of information to inform individual episodes of care as well as overarching efforts to improve health services delivery to large populations.

A learning health system approach suggests that continuous efforts to learn from available evidence and information and to apply such learning for positive changes are the pathway to improved quality, safety, and equity in healthcare. As this approach continues to gain traction throughout healthcare, the road ahead entails an emphasis on quality.

The healthcare ecosystem is rapidly changing. All indications suggest that clinical quality management and performance improvement will continue to be embedded in all that is done throughout healthcare. As healthcare changes and more patients access health services through a variety of avenues, emerging professionals must be prepared to identify new and innovative approaches to improving the quality of care provided to patients.

Check Your Understanding 21.4

Instructions: **Answer the following questions on a separate piece of paper.**

1. Which of the following terms can be defined as: "occurs when two or more professions learn about, from, and with each other to enable effective collaboration to improve health outcomes"?
   A. Interprofessional education
   B. Collaborative practice
   C. Medical staff credentialing
   D. Interprofessional collaborative practice

2. A nursing home compares fall rates among five of its nursing units. This is an example of which of the following?

   A. External benchmarking

   B. Accreditation

   C. Internal benchmarking

   D. Interprofessional education

3. Which of the following is true about the PDCA cycle?

   A. It is cyclical

   B. It is continual

   C. It is used in crisis situations

   D. Both A and B are correct

4. The concept of tracer methodology was created by which organization?

   A. CMS

   B. Joint Commission

   C. AHIMA

   D. IOM

5. The CPHQ certification exam is offered by which organization?

   A. American Board of Quality Assurance and Utilization Review Physicians

   B. American Hospital Association

   C. National Association for Healthcare Quality

   D. Joint Commission

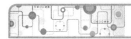 # References

Accreditation Association for Ambulatory Health Care. 2015. A History of the AAAHC. http://www.aaahc.org/about/history/

Accreditation Council for Pharmacy Education. 2015. Accreditation Standards and Key Elements for the Professional Program in Pharmacy Leading to the Doctor of Pharmacy Degree. Chicago: ACPE. https://www.acpe-accredit.org/pdf/Standards2016FINAL.pdf

Agency for Healthcare Research and Quality. 2015a. AHRQ quality indicators. http://www.qualityindicators.ahrq.gov/

Agency for Healthcare Research and Quality. 2015b. *AHRQ Quality Indicators—Inpatient Quality Indicators:* Revision 5.0 AHRQ Pub. No. HHSA290201200001C . Rockville, MD: AHRQ. http://www.qualityindicators.ahrq.gov/Downloads/Modules/IQI/V50/Version_50_Benchmark_Tables_IQI.pdf

Agency for Healthcare Research and Quality. 2015c. *AHRQ Quality Indicators—Patient Safety Quality Indicators:* Revision 5.0 Benchmark Data Tables AHRQ Pub. No. HHSA290201200001C. Rockville, MD: AHRQ. http://www.qualityindicators.ahrq.gov/Downloads/Modules/PSI/V50/Version_50_Benchmark_Tables_PSI.pdf

Agency for Healthcare Research and Quality. 2015d. *AHRQ Quality Indicators—Prevention Quality Indicators:Benchmark Data Tables.* Revision 5.0. AHRQ No. HHSA290201200001C. Rockville, MD: AHRQ. http://www.qualityindicators.ahrq.gov/Downloads/Modules/PQI/V50/Version_50_Benchmark_Tables_PQI.pdf

Agency for Healthcare Research and Quality 2015e. Care Coordination. http://www.ahrq.gov/professionals/prevention-chronic-care/improve/coordination/

Agency for Healthcare Research and Quality. 2012. *HCUPnet, Healthcare Cost and Utilization Project.* Rockville, MD: AHRQ.

Agency for Healthcare Research and Quality. n.d(a). Evidence-Based Practice. http://effectivehealthcare.ahrq.gov/index.cfm/glossary-of-terms/?termid=24&pageaction=showterm

Agency for Healthcare Research and Quality. n.d(b). National Guideline Clearinghouse. http://www.guideline.gov/

Agency for Healthcare Research and Quality. n.d(c). Patient-Centered Medical Home Resource Center. https://pcmh.ahrq.gov/

Alexander, J.W. 1985. The contributions of infection control to a century of surgical progress. *Annals of Surgery* 201(4). http://www.ncbi.nlm.nih.gov/pmc/articles/PMC1250728/pdf/annsurg00110-0033.pdf

American Board of Quality Assurance and Utilization Review Physicians. n.d. Overview of the HCQM Certification. http://www.abqaurp.org/ABQMain/Certification/Overview_of_HCQM_Certification/ABQMain/Certification.aspx?hkey=b6edc3b2-6da9-49d0-a824-3399badf629e

American College of Radiology. n.d. Accreditation. http://www.acr.org/Quality-Safety/Accreditation

American Health Information Management Association. 2014a. *Pocket Glossary of Health Information Management and Technology*, 4th ed. Chicago: AHIMA.

American Health Information Management Association. 2014b. Enabling consumer and patient engagement with health information. *Journal of AHIMA* 88(2).

American Health Information Management Association. 2014c. Information governance offers a strategic approach for healthcare. *Journal of AHIMA* 85(10).

American Hospital Association. n.d. The Patient Care Partnership. http://www.aha.org/advocacy-issues/communicatingpts/pt-care-partnership.shtml

American Medical Association. n.d. Medical Peer Review. http://www.ama-assn.org/ama/pub/physician-resources/legal-topics/medical-peer-review.page

Best, M. and D. Neuhauser. 2004. Heroes and martyrs of quality and safety: Ignaz Semmelweis and the birth of infection control. *BMJ Quality and Safety* 13:233–234. http://qualitysafety.bmj.com/content/13/3/233.full

Bowling, A, G. Rowe, N. Lambert, M. Waddington, K.R. Mahtani, C. Kenten, A. Howe, and S.A. Francis. 2012. The measurement of patients' expectations for health care: A review and psychometric testing of a measure of patients' expectations. *Health Technology Assessment* 16(30). http://www.ncbi.nlm.nih.gov/pubmed/22747798

Carroll College. 1992. A Patient's Bill of Rights. http://www.carroll.edu/msmillie/bioethics/patbillofrights.htm

Case Management Society of America. n.d. What is a Case Manager? http://www.cmsa.org/Home/CMSA/WhatisaCaseManager/tabid/224/Default.aspx

Centers for Medicare and Medicaid Services. 2015a. Clinical laboratory improvement amendments (CLIA). https://www.cms.gov/Regulations-and-Guidance/Legislation/CLIA/index.html?redirect=/clia/

Centers for Medicare and Medicaid Services. 2015b. Hospital Compare. https://www.cms.gov/medicare/quality-initiatives-patient-assessment-instruments/hospitalqualityinits/hospitalcompare.html

Centers for Medicare and Medicaid Services. 2013. Conditions for Coverage and Conditions of Participation. http://www.cms.gov/Regulations-and-Guidance/Legislation/CFCsAndCoPs/index.html

Centers for Medicare and Medicaid Services. 2012. Emergency Medical Treatment and Active Labor Act (EMTALA). https://www.cms.gov/Regulations-and-Guidance/Legislation/EMTALA/

Centers for Medicare and Medicaid Services. 2009. National Summary Statistics for RHQDAPU Clinical Process Measures as Reported on Hospital Compare March 2009. https://www.cms.gov/Medicare/Quality-Initiatives-Patient-Assessment-Instruments/HospitalQualityInits/Downloads/HospitalNationalLevelPerformance.pdf

Centers for Medicare and Medicaid Services. 2008. CMS Manual System. Pub. 100-07 State Operations. Provider Certification. https://www.cms.gov/Regulations-and-Guidance/Guidance/Transmittals/downloads/R37SOMA.pdf

Commission on Accreditation of Rehabilitation Facilities. 2015. Accreditation. http://www.carf.org/Accreditation/

Darling v. Charleston Community Memorial Hospital, 33 Ill.2d 626, 211 N.E. 2d, 253 (1965).

Dartmouth Medical School Center for the Evaluative Clinical Sciences. 2011. *Dartmouth Atlas of Health Care*. Hanover, NH: CECS. http://www.dartmouthatlas.org.

Donabedian, A. 1966. Evaluating the quality of medical care. *Milbank Memorial Fund Quarterly: Health and Society* 44(3):166–203.

Fahrenholz, C.G. 2013. Purpose of health record documentation. Introduction in *Documentation for Health Records*. Edited by C.G. Fahrenholz and R. Russo. Chicago: AHIMA.

Gerber, A. and K. Lauterbach. 2005. Evidence-based medicine: Why do opponents and proponents use the same arguments? *Health Care Analysis* 31(1).

Haddad, S. 2010. Clinical Pathways: Effects on Professional Practice, Patient Outcomes, Length of Stay and Hospital Costs. World Health Organization Reproductive Health Library. http://apps.who.int/rhl/effective_practice_and_organizing_care/cd006632_haddadsm_com/en/

Haskell, H. 2014 (June). Patient Advocacy in Patient Safety: Have Things Changed? *Perspectives on Safety*. http://webmm.ahrq.gov/perspective. aspx?perspectiveID=160

Health Resources and Services Administration. n.d.(a). NPDB e-Guidebook. http://www.npdb.hrsa.gov/resources/aboutGuidebooks.jsp

Health Resources and Services Administration. n.d.(b), Critical Pathway: Colorectal Cancer Screening—Appendix with Supporting Tools. http://www.hrsa.gov/quality/toolbox/measures/colorectalcancer/colorectalpathwayappendix.html

Health Resources and Services Administration. n.d.(c). Telehealth. http://www.hrsa.gov/ruralhealth/about/telehealth/

Healthcare Quality Improvement Act of 1986. Public Law 99-660.

Hughes, R.G. 2008. Tools and strategies for quality improvement and patient safety. Chapter 44 in *Patient Safety and Quality: An Evidence-Based Handbook for Nurses*. Edited by R.G. Hughes. Rockville: Agency for Healthcare Research and Quality. http://www.ncbi.nlm.nih.gov/books/NBK2682/

Institute for Healthcare Improvement. 2015a. Focus Areas. http://www.ihi.org/Pages/default.aspx

Institute for Healthcare Improvement. 2015b. Triple Aim. http://www.ihi.org/Topics/TripleAim/Pages/default.aspx

Institute of Medicine. 2013. *Better Care at Lower Cost: The Path to Continuously Learning Health Care in America*. Washington, DC: National Academies Press.

Institute of Medicine. 2003. *Health Professions Education: A Bridge to Quality*. Washington, DC: National Academies Press.

Institute of Medicine. 2001. *Crossing the Quality Chasm: A New Health System for the 21st Century*. Committee on Quality of Health Care in America. Washington, DC: National Academies Press.

Joint Commission. 2015. About the Joint Commission. http://www.jointcommission.org/about_us/about_the_joint_commission_main.aspx

Joint Commission Quality Check. 2015. Find a Healthcare Organization. http://www.qualitycheck.org/consumer/searchQCR.aspx

Joint Commission. 2014. Facts About the Tracer Methodology. http://www.jointcommission.org/facts_about_the_tracer_methodology/

Kohn, L.T., J.M. Corrigan, and M.S. Donaldson. 2000. *To Err is Human: Building a Safer Health System*. Washington, DC: National Academies Press.

Ladapo, J. and D. Chokshi. 2014. Continuity of Care for Chronic Conditions: Threats, Opportunities, and Policy. *Health Affairs Blog*. http://healthaffairs.org/blog/2014/11/18/continuity-of-care-for-chronic-conditions-threats-opportunities-and-policy-3/

Lateef, F. 2011. Patient expectations and the paradigm shift of care in emergency medicine. *Journal of Emergencies, Trauma, and Shock* 4(2). http://www.ncbi.nlm.nih.gov/pmc/articles/PMC3132352/

Leapfrog Group. 2015. http://www.leapfroggroup.org/

National Association for Healthcare Quality. n.d.(a). Commitment to quality. Commit to the CPHQ. http://www.nahq.org/certify/content/index.html

National Association for Healthcare Quality. 2015 (b). 2015 Candidate Examination Handbook. http://www.nahq.org/uploads/HQCC15_CPHQ_Cert_Handbook_V6.pdf

Medicare Prescription Drug, Improvement, and Modernization Act of 2003. Public Law 108-173.

Monteiro, L.A. 1985. Florence Nightingale on public health nursing. *American Journal of Public Health*. 75(2). http://www.ncbi.nlm.nih.gov/pmc/articles/PMC1645993/pdf/amjph00278-0075.pdf

Naghibi, M. and H. Baban. 2011. Strategic change management: The challenges faced by organizations. *Proceedings of the 2011 International Conference on Economics and Finance Research*, Vol. 4. pp. 542–544. Singapore.

National Center on Vital and Health Statistics. 2009. Health Data Stewardship: What, Why, Who, How—a NCVHS Primer. http://www.ncvhs.hhs.gov/wp-content/uploads/2014/05/090930lt.pdf

Overland Park Regional Medical Center. 2015. About Us. http://oprmc.com/about/

Oxford Dictionaries. 2015. Performance. http://www.oxforddictionaries.com/us/definition/american_english/performance

Patient Protection and Affordable Care Act of 2010. Public Law 111-148.

Rotter, T., L. Kinsman, E.L. James, A. Machotta, H. Gothe, J. Willis, P. Sno and J. Kugler. 2010. Clinical pathways: Effects on professional practice, patient outcomes, length of stay, and hospital costs (review). *The Cochrane Library* 7. http://apps.who.int/rhl/reviews/CD006632.pdf

Rowley, J. 2007. The wisdom hierarchy: Representations of the DIKW hierarchy. *Journal of Information Science* 33(2):163–180.

Scholl, R.W. 2003. Leadership Overview. http://www.uri.edu/research/lrc/scholl/webnotes/Leadership.htm

Schyve, P.M. 2009. Leadership in Healthcare Organizations: A Guide to Joint Commission Leadership Standards. http://www.jointcommission.org/assets/1/18/WP_Leadership_Standards.pdf

Social Security Administration. 1974. Notes and Briefs Report: Health Maintenance Act of 1973. http://www.ssa.gov/policy/docs/ssb/v37n3/v37n3p35.pdf

United Kingdom National Archives. n.d. Florence Nightingale. http://www.nationalarchives.gov.uk/education/resources/florence-nightingale/

US Department of Health and Human Services. n.d. HITECH Act Enforcement Interim Final Rule. http://www.hhs.gov/ocr/privacy/hipaa/administrative/enforcementrule/hitechenforcementifr.html

US Department of Health and Human Services. 2015. NPDB Guide Book. http://www.npdb.hrsa.gov/resources/NPDBGuidebook.pdf

Vyas, D. and A. Hozain. 2014. Clinical peer review in the United States: History, legal development, and subsequent abuse. *World Journal of Gastroenterology* 20(21).

W. Edwards Deming Institute. 2015. The PDSA Cycle. https://www.deming.org/theman/theories/pdsacycle

Wiet, M.J. 2005. *Darling v. Charleston Community Memorial Hospital* and its legacy. *Annals of Health Law* 14(2). http://lawecommons.luc.edu/cgi/viewcontent.cgi?article=1196&context=annals

World Health Organization. 2010. Framework for Action on Interprofessional Education and Collaborative Practice. http://whqlibdoc.who.int/hq/2010/WHO_HRH_HPN_10.3_eng.pdf

PART V
Management Tools and Strategies

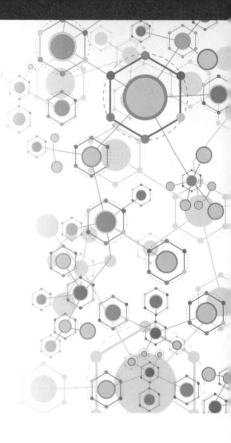

22

Managing and Leading During Organization Change

David X. Swenson, PhD, LP

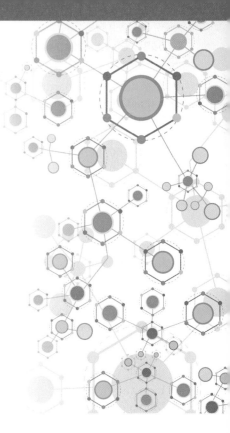

Learning Objectives

- Examine the management discipline, the evolution of management thought and theories, and the key functions and skills of management
- Identify the functions and roles of a manager
- Evaluate the relationship between management functions and skills and levels of management
- Identify different approaches to problem solving and decision making
- Compare the differences between managers and leaders

- Examine the key ideas of prominent leadership theories
- Adjust the leadership approach to various situations
- Identify the traits related to leadership effectiveness
- Assess the stages and impact of organizational change
- Determine how to facilitate a transition in order to minimize stress to people and production

Key Terms

85/15 rule
Administrative management theory
Authority
Autocratic leadership
Balanced scorecard (BSC)
Brooks' Law
Bureaucracy
Business process reengineering (BPR)

Champion
Change agent
Change driver
Cognitive complexity
Complex adaptive system
Conceptual skills
Consideration
Contingency theory of leadership
Controlling
Critic

Delegation
Democratic leadership
Discipline
Early adopter
Early majority
Emotional intelligence (EI)
Ergonomics
Esprit de corps
Evidence-based management
Exchange relationship

Executive dashboard
Expectancy theory of motivation
Gantt chart
Goal
Great person theory
Groupthink
Hawthorne effect
In-group
Initiating structure
Innovator
Interpersonal skills
Inventor
Laggard
Late majority
Leader–member exchange (LMX)
Leader–member relations
Leading
Least preferred coworker
   (LPC) scale
Line authority
Management by objectives
   (MBO)
Maslow's Hierarchy of Needs
Mission statement

Nonprogrammed decision
Normative decision model
Operational plan
Operations management
Organizational chart
Organizational culture
Organizational development
   (OD)
Organizing
Out-group
Path–goal theory
Piece-rate incentive
Planning
Position power
Program evaluation and review
   technique (PERT)
Programmed decision
Refreezing
Role theory
Scalar chain
Scientific management
Self-monitoring
Servant leadership
SMART goals

Span of control
Sponsor
Staff authority
Stages of grief
Strategic plan
Systems thinking
Tactical plan
Task and bonus plan
Task structure
Technical skills
Theory X
Theory X and Y
Theory Y
Time and motion studies
Total quality management
   (TQM)
Trait approach
Unfreezing
Unity of command
Values-based leadership
Values statement
Vertical dyad linkage
Vision statement
Worker immaturity–maturity

Models for management were originally based on traditional ways of organizing people to accomplish tasks. For thousands of years, these typically involved small family cottage industries, military organizations, or church-directed structures. With the advent of the Industrial Revolution, migration to cities, and specialization of labor, the former methods of management no longer worked effectively. Workers did not necessarily carry on family traditions, could not be commanded to comply with orders, or did not serve out of dedication to some larger corporate value. New ways of thinking about management were needed.

Management theories are not just academic exercises; they are ways of describing how managers think about the way organizations work, which in turn influence their decisions and direct their efforts and behavior. The theories described in this chapter reflect the development of management theories from the early 1900s to present, as well as newer, developing approaches. Many elements of even the early theories are still practiced widely. By identifying working theories, managers are better able to evaluate how appropriate these theories are for the setting and how they can be revised to work better.

A key idea in management is the recognition that management theories and practices grow out of the unique constellation of forces or **change drivers** that operate at the time. Change drivers are large-scale forces such as demographic, social, political, economic, technical, and more recently, global and informational factors that require organizations to revise how they operate. In a turbulent and competitive environment, management theories assist leaders to more effectively and efficiently allocate resources to respond to these changes.

In this first section of the chapter, some of the key historical and theoretical developments in management are summarized, many features of which are still used today in organizations. The functions, skills, and roles of managers are identified, along with trends in management theory related to problem solving. Finally, leadership of the organization will be examined through the evolution of leadership theories and how transition can be facilitated during organizational change.

Landmarks in Management as a Discipline

Management, as a **discipline**, is a field of study characterized by a knowledge base and perspective that are distinctive from other fields of study. The knowledge base and perspective form a foundation for the discipline's practices. Over time, changing social conditions and growing technological innovations have contributed to the way that the management discipline has evolved and management theories are framed.

Scientific Management

The late 19th and early 20th centuries marked the emergence of scientific management concepts. **Scientific management** was an early effort to apply scientific principles and practices to business processes. The individuals profiled in the following subsections were key players in that development.

Max Weber

Management theory emerged with the onset of the Industrial Revolution in the mid-19th century and initially took the form of scientific management. During this period, Max Weber (1864–1920) began formulating his ideas for the ideal organization. Recognizing the variability in standards that lead to inefficiencies, he proposed that organizations be structured as a **bureaucracy**. This form of organization was typified by clear hierarchies of relationships, rules, and regulations to standardize behavior, and the use of trained specialists for jobs. Consequently, the subjective judgment and favoritism could be eliminated, and planning could be based on the position and task rather than the person and personal preferences. Large organizations are often structured as bureaucracies in which authority is hierarchically organized—with a rigid division of labor, rigid rules and regulations, and impersonal culture. In the modern marketplace, including the healthcare market, where competitive advantage is maintained through innovation, such bureaucracy has come more often to refer to slow decision making, unresponsiveness, lack of appreciation for the uniqueness of individuals, and rules without reasons. This slowness is often due to the complexities in managing large healthcare organizations, dealing with huge databases, changing regulations, and diverse stak holders.

Frederick Taylor

About the same time that Weber was forming his ideas about bureaucracy, Frederick W. Taylor (1856–1915) discovered that his company and most others had tremendous unused potential. Pay and working conditions were poor, waste and inefficiency were prevalent, and management decision making was unsystematic and not based on research of any sort. Taylor introduced new practices, the success of which led to his being called the Father of Scientific Management (Copley 1923). Although many of his ideas are commonly accepted today, they were revolutionary at the time. He proposed that organizations observe and study how jobs were performed and then streamline the actions to be more efficient. He conducted **time and motion studies** in which tasks were subdivided into their most basic movements. Detailed motions were timed to determine the most efficient way of carrying them out. After the "one best way" was found, the best worker match for the job was hired, tools and procedures were standardized, instruction cards were written to guide workers, and breaks were instituted to reduce fatigue. A **piece-rate incentive** system was also developed by Taylor in which workers received additional pay when they exceeded the standard output level for their task, or in early industrial terms, they produced more "pieces" of a work product than the set objective.

The impact of Taylorism on healthcare has been mixed (Rastegar 2004). On the one hand, it enabled the analysis of tasks into their relatively simple components to find the one best way to complete those tasks. On the other, it contributed to the fragmentation of work, including healthcare specialties, multilayering of organizations, and problems with communication across boundaries. Today the legacy of Taylorism remains in task analysis and specialization, but there is also an awareness that organizational layers and professions must communicate more efficiently.

Frank and Lillian Gilbreth

In the early 1900s, the Gilbreths were a husband and wife team who developed many of the early ideas of ergonomics—the study of people working efficiently. Conducting time and motion studies on bricklaying, the Gilbreths divided the process into detailed individual motions they called "therbligs" (Gilbreth nearly spelled backward) to identify unnecessary or inefficient motions. Seeking the single best way to perform the tasks, they reduced the number of motions for bricklaying from 18 to 4.5, which resulted in much higher productivity, less fatigue, and better planning. Lillian was known for her studies on finding innovative ways to design efficient kitchen and home living areas for patients with cardiac-limited conditions. Work by the Gilbreths became the foundation for hospital quality assurance, surgical best practice, and lean healthcare (Towill 2009). Time and motion studies have been more recently used to assess health information technology (IT) implementation to ensure standard procedures (Zheng et al. 2011).

Henry Gantt

Henry Gantt (1861–1919) worked for Taylor and was known for his promotion of favorable psychological work conditions. He may be best remembered for his development of the Gantt chart, which is still used for project management and healthcare operations management to show how the components of a task are scheduled over time (Langabeer and Helton 2016). See figure 22.1 for an example of a basic Gantt chart showing an initial electronic health record (EHR) implementation timeline. His chart contributed to development by the US Navy in the late 1950s of the program evaluation and review technique (PERT), in which the sequence and timing of activities required to complete a task are graphically organized so they can be analyzed for efficiency. He also contributed his task and bonus plan to management, which provided bonus payment for workers who exceeded their production standards for the day.

Administrative Management

Attempting to compensate for the theory of scientific management's exclusion of senior management, the administrative management theory proposed a rational approach to designing organizations, with formal structure, clear division of labor, and use of delegation. It argued that management was a profession and could be learned. The following subsections profile three individuals who played key roles in describing management functions.

Figure 22.1. Gantt chart showing sequence of initial EHR implementation timeline

Tasks	Time to implement					
	6/1	6/6	6/11	6/16	6/21	6/26
EHR set up hardware	▮					
Apply software	▮					
Test system connectivity		▮				
Front desk staff training			▮			
Billing staff training			▮▮			
Management training		▮▮▮▮▮				

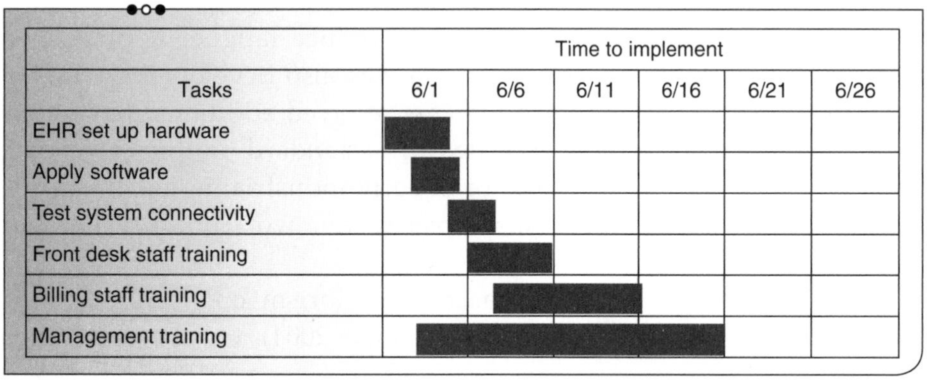

Henri Fayol

Henri Fayol (1841–1925) was a French mining engineer whose major contribution includes a description of the key functions of management and 14 principles for organizational design and administration.

Fayol's management functions have persisted with some variation into modern organizations, including healthcare, and identify key functions that define the manager's role. Fayol's managerial functions were the following (McConnell 2015):

- **Planning** consists of examining the future and preparing plans of action to attain goals.

- **Organizing** is the way in which the managed system is designed and operated to attain the desired goals. It involves the way that tasks are grouped into departments and resources are distributed to them.

- **Leading** (sometimes also called directing) is the process of influencing the behavior of others. It involves motivating, creating shared culture and values, and communicating with all levels of the organization.

- **Controlling** refers to the monitoring of performance and use of feedback to ensure that efforts are on target toward prescribed goals, making course corrections as necessary.

Fayol also formulated 14 principles of management (Fayol 1917) to guide managerial activities within the total organization (see figure 22.2). Like his four managerial functions, most have been incorporated into modern organizations and are widely accepted today. For example, **authority** was proposed as the right of an executive to give orders and expect obedience. **Unity of command** meant that each employee reports to only one boss. The **scalar chain**, or line of authority, ensured that everyone in the organization appears in the chain of command and reports to someone. **Esprit de corps** emphasized the work climate in which harmony, cohesion, and high morale promoted good work.

Chester Barnard

Chester Barnard (1886–1961), an American business executive and public administrator, elaborated on the role of top executives. He proposed that the leader receives information from those below, that the communication system be designed and implemented by the executive, and that the role of middle management is to implement plans and solve problems. In his classic book *Functions of the Executive* (1938), he emphasized formulating organizational objectives, establishing a system of essential services, and even envisioning an early version of evidence-based management (Barnard 1938). His theories of authority and incentives

Figure 22.2. Fayol's 14 principles

1. *Specialization of labor:* Work allocation and specialization allow concentrated activities, deeper understanding, and better efficiency.
2. *Authority:* The person to whom responsibilities are given has the right to give direction and expect obedience.
3. *Discipline:* The smooth operation of a business requires standards, rules, and values for consistency of action.
4. *Unity of command:* Every employee receives direction and instructions from only one boss.
5. *Unity of direction:* All workers are aligned in their efforts toward a single outcome.
6. *Subordination of individual interests:* Accomplishing shared values and organizational goals take priority over individual agendas.
7. *Remuneration:* Employees should receive fair pay for work.
8. *Centralization:* Decisions are made at the top.
9. *Scalar chain:* Everyone is clearly included in the chain of command and line of authority from top to bottom of the organization.
10. *Order:* People should clearly understand where they fit in the organization, and all people and material have a place.
11. *Equity:* People are treated fairly, and a sense of justice should pervade the organization.
12. *Tenure:* Turnover is undesirable, and loyalty to the organization is sought.
13. *Initiative:* Personal initiative should be encouraged.
14. *Esprit de corps:* Harmony, cohesion, teamwork, and good interpersonal relationships should be encouraged.

Source: Fayol 1917.

rested on principles of communication: common knowledge and access to communication channels, personal competency, and accuracy in direct communication.

Mary Parker Follett

Another major contributor to the administrative approach was Mary Parker Follett (1868–1933), and with Lillian Gilbreth was one of the first women pioneers in management theory. In contrast to what was often considered a mechanistic view by Taylor, she was interested in broader social ideas and championed the role of relationships and conflict in organizations. Although she drew mixed attention in the late 1920s, she foresaw the development of a systems view of business, the role of empowered employees in organizational development, and the use of workgroups to implement solutions. Follett promoted using teamwork and creative group effort, involving people in organizational development, and integrating the organization, which involved many elements of systems management theory (Parker 1984).

Humanistic Management and the Human Relations Movement

Although the United States has always touted itself as the home of democracy, the equity of power in the workplace has not always existed between workers and management. By the early 1900s, there were growing social pressures to treat workers in a more enlightened manner. Building on Barnard's and Follett's ideas that people should be treated fairly and that effective controls come from individual workers, the stage was set for a shift in management thought stimulated by an experiment at an electric power plant.

The Hawthorne Studies

Between 1927 and 1932, Elton Mayo, Franz Roethlisberger, and others from Harvard University conducted a series of experiments at the Western Electric Hawthorne Works in Chicago. The studies originally were designed to explore how fatigue and monotony affected job productivity and how these might be mitigated by breaks, variable work hours, temperature, humidity, and lighting. Although performance increased when desirable conditions were increased; unexpectedly, performance also improved when these conditions were reduced. The researchers concluded that it was the human factors that made a difference: attention during the study, freedom of participation, and feeling important by being singled out for participation in the project—the so-called Hawthorne effect (Landsberger 1958). Only in later reviews of the study was it also discovered that the participants were motivated by financial incentives. Nonetheless, this popularized study gave strong impetus to the consideration of social factors at work. In healthcare, the **Hawthorne effect** (also called the observer effect) is based on the principle that what gets attention and measured is what gets improved, and that is a key concern to increasing patient satisfaction (Hirsch 2011).

Human Resources Management

In the 1950s, the field of psychology in the United States was just coming into its own prominence, as were theories of motivation. Observing that many problems were derived from an inability to meet needs, Abraham Maslow (1908–1970) suggested that an understanding of employees' needs might help to explain behavior and provide guidance for managers on how to better motivate workers. **Maslow's Hierarchy of Needs** began with physiological existence needs and progressed through safety, social belongingness, self-esteem, and finally self-actualization or creativity needs. This developmental view of needs meant that to motivate people, lower-order needs should be satisfied before higher-order needs could serve as motivators (Maslow 1943).

Douglas McGregor

Douglas McGregor (1906–1964), a Sloan Management Professor at MIT, recognized the shift in conceptual models from assumptions that workers were incapable of independent action to beliefs in their potential and high performance. He formulated the contrasting views as theory X and Y (McGregor 1960). **Theory X** presumed that workers inherently disliked work and would avoid it, had little ambition, and mostly wanted security; therefore, managerial direction and control were necessary. **Theory Y** took a more enlightened view and assumed that work was as natural as play, that motivation could be both internally and externally driven, and that under the right conditions people would seek responsibility and be creative. Theory X found more application in situations where workers were typically immature, less educated, or uninterested in the work, while Theory Y found more applications in situations where workers were more mature, educated, motivated and creative workers.

Operations Management

Operations management emerged after World War II as an application of statistical, mathematical, and quantitative methods to decision making in the business setting in order to better understand how products and services could be manufactured and delivered. Techniques such as forecasting, linear programming, break-even analysis, queuing theory, logistics, and more recently data mining emerged from this emphasis on statistical control.

Contemporary Management

Although many aspects of older theories of management are still widely practiced in most organizations, research and practical experience have led to many refinements and new developments in the field. More contemporary approaches to management include management by objectives (MBO), total quality management (TQM), and an emphasis on excellence in quality and performance. Each of these has made a contribution to better understanding how effective management works, but none of them alone has yet succeeded in producing a comprehensive solution for managing organizations.

Management by Objectives

Often referred to as the Father of Modern Management (Starbuck 2013), Peter Drucker (1909–2005) revolutionized the role of business strategy by wrestling it from the hands of top management and making it everyone's job, helping workers understand how mission, strategy, goals, and performance were related. Because strategy was action-oriented, starting in the 1950s, Drucker elaborated on the technique of **management by objectives (MBO)**, in which clear target objectives could be stated and measured and could direct behavior (Drucker 1986). Drucker's MBO approach was further developed by his promotion of the ideas that workers should be considered assets rather than liabilities, the corporation is an interpersonal community, and business is customer centered (Byrne 2005). A comprehensive literature review of MBO research showed that the medical sector was the most common user, with healthcare, nursing, hospital management, and hospital pharmacy accounting for about 40 percent of the applications (Kyriakopaulos 2012).

Total Quality Management

Total quality management (TQM) claimed to overcome the limitations of MBO, criticizing the use of quotas because workers often spent too much time trying to look good or protect themselves by seeking short-term objectives and ignoring long-term and critical outcomes. TQM offered a way to build in high performance by maximizing employee potential and continuous improvement of process. The **85/15 rule** of TQM proposes that 85 percent of problems encountered are the result of faulty systems and only 15 percent are due to unconscientious or unproductive employees. The manager's job, then, becomes one of anticipating and removing barriers to high employee performance.

From the late 1970s to the mid-1980s, the United States was beset with a series of economic setbacks. Serious recessions, a growing trade deficit, government deregulation, and huge operating losses led to the downsizing of hundreds of thousands of workers. Quality became the focus as a means of increasing competitive position, and much of the idea was derived from W. Edwards Deming (1900–1993), an American statistician. Deming had initially developed his ideas in the 1940s (Walton 1986), but the American economy was booming at the time and seemed to believe it had found Taylor's one best way to do things.

Consequently, American industry was inattentive to Deming's ideas about improvement and his statistical control procedures for monitoring quality. However, the Japanese were suffering from an all-but-destroyed economy and were eager to hear new ideas about production. They quickly adopted the concept and his 14 points of total quality management (see figure 22.3) (Deming 1986; Taplan 2003).

TQM continues to be a popular and effective approach to change management and has been widely used in healthcare. In an effort to more clearly identify leadership traits associated with effective application of TQM, a survey of 50 healthcare CEOs from the British National Healthcare System, was conducted (Nwabueze 2011). The survey found that Fayol's four management functions (planning, organizing, leading, and controlling) were highly relevant, and researchers were able to prioritize a list of leadership traits. From a list of 50, the following traits were ranked from high to low by the CEOs: good communicator, good commander, good planner, hands-on, enthusiastic/highly committed, strong minded, good listener, good organizer, high integrity, and good controller. The hands-on nature of leadership was consistently cited as an essential behavior for leaders successfully implementing TQM.

Business Process Reengineering Growing in popularity in the mid-1990s and fostered by Hammer and Champy's book, *Reengineering the Corporation* (1993), **business process reengineering (BPR)** (also known as business transformation and process change management) seeks radical redesign of the organization and its business processes in order to reduce costs, streamline operations, and improve quality of service. BPR responds to a need in the business environment to rapidly adapt to changing situations brought about by computing technology in the workplace. In some ways harkening back to Taylor's best way, business process reengineering (BPR) attempts to find the best work processes to maximally improve cost, quality, service, and speed. Like TQM it emphasizes ongoing improvement and use of information technology to provide real-time information about customers, competition, and change. However, in contrast

Figure 22.3. Deming's 14 principles

1. Create a constancy of purpose toward continual improvement of products and services, with the objectives to stay in business, be competitive, and provide jobs.
2. Adopt the new philosophy for a new economic age by correcting superstitious learning, calling for a major change, and looking at the customer rather than competition.
3. Cease dependence on inspection to achieve quality by eliminating emphasis on mass inspection and building quality in from the beginning.
4. Do not award business based on price tag alone, and minimize total costs by developing trusting and loyal long-term relationships with single suppliers.
5. Constantly and continually improve production and service systems and thereby improve quality and decrease costs.
6. Institute training on the job, where barriers to good work are removed and managers provide a setting that promotes worker success.
7. Institute leadership with the aim of revising supervision to better help people, machines, and processes do a better job.
8. Drive out fear so everyone can work effectively toward company goals.
9. Break down barriers between departments so that various departments can work as a team and anticipate problems of production or use of a product or service.
10. Avoid asking for new levels of productivity and zero defects through slogans and targets because most problems of low productivity lie with the system rather than the worker.
11. Replace work standards such as quotas, numerical goals, and MBO with good leadership.
12. Remove barriers that rob people at all levels of their pride of workmanship; shift from numbers to quality.
13. Institute a program of education and self-improvement by emphasizing lifelong learning and employment.
14. Transformation of the workplace occurs through everyone's action.

Source: Deming 1986.

to TQM's incremental and top down approach, BPR has been adopted in healthcare emphasizing extensive redesign from scratch and empowering individuals and teams to be involved in developing the change (Patwardhan and Patwardhan 2008). Process improvement and work redesign is discussed further in chapter 25.

The Search for Excellence

Although elements of most major theories can be found within the practices of successful managers, developments and refinements in thinking have continued to become part of management practice and history. In 1982, Tom Peters and Robert Waterman published *In Search of Excellence.* Based on a sample of highly successful business firms, they described the management practices that led to their success. Eight characteristics were described that became the rage in management circles for a time, with managers hoping to reproduce in their own organizations what top firms had done (Peters and Waterman 1982) (see figure 22.4). Although the eight practices are very important, a follow-up of the same organizations four years later showed disappointing results. In that short time, 66 percent had fallen from a top position and 19 percent were in a troubled position (Pascale 1990). The fall from excellence was largely due to those organizations refocusing on their temporary success and not attending sufficiently to the dynamic and strategic processes that were required

to keep them there.

Although researchers continue to search for the essential ingredients that will make firms most successful, the lesson from the excellence studies highlights some important principles, including the following:

- Whether you succeed or fail, try to understand what brought about that result.

- When you succeed, recognize that the success factors are not static but, rather, are continually changing.

- Do not let past success strategies keep you from discovering new ones for the future.

- What may contribute to the success of one type of organization or competitive setting may not be as useful to other types and settings or at other stages of organizational development.

The history of management reflects much development in our understanding of how people work and how that work can be more effectively organized. From Taylor's and Fayol's early efforts to create structured work systems to more contemporary views on the importance of integrating human factors with work conditions, management theories continue to evolve and tend to focus on adapting to and leading organizational change (see table 22.1).

Figure 22.4. Characteristics of highly successful firms

1. *A bias for action:* They establish a value for action and implementation rather than overanalyzing and delaying with endless committees.
2. *Close to the customer:* They listen and respond to customers to satisfy their needs.
3. *Autonomy and entrepreneurship:* They empower people and encourage innovation and risk taking.
4. *Productivity through people:* They increase employees' awareness that everyone's contributions lead to shared success.
5. *Hands on, value driven:* Their managers should be visible, involved, and know what is going on.
6. *Stick to the knitting:* They stay with the core business, what they do well, and avoid wide diversification.
7. *Simple form, lean staff:* They have fewer administrative layers and keep the structure simple.
8. *Simultaneous loose–tight properties:* They maintain dedication to core principles but encourage flexibility and experimentation in reaching goals.

Source: Adapted from Peters and Waterman 1982.

Table 22.1. Foundations of management timeline

Scientific management 1880–1920	Administrative management circa 1920s	Humanistic management circa 1924	Operations management 1941–present	Contemporary management 1960–present
Max Weber: Bureaucracy	Henri Fayol: Four management functions and 14 principles	Elton Mayo and Franz Roethlisberger: Hawthorne studies	WWII logistics for troops and materiel	Contingency theory
Frederick Taylor: Best way to perform a job	Chester Barnard: Effectiveness and efficiency, theory of authority, theory of incentives	Abraham Maslow: Hierarchy of needs	PERT and critical path analysis	Managing by objectives
Frank and Lillian Gilbreth: Time and motion studies	Mary Parker Follett: Power sharing, conflict resolution	Douglas McGregor: Theory X and Y	Routing and supply chain management	Total quality management
Henry Gantt: Gantt chart and project management			Scheduling and queuing systems	Business process redesign
			Data mining	Systems theory

Check Your Understanding 22.1

Instructions: **Answer the following questions on a separate piece of paper.**

1. Why have some management ideas been rapidly accepted while others have required years to become popular?

2. How have management theories changed over the years and what are some factors that have contributed to such change?

3. What are some reasons why the top companies in Peters and Waterman's *In Search of Excellence* dropped from their top position within a few short years? How might that have been prevented?

4. Using the example of the Gilbreth time and motion study, identify some complex activity you engage in (such as packing for a trip, dressing in the morning, or such) and see how you can streamline the sequence to become more efficient.

5. Think of a small project you have to complete, such as writing a paper. Draw a Gantt chart, breaking down each step of writing a paper and plot each step over time to completion.

Functions and Principles of Management

Fayol identified the key functions of management. There are certain categories of skills that are needed to carry out these functions.

Managerial Functions

As theories of management began to be refined, so too did the formal nature of the manager's role. As organizations increased in diversity, complexity, and size, managers often shifted their expertise from expert knowledge in doing a task to expert knowledge in managing other people. As Mary Parker Follett is reputed to have said, "Management is the art of getting things done through people" (Stoner and Freeman 1989). Specific functions of management were defined, as were a range of skills and subroles that contribute to successful problem solving.

Planning

Planning is the first step in management and involves determining what should be accomplished and how. Although planning occurs at all levels, top-level or strategic planning is most critical in formulating the mission and providing direction for change. When these strategies are defined, they can be implemented at the lower levels of the organization. High-quality planning and implementation capability provide competitive advantage over those who minimize the importance of planning, as reflected in higher levels of performance such as profits (Hahn and Powers 2010).

Plans are usually organized hierarchically into planning levels, with a **mission statement** driving the enterprise by defining exactly the purpose of the organization; that is, what business it is in. The mission may also incorporate or be accompanied by a **values statement** that reflects the social and cultural beliefs an organization wishes to support among its members. For example, the Benedictine Health System acknowledges "hospitality, stewardship, respect and justice" as its core values (Benedictine Health System 2015). A **vision statement** describes the ideal and desired future state toward which an organization is directed, in contrast to the mission statement, which is current and realistic. The **strategic plan** follows from the mission. It is formulated by top management, sets the priorities and positioning of the organization for a time period, and is based on the internal strengths and weaknesses and external opportunities and threats. These are translated through the lower levels of the organization by middle management in formulating **tactical plans**, which are strategic plans for the organization's major divisions. At the lower departmental levels, these finally become **operational plans** that are implemented as daily activities (see figure 22.5).

Plans are usually expressed in terms of goals. **Goals** are statements of intended outcomes that provide a source of direction and motivation as well as a guideline for performance, decision making, and evaluation. Good goals cover key result areas of the strategy, and have the characteristics of being **SMART goals**—specific, measurable, achievable, realistic, and time-bound.

Organizing

After the goals have been specified, the task changes to deciding how resources can be allocated

Figure 22.5.   Planning levels

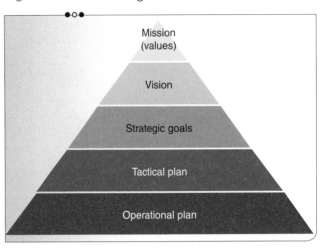

to achieve them. Traditionally, division of labor has been used to divide work into separate jobs. This specialization allows for development of greater expertise and standardization of tasks and for clear selection and training criteria. However, too narrow or specialized a task, as in data entry and some laboratory work, may produce boredom from routine affecting productivity. The emerging economy with downsized and flatter organizations (that is, with fewer levels of management) often requires workers to take on multiple roles and, consequently, to have portfolios of skills rather than highly defined job descriptions (Bridges 1994). Such skill and role portfolios are often found in healthcare, where downsizing and staff shortages occur, resulting in remaining staff assuming a broader range of duties (Apker 2001; Helseth 2007).

Jobs are most often organized by positions, and the positions are arranged hierarchically in the business by an organizational chart. (An example of a typical hospital organizational chart is shown in figure 22.6.) The **organizational chart** graphically represents the formal structure of an organization, often includes departmental subdivisions, and follows the scalar principle and unity of command discussed earlier. The vertical structure of the organization refers to the formal design of positions within departments and divisions, the lines of authority and responsibility, and the allocation of resources to them. Two kinds of authority are found in organizations.

Figure 22.6. Sample hospital organizational chart

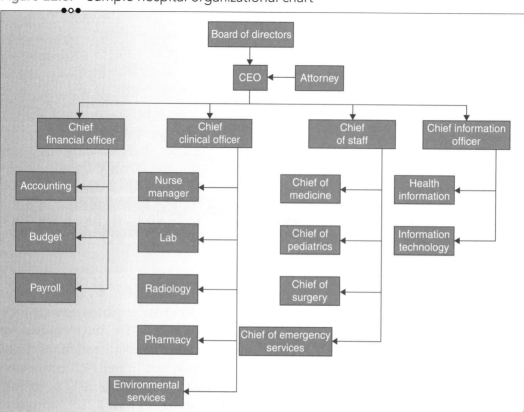

Line authority is the right of managers to direct the activities of subordinates under their immediate control; **staff authority** is related to the expert knowledge of specialists in the organization and involves their ability or right to advise and recommend courses of action.

Each supervisor has a certain number of people who report to him or her, which is referred to as the span of management or the **span of control**. Although span of control is often determined by tradition or accident, there are several factors to consider in optimally balancing the span of control. In general, the span of control is larger when work is routine and homogeneous, workers have similar tasks, rules and guidelines are available, people are well trained and motivated, workers are located together, and task times are short (Meyer 2008). Deciding how a combination of factors leads to a particular span has been facilitated by technology. For example, the Healthcare Management Council (HMC), a hospital performance management company, provides a comprehensive measurement of organizational factors leading to a span of management recommendation. The HMC span of control analysis considers organizational flatness, number of managers and supervisors, departmental fragmentation, and layers of management using organizational charts. The HMC report can be used by managers to optimize organizational structure, set staffing and financial targets, and determine needs (HMC 2013).

Related to span is **delegation**, in which managers transfer authority to subordinates to carry out a responsibility. With an increasing focus on customers and rapid response, frontline employees are trained to make decisions that once were made levels above them. When authority and responsibility move from the organization's top levels to its lower levels where they can be competently exercised, centralized decision making becomes decentralized or distributed more widely throughout the organization. Although decentralization enables top managers to take on new responsibilities or spend time with other priorities, it places an additional burden on workers.

Directing and Leading

The third managerial function accomplishes goals by influencing behavior and by motivating and inspiring people to high performance. For much of the history of management, an autocratic and centralized view of leadership was considered to be appropriate, but as humanistic views have prevailed over more recent decades, leadership has become decentralized and distributed throughout the organization.

Leading is most often accomplished by communicating, directing, and motivating, all intended to influence behavior to perform well. Power—the ability to influence—is central to leadership and derives from several sources, including the following:

- *Authority* or legitimate power comes from the right of the position in the organization to direct the activities of subordinates.

- *Reward power* is based on the leader's ability to withhold or provide rewards for performance.

- *Coercive power* maintains control over punishments.

- *Referent power* exists when the leader possesses personal characteristics that are appealing to the constituency, and the constituency follows out of admiration, charismatic impact, or the desire to be like the leader.

- *Expert power* occurs when the leader has knowledge or expertise that is of value (French and Raven 1959).

- *Information power* is based on the persuasive content of the person's message, apart from personal characteristics (Raven 1983).

Leadership behaviors and most models of leadership fall into two categories: task-oriented behaviors and social or group-oriented behaviors. Task-oriented behaviors are directed toward defining tasks, creating structure and rules, ensuring production, and placing emphasis on quality and speed of output. Social orientation focuses on interpersonal behaviors that develop and maintain harmonious work relationships, encourage morale, reduce stress and conflict, and build worker satisfaction. Several models of leadership, such as the Blake-Mouton managerial grid, use these two dimensions and are discussed later in this chapter.

Controlling and Evaluating

The final managerial function refers to the monitoring of performance—determining whether it is on or off course in achieving the goals, and making course corrections as needed. Managers are obligated to ensure that progress is made toward achieving goals, and while some organizations allow experienced and responsible employees to self-monitor, technology has enabled remote monitoring of performance. With so many tasks requiring computer input, it is possible to analyze aspects of performance, such as rate of entry, number of patients seen, or tasks completed. The employee can view personal performance compared to required levels or to a standard, and high and low performers may come to the attention of a manager.

Significant breakthroughs have occurred in control with the development of the executive dashboard and balanced scorecard introduced in 1992 (Kaplan and Norton 1996). The **executive dashboard** is often characterized as a manager's version of a pilot's cockpit dashboard; it contains all the critical information for leading the organization. The dashboard typically contains regularly updated information on key strategic measures such as forecasts, customer satisfaction, billings, profit, and so on. An example of the effective use of dashboards is their application at St. Joseph Mercy Oakland Hospital in Pontiac, Michigan. Monitors displaying results of key performance indicators (KPIs) were located throughout the hospital emphasizing the importance and transparency of monitoring. Over a two year period from 2012 to 2014 performance significantly improved in tracking average length of stay, patients who left the ER without being seen, and radiology turnaround time (Weiner et al. 2015). Refer to chapter 18 for an example of an executive dashboard.

The **balanced scorecard (BSC)** is an extension of strategic planning in which key performance indicators are measured at all levels of the organization. The BSC shows progress related to meeting the key performance indicators and offers workers and management ongoing feedback. Categories of feedback usually include financial information, customer satisfaction, internal processes (for example, quality or response time), and learning and growth. For example, using the BSC helped university and hospital clinics in Holmes County, Mississippi, move much closer to break-even in its revenues, while Harrisburg Medical Center in Illinois reported achieving a consistent 4 percent profit over a four-year period (Rural Health Resource Center 2008).

Levels of Management

The four functions of management vary in emphasis according to the level of management involved (see figure 22.7). In general, as one moves from first-line (supervisory) to middle management to top managers, planning increases, organizing increases, directing decreases, and controlling stays about the same (Jones and George 2006; McConnell 2015).

Larger organizations often have three levels of management—supervisors, middle managers, and executives; in addition they have a board of directors. These different levels of management within organizations also have different levels of leadership functions.

Supervisory managers are hands-on managers of daily operations over a unit or division within a department. They ensure that staff meet

pre-established standards of performance, policy, and procedures. They often have high-level technical skills, but may have limited hiring and financial authority.

Middle managers have a broader scope of responsibility than supervisory managers, often overseeing all functions in a department, such as the health information management (HIM) department, the admission and registration department, and others. They also are in a position to facilitate the work of positions above and below them, both supervisory and executive. More specifically, their responsibilities often include:

- Developing, implementing, and revising the policies and procedures of the organization under direction by the executive level
- Carrying out organizational plans that have been developed at the executive and board level
- Communicating operational information to executives so they can continue ongoing planning

In an HIM department, middle managers can modify department-level policies and procedures as needed and can analyze information to get at a root cause of a problem and use discretion in dealing with it. They may also track quality of clinical databases, oversee compliance programs, participate on interdisciplinary committees, and conduct risk and quality audits. Middle managers typically report to an executive manager, who could include the chief operating officer (COO), chief information officer (CIO), chief financial officer (CFO), or chief executive officer (CEO).

At the highest level of the organization are executive managers and the governing board. Executives are mostly responsible for formulating the strategic plan, ensuring consistency in the direction of the organization with its vision and mission, and allocating assets and resources toward that end. They establish policies and lead the organization toward quality improvement and compliance. In the typical "C-suite" of a large healthcare organization, there is commonly a chief operations officer (COO), a chief financial officer (CFO), a chief

Figure 22.7. Relative degree of managerial function by level in the organization

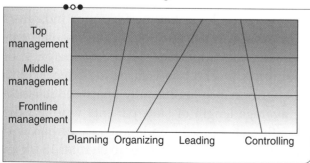

nursing officer (CNO), a chief information officer (CIO), and a chief medical officer (CMO), all of whom report to the chief executive officer (CEO). The CEO reports directly to the board of directors, also called the board of trustees or governing board.

Governing boards are legislated to be responsible for the operation of the entire organization. They are the final authority when it comes to the approval of the strategic plan and mission, vision, ethics, and values statements, and are accountable for quality and finances. In healthcare a board is usually made up of a chairperson and internal directors, and 12 to 15 board members who bring legal, insurance, business, and other expertise (Danner 2005).

Managerial Skills

The categories of skills required to perform the four management functions are conceptual, interpersonal, and technical skills (Buhler 2007; Katz 1974). As management has become increasingly complex, the requisite skills for carrying out the four managerial functions also vary by level in the organization. For example, figure 22.8 shows that technical skills are most pertinent for frontline management while conceptual skills are most relevant for top management. Interpersonal skills are used largely in middle management.

Conceptual Skills

The need for conceptual skills has increased significantly over the years. Where it once was important only to have effective technical skills, now a successful manager must be able to understand

Figure 22.8. Relative degree of functional skills by level in the organization

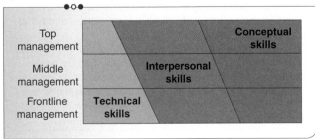

diverse fields and deal with complex situations. **Conceptual skills**, especially at the higher levels of the organization, include such competencies as visioning the organization, planning, decision making, problem solving, creativity, and conceptualizing the connections among parts of a complex organizational system, or systems thinking. **Cognitive complexity**—the ability to see the many parts of a problem, process conflicting information, and integrate that diversity into a coherent picture—is very important for top managers (Houghton et al. 2009). For example, electronic health records involve high levels of information complexity and inattention to the demands this places on providers can lead to higher patient care risks (Roberson et al. 2009; Stephenson and Schwartz 2014). Conceptual skills are needed to consider the resulting effects of making a change. In another example, computer-assisted clinical ordering reduces variation in orders thereby reducing risks (Horsky et al. 2003). In this example, conceptual skills have been used to develop solutions to the existing issue of variation.

Interpersonal Skills

Interpersonal skills involve the ability to work with and through others to accomplish goals. Depending on the nature of the work and the level of interaction needed among individuals, interpersonal skills may or may not be critical for employee success. However, managers need to cultivate impeccable interpersonal skills in their interactions with employees and with each other.

Interpersonal competency is based on self-awareness and understanding, and the best managers are those who can articulate both their strengths and weaknesses. Interpersonal communication skills have been rated as one of the five top skills for healthcare managers (Kronenberg 2014). Yet, self-awareness is not enough, and consistently high performers also demonstrate self-monitoring (Riggio and Reichard 2008). **Self-monitoring** refers to the ability to observe the reactions that one's behavior has on others and then adjust one's behavior to improve the relationship and quality of care (Epstein et al. 2008). Other important interpersonal skills include communicating, motivating and influencing, managing conflict, and complementing different ways of interacting.

Emotional intelligence (EI) is currently a widely discussed topic in management and healthcare. **Emotional intelligence** is the sensitivity and ability to monitor and revise one's behavior based on the needs and responses of others (AHIMA 2014). Advocates of EI believe that awareness and use of feelings complement rational intelligence and experience, and it is the combination of these that is the key to more effective care (Gamble 2013)(see figure 22.9). Studies examining an array of management skills conclude that people management skills are often more important to performance than are intellectual abilities (Carmeli and Tishler 2006; Hammerly et al. 2014). Other studies support the contention that interpersonal skills are strongly related to overall performance (Howard and Silverstein 2014), successful conflict management (Gerardi 2015), and team performance (Harper and White 2013); and that such skills can be enhanced (Hammerly et al. 2014).

Technical Skills

Understanding and mastering the technical information, methods, and equipment involved in a discipline constitute the **technical skills**. Although most important at the employee level of the organization, technical skills are still required for upper management so that there is a comprehensive understanding of the workings of the organization. However, conceptual and interpersonal skills are more useful in obtaining promotion in most organizations. This is true because, at higher levels in organizations, these types of skills are used more often and are more important than technical skills. Conceptual skills are more useful in the leading and planning functions because they involve understanding the systems view of the total organization. For example, as healthcare information systems shift from decentralized to more centralized operations, poorly thought out design can compromise information integrity, endanger safety, decrease quality of care, and increase fraud (Bowman 2013). The ability to understand complex connections among information centers, recognize gaps in continuity of information, and anticipate unintended consequences can do much to reduce these errors.

Managerial Activities

The activities of managers and leaders are typically organized around several roles. A role refers to a set of expectations about how a person is to behave from the perspective of oneself, peers, superiors, subordinates, consumers (patients), and others (such as legislators). **Role theory** has been a prominent framework for examining behavior in the field of sociology for decades, and it has been applied in management to clarify the wide range of responsibilities held.

Mintzberg's Role Studies

Henry Mintzberg, Cleghorn Professor of Management at McGill University, completed his dissertation at Massachusetts Institute of Technology on the roles of managers. In practice, Mintzberg (1992) found that most chief executives spent

Figure 22.9. Attributes of emotional intelligence

- *Self-awareness:* The ability to monitor, notice, and label one's feelings as they occur. This allows one to be more certain about feelings and to identify early vague feelings.
- *Self-regulation:* The ability to manage one's emotions and impulses. A person with this skill is often viewed as being reflective, comfortable with change and ambiguity, and able to control impulsiveness.

- *Motivation:* Being highly motivated is essential for focusing attention, mastering situations, showing creativity, and being productive and successful.
- *Empathy:* The ability to recognize emotions in others. This is important for teamwork as well as for helping adjust one's behavior to the emerging reactions of others.
- *Social skills:* The ability to handle relationships with others is central to being perceived as popular, effective with others, and having the qualities of a leader.

Source: Adapted from Goleman 1998.

less than 10 minutes on any activity and that the supervisor in industry averaged one activity every 48 seconds. Mintzberg summarized his findings by saying that managers completed a great deal of work at an unrelenting pace, but the activities were characterized by variety, fragmentation, and brevity. Two decades later, the pace for managers has been unrelenting, with information overload and multitasking continuing to pose challenges.

Mintzberg's subsequent research with managers showed that their activities could usually be described by 10 roles organized into three categories (table 22.2):

- *Interpersonal activity* arises from the manager's formal authority in the organization and is supportive of the informational and decisional activities. It includes the roles of figurehead for ceremonial and formal occasions, of leader for motivating and using power, and of liaison to link and network for information and support.

- *Informational activity* includes the roles of monitor of performance information, disseminator of values and information, and spokesperson for the organization with outside groups.

- *Decisional activity* includes the roles of entrepreneur to promote improvement

and change, disturbance handler to deal with disruptions, resource allocator for overseeing resources and setting priorities, and negotiator for making arrangements with other organizations. (Mintzberg 1992)

Six of the 10 roles have been found to characterize the activities of healthcare managers: leader, liaison, monitor, entrepreneur, disturbance handler, and resource allocator (Guo 2003). These roles are intricately intertwined and not easily separated by a particular problem when it comes to team management, where responsibilities are often distributed among team members. However, they provide a realistic portrayal of the wide range of skilled behaviors required of effective managers.

In healthcare, as well as other fields of management, decisions tend to be based more often on political and value considerations than on empirical sources. However, with the increased interest in alternative approaches to healthcare (for example, acupuncture and nutrition) and to healthcare delivery in order to reduce errors, decrease costs, improve outcomes of care, and reduce liabilities; an emphasis on **evidence-based management**, or information-based management, is emerging in which more informed decisions are made based on the best clinical and research evidence that

Table 22.2.   Mintzberg's managerial roles

Managerial activity	Related roles
Interpersonal	- *Figurehead:* The manager represents the organization and is a symbol for ceremonial, social, legal, and inspirational duties. - *Liaison:* The manager maintains networks of relationships outside his or her organizational unit to gather information and favors. - *Leader:* The manager directs, guides, motivates, and develops subordinates.
Informational	- *Monitor:* The manager oversees internal and external information sources. - *Disseminator:* The manager communicates facts and values to others in the organization. - *Spokesperson:* The manager communicates with others outside the organization.
Decisional	- *Entrepreneur:* The manager promotes development and planned change in the organization. - *Disturbance handler:* The manager resolves crises and unexpected problems. - *Resource allocator:* The manager uses authority to allocate budget, personnel, equipment, services, and facilities. - *Negotiator:* The manager resolves dilemmas and disputes and determines the use of resources.

Source: Mintzberg 1989.

proposed practices will work. For example, a project at the Visiting Nurse Service of New York (VNSNY) developed a new model integrating separate evidence-based and practice improvement models. The researchers found that too often evidence-based information was collected but not disseminated nor applied adequately. At the same time, the practitioner model, while eager to implement improvement, often did not utilize current and comprehensive information. The blending of these models enabled a decrease in patients' pain levels, improved quality of life, improved nurse–physician communication, and improved case management (Levin et al. 2010).

Check Your Understanding 22.2

Instructions: **Answer the following questions on a separate piece of paper.**

1. Consider a job description for a position you have held or are working toward. What is the distribution of conceptual, interpersonal, and technical skills required?

2. Draw an organizational chart of your college, a hospital, or some other organization with which you are familiar. Be sure to designate both line and staff positions.

3. *Quality* is a term that is widely used and can have many meanings. What does quality mean in your work? Identify several tasks you perform, define quality for each task, and consider how you would measure it.

4. Discuss reasons for the four management functions changing in emphasis over the three levels of management. Why do you think leadership functions, usually reserved for the top, are now emphasized more for front line managers?

5. Interview a manager regarding daily and weekly activities they engage in. Then, categorize the activities into Mintzberg's 10 managerial roles.

Trends in Management Theory

As change drivers have an impact on the healthcare marketplace, organizations must adapt in order to survive and thrive. Management theories become a guide for thinking about the structure and processes by which business is conducted. As the marketplace changes, old theories may lose their explanatory power and be replaced with more relevant theories and principles for managing the organization. In general, there has been a shift in paradigm from more traditional hierarchical, centralized, and uniform approaches, to those that are more flexible, adaptive, and that utilize the advantages of technology. Table 22.3 differentiates the factors in a traditional management paradigm with the factors in the new management paradigm. At the same time, as managers become accustomed to, and develop expertise with, a certain viewpoint, they may become biased in its use and fail to see exceptions to it. A requisite skill for managers is to know when to use a particular framework and when to change it.

Although managers at the turn of the 20th century faced a host of changes, the unrelenting pace of change is even more constant for managers today. The successful manager must be able to see patterns of change and prepare others to respond to them.

Problem Solving and Decision Making

Problems are impediments to the attainment of goals. While some managers view problems as

Table 22.3. Paradigm shift in management

Traditional management paradigm	New management paradigm
Multilevel hierarchical organization	Flatter, distributed organization
Centralized decision making	Decentralized decision making
Status measured by amount of turf controlled	Status measured by success in achieving outcomes
Funding inputs and intentions	Funding outcomes
Face-to-face interaction	Telecommunication and virtual interaction
Homogenous staffing	Workforce diversity
Job description	Skill portfolio
Annual strategic plan	Learning organization
Financial bottom line	Triple bottom line
Efficiency and stability	Ongoing innovation
Mass services	Market segmentation
Work at central office	Work at satellite and home offices

negative and something to be avoided, problem solving can also be viewed as an opportunity for managers and organizations to build experience and resilience. Solving problems requires that they be framed or defined in useful and understandable ways. Problem solving involves understanding and resolving the barriers to goal attainment, while decision making refers to making the best choices from among available alternatives.

Two primary responsibilities of managers are solving problems and making decisions. In the early years of management practice, these activities were often based on personal preferences and limited experience, with little regard for long-term consequences. Since then, however, formal models of dealing with issues have been developed, and managers are encouraged to proceed systematically through several stages, including:

1. Defining the problem and the desired outcome
2. Analyzing and understanding the nature of the problem
3. Generating alternatives
4. Selecting desired alternatives (decision making)
5. Planning and implementing the alternative
6. Evaluating and gathering feedback about the attained outcome

At each step in the problem-solving model, decisions need to be made that lead to the final choice of how to implement a means for solving the problem. However, given the changing circumstances of the modern healthcare marketplace, as well as complexity of large organizations and ambiguity of many health conditions, it is not always possible to arrive at high certainty in decisions. Frequent review of procedures, reliance on best practices and evidence-based information, and integration of multidisciplinary sources contributes to the best available decisions.

Programmed and Nonprogrammed Decisions

Decisions can be programmed or nonprogrammed. **Programmed decisions** are those in which a problem is so predictable, uniform, and recurring that rules have been developed to standardize or automate the procedure (Stair and Reynolds 2012). Such rules enable managers to delegate authority to others to make decisions using predetermined criteria or to develop expert systems in which computers can make decisions. An example of such automation is an inventory system that automatically requests an order for restocking by a supplier when stock reaches a certain level.

Nonprogrammed decisions involve situations that are unpredictable, extremely complex, ill-defined or that are not easily quantified (Stair and Reynolds 2012). These situations defy simple decision criteria and usually require careful deliberation, often in consultation with others. Examples of nonprogrammed decisions include those found in developing training for new employees with variable skill levels, revising food choices in the hospital cafeteria, and whether to rebuild a hospital that has been damaged by tornado or flood.

Groupthink: The Hazards of Team Decision Making

Groupthink refers to the tendency of a highly cohesive team to seek consensus, often at the detriment of sound decision making. Research has shown this tendency to be relatively widespread and occurs when a team is very cohesive, there is high external pressure to perform, and few mechanisms are in place to correct for poor decision making (Janis 1972). It has been found to occur across diverse fields including healthcare, business, politics, law, education, and financial institutions.

Most work teams desire to have high cohesion: close familiarity and homogeneity of styles, strong pride in and commitment to the team, and a shared mission and vision (Michalisin et al. 2004). The problem arises when cohesion is so high and pressure to succeed so great that interpersonal pressure is exerted on members to conform to team processes that can result in poor decisions. Research suggests that some of the precipitating factors that contribute to groupthink are not as strong as once believed; nonetheless, the effects of group conformity on decision making is everpresent (Baron 2005; Snell 2010).

Conditions for the Emergence of Groupthink

There are eight symptoms of groupthink and they are clustered around three risky tendencies:

- *Overconfidence* in the team's prowess can manifest as an illusion of invulnerability that leads team members to be overconfident and take excessive risks. They develop a collective rationalization that is used to discount warnings that would otherwise lead them to reconsider their underlying assumptions.
- *Tunnel vision* restricts the range of factors considered and can lead to a belief in the inherent morality of their cause, thereby

allowing decision makers to ignore the ethical consequences of their decisions. Outsiders are often viewed in stereotypical ways in which their threats are minimized.

- *Team pressures* further contribute to groupthink. Loyal members will disapprove of a member who questions the team and bring sanctions until he or she again conforms. Members also may self-censor when it appears that there is silent consensus, tunnel vision for viewing the problem, and group pressure to conform. (Janis 1972)

Figure 22.10 elaborates further on the symptoms of groupthink categorized around these three areas.

Consequences of Groupthink

The pressures to conform in groupthink often result in the restriction of information and the risk of poor decision making. Such restrictions can limit considerations of objectives, information search, alternative courses of action, examination of the risks of the preferred choice, and reassessment of the preferred choice. Moreover, they can bias the discussion and processing of the problem-solving process and lead to a level of confidence that results in contingency plans being ignored or minimized.

Countermeasures for Groupthink

The conditions that contribute to groupthink are widespread, and it requires deliberate action by the team to minimize their adverse effects. By being aware of the risk of groupthink, alert to the symptoms, and intentionally implementing countermeasures, the team can maintain adequate cohesion without sacrificing decision quality. Instruments such as the Groupthink Profile (Swenson 2003) and Predictors of Groupthink Survey (Baptist 2015), enable the team to better assess and discuss the implications of team cohesion, organizational self-correcting processes, pressure on the team, symptoms of groupthink, and countermeasures.

The use of countermeasures is especially important, and they can be internal or external to team operation. Internal procedures used by the team to reduce risk include using brainstorming, revisiting important decisions, monitoring the degree of consensus and disagreement, rotating the devil's

Figure 22.10.   Symptoms of groupthink

Team's overestimation of its own power and morality
- *Illusion of invulnerability*. The illusion that they cannot go wrong leads to excessive optimism and risk taking.
- *Unquestioned belief in team's inherent morality*. Members believe their actions are correct, leading them to ignore moral and ethical implications.

Closed-mindedness
- *Team rationalization to discount warnings*. Team members collectively minimize indications that would otherwise lead them to reconsider their assumptions and commitments.
- *Stereotypes of the opposition*. Outsiders are viewed as negative, evil, or stupid to justify negotiations or to consider they could counter the team's efforts.

Pressure toward uniformity
- *Self-censorship*. Members tend to minimize and withhold expression of their dissenting views and counterarguments.
- *Illusion of shared unanimity*. Self-censorship and the false belief that silence means consent lead to the shared illusion that everyone agrees with the decision.
- *Pressure to conform*. Members who deviate from team norms by expressing doubts or arguing against the team's position are implicitly and explicitly pressured to conform.
- *Self-appointed "mind guards."* Some members appoint themselves to protect the team from adverse information that might challenge their illusions.

Source: Adapted from Janis 1972.

advocate's role among members, actively seeking contradictory information, and developing norms to challenge and question each other. In addition, the leader can refrain from stating an opinion that might affect others' opinions too early, and the team might be divided into subgroups to encourage different conclusions. External procedures that utilize resources outside the team include discussing decisions with outside experts and non–team members and inviting external observers to provide feedback on meetings, decisions, and team processes. Such procedures increase awareness of group processes and enhance skills at arriving at better decisions.

Check Your Understanding 22.3

Instructions: **Answer the following questions on a separate sheet of paper.**

1. What are some indications that cohesion has become excessive (for example, signs of groupthink)?

2. What are the advantages and disadvantages of having a highly homogeneous and cohesive team tasked with creating innovative strategy?

3. What are five key points in forming a diverse team membership?

4. Think of a highly cohesive team of which you have been a member. What are some events and activities that created and enhanced the cohesion felt?

5. Assume you are called in by an executive who is concerned about a team that is too cohesive and experiencing groupthink. What are some suggestions you can make to reduce the groupthink of the team?

Trends in Leadership Theory

The purpose of a theory is to serve as a guide for examining a phenomenon, such as leadership. The theory labels important features, then uses them to describe, explain, and help predict what might happen if certain actions were pursued. The idea that leadership makes a difference is undisputed, but exactly how and why it makes a difference is still not well understood, and research reflects an inconsistent picture. For example, leadership has been found to be related to formation of employees' values, commitment (Lee 2005), empowerment and team effectiveness (Ozaralli 2003), cohesion, commitment, trust, and motivation (Zhu et al. 2004). The work climate of an organization has been found to account for 30 percent of variance in financial performance, and leadership style accounts for 50 to 70 percent of variance in climate (Hay Group 2010). In a study of nearly 18,000 hospital employees, it was found that the higher leader effectiveness was rated, the higher the healthcare organization was rated, and the fewer patient complaints (Shipton et al. 2008).

The Accountable Care Act has reinvigorated emphasis on the role of leadership in healthcare. The titles of senior managers in organizations has been relabeled as "leaders," and such titles have been shifted downward to middle managers as well. The point of these title and role shifts is to recognize the importance of strategic thinking throughout healthcare, not just at the top (Lindsey and Mitchell 2012). However, a Center for Creative Leadership study (2011) of nearly 35,000 healthcare professionals identified gaps between current leadership strengths and areas of need. Leaders were rated low on several important abilities including the ability to lead employees, confronting problem employees, building and mending relationships, and participative management. Another study showed that a gap remains for women in leadership roles in healthcare, despite their having more of a collaborative leadership style that is much needed (McDonough et al. 2014).

Classical Approaches to Leadership Theory

Classical leadership theories tended to focus on the principled and effective use of authority. This emphasis began to change with the many social changes emerging in the early to mid-1900s. Inventions and innovations in manufacturing increased competition, which made managers more open to new ideas. Workers became increasingly better educated and skilled, thereby requiring managers with authoritative styles to adopt more democratic approaches. The workforce also became increasingly diverse, much like today, and this required a broader understanding of different cultures and motivational approaches.

Great Person Theory

The course of human history is marked with the contributions of great people. **Great person theory** is based on the belief that such outstanding individuals originally led to the conception of leadership as an inborn ability, sometimes passed down through family, position, or social tradition, as in the cases of royal families in many parts of the world. The problem with the great person theory is that some of those who took positions of such greatness were terribly lacking, as in the case of such historical notables as Caligula in ancient Rome, Stalin in Russia, and Kim Jung Il in North Korea. In the United States, there have been people who were leaders in one sphere but who failed in others. For example, General Ulysses S. Grant excelled as a general, which largely got him elected president, a role in which he performed poorly (Waugh 2009).

Trait Approach

The **trait approach** gradually replaced the great person model and proposed that leaders possessed a collection of traits or personal behaviors and attributes that distinguished them from nonleaders. During the 1930s and 1940s, hundreds of studies on the trait approach to leadership were conducted, and as many as 18,000 traits were identified (Allport and Odbert 1936). Traits were often grouped into categories related to physical needs, values, intellect, personality, and skill characteristics. Some researchers have organized traits on the three leadership requirements of conceptual, interpersonal, and technical skills. Others add a fourth category—administrative skills—which includes the four managerial functions of planning, organizing, directing, and controlling (Yukl 2006).

Unfortunately, in much of the early research, only a weak relationship was discovered between traits and individuals who would emerge as leaders, and many leaders did not share all the traits in common. During later studies in which traits and skills were correlated with leader effectiveness rather than leader emergence, stronger connections appeared. Some of the more important traits included adaptability, social alertness, ambition, assertiveness, cooperativeness, decisiveness, dominance, energy, stress tolerance, and confidence. Skills included intelligence and conceptual abilities, creativity, tact, verbal fluency, work knowledge, organization, and persuasion (Stogdill 1974). Despite this extensive work, it appears that no single traits are absolutely required for leadership. Having certain traits and skills leads to a greater likelihood that such attributes may be more helpful in some situations and to leader effectiveness in them.

Autocratic vs. Democratic Leadership

In McGregor's formulation of **theory X and Y**, two types of environments and leaders corresponded to autocratic and democratic behaviors (McGregor 1960). Robert White and Ronald Lippitt (1960), researchers at Iowa State University, conducted studies on democratic and autocratic leaders. They found that groups under **autocratic leadership**, where the manager made decisions without others' input and gave very specific direction, performed well as long as they were closely supervised; although levels of member satisfaction were low. In contrast, **democratic leadership** that involved members in decision making led members to perform well whether the leader was present or absent, and members were more satisfied. This kind of research led to the emphasis on participative management in many organizations. The autocratic–democratic dimension was useful for understanding a range of managerial behavior that could be applied across different settings.

Based on the autocractic–democratic dimension, Robert Tannenbaum and Warren Schmidt (1973) designed a continuum that described seven degrees of leader involvement in decision making (see figure 22.11). At one end (autocratic) of the continuum, the leader makes a decision alone and announces it; at the other end (democratic), the leader encourages his or her employees to make their own decisions within prescribed limits. This model was new in that it reflected a shift from looking at the leader in isolation or in terms of a rigid or permanent style and suggested that a person had available a range of behaviors depending on the situation. But what behaviors made leaders successful?

Figure 22.11. Tannenbaum and Schmidt's leadership continuum

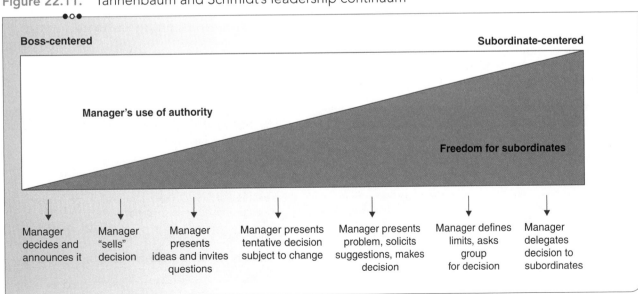

Source: Tannenbaum and Schmidt 1973.

Behavioral Theories of Leadership

While earlier theories focused on what leaders *should* do and what was expected of them, emerging behavioral theories describe what managers *actually* do. The emerging theories clearly emphasize a leader's orientation toward both tasks and people and enabled leaders to describe a variety of styles rather than just the "right" style.

Figure 22.12. Normative decision tree

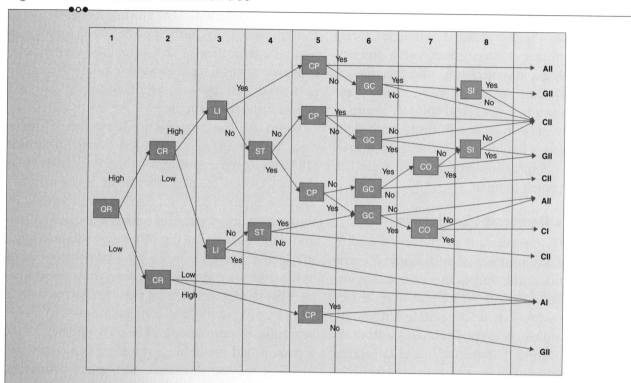

At each step in the process, a question is asked and the response determines the next branch and question. Each node of the tree has a critical criterion for determining the outcome, including:

- *Quality requirement (QR):* How important is the technical quality of the decision?
- *Commitment requirement (CR):* How important is subordinate commitment to the decision?
- *Leader's information (LI):* Do you (the leader) have sufficient information to make a high-quality decision on your own?
- *Problem structure (ST):* Is the problem well structured (for example, defined, clear, organized, lends itself to solution, time limited)?
- *Commitment probability (CP):* If you were to make the decision by yourself, is it reasonably certain that your subordinates would be committed to it?
- *Goal congruence (GC):* Do subordinates share the organizational goals to be attained in solving the problem?
- *Subordinate conflict (CO):* Is conflict among subordinates over preferred solutions likely?
- *Subordinate information (SI):* Do subordinates have sufficient information to make a high-quality decision?

Decision outcome	Description
Autocratic I (AI)	Leader solves the problem alone using information that is readily available.
Autocratic II (AII)	Leader obtains additional information from group members, then makes decision alone. Group members may or may not be informed.
Consultative I (CI)	Leader shares problem with group members individually and asks for information and evaluation. Group members do not meet collectively, and leader makes decision alone.
Consultative II (CII)	Leader shares problem with group members collectively but makes decision alone.
Group II (GII)	Leader meets with group to discuss situation. Leader focuses and directs discussion but does not impose will. Group makes final decision.

Source: Decision Methods for Group and Individual Problems and Decision-Process Flow Chart for Both Individual and Group Problems from *Leadership and Decision-Making*, by Victor H. Vroom and Philip W. Yelton, ©1973. Reprinted by permission of the University of Pittsburgh Press.

Normative Decision Tree

Using a continuum similar to Tannenbaum and Schmidt's, Victor Vroom and Philip Yetton (1971) developed the **normative decision model** in the early 1970s. They identified a series of intermediate questions and decisions that could be answered yes or no and that would lead to each outcome. See figure 22.12 for an example of the normative decision model. Crucial aspects of the situation related to the quality of the decision required, the degree of subordinate support for the decision, the amount of information available to leaders and followers, and how well structured or defined the problem was. A decision made exclusively by the leader without member input (autocratic) could create problems in acceptance, just as delegating a decision to a group (democratic) could be costly in time and effort, if unnecessary. The Vroom-Yetton model enables a manager to decide on the level of decision-making involvement (autonomous, consultative, or delegative) to seek out when approaching a decision situation.

Ohio and Michigan Studies

During the 1950s and 1960s, researchers at The Ohio State University examined the behavior of leaders in several hundred studies and reduced them to two categories: consideration or relationship orientation and initiating structure or task orientation (Shartle 1979). **Consideration** referred to attention to the interpersonal aspects of work, including respecting subordinates' ideas and feelings, maintaining harmonious work relationships, collaborating in teamwork, and showing concern for the subordinates' welfare. **Initiating structure** was more task focused and centered on giving direction, setting goals and limits, and planning and scheduling activities. During the same period, researchers at the University of Michigan developed a similar model. Comparing effective and ineffective managers, they found that a key difference was that the effective employee-centered managers focused more on the human needs of their subordinates whereas their less effective task-oriented managers emphasized only goal attainment (Likert 1979). This distinction led to the development of several assessment tools or inventories that helped identify a manager's preference or managerial style.

Leadership Grid

Building on the Ohio State and Michigan studies, Robert Blake and Jane Srygley Mouton (1976) at the University of Texas identified the same two dimensions: concern for people (consideration) and concern for production (initiating structure). Their leadership grid marked off degrees of emphasis a leader may have toward people or production using a nine-point scale and finally separated the grid into five styles of management based on the combined people and production emphasis. For example, a score of 9,9 (emphasizing both people and production) was called "Team Management." Blake and Mouton considered it the best orientation, or preference, because it emphasized harmonious cooperation in production to achieve goals. A score of 9,1, an "Authority-Compliance" orientation with an emphasis on production and operational efficiency, afforded little attention to human needs. The 1,9 "Country Club" orientation emphasized group harmony, esprit de corps, and cooperation over production. The 1,1 "Impoverished" orientation reflected inattention toward both relationships and work production. A mix of both dimensions, but less than a team orientation, is the 5,5 "Middle-of-the-Road" approach, which tries to balance the two (see figure 22.13 for an example). Although this model has been considered a key theory and it clearly presents a collaborative or team management approach as the ideal approach, subsequent contingency theories show that there are situations in which other emphases may be as effective. Like the Ohio and Michigan inventories, the managerial grid was widely used for leadership training and development.

Contingency and Situational Theories of Leadership

Most of these early theories of leadership have emphasized identifying a cluster of traits or a single style or orientation for leadership. As research in leadership has continued, it has become apparent that successful leadership does not de-

Figure 22.13.   Leadership matrix models

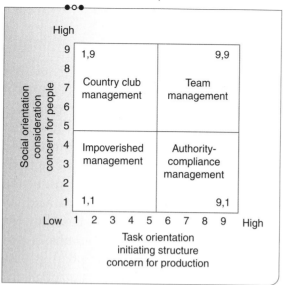

Source: Blake and Mouton 1976.

- **Task structure** is related to task dimension described by other theories and refers to how clearly and how well defined the task goals, procedures, and possible solutions are.
- **Position power** refers to the authority the leader has to direct others and to use reward and coercive power. (Fiedler 1967)

In general, the **contingency theory of leadership** contends that the greater the favorability toward the leader, the more the subordinates can be relied on to carry out the task and the fewer challenges to leadership. Situations more favorable to leadership are those in which leader–member relations are positive, task structure is high, and position power is high. Situations in which these factors are reversed are considered unfavorable to leaders because they have less leverage to influence their followers.

pend on style or skills alone but, rather, on matching a leader's style with the changing demands or contingencies of a specific situation.

Fiedler's Contingency Theory

Fred Fiedler (1967) a management psychologist at the University of Illinois designed his contingency model of leadership to compensate for the limitations of the classical and behavioral theories of leadership. Fiedler kept the social-task orientation as the cornerstone of his theory and designed a brief test, the **least-preferred coworker (LPC) scale**, to assess the degree to which a manager was task or relationship oriented. This information was used to help determine if that style was most appropriate or favorable for the situation in which leaders found themselves.

The second aspect of Fiedler's model was the favorability of the situation in which the leader would operate. Because contingency means "depends on," the favorability or fit of a leader depends on the following three situational factors:

- **Leader–member relations**, or "group atmosphere," is much like social orientation and includes the subordinates' acceptance of, and confidence in, the leader as well as the loyalty and commitment they show toward the leader.

Hersey and Blanchard's Situational Theory

One of the more popular leadership models still widely used for training, and one that has attempted to integrate other ideas from management, is Paul Hersey and Kenneth Blanchard's **situational theory of leadership** (Hersey et al. 1996). *Situational* in this case refers to the idea that the leader's style should be adjusted to different situations and employees encountered.

To the already widely used task and social dimensions, Hersey and Blanchard added a third: the maturity of the followers. **Worker immaturity–maturity** is a concept that suggests that job maturity and psychological maturity of subordinates also influence leadership style. Job maturity refers to how much work-related ability, knowledge, experience, and skill a person has; psychological maturity refers to willingness, confidence, commitment, and motivation related to work. Behaviors associated with maturity include initiative, dependability, perseverance, receptiveness to feedback, goal orientation, and minimal need for supervision. To apply a directive approach with mature workers can result in stifling their maturity and even in forcing them back to lower levels of maturity

Figure 22.14. Worker immaturity–maturity continuum

Immature	Mature
Passive	Active
Dependence	Independence
Few behavior choices	Diverse behavior
Limited interests	Deep and varied interests
Short time perspective	Past and future perspective
Subordinate position	Superordinate position
Lack self-awareness	Self-awareness and control

Source: Adapted from Argyris 1957.

(Argyris 1957). Hence, adjusting leadership style to worker maturity is an important consideration (see figure 22.14).

Hersey and Blanchard also adapted the grid format of their predecessors and structured it in a developmental sequence. Borrowing the idea that teams and organizations progress through developmental stages of a life cycle (Edison 2008) (Hwang and Park 2007), they suggested that leadership style should be adjusted to the stage of team development. For example, their Situation-1 (S1) involves high-task but low-social emphasis, thereby indicating that the leader should focus on task duties such as setting goals, identifying resources and constraints, and so on. As the team moves to Situation-2 (S2), task and social functions of the leader are both involved as members attempt to influence each other and to explore how their styles may conflict with or complement each other. In Situation-3 (S3), members clearly know the task and need little direction, but social interaction around team norms may require intervention and guidance. Finally, Situation-4 (S4) is the stage of high team performance in which both task and relationships require little intervention by the leader. Worker maturity is high, and the leader may be active only in encouraging higher performance and removing barriers to performance.

Path–Goal Theory

Another model of leadership, initially introduced by Robert House in 1971 and revised in 1996, is path–goal theory. While other theories have focused on the motivation of the leader, the path–goal theory (House 1996) examines the motives and needs of the subordinates and how the leader can respond to them. This theory was based on the **expectancy theory of motivation**, which proposes that one's degree of effort is influenced by the expectation that the effort will result in the attainment of desired goals and meaningful rewards. **Path–goal theory** states that a person's ability to perform certain tasks is related to the direction and clarity available that lead to organizational goals. For example, if a worker is unclear about what a task involves and what should be done, performance will be improved when clear instructions are given. The role of leaders, then, is to facilitate the path toward the goal by removing barriers to performance.

Path–goal theory identifies four different situations, each requiring a different facilitative response from leadership (see figure 22.15). When workers lack self-confidence, leaders provide support by being friendly, approachable, concerned about needs, and equitable. This increases the worker's confidence to achieve the work outcome. When the worker has an ambiguous job, the leader is more forthright in providing the worker with direction, schedules, rules, and regulations that clarify the path. When workers do not have sufficient job challenge, the leader uses an achievement approach by setting challenging goals, continually seeking improvement, and expecting high performance. Finally, when the reward is mismatched with worker needs, the leader takes a more consultative or participative role in which workers share work problems, make suggestions, and are included in decision making to ensure more appropriate rewards. All four strategies result in improved task performance and satisfaction—again, the task and social dimensions.

The path–goal theory is clearly applicable in the area of healthcare. The healthcare industry, including the role of HIM, is constantly changing requiring new job responsibilities for HIM staff. If a release of information specialist now needs to look into the new document imaging

Figure 22.15. Path–goal theory

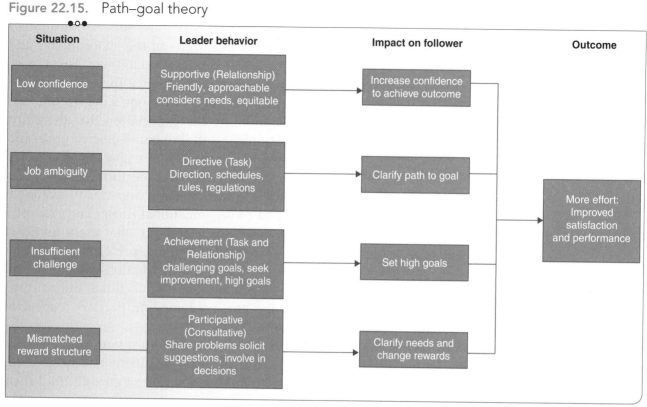

Source: Adapted from House 1996.

system for health records, clear direction on how to find records in that system is critical or some portions of a patient's record may inadvertently be omitted when filling the request for information. There are many examples of change related to new regulations and technology in HIM work that require clear and comprehensive direction for staff to be effective, such as transcriptionist roles moving from transcribing to auditing, coders requiring full knowledge of where all parts of the health record can be found in the electronic health record (EHR), or registration staff understanding enhanced procedures for patient identification.

Dyadic Relationship Theory

Some leadership theories are macro theories and attempt to explain leadership across large domains, but there also are micro theories that focus on a specific context for leadership. Leader–member exchange (LMX) (Graen and Skandura 1987) and

closely related vertical dyad linkage (VDL) represent micro theories that focus on dyadic relationships, or those between two people or between a leader and a small group. More specifically, they explain how in-group and out-group relationships form with a leader or mentor and how delegation may occur.

Vertical dyad linkage (VDL) was first formulated in 1975 (Dansereau et al. 1975) to describe the single-person mentoring relationships that occur in organizations and was later supplemented by **leader–member exchange (LMX)** theory, which applied the same idea to the leader's relations with groups. In these situations, leaders look for subordinates with high-performance and leadership potential that distinguishes them from subordinates with less potential. The best predictors of being selected for in-group, in addition to competence, include compatibility of the subordinate with the leader, interpersonal liking for each other, and being extraverted. Once identified, the leader and subordinate form an **exchange relationship**, in which a leader offers greater opportunities and privileges to a subordinate in exchange for loyalty, commitment, and assistance. The leader may delegate special responsibilities, offer interesting and desirable tasks, give opportunities for highly visible or skill-building projects, and provide mentoring.

Those subordinates who form a group around the leader are referred to as the **in-group**; those subordinates not included form the **out-group**. Being in the in-group may sound attractive, but it involves performance beyond the call of duty. In-group members may spend longer hours, take work home or work during off-hours, and take on more difficult tasks compared to members in the out-group. The out-group expects to be treated fairly by the leader, and as long as the exchanges are viewed as fair, there is little or no conflict between the in- and out-groups; they can remain fairly stable over time. However, when the out-group perceives that the in-group is receiving greater privileges for doing the same work as the out-group, the latter can feel resentment, alienation, and hostility and show lower performance. The leader must ensure fair treatment and clear expectations for both groups. In addition, leaders can promote high-quality relationships with all employees by speaking with people personally, using active listening, not imposing the leader's view on issues discussed, and sharing expectations about the job and working relationship. A 2008 study of the theory supported its key hypothesis that when there was variance in employees' perceptions of equity and fairness, this negatively affected job satisfaction and feelings of well-being (Hooper and Martin 2008).

LMX theory is somewhat different from other leadership theories in that it emphasizes the interaction and quality of the relationship between leader and follower rather than just leadership behavior alone or the same approach applied to everyone. In a review of LMX literature related to HIM, favorable benefits to both leaders and followers were found (Hunt 2014).

These included enhanced group performance, self-efficacy, more initiative, reasonable risk taking, lower turnover, job satisfaction, higher trust levels with supervisors, and career advancement (Hunt 2014).

Aspects of the personality of the leader are projected into one's leadership style, the latter of which may have some variance from situation to situation. This style is perceived by and interacts with employee attitudes and team functioning to facilitate the performance of others. This performance is finally expressed in organizational performance and its success or failure (Hogan and Kaiser 2004).

Values-Based Leadership

At the core of healthcare are strong values for caring, compassion, and service, especially to persons in high need or disadvantaged (Faith 2013). Values are core beliefs that guide and motivate attitudes and actions and both form and express an organization's culture. Values make a difference to most people, and ethical leaders tend to promote more trust and loyalty among their employees (Sanford 2006; Verbos et al. 2007).

Role of Values

"Everything a leader does sets a tone," especially regarding ethics, according to a National Business Ethics Survey (Ethics Research Center 2015). Both top leaders as well as direct supervisors were found to have an important role in modeling and supporting ethical behavior and corporate values. Employees who believe managers and leaders are transparent and honest in their communication are more likely to conduct themselves ethically as well as report bad behavior.

However, one of the significant consequences of the organization and its leaders not being perceived as highly ethical is that employees feel less loyalty and commitment and tend to leave the organization (Trevino and Nelson 2011). In a 2015 survey of over 80,000 people on employee engagement, the Gallup polling organization reported that slightly less than a third of employees nationally were enthusiastic about and committed to their jobs and workplace (Adkins 2015).

Value-based healthcare is replacing volume-driven organizations, but is a challenging transformation to shift from fee-for-service to outcomes, patience satisfaction, and quality; and perceptions of culture are important for morale and quality. Organizations that make efforts to build an ethical culture have lower levels of staff turnover (Simha and Cullen 2012), and savings in cost and resources (Guerci et al. 2015). To retain talented people as well as to maintain a competitive position, organizational leadership must reestablish and promote ethical behavior and a culture of strong, consistent, and compatible values.

Many organizations believe that merely sending managers off to training will provide sufficient skill in ethical management. However, to fully effect change, managers and leaders must not just learn about but implement the values to be developed in an organization into their own behavior.

That ethics is increasingly a high priority and visible issue is shown by the Ethisphere 2015 report on and promotion of the "World's Most Ethical Companies." For this recognition they defined *ethical performance* as proactive engagement in the communities they serve; investment in quality and innovative, sustainable business practices; and efforts made to influence and change the industry and profit fairly. In healthcare, they recognized Baptist Health South Florida, Cleveland Clinic, Hospital Corporation of America, Northshore-LIJ Health System, and University Hospitals. Novation LLC and Premier, Inc., were other US healthcare services identified with notable ethical practices (Ethisphere 2015).

Yet such awards are bittersweet, as the 2011 National Business Ethics Survey shows. The good news is that well-implemented ethics programs dramatically increase reports of misconduct, and in 2011 the percentage of employees who witnessed misconduct at work fell to a new low of 45 percent compared to 49 percent in 2009 and the record high of 55 percent in 2007. The bad news is that

> the share of companies with weak ethics cultures climbed to near record levels at 42 percent, up from 35 percent in 2009. The percentage of employees who perceived pressure to compromise standards in order to do their jobs climbed five points to 13 percent, just shy of the all-time high of 14 percent in 2000, and retaliation against employee whistle-blowers rose sharply. More than one in five employees (22 percent) who reported misconduct say they experienced some form of retaliation in return... compared to 12 percent who experienced retaliation in 2007 and 15 percent in 2009. (Ethics Resource Center 2012, 12)

To remedy these problems in ethical leadership, reinforcement of ethical practices at all levels of management and peer commitments to ethical practices are required so these practices become embedded in the organization's culture.

Servant Leadership

Values-based leadership refers to leadership behaviors that emphasize moral, authentic, and ethical orientations to how the organization and employees function (Copeland 2014). The values-based leadership theories are similar to Burns's (1978), transformational leadership in which an inspired and enthusiastic leader engages employees to strive toward higher vision for the organization and ethical performance for themselves. This is also similar to other contingency theories such as path–goal leadership in which the leader's role is to empower and facilitate employee satisfaction and productivity.

Prominent among values-based approaches is Robert Greenleaf's concept of **servant leadership** (Greenleaf 1991) in which the leader's role is viewed as serving others. Robert Greenleaf was director of management research at AT&T for 38 years, as well as a Quaker with a strong contemplative orientation. To Greenleaf, servant leaders are those who put the needs, interests, and aspirations of others above their own. A review of more than 100 characteristics of servant leadership in the literature has been condensed to 12 key values:

1. Valuing and being committed to people for who they are, not just what they bring to the organization

2. Humility by putting others first

3. Nonjudgmental listening to and understanding of others

4. Trusting others and being trustworthy through example

5. Showing caring, kindness, and concern for others

6. Integrity and consistency in living one's values

7. Service to others

8. Empower others and expect accountability

9. Serve others before self

10. Collaboration and building community

11. Love (for example, composite of acceptance, caring, appreciating, believing in the worth of others)

12. Continuous learning and personal growth (Focht and Ponton 2015)

Although servant leadership has mixed evidence to support its effectiveness largely due to its vague definition, its popularity has spread worldwide as well as to many of the best companies in the United States. It has also been explored in healthcare. Servant leadership has been found to impact the quality of relationship between healthcare leader and employees (Hanse et al. 2015), job satisfaction (Gunnarsdottir 2014), teamwork and patient outcomes (Trastek et al. 2014), customer satisfaction and financial performance (Jones 2012).

Complexity Leadership and Systems Thinking

Management guru, Peter Drucker gave the opinion that healthcare workplaces were "the most complex human organization(s) ever devised" (Drucker 2002). Healthcare organizations can be thought of as **complex adaptive systems** that refer to the complexity of structures and processes involved in healthcare, and the ongoing changes and rearrangements of these structures and processes. Such systems tend to have diverse values, individuals, and rules, and the parts and relationships reorganize as they continually learn about demands that impact them. An example might be a community health system comprised of many hospitals and clinics, pharmacies, long-term care facilities, online resources, and social networking (Martinez-Garcia and Hernandez-Lemus 2013). The interconnections among these and how they influence behavior and decision making can be mind-boggling and a source of emerging unexpected consequences, Healthcare leaders need to be able to tolerate the ambiguity that goes with such dynamic change, collaborate with diverse thinkers to help conceptualize and plan services, and identify feedback loops that can be used to anticipate change.

For example, although monitoring financial conditions have been the primary focus for generations, more currently there has been a recognition that considering additional factors should be included as criteria for healthcare performance success. For example, the balanced scorecard, triple bottom line, triple aim, and the Malcolm Baldrige Award all acknowledge the importance of interrelated and multi-criteria approach to evaluation. The balanced scorecard emphasizes the interaction among financial, operational, customer, and staff development factors. The triple bottom line goes beyond the traditional focus on finances and includes social and environmental factors. The triple aim focuses on improving the healthcare experience, improving the health of the population, and decreasing the cost. Finally, the Malcolm Baldrige National Quality Award is an annual presidential award for excellence based on the complex interaction of leadership, strategic planning, customer focus, analytics and knowledge management, workforce focus, operations focus, and results (Baldrige 2011).

The significance of these broader criteria underline the focus required for change leadership. Leaders must have an understanding of complex systems and how they interact to produce outcomes. Change strategies must include not only sound financial reasoning to reduce costs, but also create patient satisfaction and employee development, produce evidence-based outcomes, and demonstrate concern for impact on the environment.

Decision makers often focus on the immediate problem as defined and seek to find a single solution to that problem without seeking to understand the broader system that has enabled the problem to emerge in the first place. In addition, many problems are considered only in the context or department in which they occur, and the stream of events that have led to the problem may not have occurred within that department.

Furthermore, a solution may work within that department, but may cause more or worse problems downstream in other departments. Correcting this issue involves viewing more than just the simple cause and effect relationship between problem and solution, and it also needs to go further than just considering the immediate context or situation.

Systems thinking is based on understanding that a system refers to the interconnections among many components that make up a whole. In healthcare, systems thinking can involve many levels of people and actions involved in a single event, or it can involve an evolving complex of connections over time. Not taking time to understand the systemic connections can lead to neglecting factors that may be critical to patient care. For example, well-intentioned healthcare IT has sometimes produced complex system-related unintended consequences that has led to misinformation, used critical resources, and jeopardized patient safety (Ash et al. 2004).

One of the important concepts in systems thinking is that of feedback loops or causal loop diagrams (Maccoby et al. 2014). While we typically think of events as a linear series of actions, in many cases each action can have nonlinear spin-off events or lead back to the previous action, thereby making the series of events much more complex in determining what the outcome will be. For example, in a given community there are a certain number of potential healthcare users available (refer to figure 22.16). From this population, certain numbers of patients can be admitted for care who then occupy a limited number of available beds. Their occupancy and favorable treatment contributes to perceived hospital quality that in turn leads to more patients seeking admission. At the same time, there is a feedback loop resulting from long-term occupancy that limits new admissions. If this occurs too often, it could have the delayed negative effect on reputation of availability and therefore perceived hospital quality (see dotted line in figure 22.16).

Another slightly more complex situation is shown in figure 22.17. Imagine a situation in which the healthcare pressures to implement information systems combine with an organizational culture that is highly competitive and focused on tight timelines and high productivity. They have assigned the task of developing a data management system to a project team. Most projects cannot accurately estimate all of the requirements at the beginning, and often external stakeholders will add new requirements or change existing ones as needs become clearer. Such demands can lead to project teams taking on multiple and large projects with tight time frames and resulting in overtime.

Multitasking tends to lead teams to have changing membership (due to turnover and other team obligations), and adding more people to a team late in the task. Adding new team members reflects **Brooks's Law**, which states adding people actually slows down team productivity due to different work styles, low team cohesion, and learning curve or orientation to the task time (Brooks 1995). Multitasking also reduces work efficiency since it takes time to shift thinking between tasks. The combination of Brooks's Law and lower work efficiency leads to project delays. It is common in many organizations that when work falls behind, overtime is required and this is especially true of IT and project management teams. The extended overnight work on behind schedule tasks leads to fatigue and tension in team relationships as well as a greater number of errors. These in turn contribute to lower team morale that is critically needed on these kinds of projects and can likewise affect job satisfaction and even family relationships. In severe cases, this can lead to more team turnover. For what started as a well-intentioned strategic goal of taking on multiple projects and implementing a sound data management system, the actual results of multitasking, team dynamics, and fatigue unintentionally created more errors, delays, and perhaps lower patient care.

This scenario of unintentional consequences is a relatively common outcome from approaching complex problems with a simple solution mindset. Systems thinking is requisite for healthcare leaders that should be a cornerstone of strategic thinking and a shared skill among all leadership in the organization (de Savigny and Adam 2009; Trbovich 2014).

Figure 22.16. Causal loop systems view of hospital occupancy

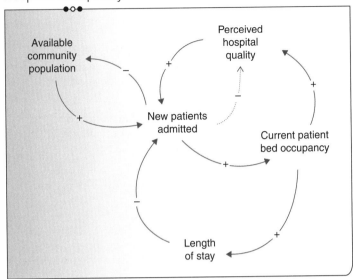

Note: Plus (+) signs indicate that a node increases the subsequent node; a negative (–) sign indicates it has a decreasing or inhibitory effect on the subsequent node.

Figure 22.17. A systems view of overtime effects

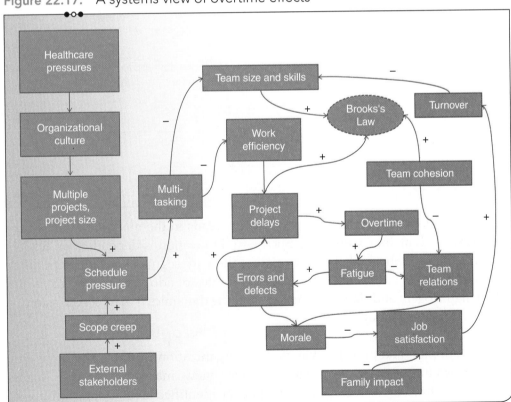

Note: Plus signs indicate that the next task is increased, while a minus sign indicates a decrease.

Source: Swenson 2014 .

Check Your Understanding 22.4

Instructions: **Answer the following questions on a separate piece of paper.**

1. Make a list of your traits and skills. Rank them in order of how effective they would make you as a leader in a given situation. Change the leadership situation and see which traits and skills might also change to give you an advantage or which ones might unexpectedly become a disadvantage. How could you develop these skills further?

2. Imagine you have been asked to be a consultant to an aspiring political or managerial figure. You are asked to recommend how this person should appear in order to increase his or her chances for election or promotion. What behaviors would you advise for and against? What ethical issues are involved in this type of image building?

3. Think of situations where you have noticed effective and ineffective leaders. What makes them different from each other? Consider their personalities, limitations in skills or adaptability, and changes in the situation, as well as what is required of them.

4. What are some work situations in which an autocratic style might be effective and appropriate?

5. Think of a decision that was made with good intentions but it produced some unintended consequences. See if you can draw a causal loop model of the sequence of events. If this sequence had been identified at the time of the decision, how might that have affected the plan?

6. Think of a decision you might have to make as a supervisor at work, such as assigning a complex and important project to an employee. Use the Vroom-Yetton decision tree to trace how you might choose whether to make the decision yourself, consult with others, or delegate the decision making to someone else.

7. Identify a project you have worked on that fell behind schedule. According to Brooks's Law, adding people would delay it further rather than speed progress. Why is that?

8. Think of people with whom you have worked who are at different stages of worker maturity. What are the behaviors that led you to place them along the immaturity–maturity continuum? What style would you use with them as a supervisor given their maturity levels? Explain what might happen if your style mismatches what they need at these stages.

9. Many problems are not as simple as they appear, and may have complex connections that appear overwhelming to people. What are some arguments you could make to encourage people to think more thoroughly and complexly about problem solving?

Diffusion of Innovations

Innovations have occurred throughout history, but little attention was given to exactly how they were adopted until Everett Rogers and Floyd Shoemaker (1971) clarified the process in their book, *Communication of Innovations.* Although Rogers and Shoemaker were not the first to develop ideas about how ideas were diffused and adopted, their presentation of the categories of innovation adopters and the diffusion curve came at a time when businesses were eager to understand consumer behavior. As organizational change is considered and innovations such as the EHR are introduced, understanding diffusion, or the way and rate of speed in which a new concept spreads in the market, becomes critical. Successful innovation is dependent on leaders appreciating the way segments of adopters differ, the stages and rates of adoption of new ideas and practices, and the dynamics that affect diffusion.

Categories of Adopter Groups

Viewing the organization in much the same way that marketers view market segments, Rogers and Shoemaker identified five adopter groups of an innovation that generally fits the normal curve (see figure 22.18 for a summary of the characteristics of each group). The percent of adopters in each group is estimated but is generally consistent across many types of organizations.

- **Innovators:** This venturesome group comprises about 2.5 percent of the organization and are individuals who are eager to try new ideas. These individuals tend to be more worldly and sophisticated, seek out new information in broad networks, and are more willing to take risks (Rogers 1995; Shoemaker 2010).

- **Early adopters:** This respectable group accounts for about 13.5 percent of the organization. The individuals in this group have a high degree of opinion leadership. They are more localized than worldly, and often look to the innovators for advice and information. These are the leaders and respected role models in the organization, and their adoption of an idea or practice does much to initiate change (Rogers 1995; Shoemaker 2010).

- **Early majority:** This group comprises about 34 percent of the organization. Although

usually not leaders, the individuals in this group represent the backbone of the organization, are deliberate in thinking about and accepting an idea, and serve as a natural bridge between early and late adopters (Shoemaker 2010)(Rogers 1995).

- **Late majority:** This skeptical group comprises another 34 percent of the organization. The individuals in this group usually adopt innovations only after social or financial pressure to do so (Rogers 1995; Shoemaker 2010).

- **Laggards:** The traditional members of this group are usually the last ones to respond to innovation and make up as much as 16 percent of the organization. The laggards are often characterized as isolated, uninformed, and mistrustful of change and promoters of change, but they may serve a function by keeping the organization from changing too quickly (Shoemaker 2010)(Rogers 1995).When planning a change, each of these groups should be considered as an internal market segment whose needs must be responded to by leaders. In general, people who are more receptive to innovation are better educated and more literate and have stronger aspirations. In addition, they have higher socioeconomic status, higher occupational prestige, more income, and greater social mobility. Moreover, they are better socially networked, cosmopolitan, diverse in interests, and well integrated into the organization and the community (Shoemaker 2010).

Diffusion Curve

Each of the adopter categories engages innovation at a different time and a different acceptance rate, as shown by the diffusion of innovation S curve (see figure 22.19). Note that during the early stages of diffusion, there is a shorter period between becoming aware of an innovation and adopting it. Over time, each adopter category becomes aware of the innovation but increasingly takes longer periods to adopt it, which can affect how well an innovation is introduced into the marketplace

Figure 22.18. Characteristics of innovation stakeholders

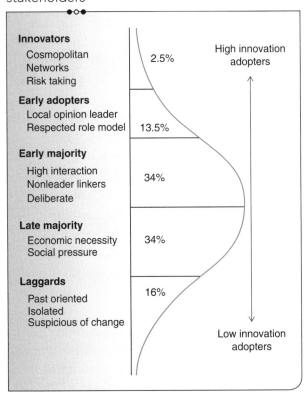

Source: Adapted from Shoemaker 2010.

Figure 22.19. Diffusion S curve

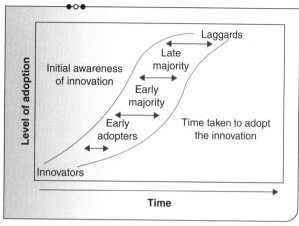

Source: Adapted from Rogers 1995.

or how fully it is practiced in the organization. In addition, how quickly an innovation is accepted is based on a number of factors, including whether it offers an advantage relative to its alternative, its compatibility with the potential adopters' values and lifestyles, how easy it is to understand and use, the degree to which it can be experimented with, and the degree to which the results are visible to others (Shoemaker 2010). These diffusion patterns are relatively consistent for a variety of healthcare innovations, including patient acceptance and use of consumer e-health innovations (Zhang et al. 2015), adoption of the EHR by physicians (Castillo et al. 2010), and consumer adoption of web-based health information portals (Baird et al. 2012).

Dynamics Affecting Innovation Diffusion

Innovations are often difficult for people to adopt, but they can be made more attractive when they meet certain conditions. In general, people are more responsive when a change is presented with consideration to these factors which include:

1. *Relative advantage.* Innovations are defined as having some advantage over what a person is already doing, and identifying improvements and advantages to work can help accept a change. For example, with a new technology, is it more secure, mobile, or easy to use over current technology? For an adopter, does the EHR provide an advantage over paper records?

2. *Compatibility.* This refers to how well the innovation matches or fits in with the adopter's needs, work pattern and style, personality, values, and other personal requirements.

3. *Simplicity.* Some innovations are too complex and easily overwhelm people, and EHRs are no exception. If they can first be presented simply and with fewer choices, they can be expanded to greater complexity later.

4. *Trialability.* Being able to try or experiment with an innovation can reduce the anxiety of making an initial commitment. Working with smaller parts of an innovation or implementing in stages can enable people to become more comfortable with the change.

5. *Observability.* If the advantages of an innovation are readily observable to oneself and others, it is more likely to be adopted. Unfortunately, many EHR implementations are not particularly eventful, but satisfaction and successes should be shared among users.

6. *Communication channels.* Identifying the pathways that are used by opinion leaders to influence adoption can improve the diffusion.

7. *Homogeneous groups.* Innovations tend to spread faster among groups who share similar characteristics, as opposed to heterogeneous groups who differ in important ways.

8. *Pace of innovation/reinvention.* Some innovations are relatively stable over time, while others are more dynamic and may be changed by adopters as they are used.

9. *Norms, roles, and social networks.* The culture, climate, norms, and social rules tend to shape and modify innovations to fit that system. Culture usually wins out over strategy.

10. *Opinion leaders.* The pace of diffusion can be affected by the influence of leaders and other respected and key persons.

11. *Infrastructure.* Adoption can be further influenced by the support structures available such as technologies that are related to the innovation (Cain and Mittman 2002; Shoemaker 2010).

The more these factors can be identified and used to plan, communicate, and execute change, the greater the likelihood there will be fewer barriers, more acceptance, and more successful outcomes. Diffusion theory also accounts for why some innovations are accepted rapidly while others are delayed regardless of substantial evidence supporting their benefits (Sanson-Fisher 2004).

Innovator Roles

In the late 1960s and early 1970s, the literature reflected a new interest in the roles of innovators within organizations who become gatekeepers or nodes for the flow of information (Allen and Cohen 1969). Four roles have been identified for the successful implementation of an innovation:

- **Inventor** (innovator): The individual who develops a new idea or practice in the organization. However, it is not sufficient to merely originate and understand the new idea. Rather, the idea must be facilitated by several other roles in the organization before it is adopted or brought to market.

- **Champion:** Someone in the organization who believes in the idea, acknowledges the practical problems of financing and political support, and assists in overcoming barriers.

- **Sponsor:** Usually a high-level manager who approves and protects the idea, expedites testing and approval, and removes barriers within the organization.

- **Critic:** A crucial but sometimes overlooked role. This role is essential in challenging the innovation for shortcomings, presenting strong criteria, and, in essence, providing a reality test for the new idea. (Daft and Marcic 2011; Roberts 2007)

In an innovative environment, all of these roles are important and exemplary of how role responsibilities are distributed in an organization.

Check Your Understanding 22.5

1. Why are all four innovator roles important for establishing innovations?

2. Think of some innovation you have adopted in your personal life—a technical device, appliance, clothing, or the like. What were the factors that influenced your adoption (for example, trialability, advantage, compatibility, simplicity, and such)?

3. Explain why identifying each of the adopter groups is important during an innovation.

4. In what way might laggards be valuable?

5. Why is there a gap between awareness of an innovation and its adoption?

Change Management

A more global role for practitioners of organizational change is often referred to as the change agent. The **change agent** is a specialist in organizational development who facilitates the change brought about by the innovation. He or she may be internal or external to the organization, as in the case of a consultant specifically hired to assist with the change. **Organizational development (OD)** is the process in which an organization reflects on its own processes and consequently revises them for improved performance. OD is "an effort planned, organization-wide, and managed from the top, to increase organization effectiveness and health through planned interventions in the organization's processes, using behavioral-science knowledge" (Beckhard 1969, 9).

Differences Between Leaders and Managers

Traditionally terms *manager* and *leader* are often used interchangeably (Schyve 2009), but technically they refer to different role functions in the organization. Managers tend to focus on the present situation, maintain efficiency of the status quo, direct others to follow the rules, control risks, carry out requirements to reach the vision through others, and focus more internal to the organization. In contrast, leaders focus on distant opportunities, challenge the status quo, make and break rules by doing things right, inspire, and focus more externally (see table 22.4). These roles tend to become blurred as organizations become flatter, decisions are driven downward, employees are more empowered, and initiative is encouraged. However, since organizations differ in culture, the roles should be explicitly clarified for those new to the position.

Leaders involved in implementing change are most active at three critical points: during the initial stage of change when they explain the reasons for change and offer the vision; during transition when people struggle and need encouragement; and finally as the change becomes accepted, success is acknowledged, and the changes need to be stabilized. Managers work closely with people to reduce errors and ensure understanding, provide encouragement and support during transition, and reward behavior that reinforces the new status quo. In some ways the roles of managers and leaders have become blurred as have the stages since there is rarely a plateau when change is not occurring in modern organizations, and change seems continuous. It is during these long transitions that expert facilitators, from inside or outside the organization, can be of great assistance.

Organizational Development Change Agent Functions

The concept of an agent for change has moved from the narrow specialty of organization development (OD), to permeate most professions, including healthcare. Although managers may perform change agent functions, generally managers are viewed as helping maintain efficiency and the status quo. Change agents are more like leaders in that they encourage and facilitate change by thinking

Table 22.4. Differences between managers and leaders

Manager	Leader
Administers	Innovates
Reproduces/replicates	Originates
Maintains	Revises
Plans short view	Plans long term
Bottom line	Horizon
Works with the status quo	Challenges the status quo
Does things right	Does the right thing
Limited focus	Systemic focus
Directs	Inspires
Follows the vision	Delivers the vision
Controls risks	Seeks opportunities
Focus on "what"	Focus on "why"
Rules oriented	Outcome oriented
Transactional	Tranformational

about what can be better. OD change agents perform a range of five functions with management:

- *Acceptant function* uses counseling skills to help the manager sort out emotions to gain a more objective perspective of the organization
- *Catalytic function* helps collect and interpret data about the organization
- *Confrontation function* challenges the manager's thinking processes and assumptions
- *Prescriptive function* tells the manager what to do to correct a given situation
- *Theory and principle function* involves helping the client system internalize alternate explanations of what is occurring in the organization (Blake and Mouton 1976)

These functions are essential for HIM professionals who are leading change in healthcare, such as facilitating the transition from ICD-9 to ICD-10. For this and other challenges, leaders will need to use their expertise and understanding of data content standards and organization requirements for effective data management and help mobilize people to participate in the change (Cassidy 2013).

Internal and External Change Agents

Change happens on its own but is usually most desirable when it is intentionally directed toward the benefit of the organization and its members. The role of the change agent is to facilitate this change process by utilizing reflective learning: drawing attention to important processes, helping people understand what the processes mean, and considering and implementing plans of action. Exactly who performs this role can be critical (Weick and Quinn 1995; Westcott 2005). There are advantages and disadvantages to using change agents from within the organization as well as from outside the organization (Swenson 2001) (see table 22.5).

Internal Change Agents

Internal change agents have the clear advantage of being familiar with the organization and its history, subtle dynamics, secrets, and resources. Such people are often well respected, are securely positioned, and have the strong interpersonal relationships to foster change. Moreover, there is an advantage to recognizing the internal expertise of employees, maintaining confidentiality of the process, and using people who are invested in the success of the outcome.

Yet, the strengths of internal change agents can also be weaknesses. Coming from the inside, however reputable they are, their previous relationships with others in the organization could lead to accusations of bias. As a product of the organizational culture, internal change agents may be as blind to certain problems as those they seek to facilitate. Another disadvantage is that they are taken away from their regular duties to conduct the facilitation or perhaps become overextended in trying to handle both responsibilities. Finally, internal change agents may be subject to pressures and sanctions regarding the outcome, whereas an external change agent would have no such obligations.

External Change Agents

The external change agent has the advantage of providing a fresh, outside view as well as having the knowledge base to compare performance across organizations. Not having direct connections to the organization, he or she usually feels more comfortable challenging norms and culture, questioning unusual or unfair practices, and generally noting events that others may be reluctant to comment on. Being from the outside, he or she may be seen as having new skills and being more objective, or at least less biased than an internal agent.

The weaknesses of the external agents include not having a history with their client organization that could enhance their awareness of important dynamics. Becoming familiar with the organization takes time, and during a crisis they may move too quickly to conclusions based on limited information. Additionally, external change agents may be strongly influenced by the viewpoint of the administrators who contracted with them. External change agents must thoroughly evaluate the relevant people and processes of the organization. Moreover, external agents can be expensive, charging tens to hundreds of thousands of dollars for their consultation. Finally, a highly charismatic, directive, and

Table 22.5.   Advantages and disadvantages of internal and external change agents

	Internal change agent	External change agent
Advantages	1. Knows the environment, culture, people, issues, and hidden agendas	1. Provides fresh, outside, objective perspective
	2. Develops and keeps expertise and resources internal	2. Is willing to assert, challenge, and question norms
	3. Creates and maintains norms of organization renewal from within	3. May have more legitimacy to insiders by not taking sides
	4. Provides higher security and confidentiality	4. Brings skills and techniques not available from within organization
	5. May have trust and respect of others	5. Brings diverse organizational experiences to bear; benchmarks comparisons
	6. Has strong personal investment in success	
Disadvantages	1. May be biased; has already taken sides, or may be disliked or mistrusted by some stakeholders	1. May or may not be available when needed by the organization; may split time and commitments with other clients
	2. May have previous relationships that contribute to subgrouping or fragmentation	2. Incurs high expense
	3. Takes change agent away from other duties	3. Takes time to become familiar with the system
	4. May be enculturated and is part of the problem or does not see it	4. May create codependency or may abandon the system
	5. Is subject to organizational sanctions and pressures as an employee	

Source: Swenson 2001

successful agent could foster dependency with a client organization, leaving the organization reluctant to learn to manage its own change processes.

Use of Internal Versus External Change Agents

Deciding on the change agent to use can be a difficult decision, and the wrong decision can delay the process or discourage participants from the effort. When an organization plans to use internal or external change agents, it should consider several questions, including the following:

- How confidential and proprietary is the information involved? Would either type of agent present a disclosure or confidentiality risk?

- Are there conflicts of interest? Is the external agent working with any competitor or internal agent loyal to conflicting parties?

- What level of commitment and availability is required? What is the potential effect of an external agent with many other clients or an internal agent with other work obligations?

- What skills are required for a successful change effort? What constellation of experience and skills do the external and internal agents offer?

- How important is it that stakeholders view the agent as being objective, fair, and neutral? Which type of agent would best be viewed this way?

- To what extent does the culture of the organization require changing? Which type of agent is better positioned to influence the change?

There are many factors to consider when deciding to use an internal or external change agent.

This decision is critical for gaining acceptance and cooperation to work toward an effective change in the organization.

Stages of Change

People and organizations move through stages of transition in response to change, and as they do, they have different needs and require different skills from the leader. Change is difficult for most people even when parts of the change are desirable, and resistance should be expected as a normal response to doing things differently. Understanding the reasons for resistance to change as well as various stages of the change can help change agents facilitate this process.

Resistance to Change

Kurt Lewin, one of the founders of organization development, said "If you wish to understand something, try changing it" (Lewin 1951). When one attempts to change a system, the mechanisms that maintain it spring to its defense. Change does not come easily to most people, and in organizations, "resistance to change is experienced at almost every step" (DeWine 1994, 281). The first step for leaders who are trying to reduce resistance to change is to understand its source.

Resistance to change occurs for a number of reasons, including self-interest and anxiety about the unknown, different perceptions, suspiciousness, and conservatism. When confronted with change, the first thing many workers want to know is how it will affect them and their jobs (Quast 2012). Because the turbulence of the marketplace makes many changes uncertain, workers may not receive satisfactory answers to their questions. Those who have attained expertise and status from their positions now may face new job descriptions or expanded or new duties. For example, many managers in downsized organizations have been reassigned as coaches to newly formed teams. This new role raises questions about their authority, status, and responsibility.

Other workers may resist change simply because they perceive the situation differently and believe the proposed change is unjustified. The result of ongoing change is to make many people uneasy about, and even mistrustful of, any innovation. Some people view all change as just another fad based on the whim of management rather than a survival strategy for the organization. And finally, some people are very conservative in their beliefs, are isolated in their social networks and information, and dislike the inconvenience of change.

Resistance can distract workers from their tasks, preoccupy them with gossiping, and contribute to stress and workplace violence. To confident change leaders, indications of resistance can be viewed as useful information about what stakeholders need before the transition can continue.

When change is resisted, continued efforts to implement the change are often presented as "overcoming" resistance to change. However, this way of thinking about change implies an adversarial approach rather than collaborative one. Early on in change theory, Lewin (1951) recognized the importance of understanding resistance as a way of reducing it, and offered a tool called the Force Field Analysis as a way of describing the opposing forces and how they could be reconciled. Change efforts are described as an interaction between driving forces for change and those that resist or restrain change. These can be represented as opposing arrows that maintain a status quo, each arrow having an estimated magnitude representing how much it is perceived as driving or resisting change. Rather than increase the driving forces that often result in eliciting a counter-reaction from the restraining forces, Lewin suggested understanding the restraining forces and finding ways to reduce them. When they are reduced, change can occur without as much adversity or conflict.

For example, a hospital is planning to implement a balanced scorecard to track key performance indicators, and the administration suspects that it may not be easily accepted. They bring in a consultant to help identify issues on the topic and discover that while there are several driving forces, there are also several resistances that would complicate, delay, or perhaps defeat the effort (see figure 22.20). On the driving side there is administrative support, incentives, vendor support, demands of consumers, and legislative requirements. These vary in strength and

Figure 22.20. Force field analysis of forces for and against implementing the balanced scorecard

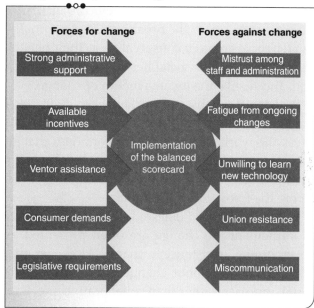

are opposed by several resistors including a climate of mistrust, fatigue from too many changes already, unwillingness to learn new skills, union support for resistance, and frequent miscommunication. Trying to push the change without appreciating the resistance factors would be problematic. Instead, strategic change would involve asking staff more about their resistances and listening and understanding their reasoning. Once staff feels understood, leaders may be able to find ways to reduce each of the objections. More transparency and involvement of representative staff in the planned change may reduce mistrust and miscommunication. Training periods and pay for training might reduce anxiety about new skills or time pressures. While there is no guarantee that all forces against change can be reduced, this broad view can at least identify those factors that are more responsive.

Facilitation of Change

The purpose of transition management is to make the potential upheaval and chaos posed by planned changes less disruptive to the people and processes of healthcare. It is helpful to think of a transition as a series of stages through which people move as they adjust to changes. Each stage has

its own set of challenges and tasks to master, the successful completion of which forms the foundation for moving on to the next stage. Kubler-Ross (1969) has described the emotional responses of people as they move through stages of grieving a loss, and this has been widely applied to losses during organizational transition. Lewin described a seminal three-stage model for organizational change that Bridges expanded in more detail. Finally, Kotter elaborated on Lewin again with emphasis on actions and pitfalls in implementing change. These models of transition and change are important to the HIM professional as they maneuver through numerous changes in technology, work processes, and regulations.

Stages of Grieving Elizabeth Kubler-Ross (1969) examined the stress of change in her classic study of the **stages of grief** experienced by terminally ill patients and their families. These stages are descriptions of the more common sequence of grief reactions that people experience due to a loss, whether loss of a close relationship or loss of one's role or usual way of working. Change in the healthcare system often involves mergers, acquisitions, downsizing, and other transitions that usually involve losses and grief. The five-stage model has become useful in anticipating and working with people in a dramatic transition, including organizational change (Shoolin 2010). As shown in figure 22.21, the five stages of the model are:

1. *Shock and denial:* Workers have difficulty believing the proposed transition. They may deny that change is imminent and go about business as usual rather than prepare for the adjustment. News of the change also may stun workers to the extent that they cannot concentrate or work efficiently, and they may isolate themselves.

2. *Anger:* Workers begin to understand the inevitability of the change. They may direct their resentment at the organization or the managers for allowing it to happen. In addition, they may engage in unproductive complaining, organize resistance, or even sabotage operations in attempts to reduce the threat.

Figure 22.21. Adaptation of Kubler-Ross's stages of grief

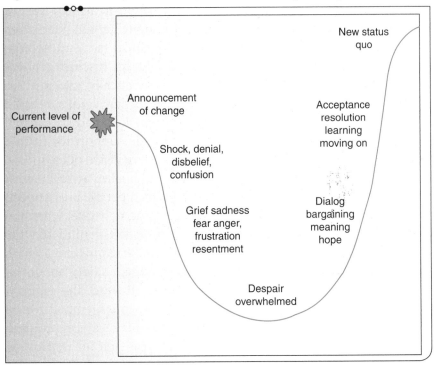

Source: Adapted from Kubler-Ross 1969.

3. *Despair:* Workers may lose their self-esteem and be unresponsive to encouragement.

4. *Bargaining:* Workers make a final attempt to avoid the change. They may actually try to bargain with managers to delay the change or work intensively to prove their value and reduce the risk of loss.

5. *Acceptance:* Workers begin to redirect their energy toward the new organization and new status quo.

During the disruption of transition, each of the stages of change requires leadership to recognize, explain, and facilitate movement onward. During the initial shock stage, employees need accurate and timely information about the change and what it will entail. Support, reassurance, and clear directives can be helpful in easing some of the initial anxiety. As people move into stage 2 with more emotional reactions, it is important for their feelings to be accepted and validated, clear communication and updates given as the change unfolds, and information offered on effective coping. Stage 3 involves attempts to bargain, negotiate,

or compromise on the inevitable change. It is important during this stage for leadership to remain consistent and reiterate the rationale for moving forward. During stage 4 when people can feel most discouragement, leadership should provide additional encouragement. Despite the popularity of the Kubler-Ross model, it is important to remember that people may not always follow these stages in exact order, and they may sometimes return to previous stages. It is therefore important to recognize and acknowledge what the person is experiencing, rather than assume they are progressing through each stage in order and in a timely manner. In addition, while the model describes emotional reactions to change, it does not specifically describe the more complex emotional–cognitive–behavioral reactions to organizational change that the following models do.

Lewin's Stages of Change Lewin's model of stages of change, identified the initial stage of change as **unfreezing** or disrupting the status quo, often by presenting the discrepancies between the status quo and the desired goals. Unfreezing often creates a state of cognitive dissonance, which is an uncomfortable awareness of two incompatible perceptions or beliefs, in this case, the discrepancy. An emerging and effective approach to unfreezing is the socioeconomic approach to management or SEAM (Buono and Savall 2007). This approach, popular in Europe, is beginning to find support in the United States and find application in healthcare (Kister 2014). Many people are hesitant to engage in change because they believe the risks are too great and costs (and losses) are too much. SEAM helps identify the hidden costs of current inefficiencies, in terms of financial, time, and emotional or intangible costs. The evidence of hidden costs that are real compared to potential costs of change is often sufficient to unfreeze them and motivate change.

The second stage of change is transition, and it involves actually making plans and efforts to revise the way work is done. This transition stage involves introducing the new practices and operations, building skills and providing reassurance, and dealing with residual resistance to change.

In the final stage of **refreezing**, the new behaviors are reinforced to become as stable and institutionalized as the previous status quo. Lewin originally conceptualized this three-stage process as one in which the organization would plateau and stabilize for a time before the next change was required. More recent beliefs about organizational change characterize the change process as continuous with little respite for workers, managers, or leaders. The status quo has become one of dealing with ongoing change, which can be stressful as people learn to let go of past practices and make efforts to learn new ones on a nearly continuous basis.

Bridges's Model for Managing Transitions William Bridges, an organization consultant, integrated Lewin's stages of change with Kubler-Ross's stages of grieving losses to create his stages of transition model (Bridges 2004, 2009). Stage 1 is a recognition of initial ending, losing, and letting go. People must accept the ending before they are ready to accept a change. During this period, initial resistance should be accepted, understanding that those impacted by the change will feel fear, denial,

anger, sadness, frustration, uncertainty, and sense of loss. It is important for leaders to explain reasons for the ending and indicating what will not change in an effort to alleviate the initial fear and trepidation. They should also encourage discussion about these reactions, listen empathetically, and provide open communication. The leader should describe how employees can use their skills and knowledge following the change, provide support for further training, and describe a positive vision of the future.

Stage 2 is the neutral zone, similar to Lewin's transition stage, during which people are between the old way and the emerging new one; when the old ways have largely been left behind but the new ones not fully accepted. Reactions can include resentment toward the change, anxiety about the ambiguity, and skepticism toward the change. Leadership guidance and encouragement is particularly important at this stage since progress may not yet be apparent. It is helpful to provide clear direction, meaningful goals, opportunities for more discussion, and feedback. Morale can also be boosted by showing how their efforts are linked to success of the change, helping them manage workloads more effectively, and encouraging innovative ideas about how to move forward with the new organization.

Stage 3 marks a new beginning where the change has been accepted, early wins are evident and encouraging, and morale and energy is high. During this final stage, it is important to again show how individual and team performance is linked to the new way in order to sustain the change efforts. Success stories should also be communicated as a way of recognition in addition to other rewards. New goals are created to provide direction; attitudes and behaviors that support the new beginning are recognized and reinforced. People progress through these stages at different rates, and it is important to be alert to laggards who may regress if they believe the change is not working as planned.

Kotter's Phases for Implementing Change In 1996, Harvard Business School professor John Kotter introduced his approach to change, expanding on the work of Lewin and Bridges. He based his model on 10 years of assisting over

100 organizations through transformations and identifying eight major errors resulting in failures and how to prevent them (Kotter 2007).

While Lewin and Bridges describe a three-stage model for change, Kotter (2007) elaborates on these with emphasis on eight underlying process steps related to success in transformation (see table 22.6 for a visual of these process steps). Similar to Lewin's unfreezing and Bridge's ending stage, Kotter proposes phase one for developing a climate for the change process to occur. This involves three steps starting with a sense of urgency by noticing market drivers and discussing related potential crises, threats, and opportunities. Kotter believes it is important to convince at least three-quarters of managers that the status quo is more dangerous to survival than the change (2007). Step two involves developing a coalition of power vendors who can work together and lead the change efforts. Creating a compelling vision of the future is step three

Table 22.6. Kotter's phases of change

Phase	Step of change	Required actions	Potential pitfalls
Phase 1: Develop a climate for change	1. Develop a sense of urgency for change	• Identify market drivers and pressures for crises and potentials • Convince 75% of managers that the status quo is more dangerous than change	• Underestimating the challenge of creating urgency, overestimating success, lacking patience, paralyzed by complexity
	2. Establish a powerful guiding coalition	• Convene a leadership group with shared commitment and power • Work as a team outside the traditional hierarchy	• Insufficient teamwork experience • Relegating team leadership to someone lower than senior line manager
	3. Create a compelling vision	• Formulate a clear vision to direct change • Develop strategies for accomplishing the vision	• Presenting an unclear or overly complicated vision that cannot be communicated
Phase 2: Enable and engage participation for change	4. Communicate the vision	• Use many channels for communicating the vision and strategies • Demonstrate new behaviors exemplifying the vision	• Undercommunicating the vision or acting in ways inconsistent with it
	5. Empower people to act on the vision	• Remove system or structural barriers to accomplishing the vision • Encourage risk taking and nontraditional ideas and actions	• Not removing individuals who resist or are barriers to change
	6. Plan and create short-term successes	• Make improvements visible • Recognize and reward employees who contribute to improvements	• Leaving short-term wins to chance • Failing to achieve early successes 1 to 2 years into the change
Phase 3: Implement and sustain change	7. Consolidate improvements and generate more change	• Use early credibility to continue to remove barriers to the vision • Hire, develop, and promote employees who are aligned with the vision • Continue to invigorate change with new projects and change champions	• Announcing success prematurely • Allowing resistors to convince others that the effort is complete
	8. Institutionalize the changes into the culture	• Show connections between behaviors and organization success • Develop leadership and succession plans that support the new approach	• Not forming new norms and shared values consistent with the change • Promoting people who are not congruent with the new approach

Source: Adapted from Kotter 2007.

that helps formulate strategies for directing and achieving the change effort.

Phase two engages and enables the organization to participate in and drive the change. Step four involves using multiple vehicles to communicate the new vision and use the coalition to role-model new behaviors. Some consultants recommend overcommunicating by delivering the message at least seven times to make the change clear (Israel 2013). Step five empowers others to act by removing obstacles, changing structures and systems that undermine the vision, and encouraging risk taking and innovative ideas and actions. Step six plans and creates short-term wins that are visible, demonstrate improvements, and reward employees for improvements.

Phase three consists of ways to implement and sustain the change. Step seven consolidates what has been improved already and encourages more change. This is accomplished by using earned credibility to change systems that are not yet compliant with the vision, mobilizing employees who implement the vision, and reinvigorating the process by introducing new themes, projects, and change agents. Step eight integrates the changes into the newly emerging culture by showing connections between behaviors and success and ensuring leadership development and succession throughout the organization.

The more carefully and thoroughly an organization proceeds through these stages, the greater the chances for success, while mistakes at any stage can jeopardize the transition (Kotter 2007). Over half of the organizations Kotter has consulted with have failed during phase one (Kotter 2007). This has often been due to leaders underestimating the difficulty of creating urgency, overestimating the ease of success, lacking patience for what will likely take years, or becoming paralyzed with the complexity of the situation. Kotter's model has been promoted for use during the implementation of the EHR and provides a detailed and unique approach (Neumeier 2013).

Vision is the center piece of Kotter and others' change strategy, but "vision" is not just an imagined favorable view of the possible future. The current strategic situation for an organization is a resolution of multiple forces and change drivers operating in the environment. Although it is unlikely that any imagining of the future can be completely accurate, especially during turbulent change, any envisioning should be framed around projections of how change drivers will shape the business environment of the future. Vision for the organization becomes more accurate the more that leaders have a sound understanding of trends and patterns among the change drivers that shape the current and emergent environment.

Leading Through Cultural Change

Organizational culture refers to an organization's norms, beliefs, and values, or generally "how we do things here." A 2013 survey emphasized the importance of culture, with 60 percent stating that considering the impact of culture is more important than strategy during change efforts (Aguirre et al. 2013).

A significant trend in healthcare is the pressure for mergers and acquisitions among healthcare systems, pharmaceuticals, and health insurance companies (Daly 2015; Plank and Cervantes 2015). The pace of these has increased substantially, in part to the pressures of the Accountable Care Act. Combining resources enables healthcare organizations to benefit from consolidating leadership, organizational structure, and reducing unnecessary duplication in skills. Merging organizations that were previously separate entities can be a major issue in trying to merge their different cultures—like trying to merge two different personalities (Plank and Cervantes 2015). These have taken the form of mergers and acquisitions as well as strategic alignments, joint operation agreements, and clinical affiliations. A merger is the combining of two or more companies to form a new one, while an acquisition is where one company purchases another, absorbing it into the parent company.

However, a study of 219 facilities and systems in the 10-year period between 1998 and 2008 by Strategy& showed that only 41 percent outperformed their market peer group, and nearly one in five actually had negative margins within a two-year period following the merger (Saxena et al. 2013). The causes of such failure are many, but primary causes include lack of a fit among capabilities between the organizations, inexperienced buyers and sellers who negotiate the consolidation, and insufficient due diligence regarding financial, operational, and cultural factors. Each of these would require extensive explanation, but culture is of most relevance regarding transition management among employees and other stakeholders.

Culture and people-related problems following the merger are two of the leading issues affecting success (Schroeder 2015). Mergers between healthcare systems, facilities, and even departments require a well thought out and agreed on alignment that cover several areas of operations (Gelineau and Brown 2015). Governing boards must be blended and they may have different styles of decision making and doing business. The executive committee and full board may also have difficulty balancing the authority between them. There are often different approaches for alignment with medical staff members, and failing to find the best combination of physicians can suboptimize operations, clinical services, and market potentials. Finally, leaders should have a candid discussion of the integration of visions for the unified system.

Merged organizations need to commit time and effort to rebuilding a new culture from the merged organizations. The stages of culture change are very similar to the stages of transition already considered. However, the initial stages for defining the emerging desired culture are worth detailing. Stage 1 typically involves a culture task force or other designated group that starts by describing the pre-existing cultures from which the organization originated. This shows respect for the previous cultures as well as clarifies differences and similarities that must be considered. Both positive and negative perceptions of the two cultures are also openly identified and discussed to surface potential conflicts and establish a norm of openness (Trimnell et al. 2015). The resulting data from stage 1 is organized during stage 2 into a meaningful conceptual framework comprised of seven attributes:

1. Physical environment—décor, symbols, artifacts, design

2. Beliefs and values—recognitions, ceremonies, stories, traditions

3. Communication process and styles—language, blogs, newsletters, memos

4. Social environment—events, interactions, ceremonies, rewards

5. Work attributes—attendance, punctuality, work ethic, retention

6. Management attributes—leadership styles, opportunities for advancement

7. Emotional environment—humor, conflict resolution styles, climate (Trimnell et al. 2015)

In stage 3 the change team generates a list of desirable culture characteristics that will be carried into the new culture, and those that will be left behind. This can produce a very large list as well as provide clarity to Bridge's ending phase. Stage 4 takes the list, makes brief definitions or descriptive phrases of each, and then reduces it to the top 10 most desirable culture characteristics. Discussion then focuses on the enablers and constraints that operate on the top 10 in preparation for the implementation plan.

Stage 5 prepares a synthesis of the top 10 most desirable characteristics into a draft of the culture and recommendations on how they can be implemented. Development of the statement by a widely representative team and sanctioned by top leadership ensures more widespread ownership. It is important that the higher level culture descriptors are translated down to individual behavior where people are engaged and accountable.

Response to Change

As much as individuals differ in their responses to change, it should not be surprising that various departments, units, and professions as well as other stakeholders also can vary in their responses. The level of perceived impact on organizational and unit culture as well as effect on work styles and turf can dramatically affect responses. For example, in some departments where there is little direct impact, staff may experience minor disruption of daily work and status quo. On the other hand, those who are more affected may show a decline in productivity, have lower morale, and express more complaints. Those who feel violated may actively defy the change or seek employment elsewhere, resulting in job gaps, loss of important knowledge and expertise. The more such reactions can be anticipated and people from all levels engaged in transition planning, the less the adverse impact on individuals, departments, and organization as a whole. As shown in figure 22.22, different departments may react differently depending on how they perceive the impact of change. Their reactions may also have different trajectories, increasing and decreasing over time.

One should think of these theories as lenses through which organizational change and innovations can be viewed. Each organization is different and change agents may need to customize the transition management model they are using. Nonetheless, each of the frameworks presented in this chapter are a helpful toolkit for leaders in the turbulent environment of healthcare.

Figure 22.22. Variable impact of change on different stakeholders

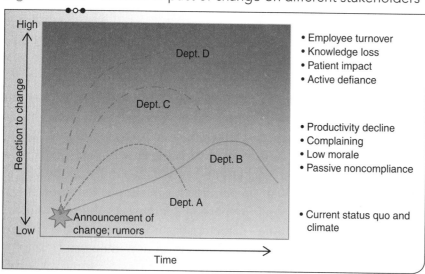

Source: Adapted from the Prosci Flight-Risk Model 2004.

 Check Your Understanding 22.6

Instructions: **Answer the following questions on a separate piece of paper.**

1. Make a list of reasons that people resist change. For each reason, suggest a way to reduce resistance.

2. Think of a significant change you have gone through, such as a change in job or position, moving to a new location, or coping with a health problem. Describe the stages you experienced related to unfreezing, change, and refreezing.

3. If you were informed that your position was being eliminated due to reorganization but that you could reapply for a new position, how would you react? What would you want from management to help cope with the stress of this change?

4. Assume you are an organizational change consultant, what are some of the issues you would explain to an executive team about the organization going through transition? What should they expect?

5. Describe the work cultures of two different departments in an organization with which you are familiar. Consider the implications of these differences and how they could be merged if necessary. Consider what common core they share (for example, values, outcomes, and such).

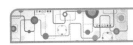

References

Adkins, A. 2015. Majority of US Employees Not Engaged Despite Gains in 2014. *Gallup.* http://www.gallup.com/poll/181289/majority-employees-not-engaged-despite-gains-2014.aspx

Aguirre, D., R. von Post, and M. Alpern. 2013. Culture's role in enabling organizational change. *Strategy&.* http://www.strategyand.pwc.com/media/file/Strategyand_Cultures-Role-in-Enabling-Organizational-Change.pdf

Allen, T.J. and S.I. Cohen. 1969. Information flow in two R&D laboratories. *Administrative Science Quarterly* 14(1):12–19.

Allport, G.W. and H.S. Odbert. 1936. Trait-names: A psycho-lexical study. *Psychological Monographs* 47:171–220.

American Health Information Management Association. 2014. *Pocket Glossary of Health Information Management and Technology.* Chicago: AHIMA

Apker, J. 2001. Role development in the managed care era. *Journal of Applied Communication Research* 29(2):117–136.

Argyris, C. 1957. *Personality and Organization.* New York: Harper & Row.

Ash, J. S., M. Berg, and E. Coiera. 2004. Some unintended consequences of information technology in healthcare: The nature of patient care information system-related errors. *Journal of the American Medical Information Association* 11(2):104–112.

Baird, A., M. Furukawa, and T. Raghu. 2012. Understanding contingencies associated with the early adoption of customer-facing web portals. *Journal of Management Information Systems* 29(2):293–324.

Baldrige Performance Excellence Program. 2011. 2011–2012 Health Care Criteria for Performance Excellence. http://www.nist.gov/baldrige/publications/upload/2011_2012_Health_Care_Criteria.pdf

Baptist, R.W. Measuring Predictors of Groupthink: Instrument Development and Validation [Master's thesis]. Normal, IL: Illinois State University; 2015.

Barnard, C. 1938. *The Functions of the Executive.* Cambridge, MA: Harvard University Press.

Baron, R.S. 2005. So right it's wrong: Groupthink and the ubiquitous nature of polarized group decision making. *Advances in Experimental Social Psychology* 37:219–252.

Beckhard, R. 1969. *Organization Development: Strategies and Models.* Reading, MA: Addison-Wesley.

Benedictine Health System. 2015. About BHS: Service Rooted in Faith. http://www.bhshealth.org/about

Blake, R.R. and J.S. Mouton. 1976. *Consultation.* Reading, MA: Addison-Wesley.

Bowman, S. 2013. Impact of electronic health record systems on information integrity: Quality and safety implications. *Perspectives In Health Information Management* 10(Fall):1c.

Bridges, W. 2009. *Managing Transitions: Making the Most of Change.* New York, NY: De Capo.

Bridges, W. 2004. *Transitions: Making the Most of Change.* New York: Basic Books.

Bridges, W. 1994. *Job Shift: How to Prosper in a Workplace without Jobs.* Reading, MA: Addison-Wesley.

Brooks, F.P. 1995. *The Mythical Man-Month: Essays on Software Engineering.* Boston: Addison-Wesley.

Buhler, P.M. 2007. Managing in the new millennium: Interpersonal skills. *Supervision* 68(7):20–22.

Buono, A.F. and Savall, H. 2007. *Socio-economic Intervention in Organizations.* Charlotte, NC: Information Age.

Burns, J.M. 1978. *Leadership.* New York: Free Press.

Byrne, J.A. 2005 (Nov. 28). The man who invented management. *Business Week* 97–106.

Cain, M. and R. Mittman. 2002. Diffusion of Innovation in Healthcare. Prepared by Institute of the Future for the California HealthCare Foundation. http://www.chcf.org/~/media/MEDIA%20LIBRARY%20Files/PDF/D/PDF%20DiffusionofInnovation.pdf

Carmeli, A. and A. Tishler. 2006. The relative importance of the top management team's managerial skills. *International Journal of Manpower* 27(1):9–36.

Cassidy, B.S. 2013. The next HIM frontier: Population health information management presents a new opportunity for HIM. *Journal of AHIMA*, 84(8), 40-46.

Castillo, V.H., A.I. Martinez-Garcia, and J.R.G. Pulido. 2010. A knowledge-based taxonomy of critical factors for adopting electronic health record systems by physicians: A systematic literature review. *BMC Medical Informatics and Decision Making* 10:60.

Center for Creative Leadership. 2011. Addressing the Leadership Gap in Healthcare. http://www.ccl.org/leadership/pdf/research/addressingleadershipGapHealthcare.pdf

Copeland, M.K. 2014. The emerging significance of values-based leadership: A literature review.

International Journal of Leadership Studies 8(2):105–135.

Copley, F.B. 1923. *Frederick W. Taylor, Father of Scientific Management.* New York, NY: Harper and Brothers.

Daft, R.L. and D. Marcic. 2011. *Understanding Management.* Mason, OH: South-Western Cengage.

Daly, R. 2015. Healthcare deals surge in 2015. Healthcare business news, Healthcare Financial Management Association. http://www.hfma.org/Content.aspx?id=29451

Danner, M. 2005. Duties of not-for-profit directors and officer and the role of the health care risk manager. *Readings in Healthcare Governance.* The Chubb Group. http://www.chubb.com/businesses/csi/chubb3821.pdf

Dansereau, F., G. Graen, and W. Haga. 1975. A vertical dyad linkage approach to leadership within formal organizations: A longitudinal investigation of the role-making process. *Organizational Behavior and Human Performance* 13:46–78.

de Savigny, D. and T. Adam. 2009. *Systems Thinking for Health Systems Strengthening.* Alliance for Health Systems Policy and Research, World Health Organization. http://whqlibdoc.who.int/publications/2009/9789241563895_eng.pdf

DeWine, S. 1994. *The Consultant's Craft: Improving Organizational Communication.* New York: St. Martin's Press.

Deming, W.E. 1986. *Out of the Crisis.* Cambridge: Massachusetts Institute of Technology, Center for Advanced Engineering Study.

Drucker, P. 2002. *Managing in the Next Society.* New York, NY: St. Martin's Griffin.

Drucker, P. 1986. The appraisal of managerial performance. *Management Decision* 24(4):67–78.

Edison, T. 2008 (May–June). The team development lifecycle. Team dynamics. Defense AT&L. http://www.dau.mil/pubs/dam/2008_05_06/edis_mj08.pdf

Epstein, R.M., D.J, Siegel, and J. Silberman. 2008. Self-monitoring in clinical practice: A challenge for medical educators. *Journal of Continuing Health Professions* 28(1):5–13.

Ethics Research Center. 2015. Ethical Leadership. http://www.ethics.org/newsite/research/eci-research/nbes/nbes-reports/ethical-leadership

Ethics Resource Center. 2012. 2011 National Business Ethics Survey: Workplace Ethics in Transition. http://www.ethics.org/nbes/files/FinalNBES-web.pdf

Ethisphere. 2015. 2015 World's Most Ethical Companies. http://web.ethisphere.com/worlds-most-ethical/

Faith, K.E. 2013. The role of values-based leadership in sustaining a culture of caring. *Healthcare Management Forum* 26(1):6–15.

Fayol, H. 1917. *Administration Industrielle et Générale; Prévoyance, Organisation, Commandement, Coordination, Controle.* Paris: H. Dunod et E. Pinat.

Fiedler, F.E. 1967. *A Theory of Leadership Effectiveness.* New York: McGraw-Hill.

Focht, A. and M. Ponton. 2015. Identifying primary characteristics of servant leadership: Delphi study. *International Journal of Leadership Studies* 9(1):44-61.

French, J.R.P. and B. Raven. 1959. The bases of social power. In *Studies in Social Power.* Edited by D. Cartwright. Ann Arbor, MI: Institute for Social Research.

Gamble, M. 2013. How and Why Emotional Intelligence is Affecting Hospitals' Bottom Lines. Becker's Hospital Review. http://www.beckershospitalreview.com/hospital-management-administration/how-and-why-emotional-intelligence-is-affecting-hospitals-bottom-lines.html

Gelineau, S. and G. Brown. 2015. Preventing a Merger Fail. Hospitals and Health Networks Daily. http://www.hhnmag.com/articles/3769-preventing-a-merger-failGerardi, D. 2015. Conflict engagement: Emotional and social intelligence. *American Journal of Nursing* 155(8):60–65.

Goleman, D. 1998 (Nov–Dec). What makes a leader? *Harvard Business Review* 74(6):92–102.

Graen, G. and T.A. Skandura. 1987. Toward a psychology of dyadic organizing. *Research in Organizational Behavior* 9:175–209.

Greenleaf, R.J. 1991. *Servant Leadership.* Mahwah, NJ: Paulist Press.

Guerci, M., G. Raedelli, E. Siletti, S. Cirella, and A.R. Shani. 2015. The impact of human resource management practices and corporate sustainability on organizational ethical climates: An employee perspective. *Journal of Business Ethics* 126(2):325–342.

Gunnarsdottir, S. 2014. Is servant leadership useful for Nordic health care? *Nordic Journal of Nursing Research and Clinical Studies* 34(2):53–55

Guo, K.L. 2003. An assessment tool for developing healthcare management skills and roles. *Journal of Healthcare Management* 48(6):367–376.

Hahn, W. and T.L. Powers. 2010 (Jan.). Strategic plan quality, implementation capability, and firm performance. *Academy of Strategic Management* 9(1):63–81.

Hammer, M. and J. Champy. 1993. *Reengineering the Corporation.* New York: Harper.

Hammerly, M.E., L. Harmon, and S.D. Schwaitzberg. 2014. Good to great: Feedback to improve physician emotional intelligence. *Journal of Healthcare Management* 59(5):354–365.

Hanse, J.J., U. Harlin, C. Ulin, and J. Winkel. 2015. The impact of servant leadership dimensions on leader-member exchange among health care professionals. http://socav.gu.se/digitalAssets/1524/1524513_johansson-hanse-et-al.2015-150416.pdf

Harper, S.R. and C.D. White. 2013. The impact of member emotional intelligence on psychological safety in work teams. *Journal of Behavioral and Applied Management* 15(1):2–10.

Hay Group. 2010. Growing Leaders Grows Profits. https://www.haygroup.com/downloads/fi/Belron%20report.pdf

Healthcare Management Council. 2013. http://www.hospitalspanofcontrol.com/index.php.html

Helseth, C. 2007 (Summer). Recruiting local people to fill health care needs. *The Rural Monitor*. http://www.raconline.org/newsletter/web/summer07.php

Hersey, P., K.H. Blanchard, and D.E. Johnson. 1996. *Management of Organizational Behavior: Utilizing Human Resources*, 7th ed. Upper Saddle River, NJ: Prentice-Hall.

Hirsch, L. 2011. What the Heck is the Hawthorne Effect and How Can It help Hospital and Healthcare Marketing? Healthcare Success. http://www.healthcaresuccess.com/blog/healthcare-marketing/hawthorne-effect.html

Hogan, R. and R.B. Kaiser. 2004. What we know about leadership. *Review of General Psychology* 9(2):169–180.

Hooper, D.T. and R. Martin. 2008. Beyond personal leader-member exchange (LMX) quality: The effects of perceived LMX variability on employee reactions. *Leadership Quarterly* 19(1):20–30.

Horsky, J., D.R. Kaufman, M.I. Oppenheim, and V.L. Patel. 2003. A framework for analyzing the cognitive complexity of computer-assisted clinical ordering. *Journal of Biomedical Informatics* 36(1-2):4–22.

Houghton, S.M., A.C. Stewart, and P.S. Barr. 2009. Cognitive complexity of the top management team: The impact of team differentiation and integration processes on firm performance. *Current Topics in Management* 14:95–118.

House, R. 1996. Path-goal theory of leadership: Lessons, legacy, and reformulated theory. *Leadership Quarterly* 7(3): 323–352.

House, R.J. 1971. A path–goal theory of leader effectiveness. *Administrative Science Leadership Review Quarterly* 16:321–339.

Howard, D.M. and D. Silverstein. 2014. The interpersonal skills of recent entrants to the field of healthcare management. *Journal of Hospital Administration* 3(3):33–43.

Hunt, T.J. 2014. Leader-member exchange relationships in health information management. *Perspectives in Health Information Management* 11(Spring):1–8.

Hwang, Y-S. and S.H. Park. 2007. Organizational life cycle as a determinant of strategic alliance tactics: Research propositions. *International Journal of Management* 24(3):427–435.

Israel, R. 2013. Change Management Critical to Accepting New Health-Care IT. Curaspan Health Group. https://connect.curaspan.com/blog/change-management-critical-accepting-new-health-care-it/

Janis, I.L. 1972. *Groupthink: Psychological Studies of Policy Decisions and Fiascos.* Boston: Houghton Mifflin.

Jones, D. 2012. Servant leadership's impact on profit, employee satisfaction and empowerment within the framework of a participative culture in business. *Business Studies Journal* 4(1):35–49.

Jones, G.R. and J.M. George. 2006. *Contemporary Management*, 4th ed. New York: McGraw-Hill Irwin.

Kaplan, R.S. and D.P. Norton. 1996. *The Balanced Scorecard.* Boston: Harvard Business School Press.

Katz, R.L. 1974. Skills of an effective administrator. *Harvard Business Review* 52:90–102.

Kister, A. 2014. Causes and sources of hidden costs in a medical facility. *Revue de Management et de Strategie.* 2(11):14–25.

Kotter, J.P. 2007 (March–April). Leading change: Why transformation efforts fail. *Harvard Business Review.* 85(1): 96–103.

Kronenberg, M.A. 2014. Evaluating important healthcare competency areas and preparation for healthcare reforms. *International Journal of Business and Public Administration* 11(2):31–40.

Kubler-Ross, E. 1969. *On Death and Dying.* New York: Simon & Schuster/Touchstone.

Kyriakopaulos, G. 2012. Half a century of management by objectives (MBO): A review. *African Journal of Business Management* 6(5):1772–1786.

Landsberger, H.A. 1958. *Hawthorne Revisited.* The New York State School of Industrial and Labor Relations: Ithaca, NY.

Langabeer, J.R. and J. Helton. 2016. *Health Care Operations Management: A Systems Perspective.* Burlington, MA: Jones & Bartlett.

Lee, J. 2005. The effects of leadership and leader-member exchange on commitment. *Leadership and Organization Development Journal* 26(8):655–672.

Levin, R.F., J.M. Keefer, J. Marren, M. Vetter, B. Lauder, and B. Sobolewski. 2010. Evidence-based practice improvement: Merging two paradigms. *Journal of Nursing Care Quality* 25(2):117–126.

Lewin, K. 1951. *Field Theory in Social Science.* New York: Harper and Brothers.

Likert, R. 1979. From production- and employee-centeredness to systems 1–4. *Journal of Management* 5:628–641.

Lindsey, J.S. and J.W. Mitchell. 2012. Tomorrow's Top Healthcare Leaders: 5 Qualities of the Healthcare Leader of Tomorrow. *Becker's Hospital Review.* http://www.beckershospitalreview.com/hospital-management-administration/tomorrows-top-healthcare-leaders-5-qualities-of-the-healthcare-leader-of-the-future.html

Lowry, R. 2014. How stand along hospitals can continue as a community healthcare asset. Warbird Consulting. http://www.healthcarewriter.com/wp-content/uploads/2014/09/Robert-Lowry-Warbird-white-paper-SAMPLE.pdf

Maccoby, M., C. Norman, C. Norman, and R. Margolies. 2014. *Transforming Healthcare Leadership: A Systems Guide to Improve Patient Care Decrease Costs, and Improve Population Health.* New York, NY: John Wiley and Sons.

Martinez-Garcia, M. and E. Hernandez-Lemus. 2013. Health systems as complex systems. *American Journal of Operations Research* 3:113–126.

Maslow, A.H. 1943. A theory of human motivation. *Psychological Review* 54:370–396.

McConnell, C.R. 2015. *The Effective Healthcare Supervisor.* Burlington, MA: Jones & Bartlett.

McDonough, K., P. Bobrowski, M.A. Keogh-Hoss, N.M. Paris, and M. Schulte. 2014. The leadership gap: Ensuring effective healthcare leadership requires inclusion of women at the top. *Open Journal of Leadership* 3(2):20–29.

McGregor, D. 1960. *The Human Side of Enterprise.* New York, NY: McGraw Hill

Meyer, R.M. 2008. Span of management: Concept analysis. *Journal of Advanced Nursing* 63(1):104–112.

Michalisin, M.D., S.J. Karau, and C. Tangpong. 2004. Top management team cohesion and superior industry returns: An empirical study of the resource-based view. *Group and Organization Management* 29(1):125–140.

Mintzberg, H. 1992. The manager's job: Folklore and fact. In *Managing People and Organizations.* Edited by J.J. Gabarro. Boston: Harvard Business School.

Mintzberg, H. 1989. *Mintzberg on Management: Inside Our Strange World of Organizations.* New York, NY: Free Press.

Neumeier, M. 2013. Using Kotter's change management theory and innovation diffusion theory in implementing the electronic health record. *Canadian Journal of Nursing Informatics* 8(1-2). http://cjni.net/journal/?p=2880

Nwabueze, U. 2011. Implementing TQM in healthcare: The critical leadership traits. *Total Quality Management* 22(3):331–343.

Ozaralli, N. 2003. Effects of transformational leadership on empowerment and team effectiveness. *Leadership and Organization Development Journal* 24(6):16–47.

Parker, L.D. 1984. Control in organizational life: The contribution of Mary Parker Follett. *Academy of Management Review* 9:736–745.

Pascale, R.T. 1990. *Managing on the Edge.* New York: Simon & Schuster.

Patwardhan, A. and D. Patwardhan. 2008. Business process reengineering—Savior or just another fad? *Journal of Healthcare Quality Assurance* 21(3):289–296.

Peters, T.J. and R.H. Waterman. 1982. *In Search of Excellence: Lessons from America's Best-Run Companies.* New York: Harper & Row.

Plank, W. and A. Cervantes. 2015. What's driving merger and acquisition activity? *Wall Street Journal.* http://www.wsj.com/articles/whats-driving-merger-and-acquisition-activity-1441846542

Prosci Flight and Risk Model. 2004. http://www.change-management.com/tutorial-flight-risk.htm

Quast, L. 2012. Overcome the five main reasons people resist change. http://www.forbes.com/sites/lisaquast/2012/11/26/overcome-the-5-main-reasons-people-resist-change/

Rastegar, D.A. 2004. Healthcare becomes an industry. *Annals of Family Medicine* 2(1):79–83.

Raven, B.H. 1983. Interpersonal influence and social power. In *Social Psychology.* Edited by B.H. Raven and J.Z. Rubin. New York: John Wiley & Sons.

Riggio, R.E. and R.J. Reichard. 2008. The emotional and social intelligences of effective leadership: An emotional and social skill approach. *Journal of Managerial Psychology* 23(2):169–185.

Roberson, D., S.M. Connell, K. Dillis, R. Gauvreau, E. Gore, K. Heagerty, L. Jenkins, A. Ma, A. Maurer,

J. Stephenson, and M. Schwartz. 2014. Cognitive complexity of the medical record is a risk factor for major adverse events. *The Permante Journal*. 18(1), 4-8.

Roberts, E.B. 2007 (Jan–Feb). Managing invention and innovation. *Research Technology Management*. http://www.iriinc.org/Content/ContentGroups/Research_Technology_Management/Volume_50_2007/Issue_Number_1_January_February_20071/Articles21/MANAGING_INVENTION_AND_INNOVATION.htm

Rogers, E. 1995. *Diffusion of Innovations*, 4th ed. New York: Free Press.

Rogers, E. and F.F. Shoemaker. 1971. *Communication of Innovations: A Cross-Cultural Approach*. New York: Free Press.

Rural Health Resource Center. 2008. Balanced Scorecard Experiences. http://www.ruralcenter.org/?id=res_bscxp

Sanford, K. 2006. The ethical leader. *Nursing Administration Quarterly* 30(1):5–10.

Sanson-Fisher, R.W. 2004. Diffusion of innovation theory for clinical change. *The Medical Journal of Australia* 180(6 suppl):s55.

Saxena, S. B., A. Sherma, and A. Wong. 2013. Succeeding in hospital and health systems M&A: Why so many deals have failed, and how to succeed in the future. Strategy&. http://www.strategyand.pwc.com/global/home/what-we-think/reports-white-papers/article-display/succeeding-hospital-health-systems

Schroeder, H. 2015. The Art and Science of Post-Merger Integration. Association for Corporate Growth. http://www.acg.org/global/theartandscienceofpostmergerintegration.aspx

Schyve. 2009. *Leadership in Healthcare Organizations: A Guide to Joint Commission Leadership Standards*. San Diego, CA: The Governance Institute.

Shartle, C.L. 1979. Early years of the Ohio State University leadership studies. *Journal of Management* 5:126–134.

Shipton, H., C. Armstrong, M. West, and J. Dawson. 2008. Impact of leadership and quality climate on hospital performance. *International Journal for Quality in Healthcare* 20(6):239–245.

Shoemaker, E.M. 2010. *Diffusion of Innovations*, 4th ed.. New York, NY: Simon and Schuster.

Shoolin, J.S. 2010. Change management—Recommendations for successful electronic records implementation. *Applied Clinical Informatics* 1(3):286–292.

Simha, A. and J.B. Cullen. 2012. Ethical climates and their effect on organizational outcomes: Implications from the past and prophecies for the future. *The Academy of Management Perspectives* 26(4):20–34.

Snell, M.J. 2010. Solving the problems of groupthink in healthcare facilities through the application of practical originality. *Global Management Journal* 2(2):74–84.

Stair, R. and G. Reynolds. 2012. *Fundamentals of Information Systems*. Boston: Cengage.

Starbuck, P. 2013. Peter F. Drucker. In *The Oxford Handbook of Management Theorists*. Edited by M. Witzel and M Warner. Oxford, UK: Oxford University Press.

Stephenson, J. and M. Schwartz. 2014. Cognitive complexity of the medical record is a major risk factors for adverse events. *Permanente Journal* 18(1):4-8.

Stogdill, R.M. 1974. *Handbook of Leadership: A Guide to Understanding Managerial Work*. Englewood Cliffs, NJ: Prentice-Hall.

Stoner, J.A.F. and R.E. Freeman. 1989. *Management*. Englewood Cliffs, NJ: Prentice-Hall.

Swenson, D.X. 2014. A systems model of overtime effects on software development team effectiveness. Thesis completed for Master of Arts in Information Technology Leadership, College of St. Scholastica, Proquest database, http://search.proquest.com/docview/1554342784

Swenson, D.X. 2003. The Groupthink Profile. http://www.behaviortrends.com

Swenson, D.X. 2001. Change Agents: The Good, the Bad, and the Ugly. http://faculty.css.edu/dswenson/web/6300-OBOD/CArole.htm

Tannenbaum, T. and W. Schmidt. 1973 (May–June). How to choose a leadership pattern. *Harvard Business Review*. No. 73311. First published in 1958 (March–April) *Harvard Business Review* 36:95–101.

Taplan, R. 2003. *Decision Making and Japan*. New York, NY: Routledge.

Towill, D.R. 2009. Frank Gilbreth and health care delivery method study driven learning. *International Journal of Healthcare Quality Assurance* 22(4):417–440.

Trastek, V.F., N.W. Hamilton, and E.E. Niles. 2014. Leadership models in healthcare—A case for servant leadership. *Mayo Clinic Proceedings* 89(3):374–381.

Traveno, L. K., and Nelson, K. A. (2011). Managing business ethics. New York, NY: John Wiley & Sons

Trbovich, P. 2014 (Fall). Five ways to incorporate systems thinking into healthcare organizations. *Horizons* 48(s2):31–36.

Trimnell, J., D. Butterill, W. Skinner, G. Golyea, L. Yue-Chan, and D. MacFarlane. 2015 (May). Rebuilding organizational culture in the wake of a merger. *Healthcare Management Forum* 14(3):11–23e.

Verbos, A.K., J.A. Gerard, P.R. Forshey, C.S. Harding, and J.S. Miller. 2007. The positive ethical organization: Enacting a living code of ethics and ethical organization identity. *Journal of Business Ethics* 76(1):17–33.

Vroom, V. and P. Yetton. 1971. *Leadership and Decision Making.* Pittsburgh: University of Pittsburgh Press.

Walton, M. 1986. *The Deming Management Method.* New York: Perigee Books.

Waugh, J. 2009. *U.S. Grant: American Hero, American Myth.* Chapel Hill, NC: University of North Carolina Press.

Weick, K.E. and R.E. Quinn. 1995. Organizational change and development. *Annual Review of Psychology* 50:361–386.

Weiner, J., V. Balijepally, and M. Tanniru. 2015. Integrating strategic and operational decision making using data-driven dashboards: The case of St. Joseph Mercy Oakland Hospital. *Journal of Healthcare Management* 60(5):319–330.

Westcott, R.T. 2005. *The Certified Manager of Quality/ Organizational Excellence Handbook.* Milwaukee, WI: American Society for Quality.

White, R.K. and R. Lippitt. 1960. *Autocracy and Democracy: An Experimental Inquiry.* New York: Harper.

Yukl, G. 2006. *Leadership in Organizations,* 6th ed. Upper Saddle River, NJ: Prentice-Hall.

Zhang, X., P. Yu, J. Yan, and I.T.A.M. Spil. 2015. Using diffusion of innovation theory to understand the factors impacting patient acceptance and use of consumer e-health innovations: A case study in a primary care clinic. *BMC Health Services Research* 15:71.

Zheng, K., M.H. Guo, and D. Hanauer. 2011. Using the time and motion method to study clinical work processes and workflow: Methodological inconsistencies and a call for standardization research. *Journal of the American Medical Information Association* 18(2011):704–710.

Zhu, W., I.K.H. Chew, and W.D. Spangler. 2004. CEO transformational leadership and organizational outcomes: The mediating role of human-capital-enhancing human resource management. *Leadership Quarterly* 16(1):39–52.

23
Human Resources Management

Madonna M. LeBlanc, MA, RHIA, FAHIMA

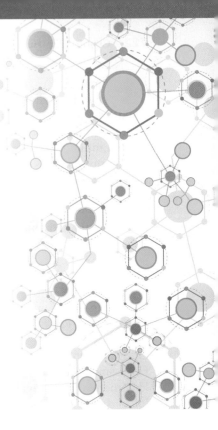

Learning Objectives

- Identify the activities associated with the human resources (HR) management function in an organization
- Apply key federal legislation with each of the human resources management activities
- Develop position descriptions, performance standards, staffing structures, and work schedules for use as tools in human resources management
- Identify how job descriptions are used in employee recruitment and selection
- Select effective steps for conducting an interview
- Evaluate the roles that employee orientation and communication plans play in the retention of staff
- Examine the benefits of teamwork in an organization
- Identify and differentiate among the four methods of job evaluation

- Analyze the relationship among performance standards, performance review, and performance counseling
- Identify the key steps a manager should take in performance counseling and disciplinary action
- Select the appropriate conflict management technique to use in each specific conflict situation
- Determine the process for handling employee complaints and grievances
- Identify the obligations an organization has to maintain the security of employee information and records
- Evaluate the impact of current workforce trends on the organization's human resources management activities

Key Terms

Age Discrimination in Employment Act (1967)
Americans with Disabilities Act (ADA) (1990)
Arbitration

Authority
Behavioral description interview
Civil Rights Act, Title VII (1964)
Civil Rights Act (1991)
Compensable factors

Compromise
Conflict management
Constructive confrontation
Control
Delegation

Discrimination
Employment-at-will
Equal Employment Opportunity Act (1972)
Equal Employment Opportunity Commission
Equal Pay Act (EPA) (1963)
Exempt employees
Exit interview
Factor comparison method
Fair Labor Standards Act (FLSA) (1938)
Family and Medical Leave Act (FMLA) (1993)
Genetic Information Nondiscrimination Act (2008)
Grievance
Grievance procedures
Harassment
Hay method of job evaluation
Job classification method
Job evaluation

Job ranking
Job specification
Labor-Management Reporting and Disclosure Act of 1959 (Landrum-Griffin Act)
Labor-Management Relations Act (Taft-Hartley Act)
Labor relations
Layoffs
Mediation
National Labor Relations Act (Wagner Act)
Nonexempt employees
Occupational Safety and Health Act (OSHA) (1970)
Orientation
Panel interview
Performance review
Performance standards
Point method
Policy
Position (job) description

Pregnancy Discrimination Act (1978)
Procedure
Progressive discipline
Recruitment
Reference check
Reliability
Responsibility
Retention
Structured interview
Team building
Termination
360-degree evaluation
Uniformed Services Employment and Reemployment Rights Act (1994)
Union
Validity
Workers' Adjustment Retraining and Notification (WARN) Act

The process of management cannot be practiced or examined meaningfully outside the social, cultural, and ethical contexts in which human organizations of all kinds operate. In modern industrial societies, human resources are every organization's most valuable asset.

Healthcare organizations are extremely complex. They must operate as effective and efficient businesses in a very tight financial environment. They also must employ a variety of well-educated technical specialists and professional employees to provide or support increasingly sophisticated healthcare services. Contemporary healthcare managers work in a unique environment that is characterized by the need to control costs and, at the same time, meet the needs of healthcare consumers and healthcare workers.

Managers work at many levels within healthcare organizations—as supervisors of functional units, as middle managers of departmental units or service lines, and as executive managers of multiple departmental units or service lines. At each level of management, the practice of managing the human resources within the prescribed scope of authority and responsibility is critical to the manager's success and the success of the entire organization.

Managing human resources (HR) is both an art and a science. Managers can learn much in this arena by partnering with HR management specialists, observing experienced colleagues, reflecting regularly on their own experiences, and continuing to develop their competencies throughout their careers.

This chapter is not meant to provide a comprehensive background in human resources management. The purpose of this chapter is to present a general introduction to the subject of managing human resources within the context of health information management (HIM) operations. The chapter begins with a brief overview of the principles and nature of organizations and a discussion of the roles of the various levels of management. Its primary focus is the interrelationship of HIM managers and HR professionals and the roles of the supervisor and middle manager as frontline implementers of the HR policies and practices of healthcare organizations.

Role of the Human Resources Department

Payroll and benefits consume the majority of most healthcare organizations' financial resources (Dunn 2010). Therefore, adequate time and attention must be paid to the management of human resources. Effective HR management is also important for reasons beyond financial impact. HR management factors affect the attitudes and morale of healthcare workers and other employees and, therefore, affect their ability to perform their work effectively as well. Employee morale becomes important when the work involves caring for patients directly or indirectly supporting those who provide hands-on care.

Entities such as hospitals, large physician groups, and integrated health systems commonly have a dedicated HR department that acts as a reference and support for managers at all levels. However, every manager must have an understanding of the principles of HR management in order to implement them effectively within the scope of the manager's authority and responsibility. Every manager must also know how to appropriately and effectively work with the organization's HR department.

The HR department is responsible for several types of interrelated activities. HR management is a set of closely related activities focused on contributing to an organization's success by enhancing its productivity, quality, and service. Each of these interrelated activities is shown in figure 23.1, which illustrates the extensive factors involved in creating a desirable, functioning employee environment. The importance of performing HR activities with the organization's unique mission, culture, size, and structure as well as the greater social, political, legal, economic, technological, and cultural environment in which it operates is also important (Mathis and Jackson 2011).

Human Resources Planning and Analysis

HR planning and analysis ensure the long-term health of the organization's human assets. Internal trends such as the aging of the workforce or the changing nature of the skill mix required to handle the organization's evolving product lines must be addressed.

One-third of the total US workforce are 50 years or older. By 2050, the US Census predicts that 19.6 million American workers will be age 65 or older (Harrington and Heidkamp 2013). This aging workforce requires healthcare employers to evaluate current HR policies and practices to determine if they are effective in retaining older staff, creating job opportunities for new trainees of all ages, and planning for a large turnover in staff and potential workforce shortage due to upcoming retirements (Harrington and Heidkamp 2013).

In addition to planning for a change in workforce numbers, there is also a shift in skills needed in the HIM profession. The growing role of information technology within healthcare has created a strong need for continuing education for current HIM professionals as processes undergo dramatic change with more technology solutions, requirements, and regulations to manage. As the complexity and sophistication of healthcare continues, the need for highly skilled professionals also increases (McNickle 2012). The HIM profession has experienced and will continue to experience rapid and significant change driven by the increased use of healthcare technology and the many government programs and regulations that impact the delivery of healthcare and the creation, use, and maintenance of health records. These changes will drive the HIM workforce to require more advanced technical skills, more advanced conceptual and analytical skills, and greater communication skills (The Caviart Group 2014). HR professionals and HIM managers need to collaborate to ensure intentional employee retention strategies, continuing education programs, and strong recruitment

Figure 23.1.   HR management activities

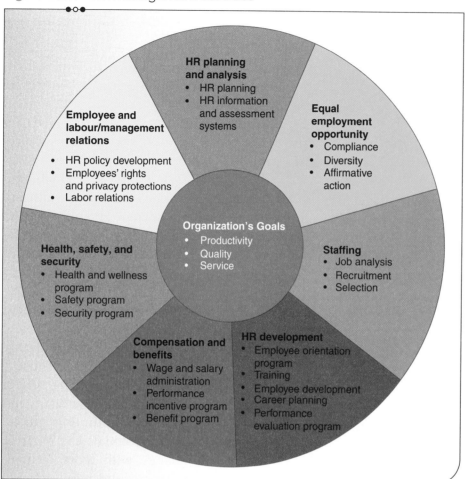

Source: Adapted from Mathis and Jackson 2011.

plans to meet both the short-term and long-term workforce needs.

Equal Employment Opportunity Practices

The HR department takes the lead in ensuring that the various laws and regulations associated with equal employment opportunity (EEO), affirmative action, and the US Department of Labor (DOL) are scrupulously applied in the organization's hiring and promotion practices. Federally enacted DOL and EEO legislation includes the following:

- Age Discrimination in Employment Act (ADEA) of 1967

- Americans with Disabilities Act (ADA) of 1990

- Civil Rights Act, Title VII (1964) and the Civil Rights Act (1991)

- Equal Employment Opportunity Act of 1972

- Family and Medical Leave Act (FMLA) of 1993

- Genetic Information Nondiscrimination Act of 2008

- Pregnancy Discrimination Act of 1978

- Uniformed Services Employment and Reemployment Rights Act (USERRA) of 1994

The Equal Employment Opportunity Commission (EEOC) was created by Title VII of the Civil Rights Act of 1964 as the agency responsible for investigating discrimination claims emanating from the Civil Rights Act of 1991, finally giving legal voice to a process that formally had none.

Discrimination and harassment are two important concepts related to fair employment practices. Discrimination refers to practices that result in people being treated differently based solely on their personal distinctions. Harassment refers to practices that create a hostile work environment that can include physical, verbal, or emotional harassment. Both are illegal under the EEO laws and the EEOC recommends the following best practices to create an anti-harassment environment: adopt a rigorous anti-harassment policy, routinely train each employee on its contents, and stringently adhere to and enforce it. The policy should include:

- "A clear explanation of prohibited conduct, including examples;
- Clear assurance that employees who make complaints or provide information related to complaints will be protected against retaliation;
- A clearly described complaint process that provides multiple, accessible avenues of complaint;
- Assurance that the employer will protect the confidentiality of harassment complaints to the extent possible;
- A complaint process that provides a prompt, thorough, and impartial investigation; and
- Assurance that the employer will take immediate and appropriate corrective action when it determines that harassment has occurred" (EEOC n.d.(a)).

It is important for both managers and employees to know these policies so that employers can ensure a safe work environment free of discrimination and harassment and so that employees are not fearful to report when these issues occur.

Rights of Employees and Employers

Although many of the basic rights of employees are defined in law, others are expectations that may be debated within organizations. For example, employment-at-will is a well-established concept—either an employer or an employee can terminate an employment relationship without providing either notice or reason. Other issues are less clear. What are the privacy rights of employees? Can an employer monitor employees' e-mails and voicemails? Organizations are well advised to address the rights of employees and the rights of the employer in an employee handbook to clarify expectations for employees and supervisors. A well-developed employee handbook also improves the organization's legal position should the organization be called on to defend its actions in a court proceeding.

Staffing

The HR department also helps managers to define staffing needs; develop job descriptions; and recruit, screen, and select staff. After an employee is brought into the organization, the HR department plays a significant role, in partnership with the employee's direct supervisor, by spearheading the employee's immediate orientation to the organization's policies, practices, and procedures. The HR department is also active in addressing the employee's ongoing training and development requirements; for the HIM department, that could include ongoing education regarding new technology, new software programs, or the likes of the ICD-10 mandate. Refer to chapter 24 for further information related to employee orientation, training, and development.

Compensation and Benefits Program

The organization's compensation and benefits program is the most prominent activity associated with HR management because it is so directly connected to the employee's financial status. This activity involves the establishment of basic definitions of employment and compensation status for the organization (for example, full-time versus part-time, temporary versus permanent, independent contractor versus employee, wage versus salary). The **Fair Labor Standards Act (FLSA)** of 1938 and the **Equal Pay Act (EPA)** of 1963 serve as fundamental legislative mandates in this area. Social Security, unemployment compensation, and workers' compensation are three benefits organizations are required to offer (SBA n.d.). Other common benefits offered to employees voluntarily by the organization are health insurance, retirement plans, wellness programs, holidays (time off with pay), vacation time, and employee assistance programs. The HR department also leads the development and administration of the organization's job evaluation and classification systems, wage and salary systems, and incentive pay systems.

Health and Safety Program

The HR department is also involved in activities designed to protect the health, safety, and security of the workforce. Healthcare organizations have given substantial attention to safety management since the enactment of the **Occupational Safety and Health Act (OSHA)** of 1970. Its intended purpose is "to assure safe and healthful working conditions (the environment and surroundings in which work is performed) for every working man or woman by setting and enforcing standards by providing training, outreach, education and assistance" (OSHA n.d.). This act established a national reporting system for accidents and injuries on the job and led to the development of specific safety management programs in most businesses. Health-related hazards associated with the use of technology or chemical substances in the workplace, injuries due to workplace violence, and employee security concerns continue to receive special attention by HR professionals (Anthony et al. 2010). For the HIM manager, concerns may include ventilation, workstation ergonomics, lighting, and fire hazards.

Labor Relations

Employee, labor, and management relations are established through the day-to-day interactions between employees and their managers. However, the organization's managers and employees often seek leadership and support from the HR department. The HR department sets the stage for developing and sustaining the quality of these critical relationships by establishing and communicating to both managers and employees the contracts, policies, practices, and rules that constitute the organization's expectations of its employees.

HR management activities associated with unions and collective bargaining are referred to as **labor relations**. Labor organizations (**unions**) enter into negotiations with employers on behalf of groups of employees who have elected to join a union. The negotiations relate to compensation and safety and health concerns. In a unionized environment, three laws came into existence over a period of 25 years (1935 through 1960) and constitute a code of practice for unions and management. HR departments pay strict attention to these three acts:

- **National Labor Relations Act (Wagner Act)** (1935)
- **Labor-Management Relations Act (Taft-Hartley Act)** (1947)
- **Labor-Management Reporting and Disclosure Act (Landrum-Griffin Act)** (1959) (Anthony et al. 2010; Mathis and Jackson 2011)

For the manager who oversees a group of employees covered by a union contract, these laws represent the basic rules for their interactions with employees in the areas of pay, benefits, safety, health, and performance evaluation. (See table 23.1 for an inclusive list of employment laws.)

Table 23.1. Labor legislation

Legislation	Concern or content	Administrative or enforcement agency
National Labor Relations Act of 1935 (Wagner Act)	Encouraged collective bargaining	National Labor Relations Board (NLRB)
Fair Labor Standards Act of 1938	Addressed the need for minimum wage, overtime pay, and record keeping	US Department of Labor
Fair Employment Act of 1941	Prohibited discrimination	Committee on Fair Employment Practices
Labor Management Relations Act of 1947 (Taft-Hartley Act)	Amended provisions of the Wagner Act; restricted activities and power of labor union	National Labor Relations Board
Labor-Management Reporting and Disclosure Act of 1959 (Landrum-Griffin Act)	Required financial disclosures of labor organizations	US Department of Labor
Equal Pay Act of 1963	Discouraged compensation relative to the sex of a worker	Equal Employment Opportunity Commission (EEOC)
Title VII of the Civil Rights 1964	Removed bias related to sex, color, race, religion, and national origin	Equal Employment Opportunity Commission
Age Discrimination in Employment Act of 1967 (amended in 1978)	Prohibited discrimination due to age (protection for those 40 to 70 years old)	Equal Employment Opportunity Commission
Occupational Safety and Health Act (OSHA) of 1970	Established regulation around workplace safety	Occupational Safety and Health Administration
Equal Employment Opportunity (EEO) Act of 1972	Promoted equal employment opportunities for all Americans	Equal Employment Opportunity Commission
Rehabilitation Act of 1973	Prohibited discrimination against people with disabilities	US Department of Labor
Employee Retirement Income Security Act of 1974	Established pension and healthcare plan rules	US Department of Labor
Pregnancy Discrimination Act of 1978 (amendment to Title VII of the Civil Rights)	Prohibited discrimination due to pregnancy, childbirth, or related medical conditions	Equal Employment Opportunity Commission
Immigration Reform and Control Act of 1986	Established employment eligibility verification	US Department of Labor
Employee Polygraph Protection Act of 1988	Prohibited use of polygraphs by most private employers	Secretary of Labor
Americans with Disabilities Act 1990	Prohibited discrimination against people with disabilities	Equal Employment Opportunity Commission
Civil Rights Act of 1991	Established provisions for damages for intentional employment discriminations	Equal Employment Opportunity Commission
Uniform Services Employment and Reemployment Rights Act (USERRA) of 1994	Protected veterans civilian jobs	Department of Labor
Family Medical Leave Act (FMLA) of 1996	Permitted unpaid leave for certain healthcare reasons related to family or self	Employment Standards Administration
Health Insurance Portability and Accountability Act (HIPAA) of 1996	Established regulation around securing health insurance coverage	US Department of Labor
Nursing Relief Disadvantaged Areas Act of 1999	Permitted temporary employment of alien or foreign RNs	US Department of Labor
Genetic Information Nondiscrimination Act 2008	Prohibits genetic information discrimination against employees or applicants.	Equal Employment Opportunity Commission

Source: Adapted from Dunn 2010; DOL OS n.d.; EEOC 2015

Check Your Understanding 23.1

Instructions: **On a separate piece of paper, indicate whether the following statements are true or false (T or F). If the statement is false, explain why it is false.**

1. Internal and external environmental trends are significant factors in HR planning and analysis.

2. The Fair Labor Standards Act is one piece of the EEO legislation package passed in the early 1960s.

3. A national system for reporting workplace accidents and injuries was mandated by the Americans with Disabilities Act.

Instructions: **Answer the following questions on a separate piece of paper.**

4. Orientation for new employees and the ongoing training of employees are the responsibility of which department?

5. The Fair Labor Standards Act, the Wagner Act, and the Equal Pay Act provide key guidelines for managing what HR program?

Role of the HIM Manager in Human Resources

Because the day-to-day management of the organization's human resources is the responsibility of supervisory, middle, and executive managers, every manager is responsible for many of the same HR activities as the HR professionals. In an HIM department, for example, the supervisor of coding services would be responsible for the day-to-day management of clinical coding specialists. Managers at all levels can use any of a variety of HR tools and processes to handle these responsibilities efficiently and effectively.

Tools for Human Resources Planning

Several tools may be used to plan and manage staff resources. Position descriptions, for example, outline the work and qualifications needed to perform a job. Performance standards establish the organization's expectations of how well a job must be done and how much work must be accomplished. Position descriptions and performance standards should be aligned with the mission and goals of the organization. Routine staff meetings and regular written communications (via departmental websites, bulletin boards, and newsletters, for example) establish a routine process for up-to-date information flow for employees.

Staffing Structures and Work Scheduling

Managers establish staffing structures (the arrangement of staff positions within an organization) and use work schedules to ensure that there is adequate coverage and staff to complete the required work. Schedules are developed to provide adequate coverage during the hours the organization or department is open for business.

In hospitals, it is possible to find some part of the HIM department open 24 hours a day, seven days a week. This schedule ensures that HIM staff will be available to provide information for admissions to the hospital and emergency department, support patient discharges and transfers, and handle other HIM functions such as the creation or transcription of a critical report. In some healthcare organizations, the demand for HIM services outside regular business hours is limited. In such cases, HIM functions can be provided by business office staff, nursing staff, or emergency department staff who have been cross-trained to perform basic HIM tasks, such as chart retrieval or faxing of patient health information.

Another scheduling consideration is space. Space limitations on the number of workstations in the department or the number of employees who can work in the file room may require that employees work in shifts or on weekends.

In addition, staff preferences need to be considered in creating the work schedule. Balancing the demands of the organization with individual requests for flexible start times makes scheduling an important part of the manager's responsibility. Organizations are commonly establishing flexible work schedules to accommodate employee needs to adjust work schedules to lifestyles, such as allowing for telecommuting for certain days or hours of the day or working a split shift in early morning and later evening to meet the demands of young families or employees who are caregivers to elderly parents.

Written policies and procedures that explain the department's staffing requirements and scheduling procedures help the manager to remain fair and objective and help the staff to understand the rules. The amount of personal time off, such as sick leave or vacation, also factors into the development of a staff schedule and the overall assessment of the number of staff positions required. (Refer to chapter 25 for more detail on considerations for work scheduling)

Position Descriptions

A **position (job) description** outlines the work to be performed by a specific employee or group of employees with the same responsibilities. Position descriptions generally consist of three parts: a summary of the position's requirements and purpose, its functions, and the qualifications needed to perform the job. Position descriptions also include the official title of the job and to whom (position) the employee will directly report. While working and collaborating with a variety of positions, it is essential to define the person ultimately responsible for the employee; for example a scanning/indexing clerk who reports to the clerical supervisor. It is critical that

the employee have one person to whom they report and that the reporting relationship is very clear, ensuring there is no confusion about from whom the employee should take direction. See figure 23.2 for a job description template that demonstrates important components of the job description.

A **job specification** is a document (or a section of the job description document) that is focused on the knowledge, skills, abilities, and characteristics required of an individual in order to perform the job. These specifications may include the following:

- Educational level and professional certifications
- Experience
- General characteristics (team player, effective writing skills)
- Specific knowledge (foreign language proficiency, software program proficiency) (Dunn 2010, 370)

Position descriptions, including the job specification, are used during the recruitment process to explain the work to prospective candidates. They also enable managers and HR staff to set appropriate salaries and wages for various positions. Moreover, they may be used to resolve performance problems. For this reason, it is essential that position descriptions are written in a criteria-based language that correlates directly to the established job functions. The manager can use the position description to clarify the tasks the employee is expected to perform.

Generally, job descriptions are needed in the following circumstances:

- When an entirely new kind of work is required
- When a job changes and the old description no longer reflects the work
- When a change in technology or processes dramatically affects the work to be accomplished
- When employee job performances are evaluated, either during probationary periods or annually

Figure 23.2. Job description template

Job title: Department:

Reports to: Cost center:

Job category: Salary (exempt) or Hourly (non-exempt)

Job type: Full-time or Part-time

Job summary:

Description of the job:

Required employment qualifications: Knowledge, skills, abilities, mental capacity, education, experience, and licensure or credentials required for the job.

Preferred employment qualifications: Knowledge, skills, abilities, mental capacity, education, experience, and licensure or credentials preferred but not required for the job.

Physical demands/safety requirements/working conditions: Lifting, standing, sitting, walking, and reaching requirements; keyboarding and use of computer monitor, noise, smells, use of chemicals, and any other physical demands and safety considerations that are part of the working conditions.

Job responsibilities and functions/competencies: All required job functions and responsibilities, can include the weight of each job function.

Mission/values/behavioral expectations: Mission and stated values of the organization including behavioral expectations for this job.

Decision-making authority: Decision-making authority required of this job role, if any.

Supervisory and/or budget responsibilities (if applicable): Supervisory responsibilities or budget responsibilities, if any.

Date Reviewed: Last date job description was reviewed for accuracy and relevance.

Sometimes top performers outgrow their job descriptions. They may find more efficient ways of doing part of their assigned tasks and want more interesting or meaningful work. The job description may need to be updated to better reflect additional assigned responsibilities to support an increase in salary and benefits or a change in title.

When writing new position descriptions, managers may use existing descriptions of other, related jobs or interview staff who are currently performing some of the tasks intended for the new job. They also might assign staff members a work measurement technique to record how they spend their time on the job for a period that reflects a comprehensive cycle of their work. Staff with more repetitive daily activities may only need to record their activities for a short period of time (for example, a week). In contrast, staff with more diverse tasks may need more time, perhaps a month, to document the scope of their duties. More information on work measurement techniques can be found in chapter 25.

Performance Standards

In addition to a position description, **performance standards** are often developed for the key functions of the job. These standards indicate the level of acceptable execution for each function. Performance standards are usually set for both quantity and quality and should be as objective and measurable as possible.

Some organizations establish measures that reflect various levels of performance. For example, one measure of a coder's performance might be coding a specified number of charts per day, perhaps no fewer than 20 charts per day. Other organizations might establish several levels of expected performance, for example:

30 to 35 charts per day	Outstanding
25 to 29 charts per day	Exceeds expectations
20 to 24 charts per day	Meets expectations
15 to 19 charts per day	Needs improvement
Fewer than 14 charts per day	Unsatisfactory

The following example shows how a quality standard might be used as a performance indicator of coding accuracy:

96 to 100% accuracy	Outstanding
92 to 95% accuracy	Exceeds expectations
89 to 94% accuracy	Meets expectations
84 to 88% accuracy	Needs improvement
Less than 84%	Unsatisfactory

In the preceding example, a definition for coding accuracy might be helpful. For example, accurate coding includes capturing correct codes and sequencing them appropriately for all diagnoses and procedures that affect reimbursement.

Standards that are measurable and relevant to an employee's overall performance are helpful in setting clear expectations. They also are useful in providing constructive feedback. (See chapter 25 for a full discussion of performance standards and measurement.)

Policies and Procedures

Policies and procedures are critical tools that may be used to ensure consistent quality performance. A **policy** is a statement about what an organization or department does. For example, a policy might state that patients are allowed to review their health records under certain conditions such as when a clinical professional is present or in the HIM department. Policies should be clearly stated and comprehensive. They must be developed in accordance with applicable laws, and they must reflect actual practice. And because they may be used as documentation of intended practice in a lawsuit, policies should be developed very carefully. Organization and departmental policies are often found on the organization's internal network or intranet.

A **procedure** describes how work is to be done and how policies are to be carried out. Procedures are instructions that ensure high-quality, consistent outcomes for tasks done, especially when more than one person is involved. One of the benefits of developing a procedure is that time is taken to analyze the best possible method for completing a process. A detailed procedure is also useful in training new staff or in providing instructions to anyone needing to perform a task in the regular employee's absence.

Several tools may be used to effectively communicate the purpose, scope, and details of the work done by employees in the organization. As written, the procedure should also have any sample forms utilized in the task attached, completed, or filled out to indicate the proper processing. (See chapter 25 for more information regarding work procedures.) The manager is responsible for developing and maintaining these tools. However, the manager's role does not end here. Given the tools described so far, he or she is ready to hire, train, and interact with employees.

Tools for Recruitment and Retention

Armed with a position description, the manager is ready to begin recruiting candidates for a new or open position. **Recruitment** is the process of finding, soliciting, and attracting new employees. However, the manager should be sure to understand the organization's recruitment and hiring policies and to seek the assistance of the HR department before the vacancy is publicized. This preparation ensures that the organization's legal obligations and policies and procedures are followed throughout the recruitment, selection, and hiring process.

Recruitment

The first thing to consider in recruiting candidates to fill a staff opening is whether to promote someone from inside the organization or to look for candidates outside the organization. The advantage of promoting from within is that the practice often motivates employees to perform well, learn new skills, and work toward advancement. To advertise a vacancy internally, the organization might post it on facility bulletin boards or list it in the organization's newsletter or intranet. The department manager may announce an opening at a routine staff meeting or use any other communication channels available. Initial communication of job opportunities internally presents the underlying message that internal candidates are considered first whenever possible.

When the position cannot be filled from within, however, there are several ways to advertise externally. For example, the organization might place an ad in a newspaper or professional journal, post the job on the organization's employment site or on external Internet recruitment sites, announce the opportunity at professional meetings, contact people who have previously applied or expressed interest in working at the organization, or work through a professional recruiter.

In most cases, the approach used depends on the nature of the open position. For example, the facility might run an ad for a clerical position in a local newspaper or on an Internet recruitment site, but not in a professional journal because the market for entry level positions is often strong locally. Alternately, the facility might turn to a professional recruiter when trying to fill a department director or experienced coding position because the number of qualified candidates for these positions is more limited.

As in every industry, job seekers looking for professional-level healthcare positions submit detailed resumes. A resume describes the candidate's educational background and work experience and usually includes information on personal and professional achievements. Candidates often submit a cover letter describing the type of position in which they are interested along with their resume. Today, it is common for candidates to submit, and organizations to accept, application letters and resumes via electronic systems, including email and employer websites.

Applications are formal documentation that job seekers complete to give prospective employers their chronological work history, current status, and the specifics of their skill sets. People seeking entry-level positions may be asked to complete an application rather than to submit a resume. In many cases, completion of applications can be done online. It is imperative that job descriptions used in the job postings are comprehensive and up to date so the best qualified candidates are not excluded. It is equally important that applicants are as specific as possible in their applications while highlighting their skill sets so, in turn, they are not excluded by an electronic HR management system that uses keyword matches to determine eligible applicants. These systems are designed to compare key skills and knowledge from the job description requirements to those identified skills and knowledge included in the employee application or resume; when the terms match between the two, that person becomes a candidate for the position.

Selection

When a sufficient pool of applicants has been recruited, the selection process can begin. The goal of the selection process is to identify the candidate most qualified to fill the position.

Testing and interviewing applicants are the two basic tools employed in the selection process.

Employment testing is commonly conducted during the applicant's first visit to the facility. **Reliability** of a test refers to the consistency with which a test measures an attribute. **Validity** refers to a test's ability to accurately and consistently measure what it purports to measure. Testing practices are under increasing legal scrutiny, which places a special burden on organizations to ensure that tests used are clearly job related. Use of tests as a selection procedure violates federal anti-discrimination laws if used to exclude people based on race, color, sex, national origin, disability, religion, or age (EEOC 2010). HR professionals are generally familiar with a variety of ability (achievement) tests that assess applicants' current skills, aptitude tests, mental ability (cognitive) tests that assess applicants' reasoning capabilities, personality tests, and honesty (integrity) tests that are designed to evaluate honesty via a series of hypothetical questions that are suitable for use in the organization (Anthony et al. 2010; EEOC 2010). Many healthcare organizations also perform routine drug testing on candidates for employment in order to create a drug-free work environment.

The interview is generally considered the most important phase of the selection process, and there are three effective interview formats:

- **Structured interview** uses a set of standardized questions that are asked of all applicants. Figure 23.2 offers an example of a tool that can be used to ensure that the same questions based on predetermined selection criteria are asked of and evaluated for each applicant.

- **Behavioral description interview** requires applicants to give specific examples of how they have performed a specific procedure or handled a specific problem in the past. The worksheet in figure 23.3 also allows a space for documenting specific information from the applicant for each criteria.

- **Panel interview** includes a team of people who interview applicants at one time. (Mathis and Jackson 2011)

Interviewing is one of the most important skills that managers need for selecting new staff. Unfortunately, many managers receive little formal training in interviewing techniques or have little practical experience. This shortcoming can be overcome through self-education, mentoring by more experienced managers, or instructional sessions with HR professionals in the organization.

Failure to adequately prepare for conducting the interview has consequences that are very serious for the organization and the applicant. Reviewing the position description, reading the applicant's resume and application form, and preparing appropriate and relevant questions are important steps to take before beginning an interview.

The interview itself has four basic purposes:

- Obtain information from the applicant about his or her past work history and future goals

- Give information to the applicant about the organization's mission and goals and the nature of the employment opportunity

- Evaluate the applicant's work experience, attitude, and personality as a potential fit for the organization

- Give the applicant an opportunity to evaluate the organization as a potential fit for his or her current and future employment goals

EEO regulations dictate the types of questions that may be asked during interviews and on employment applications. For example, questions pertaining to age, religious affiliation, and marital status should be avoided (EEOC n.d.(b)). These regulations apply during all activities associated with the interview, including during formal interview sessions and during less formal lunches, dinners, or hallway and elevator small talk, when it is very easy to inadvertently lapse into discussions on these topics. Managers should always seek the advice of HR professionals when they are uncertain about which questions to ask.

Figure 23.3. Interviewing and selection worksheet

Selection criteria	Information on: [applicant name]	Score rate 1–10	Information on: [applicant name]	Score rate 1–10	Information on: [applicant name]	Score rate 1–10

Healthcare organizations, like other employers, must be certain to conduct careful background checks of potential employees. Managers or HR professionals also check the references of candidates and communicate with the past employers of candidates via telephone or correspondence. Checking references involves confirming the information provided by applicants on resumes and applications. **Reference checks** or a background investigation should also be conducted specifically to assess the applicants' fit with the position and to validate the accuracy of information the applicants provide on their applications and during the interview. A survey of employers revealed that the false information furnished most commonly by candidates for employment dealt with past lengths of employment, salary history, criminal record, and job titles (Mathis and Jackson 2011, 73).

Hiring

After all the internal and external interviews, tests, and reference and background checks are complete, the hiring manager usually has enough information to make a hiring decision. A tool that can assist with the making a hiring decision is the decision matrix in figure 23.4. In this figure, the decision analysis matrix is designed for hiring an inpatient coder. The MUST criteria is the criteria required for the applicant; this criteria has to be

Figure 23.4.   Decision analysis matrix

DECISION: Applicant to select for inpatient coder position.

Evaluate each applicant (A, B, and C) based on the criteria specified in the job description by applying the decision analysis technique.

Criteria	A	B	C
MUSTS (required)			

Place an X across from each MUST criteria the applicant meets. All MUST criteria must be met before evaluating the WANT criteria.

	A	B	C
1. Two years inpatient coding experience	____	____	____
2. Coding credential (CCS, CPC, CIC)	____	____	____
3. Experience using an encoder	____	____	____
4. Ability to communicate clearly	____	____	____

WANTS (desired)

Each WANT criteria is weighted with the number in parentheses after it. If the applicant meets the criteria and expectations fully, assign that weight as noted. If not, give them a 0. Only rate the WANT criteria if all the MUST (required) criteria are met.

	A	B	C
1. Responsible, dependable (5)	____	____	____
2. Neat appearance (3)	____	____	____
3. Experience with CAC (2)	____	____	____
4. RHIA credential (3)	____	____	____
Total Points	____	____	____

Comments:

present to the hiring manager's satisfaction for it to be met. The WANT criteria is desired criteria. This criteria would not be considered if all the MUST criteria is not met. The WANT criteria has a weight of importance noted in parentheses after each criteria. If the criteria is met to the hiring manager's satisfaction, that weight is assigned to the criteria for the applicant. If not, a zero is given. This is an all or nothing scoring. A manager may decide to use a range between zero and the weighted score as another methodology. The total at the bottom of the matrix is the total of the WANT or desired criteria for each applicant.

In some organizations, the manager shares the hiring decision with key department staff, HR staff, and executive staff, depending on the level of the position.

When the details of the job offer have been approved by the HR department, a formal job offer should be made. The HR department should prepare a letter that describes the duties and responsibilities of the position, states the employment start date, and explains the salary and benefits package. In addition, the hiring manager may choose to communicate the offer to the candidate through a personal telephone contact, which is subsequently confirmed by an official letter (Anthony et al. 2010).

Workforce Retention

According to the Bureau of Labor Statistics, a certain level of staff turnover is expected; current variable rates for healthcare are at 2.5 percent (BLS 2015). Employees move, retire, or seek other careers. A manager can do little to prevent turnover resulting from changes in the personal lives of employees. However, the actions of managers and the policies of the organization can have an impact, either positive or negative, on staff retention. **Retention** is the ability to keep valuable employees from seeking employment elsewhere.

The following questions when assessing employee retention should be considered:

- Is there a comprehensive new employee orientation and training program giving the employee the resources needed to be successful? (Refer to chapter 24 for a full discussion of orientation and training programs).

- Does the organization support continued education either financially or through flexible work schedules?

- Do employees have opportunities to advance their careers within the organization?

- Are salaries and benefits competitive with similar organizations?

- Do working conditions provide a comfortable and safe environment?

- Does the manager treat employees fairly and follow employment regulations and guidelines?

- Is there frequent and clear communication between management and employees?

Although individual managers may have limited influence on some of these factors, they must always be aware of the impact that broader organizational HR policies and practices have on employees. Gone unnoticed or left unaddressed, concerns in these areas are often what make employees look for other jobs. For example, employees can become dissatisfied when they feel that they are being treated unfairly or that HR practices are needlessly rigid. In some cases, employees become dissatisfied simply because they do not know the rationale for a particular HR policy or because a concern they have voiced about an unsafe condition in their work area is not acted on by the manager. The challenge to the manager is to anticipate or, at the very least, to find ways to be informed as soon as possible when employees express an HR-related concern.

Staff turnover is expensive in terms of both lost productivity and recruitment and training costs. To ensure effective management, turnover should be monitored across time and benchmarked with the rest of the organization and other organizations in the community or geographic area. Routine employee satisfaction surveys can help provide information about how employees feel about their jobs and insights into how the facility might improve working conditions. Conducting routine **exit interviews** with employees who leave the organization is another way to obtain information on how employees feel about their jobs and what issues cause them to leave.

Tools for Effective Communication

Maintaining regular and effective communication with staff is one of the ongoing challenges in managing human resources. Communication is important because it contributes significantly to the morale of the staff and their ability to contribute to the department's operations as a whole. To address this challenge, a manager should establish a communication plan that includes routine and timely opportunities for both verbal and written information sharing within the department or workgroup. The plan should include, as appropriate, the following types of communication:

- Daily personal contact with every employee to maintain a sense of connectedness and, as necessary, to create opportunities for casual discussions of emerging work-related changes or issues

- Web-based or traditional bulletin boards located in an area convenient to staff to publicize official announcements, permissible personal news, written status updates, and written highlights from departmental meetings

- Weekly status meetings with the staff for each functional unit in the department in larger organizations or the entire department in smaller organizations

- Monthly departmental meetings with highlights recorded for posting

- Quarterly performance discussions with individual employees

- Ad hoc verbal or electronic (e-mail) status updates, as appropriate, to alert staff to information of interest from organizational meetings

On a day-to-day basis, when problems emerge that require resolution within the department or when decisions are made that affect the employees in the department, the management team is responsible for establishing a unique communication plan that conforms to the situation. Such a plan identifies the full range of employees affected by the problem or the decision and defines the specific approach that managers will take to engage or inform each person appropriately.

In general, keeping staff well informed is a key factor in developing and sustaining a healthy level of trust in the relationship between employees and managers. Communication plans are simple tools that managers can use to ensure that this critical aspect of their responsibilities is handled with the level of routine and regular attentiveness it requires.

Tools for Employee Empowerment

Creating an environment that encourages and allows employees to use and develop their problem-solving and decision-making competencies is an established HR management practice that has many benefits. For example, it increases the manager's capacity and productivity, improves the quality and timeliness of decision making, enhances employee morale, and contributes to improved employee retention.

Team Building

People today need to work collaboratively with others; thus, the need for **team building**—the process of organizing and acquainting team members. The team may consist of people who perform the same function within the same department, for example, a coding team. The team may bring together people who perform different functions within the same department to solve a shared problem or people from across the organization with different expertise to implement a new computer system or to study an issue that would affect the overall organization (for example, improvements in the employee evaluation system).

At their best, teams increase the creativity and improve the quality of problem solving. Often team-based decisions are more widely accepted than managerial decisions because team members enlist support for the decisions from their peers and coworkers. In addition, teams can use their collective energy to produce more work than individuals can. Moreover, teamwork establishes strong relationships among employees. Teamwork also can enrich jobs and provide variety in work assignments. Finally, teams can develop new leaders and expose employees to issues that would not be within the usual scope of their jobs.

One thing that binds team members together is having a common purpose. The purpose for an ongoing work team, for example, might be to ensure cross-training, improve procedures, and monitor quality and productivity. In other cases, teams are created for a specific purpose. Some teams exist for long periods of time because they have an ongoing reason to exist. Other teams function for limited periods of time and disband after their purpose has been fulfilled.

However, having a common purpose is only one element of an effective team. The team also must have an effective leader. This individual must be able to create agendas and organize meetings, lead discussions, and ensure that the work moves forward. The team may either appoint or elect its leader, depending on its purpose and the experience and expertise of its members.

In addition, effective teams set ground rules. For instance, team members might decide that all meetings will start on time, minutes will be recorded, decisions will be reached by consensus, and everyone will participate in discussions. The early establishment of rules can reduce conflict as the team moves forward. Team strength lies in engaging the collective brainpower of all members, and so the team leader should use techniques that effectively engage every member of the team.

Not all teams are effective, and the causes for problems vary. A team without a clear purpose could create a product that does not accomplish the work it was designed to accomplish; for example, a request to improve the release of information process without knowing the

issues or problems will likely lead to the team not meeting the expected goal. A leader who dominates the team could reduce its effectiveness and frustrate its members. Members who do not participate, have insufficient expertise, or are unconcerned with the team's success could cause the team to fail. And members who work outside the team or do not support its decisions can create dissension and reduce support for the outcome.

Managing staff teams is an important aspect of every manager's responsibilities. Careful consideration should be given to developing the team's purpose and composition. Team members need to feel that their work is important and that their contributions make a difference. A well-run team can be an effective and productive force. A poorly run team can waste time and frustrate and demoralize its members.

Delegation

Managers have specific responsibilities and the authority to act within the scope of that responsibility. **Responsibility** is the accountability required as a part of one's job. A manager's responsibilities cannot be delegated to another person; that is, the manager always remains the one accountable for outcomes in areas within his or her designated scope even if duties have been delegated to others. However, with appropriate preparation and decision-making guidelines in place, managers can and should delegate the authority to make and act on decisions to employees as individuals or teams. **Delegation** is the process by which managers distribute work to others along with the **authority**, or right, to make decisions and take action. This delegation of authority expands the manager's capacity, improves the timeliness of decisions, and develops the competencies of other staff members.

When delegating authority, managers make it possible for staff to succeed by preparing them in advance as follows:

- Explaining exactly what needs to be done
- Describing clear expectations
- Setting clear deadlines

- Granting authority to make relevant decisions
- Ensuring appropriate communication and outcomes reporting
- Providing the resources needed to complete the assigned task

Once ensuring the manager has prepared the employee, it is important to verify that the employee is still comfortable with the assigned duties. See chapter 24 for an expanded discussion of empowerment and delegation as employee development strategies.

Check Your Understanding 23.2

Instructions: **On a separate piece of paper, indicate whether the following statements are true or false (T or F). If the statement is false, explain why it is false.**

1. To lead effectively, every manager should have an understanding of HR management principles.

2. Performance standards are developed to indicate who executes each function of a job.

3. In healthcare organizations, individuals applying for entry-level positions must submit a resume and a cover letter.

4. The interview process is intended to give the applicant an opportunity to evaluate the organization as a potential fit for his or her current and future employment goals.

5. Staff turnover is expensive in terms of lost productivity and recruitment and training costs.

Instructions: **Answer the following questions on a separate piece of paper.**

6. What is enhanced between managers and employees by keeping employees well informed?

7. In terms of responsibility and authority, which can managers delegate and which cannot be delegated?

Compensation Systems

Employee compensation systems serve to reward employees equitably for their service to the organization. Organizations also use compensation systems to enhance employee loyalty and encourage greater productivity.

The Fair Labor Standards Act (FLSA), the Equal Pay Act (EPA), and several of the EEO laws (for example, Title VII of the Civil Rights Act, Age Discrimination in Employment Act, and the ADA) all have provisions that affect compensation systems. Provisions of the FLSA, for example, cover minimum wage, overtime pay, child labor restrictions, and equal pay for equal work regardless of sex (WHD n.d.). Federal regulations specify exemptions from some or all of the FLSA provisions for a number of groups of employees

(Myers 2011). These groups are referred to as **exempt employees** and are paid a salary per pay period. Covered groups are referred to as **nonexempt employees** and are paid an hourly wage.

Managers who control employee work schedules and process employee timecards at the close of each pay period become quite familiar with the provisions of the FLSA that relate to overtime pay. In general, the FLSA requires that employers pay one and a half times the employee's regular rate for all hours that a covered (nonexempt) employee works in excess of 40 per week (WHD n.d.). Some organizations institute overtime pay for all worked hours in excess of 8 hours per day and others when employees work in excess of 40 hours per week or 80 hours per 2-week pay period. In calculations of worked hours, the FLSA specifies that rest periods of up to 20 minutes each be counted as worked time, but meal periods of thirty minutes or more are not counted as worked time (WHD n.d.). Time spent in mandated job-related training is considered worked time, and significant travel time (beyond the usual time required to commute to and from work) associated with a work-related event is counted as worked time. Compensatory time, taken in lieu of overtime pay, may be used when it is part of the organization's compensation plan (Myers 2011).

Because of the complexities and sensitivities associated with compensation issues, HR professionals are a manager's best advisor when questions related to compensation regulations and practices arise.

Compensation Surveys

The HR department routinely consults compensation surveys published by government agencies and professional and trade associations to ensure that pay for the organization's employees is fair, equitable, and aligned with other organizations. This is important for effective employee recruitment and retention. In some cases, an HR department may choose to conduct an independent survey to obtain data more specific to the organization's needs. Often consultants experienced with survey design and data analysis are employed by the organization to either assist in or do the survey project to ensure a successful outcome from this costly activity. Compensation surveys provide benchmark data that the organization can use to evaluate or establish its compensation system for unique jobs within the organization or for jobs throughout the organization (Myers 2011).

Job Evaluations

Job evaluation projects are undertaken by an organization to determine the relative worth of jobs as a first step toward establishing an equitable internal compensation system. **Job evaluation** is the process of applying predefined compensable factors to jobs to determine their relative worth. A **compensable factor** is "a characteristic used to compare the worth of jobs" and "the EPA requires employers to consider [several] compensable factors in setting pay for similar work performed by both females and males" (Myers 2011, 691). These factors include skill, effort (mental and physical exertion required to perform job-related tasks), responsibility, and working conditions.

Four job evaluation methods are commonly used:

- **Job ranking** is the simplest and the most subjective method of job evaluation. It involves placing jobs in order from highest to lowest in value to the organization.

- **Job classification method** involves matching a job's written position description with a description of a classification grade. Jobs in the federal government are graded on the basis of this method of job evaluation.

- **Point method** is a commonly used system that places weight (points) on each of the compensable factors in a job. The total points associated with a job establish its relative worth. Jobs that fall within a specific range of points fall into a grade associated with a specific wage or salary.

- **Factor comparison method** is a complex quantitative method that combines elements of both the ranking and point methods. Factor comparison results indicate the degree to which different compensable factors vary by job, making it possible to translate each factor value more easily into a monetary wage (Mathis and Jackson 2011).

The Hay method of job evaluation is another system used. The **Hay method of job evaluation** is a modification of the point method that numerically measures the levels of three major compensable factors: the know-how, problem-solving, and accountability requirements of each job (Mathis and Jackson 2011; Myers 2011).

In addition, most healthcare organizations establish some type of job classification system that combines jobs with similar levels of responsibility and qualifications into job grades that determine salary ranges and benefit packages. For instance, all supervisory-level managers might be classified into one salary and benefit category, but each would have a unique job description. Job classifications also may determine whether an employee belongs to a union or is a candidate for unionization at the time a union attempts to organize the workforce, as may be the case if clerical staff is organized.

Performance Management

Most organizations use some form of **performance review** system to evaluate the performance of individual employees. Figure 23.5 offers an example of a performance appraisal form illustrating the appraisal ratings, criteria for evaluation, strengths, areas for improvement, and goals. This type of format supports a uniform approach to assessing each employee. Although performance reviews should be a part of regular communications between managers and employees, formal performance review discussions are routinely held on an annual or biannual basis. The functions of performance reviews include the following:

- Assessment of the employee's performance compared to performance standards or previously set performance goals
- Development of performance goals for the future year
- Development of a plan for professional development

Performance reviews also may include employee self-assessments. In some organizations, other employees may contribute information to the reviews of colleagues and co-workers. In the case of a supervisory manager, his or her staff may participate in the evaluation. This form of evaluation to which managers, peers, and staff contribute is called a **360-degree evaluation**.

Many organizations' base pay increases on the results of annual performance reviews. Whether or not the evaluation affects salary, the annual review is an opportunity to formally discuss past accomplishments, career development, and expectations for future performance.

Performance management is an ongoing challenge. Information about performance should be collected regularly and shared with employees, whether their jobs involve coding clinical records or directing a department. Good performance results should be shared to encourage and reward ongoing success. Performance issues are rarely resolved by ignoring them. Understanding the causes of problems and working with employees to resolve them are important management tasks. Actions that can be taken to improve performance include retraining, streamlining responsibilities, reestablishing expectations, and monitoring progress.

Performance Counseling and Disciplinary Action

When actions taken to improve performance are unsuccessful, more formal counseling and even disciplinary action may be required, such as suspension without pay, demotion, or less pay. Most organizations have formal processes in place to ensure that all staff is treated fairly and that employment laws are followed. Managers should consult with the HR department to ensure that any disciplinary actions comply with approved procedures. Refer to table 23.1 for references to common employment law.

The steps described in establishing performance standards, hiring and training employees, and conducting routine performance reviews are all necessary before doing performance counseling or taking disciplinary action. Moreover, steps to improve performance should be taken in all cases.

Performance counseling usually begins with informal counseling or a verbal warning. No record of these actions is typically required in the employee's

Figure 23.5. Performance appraisal form

PERFORMANCE APPRAISAL   Date: _____

Employee name: _____   Title: _____

Department: _____   CC: _____   Emp. No. _____   DOH: _____

Appraisal period: _____ to: _____

Instructions: Carefully evaluate employee's work performance in relation to current job requirements. Check rating box to indicate the employee's performance. Indicate N/A if not applicable.

DEFINITION OF APPRAISAL RATINGS:
Exemplary (E): Performance is exceptional in all areas and is recognizable as being superior to others.
Proficient (P): Results clearly meet most position requirements. Performance is of high quality and is achieved consistently.
Novice (N): Competent and dependable level of performance. Meets performance expectations of the job.
Unsatisfactory (U): Results are generally unacceptable and require immediate improvement.
N/A: Not applicable to this person's job.

APPRAISAL FACTOR	**RATING**
Applies past experiences to new problems	
Retains information; does not repeatedly ask the same questions or make the same mistakes	
Follows instructions and takes notes when necessary	
Has gained the skills necessary to navigate the computer system for the functions for which he or she is responsible	
Takes care of equipment	
Uses supplies wisely; exercises apparent stewardship	
Follows department procedures	
Completes assigned work accurately	
Completes volume required	
Makes efficient use of time	
Meets accuracy requirements	
Completes assigned work with little or no dependence upon others	
Handwriting is legible	
Does not transpose numbers	
Willing to work with overtime	
Requires minimum supervision	
Improved in all areas that were marked "improvement needed" or "unsatisfactory" in last evaluation	
Achieved goals outlined in last evaluation	
Maintained strengths in same areas as last evaluation	
Days of absence	
Tardies	
Area(s) for improvement:	
Strengths:	
Goals: 1. Target Date: _____ Employee's initials: _____ 2. Target Date: _____ Employee's initials: _____	
Employee Comments: Employee's initials: _____	

Employee's Signature: _____ Date: _____

Supervisor's Signature: _____ Date: _____

Manager's Signature: _____ Date: _____

official file, however a manager may choose to include it. The progressive discipline process begins with a verbal warning that may or may not be a part of the employee's file depending on organization policy and the severity and frequency of the offense. When the next offense occurs, the process progresses to a written reprimand with formal documentation of the problem and delineation of the steps needed to correct it. This and any further related action is typically a part of the employee's official HR file. Employees may be required to submit a step-by-step action plan to resolve issues and improve their performance. The next offense often result in suspension, with further related infractions resulting in dismissal.

In some environments, disciplinary actions include suspension from employment without pay or demotion to a job with lower expectations and less pay. In some cases, more than one of these actions may be taken. Generally, however, suspension and demotion are less popular than the use of binding performance improvement plans because suspension and demotion create a punitive atmosphere. Such punitive actions also affect the morale of other employees and staff. Empowering employees to create a plan of action places the responsibility for performance improvement in their own hands.

Regardless of the counseling and disciplinary actions mandated by the organization, managers should take some key steps of their own, including:

- Discussing performance problems and consequences for poor performance with the employee in a clear and direct manner
- Supporting the employee's efforts to improve performance or resolve performance issues
- Documenting the steps taken to improve performance
- Carefully following the organization's HR policies
- Consulting HR professionals before taking action
- Keeping performance issues confidential
- Following the same process for all employees

By following these steps in a timely, impartial and considerate manner, managers will construct a consistent disciplinary message and hopefully coach the employee to job performance improvement. Documentation of the steps taken in the progressive discipline process is critical in the event that performance does not improve, necessitating advanced actions up to suspension or termination. This documentation may be critical in the event of employee denial, grievance, or litigation.

Termination and Layoff

One of the most difficult duties of a line manager is delivering the notification of termination (ending of a job) to an employee. The HR department is a vital resource for advising and supporting the manager through this process to ensure that accepted HR practices as established by the organization are adhered to. The general guidelines to use when terminating an employee are:

- Determine the most appropriate location to hold the discussion privately
- Review the employee file and the progressive discipline process that has occurred
- State position quickly and concisely and end the discussion
- Be sensitive to appropriate timing for the discussion
- Be prepared with all of the appropriate severance information
- Treat the employee with dignity and respect (Delpo 2015)

Layoffs are similar to terminations except that they are essentially unpaid leaves of absence initiated by the employer as a strategy for downsizing staff in response to a change in the organization's status (for example, an unexpected or a seasonal downturn in business volume). In many cases, unlike termination, employees are called back to work at some future date.

The Workers' Adjustment Retraining and Notification (WARN) Act requires that organizations employing more than 100 people give the employees and the community a 60-day notice of its intent to close the business or to lay off 50 or more members of its workforce (DOL n.d.). The intent of the Act is to provide time for employees and their families to adjust to an impending unemployment event and seek new skills to be competitive in the current job market. Managers need to understand this requirement so they can plan accordingly for that time should they be in a position where employee layoffs are imminent. It is important to plan for a potential downturn in employee morale and productivity during this time.

Conflict Management

Sometimes problems arise because of conflicts among employees. It is common for people to disagree, and sometimes a difference of opinion can increase creativity. However, too much conflict can also waste time, reduce productivity, and decrease morale. When taken to the extreme, it can threaten the safety of employees and cause damage to property.

Conflict management focuses on working with the individuals involved in a disagreement to find a mutually acceptable solution. There are three ways to address conflict.

- **Compromise**: In this method, both parties must be willing to lose or give up a piece of their position. One scenario in which this approach may be well served is job sharing where one position (FTE) is split between two employees. If only one set of benefits apply to a position, the employees will need to determine who will enjoy the insurance benefits and who receives the paid time off (PTO). The outcome of this decision will require each employee to give up something in order for the job sharing arrangement to work.

- **Control**: In this method, interaction may be prohibited until the employees' emotions are under control. The manager also may structure their interactions. For example, the manager can set ground rules for communicating or dealing with specific issues. Another form of control is personal counseling. Personal counseling focuses on how people deal with conflict rather than on the cause of specific disagreements.

- **Constructive confrontation**: In this method, both parties meet with an objective third party to explore their perceptions and feelings. The desired outcome is to produce a mutual understanding of the issues and to create a win-win situation. For example, there are two registry abstracters sharing a desk space on their respective back-to-back shifts that are at odds, each perceiving their method of organization is most beneficial. The opposing methods of processing is creating tension that is reported to be exacerbating their anger with each other, rather than being resolved during attempted one-on-one encounters. With appropriate moderating between the two employees and a third party, often the parties at odds can receive a new understanding of a coworker's perspective.

Conflict is an expected part of working with others, but managing and resolving conflict is crucial to an effective work unit.

Grievance Management

Employees have the right to disagree with management and can express their opinions or complaints in a variety of ways. They should be encouraged to bring problems and concerns directly to their manager. When they do not achieve satisfaction at that level, the manager should explain other options to the employee. For example, dissatisfied employees should understand that they can either take their issues to the next management level or discuss them with HR staff.

Organizations establish **grievance procedures** that define the steps an employee can follow to seek resolution of a disagreement they have with management on a job-related issue. A complaint becomes a **grievance** when it has been documented in writing and brought to the attention of management or union representatives. At that point, the formal grievance procedure is set in motion. Depending on organizational policy or a union contract, the grievance procedure may vary.

Employees who belong to a union should follow the grievance procedures set by their union. Union contracts usually specify the types of actions employees can take, the time frames for filing grievances, and define the formal process for elevating the consideration or resolution of a grievance. Grievances taken to the highest levels will likely have to be resolved through mediation or arbitration. **Mediation** is when an objective third party unrelated to the dispute is invited to bring the parties to mutual agreement. **Arbitration** is when an objective third party is brought in to make a binding decision in a case where the parties cannot come to agreement.

Each of these steps takes time and can cost money. Therefore, managers should try to avoid grievances by maintaining open and effective communication with their staff.

Maintenance of Employee Records

Official documentation about an employee's job performance, must be maintained under the control of the HR department. Any employee records maintained under the control of the manager must be kept secure at all times.

Federal legislation such as Title VII of the Civil Rights Act of 1964, the Age Discrimination in Employment Act, the Immigration Reform and Control Act, and the FLSA place numerous recordkeeping and reporting requirements on the HR department. The Environmental Protection Agency (EPA) and the Occupational Safety and Health Administration (OSHA) also have recordkeeping requirements. Several of these additional recordkeeping obligations are as follows:

- Employers must protect the confidentiality of personnel records and files.
- Employers must protect the health records of employees.

- Employers must avoid intruding into the personal lives of employees, such as their other associations, alcohol use, spending habits, and financial obligations unless there are valid job-related reasons for making such intrusions.
- Employers must prevent the public disclosure of personal information that may be embarrassing to an employee.
- Employers must protect the results of employment-related tests, including written tests used in making selection decisions, and the results of both pre-employment and random drug testing. (Myers 2011, 125–26)

Employers must have consistent and stringent recordkeeping processes to protect the privacy of employees. This is a legal and ethical obligation.

Current Human Resources Trends and Practices

According to the US Department of Labor (2011a), on the heels of the 2010 US Census, the following workforce trends in employment are likely to affect the labor market in the United States during the first decades of the 21st century:

- Women will constitute a greater proportion of the labor force than in the past, with 58.6 percent of all US women in the workforce in 2010. In the healthcare industry, women are more than 50 percent of the workforce. Slightly over 71 percent of the women in the workforce have children under the age of

18, and 36 percent of women in the workforce hold college degrees.

- Minority racial and ethnic groups will account for a growing percentage of the overall labor force. Immigrants will expand this growth.
- The average age of the US population will increase, and more workers who retire from full-time jobs will work part-time.
- As a result of these and other shifts, employers in a variety of industries will face shortages of qualified workers.

From this information, employers must be prepared to function with an increasingly diverse workforce in terms of gender, age, health status, race, and ethnicity. In general, the management of an increasingly diverse workforce is receiving considerable attention in the HR literature, and some organizations are initiating diversity training programs. Three content areas that are often included in diversity training programs include:

- *Legal awareness:* Federal and state laws and regulations on equal employment opportunity and the consequences of violating these laws and regulations
- *Cultural awareness:* Attempts to deal with stereotypes, typically through discussions and exercises
- *Sensitivity training:* Attempts to sensitize people to the differences among them and how their words and behaviors are perceived by others (Mathis and Jackson 2011)

There is still work to be done within healthcare organizations and HIM departments to prepare for the anticipated growth in the multicultural profile of human assets over the coming decade (see chapter 24 for more discussion related to diversity, sensitivity, and anti-harassment training).

The Department of Labor (2011b) data also indicate that employees will increasingly seek ways to gain more control over their time. The time pressure associated with trying to balance work and personal lives (especially when both parents are working outside the family home) coupled with the time pressure associated with increasingly long commutes appear to be driving this concern to the surface in HR management. Flextime, job sharing, and home-based (telecommuting) staffing options are emerging as viable solutions to the workforce retention issue. Within transcription and coding work units in HIM services, flextime and home-based staffing options are being implemented to address the labor shortages already affecting departmental operations. The advancement of technology is playing a key role in the increased availability of staffing options and growing opportunities for work and personal life balance.

Effective management of human resources begins with attention given to the adoption of appropriate policies, procedures, and practices in each of the seven HR activity areas: HR planning and analysis; equal employment opportunity; staffing; HR development; compensation and benefits; health, safety, and security; and employee and labor management relations. HIM professionals working in close partnership with the organization's HR department hire and retain qualified employees by following these employment guidelines and fostering effective working relationships between employees and management.

Effective recruitment, selection, and hiring practices involve the consistent use of the tools designed to identify the best-qualified candidates for each position. Once hired, ensuring that employees are well-oriented and trained is the critical first step toward a successful long-term outcome. Subsequently, maintaining open and meaningful communications with employees, setting realistic performance expectations for employees, engaging employees in ways that give them appropriate control of their work schedule and environment, delegating appropriate levels of decision-making authority, and providing them with opportunities for ongoing staff development all serve to enhance employee morale and increase job satisfaction.

Managing human resources is both a science and an art. As such, it is learned through a combination of study and observation. Published HR management resources are readily available to provide the knowledge foundation associated with this field. In the workplace, HR professionals are available to serve as advisors to HIM managers who want to handle this complex aspect of their management responsibilities knowledgably and artfully.

Check Your Understanding 23.3

Instructions: On a separate piece of paper, indicate whether the following statements are true or false (T or F). If the statement is false, explain why it is false.

1. Employee compensation systems are used to enhance employee loyalty.

2. Minimum wage and overtime policies are impacted by the Taft-Hartley Act.

3. All employees are subject to the provisions of the Fair Labor Standards Act.

4. Trade associations and government agencies are routine sources for compensation benchmark data.

5. The Equal Pay Act requires employers to consider compensable factors when setting pay for similar work performed by both females and males.

6. Job ranking is a complex method for conducting job evaluations.

7. The first step in a progressive disciplinary process is a verbal, undocumented warning.

Instructions: Answer the following questions on a separate piece of paper.

8. Name a method of conflict resolution with the goal of arriving at a win-win outcome.

9. Grievance taken to the highest levels for resolution will likely be resolved through what methods?

10. What staffing alternatives are being employed in health information services to address labor shortage issues?

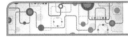 # References

Anthony, W.P., P.L. Perrewe, and K.M. Kacmar. 2010. *Human Resource Management: A Strategic Approach,* 6th ed. Boston, MA: Cengage Learning.

Delpo, A. 2015. What to Say When You Fire an Employee. http://www.nolo.com/legal-encyclopedia/what-to-say-fire-employee-36140.html

Dunn, R.T. 2010. *Dunn and Haimann's Healthcare Management,* 9th ed. Chicago: AUPHA.

Harrington, L. and M. Heidkamp. 2013. The Aging Workforce: Challenges for the Health Care Industry Workforce. *The NTAR Leadership Center* [Issue brief]. https://www.dol.gov/odep/pdf/NTAR-AgingWorkforceHealthCare.pdf

Mathis, R.L. and J.H. Jackson. 2011. *Human Resource Management: Essential Perspectives,* 6th ed. Cincinnati, OH: South-Western Publishers.

McNickle, M. 2012. 8 Trends for a Changing Healthcare Workforce. *Healthcare IT News.* http://www.healthcareitnews.com/news/8-trends-changing-healthcare-workforce?page=0

Myers, D.W. 2011. *U.S. Master Human Resources Guide.* Chicago: CCH.

The Caviart Group. 2014. A Workforce Study of the Future Direction and Skill Set for HIM Professionals [Results of the AHIMA 2014 Workforce Study]. http://bok.ahima.org/PdfView?oid=300801

US Department of Labor (DOL). n.d. The Worker Adjustment and Retraining Notification Act (WARN). http://www.dol.gov/compliance/laws/comp-warn.htm#applicable_laws

US Department of Labor Bureau of Labor Statistics (BLS). 2015 (Nov.). Job Openings and Labor Turnover—October 2015. http://www.bls.gov/news.release/pdf/jolts.pdf

US Department of Labor Bureau of Labor Statistics (BLS). 2011a. Women in the Labor Force: A Databook. http://www.bls.gov/cps/wlf-intro-2011.pdf

US Department of Labor Bureau of Labor Statistics (BLS). 2011b. BLS Spotlight on Statistics: Women at Work. http://www.bls.gov/spotlight/2011/women/pdf/women_bls_spotlight.pdf

US Department of Labor Occupational Safety and Health Administration (OSHA). n.d. About OSHA. https://www.osha.gov/about.html

US Department of Labor Office of the Secretary (DOL OS). n.d. Summary of the Major Laws of the Department of Labor. http://www.dol.gov/opa/aboutdol/lawsprog.htm

US Department of Labor Wage and Hour Division (WHD). n.d. Compliance Assistance—Wages and the Fair Labor Standards Act (FLSA). http://www.dol.gov/whd/flsa/

US Equal Employment Opportunity Commission. n.d.(a) Best Practices for Employers and Human Resources. http://www.eeoc.gov/eeoc/initiatives/e-race/bestpractices-employers.cfm

US Equal Employment Opportunity Commission. n.d.(b) Prohibited Employment Policies/Practices. http://www.eeoc.gov/laws/practices/

US Equal Employment Opportunity Commission. 2015. Laws Enforced by EEOC. http://www.eeoc.gov/laws/statutes/index.cfm

US Equal Employment Opportunity Commission. 2010. Employment Tests and Selection Procedures. http://www.eeoc.gov/policy/docs/factemployment_procedures.html

US Small Business Administration (SBA). n.d. Required Employee Benefits. https://www.sba.gov/content/required-employee-benefits

24

Employee Training and Development

Karen R. Patena, MBA, RHIA, FAHIMA

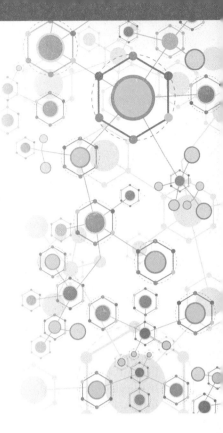

Learning Objectives

- Examine the roles that employee orientation and communication plans play in the development and retention of staff
- Manage the continuum of employee training and development
- Develop an orientation program for new employees
- Examine the role of staff development in retaining a competent workforce
- Compare various learning styles and match appropriately to the needs of adult learners
- Evaluate and respond to the needs of a culturally diverse workforce as well as the needs of employees with disabilities
- Apply appropriate delivery methods to various training needs

- Prepare and conduct appropriate in-service education programs for various healthcare employees
- Educate employees for current and future e-HIM roles
- Prepare a training and development plan for a health information management department
- Select appropriate methods for developing employee potential
- Facilitate employee development of a personal leadership style
- Assess the needs of current employees for continuing education
- Evaluate the quality and usefulness of internal and external training programs
- Interpret the requirements of laws and regulations affecting workforce training

Key Terms

Accountability
ADDIE model
Americans with Disabilities Act (ADA) of 1990

Asynchronous
Audioconferencing
Authority
Avatar

Big data
Blended learning
Blog
Career plan

Case studies
Coaching
Competency
Computer-based training
　(CBT)
Continuing education (CE)
Cross-training
Curriculum
Delegation
Development
Diversity training
e-learning
Electronic performance
　support system (EPSS)
Employee handbook
Empowerment
Ethics training
Group discussion
Incentive pay
In-service education
Intranet
Job rotation

Just-in-time training
Learning
Learning content management
　system (LCMS)
Learning curve
Learning management
　system (LMS)
Lecture
M-learning
Massed training
Massive Open Online Course
　(MOOC)
Mentor
Motivation
Multiuser virtual environment
　(MUVE)
Needs assessment
Occupational Safety and Health
　Act (OSHA) (1970)
Offshoring
Onboarding
One-on-one training

On-the-job training
Programmed learning
Programmed learning module
Promotion
Reinforcement
Responsibility
Reverse mentoring
Role playing
Simulation
Socialization
Spaced training
Strategic management
Succession planning
Synchronous
Task analysis
Team building
Train the trainer
Training
Virtual reality
Videoconferencing
Webinar
Wiki

As a service industry, healthcare relies on the availability of competent workers. The growth of new technologies, the increasing amount of **big data** (data sets so large and complex that new tools for analysis are required), the application of new vocabulary and processes, and the decreasing numbers of employees with adequate skills to respond to this new environment mean that healthcare organizations must frequently assume responsibility for preparing and developing their own labor pool, unless they choose to outsource or use employees overseas. Health information management (HIM) professionals educated many years ago need to acquire skills in emerging competencies taught in today's HIM classroom, such as public health informatics and enterprise information management (Butler 2015, 21). Providing the necessary training to workers is costly in terms of both money and time. Using overseas workers creates its own training needs in areas such as ethics or the English language. Moreover, after the organization has made the investment, it must do what it can to protect its investment by retaining its workforce.

Human resources are the healthcare institution's most valuable asset. Managing employees requires recognizing and meeting the needs of the employees as well as those of the organization. Healthcare organizations must provide employees with the tools for career success and personal achievement if they are to win the long-term commitment of staff.

This chapter focuses on training and retaining employees in the healthcare organization. It describes the orientation process and methods for training new employees as well as developing current employees for more advanced job responsibilities. It discusses adult learning strategies, techniques for delivering employee training including e-learning methods, and ways that training and development programs can enhance job satisfaction, personal career growth, and discovering one's own leadership style. Special training issues, such as diversity, the training of overseas workers, and preparation for future e-HIM roles, are addressed. Finally, the chapter describes how to implement a departmental employee training and development plan.

Training Program Development

Traditional management theory differentiated between training, or providing entry level skills required to begin a job for lower-level, technical employees, and development—maintaining or upgrading competencies for management staff who needed to improve skills such as decision making and interpersonal communication. However, this distinction has become outdated in the 21st century as organizations take a more comprehensive approach to improving employee performance. Today, the terms *training* and *development* are often used interchangeably with the primary goal of improving knowledge, skills, abilities, attitudes, and social behavior of workers at all levels. As employees who make up the organization grow, so does the organization.

Training programs should accommodate all employees. Examples of accommodation include providing instructions in another language for employees who are non-English speakers or making equipment and locations accessible to those with disabilities. In addition, the organization should develop diversity training programs. Diversity training facilitates an environment that fosters tolerance and appreciation of individual differences within the organization's workforce.

Training and development programs should be viewed as a vital part of strategic management, or creation and implementation of the long-term, major direction of healthcare institutions. The standards of accreditation organizations as well as health plans require the demonstration of high-quality, efficient healthcare delivery. To remain financially viable, healthcare organizations must emphasize productivity, performance, and profitability. Managers should identify goals and objectives first for their departments and then individual employees; next they should define the skills and knowledge necessary to achieve the objectives. This goal-oriented approach should challenge and encourage the workforce to achieve organizational goals while helping individual employees reach their highest potential.

Investment in training programs helps the organization to accomplish goals on an individual,

group, and organizational level. Other important reasons for providing employee training and development include:

- Introducing new employees to the organization
- Providing a path for employee promotion and retention
- Improving employee performance and productivity
- Updating skills for employees in new or restructured positions resulting from organizational or technological change
- Reducing organizational problems caused by absenteeism, turnover, poor morale, or substandard quality
- Delivering high-quality healthcare within budgetary constraints

As presented in table 24.1, one way to view training and development needs is as a continuum of five conceptual areas: orientation, on-the-job training, staff development through internal in-service education programs, staff development through external and professional continuing education programs, and personal career development beyond the current job (Fottler et al. 1998, 201). Each concept differs in objectives, diversity of skills, degree of emphasis on career development, training location, and frequency of delivery.

Healthcare organizations are unique—so their development programs should be unique as well. A 50-bed long-term care facility has very different staffing and training needs than a large acute-care academic medical center does. The training program and methods used should fit the context of the institution.

Investment in employee development does not end with training. Organizations need to find ways to gain the commitment of employees so that they will remain productive. Retaining good employees and developing their potential is an area of great importance, particularly in an industry that has a shortage of qualified workers.

Table 24.1.   Employee development continuum

Concept	Objectives	Scope of skill diversity	Emphasis on personal and career growth	Training site	Frequency
Orientation training	To introduce staff to the mores, behaviors, and expectations of the organization	Narrow ↑	Narrow ↑	Internal	Single instance
Training	To teach staff specific skills, concepts, or attitudes			Internal	Sporadic
In-service education	To teach staff about skills, facts, attitudes, and behaviors largely through internal programs			Internal	Continuous
Continuing education	To facilitate the efforts of staff members to remain current in the knowledge base of their trade or profession through external programs designed to achieve external standards	↓	↓	External	Continuous
Career development	To expand the capabilities of staff beyond a narrow range of skills toward a more holistically prepared person	Broad	Broad	Internal and external	Continuous

From Fottler/Hernandez/Joiner. *Essentials of Human Resource Management in Health Service Organizations*, 1E.
© 1998 Delmar Learning, a part of Cengage Learning, Inc. Reproduced by permission. www.cengage.com/permissions

Departmental Employee Training and Development Plan

Every healthcare organization and every HIM department have unique training needs. The level of education and experience of the employees, the tasks they perform, and the resources available will change the focus of training efforts. As table 24.1 shows, employee development is a continuum of concepts. The content, objectives, and frequency of a training program are all dependent on the specific situation that exists in an organization.

Training and Development Model

Several models for designing training and development programs have been developed. Each organization needs to review their needs using a systematic approach to instructional systems design. A model frequently used is the **ADDIE model**: Analyze, Design, Develop, Implement, Evaluate (Fried and Fottler 2011, 140). This method emphasizes the how, what, why, where, who, and when of training. Begin with an analysis or needs assessment that identifies what training is required. Next, design the training program by defining the objectives and methods that will be used. In the third step, the program is developed and pilot tested. Then the program is rolled out with the support of the management for successful delivery. After the program is delivered, it is important to evaluate whether the program achieved the objectives identified in the needs assessment. Figure 24.1 displays this model.

The following is a step-by-step training and development plan that expands upon the ADDIE model and can be applied on various levels to help an organization's HR department or a health information manager identify and fulfill the training and development needs of his or her employee group. The plan includes the following steps:

1. Perform a needs analysis
2. Set training objectives
3. Design the curriculum

Figure 24.1. ADDIE model

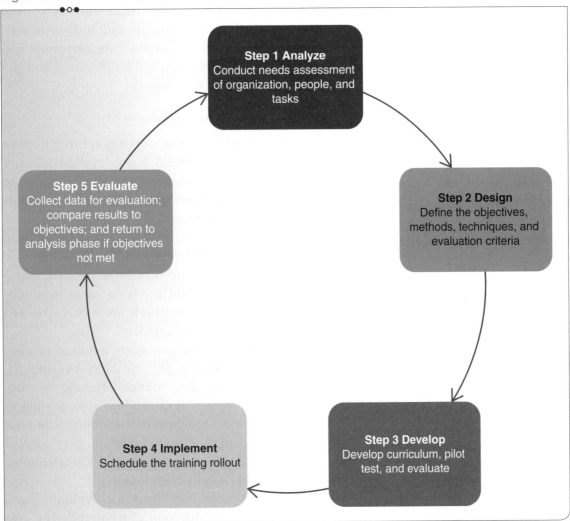

Source: Adapted from Fried and Fottler 2011, 141.

4. Determine the location and method of delivery
5. Pilot the program
6. Implement the program
7. Evaluate the effectiveness of the program
8. Make changes as needed
9. Provide feedback to interested groups

The plan should be approved and supported by upper management. Implementing a training program requires a substantial investment of time, money, and personnel. Developing a curriculum based on a systematic evaluation of needs is a much wiser investment than creating a program around the latest hot topic.

Perform a Departmental Training Needs Analysis

The needs analysis is critical to the design of the plan. This approach typically focuses on three levels: the organization, the specific job tasks, and the individual employee. The outcome of the needs analysis is an understanding of where training is needed in the organization (entry-level, remedial, or management development), based on the firm's strategic mission and goals. In addition, a list of the tasks to be learned at each level (based on the job description, job specification, and the specific skills and knowledge required) and an analysis of the deficiencies in knowledge and skills between the desired level and the current level of each employee should be completed.

This information can be obtained through observation, employee and manager interviews, surveys, tests, and task analysis of the job descriptions and job specifications.

Set Training Objectives

After the needs have been established, specific, measurable training objectives should be set. Objectives stipulate what the employee should be able to accomplish upon completion of the training program. These are based on the deficiencies that have been identified between the desired and current performance levels. It is important to set objectives before starting the program so that the results can be evaluated following completion of training.

Design the Curriculum

The curriculum is the subject content of the program that will be taught, including the sequence, activities, and materials. A budget needs to be prepared that identifies costs and available resources. Examples of training resources include trainers, off-the-shelf computer-based modules or printed textbooks, and web-based learning management systems.

After these decisions are made, the curriculum must be organized into a program that supports adult learning and the stated objectives. All program elements need to be carefully prepared to ensure quality and effectiveness.

Determine the Location and Method of Delivery

Where and when the program should be delivered is an important part of the training plan. When space is available and the instructor and materials are available internally, a classroom setting might be suitable. On the other hand, when employees work over several shifts and days or in remote locations, computer-based courses and web-based delivery might permit the employee to more readily achieve the training objectives.

Pilot the Program

It is important to validate the program by introducing it to a test audience. When computer technology is part of the program delivery, all computer programs should be tested to make sure they work with a variety of hardware and web browsers. Following completion of the program by a few employees, feedback should be obtained and the program revised, if necessary.

Implement the Program

The tested program now can be given to the entire audience for which it has been developed. When necessary, train-the-trainer workshops should be conducted for instructors who may not have formal training experience.

Evaluate the Effectiveness of the Program

Two issues should be addressed in evaluating training programs. The first is selecting the method of evaluation; the second is identifying the outcomes that will be measured.

Evaluation is most frequently assessed using a survey (refer to figures 24.3 and 24.5 for examples). Opinions obtained immediately after the training, and again after a period of time, are valuable in assessing the effectiveness of the program for both trainees and managers. In addition, pretests and posttests help identify the level of knowledge or skill that has actually been learned.

When possible, a method for evaluating the training program is to conduct a controlled experiment. A control group that receives no training is compared to a group that received training. Data are obtained from both groups before and after training. It is then possible to determine the extent to which the training program caused a change in performance in the training group.

Four outcomes can be measured in evaluating effective training programs:

- *Reaction:* What is the reaction of the trainees immediately after the program? Are they excited about what they learned?
- *Learning:* What have the trainees actually learned? Can they now use a new software program?
- *Behavior:* Have supervisors noticed a change in employee behavior? Has morale improved?

- *Results:* How does the actual level of performance compare with the established objectives? Can the employees assign codes more accurately? (Dessler 2015, 246)

Evaluating these outcomes will determine whether the training has been successful, connecting back to the gaps identified in the initial needs analysis, or whether modifications to the training program are required.

Make Changes as Needed

When the results of the evaluation show less-than-expected results, it is important to determine where changes may be helpful. This may include a change in the materials, location or time of program delivery, or subject content. In any case, it is important to adjust if needed. A program that is not meeting the desired objectives is costly.

Provide Feedback to Interested Groups

After tallying the results of the evaluations and making any needed adjustments, it is important to provide feedback to the course developers, managers and supervisors of the involved departments, and trainees. Communication is vital to maintaining interest in and support for the training program. Feedback demonstrates a desire to respond to the needs of everyone involved in this important activity.

Check Your Understanding 24.1

Instructions: **Answer the following questions on a separate piece of paper.**

1. Differentiate between the terms *training* and *development*.
2. What are the five steps in the ADDIE instructional design model?
3. What are three items to consider in designing a training program?
4. What is the relationship between setting objectives and evaluating a training program?
5. What are the three outcomes of a needs analysis?
6. What are four outcomes that should be measured in program evaluation?
7. Why is feedback important following the evaluation of the program?

Elements of Workforce Training

The goal of any institution's training program is to provide employees the skills they need to perform their jobs. Because employees are at different stages in their career development, the training program must be flexible and able to adapt to meet many needs. At any given time, new employees will need to know basic information about the organization and their specific job function, and long-term employees will want to improve their ability to contribute at higher levels within the organizational structure through developing new proficiencies.

Today's workforce needs both technical skills and soft skills, such as critical thinking and **team building**—enhancing productivity through collaborative work with others. For example, information governance is increasingly becoming an integral part of the healthcare work setting. No matter what primary task they perform, most employees will need to develop competencies to ensure data integrity.

New Employee Orientation and Training

One of the key ingredients in employee satisfaction is the feeling of being knowledgeable about the organization and competent in the job. This feeling begins with an effective orientation and training program for new employees. Just as a manager prepares for the interview and selection of a new employee, he or she must plan how the new employee will learn about the organization, department, and job.

New Employee Orientation

Most large organizations have a formal new employee orientation, or onboarding process. This process, which includes a series of activities designed to acclimate the new employee to the organization and job, may involve a one-on-one session with an advisor from the human resources department, group training with new employees from across the organization, and/or some form of individual computer-based training.

In addition to the basic skills needed to do the job, the employee needs to experience a period of socialization in which he or she learns the values, behavior patterns, and expectations of the organization. The manager must be very patient during the employee's first days and schedule adequate time to spend with the new hire. Everyone learns in different ways and at a different pace. The first days not only establish how the employee will do the job but also contribute to the employee's ongoing relationships with the manager and other staff.

In a large facility, new employee orientation is usually coordinated by the human resources (HR) department; in a small facility, it may be performed entirely by the employee's supervisor. The orientation may consist of a brief and informal presentation, or it may be a formal program that takes place over several days on a regularly scheduled basis.

Formal programs typically begin with presentations by HR and other department heads before the new employee is introduced to his or her immediate supervisor. The program usually addresses organization-specific information such as the organization's mission and vision, goals, and structure; employee relations practices; and employee-centered information such as compensation and benefits.

The supervisor then continues the orientation process within the employee's assigned department.

The employee is introduced to the department or workgroup and the specific job he or she will be performing. Orientation also may include a tour of the facility and cover computer access and responsibilities. When the organization provides this type of orientation, the manager must understand the material covered by others and feel comfortable answering any questions or directing the new employee to the appropriate resource for follow-up.

Needs Assessment for New Employee Orientation

As with all training programs, the orientation must be customized to the particular employee through needs assessment. The purpose of a needs assessment is to evaluate the employee's current level of knowledge as well as future expectations, and determine any gap(s) that must be addressed. The gap(s) should be reviewed at the organization, department, and work unit level (Fottler et al. 1998, 210). New employees will require a more in-depth orientation about items like the organization structure, policies and procedures, and benefits, than current employees who are starting a different position within the same institution and may need to spend time developing skill sets demanded by their new job function.

To develop an orientation program, it is helpful to begin with a task analysis to determine the specific skills required for the job. The job description and job specification are excellent sources for this part of the process. Beyond specific tasks, all new employees need to understand matters common to the institution such as personnel policies, benefits, and safety regulations. Federal and state governments and accreditation organizations also may require certain subjects to be included in the orientation program.

Requirements for New Employee Orientation

Although the orientation program is typically done at a single point in time, a new employee may not feel completely competent at first, depending on the amount of new learning required. The program should attempt to make employees feel that they made the right choice in accepting the position. For this to happen, they should feel welcome, comfortable in their new environment, positive about their supervisor, and confident that they are learning the skills they need to do the job. An orientation program should not just be for completing paperwork.

An effective tool used in familiarizing new workers is the orientation checklist (figure 24.2), which helps the employer know that the employee is receiving the information he or she needs to begin the job and serves as an agenda for presenting the information in a logical manner. Rather than presenting everything the new employee needs to know all at once, it is helpful to spread the orientation over several days.

In addition, it is helpful to present policies and requirements that all employees must know—insurance programs, payroll requirements, and personnel policies—in an **employee handbook** given to new employees during the orientation. The handbook provides a convenient reference after the immediate orientation period has ended. However, the facility must be careful not to include content that expresses or could imply conditions of an employment contract. If the employee views the handbook as a contract, it becomes a legally binding agreement. In this case, the employer or employee could be held liable if any conditions set out in the handbook are not strictly followed. Thus, the employee handbook should be viewed as advisory in nature and not as a legal document.

The requirements of an orientation program may be expressed on three levels: organizational, departmental, and individual.

Figure 24.2. Sample orientation checklist

Orientation checklist

Supervisor _____ Date _____
Employee _____ Department _____

Before worker arrives
(Check off tasks when completed.)
__ 1. Prepare other employees.
__ 2. Have desk and supplies ready.
__ 3. Arrange for luncheon escort.

First day
__ 1. Ensure attendance at hospital orientation program.
__ 2. Review employee handbook and (if applicable) union contract information.
__ 3. Review benefit information.
__ 4. Review safety and security regulations, including infection control procedures.
__ 5. Introduce to immediate associates.
__ 6. Introduce to the workplace.
__ 7. Give overview of the job.
__ 8. Ask whether new employee has any questions.

Second day
__ 1. Discuss confidentiality policy.
__ 2. Give job instructions.
__ 3. Review compensation.
__ 4. Explain hours of work.
__ 5. Discuss attendance requirements.
__ 6. Explain performance review.
__ 7. Explain quality and quantity standards.
__ 8. Encourage employee to ask questions.
__ 9. Explain where to store work overnight.

Third day
__ 1. Explain telephone system, computer system, and fax and copy machines.
__ 2. Explain reasons for rules and policies.
__ 3. Explain insurance plans.
__ 4. Ask whether the new employee has any questions.

Fourth day
__ 1. Give employee opportunity to describe how he or she is getting along.
__ 2. Discuss departmental policies in addition to hospital policies.
__ 3. Explain hospital continuing education program.

Fifth day
__ 1. Describe vacation system.
__ 2. Explain use of social media policy.

Sixth day
__ 1. Encourage employee to talk to supervisor when necessary.
__ 2. Administer post-orientation assessment.
__ 3. Give orientation evaluation form to employee to complete.

Orientation completed _____ (Date)
Signature of employee _____
Signature of supervisor _____

From Keeling and Kallaus. *Administrative Office Management*, 11E. © 1996 Delmar Learning, a part of Cengage Learning, Inc. Reproduced by permission. www.cengage.com/permissions

At the organizational level, the orientation program provides the information that every employee who works for the company needs to know. This information typically includes:

- Background and mission of the organization
- Policies and procedures that apply to all employees, such as confidentiality agreements or infection control procedures
- Ethics training, including how to recognize ethical dilemmas and draw upon codes of conduct to resolve problems
- Cultural diversity, sensitivity, and anti-harassment training
- Employee benefits (such as paid time off, insurance coverage)
- Performance appraisal process
- Health, safety and security regulations
- Employee orientation handbook
- Tour of the facility (Fried and Fottler 2011, 148)

At the departmental level, orientation information typically includes:

- Departmental policies and procedures
- Introduction to other employees
- Tour of department
- Work hours
- Time sheet requirements
- Training in operation of equipment (for example, photocopying machines or computers)
- Safety regulations specific to the department (Fried and Fottler 2011, 148)

At the individual level, the new employee learns specific job tasks that, at a minimum, should include:

- Specific, measurable objectives for productivity and performance
- An explanation of each job task by the supervisor, followed by a demonstration and an opportunity for the employee to demonstrate the task (Fried and Fottler 2011, 148)

The new employee's individual orientation is usually the longest portion of the orientation program.

Components of an Orientation Program

An orientation program should be developed with input from HR, other department heads, and the employee's supervisor. For a typical new employee in the HIM department of an acute-care hospital, the orientation program might follow the schedule shown in figure 24.2. The first portion of the program introduces the employee to the institution and is typically led by the director of education or the director of HR. The employee is given a handbook and any required forms to complete for payroll and insurance. The director of safety and security also introduces safety regulations.

To introduce the employee to the individual job setting as quickly as possible, the general portion of the orientation could be completed within the first half-day. The employee then could meet the immediate supervisor and be matched with a buddy to escort him or her to lunch and back to the department. Ideally, the buddy should have the same job as or work closely with the new employee. In addition to providing guidance to the new person, this experience offers an opportunity for further development of the experienced employee serving as the buddy (McConnell 2013, 362). On the afternoon of day one, the new worker should be introduced to coworkers, given a tour of the department, and shown his or her workstation. The first day could end with a basic overview explanation of the job's duties, including an opportunity for questions.

The individual portion of the orientation should continue as described in the suggested schedule with some portion of each day devoted to job training and work rules so that the new employee can gradually understand the requirements of the job and become socialized to the work environment. As the new employee is trained and tested in each important aspect of the job, the supervisor should document his or her demonstrated competency. This documentation will help the organization to comply with the standards of the Joint Commission, required for institutional accreditation.

Orientation of Overseas Workers

The demand for health information technicians to fill positions in functions such as transcription or coding exceeds the current US supply.

Also, pressure to reduce cost continues to mount on healthcare providers. As with many other industry sectors, US healthcare providers have discovered there are many benefits to be gained as a result of moving some of their work to employees who live overseas (often referred to as **offshoring**). Most often these employees are located in countries where English is frequently spoken, however, this has resulted in some unique requirements for training.

In addition to the requirements for orientation of all new employees, orientation training for overseas workers may include English proficiency, American etiquette, and cultural differences. Specific training requirements should be included in a service agreement. For those in the United States supervising the workers, issues of cultural competence are essential to be addressed. For example, holidays in different countries may result in varying days off, including days that are not official holidays in the United States.

Quality control is an important issue. Tasks to be performed, acceptable turnaround times, quantity and quality standards, and how the performance measures will be tracked and reported should be very clear. It is especially important to specify accountability for confidentiality because data are at risk when they are transmitted overseas. HIPAA requirements, including those pertaining to business associate contracts, may be applicable to overseas workers and should be included in the orientation and training.

Assessment of the New Employee Orientation and Training Program

After the orientation process, all the participants should be asked for feedback. A form should be developed by HR and completed by the new employee. Figure 24.3 presents an example of a form for evaluating the general portion of the orientation program. Typical questions include the following:

- Was the program relevant to your job and needs?
- What part of the program was most useful to you?
- What part of the program was least useful to you?

In addition, supervisors should be asked to evaluate the effectiveness of the orientation process. For example, they should be asked for feedback on the employee's ability to apply his or her newly acquired job skills and for an assessment of the employee's comfort level with the department.

On-the-Job Training

Preparing staff to carry out the tasks and functions of their particular jobs should be an ongoing effort for both new and experienced employees. A variety of methods are available to employers. Effective training programs begin with a needs assessment and an appropriate combination of methods, media, content, and activities into a curriculum that is matched to the specific education, experience, and skill level of the audience.

Definition of On-the-Job Training

On-the-job training is a method of teaching an employee to perform a task by actually performing it. Along with teaching basic skills, on-the-job training gives employees and supervisors opportunities to discuss specific problem areas and initiates socialization among the new employees and their coworkers. On-the-job training offers a number of advantages, including its relatively low cost compared to outside training programs and the fact that work is still in progress while the employee is being trained. However, employees may feel burdened if they are held responsible for work they do not accomplish during the training period, and the learning process may be less than optimal if the work setting is disrupted by ongoing distractions and pressures.

Training may be performed by either a supervisor or a coworker with particular expertise. The selection of an appropriate trainer is critical to the success of this method. Even though they are very capable at performing the job being taught, some employees may not be effective teachers and may omit vital steps if not motivated to teach. Ensuring the willingness of the employee asked to perform the training is important. If that cooperation is not present, discussing the importance and benefits of being a trainer needs to occur or, if possible,

Figure 24.3.   Sample orientation evaluation form

Employee orientation program evaluation form

Date:

Job title:

1. Please rate each of the following items to indicate your reaction to the session. If ranking is less than agree, please comment below.

Item	Poor	Strongly disagree	Disagree	Agree	Strongly agree
Objective 1: The program explained my job responsibilities.	_____	_____	_____	_____	_____
Objective 2: I was able to practice using technology needed to perform my job.	_____	_____	_____	_____	_____
Objective 3: I was able to interact with other participants.	_____	_____	_____	_____	_____
Objective 4: The program length was appropriate for the content.	_____	_____	_____	_____	_____

Comments:

2. Describe the part of the program that was most useful for you.
3. Describe the part of the program that was least useful to you.
4. Please use the following scale to comment on the instructor's ability to lead the program, where

1 = Needs improvement   2 = Adequate   3 = Good   4 = Excellent

Item	Instructor rating
Organization and preparation of content	1 2 3 4
Presentation of content	1 2 3 4
Clarity of instructions	1 2 3 4
Appropriate use of time	1 2 3 4
Connected content to your job functions	1 2 3 4
Stimulated interaction with other participants	1 2 3 4

5. How would you rate your level of skill/knowledge:

   a.   Before the program?   1 2 3 4
   b.   After the program?   1 2 3 4

6. What changes do you recommend to the program?
7. Other comments:

Source: Adapted from Dessler 2015, 176.

finding another qualified employee to do the training may be necessary.

Needs Assessment and Job Requirements

The training program should begin by reviewing the job description and the job specifications. Job descriptions and specifications should include a list of tasks performed; the skills, ability, and knowledge required; and the expected standards of performance for quality and quantity. Next, a performance analysis should be completed to assess the gap between expected performance and the employee's current performance level. In the case of a new employee, this may be verified through a written **competency** assessment, which assesses the employee's current level of ability to do the task. What the employee does not know or cannot do becomes the basis for on-the-job training. The requirements may include any of the following:

- Physical skills (for example, operation of equipment)
- Academic knowledge (for example, medical terminology or English spelling and grammar)
- Knowledge of institutional policies (for example, safety regulations)
- Technical skills, which may include both physical and mental skills (for example, use of computer software)

After the specific requirements for training are identified the appropriate delivery methods for training can be matched to the topic.

Components of On-the-Job Training

On-the-job training methods can be used individually or in combination and should be adapted to each learner. On-the-job training offers a variety of delivery options, including:

- One-on-one training by a supervisor or an experienced peer
- Job rotation
- Computer-based training
- Coaching or mentoring
- Informal learning during meetings or discussions with supervisors and peers

One-on-one training is the technique used most often. In this type of training, the employee learns by first observing a demonstration and then performing the task. For this type of training to be effective, organizations may offer **train the trainer** workshops in which the trainer—either manager or employee—learns skills in communication and instruction in order to train others on content. It is important to select a person to serve as a trainer who is not only competent in the job content, but also able to teach and interact effectively with the trainee. One-on-one training by the supervisor gives the supervisor an opportunity to observe how the trainee is doing and to make adjustments

to meet the employee's skill level. A trainee who learns quickly can move through the steps at a faster pace; a trainee who learns slowly may need an opportunity for additional practice or a second demonstration.

In **job rotation**, the employee moves from job to job at planned intervals, usually three to six months. This method is most useful for supervisory positions, where the employee needs to learn a variety of tasks performed by several different employees, as well as their interrelationships. In **cross-training**, the employee learns to perform the jobs of many team members. Cross-training provides opportunity for competent employees to experience greater task variety in their jobs and affords flexibility in shifting resources for workload or attendance fluctuation. This method is most useful when work teams are involved.

Computer-based training, including web-based training, provides an opportunity to supplement job task performance with additional knowledge and simulation. It is effective in situations where repetition aids learning; for example, with medical terminology and tasks that cannot be duplicated entirely in the practice session, such as role playing with different cases where employees are requested to release patient information.

After the trainee has demonstrated the ability to do the job, **coaching** should continue by the supervisor or an expert peer on a continuous basis. The experienced worker observes or reviews the work of the employee in a nonthreatening manner, offering advice and suggestions for revising techniques to improve productivity and efficient work performance. In a formalized arrangement in which a specific person is assigned to follow up on a regular basis, the coach is referred to as a **mentor**. In this scenario, the mentor meets with the trainee on a regular basis and often gives advice on personal career growth and development within the organization. In **reverse mentoring**, the new employee mentors a senior person on subjects in which he or she may have more expertise, such as use of social media or digital technologies. This provides an opportunity for the newer employee to gain an important sense of belonging and contribution (Schermerhorn 2013, 246).

It is estimated that approximately 80 percent of training actually results from informal interactions between the employee and his or her coworkers (Dessler 2015, 230). Learning occurs even though it is not formally designed or monitored by the organization; for example, during hallway conversations or on lunch breaks when a work topic is discussed and other employees or supervisors offer suggestions or corrections.

Training Overseas Workers

Training overseas workers on the job may be performed by a combination of remote web-based training provided from the United States and on-site group or one-on-one training. The trainer may be brought overseas from the United States or based in the country. Areas of training for overseas workers may include workshops to improve proficiency in English writing and verbal communication, medical terminology, coding, and data quality control. Instruction in the technology and equipment related to the job, such as voice recognition technology for transcriptionists or computer-assisted coding, may be provided. For those desiring career advancement, topics such as leadership development and supervision should be added.

Assessment of On-the-Job Training Program

By its nature, on-the-job training provides an opportunity for immediate assessment of its effectiveness. The trainer can observe the employee's skills as part of the performance tryout and can question the employee on his or her knowledge of policies, procedures, and other academic knowledge that may be required. If the assessment reveals areas of weakness, the training can be adjusted to reinforce knowledge or repeat steps performed incorrectly.

When the employee is working on his or her own, the supervisor should check the quantity and quality of the employee's work against performance standards as appropriate for the particular job and level of employee expertise. It could be daily for an entry-level employee to weekly or monthly or more for a more experienced employee. If the employee's performance is below standard, the training can be repeated before poor performance becomes a habit.

Finally, the employee should be encouraged to ask questions both during and after the training and should receive positive and negative feedback as appropriate. Following the training program the employee should be asked for feedback on the training program and any changes that may be helpful.

Staff Development through In-Service Education

The healthcare industry grows and changes constantly. Whether it is a new law passed by the state or the federal government, new reimbursement regulations, updates to ICD or CPT codes, new or revised accreditation standards, or future HIM roles, change is a permanent factor. Preparing workers for such changes requires continuous training and retraining.

Definition of In-Service Education

In-service education is the third step in the employee development continuum (refer to table 24.1), which is a continuous process that builds on the basic skills learned through new employee orientation and on-the-job training. In-service education is concerned with teaching employees specific skills and behaviors required to maintain job performance or to retrain workers whose jobs have changed. Although in-service education may include external programs, it is primarily developed and delivered at the work site or through computer-based training.

Needs Assessment for In-Service Education

The need for in-service education may be triggered by many events, including:

- A restructuring of the department or organization
- Updates to coding or reimbursement requirements
- Implementation of electronic health records
- A decline in productivity or morale or an increase in absenteeism
- A new organizational policy or procedure
- An external requirement imposed by accreditation or licensing organizations, such as an annual renewal of CPR certification or

retraining in infectious disease precautions or safety procedures

- Regulatory changes, such as required by HIPAA or Health Information Technology for Economic and Clinical Health (HITECH) legislation (McConnell 2010, 22)

The amount of in-service education needed varies with the event and the education and experience of the employee. Downsizing or reorganizing structure often causes changes in an individual employee's job responsibilities. Employees may need to learn other job functions within the workgroup or may even be placed in a new department. This can require a series of formal training sessions, including on-the-job training.

Renewal of training required by external organizations may be subject to defined content and duration, often including a test or demonstration of the employee's competence. On the other hand, implementation of a new policy or procedure may simply include distributing the information accompanied by a short meeting.

Decisions need to be made regarding the appropriate format of the in-service education. The following types of questions may help with the determination of format.

- Should the instruction be given as **massed training** (training in a highly concentrated session) or as **spaced training**, which occurs in several shorter sessions?
- Should the task be broken down into parts or be taught as a single unit?
- How will competence be assessed? Is the topic a skill that needs to be demonstrated by the learner, or is it a level of knowledge that should be tested with a written assessment?

As with other training categories, periodic analysis of actual vs. desired job performance will create a list of topics that should be addressed with in-service education.

Requirements for an In-Service Education Program

Unlike orientation programs, which are delivered primarily at one point in time, in-service education programs need to be available on an ongoing basis. Depending on the size of the organization, some programs (such as a refresher on the response to the institution's disaster plan) may be offered on a monthly basis. The HR department may coordinate programs on topics that affect the organization as a whole. Programs specific to health information management, such as a coding update, are more likely to be developed by a supervisor or manager in the HIM department.

Finally, some topics serve the needs of more than one department. For example, a program on ICD-10-CM coding may be given by the coding supervisor to employees from the HIM, patient accounting, and physician billing departments. This type of program probably would take place in a more formal setting and require coordination with other department managers.

Examples of in-service education topics and the individuals within the organization who are likely to have responsibility for them are shown in figure 24.4.

Steps in Conducting In-Service Education

Presenting an effective in-service program requires planning. The time frame depends on the complexity of the material and the number of participants but should include enough time to prepare materials and publicize the event. Generally, a formal in-service program should follow these steps:

1. *Set objectives.* Is the purpose of the program to teach a new job task to an individual or to improve morale within the department?
2. *Understand the audience.* Is the training intended for one employee or 50 employees? Are the participants from the same department or from several departments? Are they in the same location or dispersed?
3. *Decide whether the content should be delivered as a unit or in parts (massed or spaced).* This may be resolved by the availability of the employee as well as the topic.
4. *Determine the best method of instruction.* The education and experience of the audience, time available, and cost of preparing and delivering the instruction should all be taken

Figure 24.4. Examples of responsibility for in-service education

Organization-wide: The human resources department typically assumes responsibility for the following topics and may include staff from other departments in the planning and presentation:
- Fire and safety awareness
- Disaster plan implementation
- Infectious disease/universal precautions
- Diversity training
- Team building
- HIPAA training

Multiple departments: The health information manager may work with managers of several departments to coordinate presentation of the following topics:
- ICD or CPT annual updates
- Medical terminology training
- Use of office productivity software for employee productivity measurement
- Health record documentation

Health information management department: The health information manager may develop in-service training within the department for the following topics:
- Release of information
- Fire and safety procedures
- Record security in the event of disaster
- EHR implementation
- Data analysis

into consideration. Is there a qualified expert in-house? Are DVD or computer-based materials available for rent or purchase? Is space available to train a large group at one time? (See the discussions of adult learning strategies and delivery methods later in this chapter.)

5. *Prepare a budget.* If a specific amount has been allocated, the plan should be compared to the predetermined budget and revised, if necessary. Approval should be obtained if the proposal is a new one. In addition, the proposal should include the costs of photocopying materials, speaker fees, and training resources.

6. *Publicize the program.* Flyers or electronic notices should be posted to announce the program and should include the date, time, location, topic, and a summary of the content. When it is important to know the number of attendees in advance, the notice should include a method for RSVP.

7. *If appropriate, prepare handout materials.* Handouts would include materials to be used for instruction as well as documents to reference following the program. At a minimum, an agenda of the topics and a schedule should be developed.

8. *Practice, practice, practice!* The person presenting the program should be adequately prepared and comfortable with the content. Also, a training room should be scheduled ahead of time and any needed equipment should be checked to ensure that it is available and in good working order. Anyone planning to use a computer or a projector should know how to operate it.

9. *Use a variety of methods and be alert to your audience.* In addition to the lecture, the presenter should engage the audience through interactive questioning and activities. People learn by doing. Opportunities should be provided from time to time for questions and periodic breaks when the program lasts more than two hours.

10. *Obtain feedback from the audience.* It is important to give the participants an opportunity to document their reactions to the training. To that end, an evaluation form should be created and distributed. A sample in-service education evaluation form is shown in figure 24.5.

Figure 24.5.   Sample in-service education evaluation form

In-service education evaluation form

To help us improve the quality of future programs, please complete the following evaluation of today's session. Please use the following scale to answer questions 1 through 6:

1 = Needs improvement   2 = Satisfactory   3 = Excellent

1.   How satisfied were you with the content of the presentation?   1   2   3
2.   How would you rate the organization of the presentation?   1   2   3
3.   How would you rate the effectiveness of visual media used in the presentation?   1   2   3
4.   How would you rate the delivery of the presentation?   1   2   3
5.   How well did the presenter meet the learning goals of the program?   1   2   3
6.   How satisfied were you with the following aspects of the program?

    a.   Meeting location   1   2   3
    b.   Parking   1   2   3
    c.   Accessibility   1   2   3
    d.   Registration process   1   2   3
    e.   Meeting room setup and seating   1   2   3
    f.   Handout materials   1   2   3

7.   What is one thing you learned that you did not know prior to attending?
8.   What would you like to have learned more about?
9.   Please provide any additional comments that could improve future programs.

Assessment of In-Service Education

Because some amount of cost, in terms of both time and resources, is usually involved with in-service training, it is important to determine whether its objectives have been met. The organization's administrative staff will want evidence that the training was cost-effective and there was return on investment in terms of increased productivity and employee development. Three methods for assessing the impact of in-service education are as follows.

- *Completion of an evaluation form at the conclusion of the program.* Immediate feedback provides an assessment of the effectiveness of the delivery methods. Is the employee energized and ready to put the material to use, or was the material overwhelming?

- *Formal or informal feedback from the employee's supervisor.* Within a few days of the program, the supervisor should be contacted to determine whether the learner has applied the new skills and knowledge on the job.

- *Follow-up with the employee at a later time.* Thirty days after the in-service program, the attendees should be asked to validate the value of the program. Are they able to perform their job better? Is there something they feel they did not learn that should have been included? This may be accomplished easily via an e-mail message.

Special Issues for Staff Development

Several issues must be considered in training programs that apply to all levels, from orientation programs to staff development. Employees bring differing cultural norms, experiences, skills, and expectations to the workplace and the employer must help these individuals coexist. In addition to appreciating diversity, team building exercises can enhance the productivity of the work unit and prepare them for evolving roles in HIM.

Diversity, Sensitivity, and Anti-harassment Training

The increasing frequency of terrorist attacks has had a profound effect on training in the United States. Awareness of the impact of culture on the workforce has become an important issue, yet people are afraid to discuss differences for fear of offending others. Organizations find it is important to learn about issues such as the effect of culture on communication and learning styles.

Diversity training attempts to develop sensitivity among employees about the unique challenges facing diverse religious, ethnic, and sexual orientation groups, as well as those with disabilities, and strives to create a more harmonious working environment. It is important to help all employees from diverse backgrounds feel included and respected as part of the team, remain committed and productive, and understand how to respond appropriately to other employees, customers, or patients (Bagshaw 2004, 156). The emphasis should be on learning from each other's viewpoints. Training should be provided for the entire organization, with additional specific training for management staff.

A suggested training course about ethnic minorities might begin with a review of various cultures from a social studies perspective (that is, location of the country, climate, customs, or food preferences). Other topics to include later would be cultural norms, such as communication styles (strong eye contact or standing close when conversing), use of first vs. formal names, or tolerance of jokes. Behavior that may be offensive or inappropriate in one culture but not another should be discussed and acceptable alternatives presented. Of particular importance to the HIM employee is the perspective of some cultures on the issue of privacy, which may require that permissions be obtained to comply with HIPAA.

Another option would be to create a booklet about each group that provides knowledge of the culture, communication help, and tips for nonjudgmental respect. Employees would be advised to read the material and then follow up with a discussion. When the training course has been completed, an ongoing employee advisory group could be formed to advise management staff regarding barriers and issues of concern to diverse employees. Posting a calendar with various cultural and religious celebrations on the company intranet would be informative to all employees.

For those employees needing training in the English language and American culture, topics might include English reading and writing skills, focusing on general as well as medical terms. Interpersonal skills, customer service, and the US corporate culture are also helpful training topics.

Employee harassment is prohibited under Title VII of the Civil Rights Act. Anti-harassment training must cover all types of unlawful harassment based on sex, race, religion, national origin, disability, or sexual orientation (Civil Rights Act 1964). It should be included in new employee orientation and repeated periodically with other training required by accreditation or law. The trainer should be a carefully chosen expert in discrimination laws. The training must be substantial to be effective (that is, the requirement may not be met by simply requiring employees to view a video). Suggested stages for diversity training include:

- Anti-harassment and sensitivity training
- Cultural awareness and competence
- Development of multicultural teams
- Full inclusion of minority groups into every level of the organization (McConnell 2010, 256)

Many companies produce materials to help with diversity training including videos, facilitator materials, printed materials, and cases for role playing.

Working in Teams

Team-building training helps employees learn to work in groups that have the authority to make decisions. Emphasis is on the group rather than individual achievement. Skills are taught that help members diagnose and devise solutions to problems. Exercises such as constructing items within a group encourage creativity. Conflict-resolution training is an aspect of working in teams that focuses on communication skills needed to resolve gridlock. Facilitators may work with a group, asking group members and leaders to identify problem issues at the beginning of the session. The group then ranks the themes identified and that becomes the agenda for problem solving. A by-product of team training is improved employee attitudes and satisfaction.

Preparing the HIM Staff for Future Roles

HIM professionals must continuously transform their knowledge, skills, and abilities to keep pace with the competencies needed for the new roles. Competencies are needed in areas such as data analysis, data integration, privacy and security, information governance, clinical vocabulary development and maintenance, and public health surveillance.

In 2011, the American Health Information Management Association (AHIMA) Board of Directors, together with input from AHIMA members and industry experts, announced the Core Model to describe the roles and functions of current as well as future HIM professionals. The core model focuses on the following five functional areas of health information:

- Data capture, validation, and maintenance
- Data and information analysis, transformation, and decision support
- Information dissemination and liaison
- Health information resource management and innovation
- Information governance and stewardship (AHIMA Board of Directors 2011)

The Caviart Group, LLC, was commissioned to conduct a study of the roles and skills needed by HIM professionals both currently and in the future. The results of this study (published in March 2015) indicate the knowledge, education, and credentials needed by the HIM workforce of the future will be broader and more diverse than currently required (AHIMA 2015). As traditional coding tasks decline in volume and importance, leadership and analysis skills that build on that background will increase in volume and importance (Sandefer et al. 2015, 25). The most important tasks of the future—managing electronic health records and ensuring information privacy and security—will require more advanced technical skills, more advanced conceptual skills, and greater communication skills.

The top 10 most important skills for the future are as follows:

1. Electronic health records management skills
2. Skill in managing information privacy and security
3. Analytical thinking skills
4. Critical thinking skills
5. Skill in ensuring data integrity
6. Problem-solving skills
7. Communication skills (written, spoken, and presentation)
8. Clinical documentation improvement skills
9. Leadership skills
10. Skill in analyzing big data (AHIMA 2015, 10)

Providing training for these topics should become a focus of the HIM department's training and development plan for all employees (Sandefer et al. 2015, 39). As an example, AHIMA has developed the *Health Information Management Staff Transformation Toolkit* to assist HIM department managers in training their nonprofessional staff for working with electronic health records (AHIMA 2012, 4). Transformation gap analysis, skills assessment, functions assessment, and other tools are included to assist the manager with assessing training and development needs.

Check Your Understanding 24.2

Instructions: **Answer the following questions on a separate piece of paper.**

1. What are the purposes of an employee orientation program?

2. When is job rotation a useful training technique?

3. What are two topics to be included in orientation training for overseas workers?

4. What is the purpose of in-service education?

5. What are the top two skills required for the future HIM workforce?

6. What topics should be included in diversity training programs?

Adult Learning Strategies

Training refers to the process of providing individuals with the materials and activities they need to develop the knowledge, skills, abilities, attitudes, and behaviors desired for a new role or function in the workplace. **Learning** is what occurs in the individual to achieve the changes in behavior, knowledge, attitudes, abilities, and skills desired. In the healthcare work environment, learning translates into achieving the goals of the institution, including improved job performance. The objective is for employees to develop effective work habits. To accomplish this objective, it is important to understand how employees learn and the factors that affect the learning environment.

Characteristics of Adult Learners

One of the most difficult tasks faced by employees is achieving balance. Ideally, people shift their time between the demands of work, demands of home, and their own needs and desires to accomplish more with fewer and fewer hours. Too much stress can lead to burnout. Therefore, training must be viewed as an integral part of the work environment and not as an additional requirement. The individuals responsible for training need to understand that time is a very valuable resource.

Because time is scarce, employees need to see relevance in the activities that consume their time. They will be more willing to accept tasks that can be accomplished quickly, provide satisfaction or tangible benefits, and can be completed within short time frames.

Three fundamental concepts in helping adults learn are motivation, reinforcement, and knowledge of results.

Motivation

Motivation is the inner drive to accomplish a task. At different stages in life, adults are motivated by specific needs. Understanding that employees differ in the relative importance of these needs at any given time is important in designing a training program. For example, a newly credentialed health information technician in his early 20s with no dependents may be interested in working long hours. He may demonstrate an eagerness to devote extra hours to training that will advance his career. On the other hand, a young parent may value time to attend his or her children's school activities and want to limit time spent away from home.

Employees will be more motivated when they perceive a need for the training. The trainer should call attention to the important aspects of the job and help employees understand how to perform these tasks efficiently and effectively. The manager should help the employee know the answer to the question, What's in it for me? (McConnell 2013, 364).

Moreover, employees should see a direct connection between the knowledge learned and the work goal. Factors that truly motivate are found within the work itself, with the strongest factors finding the work interesting and challenging, and providing an opportunity to grow (McConnell 2013, 360). It is helpful when the trainer explains the reason for performing a task in a certain order and relates policies to objectives. For example, coders may be instructed to review a record in a specific order, beginning with a discharge summary and then lab reports. It is helpful when the trainer explains that the purpose of this process is to ensure appropriate evidence of diagnoses to comply with reimbursement requirements.

Reinforcement

Reinforcement is a condition following a response that results in an increase in the strength of that response. It is associated with motivation in that the strength of the response is a factor of the perceived value of the reinforcement. For example, additional pay after an employee attends a training course that requires extra work hours would serve as a positive reinforcement for the new health information technician. However, the young parent may feel negatively reinforced by the additional work hours required. Reinforcement is most effective when it occurs immediately after a correct response. This connects the reinforcement with the response and more likely results in the desired effect.

Incentive pay systems are a form of positive reinforcement. The higher the quality and quantity of work, the better the pay increase given. For example, transcriptionists might be compensated based on the number of lines correctly transcribed rather than an hourly rate.

Knowledge of Results

Many adults prefer feedback on their performance. It is important to understand the concept of the **learning curve**. As shown in figure 24.6, when a new task is learned productivity may decrease while a great deal of material is actually being learned. Later, there is little new learning but productivity may increase greatly. Either situation can be frustrating, so guidance and feedback are important to help employees understand what they have accomplished. It is important to provide encouragement when new tasks are mastered, even though the quantity of work may not be at the level desired. In addition, it is important to explain that the employee may reach a plateau where improvement slows or levels off, and that this is normal.

Education of Adult Learners

When an organization wants its workers to improve their work habits, it must demonstrate that it values the effort behind the improvements. The organizational climate must support the continued learning and growth of its employees. Some actions the administration might take to indicate this commitment include:

- Providing training during work hours rather than outside the employees' regular work schedules
- Conducting the training off-site to avoid interruptions from day-to-day activities
- Compensating voluntary education with incentives such as bonuses and promotions

Adults tend to remember and understand material that is relevant and has value to them. Therefore, it is important to present an overall picture along with the objectives they are expected to accomplish. Performance standards should be realistic and attainable. Setting artificially high standards reduces motivation and results in feelings of frustration, anxiety, and stress. Employees should feel challenged, but not overwhelmed.

Consideration should be given to the importance of motivation, reinforcement, and knowledge of results. Establishing individual goals that challenge employees and satisfy their particular motivators is the ideal. Training methods that allow for the design of individualized programs, such as computer-based training or print-based programmed learning modules, should be considered. **Programmed learning modules** lead learners through subject material that is presented in short sections, followed immediately by a series of questions that require a written response based on the section just presented. Answers are provided in the module for immediate feedback.

Learning is accomplished best by doing; therefore, it is important to provide as many hands-on activities as possible. In general, people recall 10 percent of what they read, 20 percent of what they hear, 50 percent of what they see and hear, and almost all of what they say while they do (McConnell 2013, 367). Therefore, the most effective training includes a combination of verbal instruction, demonstration, and hands-on experience, using multiple senses. Correct responses should be reinforced immediately. Recognition by the trainer or feedback about achievement may be just as effective as monetary rewards in providing reinforcement.

Adults want to know why they need to learn something (Murphy et al. 1999, 519). In addition, they

Figure 24.6. Learning curve

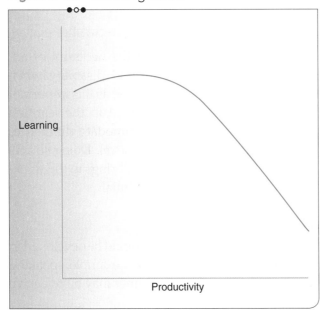

want to be in control of the situation and learn at their own pace. Where possible, training should be delivered with spaced repetition, which is the same material repeated after a lapse in time and presented in varying formats. The employee who learns quickly can move forward whereas the slower learner can devote more time to a specific activity.

Learning Styles

Just as there are varying types of personalities, there are several different ways in which people learn. It would seem appropriate, then, that the greatest amount of learning will take place if the teaching method matches the learning style of the learner. If relevancy, meaning, and emotion are attached to the material taught, the learner will learn. Learners tend to progress only as far as they need to in order to achieve their goal. Therefore, the best time to learn is when it is viewed as useful, which has made **just-in-time training** popular. Content is taught in small, relevant portions where and when the learner can use it most readily. The learner can then put the newly learned information to practice quickly.

Although an individual may have a preferred learning style, other approaches may sometimes be used. Learning styles are influenced by factors such as age, maturity, and experience, and they may change over time. In general, active learning is more effective than passive learning. Younger workers prefer concrete, sequential learning, whereas older adults prefer more ambiguity, which permits them to draw on their own experience. Following are various models for categorizing learning styles:

- *Sensory:* The learner may prefer auditory (prefers to listen), visual (prefers to read), or kinesthetic (prefers to practice) learning

- *Personality:* Various personality traits shape our orientation to the world

- *Information processing:* People differ in how they receive and process information

- *Social interaction:* Gender and social context determine learning style

- *Instructional and environmental preference:* Sound, light, structure, and learning relationships affect perceptions (Murphy et al. 1999, 518)

Various teaching techniques may be used to address different learning styles. These include:

- Individual tasks (reading, answering questions)

- Working with a partner (exchanging ideas, problem solving)

- Lecture to a group

- Working in groups (role playing, simulations)

When addressing a group with various ages and learning styles, the trainer might offer a project with broad guidelines for group completion. For example, some students might contribute text, some might create graphics, and some might build a database.

Advances in computer technology and the advent of e-learning have offered the ability to deliver content to match a variety of learning styles at relatively low cost. Some learners may prefer to read text; others may prefer to interact with graphics or solve problems. The material can be delivered in a variety of modes in a cost-efficient manner and at a pace consistent with an individual's learning style.

Additional resources for information about adult learning are provided by the American Society for Training and Development (2008), the association for workplace learning and performance professionals. Another resource is Workforce—an organization that provides a variety of human resources tools, including a magazine and an electronic newsletter (Workforce 2001).

Training Learners with Special Needs

Trainers should be aware of the necessity of addressing issues of diversity and disability when preparing training programs. Just as it is important to match the teaching technique to the learning style, it is important to accommodate differences in culture, language, and skill level. Doing so will enhance the value an employee brings to the workplace by maximizing their potential.

Diversity

Content of training programs should be developed in a culturally sensitive manner. For example, speaking in an informal or offhand manner may be offensive to some. It also is inappropriate in some cultures to question or challenge an instructor, or communal learning may be more valued than success of the individual. Males may be used to dominating a discussion; females may need to be encouraged to contribute (Dessler 2015, 543).

English as Second Language

In addition to considering cultural diversity issues when creating training programs, many healthcare institutions include employees where English may not be the primary language, either in the United States or overseas. If the number of such employees is significant, thought should be given to obtaining materials written in the primary language. Development in English proficiency in writing or oral communication should be provided if this is needed.

Disabilities

In general, employers are required to make reasonable accommodation for workers with disabilities (Zachary 2004). This may include altering training materials, modifying equipment, and making existing facilities accessible and usable. For example, employees in the HIM department may require adaptations to computer equipment.

The US Department of Education has established minimum requirements for developers of electronic and information technology to ensure accessibility for those with or without disabilities (2001). When designing training programs for use on computers, keep in mind that adjustments may need to be made so that users with disabilities are able to use the program if it requires use of a keyboard and monitor. Some programs may be developed using voice recognition software or screen readers. Web design should be compliant with requirements of the Americans with Disabilities Act. If graphics, audio, or video are to be used, a text alternative should accompany them to be accessible with a screen reader. Options for the user to control animation, flashing or blinking objects, or color contrast should be provided, as well as an option to extend time available on timed responses.

Check Your Understanding 24.3

Instructions: **Answer the following questions on a separate piece of paper.**

1. Describe the five models for categorizing learning styles.
2. Give an example of a reinforcement other than a monetary reward.
3. What role does motivation play in developing a training program?
4. Describe the concept of the learning curve.
5. What type of instruction helps learners retain the most?
6. What adaptations should be made to accommodate diversity and disability issues in training?

Delivery Methods

There are many techniques for delivering training, just as there are many purposes of training. Factors that influence selection of a training method include:

- Purpose of the training
- Level of education and experience of the trainees
- Amount of space, equipment, and media available for training
- Number of trainees and their location
- Cost of the method in comparison to desired results

- Need for special accommodation due to disability or cultural differences among the trainees

When the purpose of training is to increase the level of knowledge or to introduce new policies, a different method is appropriate than when the goal is to teach a hands-on skill. Training that requires a lot of room and equipment located near the employees' work area will require a different method than training that needs to be delivered across a distance. Instruction in essential skills or license requirements may justify a higher expenditure than instruction that is helpful, but not mandatory.

Table 24.2 presents the time and location requirements for various training delivery methods. Some subjects, such as demonstration of a new fire safety procedure, are best taught to a group of learners at the same time and place; for example, in a traditional classroom setting. Other subjects, such as use of computer software, may be taught at a time and place more effective for employees to learn, like a computer lab. Audioconferencing and videoconferencing are methods used to train people located in different offices, but at one time.

Blended learning uses several delivery methods thereby gaining the advantages and reducing the disadvantages of each method alone. Common examples are classroom lecture plus online discussion, or a combination of asynchronous discussion with synchronous webinars.

Programmed Learning

Programmed learning allows students to progress at their own pace. It presents material, questions the learner, and delivers immediate responses with either positive or negative reinforcement (Dessler 2015, 232). Giving an employee the opportunity to control the learning situation is a clear advantage. It is suitable for delivery to one or many employees and is a solution for employees who cannot attend sessions outside work hours because of home or family responsibilities.

Programmed learning was originally delivered via textbooks (Dessler 2015, 232). Although computers have replaced or supplemented them in some cases, textbooks still work well at a relatively low cost. Learners are presented with text and diagrams and then respond to questions. Answers to the questions are provided on another page in the same book for easy checking and feedback. Other advantages to using texts are that they are easily portable and may be supported by other media, for instance in an audio format. One disadvantage is that learners may not learn much more than the information in the traditional textbook, and the cost of development may not be paid back unless the book is used several times.

An example of a programmed learning subject is medical terminology. Text and diagrams of a body system are presented, and the learner is asked to label anatomical structures and to answer multiple-choice or fill-in-the-blank questions. Access codes to a publisher's website are often included with textbooks that provide the opportunity to view diagrams and listen to pronunciation of the terms via a website maintained by the publisher.

Computer-based training (CBT) is a method designed to provide individual learners with electronic training at their own pace (Dessler 2015,

Table 24.2. Location and time factors of various training methods

	Same time	Different time
Same space	Traditional with instructor:	Self-paced work station:
	Face-to-face classes	Computer or tablet
	Lectures	DVD-ROM
	Hands-on practice	Printed materials
Different space	Synchronous distance learning:	Asynchronous distance learning:
	Audioconferencing	Online courses
	Videoconferencing	Recorded multimedia
	Live webinar	Recorded webinar

Source: Adapted from Levenburg and Major 1988.

233). The students must use a computer to access the program. Similar to text-based programmed learning, the explanatory material is presented and followed by a series of questions. The text is accompanied by sounds or drawings to maintain interest and to present the material in a creative way. After each question is answered, there is an immediate response or reinforcement by the computer. In most systems, students can repeat sections of the material until they have mastered it. Students can work on different topics, at varying speeds, and in several languages. The cost of developing CBT courses may be higher than classroom instruction or texts; but once developed, the cost of delivery is less because the course can be used multiple times. It is especially useful for content that does not change frequently, such as basic medical terminology or general release of information (ROI) policies.

CBT is usually delivered locally by access to the vendor's web server, or it may be sold separately on a DVD. Both provide an excellent way to deliver text, audio, video clips, and animation; and both are particularly useful for providing simulations of work situations.

The advantages of CBT include lower training costs, reduction in travel or time away from work for workshops, and better learning retention than with traditional classroom teaching. In addition, interactive technology has been demonstrated to reduce learning time by an average of 50 percent (Dessler 2015, 233). Disadvantages are that initially it may require a cost investment, and some students prefer a live setting and instructor for interaction.

Electronic performance support systems (EPSSs) are sets of computerized tools and displays that automate training and documentation, and integrate this automation with the computer application. It is true just-in-time training—giving information at the time it is needed. These systems are especially useful for complex jobs with multiple steps. An EPSS prompts the user through a series of questions, similar to a checklist. Training time can be reduced significantly through the use of an EPSS and quality of work is enhanced. An EPSS is relatively easy to update as policies or requirements change, ensuring that the user has the most up-to-date information available.

Classroom Learning

Classroom learning is still the most popular method of instruction (Fried and Fottler 2015, 373). It enables immediate feedback and can improve communication skills. When the goal is to train a large number of employees on largely factual knowledge within a short period of time, classroom learning may be the best choice. When the intention is to convey information, this method is effective and economical. However, it is not as appropriate for developing problem-solving skills or improving interpersonal competence, unless combined with other methods.

Teaching a class used to mean solely using the **lecture** method in which the instructor delivers content and the student listens and observes primarily one-way communication. This technique usually involves little active participation by the learner. However, because students learn more by doing, today's classroom instruction frequently takes place in a "flipped" classroom—combining lecture with small group discussion, role playing, student presentations, videos, or other means where dialogue and interaction are facilitated. One method that has become popular is the use of electronic polling software, where the instructor projects a question with answers that students can review and then text their choice using a smartphone. The software then immediately presents the number of students who selected a given answer projected on a screen. Using a combination of training methods has proven to be highly effective (TrainingToday 2015). Video is useful for presenting events or demonstrations not easily accomplished in lectures, such as scenarios on interpersonal communication or conflict resolution or viewing surgical procedures. The audience can respond to the speaker using a software application on personal smartphones or using a personal response device such as a clicker. The class itself may be recorded and the video used to deliver the same material to other shifts or workers unable to attend the class.

Other techniques are frequently used in combination with the large classroom setting. **Group discussion** is effective following a lecture. Learners form smaller groups to generate ideas through interactive sharing of ideas.

Case studies are used to present opportunities for problem solving. A real or simulated situation is presented to either a group or individual to practice critical-thinking skills and formulate solutions. Depending on the issue, employees can also gain experience with communication, decision making, and negotiation (Fried and Fottler 2015, 374).

Role playing is an activity where learners are presented with a hypothetical situation they may encounter on the job, and they respond by acting out the response. It is useful for practicing tasks such as interviewing, grievance handling, team problem solving, conflict resolution, or communication difficulties.

Seminars and Workshops

Seminars or workshops offer training over the course of one or more days and usually consist of several sessions on specific topics related to an overall theme. Some sessions are large, general classes and others are small, break-out classes on topics of limited interest. The cost of workshops and seminars, especially when they are held outside the workplace, is usually high because of the costs of materials, room rental, refreshments, and speaker fees. This training is typically conducted by experts on a subject and may be held in-house or offered by professional organizations, public or private colleges, or vocational schools. It is often used to develop new skills or to retrain employees whose jobs have been affected by changes in the organization, external requirements, or new policies or procedures.

Webinars are seminars delivered via a web browser, either real-time or as a recorded broadcast. This medium reduces training costs as presenters and trainees can sit in their own offices in different locations, avoiding the need for travel. Instant messaging (IM) can add quick accessibility to responses and enhance a webinar (Fried and Fottler 2011, 145).

Simulations

Simulations are training approaches that utilize devices or programs replicating tasks away from the job site; when computer based they are known as **virtual reality** simulations. A typical simulation provides the learner with a fictional scenario of a problem, and the learner decides what action to take next, as if it were a real experience. Learning occurs in two parts. First, the learner is immersed in a true representation of an actual situation; and second, the learner is required to manage several rules and relationships involved in the process (Heiphetz and Liverman 2008). Learning is acquired through understanding the relationships among the complex processes, or learning through exploration.

Online, **multiuser virtual environments (MUVEs)**, sometimes called virtual worlds, bring a new dimension to learning. MUVEs are accessed over the Internet and can be used to simulate a work environment. Users create representations of themselves (**avatars**) and interact with other users (Heiphetz and Liverman 2008). Healthcare organizations can use a MUVE in a variety of soft skills training exercises such as interpersonal communication, decision making, and leadership. Individuals can role play to practice skills, try real-world experiences, and learn from their mistakes. Team building scenarios can be developed where avatars, working together as a team, might put together a puzzle or solve a problem. Cultural diversity sensitivity can be explored simulating scenarios that present potentially controversial situations.

MUVEs can also be used for technical training or using new equipment. Group or individual orientation for new hires in a simulation of the actual hospital or HIM department can be provided. This facilitates training of overseas workers and can be completed across different times and locations. Robotic instructors can demonstrate how to use equipment or perform procedures. "Instructors" can be asked to repeat instructions if needed, and can respond with realistic gestures, expressions, and emotion giving positive and negative feedback. Competency exams can be given through asking trainee avatars to perform demonstrations.

Other benefits of using a MUVE include the following:

- Participants can be in multiple locations, with cost savings by avoiding the need to travel to one location for training
- Hands-on, interactive learning results in faster results with higher retention

- Once a simulated environment is created, it can be stored on an organization's intranet and used repeatedly, or it can be easily changed
- The MUVE can be integrated into learning management systems

Simulation is helpful for training managers or supervisors. It is also used with group discussion and decision making within departments.

E-learning

E-learning refers to training courses delivered electronically. According to the 2015 Training Industry Report representing a variety of organizations, 26.4 percent of training hours were delivered via online or computer-based technology, down slightly from 28.5 percent the previous year (Training Magazine 2015). 31.9 percent were delivered with blended learning techniques, up a bit from 29.1 percent in 2014. Although most often used to designate web-based training, e-learning may also refer to self-directed computer-based training, video- or audioconferencing, or EPSS. There is increased demand for online training because traditional methods lack the flexibility and broad-based delivery necessary to meet the rising demand for updated skills in many areas of healthcare.

Electronic training is most successful when

- There is a large audience to train;
- Employees are geographically dispersed at several sites and work varied schedules;
- Just-in-time training is required;
- The purpose is to gain knowledge or learn applications; or
- There is a blend of solid instructional design, instructor creativity, and proven technology (Kibbee and Gerzon 2008).

Advantages of e-learning include flexibility of class time and place, consistency of delivery, reduced time and cost of training, and the ability to reuse and easily maintain content. Drawbacks include technical problems, such as connectivity or availability for large blocks of time, and learner issues with motivation or distraction. Trainers may

not be available for some time, and therefore a lag may occur between the time a problem arises and the time it can be solved. As mobile devices increase in usage, it is anticipated that the frequency of web-based training will increase. Table 24.3 shows classroom vs. e-learning advantages and disadvantages.

Audioconferencing and Videoconferencing

With audio- or videoconferencing, employees in several locations can learn together via telephone or video. For audioconferencing, all that is required is a telephone at each office. For videoconferencing, either a computer monitor with speakers or monitor and telephone is required. This enables learners to listen and respond to the same material presented by an instructor located at another site.

Audioconferencing enables students to listen to material delivered by a presenter via telephone while looking at handout material or books. At selected points in the presentation, the instructor pauses and learners interact and share comments or ask questions about the material. The advantage of audioconferencing is its relatively low cost compared to video or computer delivery. Moreover, it eliminates the time and expense of travel to the instruction site. It is useful for the same kind of purpose as the lecture method, which is to deliver specific content to a large group of people. The disadvantage is that there is little opportunity for interaction or visual demonstration by the instructor.

Interactive videoconferencing offers one- or two-way video together with two-way audio. With one-way video, students receive the image of the instructor and demonstrations and can both see and hear the presenter, but the instructor cannot see the students. Two-way video permits both parties to see each other and interact. Improved technology is enhancing the quality as well as reducing the cost of this delivery method.

Videoconferencing permits additional flexibility in delivering courses that may be enhanced through visual as well as audio presentation, such as those that include demonstrations or simulation exercises. It is useful for training employees in organizations with multiple sites, such as integrated

Table 24.3.   Classroom vs. e-learning advantages and disadvantages

	Classroom	Asynchronous web-based	Synchronous web-based
Advantages	• High-quality, personal delivery • Immediate answers to questions • All students get same info at the same time • Interactive experience	• Just-in-time training • Self-paced learning • Consistency • Training materials easy to update • Flexible time and place • Cost-effective • Measurable—test scores can be used for evaluation	• High-quality delivery • Immediate answers to questions • Rapid, low-cost content
Disadvantages	• Expensive • Training too soon or too late • Scheduling can be difficult • Effectiveness is dependent on lecturer	• Motivation can be difficult • Lack of classroom collaboration • Delay in trainer response • Not effective for teaching soft skills • Not interactive; can be boring • Requires technical expertise	• Higher cost per student than asynchronous • Instructor and students need to be available at same time
Best for	• Multiple students with similar skills • Training in single location • Interpersonal skills • Discussion is needed	• Basic training • Large number of students in multiple locations • Students are self-motivated	• Basic training • Students in multiple locations that need to convene • Highly interactive knowledge sharing • Technical support is available
Worst for	• Students of varying skill levels • Consistency across learner groups	• Observing interpersonal skills and feedback • Real-time knowledge sharing • Complex content	• Students of varying skill levels • Observing interpersonal skills and feedback

Source: Adapted from Kibbee and Gerzon 2008; Workforce 2001.

delivery networks with inpatient and outpatient facilities. The disadvantage is the high cost, but the expense is justified for large organizations that do extensive training.

Web-Based Courses

The most frequent mode of e-learning is the web-based course. Internet-based training is delivered via a universally available medium and is relatively low cost. It permits on-demand training, removing both time and space barriers. The medium is familiar to individuals and requires a minimum of instruction in the specific courseware used to deliver the course. This method provides instruction when, where, and at a pace suited to each learner. The instruction can be delivered in several forms.

Web-based courses can be delivered **synchronously**, which is real-time with employees and trainers interacting via chat rooms, whiteboards, or application sharing at a predetermined time with review of materials. This closely mimics a traditional classroom setting. Another option is **asynchronous** delivery, where learners and instructors interact through e-mail or discussion forums. It is not necessary to be online at the same time and is therefore more convenient than synchronous delivery. The discussion board format is the most frequently used, where learners post comments and then review and respond at different times. Materials also can be posted for review at the learner's convenience.

Software can be distributed simultaneously to learners via download from a website. Learners can interact with other learners and the instructor via a variety of communication tools. A common form of delivery today is to access courses developed by training organizations or universities via a website. Course authoring tools are now readily available that permit trainers to develop e-learning courses easily and quickly without professional course developers. Most rapid e-learning tools also incorporate search tools, bookmarking, and data tracking. Employees are issued a username and password to access the course. Material can be presented using a variety of methods, including text, audio, or video. Relevant material can be accessed through hypertext links embedded in the website that learners can access with the click of a mouse.

Software for delivering web-based courses is developed as **learning management systems (LMSs)** and **learning content management systems (LCMSs)**. LMSs manage the learning process, tracking grades and access, presenting the content, and collating statistics on use. LCMSs provide a technical framework to develop the content and permit sharing and reusing content. Most courseware used by colleges and universities has both components. Rapid e-learning tools can be linked to learning management systems to facilitate course development.

A **massive open online course (MOOC)** is an online course with unlimited participation and open access offered via the Internet. A number of institutions have offered content on various subjects, including data analysis techniques and human anatomy and physiology. The model offers content to a large number of students and is usually free (Educause 2015). Sometimes college credit may be offered for a fee with completion of additional assessments or assignments.

Intranets are private computer networks that use Internet technologies but are protected with security features and can only be accessed by employees of the organization. Many hospitals use intranets to distribute policies, procedures, and education courses on a variety of topics. Material can be delivered via intranets for employee self-study, as well as other customized courses for specific employee needs.

The advantages of web-based courses include the availability of the delivery medium (the Internet or intranet), which brings the course to the employee's computer at home or work, and the ability to easily update materials. Multimedia materials, including audio, video, graphics, and animation, provide an interesting way to deliver material and have been shown to result in faster learning and greater retention. They also are well suited to adult learners, meeting their needs for education on their terms of time and location. Although sometimes expensive to develop, the cost of delivering web-based courses is usually less compared to the cost of classroom or seminar courses for large numbers of employees (TrainingToday 2015).

It is important to remember to start training with an understanding of the specific performance goals to be attained. Using an authoring tool without a strong, outcomes-focused instructional design will not achieve success.

Social Networks

The increasing popularity of social networking websites provides another opportunity for e-learning. These sites provide an online community where participants can share information including file attachments, website bookmarks, or multimedia files. Web logs (**blogs**) provide a web page where users can post text, images, and links to other websites. While blogs originally started as a type of online personal diary, they are now used for a variety of purposes, including communication within organizations, and can be helpful for distributing training materials. **Wikis** are a collection of web pages that together form a collaborative website. A wiki can be modified by its users. Healthcare organizations may use wikis as a tool where trainers or supervisors can post material and employees can respond and discuss questions. Facebook and LinkedIn also may provide easily accessible tools to post documents and reminders for employee groups and provide platforms for asking questions.

M-Learning

M-learning, or mobile learning, is an electronic learning mode in which content typically delivered via the Internet to computers can be received by smartphones or tablets, thereby expanding the accessibility to a true anytime, anyplace level. Issues to consider are the type of device (small handheld vs. tablet PC) and type of connectivity. Screens on a tablet PC are larger than on a smartphone, permitting more information to be transmitted. Information can be downloaded from a PC to a mobile device and then accessed later away from the organization; or the device can be directly connected to the Internet via wireless connection. Content is easy to access and delivery permits viewing on the learner's schedule. As with any form of e-learning, effective instructional design is important. M-learning is not appropriate for very long courses with a great deal of material but is appropriate for delivering key points and short updates. It is an effective way to deliver multimedia information to a large number of people quickly. Following review of the material, participants might respond to questions or use social networking tools such as blogs or wikis, providing an interactive learning environment.

A recent study looked at the effectiveness of traditional classroom, asynchronous e-learning, and m-learning in organizational training and concluded there was no significant difference in post-assessment performance. Therefore, when considering which training method to invest in, managers should focus on convenience, cost, accessibility, development, and deployment speed (Paul 2014, 10).

Intensive Study Courses

Intensive study courses allow a great deal of material to be compressed into a small time frame. A common example is the weekend college, where learners attend 10 to 12 hours per day on Saturday and Sunday. These courses are usually delivered on a college campus or at a hotel setting and require an overnight stay. This training method is suited for teaching special skills that can best be learned in a setting away from day-to-day operations. Examples of courses include cultural awareness, training in teamwork and empowerment, and management development.

A popular exercise is to take the organization's leadership team to an outdoor setting where they learn spirit and cooperation and the need to rely on others in order to overcome physical obstacles. The process builds trust to be transferred to the work setting.

Check Your Understanding 24.4

Instructions: Answer the following questions on a separate piece of paper.

1. What factors should be considered in selecting a training method?

2. What training option can reduce costs for seminars or workshops?

3. What type of training is appropriate for delivery on mobile devices such as smartphones and tablet computers?

4. What is the difference between synchronous and asynchronous web-based course instruction?

5. What training obstacles are reduced with e-learning?

6. What is an appropriate role for case studies and role-playing in training employees?

7. How would a healthcare organization use its intranet to deliver training?

8. What is a MOOC?

9. Describe how social networks and MUVEs can be used for training.

Positioning Employees for Career Development

Developing strong healthcare leaders in an increasingly competitive market is a growing need. Successful organizations are those that have a formal process in place for leadership development.

Creating an environment that encourages and allows employees to use and develop their problem-solving and decision-making competencies is an established HR management practice that has many benefits. For example, it increases the manager's capacity and productivity, improves the quality and timeliness of decision making, enhances employee morale, and contributes to improved employee retention. Employees often look for opportunities for personal growth. A significant amount of training should be devoted to developing the ability of employees to help themselves and to realize that they are the ones responsible for their advancements. Ideally the organization strives to match individual goals with the entity's needs. Identifying what each party (the individual and the organization) requires from and contributes to the relationship, and understanding how to keep these balanced, can determine training and development needs. Career development is a partnership between the employee and the entity (May 2013, 12).

Empowerment

Empowerment is the concept of providing employees with the tools and resources to solve problems themselves. In other words, employees obtain power over their work situation by assuming responsibility. Empowered employees have the freedom to contribute ideas and perform their jobs in the best possible way. The idea of empowerment actually began as part of total quality management programs, which many organizations initiated in order to improve the quality of service provided to customers and to increase their competitiveness in the marketplace. A high-quality organization strives to understand and improve work processes in order to prevent problems.

Healthcare organizations that empower their employees believe that all employees can perform—and truly want to perform—to their highest potential when given the proper resources and environment. Because they perform jobs on a regular basis, they are intimately familiar with the steps in the process. What the employees may lack are skills in analysis and problem solving. Training sessions in skills such as data analysis, use of control charts, or flowcharting will help employees to identify problems, develop alternatives, and recommend solutions.

To perform effectively, employees also need to be given responsibility, authority, and the trust to make decisions and act independently within their area of expertise. Figure 24.7 offers suggestions on how managers can empower their employees.

Empowered employees are less likely to complain or feel helpless or frustrated when they cannot resolve a problem on their own. Moreover, they are more likely to feel a sense of accomplishment and to be more receptive to solutions that they develop themselves. In addition, they tend to demonstrate commitment and self-confidence and produce high-quality work.

One disadvantage that is frequently mentioned by managers is that empowerment involves too much time for meetings and discussion and takes employees away from their "real work." Actually, it is much more efficient to take the time necessary to prevent problems than to solve them after they occur. In the long run, empowered employees work more efficiently and productively.

Indeed, some managers are afraid to share power. They feel that they have worked hard to gain the power they have and are reluctant to give it up. But the manager who empowers others usually increases his or her own power because a high-performing unit reflects the manager's expertise.

Figure 24.7. How to empower employees

- Get others involved in selecting their work assignments and the methods for accomplishing tasks.
- Create an environment of cooperation, information sharing, discussion, and shared ownership of goals.
- Encourage others to take initiative, make decisions, and use their knowledge.
- When problems arise, find out what others think and let them help design the solutions.
- Stay out of the way; give others the freedom to put their ideas and solutions into practice.
- Maintain high morale and confidence by recognizing successes and encouraging high performance.

Source: Schermerhorn 2005, 328. Copyright ©2011, 2006, 2003, 1996 by John Wiley & Sons, Inc. All rights reserved. Reprinted with permission.

An example of empowerment in the HIM department would be to train ROI employees to solve a slow turnaround issue. The employees are probably more aware than the supervisor of problems that prevent them from filling requests for information (such as missing documents, insufficient fees, and incomplete records). With proper training in brainstorming and flowcharting, as well as a supportive environment, the employees may be able to develop a procedure that can be performed differently to prevent delays.

Delegation

Delegation is the process of distributing work duties and decision making to others. To be effective, delegation should be commensurate with authority and responsibility. A manager must assign **responsibility**, which is an expectation that another person will perform tasks. At the same time, **authority**—or the right to act in ways necessary to carry out assigned tasks—must be granted. An employee cannot be expected to perform a job for which he or she is not given authority to obtain resources. Authority should equal responsibility when work is delegated. Finally, **accountability** must be created, which is the requirement to answer to a supervisor for results. An employee must be empowered to act, given the necessary tools and skills, and held accountable for the quality of his or her work.

Successful delegation includes:

- Assigning responsibility
- Granting authority
- Creating accountability (Schermerhorn 2013, 286)

Guidelines for delegating are presented in figure 24.8. As an employee development tool, delegation can give employees the opportunity to try new tasks previously performed by someone in a higher position and leads to empowerment because employees contribute ideas and fully utilize their skills. At the same time, the manager should remain available to provide assistance and support.

Sometimes managers have difficulty delegating because they feel that only they can do the job

Figure 24.8. Ground rules for effective delegation

- Carefully choose the person to whom you delegate
- Define the responsibility; make the assignment clear
- Agree on performance objectives and standards
- Agree on a performance timetable
- Give authority; allow the other person to act independently
- Show trust in the other person
- Provide performance support
- Give performance feedback
- Recognize and reinforce progress
- Help when things go wrong
- Do not forget your accountability for performance results

Source: Schermerhorn 2005, 264. Copyright ©2011, 2006, 2003, 1996 by John Wiley & Sons, Inc. All rights reserved. Reprinted with permission.

correctly. In other cases, they feel threatened by the idea that another employee can do their tasks and perhaps do them better. This thinking can lead to poor morale and result in talented employees leaving the organization. In addition, it can lead to managers being overburdened with work that could be done by others and to employees being denied opportunities to learn new skills.

In some situations, employees may be unwilling to accept delegated responsibilities when they feel that they are unqualified to do the tasks or that they are being dumped on. Dumping can involve assigning an employee unpleasant or unpopular work that seems to have little value or asking an employee to take on work in addition to an already demanding workload. This results in resentment or anger. Employees may feel this way when they have a poor working relationship with their supervisor, know that others have refused the same task, or have been taken advantage of in the past.

To avoid these problems, employees who are either competent to perform the tasks or willing to undergo the necessary training should be selected. People are more willing to accept tasks that they understand, have a choice in doing, and recognize the value added to the organization and their personal growth. Managers should set checkpoints, monitor how the delegate is doing, and allow the opportunity for questions and feedback.

Delegation is a skill that matches the right employee with the right task. It requires communication, support, and an environment that fosters risk taking. It is essential in order to identify and develop successors and is important if a manager wishes to provide a path to advance in the organization. Effective delegation actually leads to a more efficient and productive department overall and mutually benefits the manager, employee, and institution.

Coaching and Mentoring

Both new employees and experienced employees who may be ready for a change can benefit from coaching or mentoring (Schermerhorn 2013, 334). As discussed earlier in this chapter, coaching is an ongoing process in which an experienced person offers performance advice to a less experienced person. However, coaching goes beyond teaching. A good coach is also a counselor, a resource person, a troubleshooter, and a cheerleader. Coaches deal with improving attitudes and morale, correcting performance problems, and encouraging career development in addition to giving instruction in specific tasks.

Effective coaches are dedicated leaders who display a high level of competence and are able to push or pull employees to their highest level of performance. They are role models who set a good example; show workers what is expected and how to get the job done well; provide praise or constructive feedback where appropriate; and are ready to help with routine work alongside the employee, if necessary. Department managers are well positioned to share their knowledge and expertise of the job they manage.

Coaching starts with orientation of the new employee and continues throughout his or her time with the organization. The more time the coach spends observing and listening to employees, the more opportunities there will be to support, praise, and offer advice.

Helping employees should be done in a manner that encourages self-sufficiency. For example, when an employee comes forward with a problem, a good coach does not simply give the answer but, rather, asks the employee for suggestions. In other words, the coach's response should be "What do you think?" rather than "Here's what you should do."

Coaches defend and support their employees. They are facilitators who remove obstacles and obtain resources to enable and empower their staff. It is important to praise performance above and beyond the expected; for example, when the employee completes a task ahead of schedule or offers to help a colleague. It is equally important to praise the worker who consistently meets objectives or improves in an area that was below standard—in other words, for doing what is expected. To be effective, both positive and negative feedback must be timely, specific, and in the right setting (privately or publicly, depending on the circumstance). Good coaches direct negative feedback at the behavior they wish to correct, not at the person.

However, coaching can be done poorly. This happens when criticism is overused or praise is undeserved. In addition, the approach needs to be adjusted to the employee. Good coaching takes time to allow flexibility and encourage the employee to perform correctly without jumping in too quickly with advice.

Mentoring is a form of coaching. A mentor is an experienced employee who works with other employees early in their careers, giving them advice on developing skills and career options. Several employees may be assigned as protégés to the mentor, but contact is usually one-on-one. Through the mentoring relationship, employees have an advisor with whom they can solve problems, analyze and learn from mistakes, and celebrate successes. Many organizations have formal mentoring programs where protégés are matched with potential mentors. Other managers voluntarily offer to work with up-and-coming employees. A mentor should never be forced to serve, but rather should be selected as a volunteer, willing to give the time and energy such a relationship requires, and be someone who demonstrates an interest in the development of others.

Mentors share their knowledge of management styles and teach prospective supervisors specific job or interpersonal skills. They may assign challenging projects that allow employees to explore real-life learning experiences while still under the guidance of an experienced teacher.

Successful mentoring depends on effective interaction between mentor and protégé. Mentors must be chosen who enjoy passing on their experience and knowledge to others.

Promotion and Succession Planning

Promotion may be another tool to encourage employee development and commitment. When tied to training programs, it can become a powerful incentive. **Promotion** usually refers to the upward progression of an employee in both job and salary. However, it also can mean a lateral move to a different position with similar job skills or to a change within the same job as a result of completing higher education or credentialing requirements. To attract, retain, and motivate employees, organizations should provide a career development system that promotes from within.

When tied to promotion, career development programs offer an incentive to ambitious employees. Goals can be incorporated into the performance review process. In the HIM department, clerical employees can be encouraged to take classes that would lead to an associate's degree in health information technology or a bachelor's degree in health information management, making them eligible for certification exams. In addition, employees may be encouraged to enter coding certificate programs and achieve coding certification, or achieve specialty certifications such as the certified health data analyst (CHDA).

The higher the status of the person in the organization, the more likely it is that promotion will work as a motivator. To improve employee performance, promotion should be awarded based on competence, not on seniority. In some organizations, union contracts emphasize seniority and thus restrict the organization's ability to use competence as a sole criterion.

Promotion based on performance is usually measured by appraising past performance against standards. However, past performance does not always predict future potential. Some organizations use testing instruments to assess this capability.

Succession planning is a specific type of promotional plan in which senior-level position openings are anticipated and candidates are identified from within the organization. The candidates are given training through formal education, job rotation, and mentoring so that they can eventually assume these positions. It should be considered an essential part of every manager's job to identify and develop potential successors. The goal of succession planning is to provide a basis for promotions, transfers, and movement of employees and to fill voids when these changes occur (Fried and Fottler 2015, 363).

To be effective, promotion criteria should be published in a formal policy and procedure, which usually includes job postings of open positions, so that all employees have the opportunity to apply for consideration. When promotions appear to be given to favored employees, or when the procedure is shrouded in secrecy, promotion ceases to be attractive.

Continuing Education

Continuing education (CE) is a requirement of most professionals, including those in HIM. It usually requires a person to complete a certain number of hours of education within a given time period to maintain a credential or license status. Accrediting organizations such as the Joint Commission also include CE in their standards. The HIM field is changing rapidly, primarily in the areas of technology, data analytics, e-HIM, and legal and regulatory requirements. It is important that credentialed professionals remain current in their knowledge of the profession so that they can provide high-quality skills to the organizations for which they work.

CE refers to keeping up with changes in the profession or to improving skills required to perform the same job. It is different from career development, which is geared toward preparing an individual for a new job. Sometimes this line is blurred. In HIM, management development programs may be essential for the current position when one is already a supervisor, for example. On the other hand, preparing a technical employee to assume a new management role would be considered career development. Some organizations have tuition reimbursement policies to encourage career development.

CE programs are most often provided by external organizations such as AHIMA or its component state associations. Career development, by contrast, usually includes a combination of internal methods, such as job rotation through progressively increasing job responsibilities in-house and externally taught formal classes and workshops.

As part of the formal performance appraisal process, CE goals should be set for all employees. A record should be kept in the employee's personnel file that indicates the number of CE hours earned as well as the topic, place, and person who provided the education. Management should support the individual's achievement by such activities as providing time off to attend workshops, flexible scheduling for formal classes offered at educational institutions, and financial reimbursement.

CE programs are delivered via many different formats to suit the individual learner. These include classroom as well as computer-based modules or web-based courses that all employees can access, regardless of where they live or their personal or physical limitations. Continued skill development should be an important requirement for all HIM employees.

Developing a Personal Career Plan

While an organization can use the methods discussed to assist employees with career advancement, the major responsibility still falls on the employees themselves. A **career plan** is a strategic plan for an individual, providing direction, goals, and an action plan to reach those goals. It includes the individual's own strengths, weaknesses, personal values, and interests. Successful leaders have a clear understanding of themselves and a sense of in what direction they want to go. A solid career plan will identify the skill sets and resources needed to reach one's goals, and how to better align them with those of the organization (Broscio and Scherer 2014, 62). When an opportunity for a lateral or advanced opportunity presents itself, an individual with a career plan will have developed the necessary skills, such as project management, data analytics, or leadership, and will be ready to act when called upon. A career plan needs to be flexible and updated regularly. See figure 24.9 for the key components of a career plan.

Figure 24.9.   The key components of a career plan

A strategic career plan should have these core components:

- Statement of one's personal values set and short- and long-term goals, clearly outlined but flexible based on the iterative process of building a plan to meet the needs of the individual, employer, and market
- Answers to the following questions:
  - What do I require for fulfillment in my work and life?
  - What does my current or future employer contribute that meets my requirements for fulfillment?
  - What is required of me to be successful by my current or future employer?
  - What do I contribute to my current or a future employer's success?
  - What am I doing well (and not so well) to meet my current or potential employer's needs, and what is my current or potential employer doing well (or not so well) to meet my needs?
- Analysis of gaps between one's own needs and aspirations and the current situation and market requirements
- Your value proposition today, what it should be in the future, and how this positions you to reach your goals
- Action steps to close the gaps and achieve your goals, including:
  - Market research: to stay informed
  - Learning plan: to stay relevant
  - Personal marketing: to build relationships
  - Managing risk: to eliminate career barriers
  - Identifying sources of support: to determine the need for a coach or mentor
- Process to monitor progress, gain feedback, and update the plan on an ongoing basis

Broscio, M.A. and J.E. Scherer. 2014. What's your plan? *Healthcare Executive* 29(6):60–62. Used with permission.

Social media can be helpful in finding resources for both the individual and organization. Viewing pertinent articles and blogs can provide insight on specific topics (May 2013, 18). Organizations need to maintain a presence and can use Twitter to present concise thoughts, ideas, and interests as reminders of training topics such as HIPAA regulations. Facebook and LinkedIn can be used by individuals to create profiles based on interests and work history. Organizations can post job opportunities and highlight career paths to encourage employee advancement. An appropriate mix of personal interaction and social media can be mutually beneficial to career development (Kelly 2010, 62).

AHIMA has created tools to assist HIM professionals with personal career development. The AHIMA Professional Development Inventory permits practicing HIM professionals to evaluate their own skills and knowledge in comparison to what is required for new program graduates. This information can then be used to build an individual's career plan in order to develop skill sets where gaps are identified. The Health Information Career Map illustrates jobs and career paths for HIM professionals (Sandefer et al. 2014, 42). One can select a particular HIM job title at a given educational level, view job responsibilities and salary data, and see promotional paths to other positions.

Employment Laws and Regulations Impacting Training

In developing training programs, healthcare organizations must recognize that special accommodations may be required to address the needs of both a culturally diverse workforce and employees with disabilities. Employers need to understand the requirements affecting training that are included under Title VII of the 1964 Civil Rights Act, the 1991 Civil Rights Act, and the Americans with Disability Act (ADA) of 1990. If completion of a training program is part of the selection process for a particular job, the organization must be able to demonstrate that the requirements for training are valid and do not discriminate against, or have a negative impact on, women, minorities, or disabled individuals. For example, the vocabulary in written documents used for training should match the level required for the job, and training equipment and locations should be accessible to individuals with mobility disabilities.

In order for employers to avoid liability for harassment and discrimination acts of their employees, they must not only implement antidiscrimination policies but also provide training to ensure that employees understand their rights and responsibilities. The courts interpret this as exercising reasonable care to prevent harassment. The training should cover all types of harassment, be provided for all employees shortly after they are hired and periodically thereafter, be of substantial length, and permit the employee to repeat as necessary until competence is demonstrated. Inadequate training exposes employers to potential liability for negligent training if an employee harms a third party (Johnson 2004, 121).

The **Occupational Safety and Health Act of 1970** (OSHA) was established by the federal government to ensure safe working conditions. Among its many requirements is training to reduce unsafe acts. Hospitals are required to train employees in fire safety and other job-related safety measures. If necessary, the training must be provided in the worker's native language (other than English), and the worker must be able to demonstrate proficiency following the training.

The **Americans with Disabilities (ADA) Act of 1990** requires employers to provide reasonable accommodations for physical or mental limitations with regard to many employment-related functions, including training (ADA 1990). For example, this would require that accommodations be made to computer-based training to provide accessibility through voice recognition or screen readers, if necessary. The World Wide Web Consortium's Web Accessibility Initiative publishes information about ADA Compliance for websites (WWW Consortium 2012). Section 508 of the Rehabilitation Act of 1973 provides accessibility standards for electronic and information technology.

Finally, the Joint Commission requires staff orientation and continuing education to meet requirements of a particular position and defines several topics for training, including cultural diversity sensitivity (Joint Commission 2015).

Check Your Understanding 24.5

Instructions: **Answer the following questions on a separate piece of paper.**

1. In what three ways can managers empower employees?

2. What two reasons might managers have for not empowering employees?

3. How does mentoring differ from coaching? How is it similar?

4. On what should promotion be based if it is to motivate?

5. What requirements does OSHA have related to training in healthcare organizations?

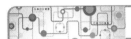

References

AHIMA Board of Directors. 2011 (Sept. 28). AHIMA Report. New View of HIM: Introducing the Core Model. http://bok.ahima.org/PdfView?oid=105304

American Health Information Management Association. 2015 (March 2). AHIMA Report. Results of the AHIMA 2014 Workforce Study. http://bok.ahima.org/PdfView?oid=300801

American Health Information Management Association. 2012 (June 2). AHIMA Toolkit. Health Information Management Staff Transformation Toolkit: A Practical Guide for Transitioning Staff to the Electronic Health Record .http://bok.ahima.org/PdfView?oid=105648

American Society for Training and Development. 2008. http://www.astd.org

Americans with Disability Act of 1990. Public Law 101–336

Bagshaw, M. 2004. Is diversity divisive? A positive training approach. *Industrial and Commercial Training* 36(4):153–157. http://site.ebrary.com/lib/uic

Broscio, M.A. and J.E. Scherer. 2014. What's your plan? *Healthcare Executive* 29(6):60–62.

Butler, M. 2015. Mind the gap: HIM rushes to bridge educational and professional gaps caused by a quickly advancing industry. *Journal of AHIMA* 86(2):20–24.

Dessler, G. 2015. *Human Resources Management,* 14th ed. Upper Saddle River, NJ: Pearson Prentice-Hall.

Educause. 2015. Massive Open Online Course (MOOC). http://www.educause.edu/library/massive-open-online-course-mooc

Fottler, H., S. Hernandez, and C. Joiner, eds. 1998. *Essentials of Human Resource Management in Health Service Organizations.* Albany, NY: Delmar.

Fried, B. and M. Fottler, eds. 2015. *Human Resources in Healthcare: Managing for Success,* 4th ed. Chicago: Health Administration Press.

Fried, B. and M. Fottler, eds. 2011. *Fundamentals of Human Resources in Healthcare.* Chicago: Health Administration Press.

Heiphetz, A. and S. Liverman. 2008. Using Robotic Avatars in Second Life Simulations and Training. https://brandonhallresearch.wikispaces.com/file/view/Using+Robotic+Avatars+in+Second+Life+Simulations+and+Training.pdf

Johnson, M. 2004. Harassment and discrimination prevention training: What the law requires. *Labor Law Journal* 55(2):119–129.

Keeling, B. and N. Kallaus. 1996. *Administrative Office Management,* 11th ed. Cincinnati, OH: South-Western.

Kelly, J.W., F.A.C.H.E. 2010. Using social media to boost your career. *Healthcare Executive* 25(1):62–65.

Kibbee, K. and J. Gerzon. 2008. MIT Training Delivery Guide. http://web.mit.edu/training/trainers/guide/deliver/train-guide-matrix.pdf

Levenburg, N. and H. Major. 1998. Distance learning: Implications for higher education in the 21st century. Originally published in *The Technology Source.* http://www.technologysource.org/article/distance_learning__implications_for_higher_education_in_the_21st_century

May, E.L. 2013. Managing your career in transformative times. *Healthcare Executive* 28(6):10-12, 14-16, 18.

McConnell, C. 2013. *The Health Care Manager's Human Resources Handbook*, 2nd ed. Burlington, MA: Jones and Bartlett Learning.

McConnell, C. 2010. *Umiker's Management Skills for the New Health Care Supervisor*, 5th ed. Sudbury, MA: Jones and Barlett.

Murphy, G., M.A. Hanken, and K. Waters. 1999. *Electronic Health Records: Changing the Vision.* Philadephia: W.B.Saunders.

Paul, T.V. 2014. An evaluation of the effectiveness of e-learning, mobile learning, and instructor-led training in organizational training and development. *Journal of Human Resource and Adult Learning* 10(2):1–13.

Sandefer, R. and E.S. Karl. 2015. Ready or not, HIM is changing: Results of the new HIM competencies survey show skill gaps between education levels, students, and working professionals. *Journal of AHIMA* 86(3):24–27.

Sandefer, R., H. DeAlmeida, R. Dilhari, M. Dougherty, D. Mancilla, D.T. Marc. 2014. Keeping current in the electronic era: Data age transforming HIM's mandatory workforce competencies. *Journal of AHIMA* 85(11):38–44.

Schermerhorn, J. 2013. *Management,* 12th ed. New York: John Wiley & Sons.

Schermerhorn, J. 2005. *Management,* 8th ed. New York: John Wiley & Sons.

The Joint Commission. 2015. *Comprehensive Accreditation Manual for Hospitals: Effective January 1, 2015.* Oak Brook.

Title VII of the Civil Rights Act of 1964. Public Law. 88-352.

Training Magazine. 2015. 2015 Industry Report. https://trainingmag.com/trgmag-article/2o15-training-industry-report

TrainingToday. 2015. The Most Effective Training Techniques. http://trainingtoday.blr.com/employee-training-resources/How-to-Choose-the-Most-Effective-Training-Techniques

US Department of Education. 2001. Requirements for Accessible Electronic and Information Technology (E&IT) Design. http://www.ed.gov/print/fund/contract/apply/clibrary/software.html

Workforce. 2001. Pros and cons of training modes. *Workforce Management Magazine.* http://www.workforce.com/articles/pros-and-cons-of-training-modes

World Wide Web Consortium. 2012. Web Accessibility Initiative. http://www.w3c.org/WAI

Zachary, M. 2004. Labor law for supervisors: Training for the disabled. *Supervision* 65(5):23–26.

25

Work Design and Process Improvement

Pamela K. Oachs, MA, RHIA, CHDA, FAHIMA

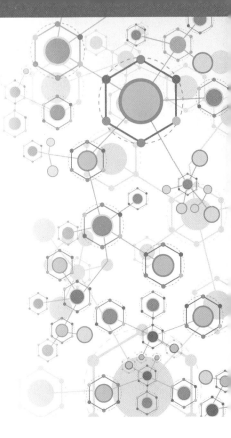

Employee self-logging
Ergonomics
External customer
Feedback control
Fishbone diagram
Flextime
Float employee
Flowchart
Force-field analysis
Goal
Histogram
Internal customer
Job procedure
Job sharing
Key indicator
Lean
Movement diagram
Multivoting technique
Narrative
Nominal group technique (NGT)

Objective
Offshoring
Open system
Outsourcing
Parallel work division
Pareto chart
Performance
Performance measurement
Playscript
Preventive control
Procedure manual
Process redesign
Productivity
Qualitative standard
Quantitative standard
Run chart
Scatter diagram
Serial work division
Service level agreement (SLA)
Shift differential

Shift rotation
Six Sigma
Special cause variation
Standard
Statistical process control (SPC)
    chart
Swimlane diagram
System
Telecommuting
Time ladder
Unit work division
Use case analysis
Volume log
Waste
Work
Work distribution analysis
Work distribution chart
Work measurement
Work sampling
Workflow

Management is getting work done through and with others. It may be thought of as both a science and an art. Management is a science because it is based on theory and principles that have been—and continue to be—tested and explored. It is an art because effective management depends on the use of sound judgment, intuition, communication, and interpersonal skills. Managers engage in specific functions, including planning, organizing, directing, and controlling, to create and facilitate effective work processes so that the desired outcome can be achieved in a cost-efficient manner.

Management of human resources is one of the most challenging and critical functions in a healthcare organization. Whether a lead staff person, supervisor, manager, or department director, to a great extent, people and performance management skills are the key factors impacting one's ability to successfully achieve organizational goals.

Performance management does not occur by accident. Careful consideration of available staff resources and how the staff resources are organized is fundamental to delivering effective and efficient HIM-related services.

This chapter introduces key concepts, tools, and techniques associated with evaluating, designing, redesigning, and implementing effective and efficient work processes within an organization. It includes discussion of various methods of work division and work scheduling; management of work procedures; components of the work environment; elements of a performance management program, including methods for establishing performance standards; and various process improvement methodologies to continuously improve or to reengineer workflow, work processes, and staff performance to accommodate changes in service requirements and fiscal limitations.

Functional Work Environment

Considering the fact that the average full-time employee spends more waking hours in the work environment than elsewhere, it would be prudent for management to create a workplace infrastructure and ambiance that evokes comfort and productivity. Whether creating new space or evaluating current space for the remote or on-site employee, developing the work environment involves consideration of these fundamental elements: workflow, space and equipment, aesthetics, and ergonomics.

Departmental Workflow

The **workflow** in a departmental setting is the established path along which tasks are sequentially completed by any number of staff to accomplish a function. Well-designed workflow is critical to achieving optimal efficiency when a function requires the coordinated activity of a group of employees. Spatial relationships among a group of people who perform tasks and the equipment required to perform them are critical factors in planning efficient workflow. In such situations, creating a layout diagram, sometimes called a **movement diagram** (see figure 25.1), helps the manager to visualize the functions and related tasks performed in a defined work area and how they are related.

Space and Equipment

Workspace design can influence the department culture including employee morale, productivity, quality, and job satisfaction. The design of efficient work space involves a number of considerations including the number of employees, physical activity of employees, workflow, equipment used, the type of environment (paper or electronic), job functions, and the need for privacy. Even in a highly electronic environment, there may still be an abundance of paper to manage, equipment to place, and workflow to manage. For example, whether health records are scanned or physically stored, there needs to be a plan for their location throughout the record processing functions that keeps them safe and secure while still being available to the employees.

Space is considered a precious and costly commodity in healthcare facilities and must be used efficiently. Department managers should understand basic facility planning techniques and know who their facility planning resources are in the organization. They must be able to consider the facility's master plan in consideration of their department or work unit needs to collaboratively develop a design for the work area.

Reorganization of a department because of changes in workforce numbers, telecommuting efforts, a shift in workforce functions, or acquisition of new functions constitutes a space planning process. Departmental reorganization in response to changes in methods or functions, such as a move to remote coding or implementation of an electronic health record (EHR), can trigger the need for revised space planning. Sometimes the basic need to improve workflow and the appearance of a department can be a pivotal reason for space planning.

Another space consideration is personal space or the area of privacy surrounding an employee. Depending on the employee's job role, confidentiality may be a concern. If the employee is in a mentoring or leadership role, privacy may be necessary when offering feedback to other employees. If the employee works directly with patients either on the phone or in person, there are also confidentiality concerns to consider.

It is also important to realize that space and equipment considerations do not go away when employees work remotely. Telecommuting will require redesign of on-site space as workers begin to vacate work areas, temporary work space may need to be designed for required on-site meetings, and employees working from home also need to have their home offices properly equipped. See chapter 23 for more information on considerations for telecommuting.

Effective space planning has the following characteristics:

- Keeping costs to a minimum
- Contributing to the quality of the work
- Contributing to employee satisfaction
- Contributing to services provided by the department

Space needs change over the course of time and should be reevaluated periodically to determine whether these characteristics as well as the needs of the department and staff are still being met.

Aesthetics

Aesthetics of the workplace are the physical surroundings of the employees' work space; they have physiological as well as psychological effects on employees. Aesthetic elements include the lighting of both the general work area and the personal workspace, the colors of the walls and furniture, auditory impacts, and atmospheric condition and temperature.

Light within the workspace should be considered in regard to brightness and diffusion for the work situation. Exposures to natural light may be easiest on the eyes, however strong direct light from any source may cause eye strain and fatigue. Desk or task lighting is more physically supportive than overhead florescent lighting alone. Many health information management (HIM) functions include computer monitors, and the degree of contrast on the screen can influence the employee's comfort level as well as the glare from light sources or computer screens. There several ways to address these issues including glare filters, placement of the computer screen, and window treatments (US Department of Labor n.d.(a)).

Color influences how people feel. For example, dark areas feel brighter or lighter when painted with light colors. Moreover, certain colors evoke a variety of sensations and feelings. Blues are cool, reds are warm, greens evoke luxury, neutral colors can have a calming effect, and so on (Cherry 2015). When choosing color schemes, it is important to consider the area, the function of the area, and who will occupy it.

Music and sound can be incorporated to improve working conditions and relieve both mental and visual fatigue. Certain kinds of music can reduce tension and make employees generally feel better. Sound conditioning and soundproofing are important considerations because a noisy office is seldom efficient. A certain level of routine office background noise is expected and usually is not irritating. However, loud or abrupt sounds can be alarming, distracting, and disruptive. Planning separate space for noisy work processes, such as copying and printing, is effective because it addresses the source of the noise. Carpeting, window coverings, and partitioning can offer noise control because they absorb significant amounts of sound.

Air conditioning and ventilation impact temperature, circulation, and moisture content. Air that is too warm or too cold is equally distracting, and a balance can be difficult to maintain. Dry air can cause eye irritation; and lack of circulation can cause stagnant, uncomfortable conditions (US Department of Labor n.d.(a)).

Ergonomics

The discipline of **ergonomics** is considered "fitting the job to the person" (US Department of Labor n.d.(b)) and has helped redefine the employee workspace with consideration for comfort and safety.

Questions to consider in workspace design include the following:

- Do staff members assume fixed working postures that remain static for the majority of the workday? For example, do they sit at a keyboard all day?
- Do staff members perform repetitive motions such as scanning, typing, stamping, hole punching, and so on?
- Has the psychological stress caused by uncomfortable workstations been taken into consideration?

In effective ergonomic planning, the designer must know the work requirements of the job and the tasks involved. The physical traits of the worker assigned to each workstation also influence ergonomic considerations. For example, height or leg length or back or waist length will determine specific needs. Another consideration is whether an individual or multiple persons share one workstation throughout the workweek. Finally, one must consider what equipment is currently available at the workstation and what equipment must be purchased to create an ergonomically correct work environment. Often, organizations employ ergonomic specialists to perform assessments on employees and their work environment. These specialists may be employees of the organization, possibly physical or occupational therapists; or they may be consultants to the organization brought in on an as-needed basis. HIM managers must collaborate with these professionals to ensure the employees' needs and work functions are understood allowing the ergonomic specialist to perform a proper evaluation and make appropriate recommendations.

When the work environment is not ergonomically sound, issues such as back and neck strain, carpal tunnel syndrome, tension headaches, and eyestrain can occur. Preventive, proactive ergonomic management includes educating staff on how to care for themselves to reduce potential ergonomic injuries or discomfort. Careful consideration and professional assessment of individual employees' work environment needs will help reduce or eliminate physical barriers to employee comfort and productivity. Preemptive, ergonomically correct practices markedly reduce employee absence and workers' compensation usage due to workplace injury.

Check Your Understanding 25.1

Instructions: **Answer the following questions on a separate piece of paper.**

1. Identify three reasons why space may need to be redesigned.
2. Explain how a movement diagram (or layout flowchart) assists a manager during an office design or redesign effort.
3. Name the fundamental elements addressed in good work environment planning.
4. Identify three symptoms that result if a workstation is not ergonomically sound.
5. Describe what types of impact aesthetic elements, such as lighting, the colors of the walls and furniture, noise, and temperature have on employees.

Methods of Organizing Work

Staffing involves the determination of which types of employees are needed, how many of each type are needed, and what kind of work schedule is needed. The types of employees needed depend on the skills, experience, and education required for the specific work that must be done. The number of employees needed depends on the volume of work and the pattern of work division that has been selected for the work setting. Work scheduling is based on when employees are needed to provide the services they are responsible to deliver within the organization.

Work Division Patterns

The method to dividing work among employees used in a process-oriented department depends in large part on the nature of the work to be performed and the number of employees available to perform it. Three basic types of work division patterns are serial, parallel, and unit work division.

Serial Work Division

The consecutive handling of tasks or products by individuals who perform a specific function in sequence is called serial work division. Often referred to as a production line, serial work division tends to create task specialists. For example, a receptionist receives a request for release of information (ROI); the request is scanned or entered into the ROI specialist work queue; an ROI specialist validates that the release is authorized, determines where the requested information can be found, identifies the records that are available electronically, and enters a request to the appropriate staff to retrieve the paper-based medical records that are not available online. The medical record is retrieved and delivered to the ROI specialist, who scans the pages into the electronic system for release; an evening clerk returns the medical record to the file room; and the ROI specialist completes the process by preparing the requested information for release to the requesting party. In this staffing model, each type of employee sequentially handles a step in the total ROI work process.

Parallel Work Division

The concurrent handling of tasks is called **parallel work division**. Multiple employees do identical types of tasks and basically see the process through from beginning to end. For instance, there are three ROI specialists in the department, and each is responsible for receiving requests for release, locating the medical record, identifying the content to be released, and preparing the content for distribution to the requestor. Thus, all three ROI specialists are expected to perform all of the tasks that comprise the release of information work process independent from the others.

Unit Work Division

Simultaneous assembly in which everyone performs a different specialized task at the same time is called **unit work division**. The tasks are all related to the same end product but are not dependent on each other. The work is specialized, but the sequence of tasks is not fixed. Unit assembly is rarely used in health information services (HIS) departments but is a typical work division pattern used in manufacturing. For example, one machinist makes metal chair legs, another molds metal chair seats, and another molds metal chair backs. One employee takes four metal chair legs, one metal chair seat, and one metal chair back and assembles them into a complete chair.

Work Distribution Analysis

Work distribution analysis is a process for evaluating the types of work functions being performed in a department, the amount of time given to those functions, who is performing each function, and the way work is distributed among the employees. It is used to document and describe the major functions of a work unit, determine whether a department's current work assignments and job content are appropriate, and identify process variation. Making time to perform this analysis can lead to one or more of the following observations:

- Large amounts of time are being dedicated to functions of minor importance
- Small amounts of time are being dedicated to functions of key importance
- There is too much or too little job function specialization
- There is duplication of efforts or functions
- Some employees are overloaded with work assignments
- Some employees do not have enough work to keep busy
- Staff are performing tasks inappropriate to their positions

Work distribution analysis can be helpful in determining whether adequate time is available and appropriate for each task and whether employees are overburdened or have time for additional responsibilities. In addition, it can help the manager assess whether the work is organized and distributed appropriately.

Basic work distribution data can be collected in a **work distribution chart** that is initially completed by each employee and includes all responsible task content as well as hours or parts of hours spent on tasks gathered over a designated period of time. Work distribution charts can be formulated in a variety of ways but frequently are tables, with work tasks forming the row headings and a double column of employee names and hours spent on tasks forming the column headings. (See table 25.1.) Actual data collection time varies depending on what is needed to get a representative sample of activities and times. When adequate data have been collected, the manager compiles them, clusters similar job tasks together, and completes the chart.

In table 25.1, four HIM department employees have identified how much time they have spent on each of the identified tasks in a 40-hour work week. Task content should come directly from the employee's current job description. In addition to

Table 25.1. Work distribution chart

Position/ employee	Supervisor/ J. Johnson		Admissions clerk/A. Jones		Discharge clerk/B. Olson		Scanning/indexing clerk/R. Smith	
Activity	Task	# of Hours	Task	# of Hours	Task	# of Hours	Task	# of Hours
Release of information	Post requests; give depositions	2 10	Photocopy/ scan	8	Certify content	15	Retrieve records	4
Analysis	Determine completion	2	Place in queue	3	Tag for incomplete	15	Collect records	5
Scanning / indexing	Audit scanned records	2	—	—	Check for scanned record for MDs	4	Prep records; scan/index records	30
Administrative overhead	Attend meetings; supervise employees	12 10	Receive visitors; typing	14 14	Generate MD letters	5	—	—
Training	Read literature	2	Attend software training	1	Attend computer training	1	Attend computer training	1
Totals	40 hours/40 hours		40 hours/40 hours		40 hours/40 hours		40 hours/40 hours	

task content, each employee tracks each task's start time, end time, and volume or productivity within a typical workweek. In the example in table 25.1, the work distribution chart shows that the supervisor spends just over half of the time doing administrative work (often in meetings), yet there is a rather large amount of time given to release of information, giving depositions in particular. The admissions clerk spends the majority of time receiving visitors and typing. The discharge clerk spends the same amount of time on release of information as analysis. The scanning/indexing clerk spends the majority of work time on prepping, scanning, and indexing records. Analysis of this chart may indicate that an unusual amount of time is spent by the supervisor in the release of information function and that there is little time left for supervising duties; or possibly the discharge clerk is distracted by a large amount of ROI activity. This information can be used to investigate these questions further to determine if a change should be made.

The results of a work distribution analysis can lead a department to redefine the job descriptions of some employees, redesign the office space, or establish new or revised procedures for some department functions in order to gain improvements in staff productivity or service quality.

Work Scheduling

After management has determined the appropriate work distribution within a department and makes adjustments accordingly, a work-scheduling system can be developed. Determining the work schedule for departmental staff involves more than simply assigning the correct number of work hours to each employee. Effective scheduling results in the following:

- A core of employees on duty at all times when services must be provided
- Enough employee hours scheduled to meet the required volume of work to be done per established performance standards
- A pattern of hours (shifts) to be worked and days off that employees can be reasonably sure will not change except in extreme emergencies
- Fair and just treatment of all employees with regard to hours assigned
- A committed workforce with high morale and a strong rate of retention

Several staffing issues should be considered when devising an effective staff schedule. Answers to the following questions will help determine the department's or work unit's course of action:

- How is the workweek defined by policy? The workweek is generally established to begin on Sunday, but organizational policy may dictate otherwise.

- What days of the week is the department open? How many and what hours and days are covered?

- What functions must be performed each day and within what time frame?

- How many full-time equivalents (FTEs) are needed to handle the work volume?

HIM departments often are on a standard Monday through Friday, eight-hour-day pattern but depending on the services the department provides may need evening or weekend coverage to handle specific functions that must be provided 24 hours per day, seven days a week. The transcription function is one function where 24-hour coverage may be necessary. Understanding the type and volume of work that needs to be done during specific time frames along with knowing the number and type of staff available is critical to effective scheduling.

Shift Rotation and Shift Differential

Employee schedules may involve **shift rotation** and shift differential depending on departmental needs. Rotation among morning, afternoon, and evening shifts is not the ideal scheduling situation but is often necessary when coverage is needed and personnel have not been specifically hired to work afternoons or evenings on a regular basis. Specific start and end times should be determined for every shift, and a reasonable amount of time should elapse between the time an individual ends one shift and begins another. An employer should allow adequate time off between shifts to avoid employee fatigue, however there is not state or federal law that requires a minimum amount of time off between shifts (Stone 2015). Time spent on the more undesirable shifts should not exceed time spent on the preferred shift. It may be prudent to adopt **cyclical**

staffing, which is the rotation of work schedule for a group of employees to allow for a fair distribution of day, evening, and weekend shifts for each person within the group. **Float employees**, staff that are cross-trained in a number of departmental functions, can often be utilized to enable this particular type of scheduling.

In situations where weekend coverage is an issue, employees should have at least alternate weekends off. Many employers pay a slightly higher hourly wage to employees who work less desirable shifts (evening, night, weekend). This is referred to as a **shift differential**. Under the Fair Labor Standards Act, an employer is not required to pay a shift differential (Society for Human Resource Management 2014) but it may be beneficial for employee morale and retention.

Mandatory work functions and the minimal staff needed to cover them should be defined by the manager when determining weekend or holiday coverage. All employees should participate in holiday and weekend rotation. Employees should be required to provide their own holiday or weekend replacements but should not be responsible for providing replacements when their absence is due to illness.

Vacation and Absentee Coverage

To keep productivity optimal, the HIM manager must plan appropriately for vacation staffing and absentee coverage. Temporary staff hired to cover for vacationing employees may be desirable, but not always financially feasible. Moreover, some positions are too complex to be filled with temporary employees. For example, it is unlikely that a temporary assistant director could be hired to fill in for an assistant director on a two-week vacation due to the complexity of that job role. In such a case, key tasks that must be performed should be identified and distributed appropriately among staff who will handle them while the employee is on vacation. Generally staff who are absent for more than a week can add undue stress on the remaining employees and adversely affect department service levels; thus, it is advisable to hire temporary help when more than one week of absence is expected.

Alternate Work Schedules

Today's work environment has accepted some work scheduling alternatives to the regular 40-hour workweek; the following are examples:

- **Compressed workweek**: A week in which more hours are combined within fewer days (for example, four 10-hour days, three 12-hour days, seven 10-hour days with seven days off [seven on/seven off], and so on). This type of scheduling has advantages but may present child care issues and psychological or physical fatigue that could reduce efficiency and productivity.

- **Flextime**: Employees choose their arrival and departure times around a fixed core work time. For example, if management feels full coverage is essential between 10 a.m. and 2 p.m., employees could start as early as 5:30 a.m. or end as late as 6:30 p.m. and still provide the department with core coverage.

- **Job sharing**: Divides one job between two part-time employees, each with partial benefits (as they apply). In some organizations, the two employees split full-time benefits (for example, one takes insurance coverage and one takes vacation time). Job sharing may work well in some cases, but it also can be problematic depending on the compatibility of the two individuals involved. And should one person terminate employment, finding a compatible new job-sharing partner could present a challenge.

In general, the benefits to employers of alternative work schedules include easier staff recruitment and better retention, increased morale, decreased absence and tardiness, and some productivity improvements. For employees, the benefits can include less home stress, reduced commuting time, and a perception of greater autonomy in the workplace. (See chapter 23 for further discussion on staffing and scheduling.)

Telecommuting

With a **telecommuting** option, employees work full- or part-time in their own homes. The first employees in HIM departments to take advantage of telecommuting were transcriptionists; they were soon followed by coders. The EHR has enabled even more employees to work remotely including employees performing discharge analysis, abstracting, and auditing. These telecommuters use computers (often provided by the facility) at home to transcribe or code information and then transmit it electronically back to the facility. The advantages to this type of work scheduling are that it saves space in the department, reduces long commutes to the workplace, retains parents who prefer to be home, and offers work opportunities to the physically challenged. On the other hand, employers may feel a loss of control when employees telecommute. And some employees in alternative work situations, such as telecommuters, need contact with other employees to avoid feeling disconnected from the department. (See chapter 23 for further discussion on telecommuting.)

Outsourcing

In some cases, flexible job arrangements may not be an option or solve a staffing issue. A potential solution to the problem of a shortage of qualified staff is **outsourcing**. In this arrangement, the organization contracts with an independent company with expertise in a specific job function. The outside company then assumes full responsibility for performing the function rather than just supplying staff. Outsourcing (domestic and offshore) provides access to staff as needed, even in a tight labor market; frees up internal resources for other things; eliminates some process or service headaches; provides access to the newest technologies quickly; and accelerates change. The disadvantages for the health information manager include less immediate control over the quantity and quality of the work, the need to know negotiation techniques and contract language, and reliance on the vendor. The Health Insurance Portability and Accountability Act (HIPAA) also requires special arrangements regarding security and confidentiality for outsourcing contractors (covered entities) (HHS 2003). In an outsourced environment, the health information manager's responsibility shifts from supervising employees to managing a vendor relationship.

Common functions that are candidates for outsourcing in the HIM department include transcription, release of information, document imaging, and coding. The outsourcing company may perform the functions either at the institution or partially or completely off-site. Advances in secure communication have resulted in many remote workers being employed by such independent companies.

When healthcare organizations decide to use outsourcing, a manager is challenged to select the most appropriate vendor to provide the services desired. Specific key factors to consider when selecting a vendor or partner include:

- Commitment to quality
- Technology
- Training
- Fees
- References and reputation
- Experience
- Cultural match
- Flexible contract terms
- Personnel policies (Bellenghi 2010)

Senior executive support is a requisite for achieving success when adopting an outsourcing vendor or contracted service. The administration's confidence in the process is essential to creating the seamlessness necessary for continued, smooth, functional operation. Administrative support can best be engaged when the manager understands the organization's goals for each outsourcing or contracted service effort being planned. Selecting the right vendor is a definite variable for successful outsourcing.

Suggestions for successful outsourcing arrangements include:

- Seeking assistance from someone skilled in negotiation when developing the contract with the vendor
- Engaging legal counsel to review the language of the contract to ensure that it complies with HIPAA and other regulatory requirements
- Requiring competitive bidding for each outsourced service at regular intervals

- Establishing quality expectations and performance standards for contractors
- Monitoring compliance with performance standards
- Performing periodic customer surveys to assess satisfaction with the service

Effective management of the relationship between the healthcare organization and the outsourcing partner includes properly constructed contracts, open communication among partners, and careful attention to personnel issues. Careful review and evaluation of the functions and performance of the outsourced staff in regard to contract requirements is critical to a successful outsourcing arrangement.

Offshoring

Offshoring is a special type of outsourcing, where employees of the company are based overseas. The major benefits are cost savings and availability of a labor pool. Employees in foreign countries are generally paid much less than those in the United States and are extremely productive. There may also be less turnover. HIM jobs such as transcription, coding, and insurance claims processing are well suited to these types of workers. Jobs most suitable for offshoring have the following characteristics:

- No face-to-face customer service requirements
- High information content
- High wage differential with workers in the destination country
- Low social networking requirement
- Little interaction with others in the organization (Bardhan and Kroll 2003)

Those countries with young populations that speak English are preferred. The country also should have reliable utilities and suitable digital and voice networks.

As in any outsourcing arrangement, quality control and compliance with privacy and security standards are important issues to be addressed in contracts and performance monitoring.

Contracting for Services

When a manager is planning to contract for staffing in a transitional situation in order to meet organizational goals, various types of arrangements can be considered, including:

- *Full service:* Contracting for staff to handle a complete function within the department; for example, release of information function
- *Project based:* Contracting for staff to focus on completion of a specific project; for example, a master patient index (MPI) clean up in which duplicate records are resolved.
- *Temporary:* Contracting for staff to cover for a temporary situation in order to keep productivity in line; for example, a coding backlog due to staff vacancy, vacations, or a learning curve on a new system or technology

Clear definitions of the work or services needed as well as the performance expectations are crucial to a successful contract for services. **Service level agreements (SLAs)** provide this detail in writing, plus price and payment terms, the reporting chain of command, terms for termination of the relationship, and privacy, security, and confidentiality expectations of the vendor and vendor staff.

Work Procedures

Management has the responsibility to develop procedures for employees that fully aid them in effectively and efficiently carrying out their job functions. A **job procedure** is a structured, action-oriented list of sequential steps involved in carrying out a specific job or solving a problem.

Rules of Procedure Writing

To be effective, procedure writing requires considerable attention to detail. The following criteria facilitate the development of well-written procedures:

- Display the title of the procedure accurately and clearly.
- Number each step of the procedure for easy reference.
- Begin each activity with an action verb.

- Keep sentences short and concise.
- Include only procedures, not policies. Policy manuals should be maintained as separate documents, though it is appropriate to include references to related policies within the procedure so the employee can easily locate the policy within the policy manual as may be necessary or desired.
- Identify logical beginning and end points to simplify directions.
- Consider the audience and construct the procedure to be of most help to that audience. For example, new staff, temporary staff, or cross-trained staff who performs these procedures only occasionally needs a basic, simplified version to ensure completion of a new or seldom-performed task.

In addition, the written procedure should provide completed samples of forms used during the procedure.

It is effective to have an experienced employee who does the job write (or at least draft) the procedure because he or she knows it best. Supervisory personnel should collect all the written procedures and determine whether they are complete and follow a consistent format. Supervisory personnel are also responsible for ensuring that procedures are reviewed at least annually and updated in a timely way when the procedure is modified.

Procedure Formats

When determining the appropriate format for a procedure, the HIM manager needs to consider the audience as well as the complexity of the task. The following are formats that can be followed for procedural documentation.

- **Narrative**: Narrative formats are the most common for procedure writing. The author details the processes of the procedure in a step-by-step descriptive method.
- **Playscript**: This format describes each player in the procedure, the action of the player, and the player's responsibility regarding the process from the start to completion of a specific task within the procedure.

- **Flowcharts**: Flowcharts are a visual illustration of the procedure using standard flowcharting symbols. These symbols are provided in various software programs to depict the steps associated with a procedure.

Sometimes a combination of formats is used. However, whatever format is chosen, all procedures should be available to employees at any time.

Procedure Manuals

A **procedure manual** is a compilation of all of the procedures used in a specific unit, department, or organization. Procedure manuals may be kept as hard copies that have been printed and bound together in a book or binder, or they may be maintained on an organization's secure website or intranet. The valuable aspects associated with procedure manuals include:

- Promoting teamwork
- Promoting consistency in the work of employees
- Reducing training time
- Establishing guidance on the standards of the work unit
- Explaining what is expected of employees
- Answering employee questions

The manual's content and format are relatively straightforward. Procedure manuals should include the following elements:

- *Title page:* Name of the facility, name of the manual, name of the department, and date
- *Foreword:* Paragraph form, purpose of manual, suggestion for use by employees
- *Table of contents:* List of all procedures in the manual referenced to page number
- *Job procedures:* Step-by-step job procedures and the forms used in each procedure, including completed forms together with explanations to ensure accurate use of forms
- *General rules and regulations:* Information that includes department- or unit-specific details often influenced by state or federal law and regulatory agencies
- *Index:* Alphabetical list of topics covered in the manual (optional)

Procedure manuals are particularly important for work units that have a variety of duties or have a variety of staff who may not do the same tasks routinely. An updated, organized procedure manual that is readily available and in a standardized format can save employees time and ensure accurate results.

Check Your Understanding 25.2

Instructions: **Answer the following questions on a separate piece of paper.**

1. Explain what information is included in a service level agreement (SLA) and why it is needed.

2. Describe three procedure formats.

3. List the potential problem areas a work distribution analysis can reveal.

4. Differentiate flextime, job sharing, and the compressed workweek as three unique alternatives to the regular 40-hour staffing schedule.

5. Differentiate serial, parallel, and unit work division.

6. Explain the four areas addressed by work distribution analysis.

Performance and Work Measurement Standards

Work is the task to be performed; **performance** is the execution of the task. Effective management involves discerning what work is to be done, what performance standards are achievable and appropriate, how performance can be measured in terms of efficiency and effectiveness, and how performance can be monitored for variances from the standards that are set. Most employees simply want to know for which tasks they are responsible, what is expected of them, and how they are performing relative to that expectation. Through performance standard-setting and measurement processes, managers can confirm the level of success of a work unit or identify opportunities for improvement.

A **standard** may be defined as a performance criterion established by custom or authority for the purpose of assessing factors such as quality, productivity, and performance. Managers are responsible for controlling all of the resources available to them, including manpower (staff), materials (supplies), machines (equipment), methods (procedures), and money (budget)—often referred to as the five Ms. Thus, managers are expected to set standards for each of these resources and then use them as ways to assess the quality, productivity, and performance of those resources. Performance standards should be aligned with the mission and goals of the organization.

Criteria for Setting Effective Standards

To create viable, significant standards, it is important to be aware of the criteria commonly considered as the foundation for developing effective standard setting. Effective standards are:

- *Understandable:* The person(s) affected by the standard knows what it means, and it makes sense to him or her.
- *Attainable:* It is reasonable to expect that the person(s) affected by the standard can actually achieve it.
- *Equitable:* If more than one person is affected by the standard, all are held accountable for it.

- *Significant:* Meeting the standard is important to the goals of the work unit or organization; the effort it takes to meet the standard is worth it.
- *Legitimate:* The standard has been formally accepted within the organization and is documented in appropriate places and ways.
- *Economical:* The standard can be met and monitored without incurring costs that are beyond the value of that which is gained by having it. In other words, achieving the standard must be worth the expense associated with achieving it.

Types of Standards

Standards are worded differently at various levels within the organization depending on whether they reflect a goal or an objective. A **goal** is a generalized statement of a unit, departmental, or organizational standard. An **objective** is a statement of the end result in measurable terms with time and cost limits, as applicable. The development of specific objectives can bring goals to a practical, working level (Liebler and McConnell 2012). For example, the HIM department might have a general standard (often called a goal) for its transcription function to support patient care through accurate and timely transcription of medical reports. The transcription function then might state a standard in objective form to make it more specific and measurable; for example, to transcribe routine history and physical, operative, and consultation dictation within eight hours of dictation. Note that this objective is related directly to the timeliness aspect of the preceding goal statement.

Qualitative and Quantitative Standards

Objective-level standards are also commonly characterized in two other ways—as quantitative standards and qualitative standards.

Qualitative standards specify the level of service expected from a function, such as:

- *Accuracy rate:* For example, assignment of diagnostic and procedure codes for inpatient records is at least 98 percent accurate.
- *Error rate:* For example, mistakes in the assignment of diagnostic and procedure codes occur in no more than 2 percent of inpatient records coded.
- *Turnaround time:* For example, dictation must be transcribed within 24 hours.
- *Response time:* For example, requests for information are responded to within seven working days of receipt.

Quantitative standards specify the level of measurable work, or **productivity**, expected for a specific function, such as:

- *Number of units of work per specified period of time*: For example, 70 records per full-time employee per day
- *Amount of time allotted per unit of work*: For example, no more than 15 minutes to code one inpatient record

Quantity standards (also called productivity standards) and quality standards (also known as service standards) are generally used by managers to monitor individual employee performance and the performance of a functional unit or the department as a whole. They are also used for planning, staffing, and budgeting purposes. To properly communicate performance standards, managers need to make the distinction between quantitative and qualitative standards and identify examples of each for the HIM functions.

Keeping the criteria for effective standards and the difference between qualitative and quantitative standards in mind, it is possible to develop standards for any of the resources under the control of management. Several examples of resource management standards are provided here.

- Standards related to manpower (staff resources)
  - Qualitative (service): Chart deficiency analyst accurately identifies chart completion status in 98 percent of charts analyzed
  - Quantitative (productivity): Coders code 25 to 30 inpatient discharges per eight-hour workday
- Standards related to materials (supply resources)
  - Qualitative (service): Monitoring strips must be printed with nonfading permanent ink
  - Quantitative (productivity): Each functional work unit in the department maintains no more than one week's volume of consumable supplies on hand
- Standards related to money (budget resources)
  - Qualitative (service): Major expense categories (salaries, supplies, postage, telephone, travel, and maintenance) must remain within plus or minus 3 percent of the budgeted amount monthly
  - Quantitative (productivity): Paid dollars per key statistic (P$PKS) must be less than $2 plus or minus the target P$PKS indicator established for the department
- Standards related to methods (procedures)
  - Qualitative (service): An employee can complete the entry of a release of information (ROI) request into the ROI tracking system with 99 percent accuracy by following the steps outlined in the documented procedure
  - Quantitative (productivity): The steps outlined for completing the entry of a release of information (ROI) request into the ROI tracking system can be completed in less than one minute per request
- Standards related to machines (equipment)
  - Qualitative (service): The copier must be functioning properly 99 percent of the time, that is, less than two hours of downtime per month.
  - Quantitative (productivity): The document imaging equipment must be able to process 30 to 40 images per minute.

Key Indicators

Key indicators are current measurement thresholds that alert a department or work unit to its existing level of service. Common key indicator examples include:

- Transcription turnaround time
- Days outstanding in accounts receivable (A/R)
- Release of information turnaround time
- Percentage of incomplete records

The following red flag indicators would move a department manager to take corrective action:

- The number and severity of complaints increase. When the number or severity of complaints increases, the circumstances surrounding the complaints need to be assessed immediately so that corrections to the process or personnel involved can be made.
- Compliance surveys to assess performance on accreditation, legal, or regulatory standards indicate that the organization has failed to comply in one or more areas. When this occurs, the organization needs to correct the variance(s) as soon as possible and return to compliance.

Key indicators allow managers to monitor critical service standards on a current and ongoing basis so they can make timely staffing or process adjustments to ensure that department service performance remains as expected.

Methods of Communicating Standards

After standards have been created, they must be communicated to staff. All of the given types of standards can be provided to staff in a number of ways:

- Written specifications: In job descriptions, performance evaluation forms, equipment specification sheets, and forms design guidelines
- Documented rules, regulations, or policies: In policy manuals, regulations or accreditation manuals, and employee handbooks
- Demonstration models: Samples, videos, and computer-based learning modules
- Verbal confirmations: In departmental or work unit meetings or individual employee counseling sessions

Whatever the method of communication deemed most appropriate, it is critical that employees are aware of departmental standards so they can be successful in meeting them.

Methods of Developing Standards

There are several methods that can be employed to develop performance standards in a work unit. Two approaches are commonly used: benchmarking comparable performance and measuring actual performance.

Benchmarking Comparable Performance

Benchmarking is based on researching the performance of similar organizations and programs (Liebler and McConnell 2012) or gathering data on standards established by national or local sources such as professional associations and standard-setting organizations. Benchmarking is a common approach to standard setting in HIM management in the past few years because this type of information is published regularly.

To engage in a benchmarking effort, the manager should first select key functions of the department that will be benchmarked (coding service, transcription service, ROI service). Relating benchmarks to the specific process is critical. Thought must be given to the types of performance measure(s) desired as indicators (for coding, payments remaining in accounts receivable due to uncoded records and payments remaining in accounts receivable due to coding disputes; for transcription, turnaround time [dictation to charting] for consultations, operative reports, history, and physicals).

When the key functional areas have been selected and the types of indicators identified, the research for benchmarks available through published sources (preferably) can begin. Investigation of benchmark standards gathered through this research must also involve a critical assessment of their relevance to the department's specific situation; then the standard can be successfully sold to the rest of the organization. Benchmarking involves the following steps:

1. Identifying peer organizations and departments that have achieved outstanding performance based on some key indicator (for example, 98 percent of health records coded within two days post discharge)

2. Studying the best practices within the organization that make it possible to achieve that performance level

3. Acting to implement those best practices in one's own organization to achieve a similar performance

Before officially adopting a benchmark standard, a manager should routinely gather performance data in the department to compare actual performance against the benchmark and then evaluate factors in department processes that must be changed to eventually move actual performance into the benchmark range.

Measuring Actual Performance

Work measurement is the process of studying the amount of work accomplished and the amount of time it takes to accomplish it. It involves the collection of data relevant to the work, such as the amount of work accomplished per unit of time. Its purpose is to define and monitor productivity.

Work measurement can support a manager in many activities, including:

- Setting production standards
- Determining staffing requirements
- Establishing incentive pay systems
- Determining direct costs by function
- Comparing performance to standards
- Identifying activities for process and methods improvement

Gathering the information available through work measurement efforts will be invaluable to the manager in making administrative decisions. But how do managers know which method of work measurement is best?

When selecting the work measurement technique that best suits the department or work unit, the manager should consider the following factors:

- Amount of financial resources available
- Availability of qualified personnel to take part in the study
- Amount of time available to devote to study
- Attitudes of employees toward participation in a study

Work measurement can be accomplished through a variety of techniques. The analysis of historical or past performance data generally uses work volume (direct or estimated) and hours paid from past records to establish the standard. When using historical data, managers are cautioned to keep in mind that volume figures are not adjusted for the level of quality and the number of hours paid is different from the number of hours actually worked.

Employee self-logging is a form of self-reporting in which the employees simply track their tasks, volume of work units, and hours worked. Employee logging incorporates a **time ladder**, which is a document used by the employee to record the amount of time worked on various tasks. It can be modified to include the number of units produced per task throughout the day. **Volume logs** are sometimes used in conjunction with a time ladder to obtain information about the volume of work units received and processed in a day by simply keeping track of the number of products produced or activities done. (See table 25.2.)

The scientific methods of work measurement include time studies and the use of pre-established time/unit standards. For example, time studies

Table 25.2.   Sample volume log

Task	Number of worked hours	Number of units
Coding	40	120 records
Loose filing	36	48 inches

The coding standard calculates at three records per worked hour for this employee (120 records/40 hours) and a filing standard of 1.3 inches per worked hour (48 inches/36 hours). It does not capture any interruptions or unworked time in the eight-hour day but is a simple way to arrive at a ballpark figure.

use a stopwatch to record and document the time required to accomplish a specified task.

Work sampling is a technique of work measurement that involves using statistical probability (determined through random sample observations) to characterize the performance of the department and its functional work units.

Each one of the varieties of work measurement techniques offers calculations of employee productivity in either unit/time or time/unit.

Check Your Understanding 25.3

Instructions: **On a separate piece of paper, indicate whether the following statements are true or false. Then correct any false statement to make it true or explain why it is false.**

1. A standard is a criterion established by custom or authority for the purpose of assessing quality, productivity, or performance.

2. Work sampling is a work measurement methodology that relies on statistical probability to characterize the performance of the functional work units in a department.

3. Turnaround times are examples of qualitative standards, and error rates are examples of quantitative standards.

4. Benchmarking does not include the use of published information.

5. Manpower (staff), money (budget), materials (supplies), machines (equipment), and methods (procedures) are the basic resources under the control of a manager.

Performance Measurement

Performance measurement is the process of comparing the outcomes of an organization, work unit, or employee to pre-established performance standards. The results of the performance measurement process generally are expressed as percentages, rates, ratios, averages, and other quantitative assessments. Performance measurement is used to assess quality and productivity in clinical services and in administrative services. Examples of performance measures maintained by acute-care hospitals in clinical services include the rate of nosocomial infection, the percentage of surgical complications, the average length of stay, and the ratio of live births to stillbirths. Examples of performance measures maintained by an administrative service such as the HIM department include transcription lines transcribed and turnaround times per report type, turnaround times for ROI requests, and days in A/R due to uncoded patient discharges.

Performance measurement is a fundamental management activity that supports two of the basic functions of management—controlling and planning. The controlling function is concerned with ensuring that the work unit or organization is doing what it should be doing in the right way. The planning function is concerned with defining the expectations of performance (standards or objectives), the processes required for achieving those expectations (procedures), and the desired outcomes of performance (goals). The goals, objectives, standards, and processes established during the planning process become the criteria used in the control process to evaluate actual performance.

Performance Controls

In the control process, specific monitors, or controls, are established for the purpose of identifying undesirable circumstances occurring in a work process that could lead to an undesirable outcome;

the intent is for appropriate intervention to be introduced into the process.

The characteristics of effective performance controls include the following:

- Flexibility refers to the fact that controls must be adaptable to real changes in the requirements of a process. For example, a budget is a control on the use of money. Money budgeted in one category (equipment) may need to be spent in another category (travel) because of a change in a program or a new law or regulation.

- Simplicity refers to the fact that those involved in the process must find the controls understandable and reasonable.

- Economy implies that controls should not cost more than they are worth. The time and money spent to implement a control should be in line with the level of risk (loss) involved if the process fails to meet performance expectations. For example, potential loss of a life calls for a significant investment in controls; potential criminal liability calls for significant investment in controls; while the potential for having to pay for a day of overtime to correct clerical errors calls for a minimal investment in controls.

- Timeliness suggests that controls should be implemented to detect potential variances within a time frame that allows for corrective action before any adverse effect has occurred. For example, the accuracy of a medical record number assignment should be confirmed at the time of registration or the coding checked before a bill is transmitted in order to avoid the adverse effects associated with errors that are then transmitted to other areas of the organization or outside the organization (for example, the insurance carrier).

- Focus on exceptions demands that controls be targeted at those aspects of a process that are most likely to vary significantly from expectations. For example, a new

transcriptionist who is likely to make more errors that could do damage to customer service ratings is generally monitored (controlled) more closely and more frequently than one who is experienced and has performed well for the past year.

There are two general types of controls—preventive (self-correcting) and feedback (non-self-correcting). **Preventive controls** are front-end processes that guide work in such a way that input and process variations are minimized. Simple things such as standard operating procedures, edits on data entered into computer-based systems, and training processes are ways to reduce the potential for error by using preventive controls.

Feedback controls are back-end processes that monitor and measure output and then compare it to expectations and identify variations that then must be analyzed so corrective action plans can be developed and implemented. Processes with feedback controls in place are also called cybernetic processes or systems. Some may be self-regulating (such as thermostatic systems), but most are non–self-regulating, meaning that they require intervention by an oversight agent (a supervisor, manager, or auditor) to identify the variance and take action to correct it. A customer survey or routine performance reviews are examples of this type of control.

Variance Analysis

In the context of performance measurement, when variations are identified (that is, actual performance does not meet or significantly exceeds expectations), further analysis is needed. Analysis of the resources involved in the work (people, procedures, supplies, equipment, and money) is conducted to help determine what, if any, changes should be made. Changes may involve activities such as additional staff training, modifications in procedures, adjustments in workflow, revision of policies, or purchases of updated equipment. As a result, the analysis and the changes to address findings may also lead to revisions in performance criteria and expectations.

Assessment of Departmental Performance

When establishing an employee performance assessment program, the steps in the control (evaluation) process include:

1. Monitoring and measuring outcomes performance
2. Comparing performance to established goals and standards
3. Evaluating variance and developing action plans
4. Taking appropriate action
5. Assessing whether the actions have corrected the variance (Dunn 2010).

It is not enough to just measure and compare the measurements to goals and standards; it is also important to evaluate any variances, develop and implement action plans, and measure again to see if positive changes have been made.

Monitoring and Measuring Performance

Monitoring and measuring performance involves taking an aggregate look at performance over a period of time. Options include operating with an employee self-reporting method such as self-logging, using computerized monitoring to audit productivity, manually auditing work samples, or relying on customer feedback to measure performance.

Effective outcomes performance monitoring depends on both employee performance measurement and management execution. The focus of the effort is on service indicators such as turnaround time, cost and revenue reports, and customer feedback. Consider this practical application of department outcomes performance monitoring. Assume that one established expectation of the department is that routine response to an authorized ROI request occurs within five working days of receipt of the request in the department.

The first step in controlling this function would be to set up a data collection and reporting activity to obtain information that can be used to monitor the time it takes the department to respond to a routine ROI. (See table 25.3.)

Next, the department should determine the kinds of controls it wants to establish. The department wants to monitor routine requests, but how are rou-

Table 25.3. ROI variance report

On June 6, 2016, total routine ROI requests in processing: 130					
Days since receipt	**6–10 days**	**11–15 days**	**16–20 days**	**>20 days**	**Summary**
Number of total requests	12 9%	15 12%	2 2%	1 1%	30 24%
Reasons					
Unable to locate record	0	2	0	1	3 10%
Incomplete record	12	12	2	0	26 87%
Issue with authorization	0	0	0	0	0
Unavailable record	0	1	0	0	1 3%
Other	0	0	0	0	0

tine requests defined? A routine request may be any request that is not urgent (that is, it does not have to be handled within minutes, hours, or some stipulated amount of time under five working days). For example, a subpoena for a record that must be handled within three days or a request for a record needed for an appointment in a clinic the next morning would not be considered a routine request.

The line related to ROI turnaround time (TAT) in the middle of the performance report shown in table 25.4 indicates the average number of days it took the HIM department to respond to routine ROI requests in January (3), February (3), March (6), and April (5).

The average turnaround time is calculated by dividing the total response days attributed to the volume of routine requests that were responded to within the reporting period by the volume of routine requests responded to. For example, if the department responded to 300 routine requests in the month of May and 100 were responded to in six days, 100 in two days, and 100 in four days, the average turnaround time in May would be four days:

$$\frac{(600\,\text{days} + 200\,\text{days} + 400\,\text{days})}{300\,\text{requests}}$$
$$= 4\,\text{days (average)}$$

Having the information on a monthly basis to include as part of the regular performance reporting

Table 25.4. Sample health information services performance report

Indicator	January 2016	February 2016	March 2016	April 2016
Discharge equivalents	5,000	5,400	5,360	5,500
Labor cost per discharge equivalent (DCE): <$10.00	$10.00	9.25	9.33	9.90
FTE budgeted at 50	50	50	50	48
Days in analysis at end of month: <2 days	1	2	2	3
Delinquency rate: <50%	35%	40%	43%	45%
Coding: Days in A/R due to uncoded records <5 days	3	5	4	5
Lines transcribed	120,000	130,000	128,000	132,000
Transcription: TAT for History & Physicals (H&Ps) <24 hours	12	16	18	26
ROI requests received	200	245	300	260
Release of info: TAT <5 days	3	3	6	5
File pull requests	2,000	2,200	2,300	2,500
Retrieval rate: >95%	94%	96%	93%	91%
Resignations: <1%	0	0	0	2/50 = 4%
Education hours	4	16	2	8
Unproductive hours (sick, vacation): <15%	10%	12%	20%	10%

within the department allows the manager to review monthly trends and identify potential focus areas for future process improvement activities.

The underlying data indicate that a considerable number of requests are not responded to within the five-working-days standard set by management (for example, 100 [or 33 percent] were responded to in six working days). In this case, the direct supervisor of the ROI function would likely want access to data of this nature more often than once a month. For example, a weekly report showing the number of routine requests in the system for five days or more that have not yet been answered would allow the supervisor or ROI clerk to identify problem requests and take corrective actions over the course of the following week.

Comparing Performance to Established Goals and Standards

The next step in monitoring and measuring outcome performance is to compare current performance against established goals (standards). Continuing with the example in the preceding section, when comparing performance against the standard performance indicator of responding to routine ROIs within five

days, the data in table 25.4 show an upward trend in March and April.

When comparisons are done, the manager should evaluate any variances and develop an action plan specific to each. Action plans can be additional staff training, modifications in procedures, adjustments in workflow, revision of policies, purchase of updated equipment and others. For example, in an evaluation of the performance variance in responding to routine ROI requests, the direct supervisor would likely begin to collect data that will provide the following types of information in order to uncover the factors that have triggered the variances (see table 25.3):

- How many open ROI requests exist with a date of receipt of more than five working days?

- What is the aging profile of those open ROI requests; that is, how many are 6 to 10 working days, 10 to 15 working days, 16 to 20 working days, or more than 20 days?

- What are the reasons the requests are still open?

- In what time increments since receipt of the requests has the requesting party been notified of the delay and the reason for the delay?

After the variances have been evaluated, an action plan can be formulated to address areas for performance improvement.

- Establish a procedure to ensure weekly contact with the requestor to determine continuing need for the information and to update the status of the request
- Flag the incomplete record with ROI REQUEST PENDING to ensure that it is routed to ROI immediately when required documentation is complete
- Hold a staff in-service to ensure all employees understand the policies and procedures impacting the turnaround time requirements

The supervisor, working with the ROI staff, will take the actions put forth in the plan and then continue to monitor the ROI function to determine if the actions taken are effective in resolving the identified performance variance.

Check Your Understanding 25.4

Instructions: **Answer the following questions on a separate piece of paper.**

1. Differentiate between preventive controls and feedback controls.
2. Identify the five characteristics of effective performance controls.
3. Define performance measurement and explain why it is a major responsibility of management.
4. Explain the purpose of monitors (or controls) placed on the functions performed in a work unit.
5. Provide examples of the types of changes or actions a manager might take to address performance issues revealed when he or she completes an analysis of performance variances in the department.

Performance Improvement

The reason managers set performance standards and routinely measure departmental performance against those standards is to ensure the department is serving its internal and external customers in ways that meet their needs and expectations. A natural outcome of any performance measurement system is the identification of variances from performance expectations and thus the opportunity to engage in performance improvement (PI) activities to bring performance back into line. As an example, the Joint Commission publishes standards that specifically require accredited organizations to have PI efforts as an integral aspect of their day-to-day operations.

The Role of Customer Service

All process improvement environments today focus on the customer and work to create a true customer orientation within the work environment by listening and responding to customers, thinking about their needs, and using that information to modify and improve the way our systems work for them.

In the process of customer orientation, management and staff should:

- Identify the key processes in the department or organization
- Identify the customers of those processes
- Define quality and expectations from a customer perspective
- Develop and collect quality measures to meet expectations for the identified key processes
- Evaluate and continuously monitor performance measures to ensure expectations are being met

Customers are the people, external and internal, who receive and are affected by the work of the organization or department. They have names and needs and are the reason(s) for the collective work of the organization.

Internal customers are located within the organization. They may be anyone within the work unit who is affected by the HIM functions. Physicians and clinical staff need high-quality, expedient patient health information in order to deliver high-quality patient care. Administrative staff members are customers of the information harvested from collective databases for use in planning facilities and services. And not least among the department's internal customers are the HIM department staff who work in each of the functional areas and rely on each other in various ways to get their work done.

External customers reside outside the organization. Patients seen by providers are considered external customers, as are payers who need information so they can reimburse their enrollees in a timely manner. Regulatory agencies look to HIM for data on conditions of accreditation or participation. Vendors assist HIM, with the department's direct input, in making optimal selections of products. Public health agencies look to HIM for information and data on the health status of the community population in order to earmark services the population needs to maintain a healthy existence.

Identification of Performance Improvement Opportunities

In a department that employs performance standards and engages in routine performance measurement, opportunities for performance improvement present themselves as a natural outcome of that effort. Even when a department is lacking a formal performance measurement program, the following can be seen as symptoms of performance problems. When they are observed, they present obvious opportunities for performance improvement efforts as well:

- Inaccuracies and errors in work
- Complaints from customers

- Delays in getting things done or lots of interruptions
- Low employee morale or high rates of absenteeism or turnover
- Poor safety records and on-the-job injuries

When inaccuracies and errors are evident in the work products of a group of employees, an investigation of the underlying cause(s) is required and appropriate actions must be taken to address them so the inaccuracies and errors are eliminated.

Customer complaints indicate that performance is not meeting expectations. Managers need to consider each complaint and determine whether it is circumstantial or a signal of something bigger that needs to be investigated and resolved through an improvement effort.

Delays in getting things done or continuous interruptions to a process can warn of roadblocks to success. Delays give time to revisit the current workflow and analyze what might be improved. If transcribed operative reports, for example, are not available in the patient's record within the prescribed time, the reason for the delay should be identified and the improvement activity planned to eliminate the delay.

Low employee morale and a high rate of absenteeism or turnover are serious indicators that something needs to be improved. While not always the case, these indicators can be a sign that there are training, procedural, or task-related problems that underlie the employees' behavior. High turnover and absenteeism are budget draining and call for an investigation followed by a defined plan of action to avert a continued pattern.

Poor safety records or injuries are indicative of urgent process improvement opportunities. Work-related injuries and accidents are management markers regarding a poorly designed or configured work environment, poor equipment, or poor training. Work injuries are a costly burden for both the individual employee and the organization.

Collecting meaningful performance data, being alert, and observing and listening to customers and key staff are all ways to identify improvement opportunities. It is a continuous process that has no tolerance for complacency. Excellence is not an accident; it is an intended outcome that requires a manager's commitment and continuous attention.

Principles of Performance Improvement

The concepts of performance improvement, work improvement, process improvement, and methods improvement are essentially synonymous. They all relate to a management philosophy that is, at its core, systems oriented, meaning that it views the work processes in an organization as being systematic in nature and seeks to constantly improve them by adjusting various components of the system.

A **system** is a set of related elements (components) that are linked together according to a plan in order to meet a specific objective to achieve desired outcomes. Systems come in manual, automated, and hybrid forms. A system is made up of the following components.

- *Input*: Resources available to system, namely manpower (staff), money, methods (procedures), machines (equipment), and materials (supplies).

- *Process:* The transformation of the inputs. What is done to or with the inputs that result in something being accomplished?

- *Output*: The finished product or the result of the process, such as an educated student, a transcribed report, a coded record, and such.

- *Controls and standards*: The expectations of what the output should be and the mechanisms in place to monitor, track, and observe how well actual performance measures up to expectations.

- *Feedback*: Information that is reported when output is compared to the standards to identify how well actual output met standards (desired output). Feedback sometimes comes in the form of customer complaints, and certainly feedback can and should come in the form of compliments to staff, as well, when performance expectations are met.

- *External environment*: Anything outside the system that affects how the system functions (for example, laws or regulations set by the local, state, or federal government). In HIM departments, examples of external factors that affect its systems include:
  - The HIPAA regulations related to patient information confidentiality and security
  - Medicare's Conditions of Participation requirements for patients' medical record content
  - Medicare severity diagnosis-related groups (MS-DRGs) and Present on Admission (POA) regulations that impact coding and reimbursement systems in hospitals
  - A tight labor market, which makes it difficult to hire well-qualified employees for specialized jobs

Open systems are those systems affected by what is going on around them and must adjust as the environment changes. These are systems that cannot function in isolation, they must consider influences outside of the system itself. For example, the healthcare system is an open system; it must adjust to external influences such as HIPAA regulations, Joint Commission standards, economic status, and patient needs. They also can be considered **cybernetic systems** because they have standards, controls, and feedback mechanisms built into them. On the other hand, a **closed system** operates in a self-contained environment; that is, it is not affected by outside factors. A mechanical system (engines, motors, and such) is the best example of a closed system.

The aim of all performance, work, method, or process improvement efforts is to increase the effectiveness, efficiency, or the adaptability of the systems that are operating within an organization. These three goals of improvement efforts are described as follows.

- *Effectiveness*: How closely the output of a system matches what is expected of it. If a department is effective, it is getting done what it is supposed to get done.

- *Efficiency*: How well the department is using its resources; that is, is the department getting the most bang for its buck, or is it wasting staff time, money, or any other of its resources?

- *Adaptability*: The ease with which the system can adjust when circumstances require it to change to meet new demands or expectations. Adaptable systems respond appropriately to changing needs.

Organizations need to accomplish their goals with the fewest number of resources while being able to adjust as needed. This is the intent of improvement efforts.

Check Your Understanding 25.5

Instructions: **On a separate sheet of paper, indicate whether the following sentences are true or false and correct any false statement to make it true or to explain why it is false.**

1. The components of an open, cybernetic system only include input, process, and output.

2. An efficient process or system is one that uses its resources wisely—does not waste staff, supplies, money, and so on.

3. The Joint Commission has standards that specifically require accredited organizations to have performance improvement efforts as an integral aspect of their day-to-day operations.

4. Internal customers are the government agencies and public health organizations who have established regulations and policies that affect the way the department does its work.

5. The three goals of performance improvement efforts are effectiveness, economic stability, and consistency.

Process Improvement Methodologies

The principle methodologies available to healthcare facilities interested in PI are continuous quality improvement and business process redesign. These approaches have the same goal and use many of the same tools. However, they differ in focus and breadth of improvement effort.

Continuous Quality Improvement

Continuous quality improvement (CQI), sometimes still referred to as total quality management (TQM) or service excellence, is a management philosophy that "emphasizes the importance of knowing and meeting customer expectations, reducing variation within processes, and relying on data to build knowledge for process improvement" (AHIMA 2014). Its focus is on improving the quality of services provided to customers, whether internal (employees) or external (patients, physicians, payers). The approach is to make efforts to meet or exceed customer expectations by conducting small tests of change aimed at improving the quality of services. Of course, not all customer expectations can be met at the same time. In fact, some customers have expectations that conflict with the expectations of other customers. However, the goal is worth pursuing, even when only partly achievable.

CQI subscribes to the theory of seeking ways to improve the system through small, incremental changes with the expectation that over time the changes that will continually improve the quality of care. CQI never stops; it ensures processes are continually improved (Faculty of Pain Medicine n.d.). To achieve this, CQI relies on the gathering and analysis of data that can be used to make informed decisions.

CQI is a way of thinking, a way of being, a way of managing, and a way of conducting business. It can be applied to individuals as well as organizations. Moreover, CQI does not seek to blame problems on individuals but, instead, suggests that systems or processes may have inherent flaws that contribute to problems.

CQI attempts to involve people in the examination and improvement of existing systems. Several principles are incorporated into the CQI philosophy, including:

- *Constancy of variation*: Systems will always produce some normal variation in their output; the manager's job is to reduce the amount of variation as much as possible so that the process can become more stable and produce a more reliable output. Managers should not assume that any variation is a defect but, rather, should monitor and measure data over time to ensure that any variation is, in fact, caused inherently by the system. This type of variation is **common cause variation**. A greater-than-expected variation is a **special cause variation**. Sometimes a change is initiated with the express purpose of producing an improvement effort, in which case it should be encouraged. Other times, changes result in negative outputs and these must be eliminated. An example of variation in HIM departments might be found in the coding of records. A coder may complete 20 records one day but only 18 the next. The variation is not due to the clerk's lack of productivity but perhaps to the size of the records that day. In other words, the change is attributed to common cause variation. A significant drop in coding might indicate that a special cause is in effect. Perhaps the coder was assigned duties that day in addition to coding.

- *Importance of data*: Far too often, decisions for improvement are based on faulty assumptions. CQI recognizes the importance of collecting sufficient data so that informed decisions can be made. An organization must continually collect and analyze data related to performance measures to improve decision-making accuracy, gain consensus when making and implementing decisions, and allow the ability to predict further (ASQ n.d. (b)).

- *Vision and support of executive leadership*: Acceptance of the CQI philosophy must funnel down from the top to truly permeate the organization's culture. Executive leadership must communicate a clear vision and mission statement that every employee can understand and share.

- *Focus on customers*: To be successful, the organization must know and understand what its customers need and want. One way to obtain customer feedback is to administer satisfaction surveys on a regular basis. Any needs that are identified should be addressed.

- *Investment in people*: The CQI philosophy assumes that people want to do their jobs well. However, some employees may need training on how they can more adequately serve their customers. Management can empower employees by giving them opportunities to learn and grow and feel more competent in performing their jobs.

- *Importance of teams*: Because CQI seeks to improve processes that may extend beyond the boundaries of individual departments, the people directly involved with the processes must work together. Teams should include individuals with different expertise and from different levels of the organization. Team members should be knowledgeable about portions of the process and be able to contribute to the improvement effort. Having members from different areas on the team brings fresh perspectives and opens communication. A good team also is able to communicate its purpose and activities to other parts of the organization.

These principles incorporate an understanding of variation, data, vision, executive-level support, customer-focus, investment in people, and teamwork for successful CQI projects.

Basic PI Tools

A number of tools and techniques are frequently used with PI initiatives (Brassard and Ritter 2010). Some of them are used to facilitate communication among employees; others are used to assist people in determining the root causes of problems.

Some tools show areas of agreement or consensus among team members; others permit the display of data for easier analysis (see chapter 18 for more on data display tools). The following section presents a brief description and discussion of the purpose of tools and techniques commonly used by improvement teams.

Movement Diagram   A movement diagram is a visual depiction of the layout of the workspace with all the furniture, equipment, doorways, and so on sketched in. Superimposed on the layout are the movements of either individuals or things (for example, documents, files, and such). The movement diagram can be used to evaluate the workflow and to redesign one that is more efficient. An inefficient workflow is depicted in figure 25.1 (top), showing long distances between connected points in the workflow, crisscrossing paths, and paths that backtrack in the work space. A redesigned movement diagram in figure 25.1 (bottom) depicts a smoother workflow resulting in improved efficiency.

Brainstorming   Brainstorming is a technique used to generate a large number of creative ideas. It encourages team members to think outside the box and offer ideas. There are some variations in using the technique—one can use an unstructured method for brainstorming or a structured method. The unstructured method involves having a free flow of ideas about a situation. The team leader writes down each idea as it is offered so all can see. There should be no evaluative discussion about the worthiness of the idea because we want to do nothing that will inhibit the flow of ideas. Each idea is captured and written for the team to consider at a later point.

Structured brainstorming uses a more formal approach. The team leader asks each person to generate a list of ideas for themselves and then, one by one, the team leader proceeds around the room eliciting a new idea from each member. The process may take several rounds. As team members run out of new ideas, they pass and the next person offers an idea until no one can produce any fresh ideas.

Brainstorming is highly effective for identifying a number of potential processes that may benefit from improvement efforts and for generating solutions to particular problems. It helps people to begin thinking in new ways and gets them involved in the process. It is an excellent method for facilitating open communication.

Affinity Grouping   Affinity grouping allows the team to organize and group similar ideas together. Ideas that are generated in a brainstorming session may be written on Post-it notes and arranged on a table or posted on a board. Without talking to each other, each team member is asked to walk around the table or board, look at the ideas, and place them in groupings that seem related or connected to each other. Each member is empowered to move the ideas in a way that makes the most sense. As a team member moves the ideas back or places them in other groupings, the other team members consider the merits of the placement and decide if further action is needed. The goal is to have the team eventually feel comfortable with the arrangement. The natural groupings that emerge are then labeled with a category. This tool brings focus to the many ideas generated. (See figure 25.2.)

Nominal Group Technique   Nominal group technique (NGT) is a process designed to bring agreement about an issue or an idea that the team considers most important. It produces and permits visualization of team consensus. In NGT, each team member ranks each idea according to its importance. For example, if there were six ideas, the idea that is most important would be given the number 6. The second most important idea would be given the number 5. The least important idea would have the number 1. After each team member has individually ranked the list of ideas, the numbers are totaled. The ideas that are deemed most important are clearly visible to all. Those ideas that people did not think were as important are also made known by their low scores. NGT demonstrates where the team's priorities lie.

Multivoting Technique   The multivoting technique is a variation of NGT and has the same

Figure 25.1. Movement diagram: Inefficient (top) and efficient (bottom)

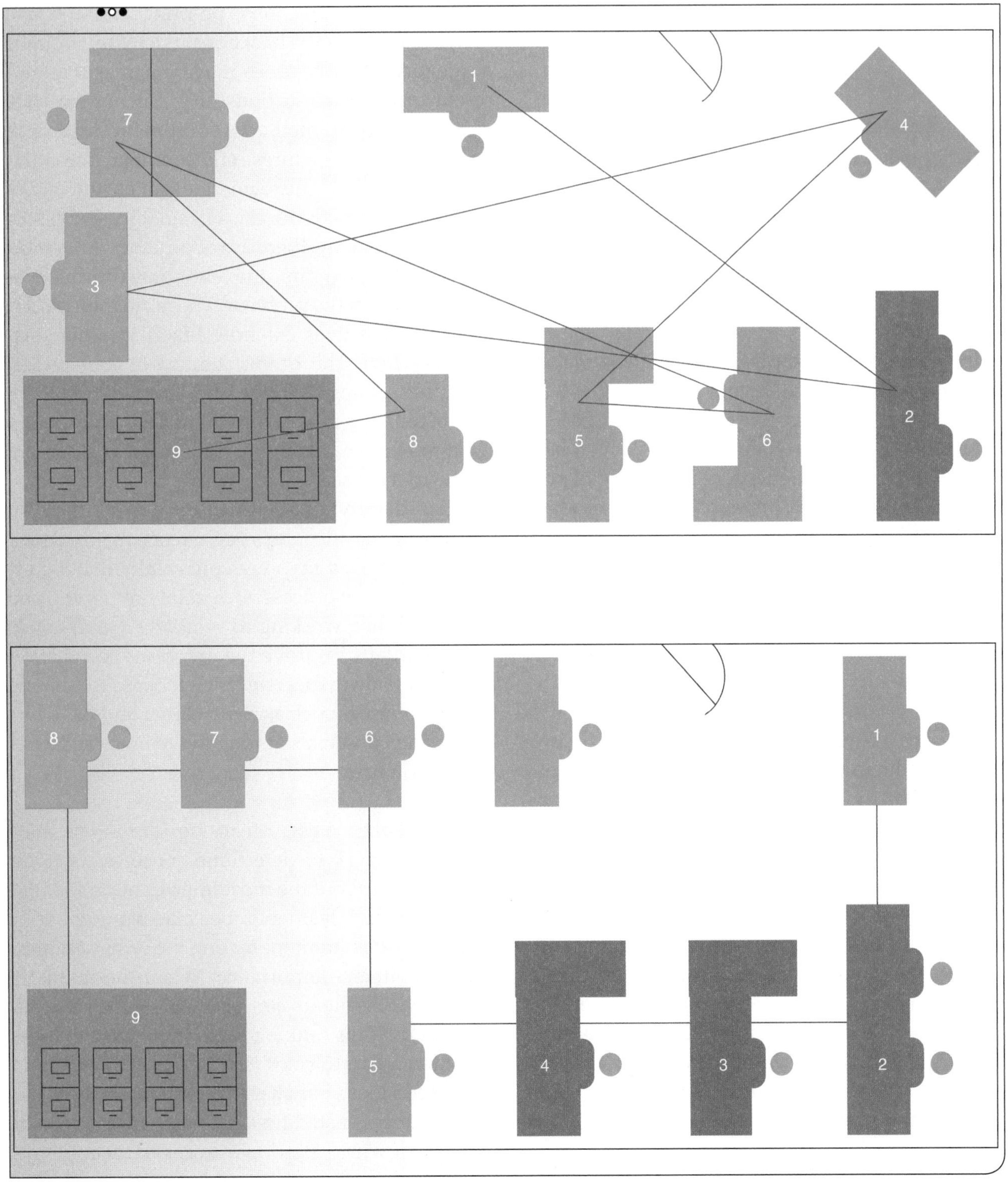

purpose. Rather than ranking each issue or idea, team members are asked to rate the issue using a distribution of points or colorful dots. Weighted multivoting is a variation of this process. For example, a team member may be asked to distribute 25 points among 10 total issues. Thus, one issue of particular importance to him or her may receive 12 points, four others may receive some variation

Figure 25.2. Affinity grouping

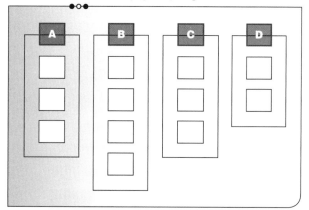

of the remaining 12 points, and five others may receive no points. After the voting, the numbers are added and the team is able to see which issue has emerged as particularly important to its members.

This process also can be done with colored dots. For example, if there are eight items on a chart, each team member may be given four dots to distribute on the four items that are most important to him or her. This method particularly enables team members to see where consensus lies and what issue has been deemed most important by the team as a whole.

Flowchart Whenever a team examines a process with the intention of making improvements, it must first thoroughly understand the process. Each team member comes to the team with a unique perspective and significant insight about how a portion of the process works. To help all members understand the process, a team will undertake development of a flowchart. (See figure 25.3.) This work allows the team to thoroughly understand every step in the process and the sequence of steps. It provides a picture of each decision point and each event that must be completed. It readily points out places where there is redundancy and complex and problematic areas.

Root-Cause Analysis (Fishbone Diagram) When a team first identifies a problem, it may use a fishbone diagram, also known as a cause-and-effect diagram, to help determine the root causes of the problem. (See figure 25.4.) The problem is placed in a box on the right side of the paper. A horizontal line is drawn (somewhat like a backbone), with diagonal bones, like ribs, pointing to the boxes above and below the backbone. Each box contains a category. The categories may be names that represent broad classifications of problem areas (for example, people, methods, equipment, materials, policies and procedures, environment, measurement, and so on). The team determines how many categories it needs to classify all the sources of problems. Usually, there are about four. After constructing the diagram, the team brainstorms possible sources of the problem. These are then placed on horizontal lines extending from the diagonal category line. The brainstorming of root causes continues among team members until all ideas are exhausted. The purpose of this tool is to permit a team to explore, identify, and graphically display all the root causes of a problem.

After identifying a number of causes of a problem, a team may decide to begin working to remove one of them. CQI involves continually making efforts to improve processes; certainly removing one cause and then working to remove another cause will eventually improve the process. The question may arise, however, about which cause to remove first. Techniques such as multivoting and NGT can help bring consensus among the team about what to work on first.

Pareto Chart When a team decides to use multivoting or NGT to determine consensus among the members about the most important problem to tackle first, each team member places a number or mark next to an item indicating his or her opinion about the item's importance. When the numbers are tallied, the items can be ranked according to importance. This ranking can then be visually displayed in a Pareto chart (see figure 25.5). A Pareto chart looks like a bar chart except that the highest-ranking item is listed first, followed by the second highest, down to the lowest-ranked item. Thus, the Pareto chart is a descending bar chart. This visualization of how the problems were ranked allows team members to focus on those few that have the greatest potential for improving the process. The Pareto chart is based on the Pareto principle, which states that 20 percent of the sources of

Figure 25.3. Release of information flowchart

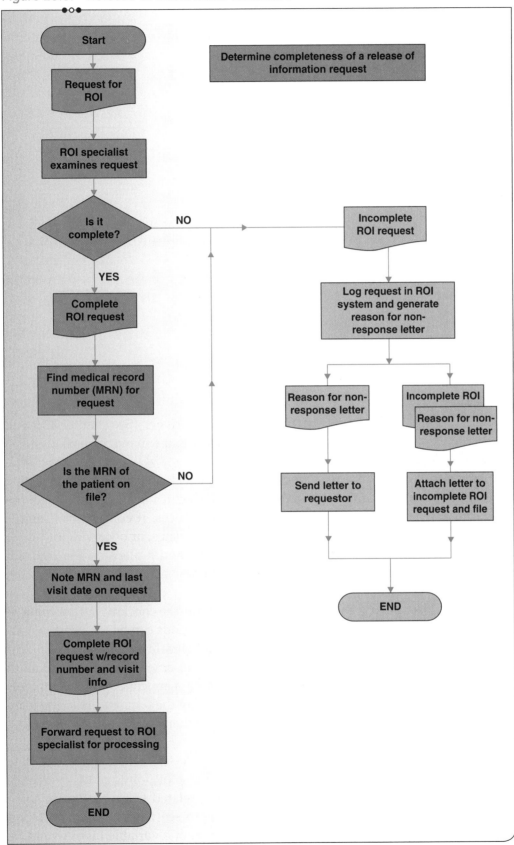

Figure 25.4.   Fishbone diagram

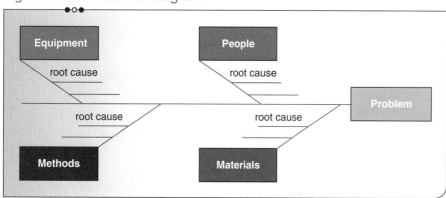

Figure 25.5.   Pareto chart

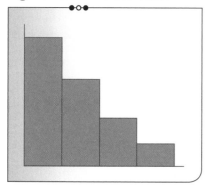

Figure 25.6.   Force-field analysis

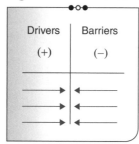

the problem are responsible for 80 percent of the actual problem (Brassard and Ritter 2010). By concentrating on the vital few sources, a large number of actual problems can be eliminated.

Force-Field Analysis   A **force-field analysis** also visually displays data generated through brainstorming. The team leader draws a large T formation on a board. (See figure 25.6.) Above the crossbar and on the left side of the T is a title related to positive drivers, such as benefits or forces for change; and above the bar and written on the right side of the T is a title related to negative drivers, such as barriers or forces against change. Team members are then asked to brainstorm and list on the chart under the crossbar the reasons or factors that would contribute to a change for improvement and those reasons or factors that can create barriers. Thus, the force field enables team members to identify factors that support or work against a proposed solution. Often the next step in this activity is to work on ways to either eliminate

barriers or reinforce drivers. (See chapter 22 for an example related to change management).

Check Sheet   A **check sheet** is a data collection tool permitting the recording and compiling of observations or occurrences. It consists of a simple listing of categories, issues, or observations on the left side of the chart and a place on the right for individuals to record checkmarks next to the item when it is observed or counted (see figure 25.7). After a period of time, the checkmarks are counted and the patterns or trends can be revealed.

A check sheet is a simple tool that allows a clear picture of the facts to emerge. It enables data to be collected. After data are collected, several tools can be used to display the data and help the team more easily analyze them.

Scatter Diagram   A **scatter diagram** is a data analysis tool used to plot points of two variables suspected of being related to each other in some way. For example, to see whether age and blood pressure are related, one variable (age) would be plotted on one line of the graph, and the other variable (blood pressure) would be plotted on the other line. After several people's blood pressures are plotted along with their ages, a pattern might emerge. If the diagram indicates that blood pressure increases with age, the data could be interpreted as revealing a positive relationship between age and blood pressure. (See figure 25.8.)

In some cases, a negative relationship might exist, such as with the variables age and flexibility or with the number of hours of training and number of mistakes made. Whenever a scatter diagram indicates that the points are moving together in one direction or another, conclusions can be drawn about the variables' relationship, either positive or negative. In other cases, however, the scatter diagram may indicate no linear relationship between the variables because the points are scattered haphazardly and no pattern emerges. In this case, the conclusion would have to be that the two variables have no apparent relationship.

Histogram A **histogram** (figure 25.9) is a data analysis tool used to display frequencies of response. It offers a much easier way to summarize

and analyze data than having them displayed in a table of numbers. A histogram displays **continuous data** values that have been grouped into categories. The bars on the histogram reveal how the data are distributed. For example, an HIM administrator may want to show the number of minutes it takes to respond to patient requests for information. Minutes may be categorized into four groupings—for example, 1 to 30 minutes, 31 to 60 minutes, 61 to 90 minutes, and more than 90 minutes. Checkmarks may be recorded indicating the category of minutes taken to respond to the request. After a period of time, the checkmarks are added and the histogram is plotted with the frequencies shown on the vertical axis, or y-axis, and the minute intervals shown on the horizontal axis, or x-axis.

The graph in figure 25.9 indicates the different intervals patients had to wait for their requests to be filled. A histogram can give an excellent idea of how well a process is performing. Thus, it can show how frequently data values occur among the various intervals, how centered or skewed the distribution of data is, and what the likelihood of future occurrences is.

Run Chart A **run chart** displays data points over a period of time to provide information about performance (see figure 25.10). Measured points of a process are plotted on a graph at regular time intervals to help team members see whether there are substantial changes in the numbers over time. For example, suppose a HIM manager wanted to reduce the number of incomplete records in the HIM department. The manager might first plot

Figure 25.7. Check sheet

	1	2	Total
A	ⅲⅲ	///	8
B	////	////	8
C	//	/	3

Figure 25.8. Scatter diagram

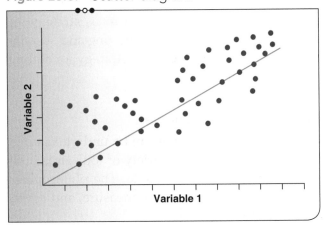

Figure 25.9. Histogram

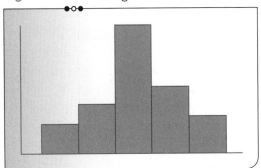

on a graph the number of incomplete records each month for the past six months and then enact a change in the processing of records designed to improve the process. Following the improvement effort, data would continue to be collected on the number of incomplete records and would continue to be plotted on the graph. If the run chart shows that the number of incomplete charts has actually decreased, the HIM manager could attribute the decrease to the improvement effort.

A run chart is an excellent tool for providing visual verification of how a process is performing and whether an improvement effort appears to have worked.

Statistical Process Control Chart A **statistical process control (SPC) chart** looks like a run chart except that it has a line displayed at the top, called an upper control limit (UCL), and a line displayed at the bottom, called a lower control limit (LCL). (See figure 25.11.) These lines have been statistically calculated from the data generated in the process and represent three units of dispersion above

and below the midline (three standard deviations) (Omachonu 1999).

Like the run chart, the SPC chart plots points over time to demonstrate how a process is performing. However, the two control limit lines enable the interpreter to determine whether the process is stable, or predictable, or whether it is out of control. Remembering the constancy of variation principle, it is easy to see the purpose of the SPC chart. The SPC chart indicates whether the variation occurring within the process is a common cause variation or a special cause variation. It indicates whether it is necessary to try and reduce the ordinary variation occurring through common cause or to seek out a special cause of the variation and try to eliminate it.

Business Process Redesign

Used extensively in the mid-1980s and early 1990s, business process reengineering (BPR) has met with resistance in the healthcare sector because of the fear it has invoked among healthcare workers. The term *reengineering* may be confused with reorganizing or downsizing, which can result in the loss of jobs (Dunn 2010). Because salaries and benefits comprise 50 to 60 percent of a healthcare facility's total expenses, a drop in personnel can have a significant impact on reducing expenditures (Society for Human Resource Management 2008). Due to negative connotations related to downsizing, restructuring, and outsourcing, the perception of reengineering went from a strategy an organization does to something that is done to the organization. Although the term *reengineering* itself is not always favorable in organizations today, **business process redesign** is still a focus strategy for rethinking and drastically improving and sustaining overall performance, not a strategy for cutting costs (Dunn 2010).

Models and Methodologies

Business process redesign can be undertaken in a variety of ways using a variety of tools; it is built around the foundation of data. The philosophies and methods used to collect, measure, and act on that data are numerous.

Figure 25.10. Run chart

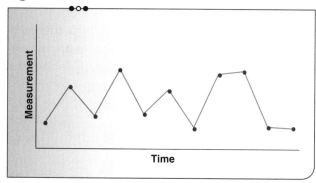

Figure 25.11. Statistical process control chart

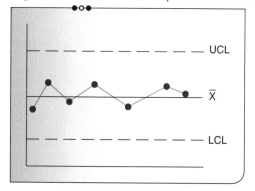

Unlike CQI, which focuses on conducting small tests of change to achieve continuous but incremental improvement over time, BPR focuses on the potential redesign of the entire process to achieve improvement. (See table 25.5 for a comparison of reengineering and quality management.) Reengineering implies making massive changes to the way a facility delivers healthcare services.

Philosophy of Reengineering

Business process reengineering has entered the healthcare sector after first being successfully applied in the wider business community. In reengineering, the entire manner and purpose of a work process is questioned. The goal is to achieve the desired process outcome in the most effective and efficient manner possible. Thus, the results expected from reengineering efforts include:

- Increased productivity
- Decreased costs
- Improved quality
- Maximized revenue
- More satisfied customers

The goal of reengineering is to develop sustained improvements and efficiencies over the long term, not just a quick fix.

Process of Reengineering

When an organization decides to use reengineering as an improvement strategy, it commits itself to looking at selected processes within the organization in fine detail. Processes are selected for reengineering based on a number of criteria, including:

- Frequency and severity of problems created by the process, such as slow turnaround time or excessive waiting time
- Impact on customer satisfaction
- Complex processes involving multiple departments, procedures, and employees
- The feasibility of actually creating improvement (McConnell 2014)

Selecting a process for reengineering raises several questions:

- What is the intended purpose of the process? Is that purpose being accomplished efficiently?
- Is the process absolutely necessary? Could any redundancies or non–value-added activities be eliminated?
- Which employees are involved in the process, and which ones are actually needed? In other words, what are the minimum qualifications and minimum number of employees needed to do the job?
- Is the process as efficient as it could be, or are there more efficient means for accomplishing the goal?
- Is the process contributing to the efficiency of other processes that may be affected by its results?
- Is there an opportunity to combine processes and to train or use employees to perform more functions than they currently perform?
- Can any steps of the process be eliminated?
- Is outsourcing a feasible and more cost-effective alternative?
- Would new equipment or new technologies improve the process?

Many of the tools and techniques used in systems analysis and CQI also are used in reengineering. In reengineering, it is essential to thoroughly understand how the process contributes to how the

Table 25.5. Reengineering compared to quality management

Reengineering		Quality management	
Rethinking and radical redesign	**Focus**	**Incremental improvements**	**Focus**
Rethink	Think outside of the box	Quality planning	Focus on the customer
Redesign	Think both process and outcome	Quality control	Measure and monitor performance
Retool	Use technology to control and define work processes	Quality improvement	Use data, eliminate boundaries, and empower work

organization functions and to determine whether a better method exists. Therefore, observation of processes, customer input, interviews with employees, and the use of cross-functional teams to discuss the current steps of the process are frequently used methods for obtaining data. Data must be collected for a sufficient period of time to actually reflect the effectiveness of the process.

In addition, the data must be analyzed appropriately, and the analysis should include the input of individuals qualified to interpret the findings. Thus, a team composed of individuals involved in various aspects of the process should be permitted access to the data and should give input about alternative strategies. Moreover, the team can investigate the acceptability of new technologies that might allow for greater efficiency. Before new technologies are adopted, however, the team should thoroughly analyze the potential benefits, costs, and feasibility of using them in the organization.

After a reengineered process has emerged, new policies and procedures must be written and distributed to the people involved in the process. In addition, employees should be thoroughly trained in the redesigned process. However, it is important that they be given adequate time to master the process. Managers play an important role in reengineering through their support, encouragement, and commitment to the process.

Factors for Success in Reengineering Efforts

One critical factor for the success of the reengineering effort is the visible and persistent commitment of senior administration. A second critical factor is management's commitment to excellence. Managers must demonstrate a can-do attitude in working through the change. In addition, the fact that change is needed to address an unacceptable problem must be effectively communicated throughout the organization. Having everyone, or almost everyone, acknowledge that a problem exists creates a great deal of buy-in. Employees, including physicians, should be encouraged to overcome any reluctance to participate in the change process due to fears about restructuring. Many healthcare organizations make the mistake of not including

their physicians in critical decision making. The likelihood of a successful reengineering effort increases when every stakeholder is involved in the process.

Reengineering takes time. The organization should realize that change cannot be achieved overnight and should avoid trying to change too many processes at one time. Instead, it should focus its efforts on a few processes at a time. A great deal of planning, information gathering, and analysis must occur before an actual redesign can be implemented. When the planning phase has been completed, the organization should revise or develop policies and procedures accordingly and distribute them throughout the organization.

Finally, implementation of the redesigned processes requires patience. Glitches may occur with any new system, but reengineering can produce significant PI with careful monitoring and persistent adjusting.

Lean   Lean is a management strategy in which the core idea is to maximize value while minimizing waste; basically creating more value with fewer resources (Lean Enterprise Institute n.d.). Lean is known for its focus on the reduction of waste and is based on the Japanese success story of Toyota. Toyota's steady growth from a small company to one of the largest automobile companies in the world through the use of Lean principles has made Lean a hot topic in management science in the 21st century.

Lean implementation focuses on eliminating waste and creating a smooth workflow. Through analysis of the process vs. a prime focus on the end goal, quality problems are exposed and waste reduction occurs naturally as a consequence. The goals of the organization remain the same; the approach toward achieving the goals differs in the Lean methodology. Lean works to eliminate non–value-added work, or waste, brought about by a lack of error detection, confused responsibilities, unnecessary work, disconnects, and workarounds. Waste can be defined "as anything that does not add value to a product or service from the standpoint of the customer" (Womack and Jones 1996). Lean is about creating a continually improving system that is capable of achieving more while using less.

Lean has been applied in many industries, not just manufacturing. It has been used in healthcare with significant improvements in quality and efficiency. The principles of removing activities that do not add value can be applied anywhere. Value in a hospital setting may be described as patient comfort, competent caregivers, or patient discharge after achieving the desired outcomes. Anything that helps treat the patient is value-added; everything else is waste. Toyota identified seven areas of waste: delay, overprocessing, inventory, transportation, motion, overproducing, and defects (Hiroyuki 1989). Examples of how these areas of waste may relate to healthcare are found in table 25.6. There are a number of Lean tools and techniques used in manufacturing; several have a strong application to the healthcare industry. The following tools seem simple, but when intentionally used, can uncover large amounts of waste (Zidel 2006).

- *The five whys*: In this technique, simply ask "why" in every situation until you discover the root cause of the problem. Usually this

process takes approximately five times before the root cause is identified.

- *The five Ss*: The five Ss are sort, straighten, scrub, standardize, and sustain. This method, simply stated, is housekeeping.
  - Sort—Remove everything that is not used or expected to be used
  - Straighten—Organize what is kept, have a place for everything, and keep everything in its place
  - Scrub—Clean the area
  - Standardize—Establish procedures to keep the area organized
  - Sustain—Maintain the gains and avoid backsliding

- *Visual controls*: The visual controls tool is used to create a workplace where all that is needed is displayed and immediately available. There are four levels of visual controls:
  - Visual indicator—Something that just informs, such as a sign on a patient's door with special instructions
  - Visual signal—An alert or alarm, such as a nurse call light
  - Visual control—A mechanism to control behavior, such as a needle box that automatically closes when full to eliminate the risk of overfilling
  - Visual guarantee—A mechanism that allows only a correct response, such as a medication dispensing machine that will not dispense a medication without proper identifiers; a visual guarantee is foolproof (Zidel 2006)

In addition, the following two tools have applicability in the healthcare setting:

- *Value stream mapping:* This is a visual method of documenting both material and information flows of a process. It is a flow diagram that identifies all the value-added and non–value-added activities in the process. This is first developed to analyze the current process and eliminate non–value-added steps; then it is developed again to illustrate the improved, streamlined process.

Table 25.6.   Seven areas of waste related to healthcare

Area of waste	Healthcare examples
Delay	Waiting for discharge order, waiting for a dictated report holding up surgery, waiting for nursing home placement
Overprocessing	Multiple requests for patient demographic information, duplicate lab tests, multiple patient signatures
Inventory	Outdated forms kept on hand, excess supplies, dictation awaiting transcription
Transportation	Transporting patients, retrieving medical records, delivering medical records, transporting medication
Motion	Searching for records in various locations, seeking physicians for documentation queries, providers giving care in different locations
Overproducing	Creating paperwork packets for potential surgery patients, preparing extra patient meal trays in case of overflow
Defects	Medication errors, assignment of duplicate medical record numbers, equipment malfunctions

Source: Adapted from Zidel 2006.

The value stream shows all the actions (both value-added and non–value-added) and related information required to bring a patient through the process from the start to the end of his visit.

- *Pull system:* This is a method of controlling the flow of resources by replacing only what the customer has consumed. Pull systems consist of production based on actual consumption, small volumes, low inventories, management by sight, and better communication. To create value, services must be in line with demand; no less, no more. Delivering services in line with demand means that work, material, and information should be pulled toward the task when needed. (Jones and Mitchell 2006)

Identifying the value streams, mapping and understanding each action in the value stream, and identifying and implementing immediate and future improvements using Lean tools and techniques are all a part of building a culture of continuous improvement in the organization.

Six Sigma   Six Sigma is a data driven methodology for removing defects in any process (AHIMA 2014). Some industry experts doubted that Six Sigma could be applied to the healthcare industry because of the human variability of patients. However, the 2000 Institute of Medicine report highlighting the alarming statistic of up to 98,000 deaths linked to medical errors soon resulted in a movement to review statistical data in the healthcare industry (IOM 2000). Both industry and healthcare are customer driven and rely on feedback regarding success and failure in relevant data. Healthcare leaders became invested in enlisting this philosophy of excellence, reducing costs, lowering lengths of stay, and raising the bar for high-quality healthcare. The healthcare industry leaders who have embraced Six Sigma are quick to share their successes as the industry continues to come to understand the richness of the data that are captured and how to understand their inherent value.

Six Sigma uses a methodology not unique. It uses a scientific methodology that involves the following steps: define, measure, analyze, improve, and control (DMAIC).

- Define the problem, improvement opportunity, goals, and customer requirements
- Measure performance
- Analyze the process to determine root causes of variations or poor performance
- Improve the process by addressing the root causes
- Control the improved process and future performance (American Society for Quality n.d.(a))

The DMAIC process is used in a variety of quality improvement initiatives, not just Six Sigma.

Six Sigma uses many of the same tools used by other quality management systems. In addition, Six Sigma uses soft tools that do not have a math basis; however, soft tools can be tricky to use because they have a subjective quality to them. Examples of some basic soft tools are a set of ground rules, a team agenda, a parking lot to track ideas not immediately pertinent, and activity or progress reports.

Six Sigma focuses on improving management and clinical processes. Statistical analysis is used to find the most defective part of a process, and rigorous control procedures are used to ensure sustained improvement. To achieve Six Sigma, a process must not produce more than 3.4 defects per million opportunities (iSixSigma n.d.).

Six Sigma can be used successfully in healthcare. It provides a systematic approach to validate data and focuses on the most meaningful improvements. Successful implementation of Six Sigma in healthcare organizations has produced benefits such as the following:

- Higher productivity
- Fewer errors and adverse effects
- Improved organizational communication
- Improved patient satisfaction
- Better physician satisfaction

- Better nursing satisfaction
- Increased patient flow
- Short patient wait times
- Better use of advanced technologies

As in other quality management concepts, the customer defines acceptable performance with the focus on delivery, quality, and cost. This parallels with the Institute for Healthcare Improvement's (IHI) Triple Aim, consisting of improving the patient experience of care (including quality and satisfaction), improving the health of populations, and reducing the per capita cost of healthcare (IHI 2015).

Lean Six Sigma The uses of Lean methods along with Six Sigma techniques have been successful. Despite numerous debates over which process improvement methodology is best, it may be that the two methods work quite well together. Lean provides tools to identify and implement value-added activities designed to streamline processes and improve efficiency as a result of waste reduction. Six Sigma focuses on reducing variation through statistical analysis, validation of data, and measuring improvements. Lean and Six Sigma complement each other with goals aimed toward overall improvement, organizational buy-in, and a culture change that promotes continuous improvement via a structured methodology and identified tools and techniques.

Workflow Analysis and Process Redesign

Whatever the methodology or strategy used, workflow analysis and **process redesign** are necessary components of overall organizational improvement. The study of workflow as "who does what when" has become a critical part of process analysis and design methodologies.

Process and Workflow Theory

The delivery of healthcare is increasingly complex; therefore, the related workflows are also increasingly complex. As the use of technology becomes critical in all aspects of patient care, understanding how the work flows within and between processes is critical. The success of information technology projects is not solely dependent on the technology, but also on the people and the process. A business process can be defined as a collection of interrelated work tasks initiated in response to an event that achieves a specific result for a customer of the process (Sharp and McDermott 2009). A process must remain customer focused; redundancy, delay, and error must be avoided. The goal of workflow analysis is business process redesign.

Workflow analysis should be done any time work involves multiple departments or functions and prior to identifying an information technology (IT) solution. It is important to ensure all the stakeholders are a part of the analysis, the entire process is considered when making improvements, the business process is accurately identified, and the team does not get stalled in overanalysis of the current process. HIM professionals are well suited for workflow analysis because they can see the big picture of the overall healthcare process, they understand how healthcare professionals work together toward quality patient care, and they understand information flow and the users of the information.

The steps in workflow analysis are described as follows:

1. Frame the process
2. Understand the current (as-is) process
3. Design the new (to-be) process
4. Develop use case scenarios (Sharp and McDermott 2009)

Outside of the actual methodology of workflow analysis, related key concepts include understanding the organizational structure and managing change.

An essential, necessary distinction in workflow analysis is the difference between a process and a function. A process, as stated earlier, is a collection of interrelated work tasks done in response to an event that achieves a specific result for a customer. A function is an occupation or a department that focuses on related activities and similar skills. See table 25.7 for an example distinguishing a process from a function. If a function is identified erroneously as a process for analysis, work methods will be defined for the benefit of the individual function, not to optimize the manner in which work flows

Table 25.7.   Process vs. function

Coding process (Interdepartmental, multiple skill sets)	Coding function (Intradepartmental, one skill set)
Register patient	Go to worklist and select case
Generate clinical documentation about patient assessment and services provided in the course of patient care	Obtain clinical documentation and charges
Enter charges	Review and determine adequacy of information
Process medical record for completeness and accuracy	Apply coding rules and select codes
Generate codes for billing and clinical databases	Enter codes into databases for billing and clinical systems
Analyze remittance advice and denials	

Source: AHIMA 2006.

through the function and through other areas of the organization as a whole. Focusing on functions and not business process perpetuates the development of functional silos or stovepipes. This should be avoided in process redesign.

Once a process is identified, framing that process is crucial in establishing and documenting the process boundaries. This will clarify the scope of the process—what is both within and outside of the scope. Documenting all the pertinent information about the process is called developing the process frame. In the process frame, one must:

- Describe the process triggers, steps, results, and stakeholders
- Understand the environment, including the mission, vision, goals, and culture
- State the case for analysis

The purpose of analysis is to understand processes to identify bottlenecks, sources of delay, rework due to errors, role ambiguity, duplication, unnecessary steps, and handoffs. This understanding of the current (as-is) process will lead to a redesigned future (to-be) process that can then be tested through a use case analysis.

Tools and Techniques

As with continuous quality improvement, there are several process mapping tools that can assist with workflow analysis and process redesign. Process mapping shows the activities of the process including the sequence and flow of the work. Tool selection will depend on the level of precision needed and the nature of the process being mapped. Tools may be simple or complex, paper based, automated, or web based. Some of these tools are the same as or similar to the CQI tools such as the workflow diagram for illustrating the movement of information (see figure 25.1) and the process flowchart for illustrating each step in a process and the sequence of steps (see figure 25.3). Other process mapping tools include the top-down process map, the swimlane diagram, and process simulation software.

Top-Down Process Map   The top-down process map identifies the least number of steps necessary in a process. The main steps are worded broadly and simply, with each step showing only three to four subtasks in more detail (see figure 25.12).

Swimlane Diagram   A **swimlane diagram** shows an entire business process from beginning to end and is especially popular because it highlights relevant variables (who, what, and when) while requiring little or no training to use and understand. The swimlane diagram is often used to identify the current (as-is) process as well as to design the new (to-be) process (see figure 25.13).

Process Simulation Software   Process simulation software can show the flow of work, individuals, or movement of information in varying existing or hypothetical situations. This software can show movement in existing situations and can show various alternative designs to help identify the most appropriate workflow.

These tools and techniques assist in analyzing current workflows to focus on facts rather than opinions, to truly understand the existing process, and to document all aspects of the process. Additionally, process maps can bring stakeholders to a common understanding to move forward with process redesign.

Use Case Analysis

A **use case analysis** is a technique to determine how users will interact with a system. It uses the

Figure 25.12.   Top-down process maps

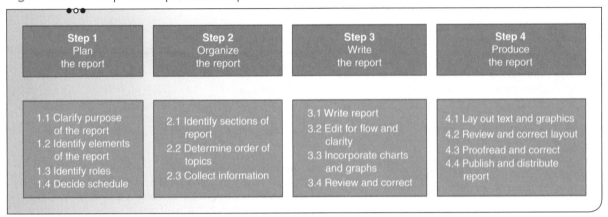

Source: AHIMA 2006.

Figure 25.13.   Sample swimlane diagram

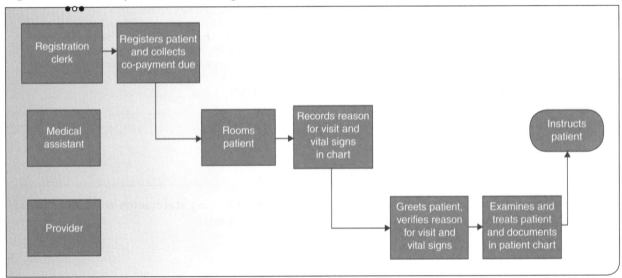

Source: AHIMA 2006.

designed future (to-be) process and describes how a user will interact with the system to complete process steps and how the system will behave from the user perspective. The purpose of use case analysis is to bridge the gap between user needs and system functionality. A use case analysis helps identify system requirements, design the user interface, facilitate documentation, create test plans, and develop training and support plans. It is critical to list all use case scenarios that impact each and every user so that no case is overlooked. Priority should go to developing use case scenarios that focus on those areas that have the most impact on the success of the project such

as those that affect workflows of multiple users (Sharp and McDermott 2009).

Identifying all potential use cases is valuable to ensure that nothing is overlooked and all users are involved. More value emerges when each use case is not only identified but also described. Basic elements of a use case description are the use case name, a description of the use case, the users of the system for that use case, preconditions that must be in place before the use case can be tested, the normal sequence of steps, the post conditions or results expected, any alternate steps as needed, and any variations or issues known to that particular use case that are important to know. (See example in figure 25.14.)

Figure 25.14.   Use case description

Use case name
Provider orders lab work for inpatient.

Description
When a provider determines a need for lab work for an inpatient, he or she will complete the ordering process for lab

Actor(s)
Care provider

Preconditions
• The patient must currently be admitted in the hospital.
• The provider has active privileges at the facility.
• The computerized provider order entry system is functioning properly.

Normal sequence of steps
1. Provider signs on to the system using a password.
   System validates the password and displays the patient search screen.
2. Provider enters the patient's medical record number.
   System verifies the medical record number and displays the patient's electronic medical record.
3. Provider selects the lab module.
   System verifies the user is allowed access to the module and displays the lab module.
4. Provider selects the lab test from drop-down list.
   System verifies the lab test name.

5. Provider enters the lab test.
   System verifies the test.
6. Provider submits the lab order by selecting the Submit button.
   System sends lab order

Postconditions
• The order is submitted to the laboratory information system.
• The lab receives electronic notification of pending order.
• A pending order is recorded in the patient's electronic medical record.

Alternative sequence of steps
• If the provider does not have the medical record number, he or she may enter the patient's last name and the first name. The system will then provide a list of patient names that the physician may choose from.
• An additional free-text field may be provided to the physician to record any additional notes or messages in relation to the lab being ordered.

Comments, issues, and design notes
• When searching for a patient's electronic medical record, it may be necessary to also be able to search by patient date of birth.
• For the lab test fields, it may be necessary to create drop-down lists that can be selected from instead of allowing free text. This will allow more control of the data entry and reduce data entry errors.

Source: Adapted from Sharp and McDermott 2009.

Check Your Understanding 25.6

Instructions: On a separate piece of paper, indicate whether the following statements are true or false. Then correct any false statement to make it true or explain why it is false.

1. The goal of CQI—to meet or exceed the expectations of all the organization's customers—is generally attainable and achievable.

2. Obtaining and using actual data to inform managers who need to make decisions is a critically important element of the CQI philosophy.

3. Lean is particularly focused on the elimination of waste.

4. A manager's job with regard to performance improvement is to seek ways to reduce the amount of normal variation that occurs within systems and processes.

5. An example of a soft tool used in Six Sigma is statistical analysis.

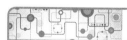

References

American Health Information Management Association. 2014. *Pocket Glossary of Health Information Management and Technology,* 4th ed. Chicago: AHIMA.

American Health Information Management Association. 2006. *Optimizing Investment in the EHR: Workflow Analysis as the Foundation for Success* [Workshop resource book]. Chicago: AHIMA.

American Society for Quality (ASQ). n.d.(a). The Define Measure Analyze Improve Control (DMAIC) Process. http://asq.org/learn-about-quality/six-sigma/overview/dmaic.html

American Society for Quality (ASQ). n.d.(b). Total Quality Management (TQM). http://asq.org/learn-about-quality/total-quality-management/overview/overview.html

Bardhan, A. and C.A. Kroll. 2003 (Oct.) The New Wave of Outsourcing. Fisher Center for Real Estate & Urban Economics Research Report Series No. 1103. http://www.haas.berkeley.edu/news/Research_Report_Fall_2003.pdf

Bellenghi, G.M. 2010. Outsourcing Release of Information Services: How to Build and Maintain a Vital Partnership [White paper]. Association of Health Information Outsourcing Services. http://www.ahios.org/pdf/AHIOS_WP_Outsourcing_ROI.pdf

Brassard, M. and D. Ritter. 2010. *The Memory Jogger II*, 2nd ed. Salem, NH: GOAL/QPC.

Cherry, K. 2015. Color Psychology: How Colors Impact Moods, Behaviors, and Feelings. http://psychology.about.com/od/sensationandperception/a/colorpsych.htm

Dunn. R.T. 2010. *Dunn & Haimann's Healthcare Management*. Chicago: HAP.

Faculty of Pain Medicine. n.d. Guidelines on Continuous Quality Improvement. http://www.fpm.anzca.edu.au/resources/educational-documents/documents/guidelines-on-continuous-quality-improvement.html#2-continuous-quality-improvement

Hiroyuki, H. 1989. *JIT implementation manual: The guide to just in time manufacturing*. Tokyo, Japan: JIT Management Laboratory Company, Ltd.

Institute for Healthcare Improvement (IHI). 2015. The IHI Triple Aim. http://www.ihi.org/engage/initiatives/tripleaim/Pages/default.aspx

Institute of Medicine. 2000. *To Err Is Human*. Washington, DC: National Academies Press.

iSixSigma. n.d. What is Six Sigma? http://www.isixsigma.com/new-to-six-sigma/getting-started/what-six-sigma/

Jones, D. and A. Mitchell. 2006. *Lean Thinking for the NHS*. A report commissioned by the NHS. http://www.leanuk.org/downloads/health/lean_thinking_for_the_nhs_leaflet.pdf

Lean Enterprise Institute. n.d. What is Lean? http://www.lean.org/WhatsLean/

Liebler, J.G. and C.R. McConnell. 2012. *Management Principles for Health Professionals*, 6th ed. Sudbury, MA: Jones & Bartlett Learning.

McConnell, C.R. 2014. *Umiker's Management Skills for the New Health Care Supervisor*. Burlington, MA: Jones & Bartlett.

Omachonu, V.K. 1999. *Healthcare Performance Improvement*. Norcross, GA: Engineering and Management Press.

Sharp, A. and P. McDermott. 2009. *Workflow Modeling: Tools for Process Improvement and Application Development*, 2nd ed. Norwood, MA: Arctech House.

Society for Human Resources Management. 2014. Shift Differential Policy. http://www.shrm.org/templatestools/samples/policies/pages/cms_022520.aspx

Society for Human Resources Management. 2008. Salaries as a Percentage of Operating Expense. http://www.shrm.org/research/articles/articles/pages/metricofthemonthsalariesaspercentageofoperatingexpense.aspx

Stone, J. 2015. Labor Law on Time Between Shifts. http://smallbusiness.chron.com/labor-law-time-between-shifts-73284.html

US Department of Health and Human Services. 2003. Business Associates. http://www.hhs.gov/hipaa/for-professionals/privacy/guidance/business-associates/index.html

US Department of Labor, Occupational Safety and Health Administration. n.d.(a). Computer Workstations eTool. https://www.osha.gov/SLTC/etools/computerworkstations/wkstation_enviro.html

US Department of Labor, Occupational Safety and Health Administration. n.d.(b). Ergonomics. https://www.osha.gov/SLTC/ergonomics/

Womack, J.P. and D.T. Jones. 1996. *Lean thinking: Banish waste and create wealth in your corporation*. New York: Simon and Schuster.

Zidel, T.G. 2006 (Jan.-Feb.). Quality toolbox: A Lean toolbox—using Lean principles and techniques in healthcare. *Journal for Healthcare Quality*—web exclusive. http://www.leanhospitals.com/downloads/JanFeb06.pdf

26

Financial Management

Rick Revoir, EdD, MBA, CPA and
Nadinia Davis, MBA, CIA, CPA, RHIA, FAHIMA

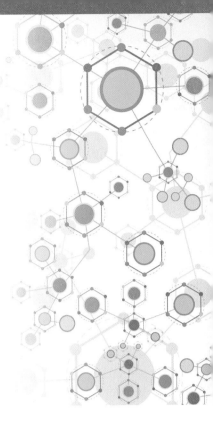

Learning Objectives

- Utilize balance sheets and income statements
- Differentiate between financial accounting and managerial accounting
- Recognize the importance of accounting to nonfinancial managers
- Calculate and identify the components of basic financial ratios
- Interpret basic financial ratio results in terms of organizational impact

- Explain the importance of internal controls and their role in financial management
- Describe the components of operational and capital budgets
- Discuss the impact of claims processing and reimbursement on financial statements
- Describe the financial management functions of HIM professionals

Key Terms

Accounting
Accounting rate of return (ARR)
Accounts payable
Accounts receivable
Accrue
Activity-based budget
Asset
Balance sheet
Capital budget
Centers for Medicare and Medicaid Services (CMS)
Conservatism

Consistency
Corporation
Cost accounting
Current ratio
Days in accounts receivable
Debt ratio
Debt service
Depreciation
Direct cost
Equity
Expense
Favorable variance

Financial Accounting Standards Board (FASB)
Fiscal year
Fixed budget
Fixed cost
Flexible budget
For-profit organization
General ledger
Generally accepted accounting principles (GAAP)
Going concern
Income statement

Indirect cost	Net present value (NPV)	Revenue Principle
Internal rate of return (IRR)	Not-for-profit organization	Securities and Exchange Commission (SEC)
Internal Revenue Service	Operational budget	
Liability	Overhead cost	Sole proprietorship
Liquidity	Partnership	Statement of cash flow
Managerial accounting	Payback period	Statement of retained earnings
Matching	Profitability	Statement of stockholder's equity
Materiality	Public Company Accounting	Total margin ratio
Net assets	Oversight Board (PCAOB)	Variable cost
Net income	Return on investment (ROI)	Variance
Net loss	Revenue	Zero-based budget

A physician treats a patient. A hospital admits a woman in labor. A professional association offers continuing education for its members. These scenarios are examples of organizations providing services for which they receive compensation. How organizations arrange to provide those services, determine compensation, and handle the flow of funds that these activities both require and generate is guided by financial management.

This chapter focuses on the concepts and tools associated with planning and controlling the financial resources required to operate a department or a work unit. It presents operations, labor, and capital budgeting processes and techniques; reviews organizational and departmental financial performance measures; and explores techniques for improving financial performance at the departmental level. Finally, the chapter acquaints readers with the language of financial and managerial accounting to enhance their understanding of the role of the health information management (HIM) professional as a manager.

Healthcare Financial Management

The process of financial management involves various players within the organization's financial arena. Table 26.1 lists and describes the roles of the financial personnel who work in hospitals. However, healthcare financial management also involves a number of players outside the financial arena. For example, HIM professionals are involved with reimbursement through the coding function. Record retention and release of information activities help support claims auditing and claims denial appeals. HIM professionals play an important role in clinical documentation improvement (CDI) activities, including clinical training to support medical necessity and reimbursement. Figure 26.1 illustrates the potential relationship between HIM and the financial personnel in a hospital.

HIM professionals are familiar with financial data as one of the components of a health record, or the data related to payers and billing. To financial managers, financial data are the individual elements of organizational financial transactions. (The term *financial* refers to money and, as is discussed later, money is the measurement of financial transactions.) A financial transaction is the exchange of goods or services for payment or the promise of payment. Financial data are compiled into informational reports for users. The degree of detail that users require depends on their needs and is largely influenced by the relationship of the user to the originator of the transaction.

Financial transactions that originate at the department level require review by that department. For example, the pharmacy department will review

Table 26.1. Financial personnel and their roles in a hospital

Position	Typical or minimum background	Financial roles
Board of directors or trustees	Depends on the needs of the facility	Ultimate responsibility for the fiscal integrity of the organization
Chief executive officer (CEO)	Master's degree prepared in public administration, hospital administration, or business administration; occasionally, clinical background	Overall responsibility for administration of the organization
Chief information officer (CIO)	Bachelor's degree and often a master's degree in information technology or a master's of business administration	Overall responsibility for information systems and HIM
Chief financial officer (CFO)	Bachelor's degree and certified public accountant (CPA) or certified management accountant (CMA)	Overall responsibility for related departments, including patient accounts, accounting, decision support, and internal auditing
Controller or accounting manager	Bachelor's degree and CPA	Oversees accounting and cash disbursement, including payroll
Patient accounts manager	Bachelor's degree	Oversees claims processing

its drug transactions, and the HIM department will review its purchases of supplies and services. On the administrative level, however, such detail is not usually required. Instead, informative summaries are often more useful. For example, an organization administrator does not usually need to know the number of cases of copier paper purchased in each department. Instead, he or she would look at the total office supply purchases and evaluate whether they were at appropriate and expected levels. Additional detail or explanation would not be required unless the purchases were unusual. The accumulation and reporting of financial data within an organization are accounting functions.

Accounting

Accounting is an activity as well as a profession. Just as there are many HIM roles and functions, so are there diverse accounting roles and functions. The accounting activity involves the collection, recording, and reporting of financial data. Accountants are both the individuals who perform these activities and many of those who use the reported data. Accounting is important because it is the language that organizations use to communicate with each other to record transactions, determine investment strategies, and evaluate performance.

The conceptual framework of accounting underlies all accounting activity and is based on the following ideas:

- The benefits of having financial data should exceed the costs of obtaining them.
- The data must be understandable.
- The data must be useful for decision making.

In other words, the data must be relevant, reliable, and comparable.

Although some of these requirements are similar to general data quality concerns, they are discussed specifically with financial data in mind.

Accounting Concepts and Principles

Concepts and principles that define the parameters of accounting activity are briefly discussed here and summarized in figure 26.2.

Concepts

An entity is a person or an organization such as a corporation or professional association. When analysis of an entity's financial data shows that the organization can continue to operate for the foreseeable future, the organization is considered a going concern. Assuming that a business is going

Figure 26.1.   Organization of the nonphysician side of the hospital

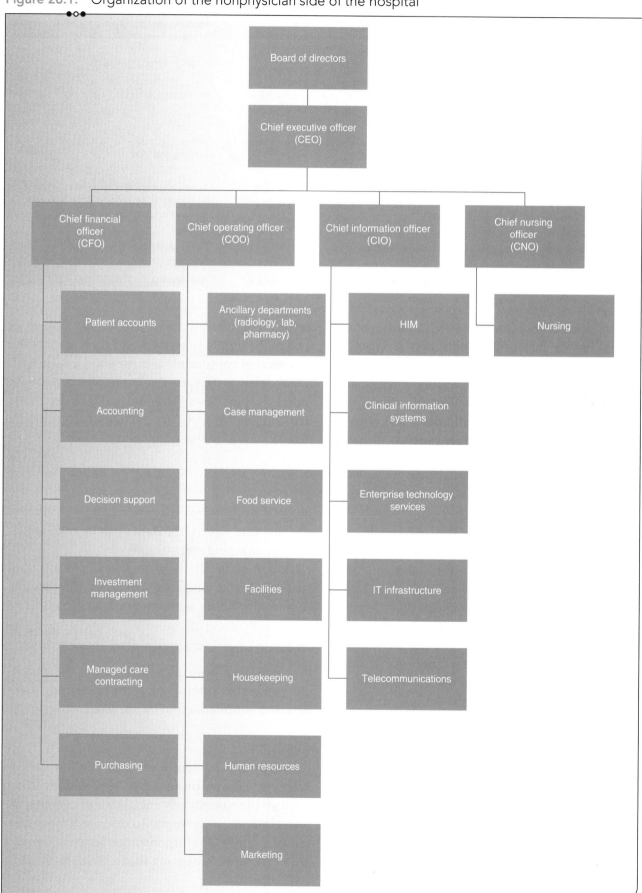

Figure 26.2. Basic accounting concepts and principles

Basic accounting concepts

- *Entity:* The financial data of different entities are kept separate.
- *Going concern:* Organizations are assumed to continue indefinitely, unless otherwise stated.
- *Stable monetary unit:* Money is the measurement of financial transactions.
- *Time period:* Financial data represent a specified time period.
- *Conservatism:* Resources must not be overstated, and liabilities must not be understated.
- *Materiality:* The financial data collected by an organization are relevant to its goals and objectives.

Basic accounting principles

- *Reliability:* Amounts represent the transactions that occurred.
- *Cost:* Transactions are recorded at historical cost.
- *Revenue:* In order to record revenue, it must be earned and measurable.
- *Matching:* Expenses are recorded in the same period as the related revenue.
- *Consistency:* When an accounting rule is followed, all subsequent periods must reflect the same rule.
- *Disclosure:* Financial reports must be accompanied by helpful explanations, when necessary.

---

to continue, projections of future activities can be made based on historical trends and assumptions about future conditions. The concept of going concern also places constraints on the organization to maintain sufficient financial and other resources to ensure future stability and growth.

All of an entity's transactions must be quantified using a standard measurement or stable monetary unit. In the United States, financial transactions are recorded in US dollars and cents.

Financial data represent transactions during a specified period of time: hour, day, week, month, quarter, year, and so on. The specific time period depends on the use of the data. The **fiscal year** (also called the financial year) is defined by the tax year. Individuals generally have a tax year that coincides with the calendar year. Organizations, on the other hand, use fiscal years that correspond to their business needs, usually their business cycle, representing the total activities of the organization. Many not-for-profit healthcare organizations have a June 30th fiscal year end.

For financial reporting purposes, a fiscal year is divided into quarters (three-month periods) and months. Because the months generally end on the last calendar day, the quarters can be of slightly different duration. For example, the first quarter of a fiscal year that begins April 1 includes April, May, and June: 91 days. The second quarter of that same fiscal year includes July, August, and September: 92 days. Over time, it is common to compare similar quarters from year to year, particularly when the business cycle has predictable peaks and valleys.

Not all financial data represent completed transactions within the period represented. Sometimes estimates are involved, or transactions are completed between periods. When amounts are estimated, efforts must be made to ensure that their use does not misrepresent the actual financial transaction. Therefore, financial data must comply with **conservatism** in that they fairly represent the financial results of the period and do not overstate or understate information in a significant (material) way.

Materiality refers to the thresholds below which items are not considered significant for reporting purposes. These thresholds may be a dollar value or a percentage of a dollar value. For example, if an organization made a $10,000 error in estimating bad debt expense, this error would be material for a company that has $100,000 in expenses but the error would be immaterial to an organization that has $1 billion in expenses. An item is material when it could affect the decision making of anyone using the financial statements. This issue arises when determining the significance of errors, potential liabilities, and the necessity for disclosures.

Principles

Accounting principles support the quality of financial data. Because they are data, financial data must possess the same data quality characteristics, such as timeliness and validity, as any other type of data. In financial data, reliability refers to whether the data actually represent what occurred and are free of material error both in the current period and over time. Transactions are recorded at their historical cost measured at the time of the transaction. For some transactions, such as the purchase of equipment or investment in marketable securities, such as stock or shares in a company, there may be a change in the actual or perceived value of the underlying asset or liability. In those cases, adjustments or disclosures are made when reporting the financial data. The Revenue Principle states that earnings as a result of activities and investments may only be recognized when they have been earned, can be measured, and have a reasonable expectation of being collected. For an organization to generate revenue, it must incur expenses; for example, payroll, rent, travel, and raw materials. Whenever possible, expenses are recorded in the same period as the associated revenue, thereby matching the expenses and revenues. Some accounting rules include variations. The principle of consistency requires that the method not change over the life of the asset. Thus, the financial data are prepared in the same way from one period to the next. In fact, organizations sometimes change their choices. Consistency then requires that financial data be restated to show the effect of the change applied to previous periods. Interestingly, some allowed financial accounting rules differ from tax accounting rules, producing different results. Sometimes the financial data alone do not provide enough information for users of the data to make informed decisions. The impact of a building fire, a potential or ongoing lawsuit, or an expiring collective bargaining agreement cannot be reflected in the financial data when no financial transaction has occurred. Therefore, notes or disclosures that help the user to make informed decisions must accompany all financial reports.

Authorities

Just as clinical data are organized and reported in predetermined formats for ease of communication, financial data also are organized and reported in specific ways. Theoretically, organizations can design their own accounting systems and reporting mechanisms. Internally, this is often the case, as will be seen with budgeting. However, organizations that want to borrow funds or attract investors must follow generally accepted rules that apply to their industry and accounting in general. Five major sources of accounting and reporting rules apply to healthcare organizations: the Financial Accounting Standards Board (FASB), Securities and Exchange Commission (SEC), Internal Revenue Service (IRS), Public Company Accounting Oversight Board (PCAOB), and Centers for Medicare and Medicaid Services (CMS).

Financial Accounting Standards Board

The **Financial Accounting Standards Board (FASB)** is an independent organization that sets accounting standards for businesses in the private sector. Its counterpart, the Government Accounting Standards Board (GASB), sets standards for accounting for government entities. The FASB makes the rules by which financial data are compiled, reported, reviewed, and audited publicly known. These rules, which include the conceptual framework, are referred to as **generally accepted accounting principles (GAAP)** and generally accepted auditing standards (GAAS).

Securities and Exchange Commission

The **Securities and Exchange Commission (SEC)** is a federal agency that regulates public and some private transactions involving the ownership and debt of organizations. The SEC sets standards regarding reporting financial data, disclosures, timing, marketing, and execution of these transactions. Public transactions take place through an exchange, such as the New York Stock Exchange (NYSE) or the National Association of Securities Dealers Automated Quotation System (NASDAQ). Organizations whose ownership interests (stocks) are traded on these exchanges are called public companies.

Internal Revenue Service

The tax status of an organization influences its administration. The **Internal Revenue Service (IRS)** regulates and collects federal taxes. Healthcare organizations fall into one of two major tax categories: for-profit and not-for-profit. The primary differences between for-profit and not-for-profit organizations are related to the level of accountability and the distribution of profits. Within these categories are several legal structures, such as sole proprietorship, partnership, and corporation. A summary of legal structures is provided in table 26.2.

Public Company Accounting Oversight Board

Historically, the accounting profession has been largely self-regulated. The FASB and GASB, although technically independent, have strong ties to the profession. Although IRS and SEC standards and regulations constrained the specific representation of financial activities, the accounting profession was free to accomplish its reporting and other activities without government intervention. However, that changed in 2002. The federal government responded to the collapse of ENRON, WorldCom, and others with the Sarbanes-Oxley Act, which restricted the professional services of independent auditors of public companies and, among other things, created the **Public Company Accounting Oversight Board (PCAOB)** that oversees the audits of companies that are publicly traded. Sarbanes-Oxley had a significant impact on the degree of scrutiny and testing of internal controls, financial reporting, and governance of organizations.

Centers for Medicare and Medicaid Services

Formerly called the Health Care Financing Administration (HCFA), the **Centers for Medicare and Medicaid Services (CMS)** is the federal agency that administers the Medicare program and the federal portion of the Medicaid program. The federal government is the largest single payer of healthcare expenses in the United States. Although CMS does not set accounting rules, it enforces the federal regulations regarding the reimbursement for Medicare and the federal portion of the Medicaid program, and sets standards for the documentation and reporting of transactions related to such reimbursement. Since CMS requires significant reporting from participant organizations, its influence on financial activities and data collection should not be underestimated.

Financial Organization

The way an entity organizes itself depends on its financing, leadership, and tax status. The three basic forms of business organization are the sole proprietorship, the partnership, and the corporation. Other organizational entities, such as trusts and variations like limited liability corporations (LLCs), are beyond the scope of this discussion.

Table 26.2. Common legal structures of nongovernmental organizations

Structure	Description	Healthcare examples
Sole proprietorship (for profit only)	One owner; all profits are owner's personal income	Solo practitioners
Partnership	Two or more owners; all profits are owners' personal income	Physician group practices
Corporation	One or many owners; profits may be either retained or distributed as dividends. Dividends are income to the owners. May be public or private. "Owners" may be individuals, other organizations, or an interest group.	Hospitals, insurance companies

- **Sole proprietorship**: An independent coding consultant who operates from home and has no employees may choose to operate as a sole proprietor. The owner, or proprietor, is the leader of the organization and is responsible for all aspects of the business. Income from the business flows through the owner's individual tax return. If the consultant's business expands, employees or subcontractors can be added without changing the organizational structure. Some physicians are solo practitioners and therefore sole proprietors.

- **Partnership**: Two or more consultants who want to be in business together may choose a partnership structure. Partners share in the responsibility for the business, and income still flows through the individuals' tax returns. Partners do not need to share equally in the financial or other business responsibilities. A partnership agreement details the contractual arrangement. Because a partnership is a separate legal and accounting entity from the individuals, a tax identification number is required for the partnership, and the partnership may be required to file its own tax returns detailing the income allocated to each partner. Partnerships survive as entities only so long as the partners remain together. A change in ownership dissolves the original partnership and a new one must be created.

- **Corporation**: A corporation is a legal entity that exists separately from its owner(s). Corporations pay their own taxes and have their own legal rights and responsibilities. In fact, the owner(s) of the corporation may have nothing to do with its leadership or day-to-day operations. A corporation is typically governed by a board of directors or trustees, and the day-to-day operations are led by one or more administrators who report to the board. The corporation's income after taxes may or may not be distributed in whole or in part to the owner(s). This after-tax distribution is a dividend and is taxable income to the owner(s). This two-tiered taxation, on the corporation and then again on the distributed dividend, is referred to as double taxation

and may make this structure less attractive to individuals.

The underlying purpose of the organization drives another consideration in the financial organization of the business. Is the purpose of the business to generate income for the owners, or is there a more altruistic foundation? The answer to this question helps to define the tax status the organization will be able to obtain.

For-Profit Organizations

For-profit organizations may be sole proprietorships, partnerships, or corporations. In this context, profits are the funds remaining after all current obligations have been met, including taxes. Inherently, the underlying goal of for-profit organizations is to increase the wealth of the owners. Increase in wealth can be accomplished through the generation of profits to be distributed to the owners or by increasing the value of the organization so that the owners' investment is more valuable. The leadership of the organization may distribute the profits to the owners or otherwise invest them as they see fit. For-profit organizations may be privately or publicly owned.

Private ownership may be by an individual, a group of individuals, or an organization. Physician practices, urgent care centers, and freestanding ancillary care organizations are often privately owned. The distribution of profits from a privately owned organization is at the discretion of the owners or as defined by contract among owners.

Public ownership means that the ownership interest in the organization may be bought and sold in the financial marketplace. For example, Tenet Healthcare Corporation (THC) is a publicly held organization with hospitals in numerous states. Its stock is traded on the NYSE under the symbol *THC*. A publicly held organization's board of directors determines the distribution of profits. Boards are constrained in these determinations by contractual obligations such as mortgage contracts and preferred stock obligations, stockholder expectations, and strategic organizational goals.

Not-for-Profit Organizations

Not-for-profit organizations are not owned but, instead, are held in trust for the benefit of the communities they serve. Many hospitals fall into this tax category. Other not-for-profit organizations include professional associations such as the American Health Information Management Association (AHIMA), charitable organizations such as the American Red Cross, and educational foundations such as the AHIMA Foundation. The IRS defines numerous types of not-for-profit organizations, some of which are summarized in table 26.3. The two categories of not-for-profit organizations discussed here are 501(c)(6) and 501(c)(3).

501(c)(6) Most professional associations are organized under 501(c)(6), which gives them some federal tax benefits and the freedom to engage in some activities unrelated to their organizational purpose. For example, organizations under 501(c)(6) may lobby and sell goods and services but are largely involved in activities that benefit their major interest group, which may be defined as paid membership. Such organizations may be subject to state sales tax, both as purchaser and seller. AHIMA and most of its component state associations are 501(c)(6) organizations.

501(c)(3) On the other hand, 501(c)(3) organizations are largely exempt from federal taxes but must confine their activities to the public benefit. Donations to 501(c)(3) organizations are generally tax deductible (for the donor) to the extent that no goods or services have been received in return. For that reason, charities are generally 501(c)(3) organizations, and many 501(c)(6)

organizations have charitable components that are separately incorporated. For example, AHIMA is a 501(c)(6) organization that has a 501(c)(3) component, the AHIMA Foundation. Organizations classified as 501(c)(3) may also be exempt from state sales tax under certain circumstances.

Tax Status Issues

It is important to understand the underlying tax status of an organization because tax status affects the organization's business decisions and long-term strategies. Undistributed profits from a for-profit organization may stay in the business and be available for investment or future distribution. There is no necessity to identify the future use for these funds, although stockholders may ultimately press for distribution when undistributed profits appear excessive. Occasionally, portions of undistributed profits are held in reserve for specific uses.

On the other hand, profits from a not-for-profit organization stay in the business. Because all such profits must be used for the benefit of the community the organization serves, the future use of these profits should be clearly defined. Excessive unrelated business income or high unrestricted reserves (effectively, too much savings) may result in the loss of not-for-profit status. For further information about tax exemptions of organizations, see IRS Publication 557 (IRS 2015).

Sources of Financial Data

Just as a health record is constructed from the data collected, financial records are also composed of

Table 26.3. Common not-for-profit tax statuses

Not-for-profit	Description	Healthcare examples
501(c)(3)	Largely exempt from taxes, donations to these organizations can be tax deductible. Underlying purpose of the organization must be charitable or educational.	Charities, AHIMA Foundation, many healthcare organizations
501(c)(6)	Partially exempt from taxes. May lobby and sell goods and services. Underlying purpose must benefit the interest group or public.	Professional associations
501(c)(4)	Business leagues	N/A
501(c)(14)	Credit unions	N/A
501(c)(19)	Veterans' organizations	N/A

data. Health records are built from medical decision making; financial records originate with financial decision making, the smallest component of which is the transaction.

Transactions

Virtually every financial transaction consists of three fundamental steps:

1. Goods or services are provided.
2. A transaction is recorded.
3. Compensation is exchanged.

Each step may require a number of additional steps, depending on the service and the industry. In addition, the steps are not always performed in the same order. Independent contractors that perform hospital coding represent a simple example. The contractor codes the charts, submits an invoice, and receives a check from the hospital. In this case, four specific steps may be needed to support the transaction: keeping a log to track the charts that have been coded, preparing an invoice to bill the hospital, keeping a list of the invoices sent, and checking the invoices off when they are received.

In a hospital, multiple individuals and departments perform services and provide administrative support for financial transactions. Four areas are of particular concern in the context of this discussion: clinical services, patient accounts, health information management, and administration.

Clinical Services Just as contract coders keep track of the records they have coded, clinical or patient care services providers also keep track of the services they perform. The documents of original entry or source documents enable the healthcare facility to verify that the services were provided and communicate to supporting departments that a transaction has been initiated. The source document includes two elements—the clinical documentation and the billing documentation.

Clinical documentation is a record of who has seen the patient, which tests or treatments were performed, and why these tests and treatment were administered; in other words, everything clinically relevant that happened to the patient during his or her interaction with the organization.

Along with the recording of clinical documentation is the capture of the associated billing information. Regardless of the reimbursement system (discussed in chapter 7), the organization must capture the billable event in such a way that the financial transaction can be completed. Therefore, when a medication is administered to a patient, the clinical record reflects the medication; dosage; time, date, and route of administration; and the clinical personnel who administered it. At the same time, the charge for the drug must be communicated to patient accounts. This detailed tracking of billable events also supports the cost accounting function, which is discussed later in this chapter.

Patient Accounts The patient accounts department is responsible for collecting recorded transactions, billing the payer (generating the claim), and ensuring the correct receipt of reimbursement. This department depends on the reliable recording of services. This means that the capture of billing information must be timely and accurate in order to complete the financial transaction efficiently. In addition to the clinical support staff and departments, the patient accounts department relies on the HIM professionals for coded data.

Health Information Management HIM professionals are responsible for identifying and recording the appropriate clinical codes to describe the patient's interaction with the organization. In some cases, this coding drives the reimbursement to the facility; in other cases, it is used to support the billing. In addition to the coding activity, HIM professionals are responsible for aggregating and maintaining the documentation that supports the reimbursement.

Administration Financial transactions occur throughout the facility. Employees are paid, equipment and supplies are purchased, and departments perform services for each other. The finance department accumulates and analyzes all of the financial data. Ultimately, the entire management team participates in the review and analysis of financial data.

Uses of Financial Data

Financial data are generated virtually everywhere in a healthcare facility. Managerial and supervisory personnel use these data for four key purposes—tracking reimbursement, controlling costs, planning future activities, and forecasting results.

Reimbursement

Healthcare facilities are service organizations that derive almost all their income from clinical activities. Therefore, a key use of financial data is to track reimbursement and ensure that the desired amount of profit is generated. In the current industry environment where payers often dictate the amount of reimbursement, the provider is increasingly unable to control pricing as a method of managing desired profit. Therefore, the cost of providing services has become the controllable factor.

Control

Controlling costs is best done at the departmental level. For example, the chief executive officer (CEO) of a hospital does not shop around for the best price on copier paper, and the chief financial officer (CFO) does not monitor employee productivity in the food services department. Each department is charged with responsibility for ensuring prudent management of financial and other resources. Departments are given this charge through the budget process, which is one of the outcomes of administrative planning.

Planning

Administrative planning reflects the organization's mission. From that mission, goals and objectives are derived that help move the organization toward achieving its mission. Financial data are used to analyze trends, develop budgets, and plan for the future. Planning cannot be accomplished by using historical data alone because the industry changes, sometimes rapidly. Therefore, the administration must forecast future scenarios.

Forecasting

Forecasting is the prediction of future behavior based on historical data as well as environmental scans. It can be as simple as predicting the profits of an organization on the basis of anticipated changes in reimbursement. It also can involve complicated predictions of consumer behavior based on market research and news reports.

Check Your Understanding 26.1

Instructions: Answer the following questions on a separate piece of paper.

1. If an insurance company representative contacted the HIM department about a claims audit, to which financial personnel should he or she be directed and why?

2. What is the tax exempt status of many healthcare organizations?

3. Big Medical Center earned a lot more revenue than expected this year but does not expect to earn as much next year. To make the financial reports more consistent, a junior accountant suggests that the hospital record some of next year's expenses this year. Would you agree or disagree that this is a good strategy? Why?

4. Explain how an organization's fiscal year may vary from a calendar year.

5. If a hospital has excess coding or transcription staff, can the hospital sell coding or transcription services to other hospitals (based on what has been covered so far in this chapter)? Why or why not?

Basic Financial Accounting

A basic understanding of the mechanics of financial accounting helps department managers to understand the impact of their financial transactions on the overall organization. The system of recording financial transactions is based on balancing the *purpose* of the transactions with their impact on the organization. For example, a facility purchases drugs with the purpose of ensuring that sufficient and appropriate drugs are on hand to treat patients. The purchase of the drugs increases the facility's pharmaceutical inventory. The impact of that purchase is the outlay of cash. After the cash is spent on drugs, it cannot be spent on something else. Recording both the increase in inventory and the outlay of cash enables the organization to understand and communicate information about its activities. Fundamental to this communication is an understanding of the components of financial data and their relationship to each other.

Assets

An **asset** is something that is owned or due to be received. In a transaction, the compensation that has been earned by providing goods or services becomes an asset as soon as it has been earned. Examples of assets include cash, inventory, accounts receivable, buildings, and equipment.

Cash

Cash consists of monetary instruments, including those instruments that can be converted into cash quickly. Those that can be converted to cash, for example Treasury bills, are often referred to as cash equivalents. Included in cash are funds that are maintained in bank accounts. It is important to remember that for accounting purposes currency and bank accounts are both considered cash. At the point of sale, such as purchasing lunch in the cafeteria, currency may be tendered. CMS, on the other hand, does not deliver reimbursement to a hospital in truckloads of currency; instead, it wires funds between financial institutions. Nevertheless,

both are considered cash to the hospital. Cash is only recorded, and becomes an asset, when it has been received.

Inventory

An organization has inventory if it maintains goods on hand that it intends to sell to a client. Drugs are part of a hospital's pharmaceutical inventory because they are effectively on hand to be sold to patients. It is important to distinguish between goods that are available for sale and goods that are used by the organization in other ways. Photocopy paper is inventory to the office supply store. To the hospital HIM department, it is used for general business purposes and is considered a supply. In this case, the hospital is the client (the consumer of the goods). Because hospitals are primarily service organizations, and the provision of goods is incidental to the services provided, hospitals tend not to have a great deal of inventory other than supplies.

Accounts Receivable

When an organization has delivered goods or services, payment is expected. Remember that the second step in a transaction is to record the transaction. Because the revenue has been earned upon delivery or a provision of the goods and services, the organization must have some way to keep track of what is owed as a result. **Accounts receivable** then is merely a list of the amounts due from various customers (in this case, patients). Payment on the individual amounts is expected within a specified period. A schedule of those expected amounts is prepared in order to track and follow up on payments that are overdue (late). Figure 26.3 shows one way to prepare a simple aged accounts receivables report. One can use this report to prioritize follow-up efforts on the accounts that are most delayed (for example, those greater than 120 days overdue) or those accounts that that are the highest dollar amount despite the aging (for example, accounts over $250 such as the two accounts noted

Figure 26.3. Aged accounts receivable

A/C #	D/C	SER	0–30 days	31–60 days	61–90 days	91–120 days	>120 days	Total A/R
46153153	04/15/16	ED					149	
46160492	07/06/16	ED				25		
46162518	07/31/16	REC			10			
46162874	08/31/16	REC			30			
46163484	08/07/16	ED					165	
46162580	07/30/16	ED				114		
46125122	06/19/16	OP					16	
46160520	07/06/16	ED				50		
46169245	10/09/16	OP	175					
46165628	09/30/16	REC		266				
46163713	08/12/16	OP			52			
46166048	09/04/16	ED		280				
46161964	07/23/16	OP				94		
46162506	07/30/16	OP				94		
46164953	08/25/16	OP			52			
46169231	10/09/16	ED	25					
46157104	05/30/16	ED					50	
46124652	06/15/15	OBN					84	
46126673	07/09/15	OP					148	
46122161	05/20/15	OP					207	
Total amounts			**$200**	**$546**	**$144**	**$377**	**$819**	**$2,086**
Total number of accounts			**2**	**2**	**4**	**5**	**7**	**20**

Source: Adapted from Schraffenberger 2011, 459.

under the 31 to 60 days column). This report could be sorted by discharge date or payer and the amounts subtotaled.

Building

Many organizations own the buildings in which they reside. These buildings are assets to the organization because they are part of its physical plant, its infrastructure. If an organization leases space for its operations, that space is not considered an asset because the organization does not own it. Buildings are considered long-term assets because they are typically owned for many years.

Equipment

Equipment is another long-term asset. Hospitals include CT scanners, computer systems, and ve-hicles in this category. Each organization decides what items are relevant to this category, depending on industry conventions and materiality. For example, a large hospital would rarely consider a $500 personal computer to be equipment, whereas an independent coding consultant might view it as a significant, long-term investment.

Purchase Price In acquiring a piece of equipment (and certain other assets), the transaction is recorded at the purchase price. For example, the hospital purchases digital mammography equipment for $200,000. The hospital then would have a $200,000 asset in equipment. However, the equipment gradually wears out from use over time. That $200,000 asset is not worth $200,000 four years after it was purchased. To provide better information about the financial value of its equipment, the organization provides an estimate of this decrease in value every year. This estimate is called **depreciation**.

Depreciation Depreciation is an example of a contra-account. This estimate of the cumulative decrease in value of an asset actually reduces the cost of the underlying asset. Thus, the mammography equipment purchased for $200,000 may have an accumulated depreciation of $75,000 after two years. At that point, its remaining book value to the organization is $125,000. The following shows this illustration:

Mammograph	$200,000
Accumulated depreciation	$75,000
Book value	$125,000

Liabilities

Liabilities are debts. They are amounts that are owed, often due to the acquisition of an asset. Examples of liabilities include accounts payable, loans payable, and mortgages.

Accounts Payable

Accounts payable is a liability that is created when the organization has received goods or services but has not yet remitted the compensation (that is, paid for the goods or services). Referring to the accounts receivable discussion, the provider of the goods and services records a receivable when payment is not received at the point of the sale. On the other side of that transaction is the organization for which the goods and services were provided. When the recipient of the goods and services does not intend to pay immediately, the amount is recorded by the recipient as an account payable. The recipient also records either the acquisition of an asset or the recognition of an expense (discussed later in this chapter).

Loans Payable

A loan is an amount an organization has borrowed that will be repaid over a specified time period. The creation of the loan may be associated with

the purchase of goods or services, and the material goods may be guaranteed by the value of specific assets (collateral). For example, the organization may need $50,000 more than it has on hand in order to purchase a CT scanner. It might take a two-year loan from the bank (or the vendor), using the scanner as collateral meaning that if the organization does not pay the loan back on a timely basis, the lender is entitled by contract to take possession of the scanner.

Mortgage

A mortgage is a liability that is created when the organization borrows money and uses a physical asset, such as a building, as collateral. Organizations may use a mortgage to finance the construction of a clinic or building. Individuals obtain a mortgage to finance the purchase of a home.

Equity and Net Assets

All financial accounting is based on an equation that pictures the organization holistically, balancing what is owned against what is owed: assets versus liabilities. **Equity** (or owner's equity) is the arithmetic difference between assets and liabilities. In a not-for-profit environment, the difference between assets and liabilities is referred to as **net assets**. These relationships can be expressed in the following equation:

$$\text{Assets} - \text{liabilities} = \text{net assets (equity)}$$

The purchase of a building illustrates this equation. The purchase of a house typically involves a deposit of cash and an assumption of a mortgage. The building is an asset whose value is, historically, the price that was paid at the time of the purchase. The mortgage is a liability. As mortgage payments are made, the amount of the mortgage owed declines. The deposit of cash is the owner's equity in the building. As mortgage payments are made, the amount of owner's equity in the building increases. For example, Dr. James purchases an office building for $200,000. She makes a down payment (or deposit) of $50,000 and assumes a mortgage of $150,000. As the mortgage is paid over 30 years, the historical value of the house remains the same, the amount of the mortgage decreases, and the owner's equity in the property increases. When the mortgage is completely paid, the owner's equity in the house equals the historical value of the house, as shown here:

	Assets		Liabilities		Equity
At purchase	$200,000	–	$150,000	=	$ 50,000
After 10 years	$200,000	–	$100,000	=	$100,000
After 20 years	$200,000	–	$ 50,000	=	$150,000
After 30 years	$200,000	–	–0–	=	$200,000

Earlier, it was stated that an equation balances what is owned and what is owed. Therefore, another way to look at the accounting equation is:

Assets = liabilities + net assets (equity)

Using the previous mortgage example, the second version of the equation proves useful. At every step in the following calculation, the equations balance. An increase in assets increases equity. A decrease in assets decreases equity. An increase in assets with an equal increase in liabilities has no impact on equity. Notice that increasing a liability reduces equity in the same manner that decreasing an asset does.

	Assets		Liabilities		Equity
At purchase	$200,000	=	$150,000	+	$ 50,000
After 10 years	$200,000	=	$100,000	+	$100,000
After 20 years	$200,000	=	$ 50,000	+	$150,000
After 30 years	$200,000	=	–0–	+	$200,000

Assets, liabilities, and equity are the components of the balance sheet (discussed later in this chapter). First, it is important to understand the revenue and expense components of financial information.

Revenue

Revenue consists of earned, known amounts. It is the compensation that has been earned by providing goods and services to the client or patient as well as amounts received or earned from other sources.

Sources of Revenue

Patient services is the main source of revenue for a healthcare facility. Indeed, depending on the nature of the facility, patient services may be its only source of revenue. Examples of nonclinical services that are a source of revenue include employee food services, donated services, monetary donations, and copy fees.

Categories of Revenue

How an organization describes its revenue depends on industry convention, materiality, and whether the revenue is recurring or unusual. Revenue from any source increases equity. A coding consultant works for a week at a client hospital and earns $1,500. He receives a check from the hospital and deposits it in his bank account. This increases his cash asset by the amount of the deposit: $1,500. The increase in the asset, absent an associated liability, increases equity by the same amount. Most organizations can group their revenue sources into at least two categories—operating and nonoperating.

Operating Revenue   A hospital considers patient services revenue to be operating revenue. Because the hospital is in the business of serving patients, patient services is its main source of revenue and thus falls under the heading of operating revenue. Consider food services. Inpatients must be fed, so food services is a patient service and thus an operating expense. The employee cafeteria also generates revenue, but the revenue it generates is unrelated to patient services. In the HIM department, small revenue streams may be generated through release of information activities or through contracting services out to other facilities. Since the pricing of these activities is generally cost based, it is more appropriately thought of as an offset or quasi-reimbursement of the underlying cost.

Nonoperating Revenue   A hospital with a large endowment that generates significant income may want to highlight this investment revenue in a separate category. Investment income is one example of nonoperating income. Other examples include gift shop sales and unrestricted monetary donations.

Expenses

It is unlikely that revenue is generated without any reduction of cash or liability being incurred. The coding consultant in the previous example must purchase coding software, travel from home to the client and back, and engage in continuing education (CE). **Expenses**, then, represent the utilization of resources by the organization in order to generate revenue. The consultant coder uses cash to purchase coding software. The software helps to generate revenue for one year, at which time it expires. Therefore, the price of the software is an expense to the coder.

The simple example that follows in table 26.4 illustrates the impact on the accounting equation of the financial transactions discussed thus far. The chart shows how one's financial transactions affect one's equity; as liabilities are subtracted from one's assets, equity or net assets is calculated. This individual began with a balance in assets of $1,500; after purchase of a codebook, payment of health insurance, attendance at a CE session, and purchase of a computer with $200 cash down, total assets equal $3,520. Subtracting $800 on credit for the computer (liability), this person has net assets or equity of $2,720.

Purchasing

As previously stated, healthcare organizations typically cannot affect revenue by raising prices, so they must attempt to control expenses as much as possible. One way to do this is through the purchasing function. Individuals responsible for purchasing activities must adhere to their facility's policies and procedures, which may vary somewhat from the basic descriptions in this section.

Organizations handle the purchasing function differently depending on their size and needs. Large organizations tend to maintain a central purchasing and distribution department that is responsible for the acquisition of supplies and equipment.

Significant savings can be obtained by purchasing supplies in bulk and distributing them as needed to departments. Central purchasing also has the benefit of minimizing the space required for storage of items on hand. Central purchasing systems should be designed to minimize the risk of loss due to misappropriation of stored items. The periodic comparison, by counting, of items on hand with the items recorded and the itemized distribution of stored items can assist in this process.

In order to obtain the benefits of purchasing in large quantities, some facilities combine their purchasing efforts. Hospital associations, for example, may offer coordinated purchasing on behalf of multiple facilities. Nevertheless, the control over the use of the items remains with the department.

Maintaining a central purchasing and distribution department results in direct administrative costs to the organization (for example, salary, facility maintenance, and administrative processing). Therefore, the control benefits of centralized purchasing must be weighed against the cost of such operations. Savings also can be obtained by limiting the source of supplies to one or two key vendors who offer discounts to the organization. In this scenario, department managers would order items as needed, but only from approved vendors.

Finally, an organization may choose to allow individual departments to make purchases independently. Although this can result in additional

Table 26.4. Impact on accounting equation

October activity					
	Assets	–	**Liabilities**	=	**Equity**
Beginning balance	$1,500	–	–0–	=	$1,500
Purchase codebook	<100>	–		=	<100>
Pay health insurance	<100>	–		=	<100>
Receive payment from client	$1,200	–		=	$1,200
Purchase computer (on credit)	<200>	–	800	=	<1,000>
Receive payment from client	$1,300	–		=	$1,300
Attend CE session	<80>	–		=	<80>
Ending balance	$3,520	–	800	=	$2,720

supply and equipment costs, there may be overall savings in not maintaining a central purchasing department. The major disadvantages of independent, or decentralized, purchasing are the need for supply storage space in the ordering department and the allocation of managerial resources to purchasing.

Regardless of the purchasing system used, controls must be in place to ensure the efficient execution of approved transactions. Purchase orders, shipping and receiving documents, and invoices are the key controls over the purchase process.

Purchase Orders The purchase order system ensures that purchases have been properly authorized prior to ordering. Authorization is often tied to dollar limits or the budget process. Purchase orders are numbered sequentially so that all orders can be verified. In a paper environment, a purchase order is a paper form on which all details of the intended purchase are reported. Purchase orders for routine, budgeted items often require only the authorization of a supervisor or manager. For large-dollar items, as specified in the organization's policy and procedure manual, additional authorization may be required. In a computer-based system, there may be no physical form; however, authorization levels are still required.

The purchase order shows that the appropriate individual with the appropriate authorization ordered the specific items. The order is then forwarded to the vendor. The originator of the order keeps a copy and another copy is sent to the accounts payable department. When there is a central receiving department, that department also should receive a copy of the order. In a computer-based system, access to the orders may suffice.

Shipping and Receiving Documents Items received from a vendor contain a packing slip, also known as a shipping and receiving document. This document lists the quantities and descriptions of the items sent from the vendor, but not usually the price. The recipient of the items must verify that the items received match the ones that were ordered. The verified shipping and receiving document is forwarded to accounts payable.

Invoices The vendor sends an invoice (bill or request for payment) directly to accounts payable. The accounts payable department matches the invoice to the shipping and receiving document and the purchase order on file. When all the documents match, the invoice can be processed and payment scheduled. Invoices generally have terms: for example, payable upon receipt or within 30 days. Some vendors offer discounts for early payment, such as "2/10, net 30," which means that the seller will grant a 2 percent discount for payment within 10 days; otherwise, the full amount is due within 30 days. Other terms may include interest charges for late payment. The facility's accounting department has to balance expected payments (receivables) with obligations (payables). Departments such as HIM often receive invoices directly; it is important to forward all invoices to the accounting department immediately upon receipt and verification so that accounting has the information it needs to make appropriate and timely decisions about payment.

Statements A statement is a list of outstanding invoices the vendor has sent but for which no payment has been received. Some companies send statements that include all activity for the period, including payment. The statement is one way the vendor lets the customer know that payments are late. Statements are not payable without supporting documentation. When there is no purchase order, receiving document, and invoice, accounts payable will not remit payment.

Statements received for which there is no underlying documentation should be treated as suspicious. Purchases may have been made without proper authorization. Additionally, there are fraudsters that send statements when no transaction has taken place in the hope that the receiving organization's controls are lax and payment will be made. This is particularly true of fraudulent subscriptions and advertising schemes.

Inventory Slips The purchase of large quantities of supplies is called supplies inventory and may be recorded as an asset at the time of purchase. Items are then removed from assets and recorded as expenses as they are used. This same system may be used to track pharmacy inventory (by patient rather than department). In a centralized purchasing system, some mechanism must be in place to track the distribution of items to other departments. The financial transaction consists of moving the responsibility for the expense of the items from the purchasing department to the requesting department. Table 26.5 shows some common accounts and what they represent.

Recording Transactions

As previously discussed, financial transactions begin with the documents of original entry or source documents. Whether the organization's transactions are recorded on paper or via computer, there must be a way to determine the origination of the transaction. The originating document details the

Table 26.5. Common accounts

Account	Description	Example
Assets		
Cash	Money. Typically, money is represented by several accounts, depending on how the money is stored (for example, in different banks).	Bank account
Inventory	Goods that are available for sale.	Pharmaceuticals
Accounts receivable	Amounts owed the organization for goods and services.	Claims to payers that have not yet been paid
Building	Permanent structures. The land on which they are built is often listed separately.	Office building
Equipment	Items that are used to generate revenue or to support the organization during more than one business cycle.	Photocopier CT scanner
Liabilities		
Accounts payable	Amounts the organization owes but has not yet paid.	Supplies purchased on credit
Loans payable	Amounts the organization has borrowed that will be paid over more than one business cycle.	Bank loan
Mortgage payable	Amounts the organization has borrowed to finance the purchase of buildings and equipment.	Building mortgage
Equity		
Capital, stock, or fund balance	In a sole proprietorship or partnership, capital is the owner's equity in the organization. In a corporation, stock is the amount invested by owners in the corporation. In a not-for-profit organization, the fund balance is the amount represented by the difference between assets and liabilities.	
Retained earnings or reserves	In a corporation, retained earnings are profits that have not been distributed. Reserves are amounts that have been designated for a specific purpose.	
Revenue	Temporary account that captures amounts earned by the organization in the current fiscal year.	The difference between revenue and expenses is net income (profits or losses). These accounts are closed at the end of every fiscal year and the net income is moved to retained earnings or reserves.
Expenses	Temporary account that captures amounts disbursed by the organization in the current fiscal year to support the generation of revenue.	

parties involved in the transaction, the amount of the transaction, the type of financial impact involved (revenue or expense, asset or liability), and the individual responsible for the transaction.

Double-Entry Bookkeeping

All financial transactions are recorded with the accounting equation in mind: assets = liabilities + net assets (equity). To simplify the recording of transactions, accountants use special terminology to reflect the maintenance of a balanced equation.

Debits and Credits Visually, transactions have two sides—left and right. Debits are shown on the left; credits are shown on the right. Each account has two sides—increase and decrease. In asset accounts, the left-hand debit side represents the natural balance of the account and debits increase the account. Conversely, credits decrease an asset account. For the accounting equation to balance, the opposite is true of liability and equity accounts. The right-hand credit side of liability and equity accounts represents the natural balance, and credits increase the accounts. Instead of using minus signs or brackets to represent the increases and decreases, debits and credits provide an additional safeguard against clerical error because every transaction must balance.

Look at the coding consultant example again in table 26.6, using debits and credits. It is shown that as assets increase with payments from clients,

that amount is placed on the left side of the asset account (debited). As the asset decreases due to purchases, that amount is placed on the right side of the asset account or (credited). As noted before, for the accounting equation to balance, the opposite is true of liability and equity accounts; the credit side of the equity account increases when accounts payables are increased. As liabilities and equities decrease (for example, when accounts payables are paid off), the liability account is debited.

Impact on Individual Accounts Assets involve multiple accounts as described previously: cash, accounts receivable, and building. Similarly, liabilities have their own accounts. Revenues and expenses fall into the equity section. This system of debits and credits enables us to understand immediately whether a transaction increases or decreases a particular account. Individual accounts increase and decrease in value; however, the overall equation always remains in balance.

Keeping Track of Transactions

Financial transactions are recorded, or posted, to the accounts described earlier, according to a system of journal entries.

Journal Entry Each journal entry contains at least one debit and one credit. For every transaction, the sum of the debits must equal the sum of the credits. Ensuring that the debits and credits

Table 26.6. Debits and credits

	October activity								
	Assets		**−**	**Liabilities**		**=**	**Equity**	
	Debit	**Credit**		**Debit**	**Credit**		**Debit**	**Credit**
Beginning balance	$1,500		−	—0—		=		$1,500
Purchase codebook		100	−			=	100	
Pay health insurance		100	−			=	100	
Receive payment from client	$1,200		−			=		$1,200
Purchase computer (on credit)		200	−		800	=	1,000	
Receive payment from client	$1,300		−			=		$1,300
Attend CE session		80	−			=	80	
Ending balance	$3,520		−		800	=		$2,720

equal is one aspect of ensuring the accuracy of financial data. Other aspects include posting to the correct accounts and in the correct time period. Table 26.7 shows the purchase of supplies on credit. The supplies are delivered on February 24, and the supplier's invoice is paid on March 15. Note that no financial transaction is recorded until the supplies are received.

The accounts payable amount is eliminated when the invoice is paid. It is common business practice to record, or **accrue**, liabilities as they are incurred. This accrual basis of accounting enables organizations to understand their total liabilities continuously and to match expenses with the associated revenue. Some organizations, such as small professional associations and sole proprietorships, only record transactions when the cash is paid or received. This cash basis of accounting is analogous to the way individuals handle their private transactions.

In the preceding tabulation, the supplies expense entry is a debit to increase that account. Expenses are temporary equity accounts that close annually. Revenue increases net income; expenses reduce net income. Therefore, revenue accounts have a natural credit balance and expenses have a natural debit balance.

It should be noted that all the financial accounting examples in this chapter relate to corporate and not-for-profit accounting. Government accounting activity, although a system of debits and credits, is significantly different in some respects. For example, a supply purchase would be recorded (encumbered) at the time the supplies were budgeted and then reduced at the time they were ordered. Government accounting is outside the scope of this discussion.

General Ledger   In a paper-based accounting system, journal entries are recorded chronologically in a general journal and their component debits and credits are posted to the individual accounts. The list of all the individual accounts is referred to as the **general ledger**. In a computer-based environment, only the original journal entry is posted. The computer stores the entries and generates summaries of the individual accounts on request.

The example in figure 26.4 is based on this chapter's original description of a financial transaction. The result of this completed transaction is an increase in cash and an increase in equity (revenue). Note that the amount in accounts receivable is eliminated when the reimbursement is received.

Nonfinancial managers are rarely required to make actual journal entries to record financial transactions. However, they do initiate the transactions and receive reports that detail them. Often the reports only show the department's side of the transaction. For example, a purchase of supplies would appear to the manager on a list of expenses and be added to a summary of all supply expenses

Table 26.7.   Journal entry for purchase of supplies

Date	Description	Debit	Credit
2/24	Supplies expense	$300	
	Accounts payable		$300
	Purchase office supplies		
3/15	Accounts payable	$300	
	Cash		$300
	Pay 2/24 office supply invoice		

Figure 26.4.   Example of a financial transaction

Service provided:

Physician sees in the office a new patient, whose chief complaint is an itchy rash.

Transaction recorded:

Clinical record: History and physical or progress note reflect examination of rash and notation that the patient encountered poison ivy while weeding his garden. Over-the-counter (OTC) topical ointment prescribed, and free sample distributed with instructions.

Billing record: Encounter form—office visit recorded

Journal entry:

	Debit	Credit
Accounts receivable—Patient X	60	
Patient service revenue		60

Reimbursement received:

Journal entry:

	Debit	Credit
Cash	60	
Accounts receivable—Patient X		60

on another report. The cash and accounts payable portions of the transaction would not show because they are controlled by the accounting department. Another example is the discharged, no final bill (DNFB) report (discussed later in this chapter). The DNFB lists individual patient accounts, which are accounts receivable to the organization. Managerial reporting activity is also discussed later in this chapter.

Financial Statements

At the departmental level, individual financial transactions are reviewed for data quality and compliance with policies and procedures. On an administrative level, the overall impact of transactions is generally of more interest than the individual transactions; therefore, summary reports are prepared. These summaries also are used to communicate with lending institutions, potential investors, and regulatory agencies. A variety of summaries are useful for analyzing an organization's financial activities. The three key reports are the income statement, statement of retained earnings, and balance sheet.

Income Statement

The **income statement** summarizes the organization's revenue and expense transactions during the fiscal year. The income statement can be prepared at any point in time and reflects results up to that point. The income statement contains only income and expense accounts and reflects only the activity for the current fiscal year.

The arithmetic difference between total revenue and total expenses is **net income**. When total expenses exceed total revenue, net income is a negative number, or a **net loss**. Net income increases equity; net loss decreases equity.

At the end of the fiscal year, all income statement accounts are closed and the net results are added to, or subtracted from, the appropriate equity account (net asset). For the purposes of periodic reporting, net assets are adjusted in this manner every time this report is prepared. However, at the end of the fiscal year, the income and expense accounts are actually closed so that the new fiscal year begins at zero.

Retained Earnings

The **statement of retained earnings** expresses the change in retained earnings from the beginning of the balance sheet period to the end. Retained earnings are affected, for example, by net income and loss, distribution of stock dividends, and payment of long-term debt. Net income and loss is carried forward from the income statement. When the income statement accounts are closed, the net income and loss is transferred to equity. The mechanics of this transaction are to take the balance in each revenue and expense account and record the opposite amount so that all of the income statement accounts have a zero balance. The net dollar amount of the debits and credits is recorded to equity. The statement of changes in retained earnings highlights this transaction. The ending balance in retained earnings is then reported on the balance sheet.

Balance Sheet

The **balance sheet** is a snapshot of the accounting equation at a point in time. Because every financial transaction affects the equation, theoretically, the balance sheet will look different after every transaction. To ensure a meaningful evaluation, the balance sheet is typically reviewed on a periodic basis (monthly, quarterly, semiannually, and annually). It is often compared to balance sheets from previous fiscal years in order to analyze changes in the organization.

The balance sheet lists the major account categories grouped under their equation headings: assets, liabilities, and equity and fund balance. Figure 26.5 shows a set of simple statements. The dollar amount shown next to each account category is the total in each category on the ending date listed at the top of the report. This figure also shows the relationship among the income statement, statement of retained earnings, and balance sheet.

Analysis Statements

A number of other types of summary statements are required by users to analyze an organization's financial activity and position. Depending on the organization and its use of the analysis statements, the additional financial statements may be required by GAAP as part of a complete financial summary report. Figure 26.6 shows a two-year

Figure 26.5. Financial statements and relationship among the income statement, net assets, and balance sheet

Sample hospital statement of revenues and expenses

	12/31/16 (000)
Revenue	
Net patient service revenue	$650
Unrestricted gifts	40
Other	95
Total revenue	$785
Expenses	
Salaries and wages	$430
Fringe benefits	95
Supplies	175
Total expenses	$700
Income from operations	$85
Nonoperating gains	
Unrestricted gifts	$15
Excess of revenues over expenses	$100

Sample hospital statement of changes in unrestricted fund balance

	2016 (000)
Beginning balance January 1	$900
Excess of revenues over expenses	100
Ending balance December 31	$1,000

Sample hospital balance sheet

	12/31/16 (000)
Assets	
Cash	$500
Accounts receivable	600
Inventory	400
Building	2,500
Total assets	$4,000
Liabilities	
Accounts payable	600
Mortgage	2,000
Total liabilities	$2,600
Fund balance	
Restricted funds	400
Unrestricted funds	$1,000
Total fund balance	$1,400
Total liabilities and fund balance	$4,000

Source: Adapted from Davis and Revoir 2013, 778.

side-by-side comparative balance sheet and three simple examples of statements that help to explain the changes from one year to the next. These statements are included for completeness of discussion and are not statements that HIM professionals usually need to analyze.

Cash Flow The **statement of cash flow** details the reasons that cash changed from one balance sheet period to another. It shows the analyst whether cash was used to purchase equipment or to pay down debt and whether any unusually large transactions took place.

Stockholder's Equity The **statement of stockholder's equity** (also called the statement of net assets) details the reasons for changes in each of the stockholder's equity accounts, including retained earnings.

Figure 26.6.   Two-year comparative balance sheet with analytical statements

Sample hospital statement of revenues and expenses	12/31/16 (000)	12/31/15 (000)	Sample hospital balance sheet	12/31/16 (000)	12/31/15 (000)
Revenue			**Assets**		
Net patient service revenue	$650	$500	Cash	$ 500	$ 650
Unrestricted gifts	40	30	Accounts receivable	600	750
Other	95	70	Inventory	400	350
Total revenue	$785	$600	Building	2,500	2,150
Expenses			*Total assets*	$4,000	$3,900
Salaries and wages	$430	$290			
Fringe benefits	95	90	**Liabilities**		
Supplies	175	180	Accounts payable	600	500
Total expenses	$700	$560	Mortgage	2,000	2,100
Income from operations	$ 85	$ 40	*Total liabilities*	$2,600	$2,600
Nonoperating gains			**Fund balance**		
Unrestricted gifts	$ 15	$ 10			
Excess of revenues over expenses	$100	$ 50	Restricted funds	400	400

Sample hospital statement of revenues and expenses	2016 (000)	2015 (000)		12/31/16	12/31/15
			Unrestricted funds	1,000	900
Beginning balance January 1	$ 900	$850	*Total fund balance*	$1,400	$1,300
Excess of revenues over expenses	100	50	*Total liabilities and fund balance*	$4,000	$3,900
Ending balance December 31	$1,000	$900			

Source: Adapted from Davis and Revoir 2013, 779.

Ratio Analysis

After the financial statements have been prepared, they are ready for ratio analysis. Financial analysts can use financial statements, particularly the balance sheet, to determine whether an organization is using its resources similarly to or differently from other organizations in the same industry. For example, hospitals compare their days in accounts receivable ratio to peer hospitals and industry averages. In any industry, one of the most common reasons to analyze financial statements is to lend money to the organization or to invest in it. Thus, the organization's use of assets compared to its liabilities is extremely important. Changes in an organization's ratios are of particular interest.

Ratios, as a comparative tool, are only meaningful within the context of the organization's industry. It is not useful to compare a ratio for a hospital against a ratio for an automobile manufacturer, except to state that one would expect the ratios to be different. Whether an organization's particular ratio is inherently good or bad depends on expected ratios for similar organizations in that industry.

Liquidity and Debt Service

A key issue to lenders and investors is the organization's ability to repay its financial obligations. **Liquidity** refers to the ease with which assets can be turned into cash. This is important because payroll, loan payments, and other financial obligations are typically paid in cash. **Debt service** is the extent to which those financial obligations are loans.

Current Ratio   An organization's ability to pay current liabilities with current assets is important to lenders. Current assets include cash, short-term investments, accounts receivable, and inventory. Current assets implicitly will be (or could be) converted to cash at some point within a year, through collections, sales, or other business activity. Current liabilities include accounts payable and the current portion of loan obligations. Again, the term *current* implies that the liability will be discharged within a year. The **current ratio** compares total current assets with total current liabilities:

$$\frac{\text{Total current assets}}{\text{Total current liabilities}}$$

From the balance sheet in figure 26.6, one can take the current assets (cash plus accounts receivable plus inventory) and divide them by the current liabilities (accounts payable) to determine the current ratio:

$$\frac{1,500,000}{600,000} = \frac{15}{6} = 2.5$$

The current ratio indicates that for every dollar of current liability, $2.50 of current assets could be used to discharge the liability. A higher current ratio is more favorable than a lower current ratio. In this example the current ratio is 2.5, which is more favorable than another organization that has a current ratio of 1.0.

Days in Accounts Receivable Ratio   A key measure for healthcare organizations to track is the **days in accounts receivable** ratio that reflects how long it takes for an organization to collect its accounts receivable. A lower ratio is preferable and it means an organization is collecting its receivables more

quickly and results in more available cash. The days in accounts receivable divides net accounts receivable by average daily net patient service revenue:

$$\frac{\text{Net accounts receivable}}{(\text{Net patient service revenue} / 365)}$$

For example, if a hospital had net accounts receivable of 90,000 and net patient service revenue for the year of 650,000 the ratio is calculated as follows:

$$\frac{90,000}{(650,000 / 365 \text{ days})}$$
$$= 50.5 \text{ days in accounts receivable}$$

In this example, patients and payers are on average paying their bills within 50.5 days. A lower ratio is preferable and indicates that the hospital is efficient at collecting its accounts receivable. A lower ratio provides organizations with more liquidity or access to cash.

Debt Ratio   Looking back to the mortgage example, the organization's building asset was purchased using 10 percent cash and 90 percent mortgage. Ninety percent of that asset was financed with debt. Looking at all the liabilities and all the assets together gives the analyst an overall picture of how the assets were acquired. The **debt ratio**, therefore, is total liabilities divided by total assets. Using the balance sheet in figure 26.6, the debt ratio is

$$\frac{2,600,000}{4,000,000} = 65\% \text{ or } 65.0$$

It is important to remember that all ratio analysis is industry specific and varies somewhat depending on the economic environment. Therefore, ratio analysis can be used to compare similar organizations at a specific point in time or the same organization at different points in time. However, a hospital ratio would never be compared with a professional association ratio.

Profitability

The preceding examples illustrate how organizations can evaluate their ability to pay their bills. Another measure of an organization's health is its profitability.

Profitability refers to an organization's ability to increase in value: how well does it invest its assets? As with other ratios, profitability measures are only meaningful as benchmarks against like organizations or in trending a single organization over time.

Return on Investment Return on investment **(ROI)** measures the increase in the value of an asset. In a savings account, this increase is measured as the amount of interest received in a period. The beginning balance in the account is the measurement of the asset. Interest received in the period is the return. Thus,

$$\text{ROI} = \frac{\text{Interest earned in the period}}{\text{Asset value at the beginning of the period}}$$

Return on individual investments can be calculated in this manner. For an entire organization, interest earned is replaced by earnings, usually after taxes. Asset value is replaced by total assets:

$$\text{ROI} = \frac{\text{Earnings (after taxes)}}{\text{Total assets}}$$

To illustrate ROI, examine the acquisition of technology to generate income:

Purchase: $100,000 (invest in document imaging system)
Liability: $90,000 (long-term loan from bank)
Net income: $30,000 (after taxes)

$$\text{ROI} = \frac{\$30,000}{\$100,000} = 30\%$$

In this example, a $100,000 investment generated an ROI of $30,000 or 30 percent. When analyzing new investments, organizations will often identify a benchmark ROI that all new investments must meet or exceed.

Additional measures of return are discussed later in the section on capital projects.

Total Margin Ratio Overall profitability of an organization is measured by the **total margin ratio**, which compares excess of revenue over expense by total revenue. The ratio is calculated as follows:

$$\frac{\text{Excess of revenue over expense}}{\text{Total revenue}}$$

From the income statement in figure 26.5 the total margin ratio is:

$$\frac{100,000}{785,000} = 0.127 \text{ or } 12.7\% \text{ or } 12.7$$

The total margin ratio indicates that for every $1.00 of revenue the organization earned a profit of 0.12 cents. A higher total margin ratio is preferable because it demonstrates an organization's profitability. It is critical for an organization to maintain profitability in order to continue to invest in new programs and facilities.

Check Your Understanding 26.2

Instructions: Answer the following questions on a separate piece of paper.

1. Calculate the total margin ratio for 12/31/15 using the income statement in figure 26.6.

2. Define the accounting equation.

3. Discuss the three key financial statements and the components of each.

4. Why is knowledge of accounting important to nonfinancial managers?

5. A lender wants to know how quickly a borrower would be able to repay a debt. What is the best ratio to use for this analysis? Why?

Basic Management Accounting

To obtain appropriate compensation for goods and services provided, the organization must understand and measure the resources used to manufacture, acquire, or otherwise produce those goods and services. The measurement of those resources is monetary and is referred to as their cost. In manufacturing and other goods-oriented businesses, sales are compared to the cost of goods sold, which are composed of raw materials and other manufacturing costs. Calculation of the manufacturing cost of goods sold, by-products, salvage, and waste is outside the scope of this discussion. In a service industry, the underlying costs consist largely of human resources, supplies, and the tools of the trade.

Management accounting focuses on the internal communication of accounting and financial data for the purpose of facility-based decision making. Management accountants use the same transaction data that are summarized in a financial statement. They also use a variety of additional data, such as prevailing interest rates and staffing levels, to provide meaningful information required by management.

Describing Costs

Cost accounting is the discipline of identifying and measuring costs and is a unique subset of the accounting profession. However, a general understanding of the terminology helps nonfinancial managers participate in and support the process. There are numerous ways to describe costs, but the most important for purposes of this discussion are included here.

Direct Costs

Direct costs are traceable to a specific good or service provided. To a hospital, the cost of a specific medication can be matched to the specific patient to whom it was administered. Room charges are another example. Similarly, to a consulting firm, the hours that a consultant coder spends coding are directly linked to the services provided to a specific facility.

Indirect Costs

Indirect costs or **overhead costs** are incurred by the organization in the process of providing goods or services; however, they are not specifically attributable to an individual product or service. The costs of providing security services at a hospital or clerical support at the call center are indirect costs with respect to patient care. To the consulting firm, the cost of continuing education (CE) for its coding staff is an indirect cost of providing services to a particular client.

The classification of costs as direct or indirect depends on the relationship of the cost to the client, department, product, service, or activity in question. Payroll in the security department is an indirect cost to patient care, but it is a direct cost to the security department. Therefore, the distinction between direct and indirect costs is important in understanding the broader financial impact of activities within the facility. In developing capital projects (discussed later in this chapter) such as the development and implementation of an electronic health record, an understanding of the associated costs (and, conversely, the cost savings) is crucial in making realistic financial estimates and projections.

Fixed Costs

For planning and analysis, it is useful to classify costs as fixed or variable. **Fixed costs** remain the same, despite changes in volume. For example, a manager's base salary does not change, regardless of patient volume or other changes in activity. Mortgage payments also are not dependent on activity. In figure 26.7, the copy machine depreciation expense does not vary, regardless of the number of requests.

Variable Costs

Variable costs are sensitive to volume. Medication is a good example. The more patients are treated, the more medication is used. Paper medical record documentation is another example. The larger the volume of patients, the more paper is used. In figure 26.8, the cost of paper used to print release of information requests rises proportionately with the number of requests.

Semi-Fixed Costs

Costs may behave in a combination of fixed and variable ways, and volume is not the only change agent. For example, consider the coding function. Base coding salaries are fixed. Increases in discharges may require a temporary coding consultant. If the consultant charges on a per chart basis, the cost of coding services rises variably with that volume. Similarly, the combination of personnel and paper costs for release of information has a combined mixed variability, as illustrated in figure 26.9.

On the other hand, nursing base salaries are also a fixed cost. However, hospitals do not staff nursing for full capacity. Therefore, increases in census require the use of part-time or per diem nurses, who are added based on established patient-to-

nurse ratios. The full cost of nursing services, then, goes up in steps. Figure 26.10 illustrates this type of personnel cost variability, as applied to the copy cost example.

Cost Reports

Prior to implementation of prospective payment systems (PPSs), Medicare reimbursement to hospitals was related directly to the costs incurred by the facilities. Individual facility cost reports were submitted to Medicare, identifying the direct and indirect costs of providing care to Medicare patients. Direct costs include nursing and radiology; indirect costs include HIM and information systems.

The expense of non–revenue-producing cost centers is allocated to revenue-producing cost centers in order to fully understand the cost of providing services. Although cost reporting is no longer used to directly determine Medicare reimbursement for prospective payment facilities, critical access hospitals were reimbursed 101 percent

Figure 26.7. Fixed cost

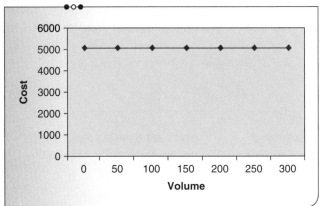

Figure 26.9. Mixed cost

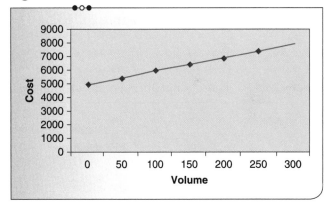

Figure 26.8. Variable cost

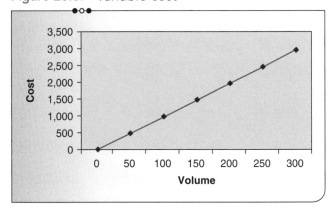

Figure 26.10. Step mixed cost

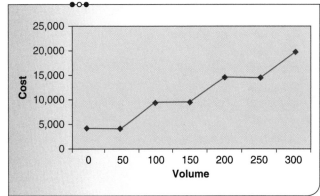

of eligible Medicare costs; however, sequestration, or reduction, by Congress has reduced the rate to 99 percent of eligible Medicare costs (Holmes and Pink 2013). In addition, CMS uses cost reports to help determine facility-specific and regional cost adjustment factors for healthcare PPSs.

Allocation of Overhead

The attribution of indirect or overhead costs to revenue-producing service units illustrates the budget concept that all activities must support the mission of the organization. There are four methods of allocation of overhead:

- *Direct method of cost allocation* distributes the cost of overhead departments solely to the revenue-producing areas. Allocation is based on each revenue-producing area's relative square footage, number of employees, or actual usage of supplies and services.

- *Step-down allocation* distributes overhead costs once beginning with the area that provides the least amount of nonrevenue-producing services. (See figure 26.11.)

- *Double distribution* allocates overhead costs twice, which takes into consideration the fact that some overhead departments provide services to each other.

- *Simultaneous equations method* distributes overhead costs through multiple iterations allowing maximum distribution of interdepartmental costs among overhead departments.

The last three methods of cost allocation listed assume that overhead cost centers (such as housekeeping) perform services for each other as well as for revenue-producing areas. Therefore, overhead costs are distributed among overhead cost centers as well as revenue-producing areas.

Although each of these methods may produce slightly different results, the ultimate goal is to allocate overhead costs appropriately. Appropriate allocation enables the facility to express the full cost of providing services.

Impact of Accounts Receivable on Financial Statements

Accounts receivable represents a current asset. Delays in processing claims cause receivables

Figure 26.11.   Direct allocation versus step allocation

	Nonrevenue-producing department		Revenue-producing department	
	HIM department	**Business office**	**Medicine**	**Laboratory**
Direct method:				
Overhead costs before allocation	$360,000	$240,000	$400,000	$250,000
Allocation				
HIM (number of discharges processed)	($360,000)		$340,000	$20,000
Business office (number of labor hours used)		($240,000)	$80,000	$160,000
Total overhead after allocation	$0	$0	$820,000	$430,000
Step method:				
Overhead costs before allocation	$360,000	$240,000	$400,000	$250,000
Allocation				
HIM (number of discharges processed)	($360,000)	$50,000	$300,000	$10,000
Business office (number of labor hours used)		($290,000)	$90,000	$200,000
Total overhead after allocation	$0	$0	$790,000	$460,000

to age. Aged receivables can negatively affect a facility's ability to borrow money. Failure to claim and collect receivables affects cash, which in turn negatively affects the facility's ability to discharge its current liabilities, the largest of which is payroll. Therefore, in a facility for which reimbursement is the largest revenue item

and payroll is the largest expense, there is a direct relationship between getting paid and paying employees. Thus, the role of HIM becomes a critical component of maintaining the facility's fiscal integrity. Strategies for effectively managing accounts receivable are further discussed in chapter 8.

Internal Controls

In any industry, internal controls must be in place to safeguard assets and to ensure compliance with policies and procedures. Internal controls may be designed to prevent the theft of cash or to ensure that a patient receives the correct medication. The three major categories of internal controls are preventive, detective, and corrective controls.

Preventive

Preventive controls are implemented prior to the activity taking place because they are designed to stop an error from happening. In financial management, pretransaction supervisory review and authorization is a preventive control. Data entry validation is another preventive control. Data entry validation prevents the user from entering "64," for example, as a day of the month. Preventive controls are sometimes more costly than their effect warrants. In those cases, other types of controls must be put in place to find and correct errors.

Detective

Detective controls are designed to find errors that have already been made. Detective controls tend to be less expensive than preventive controls and can be implemented at many levels. Quantitative record reviews and computer exception reports are examples of detective controls. In accounting, the summing of debits and credits is a detective control because the two sums must always be equal. Footing and cross-footing financial reports are another detective control. (See figure 26.12.)

Corrective

When an error or other problem has been detected, action must be taken to correct the error,

solve the problem, or design controls to prevent future errors or problems. The error or problem must be analyzed to determine the cause. When a correction can be made, it is documented and implemented. However, some errors, such as amputation of an incorrect limb, cannot be corrected. In these cases, analysis of the root cause is important so that the error can be prevented in the future. In financial management, very few errors cannot be corrected. Typical errors include posting transactions to an incorrect account, posting transactions that have not been completed, and posting incorrect amounts. Even financial statement errors can be corrected and the reports redistributed. Problems that cannot always be corrected include theft of assets and failure to invest funds on a timely basis. These problems require analysis and development and implementation of controls for the future.

Corrective controls are designed to fix problems that have been discovered, frequently as a result of detective controls. Many errors and problems occur routinely, such as failing to complete forms, making computation errors, and wrongly posting transactions. Therefore, procedures must be in place to ensure the timely and accurate correction of the error or solution to the problem. In the HIM department, the incomplete chart system is a corrective control. Incomplete charts have been detected, the source of the error identified, and the responsible individual contacted for completion of the chart. In financial management, supervisory review of transactions is typically used to detect errors and problems. The ability to correct errors in journal entries is essential.

Figure 26.12.　Footing and cross-footing financial reports

Summing of debits and credits

Cash	$1,345	
Photocopy paper		$974
Toner		$362

In this journal entry, the debit ($1,345) does not match the credits ($1,336). This means that an error has been made. Refer to the original documentation that will reveal the sales tax on the items was not accounted for.

Footing and cross-footing

	January	February	March	Year-to-date (Cross-foot)
Payroll	20,000	20,000	20,000	60,000
Benefits	6,000	6,000	6,000	24,000
Office supplies	1,000	1,000	1,000	3,000
Equipment service	400	500	600	500
				87,500?
Monthly totals	27,400 (Foot)	27,400	27,400	82,200?

The foot is the sum of the columns; the cross-foot is the sum of the rows. Notice that in this example the sums do not match. Footing and cross-footing reports that are supposed to represent arithmetic totals is a very useful detective control, particularly with manually prepared or PC-prepared reports. A simple error in creating a formula in a spreadsheet program can cause an entire report to be wrong.

Internal controls may be present at every level of the organization. In a service organization, such as a hospital, controls over expenditures are some of the most important responsibilities of individual managers. Two key methods of exerting such controls are through purchasing and analysis of budget variances.

Check Your Understanding 26.3

Instructions: **Answer the following questions on a separate piece of paper.**

1. Differentiate among direct, indirect, fixed, and variable costs.

2. How can the management of accounts receivable affect the financial statements and an organization's financial health?

3. Summarize the three types of internal controls.

4. Describe the focus of management accounting.

5. List and describe the four methods of allocation of overhead.

Budgets

Managers must have some understanding of managerial accounting in order to control the financial aspects of their departments' operations. As stated earlier, managers must work within budgets that have been developed based on their organization's goals and objectives. Therefore, it is not sufficient for a manager merely to review for accuracy the financial transactions generated by the department during the period. Rather, the transactions must be compared to the expected or budgeted transactions to ensure that the goals and objectives of both the department and the organization are being met. **Managerial accounting** is the development, implementation, and analysis of systems that track financial transactions for managerial control purposes; it includes both budget and cost analysis systems.

Types of Budgets

In addition to the most familiar budgets, operating and capital budgets, organizations develop and monitor other budgets, including financial budgets, cash flow budgets, and incremental budgets. These budgets are the responsibility of the finance department.

The development and monitoring of budgets is guided by the facility's policy and procedures manual and the management styles of the administrative and departmental management team. Therefore, it is important for department managers to understand the facility's budgeting methods, including how administration uses budgets.

A budget is a manager's best guess at the outcomes of future financial transactions. Unexpected events that influence those transactions, such as declining census, increase in interest rates, and staffing changes, create budget variances. Some budgets are specifically designed to take these fluctuations into consideration. A budget can represent virtually any projected set of circumstances. Therefore, there are many different types of budget methodologies. Common methodologies include fixed, flexible, activity-based, and zero-based budgets.

The most common type of budget is a **fixed budget**. Budget amounts are based on expected capacity. Fixed budgets do not change when expected capacity changes. For example, the HIM department would budget outsourced transcription service expense on the basis of the estimated number of discharges and historical need. When the number of discharges materially increases or declines, the outsourced transcription service expense will increase or decrease, thus creating a budget variance.

Flexible budgets are based on projected productivity. In this case, the HIM department would budget outsourced transcription service expense at several levels of discharges. As the actual discharges become known, the budget reflects the estimate at that level of activity. Used primarily in manufacturing, this method of budgeting also is useful for projecting personnel budgets in service areas, such as nursing units, where increased activity has a direct impact on staffing and supplies.

Activity-based budgets are based on activities or projects rather than on departments. Typically used for construction projects, an activity-based budget can be useful for any project that spans multiple budget lines or departments and for projects that span more than one fiscal year. Computer system installation and implementation should be controlled using an activity-based budget.

Different budget methodologies are developed to meet the needs of the organization. Fixed and flexible budgets are characteristic of operating budgets. Activity-based budgets are more often used for capital projects. All three types of budgets can be used by virtually any organization. **Zero-based budgets**, on the other hand, apply to organizations for which each budget cycle poses the opportunity to continue or discontinue services based on the availability of resources. Every department or activity must be justified and prioritized annually in order to effectively allocate the organization's resources. Professional associations and charitable foundations, for example, routinely use zero-based budgeting.

Operational Budgets

The purpose of an operational budget is to allocate and control resources in a manner consistent with the organization's goals and objectives. These goals and objectives are tied to the organization's mission. Each department also should have its own mission, goals, and objectives that identify how it contributes to the organization's overall mission. Every item in the operational budget should have a direct relationship to a departmental goal that supports an organizational goal.

The budget process begins with the board of directors or trustees, which approves the fiscal assumptions for the upcoming year. Those assumptions are quantified and communicated to the department managers, who develop budgets based on those assumptions. Typical assumptions include the desired growth in revenue and targeted cost reductions.

Budget Cycle

The operational budget cycle generally coincides with one fiscal year. The purpose of the **operational budget** is the quantification of the projected results of operations for the coming fiscal year. This process begins three to four months before the end of the current fiscal year. Projected budgets should be collected, compiled, reviewed, and approved prior to the start of the new fiscal year.

Fiscal Period An organization's budget year coincides with its fiscal year on file with the IRS. Although the actual operational budget generally only applies to one fiscal year, financial managers often project multiple years of budgets with a variety of scenarios in order to test the financial impact of current decision making.

Interim Periods Monthly budget reporting is the most common budget cycle. Any period that represents less than an entire fiscal year is an interim period. Figure 26.13 provides a sample budget report for an HIM department for May. The budgeted amounts for each item are listed next to the actual amounts for the month. As is common, the year-to-date (in this case, January through May) budget and actual amounts also are included. It is useful for budget reports to show the differences—variances—between budgeted and actual amounts. Many budget reports also show the percentage variance for each item, based on the budget. Managers may be required to explain variances that exceed a particular dollar value or a specified percentage.

In the budget report shown in figure 26.13, there is a large variance in May's budgeted expense for printer paper. By following that line item across to the year-to-date amount, it is evident that there is no year-to-date variance in the budget. This illustrates a timing difference between the expected expense and the actual expense. The budget may have placed that expense in April even though the actual expense occurred in May. These types of temporary variances are the result of normal business activities; and although they may require explanation, they are usually not of concern.

Budget Components

The components of an operational budget generally follow the format of the income statement and list revenue items and expense items. Every department is different, depending on its unique activities. However, budget reports tend to be uniform throughout the organization. Therefore, line items that do not apply to a particular department are likely to be listed with zero values rather than be omitted.

Revenues There is little, if any, revenue in the HIM department. Occasionally, a facility with excess capacity will contract or outsource transcription services. Copy fees are another potential source of revenue; however, because such fees should be cost based, they are probably more appropriately considered a reimbursement (reduction of expenses).

Expenses The HIM department budget consists primarily of expenses. Expenses may be incurred as a result of financial transactions outside or within the organization. Some departments, such as housekeeping and facilities maintenance, perform services for other facility departments. Therefore, charges from these departments may appear on the budget. Such charges are generally carried forward through the cost allocation process and usually are not estimated by individual managers.

Ordinarily, the single largest expense in a healthcare facility is payroll. This is typical for service organizations. Payroll can be a difficult expense to project because employees have different anniversary dates and different salary increases. For direct patient care departments the payroll budget is driven by patient volumes. For example, on a nursing floor a manager will multiply the number of budgeted patient days times the budgeted hours per patient. As patient days increase or decrease the number of budgeted nursing hours will change along with the payroll budget. For many

Figure 26.13. HIM department budget report for May

Description	May budget	May actual	May variance	YTD budget	YTD actual	YTD variance
Payroll	$25,000	$22,345	$2,655	$125,000	$110,321	$14,679
Fringe benefits	$8,000	$7,360	$640	$40,000	$37,870	$2,130
Contract services	$5,000	$8,000	($3,000)	$25,000	$40,000	($15,000)
Office supplies	$150	$145	$5	$750	$975	($225)
Printer paper	$100	$250	($150)	$500	$500	—
Postage	$95	$97	($2)	$475	$456	$19
Travel	$0	$0	—	$0	$0	—
Continuing education	$0	$0	—	$0	$45	($45)

indirect departments such as HIM or accounting the payroll budget is often based on the prior year's actual expenses and adjusted for any staffing changes and pay increases. Because payroll is the largest expense category there is often pressure from management to reduce payroll expenses.

The cost of employee benefits is part of payroll but is often listed separately. Facilities rarely expect department managers to calculate benefits budgets because this is a human resources–controlled line item. The cost of benefits tracks with payroll.

The next largest expense account is often supplies. Clinical supplies are a substantial item on the cardiology or radiology department budget, whereas office supplies might be a large item for HIM.

Cost of goods sold is a manufacturing concept that refers to the underlying cost of making the finished goods. This concept applies to healthcare providers in the sense that there is a cost basis for providing services. For every inpatient treated, there are payroll, utility, office supplies, pharmaceutical, and equipment costs that the facility incurs. Unlike manufacturing, in which the cost of producing items is tracked very closely, healthcare facilities historically have not been good at tracking each of the underlying costs of providing services to individual patients. The costs of providing care are often analyzed at a facility-wide level that includes total costs for all patients.

Management of the Operating Budget

When the operating budget has been developed and approved, it is the responsibility of the department management to ensure that the budget goals are met. As a general rule, in meeting goals, revenue should meet or exceed budget and expenses should meet or be less than budget. However, because expenses support revenues, an increase in revenues (perhaps due to unexpected volume) may signal an expected increase in expenses, such as variable expenses. This is particularly true when the patient census exceeds expectations. Despite the logical and expected nature of these results, managers are required to investigate and explain differences between budgeted and actual amounts on a regular basis.

Identification of Variances

A **variance** is the arithmetic difference between the budgeted amount and the actual amount of a line item. Variance analysis places accountability for financial transactions on the manager of the department that initiated the transaction.

Variances are often calculated on the monthly budget report. The organization's policies and procedures manual defines unacceptable variances or variances that must be explained. In identifying variances, it is important to recognize whether the variance is favorable or unfavorable and whether it is temporary or permanent.

Timing The problems identified by variance analysis and the action that must be taken depend largely on whether the variance is temporary or permanent. Temporary variances are generally self-limiting.

Temporary budget variances are not expected to continue in subsequent months. For example, a department may budget for a large purchase of printer paper in May. When that purchase does not actually take place until July, there will be a temporary variance in the May and July monthly report and a temporary variance in the May and June year-to-date numbers. Figure 26.14 illustrates this point. In this example, the HIM department budgeted $260 per month for department supplies, plus an additional $900 in May for printer paper. This created a temporary, favorable variance in expenditures in May and June.

In contrast, permanent budget variances do not resolve during the current fiscal year. In the preceding example, a variance still would have existed at the end of December (the close of the fiscal year) if the printer paper had been budgeted in November. The department supplies variance then would be a permanent variance during the current and subsequent fiscal year, unless the subsequent year's budget can include the purchase.

Impact In addition to identifying whether timing is an issue, the variance analysis is expected to identify whether the variance is favorable or unfavorable. This is often determined from the budget report but should be stated clearly when discussing the variance so that the information is not misinterpreted.

Favorable variances occur when the actual results are better than budget projections. Actual revenue in excess of budget is a favorable variance. Unfavorable variances occur when the actual results are worse than what was budgeted. Actual expenditure in excess of budget is an unfavorable variance. Note that the terms *favorable* and *unfavorable* refer to the impact on the organization rather than to the magnitude or direction of the variance. Sometimes the terms *negative* and *positive* are used instead. This can be confusing because a negative expense variance is favorable. Therefore, it is extremely important to ensure that the manager understands and correctly uses the language of the organization.

Explanation of Variances

The analysis of budget variances is a financial management control. Administration may review the monthly budget report first and then ask questions of the appropriate manager. In other instances, the department managers are automatically required to respond to certain variances.

In general, the reason for a temporary budget variance is the timing of the transaction. Referring to the department supplies and printer paper example in figure 26.14, there is a simple explanation for the temporary variance. In wording the explanation to administration, the department manager should state the following:

- Nature of the variance (favorable or unfavorable, temporary or permanent)
- Exact amount of the variance

Figure 26.14. Examples of budget variances

			May budget report			
Department supplies	Budget	Actual	Variance	YTD budget	YTD actual	YTD variance
	1,150	250	900	2,150	1,250	900
			June budget report			
Department supplies	Budget	Actual	Variance	YTD budget	YTD actual	YTD variance
	250	250	0	2,400	1,500	900
			July budget report			
Department supplies	Budget	Actual	Variance	YTD budget	YTD actual	YTD variance
	250	1,150	–900	2,650	2,650	0

- Cause of the variance
- Any mitigating circumstances or offsetting amounts

Understanding and explaining budget variances is an important aspect for managers to control expenses.

Amount In the analysis of variance, materiality is an issue. Rarely will a manager be required to explain a $5 variance. Clearly, the cost of a manager's time to explain such an insignificant amount far exceeds the benefit of knowing why the variance has occurred. In fact, because budgets are largely estimates, it would be quite odd if the actual amounts always matched the budgeted amounts. Therefore, dollar and percentage limits are set in the organization's policies and procedures manual. Variances that exceed these limits must be explained in detail.

Cause For the preceding printer paper variance example, the explanation might be something like the following: In department supplies, the favorable, temporary variance of $900 will resolve in July when the budgeted expenditure for printer paper is processed. For such a temporary variance, no additional explanation is usually necessary.

Temporary variances are not typically of serious concern to administrations. However, permanent variances can be a problem because management of departmental budgets is an important indicator of the competence of department managers.

Whether a variance is temporary or permanent depends on the answers to two questions:

- Are the subsequent transactions that will compensate for the variance likely to occur within the same fiscal year?
- Is it reasonably certain the transactions will occur as predicted?

If the compensating transactions are unlikely to take place during the current fiscal year, the result is a permanent variance in the current budget report. Sometimes the manager may not know when—or if—the transactions will actually take place. For example, the manager may have budgeted $2,000 for attendance at an unspecified CE conference in June. A conflict with the Joint Commission survey prevented the manager from attending the conference, creating a favorable expense variance. As long as the manager believes the amount will be spent appropriately at some time during the fiscal year, the variance is temporary. For example, the manager may be able to attend a conference later in the year. However, if the manager knows that there is no chance of attending a conference and appropriately spending the budgeted amount, the variance should be explained as permanent.

Additional explanation may be necessary for a permanent variance. An expenditure that must be deferred until the next fiscal year is particularly important. In that case, the explanation might be as follows: In department supplies, there is a favorable, permanent variance of $900 because a large order of printer paper was planned for this fiscal year but did not occur; this amount is included in next year's budget.

Circumstances Managers may have the opportunity to utilize favorable variances in one line item to offset unfavorable variances in another line item. For example, unused travel budget may be used for CE. The explanation of these circumstances will generally be carried forward through all remaining variance analyses for the remainder of the fiscal year.

The ability to work with the departmental budget as a whole as opposed to justifying line items is entirely dependent on the administration of the budget process. One typical example of offsetting variances occurs when an employee leaves and cannot be replaced immediately. Several things may happen. The vacancy may cause a favorable variance in payroll expense until the position is filled or an unfavorable variance in payroll expense if other employees are paid overtime to help fill the vacancy. Both of these variances are permanent. Alternatively, the vacancy may cause a permanent, favorable variance in payroll expense and a permanent, unfavorable variance in consulting expenses when the vacant position is outsourced. In the latter case, the two variances at least partially offset each other, which must be explained in the monthly variance report.

Capital Budget

Unlike the operational budget, which looks primarily at projected income statement activity for the next fiscal year, the **capital budget** looks at long-term investments. Such investments are usually related to improvements in the facility infrastructure, expansion of services, or replacement of existing assets. Capital investments focus on either the appropriateness of an investment (given the facility's investment guidelines) or choosing among different opportunities to invest. The capital budget is the facility's plan for allocating resources over and above the operating budget.

Funding for the capital budget may come from diverse sources. For example, donations or grants may fund a building project or retained earnings or unallocated reserves may fund equipment purchases. Federal and state government funds may be available to offset the cost of capital investments. Regardless of the source of the funds, capital investments are defined by facility policy and selected using financial analysis techniques.

Large-Dollar Purchases

From a departmental perspective, capital budget items are large-dollar purchases, as defined by facility budget policies and procedures. Capital budget items usually have a useful life in excess of one fiscal year, making them long-term assets, and a dollar value in excess of a predetermined amount, often $500 or $1,000. Common HIM department capital budget items include office furniture, photocopying and scanning equipment, and computer equipment. Some organizations maintain a separate capital budget and process for computer-related equipment and software. In addition, control over the acquisition of the related long-term assets in such cases may rest with the information technology or information systems department.

Acquisitions

The acquisition of long-term assets may be controlled by the purchasing department. The purchasing department may already have a contract with a specific vendor to provide certain types of equipment or furniture. In the absence of an existing contract, it may still be the purchasing department's responsibility to ensure the appropriate acquisition of assets through the request for proposal (RFP) process. The RFP process is a preventive control designed to eliminate bias and to ensure competitive pricing in the acquisition of goods and services. Refer to chapter 13 for more information on the RFP process.

Cost-Benefit Analysis

Cost benefit is the concept that the benefit of an action should exceed its cost. For example, an old photocopying machine breaks down at least once a week. Repair of the machine takes up to two days and is increasingly expensive. During the downtime, release of information clerks must use a machine located two floors below the HIM department and shared by three other departments. It seems obvious to HIM department personnel that a new machine is needed and including a new machine in the HIM department's capital budget request is certainly warranted. However, funding for a new machine is based on specific, detailed cost justifications and is weighed in comparison to all departments' requests. Facility administration may be forced to choose between a new copier for the HIM department and several new computers for the patient accounts department. All other factors being equal, increased efficiency and productivity in claims processing is likely to be chosen over increased efficiency in release of information. For this reason, HIM managers should include cost savings calculations in such requests.

Depreciation

As discussed previously, certain long-term assets, such as equipment and furniture, wear out over time and must be replaced. Such assets contribute to revenue over multiple fiscal periods. Therefore, the cost of these assets is not recorded as an expense at the time of purchase. Rather, the current asset—cash is exchanged for a long-term asset—equipment. A portion of the historical cost of equipment then is moved from asset into expense each fiscal year and cumulated into the contra-account—accumulated depreciation. Eventually, the cost of equipment has been expensed and equipment account value is zero. The purpose of depreciation is to spread the cost of an asset over its useful life. (See table 26.8 for sample depreciation methods.)

Note that the depreciation of long-term assets does not necessarily have a direct relationship to the activity of actually using the asset. It is common to depreciate an asset over five years and then continue to use it for another five. For example, a facility whose equipment is fully depreciated and whose current assets are heavily financed with debt obligations may be unable to reinvest in new equipment. This is another example of how ratio analysis affects lending decisions.

Capital Projects

A facility's ability to invest in capital projects is important to the continued success of its operations. Because buildings deteriorate, equipment wears out, and new technology is important to healthcare delivery, capital improvements must be implemented. Individual departments request equipment purchases and facility improvements as the needs arise. Facility administration must choose among the suggested projects to optimize use of its resources.

Table 26.8. Sample depreciation methods

Method	Description	Formula
Straight line	The cost of the asset is expensed equally over the expected life of the asset. The estimated sale value of the asset at the end of its useful life is called the residual value and is subtracted from the cost prior to depreciation. **Example:** Copy machine purchased at a cost of $5,000 Useful life = 4 years Residual value = $200 Annual depreciation $\dfrac{\$5,000 - \$200}{4} = \$1,200$ per year	$\dfrac{Cost - residual\ value}{Number\ of\ years\ (useful\ life)}$
Units of production	The cost of the asset is expensed over the expected life of the asset, measured in usage. In this case, usage would be the number of copies. **Example:** Copy machine purchased at a cost of $5,000 Useful life = 100,000 copies Residual value = $200 Depreciation rate $\dfrac{\$5,000 - \$200}{\$100,000} = \$0.048$ (4.8 cents) per copy Annual depreciation = $0.048 times the number of copies actually made	$\dfrac{Cost - residual\ value}{Number\ of\ copies\ (useful\ life)}$
Accelerated	There are several accelerated depreciation methods, all of which are designed to expense more of the asset's value early in its useful life. One such method is called double declining balance (DDB). DDB expenses the asset at double the straight-line method, based on the book value rather than on the historical cost. **Example:** Copy machine purchased at a cost of $5,000 Useful life = 100,000 copies Residual value = $200 Straight-line rate $1,200/$4,800 = 25% Annual depreciation = Book value times 50%	Book value times twice the straight-line rate Straight-line rate $= \dfrac{annual\ depreciation}{cost - residual\ value}$

Note: These examples of depreciation methods are just a few of the acceptable methods in use today for various purposes. The reader should be aware that there are other methods and that not all methods are acceptable for income tax purposes or for GAAP. Accounting for income taxes is beyond the scope of this discussion.

In addition to capital improvements, facilities may make capital investments that improve operational efficiency. Some of these capital investments require broader analysis than the cost of the equipment. Replacing a manual incomplete record tracking system with a computer-based system, for example, involves an analysis of employee time and departmental space allocations as well as the associated equipment and software costs. Medical staff relationship improvement is another factor that is difficult to quantify but should be considered.

Facility administration looks at capital projects differently than it reviews operational activities. Theoretically, operational activities contribute to the generation of revenue for the facility. For example, all hospital activities either provide healthcare services or in some way support departments that provide healthcare services. A hospital may elect to perform its own printing rather than outsource the printing function; however, it is unlikely to provide printing services to the general public. Printing forms supports clinical and administrative services internally; running a printing business does not. Therefore, the justification for operational budget amounts generally rests on the extent to which the underlying activities support the mission of the facility at the projected productivity levels. Capital projects, on the other hand, although still mission supportive, often leverage the facility to higher levels of productivity, increased efficiency, or expansion of services and capacity.

Departments acquiring capital equipment will often work with the finance department to prepare financial analysis reports that review projected revenues, costs, and cost savings and use a variety of financial analysis techniques discussed later in the chapter to determine whether the project meets predetermined levels of return. For example, if the obstetrics department wants to acquire an additional ultrasound machine, the department manager would work with the finance department to project expected patient volumes, reimbursements, and costs that a new ultrasound machine would be expected to generate and compare those returns to predetermined levels set by management.

Finally, budgeted capital funds generally must be expended in the time period for which they were approved. Even when allocated, capital budget items may be prioritized and timed so that purchases are made only with administrative approval. Actual funding may not meet anticipated levels, or unforeseen circumstances may change administrative priorities.

For capital budgets, supporting the mission of the facility is not sufficient justification. Capital projects also must satisfy predetermined levels of return on the projected investment.

Cost Justification

All departments in a facility compete for finite facility resources. Therefore, department managers must be familiar with cost justification techniques and with their facility's method of analyzing capital projects. Typical cost justifications are based on increased revenue, increased efficiency, improved customer service, reduced liability, and reduced costs. The analysis of a capital project is based on the estimated ROI, including the weight of the costs versus the benefits to be derived from the project. The specific cost-benefit analysis method used by facility administration depends on the characteristics of the project as well as the preferences of the analyst. When no specific cash inflows are expected, return may be based on depreciation or other cost savings. Sometimes the capital budget includes the allocation of resources for assets whose acquisition will attract or retain valuable personnel or physician relationships. Even in such cases, the acquisition should be analyzed financially, not just politically.

Payback Period

The **payback period** is the time required to recoup the cost of an investment. Mortgage refinancing analysis frequently uses the concept of payback period. Mortgage refinancing is considered when interest rates have dropped. Refinancing may require up-front interest payments, called points, as well as a variety of administrative costs. In this example, the payback period is the time it takes for the savings in interest to equal the cost of the refinancing:

Payback period	
Investment:	$100,000
Cash in:	$50,000 per year
Payback period:	2 years (100,000/50,000)

The advantage of using a payback period to analyze investments is that it is relatively easy to calculate and understand. For example, a payback period can be used to describe the time it takes for the savings in payroll costs to equal the cost of productivity-enhancing equipment. In the previous photocopy machine example, the payroll costs would be calculated based on downtime incurred when using a copier in another area of the building.

The disadvantage of a payback period is that it ignores the time value of money. Because the funds used for one capital investment could have been invested elsewhere, there is always an inherent opportunity cost of choosing one investment over another. Hence, there is an assumed rate of return determined by administration against which investments are compared and a benchmark rate of return under which a facility will not consider an investment.

Accounting Rate of Return

Another simple method of capital project analysis is the **accounting rate of return (ARR)**. This method compares the projected annual cash inflows, minus any applicable annual depreciation, divided by the initial investment. Consider the purchase of an ultrasound machine. Reimbursement from use of the machine is the cash inflow. Depreciation is calculated based on the initial investment. The following example shows the accounting rate of return for the purchase of a $100,000 ultrasound machine:

Accounting Rate of Return	
Investment:	$100,000 ultrasound machine
Straight-line depreciation over 5 years:	$20,000 per year
Cash in:	$50,000 per year
ARR:	30 percent [(50,000 − 20,000)/100,000]

Accounting rate of return is another example of a simple method of capital project analysis. However, it also ignores the time value of money. In addition, accounting rate of return is based on an estimate. If the analyst incorrectly projects annual cash inflows, the projected rate of return will be incorrect.

Return on Investment

Return on investment (ROI) is most frequently used to analyze marketable securities, or investments in stock, retrospectively. The increase in market value of the securities divided by the initial investment is the ROI. When an income stream is associated with the investment, the income stream is added to the market value of the securities in calculating return. In comparing the ROI among different securities, the tax implications must be considered. Long-term gains are taxed differently than short-term gains. Tax-exempt investments result in different returns than taxable investments.

With respect to capital investments, the equation is similar. Divide the controllable operating profits by the controllable net investment. Operating profits are the cash inflow minus the direct costs of operation. For instance, the return on investment for the purchase of $100,000 worth of equipment would be calculated as:

Return on Investment	
Investment:	$100,000 in equipment
Straight-line depreciation over 5 years:	$20,000 per year
Operating costs:	$5,000 per year
Cash in:	$50,000 per year
ROI:	25 percent [(50,000 − 25,000)/100,000]

As with accounting rate of return and payback period, ROI is easy to calculate and understand. Similarly, it does not consider the time value of money. Organizations will establish a benchmark ROI that is required for new investments. In this example, if the benchmark ROI is 15 percent this investment would be approved because it is projected to generate an ROI of 25 percent.

Net Present Value

To take into consideration the time value of money, the analyst must establish an interest rate at which money could have otherwise been invested. From that implied interest rate and the projected future cash inflows of the investment, the present value of the cash inflows is calculated. Present value is the current dollar amount that must be invested today in order to yield the projected future cash inflows at the implied interest rate. **Net present value (NPV)** is the calculated present value of the future cash inflows compared to the initial investment.

The advantage of using net present value to analyze investments is that it considers the time value of money. When choosing among like investments, net present values can be reliably compared to determine the financial advantages of the investment. For example, the NPV of $100,000 worth of equipment would be calculated as:

Net Present Value	
Investment:	$100,000
Cash in:	$25,000 per year (revenue minus depreciation and operating costs)
Interest rate:	7 percent
NPV:	$2,505 (based on 5 years of service)

As with other analysis tools, analysts may have to estimate the projected cash flows. However, the main disadvantage of net present value is that the interest rate is subjective. Therefore, it is best used to compare multiple investment opportunities rather than to analyze one investment alone. Another disadvantage of using net present value is that it requires some knowledge of mathematics to calculate as well as to accept its validity and understand its relevance. Fortunately, financial calculators and spreadsheet programs have made the calculation of net present value relatively simple.

Internal Rate of Return

Internal rate of return (IRR) is the interest rate that makes the net present value calculation equal zero. In other words, it is the interest rate at which the present value of the projected cash inflows equals the initial investment. IRR considers the time value of money. Both individual and multiple investments can be evaluated. As with net present value, knowledge of mathematics is helpful. The main disadvantage is that a project may have multiple

IRRs. For example, the IRR of $100,000 worth of equipment would be calculated as:

Internal Rate of Return	
Investment:	$100,000
Cash in:	$25,000 per year (revenue minus depreciation and operating costs)
NPV:	$0 (based on 5 years of service)
Interest rate:	8 percent

Profitability Index

Facilities cannot automatically invest in seemingly profitable projects. For example, a $500,000 radiology equipment investment may have a present value of cash inflows of $1,500,000, for a net present value of $1,000,000. At the same time, a $10,000 pharmacy computer system yields a net present value of $30,000. This seems to be a great investment; however, the facility's capital budget may be limited to $100,000. In this case, a profitability index helps the organization prioritize investment opportunities. For each investment, divide the present value of the cash inflows by the present value of the cash outflows. In this example, the pharmacy system has a higher profitability index, illustrated as follows:

Radiology		Pharmacy
$1,500,000	Present value of cash inflows	$40,000
$500,000	Present value of cash outflows	$10,000
3	Profitability index	4

Management roles in any healthcare facility require some knowledge of accounting and financial management. The ability to read, understand, and interpret pertinent financial reports is a desirable business skill. Because of the close ties between reimbursement and HIM, this basic skill is even more important. Although the financial accounting methodologies of compiling and analyzing financial statements may not be needed routinely, the managerial accounting skills involving budget preparation and analysis are critical. Also important is an awareness of the preventive, detective, and corrective controls that managers must implement to ensure the accuracy of financial data.

Check Your Understanding 26.4

Instructions: **Answer the following questions on a separate piece of paper.**

1. Compare and contrast financial accounting and managerial accounting.

2. Compare and contrast operational budgets and capital budgets.

3. Identify the three major categories of internal controls.

4. Explain how budget variances are used in financial management of an organization.

5. The HIM department has a YTD budget for a payroll of $100,000. The actual YTD amount is $98,000. Is this a favorable or an unfavorable variance?

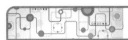

References

Davis, N. and R. Revoir. 2013. Financial management. Chapter 25 in *Health Information Management: Concepts, Principles and Practice*, 4th ed. Edited by LaTour, K.M., S. Eichenwald Maki, and P. Oachs. Chicago: AHIMA.

Holmes, M. and G.H. Pink. 2013 (Dec.). Change in Profitability and Financial Distress of Critical Access Hospitals from Loss of Cost-Based Reimbursement. NC Rural Health Research Program. http://www. shepscenter.unc.edu/wp-content/uploads/2013/12/Change-in-Profitability-and-Financial-Distress-of-CAHs-November-2013.pdf

Internal Revenue Service. 2015. Tax Exempt Status for Your Organization. Pub. 557. http://www.irs.gov/pub/irs-pdf/p557.pdf

Schraffenberger, L.A., ed. 2011. *Effective Management of Coding Services*, 4th ed. Chicago: AHIMA.

PART VI
Leadership

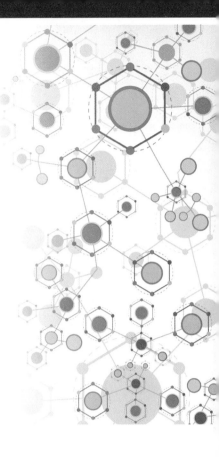

27

Project Management

Brandon D. Olson, PhD, PMP

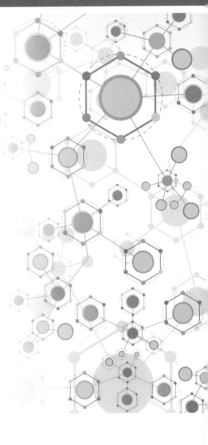

Learning Objectives

- Differentiate between project and operations activities
- Identify and explain the three sources of projects
- Describe the purpose of each of the project management process groups
- Associate the project roles with the activities in the project management process
- Identify and describe the skills and abilities needed for project management
- Explain the use of a WBS and Gantt chart in project planning
- Determine the purpose for each step in the change management process
- Differentiate among project management, program management, and portfolio management

Key Terms

Administrative supervisor
Agile approach
Balanced matrix organization
Compliance projects
Consultant
Contractor
Expense projects
Functional organization
Gantt chart
Industry knowledge
Iterative approach
Matrix organization
Operations
Organizational experience

Outsourcing agency
Process knowledge
Professional behavior
Program
Program management
Project
Project budget
Project champion
Project coordinator
Project expediter
Project failure
Project management
Project management constraints
Project management lifecycle

Project manager
Project performance
Project portfolio management
Project portfolio manager
Project scope
Project sponsor
Project stakeholder
Project team
Projectized organization
Requirements document
Revenue projects
Scope creep
Strong matrix organization
Triple constraint

Users
Variance

Waterfall method
Weak matrix organization

Work breakdown
structure (WBS)

The healthcare industry is undergoing rapid change. This change requires many systems and processes to be revised or replaced and requires people from multiple departments to work together to support these changes. The health information management (HIM) professional interacts with many functions across the healthcare organization and is called upon to participate in or lead new initiatives that enable the organization to change. These efforts taking place to support changes to the healthcare system occur while the day-to-day operations continue. As a result, a separate set of activities occurs outside of the daily work supporting patient care. These additional activities are the projects carried out in response to the changing healthcare industry.

Projects and managing projects are an important part of any industry, and given the current changing environment in healthcare, effective project management is critical to keep up with the amount of change taking place. In this chapter, projects, project management, and the role and attributes of a project manager are introduced and the methods used to lead projects are discussed. It also includes an introduction to concepts that are applied to projects and project management in order to connect the project efforts with the long-term goals of the organization.

The Project

Projects exist as a result of the organization's response to change. The need for change or reaction to change is the basis for all projects. Change may be due to the desire to offer new products or services, respond to new industry trends or regulations, or improve or automate processes. Regardless of the reason for change, projects are created to coordinate the organization's efforts and resources to ensure an effective transition from the current state of operating to a new state. In other words, projects are used to make changes in the organization.

Change has become common in the workplace and creating change is often a strategic priority for organizations. Projects and the management of these projects are considered to be key to achieving long-term goals and critical to an organization's success. A report found that in organizations that were most successful in achieving desired results from projects, 97 percent of the executives consider project management critical to the organization's performance and 94 percent believe projects enable the organization to grow (PMI 2013a). Organizations who experience the benefits from projects recognize the importance project

management plays in achieving these results and associate the projects with the change needed to increase their success in the marketplace. Projects are an effective means to institute change in the organization as a way to achieve both long-term and short-term improvement goals.

Definition of a Project

Projects are important to organizations, but it may not be clear what a project is and how it differs from the ongoing operations taking place in an organization. There are many ways to define projects and each definition offers additional characteristics to the term. Following are examples of project definitions:

- "a temporary endeavor undertaken to create a unique product, service, or result"(PMI 2013b, 3).

- "a complex, nonroutine, one-time effort limited by time, budget, resources, and performance specifications designed to meet customer needs" (Gray and Larson 2014, 5).

- "any series of activities and tasks that have specific objectives to be completed within certain specifications; have defined start and end dates; have funding limits; consume human and nonhuman resources; are multi-functional" (Kerzner 2013, 2).

Each of these definitions use different language to describe the same term and each definition centers on different characteristics. Although there is more than one definition for the term project, the collection of definitions given point out several characteristics of projects. These characteristics are:

- Temporary and one-time instance of work
- Use of resources from multiple disciplines
- Defined and specific outcome goals
- Limited resource budgets
- Targeted start and end dates

Using the characteristics of a project, a comprehensive definition can be derived. A **project** is a temporary and single instance of work involving specialized individuals working together to achieve a specific goal within resource and time limitations.

In order to better understand the concept of a project, it is important to be able to differentiate projects from operations. Projects differ from the ongoing operations in the organization. While a project is temporary and occurs only once, **operations** do not have a planned end date and the work is repeated routinely. Additionally, projects differ from operations in terms of repetition where each project differs from other projects; while operations is designed around consistency. The temporary and unique nature of projects differentiate these efforts from the ongoing operations. Table 27.1 provides examples to illustrate the differences between projects and operations.

The routine work of operations is important for the organization to carry out its mission by delivering quality products and services in a consistent manner. Operations are the ongoing and routine work that changes only when the organization's objectives can no longer be met. When these operational objectives can no longer be met, change must occur. These changes are carried out through projects. Projects are the temporary efforts carried out to meet specific objectives and enable change.

The need for change may be requested or required from within the organization or outside of the organization. As a result, a project is created to achieve the outcomes needed to allow the organization to change. These unique and temporary projects are planned and executed to accomplish specific objectives that enable the organization to change. Understanding the objectives is important to determining why the project exists. These project objectives or sources are associated with the real purpose for the need or desire to change and understanding the true purpose enables the organization to focus on the important outcomes from the project.

Project Sources

The objective or source of any project can be associated with one of three separate categories. Each project category determines the business goal of the project and describes the reason the project exists. Three sources of projects and project examples for each source are listed in table 27.2. The three separate groups include:

- Revenue: Projects with a goal of increasing the organization's income
- Expense: Projects with a goal of reducing the costs of providing goods or services

Table 27.1.   Differences between operations and projects

Operations	Project
Taking notes in class	Writing a research paper
Using an existing electronic health record system	Implementing an electronic health record system
Attending team meetings	Planning a professional conference
Practicing the piano	Organizing a community concert
Storing provider dictations	Creating a new method to integrate provider dictations into the electronic health record
Following a patient registration process	Designing a new registration workflow

Table 27.2.   Examples of categorized projects

Project type	Examples
Revenue	• Open a new clinic • Add a sports medicine practice • Extend clinic hours
Expense	• Digitize charts in warehouse • Share electronic health records across departments • Create new productivity report
Compliance	• Adopt ICD-10 coding • Upgrade all computers to a new operating system • Develop and conduct HIPAA training

• Compliance: Projects with a goal of meeting the expectations or directives set by an internal or external governing body

There are a few things to note regarding the categorization of projects. **Revenue projects** may include projects that result in new or expanded products or services. In nonprofit and government organizations, these revenue projects may not increase revenue but rather increase the quantity or capacity of its services. **Expense projects** include projects where new and improved information is created. Such projects fall into the expense reduction category since increased access to information and knowledge results in better decision making and reduced costs from inferior decisions. Finally, it should be noted that **compliance projects** include self-imposed initiatives organizations place on themselves, industry imposed compliance where organizations must meet a minimum level of stakeholder expectations, and government or regulatory compliance that organizations must meet in order to remain in business.

Understanding the categorization of a project is important as it determines the ultimate goal for the change the organization seeks to make. Some projects will have a goal to help the organization increase its revenue or services, other projects will have a goal to reduce inefficiencies and expenses, and some projects will have a goal to comply with an internal or external requirement. Whichever the purpose of the project, the goal becomes a target for the project and projects must be planned and executed to address this goal.

Check Your Understanding 27.1

Instructions: **Answer the following questions on a separate sheet of paper.**

1. Why do organizations conduct projects?

2. What are the characteristics of a project?

3. How do projects differ from operations?

4. What is the purpose of a revenue project?

5. What is the purpose of an expense project?

6. What is the purpose of a compliance project?

7. Is cost savings or revenue generation a measure for a compliance project? Why or why not?

Project Management

Projects, and various forms of managing them, have existed for thousands of years; but the modern systematic methodology and specific discipline of project management emerged in the mid-20th century. The US Navy's Polaris project of 1956 to 1961 was credited as the first project to refine and apply the project management concepts used today (Kwak 2003). Between the early 20th century and today, the evolution of project management can be broken down into four periods:

- 1900 to 1958: Transportation and telecommunications advances shortened project schedules, and initial project planning tools like the Gantt chart and work breakdown structures emerged

- 1958 to 1979: Computer systems automated processes, and advanced planning tools and project management software supported more complex project planning

- 1980 to 1994: Availability of personal computers provided greater access to processing power and increased the availability of project management software and analysis tools

- 1995 to present: The availability of the Internet to the general public connected individual team members, reduced the time for communication, and led to new tools supporting collaboration by project team members

The project management method has continued to be improved and used by almost every industry as a means to govern a project. During this time, project management became a specific discipline with professional organizations like the Project Management Institute (PMI) establishing best practices and promoting the project management field. Today there are over 471,000 PMI members in 202 countries and over 663,000 people who hold a Project Management Professional (PMP) certification (PMI 2015). Additionally, the PMI standard for best practices in project management—the Project Management Body of Knowledge—has over 5 million copies in circulation. The project management profession has grown significantly and matured with recognized best practices and professional certifications.

Project management is defined as "the application of knowledge, skills, tools, and techniques to project activities to meet the project requirements" (PMI 2013b, 5). This means that project management is both a process as well the application of previous experience and is used to guide the project activities toward achieving the project goals. Perhaps more specifically, project management is an intentional effort to plan, organize, direct, and control the organization's resources toward achieving a specific short-term objective. This short-term effort is the project; and the planning, organizing, directing, and controlling take place in the act of managing the project. Using either definition, project management requires expertise to be applied to a set of processes.

Project Management Process

Project management is achieved through the execution and integration of project processes. Based on an evolution of best practices, PMI logically grouped a set of 47 core project management processes and categorized them into groups (PMI 2013b). This formal categorization of processes are referred to as process groups, and these groups and their relationship to one another is commonly viewed as the project management process. The five process groups are: initiating, planning, executing, monitoring and controlling, and closing. Each of these process groups is required to complete a project and omitting any of these process groups from the project greatly increases the risk of failure for the project. The process groups are also connected and sequenced for a project. Figure 27.1 illustrates an example of how the process groups may be sequenced in a project.

The process groups are carried out over time and successful completion of all process groups results in a completed project. Although the sequencing may change for each project, the order of these process groups is important since the output of one process group is often needed for successful

Figure 27.1.   Sample process group sequence

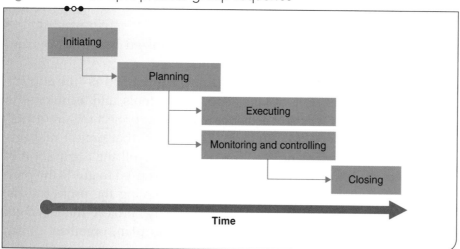

completion of the next process group. For instance, the executing process group cannot be completed without some or all results from the planning process group. The exception to the sequencing is that the executing and monitoring and controlling phases may occur simultaneously. Each of the process groups include many individual processes to create the output needed for subsequent process groups. Figure 27.1 represents the sequencing of the process groups but does not indicate the activities taking place within each group. A more detailed explanation of the activities taking place within each process group is provided later in the chapter.

Alternative Project Methodologies

Each of the process groups may also be considered a phase of a project. The collection of project phases forms the **project management life cycle**. The traditional method of completing the life cycle is in a sequential order. This sequential method of completing the project phases is commonly referred to as the **waterfall method**. In this method, the phases are structured so that one phase begins at the end or near the end of the previous phase. This method has been successfully applied for decades and ensures the output from one phase is complete and ready to serve as inputs for the next phase.

The traditional waterfall method ensures the entire project is cohesively planned and executed.

The waterfall method is a good fit for complex projects or projects having a clear understanding of the specifications for the final output. However, the downside to the waterfall method is that the sequential nature delays delivery of the final project output until the end of the project and does not offer the flexibility needed if the output or design specifications for the project are not clear. The waterfall method requires the planning to be complete prior to executing, and output from the project is not available until the very end of the project. In order to make project output available sooner, some projects are executed in releases following an **iterative approach** to the project management life cycle (figure 27.2) or through an **agile approach** (figure 27.3) where the life cycle is repeated in many iterations.

Each life cycle approach—waterfall, iterative, and agile—has been applied to many projects, but each approach may not fit all projects. There are several factors to consider when evaluating which life cycle approach to use in a project. The fluidity of the project output specifications, the familiarity of the team with alternative project methodologies, and the organization's acceptance of alternative methods are all factors that should be taken into consideration before determining the best approach to use. Regardless of the life cycle approach selected, the project must complete each phase in the life cycle to reduce the likelihood of a failed project.

Figure 27.2.   Sample iterative sequence

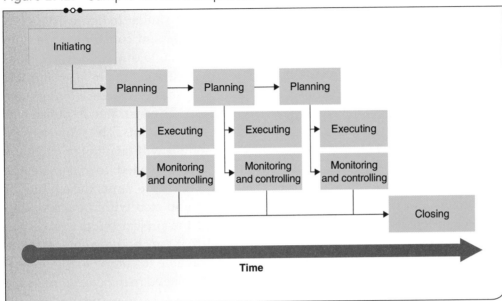

Figure 27.3.   Sample agile sequence

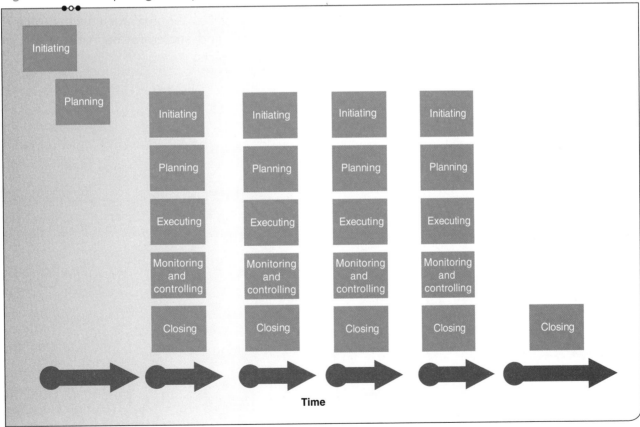

Project Management Constraints

Projects sometimes fail. Project failure can have different meanings from different perspectives, but from a basic project management perspective, **project failure** occurs when the entire scope identified is not delivered, all work is not completed before the targeted date, or all work cannot be completed while remaining within the defined resource budget. These three forms of project failure are the central concerns in project management.

At the beginning of each project, the scope of the work to be accomplished is defined for the project. The project scope is to be completed within an allocated budget and before a targeted date. For example, a project could be defined with a scope of scanning all paper medical records from the past 10 years within four months using only two analysts. These three expectations comprise the limits, or constraints, of the project. In this case, the scope constraint is scanning all paper records from the past 10 years, the time constraint is a four-month period, and the budget constraint is limiting the resources (in this case human resources) to two full-time analysts. These three constraints are commonly referred to as the **triple constraint** and expressed as a triangle similar to figure 27.4.

The **project management constraints** are typically depicted as a triangle due to the three sides representing the three constraints. The triangle also represents the connectedness of the three constraints where each constraint is dependent upon the other two constraints. The **project scope** determines how long it will take to complete the work and the budget needed to complete the project; the project schedule limits the amount of scope that can be completed within the time and given budget; and the project budget limits the amount of scope that can be delivered and the amount of time available to complete the project. A project must be managed to maximize the scope while minimizing the schedule and budget. Increased scope may cost more and take more time. Conversely, decreased resource budget or time may limit the amount of scope the project may deliver. This careful balancing of scope, schedule, and budget is the goal for effective project management, and successful balancing leads to successful projects.

Figure 27.4.   Project management constraints

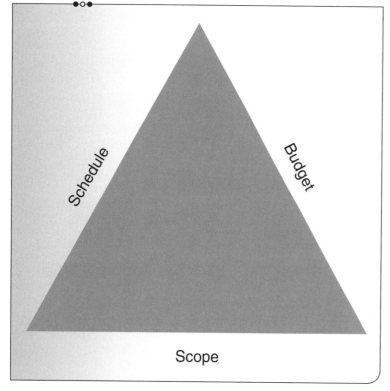

Due to the importance of the project management constraints, most project reporting will center on progress toward these three constraints. The project begins with an initial set of scope, schedule, and budget expectations. These initial expectations are the baseline for the project, and any deviation from these baseline expectations is referred to as a **variance**. As the project is underway, projects typically report the current progress and forecasted estimates of the three constraints and identify any deviation from the project baseline. In addition to reporting the status for the project in respect to these three constraints, the project is often required to make adjustments in order to correct any variances with scope, schedule, and budget to ensure the project falls within the expected baseline targets.

Project Members

There are many individuals associated with a project. Anyone with an interest in the deliverables created as part of the project is considered a **project stakeholder**. The project stakeholders frequently rely on results from the project to fulfill some of their operational needs or long-term goals. In addition to the project stakeholders, individuals directly involved in specifying, supporting, or creating the project deliverables have an interest in the project.

Projects are carried out by a number of individuals who contribute a specialized skill set or knowledge to complete the project deliverables. The specialized skills and knowledge are driven by the type of work required to complete the project scope. While roles and specialties vary across all projects, there are many roles associated with the project that are clearly defined and are required for any successful project. These roles include the project manager, project champion, project sponsor, users or recipients, and the project team members. Each of these roles are directly related to specifying, supporting, and completing the project; and are not a part of the organization's more permanent operations roles.

Project Sponsor

Every project begins with a need or desire for change. This need may originate from a functional leader or it may originate at the top level of the organization. Regardless of where the need originates, the organization must determine the functional area(s) within the organization where the project should reside. Either the functional leader expressing the need for change or a leader over the functional area most likely to be affected or benefited by the project often becomes the **project sponsor** or project owner. For example, the manager over release of information could serve as the project sponsor for a project where the release of information module is integrated within the electronic health record system. This individual may be responsible for securing the budget for the project and would provide overall direction for the project and its fit within the electronic health record system. The project sponsor secures resource commitments for the project and makes many of the decisions regarding the project objectives and scope. The sponsor is a key decision maker for the project and is responsible for ensuring the project deliverables effectively satisfy the needs of the organization.

User or Recipient

Although the project is owned by the project sponsor, it is often executed for the benefit of a group of users or recipients. The **users** are all internal and external stakeholders who are directly affected by the project deliverables. In the case of a release of information module implementation project, the staff working on release of information who are familiar with the current workflows would serve as users in the project. These individuals will be able to offer insight as to how the results from the project will affect them or their work and identify the specifications of the project deliverables so that the results fulfill their expectations. The project users must be engaged in the project to ensure they are satisfied with the project deliverables and that these products meet their needs. The project sponsor provides the overall direction for the project, but the project users provide the detailed specifications and are best able to determine the acceptability of the project deliverables.

Project Manager

Every project must have an individual responsible to ensure the work is planned, organized, assigned, directed, and monitored. The project manager is responsible for these activities as well as ensuring the project is completed within the constraints of scope, schedule, and budget. The project manager may come from within the HIM department or may be a project management specialist from another department. While planning and managing the work is an important responsibility of the project manager, communications is the most critical to project success. Project managers must ensure communications exist within the project team and between the project team and the stakeholders. Through project planning documents, standardized and structured status reports, e-mail messages, tracking logs, and project meetings, the project manager must insist that communications take place so that all project stakeholders are engaged and the project team is able to receive the information and resources needed to successfully execute the project.

Project Champion

Projects require support from the organization in order to meet the organization's needs. This support includes both the continued approval from the organization as well as sufficient resources to properly complete the project. The project champion is an executive in the organization who believes in the benefits of the project and advocates for the project. Depending on the overall impact the project has on the healthcare organization, this individual may be the manager of the HIM department or the director over the business unit where the HIM department resides, or it could be the chief operations officer (COO). The project champion is responsible for making sure the project objectives align with the organization's goals and also to ensure the project is receiving the resources needed to meet these objectives. Without the project champion, organizational support for the project would wane and the project could lose access to the budgeted resources.

Project Team

In addition to the project-specific roles, there are many skilled individuals who make up the project team. The project team consists of individuals with knowledge or skills specific to the project needs. The knowledge and skills needed are dependent upon the type of project, the industry where the project takes place, and the needs specific to the phase of the project. For example, in a paper record scanning project, a software developer may be needed to build an interface to allow scanned records to be input into the electronic health record but the developer would not be needed to scan the paper records. The knowledge and skill sets required for the project vary at different times of the project. As a result, project team members will move on and off the project throughout the entire project life cycle and return to their operational roles once their need on the project has ended.

Check Your Understanding 27.2

Instructions: **Answer the following questions on a separate sheet of paper.**

1. What is the project scope?
2. How is the project scope related to the budget?
3. What purpose does a project champion serve on the project?
4. Why are some project members only temporarily assigned to a project team?
5. Who are the stakeholders for a project?

Organizational Structures

Project team members are borrowed from functional departments across the organization to contribute specialized skills or knowledge to the project. Once the project no longer requires their contributions, they return to their role within the functional department. As a result of the temporary nature of projects, no permanent organizational structure exists for the project team. The project exists as a dynamic structure within the existing permanent or semi-permanent organizational structure. Some organizational structures support the project environment better than others. The following sections outline several common organizational structures and the corresponding fit for a project environment.

Functional Organization

The traditional hierarchy in an organization is the functional organization where each employee has a single supervisor and employees are grouped in departments by specialty or subspecialty (see figure 27.5). Each department within the functional organization operates independently of the other departments.

The specialization of the functional organization creates challenges for projects. If a project exists within a single department and only members of the department are affected by the project, a functional organization can support projects. However, many projects span multiple areas of specialty making it a challenge for the functional organization to manage coordination between departments. This cross-departmental collaboration must take place, but it is counter to the contained department-specific work typically carried out in the functional organization.

Due to the independent nature of the functional organization, the true role of a project manager does not typically exist. A project manager in this structure would have little or no authority, have limited abilities to obtain resources or budget, and would perform project manager duties in addition to department responsibilities. Rather than a true project management role, the functional organization uses what is referred to as a project coordinator to facilitate resources and collaboration across the departments participating in the project. The project coordinator, typically a HIM professional with

Figure 27.5.   Functional organization

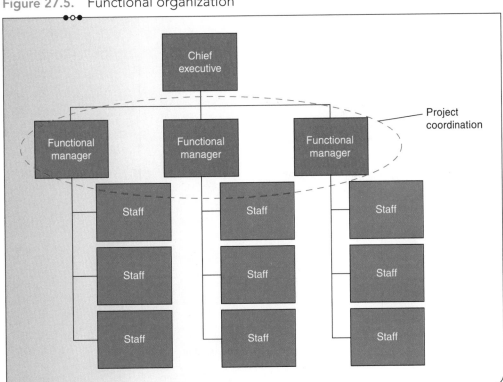

experience working with different departments within the HIM area, works with the functional manager of each department to get work completed. The functional manager maintains full authority, and the project is dependent upon the project coordinator's effective collaboration with the participating functional managers and each functional manager's direct authority over the staff completing the project work. In this case, the project coordinator does not have authority over the staff but rather work is directed by the staff's functional manager. For example, a release of information analyst may coordinate the activities of a release of information-related project but cannot prioritize the work of any of the members working on the project since these priorities are governed by the individual's respective managers.

Matrix Organization

Functional organizations can be modified to form a matrix organization by integrating a secondary project structure. In the **matrix organization**, employees report to an administrative supervisor from the original functional area to carry out their operational work but may also report to a functional supervisor to manage their work on the project. The matrix organization offers a better support structure for projects but is partially dependent upon the type of matrix organization.

A matrix organization is further classified as either a weak matrix, balanced matrix, or strong matrix. In the **weak matrix organization** (see figure 27.6), the project manager role does not exist but a **project expediter** role is used to work directly with the functional staff rather than through the functional managers. This modification from the functional organization provides a little more authority and resources for the project expediter, but the budget and resources are still managed by the functional managers. As a result, the project expediter role is part time in addition to operational responsibilities.

The role of project manager does not exist within the pure functional or weak matrix organizations due to inseparability of the project work from the operational work. Balanced matrix organizational structures provide the separation of operations and

Figure 27.6. Weak matrix organization

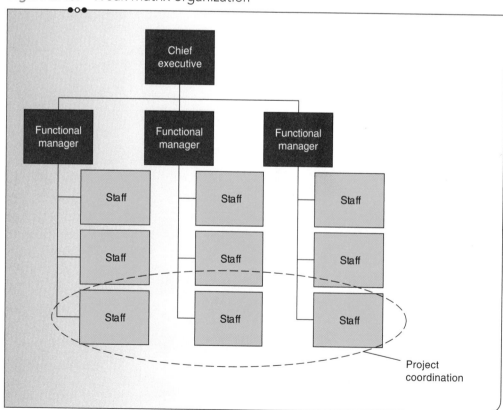

project work. In the **balanced matrix** organizational structure, a project organization exists within the existing functional hierarchy and a project manager is recruited from one of the functional departments to serve as the leader of the project. In the balanced matrix organization, the project manager has moderate authority and access to resources but must still collaborate with the functional managers to obtain these resources. The work on the project is directed completely by the project manager with the functional managers making decisions regarding project scope. The balanced matrix organizations commonly use a full-time project management role to lead the project team made up of part-time project members (see figure 27.7).

The third type of matrix organization is the strong matrix organization. The **strong matrix organization** is very similar to the balanced matrix but includes a department of project managers. In these organizations, project managers are not functional staff members assuming the role of project manager but rather project manager specialists reporting to a manager of project management. For instance,

the transcription group within the HIM department may include an individual who reports to the manager of transcription and is responsible for managing projects within the HIM department. The strong matrix organizations provide the project manager a moderate to high level of authority over the project and project resources. In many cases, the project manager in a strong matrix organization manages the budget and is a full-time project manager (see figure 27.8).

Projectized Organization

The functional and matrix organizations are designed around operational work. For this reason, they are separated by functional areas and any project structure must fit within the operational structure. Some organizations are designed around work in projects rather than operations and for these organizations a projectized structure is applied. In this **projectized organization**, the operational department structures focused on a specialty or subspecialty are replaced by multidisciplinary project teams led by a project manager. (See figure 27.9.)

Figure 27.7. Balanced matrix organization

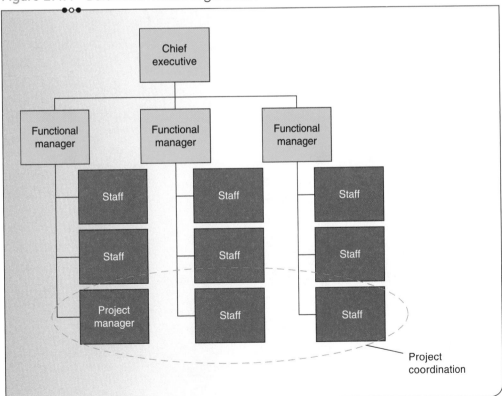

Figure 27.8. Strong matrix organization

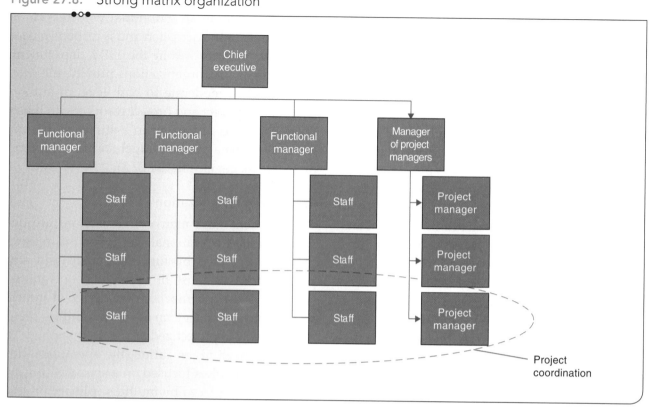

Figure 27.9. Projectized organization

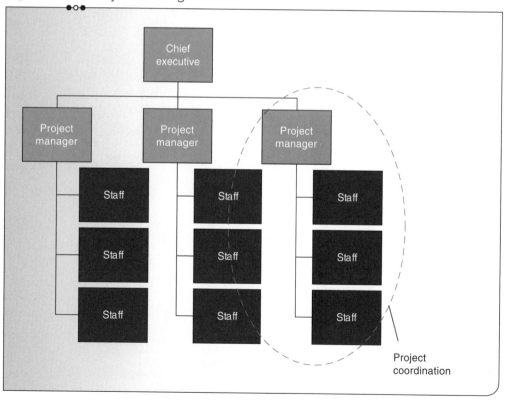

In these projectized organizations, the project manager has almost total authority over the team and access to resources as well as the project budgets. Similar to the strong matrix organizational structure, projectized structures also make the project management role full time and the project staff full time.

Summary of Organizational Structures

Each of these organizational structures serve different purposes and one or more may exist within the same organization. Also, these structures may evolve over time so any one structure may be a temporary organizational structure based on the organization's needs at the time. Table 27.3 summarizes organizational structures and the relationship to the project environment. In the context of project management, the projectized and strong matrix structures offer the most control and authority to project managers while the balanced and weak matrix organizations reduce the authority and decision making permissions. Finally, in a true functional organizational structure, project managers exist in the form of a project coordinator or a project expediter who merely coordinates the activities across departments under the direction of the individual department managers.

Organizations undergoing frequent change and wishing to promote project management practices adopt a balanced matrix or strong matrix structure to provide the ability to centralize authority of the project and encourage collaboration across departments. Organizations with infrequent change and fewer project needs may continue to adopt a functional or weak organizational structure so they remain focused on operations and the specialization of each department. The projectized structure is adopted by organizations whose work is predominantly centered around projects spanning multiple disciplines or for organizations going through significant change where projects become a focus over operations. See table 27.3 for a comparison of the various project management organizational structures.

Team Structures

In addition to the structure of the organization, the structure of the team also contributes to the project team dynamics and the role of the project manager. The project team structure characteristics include the physical location of the team members, the time allotted to the team members for the project, and the employment status of the team members. The physical location of the team influences the team communications and management of work. Additionally, the project availability of the team members determines project workload and scheduling, and the employment status may impact commitment and expertise. Each of these characteristics influence how the project team interacts and how the project manager leads the team.

Part-Time Team Members

Often project team members are assigned to a project in a part-time capacity. This is especially true in functional, weak matrix, and balanced matrix organizations. Even in strong matrix and projectized organizations project team members may not be permanently assigned to the project since the project needs vary over the duration of the project. Regardless of whether the part-time status is due to the availability of the project team member or of the needs of the project, many project team members are not fully allocated to the project.

As a result of the dynamic makeup of the project team members and their availability to work on the project, project managers must be able to shift work from one team member to another

Table 27.3. Change and organizational structure

	Functional	Weak matrix	Balanced matrix	Strong matrix	Projectized
Change frequency	Stable	Low	Moderate	High	Continual
Project manager's authority	Little or none	Low	Low to moderate	Moderate to high	High
Project manager's role	Part-time	Part-time	Part-time	Full-time	Full-time

Source: Adapted from PMI 2013b.

team member and try to capture and disseminate project knowledge between team members. As new team members are added to the project, the project manager must be able to quickly prepare the new team member with project and process knowledge and integrate them into the team so they may be effective. Project managers also must be able to capture any knowledge or information from team members transitioning off the project so this knowledge is not lost and may be transferred to other project team members.

In addition to managing the knowledge of new and transitioning team members, project managers must also properly assign work based on availability. Part-time project team members cannot be assigned the same workload as full-time team members. Additionally, members assigned to the team on a temporary basis cannot be assigned work beyond their anticipated time on the project. This work assigned must match the expected availability. Project managers must assign work based on time of day, day of week, or time of year availability and must assign work for only the time period when the team member is assigned to the team. Proper work assignment requires careful planning and revisions as plans change.

Vendor Partners

Not all project members will be employees of the organization. The organization may partner with outside vendors to bring in specialized expertise or additional expertise to supplement any shortages of employees with a specific skill set. The vendor partners work alongside the organization's employees and become a part of the project team. These vendor partnerships may fall into three separate categories—consultants, contractors, and outsourcing agencies.

An organization may add a consultant to a project team. The role of the **consultant** is to provide specialized expertise to the project that may not exist within the current employees. These consultants may offer business, process, technology, regulatory, or other knowledge relevant to the project. For example, a professional with experience implementing electronic health records may be hired to offer expert advice and direction to the project

team. The organization adds the consultant to the project team so the team may learn from the consultant's knowledge and previous experience to make the team more effective when encountering a new domain. Consultants may be added to the team for a short period of time or may be brought in for the duration of the project. The length of time the consultant is allocated to the project is based on the project needs, budget, and availability of the consultant.

Similar to consultants, **contractors** are added to a project team to fill a temporary void. Unlike consultants who are added for higher-level knowledge, contractors are added to the team for their specialized skills and detailed knowledge not available within the existing employees; or the contractors may be added to increase the work capacity of the existing project team. These contractors should be integrated with the team while their services are needed by the project team. As is the case with part-time team members, onboarding and knowledge capture and sharing should take place with all outside partners.

Consultants and contractors are brought into the project team to fill voids in skill and knowledge areas. These individuals supplement the project team. Another vendor partnership, **outsourcing agencies**, are used to offload a portion of the work rather than being brought in to work directly with the project team. For instance, an outsourcing agency could be contracted to scan and properly dispose of paper records for a digitization project. In this case, the outsourcing agency specializes in this process and could perform the work in a more efficient manner than if the organization attempted to perform the work themselves.

Co-located Teams

The traditional project team is located within the same space. This co-location allows members to carry on ad-hoc conversations and quickly and easily collaborate and share work. Additionally, this frequent interaction allows the team to develop into an effective group where each knows the working and communication styles of the other and they adjust to work as a cohesive team. Unfortunately, this means that the knowledge and skills needed for any given project must be made available in the same location. This is not always possible; especially in balanced or weak matrix organizations where the team members are not fully assigned to the project. Locating the team in a single location simplifies communication and collaboration but limits the selection of specialists who may participate in the team.

Distributed Teams

Within a more geographically dispersed workforce and national or global businesses, employees may no longer work in the same building, city, or country. It may not be possible to place all of the members of a project team together in the same location. Additionally, specialized knowledge or skills may be needed that do not exist with the employees at the firm. In these cases, consultants or contractors from vendor partners are brought in to participate on the project and these partners may not work within the same location as the rest of the project team. It is becoming more common to work in a distributed team located in many different locations. These teams enjoy the different backgrounds and experiences offered by a distributed team and the access to specialists not available at any single location. However, communications and collaboration is more challenging in the distributed team environment. In these distributed team projects, the project manager must prepare a plan to support and promote communication and collaboration so that the team will not be limited in its interactions.

Check Your Understanding 27.3

Instructions: **Answer the following questions on a separate piece of paper.**

1. Where does project coordination take place in a functional organization?
2. Where does project coordination take place in a matrix organization?
3. What is the difference between a strong matrix and weak matrix organization?
4. Name and describe the three categories of vendor partners.
5. What is a distributed team?

The Project Manager

A project manager is critical to the success of the project. This individual is responsible for planning and directing the project activities from the beginning to the end of the project and keeping all stakeholders informed and engaged throughout the project. While the project manager has responsibility to lead the project team, this functional leadership is often provided without administrative authority. With exception of projectized organizations, the project manager is a leader for the project team members while they are on the project but the team members continue to report to their **administrative supervisor** within the functional departments. The administrative supervisor is the supervisor from the functional area to where the employee reports. This supervisor has the authority to hire, fire, and promote the employee and may also remove the employee from the project team. This means the project manager often must lead and motivate a project team without the benefit of authority over the team members. As a result, the project manager must possess strong leadership attributes and soft skills in addition to technical knowledge and abilities. A set of common project management skills is listed in tables 27.4 and 27.5 and emphasizes the importance of both the technical and interpersonal skills required for a project manager.

The project manager must possess a set of technical skills in order to accomplish the work of

Table 27.4. Project manager technical skills

Technical skills	Description
Project management processes	Understanding of all project management processes, the inputs needed for each process, and the outputs resulting from each process as well as the ability to execute each process
Project management software	Expertise in using project management software and other software tools used in planning and executing the project
Project technology	Awareness of the technologies, tools, and techniques used by the project team in producing the project deliverables
Business domain	Basic understanding of the functional areas involved in and affected by the project
Budgets	Ability to plan, build, maintain, and evaluate a project budget as well as the tools for managing the budget
Cost estimates	Expertise to identify, estimate, schedule, and evaluate project costs throughout the project
Time estimates	Knowledge of multiple time estimation techniques and the ability to accurately collect and produce task and activity durations
Communication tools	Proficiency with many tools used to communicate and collaborate with the project team and project stakeholders

Source: Adapted from PMI 2013a and Brewer and Dittman 2013.

Table 27.5. Project manager interpersonal skills

Interpersonal skills	Description
Leadership	Moving a group of individuals within and outside of the project team to work together toward a common goal
Team building	Guiding the project team to form into a cohesive unit with the ability to work together to accomplish the project tasks while respecting and supporting each other
Motivation	Creating an environment where the project team achieves satisfaction through their work and rewards while having a common desire to reach the project goals
Communication	Conveying oral and written messages and meaning to the project team and project stakeholders while recognizing the proper styles, norms, relationships, and context of the communicated message
Influencing	Using interpersonal skills and shared power to obtain cooperation by the team and stakeholders to work toward the project goals
Decision making	Applying the appropriate decision method based on the decision making factors (time, trust, quality, and acceptance)
Political and cultural awareness	Understanding and appreciating the cultural and political landscape of the organization to identify and adeptly make use of the organization's power structures to accomplish the project while being sensitive to differences in organizational and individual cultures
Negotiation	Reaching agreements between parties of opposing interests through compromise and identification of mutual benefits
Trust building	Demonstrating information sharing, cooperation, and successful problem resolution to create trust across the project team and with the project stakeholders
Conflict management	Recognizing that conflict will occur, identifying when conflict is likely to occur, and helping the project team rationally work through disagreements to work toward the best results for the team
Coaching	Empowering and developing the project team and all team members to realize their potential through mentoring or training to increase skills and improve performance
Change management	Preparing the organization for the change resulting from the project as well as providing the flexibility to adjust the project based on changing business needs and shifts in the business environment
Active listening	Focusing on the speaker to understand the message and reiterating the message to ensure the message was properly understood and applying this form of listening to all project team members and stakeholders to build trust and effective communication

Source: Adapted from PMI 2013b.

managing a project. While these skills are important to the project manager, they represent only a part of the skills needed. Project managers are not only proficient in operating projects within the organization but they also need to be leaders. As a result, the project manager must possess or develop many interpersonal skills. These skills are needed to lead the project team and engage the project stakeholders while navigating the project through the challenges it will face. Table 27.5 includes several of the interpersonal skills the project manager must possess or develop to direct the project.

Comparing the two sets of skills, technical and interpersonal, it is clear that project managers must be proficient beyond the technical skills of the position. Interpersonal skills play a critical role in project management and the project manager relies significantly on these skills. Project management is more than simply assigning work and tracking the project. Project managers must be able to lead teams without having authority over the members and make organizational change without having leverage of a functional leadership position. All of these skills are needed to support the project manager as they serve multiple roles throughout the project.

Roles of a Project Manager

Project managers serve multiple roles in the project and are responsible for leading the project to successful completion. Since project management involves the planning, organizing, directing, and controlling the organization's resources to achieve the project's objectives (Kerzner 2013), the project manager takes on many responsibilities. These responsibilities can be summarized into six basic functions related to guiding the project to successful completion; that is, to manage resources, scope, quality, schedule, costs, and communications (Brewer and Dittman 2013).

Manage Resources

The project's resources must be managed to most effectively contribute to the project objectives. This means the project manager must ensure the project team is performing well and the resources for the project are planned and made available as needed without delays. These resources may include record storage space, scanning or photocopying equipment, HIM staff, and budget assigned for the project. The project manager is the steward over the human resources as well as the project materials and must ensure these resources are not wasted and are applied effectively.

Manage Scope

The project manager must first determine the scope for the project to ensure the team delivers the right deliverables so as to not deviate or fall short of the organization's needs. While the project is executed, the project manager must ensure the entire scope is delivered to satisfy project objectives. Even after the scope is determined for the project, the project manager must monitor the project scope to ensure the project plans are reevaluated in the event the scope changes. Changes to projects are common and typically lead to increased scope. These changes could include additional unplanned functionality added to the electronic health record system, increasing the number of records included in a digitization project, or adding additional departments to a workflow standardization project. While the project is underway new needs or revised needs are uncovered. For this reason, the project manager must be aware of changes in the scope so that revisions to the project plans may be made if necessary.

Manage Quality

In addition to ensuring the scope of the project is managed, the project manager must put controls in place to inspect the project output and evaluate the quality of the deliverables. The project deliverables must not only align with the scope defined for the project, but must also meet the stakeholder's quality expectations. Managing project quality at times creates conflicts with the project manager's other functions in terms of completing the project on time and within budget. For instance, adding field validation to a patient's blood type field in an EHR ensures higher quality data but requires additional development time. Producing quality deliverables or reworking deliverables to meet quality expectations require additional time and cost and, as a result, negatively affect the schedule and budget targets. Due to this conflict in priorities, project managers should attempt to plan quality into the project deliverables to reduce the risk of rework or inferior deliverables.

Manage Schedule

The timeline goals are established at the beginning of the project and these timelines drive the organization's plans for adopting the project deliverables. Due to this dependency on the deliverables, it is important that the project team complete the work based on the timelines. The project manager must prepare a schedule for the project and guide the project to produce the deliverables on time or provide early communication when they may be delayed. This project schedule and communication allows the organization to plan the adoption of the project deliverables.

Manage Costs

Similar to the schedule, the project manager must establish, maintain, and communicate the project budget. The project is given a budget and the project costs must be controlled so that they do not exceed the project budget. In the event that an overage occurs or will occur, the project manager must communicate the cost variance and attempt to secure additional funding or take other actions to reduce costs through other means.

Manage Communications

Communication is the most important function a project manager performs (Besteiro et al. 2015).

Project communication is critical both within and outside the team with all stakeholders. Project managers must make a conscious effort to communicate with the project stakeholders on a regular basis as well as ensure effective communication among the project team members and their interactions with the project stakeholders.

Communication is one of the key reasons why projects are important. Projects frequently work across multiple departments with involvement by multiple layers of management in the organization. Working with so many different groups is challenging and many organizations struggle to do this with multifunctional communications. Organizations are split in many different ways as illustrated in figure 27.10. There are layers of management where each layer views the business through a different perspective. The organization is also broken down into different units or functions. Between the organizational layers and functional units, people work on an operational island where they are focused mostly on the function and processes within their own unit and within their own management perspective.

One of the purposes of projects and project managers is to fill the gaps between operational islands so that diverse groups are able to work together. Much of this collaboration is supported by good communication. The project manager must take steps to connect all of the necessary groups together and connect these groups with the project team so that agreements can be made, expectations are clear, and the project work products are adopted. Filling the gaps between the operational

Figure 27.10.   Operational islands

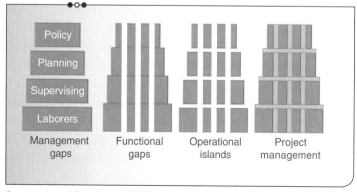

Source: Adapted from Kerzner 2013.

islands is an important factor for successfully executing the project.

Project Management Competencies

There is no such thing as a perfect project manager. Project managers must continually develop their skills and knowledge. There are many areas to master and the field evolves so that project managers always have areas to develop. Given the need for continued development, PMI proposed a framework to outline the competencies project managers must develop. This framework is referred to as the Project Manager Competency Development (PMCD) framework (PMI 2007). This framework can also be considered a set of building blocks that a project manager develops over time. Each of these blocks are connected and build upon each other to form the complete project manager. The individual blocks are personal behaviors, process knowledge, project performance, industry expertise, and organizational expertise (PMI 2007).

Figure 27.11 is a model of the project manager building blocks. Each block represents an area of development. Since project management is an applied field, the project management-specific areas of development must be based on a firm foundation of experience within the field. For example, effective project managers in the healthcare field must be familiar with healthcare processes and terminology and must have a good understanding of key decision makers and influencers in the organization in order to effectively apply project management practices. These categories are directly based on the PMCD framework but direct project management skills and knowledge are separated from supporting skills and knowledge. The industry experience and organizational experience building blocks are needed to emphasize the value of the industry and organizational nuances so that the project context is properly understood. Industry and organizational experience provide the foundational building blocks for the project management-specific blocks.

Industry Experience

Industry experience is a supporting competency for project managers. Competent project managers should have a solid foundational knowledge of the industry and some technical skills, or at least an appreciation of the technical skills, required in the industry. The industry knowledge includes awareness of regulatory and legal requirements, past and future trends within the industry, and experience with projects in the industry. For example, a project manager within the healthcare field should be familiar with HIPAA requirements, as well as history and trends in patient charting; and possess the insight gained from previous healthcare projects to understand the sources of project risk in a healthcare project (like communication, regulatory compliance, transportation logistics, and such).

In addition to the industry knowledge, a project manager must also possess the technical skills or at least an understanding and appreciation for the skills needed for the work to be carried out in a project within the industry. For example, in an IT project, the project manager should understand the level of difficulty for writing the code for a piece of software and understand the amount of time it takes to design, code, and test the software. The technical experience or technical skill appreciation helps the project manager assign the work to the properly skilled team member and evaluate the schedule needed to complete the work.

Industry experience is not always required for a project manager. Project managers may still succeed in managing a project outside of their industry expertise. However, the knowledge of the industry and the technical skills within the industry are beneficial in understanding projects

Figure 27.11. Project manager building blocks

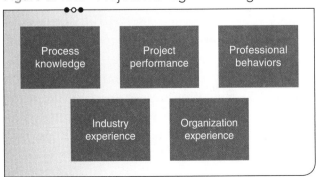

within the context of the industry. This contextual understanding of the industry enables the project manager to better communicate with the project stakeholders, better understand the sources and solutions to project risk within the industry, and improve project decision making.

Organization Experience

Similar to industry experience, organizational experience is a foundational competency for project managers. These skills and knowledge are not directly related to project management but provide the background needed for a contextual understanding of the project environment. The industry experience building block previously described represented the industry-specific experience that help project managers understand how projects are successfully executed within a specific industry. The **organizational experience**, on the other hand, provides the project manager with an understanding of how projects are executed within the context of the organization.

Organizational experience is gained from developing an understanding of the processes an organization follows, recognizing the power structures that exist within and outside of the organization and realizing who has the authority to make things happen, and observing the unwritten rules and expectations the organization has for its employees and supervisors. These organizational factors may be unique in each organization and it is beneficial for the project manager to understand these characteristics before initiating a project.

Organizational experience is an important competency to develop for project management consultants who may be experts in the project management field but may be at risk in the role due to insufficient experience with the organization. People unfamiliar with the organization will need to quickly understand the organizational context and apply it to the project.

Process Knowledge

Anyone new to the project management field will begin developing project manager competencies in the process knowledge building block. The **process knowledge** competency is developed by identifying and understanding all of the processes used across one or more project management methodologies; for instance, becoming familiar with PMI's Project Management Body of Knowledge (PMBOK), reading project management textbooks, and discovering project management tools and other resources.

Understanding the common processes and tools successful project managers use is an important step in developing as a project manager. Although the project management field is fairly new, there is a growing body of best practices available and these best practices help a project manager understand and adopt proven project management practices.

In developing the process knowledge building block, a project manager becomes familiar with common and unique processes and tools and understands how they are applied to the project setting. While the process knowledge building block is primarily developed by those new to the project management field, a project manager should continually refine their process knowledge to discover new and changing tools and processes in order to improve their own project management practice.

Project Performance

The **project performance** competency building block represents the project manager's ability to apply the project process knowledge and technical skills to the project environment. Project managers must not only know the project management processes and tools but also must be able to apply them to real projects. The project performance competency is developed by identifying the performance elements, determining target performance criteria, evaluating the individual's project performance competencies, identifying gaps between performance and target criteria, establishing a development plan, engaging in performance competency development activities, and re-evaluating the performance. The evaluation, gap analysis, development plan, and development steps are continually iterated as the project manager continues to develop project performance competency. This cycle of performance competency development should continue throughout one's career as the project manager constantly learns and gains proficiency in applying project management process knowledge. A project manager needs to determine the elements of project management that are important to evaluate, determine how to measure the performance for each of the elements, define a target goal for each element, and discover ways to improve in the lower performing elements.

Professional Behaviors

The professional behavior building block is based on the personal competencies in the PMCD framework (PMI 2007). This building block consists of the ability to manage project resources; guide a team through motivation and goal setting; communicate effectively with all project stakeholders; understand the project complexities and the external environments affecting the project; apply good judgment when evaluating the project environment leading to sound decisions; and demonstrate ethical and professional behaviors to achieve the desired project results.

The professional behavior is developed outside of project management skills and knowledge. The professional behaviors must be developed through experience, education, and mentoring. A project manager may be technically sound in the knowledge and application of the processes and tools but without developed professional behaviors the project manager will struggle in leading the team and stakeholders to achieve the desired results.

The professional behaviors building block along with all of the project manager building blocks require continual development. The project environment is always changing and a project manager can always find ways to learn new techniques or improve existing practices. These building blocks are simply a way to view the different types of skills and knowledge needed to be a successful project manager.

Check Your Understanding 27.4

Instructions: **Answer the following questions on a separate piece of paper.**

1. What is the difference between an administrative supervisor and a functional supervisor?
2. How does the functional supervision capacity of the project manager make it difficult to lead a team?
3. What are operational islands and how does project management address these islands?
4. Why is industry experience important to effective project management?
5. How does organizational experience help a project manager?

The Project Management Process

As noted in the project management competencies, knowledge of project processes is the first area of development for project managers. Understanding the processes of project management provides the foundation for becoming a project manager. Fortunately, over the decades, project management processes have matured and best practices have emerged. These best practices have been published through PMI as the Project Management Body of Knowledge (PMI 2013b). This guide outlines the processes that occur while managing a project. These processes are categorized into five separate and sequential groups—initiating, planning, executing, monitoring and controlling, and closing. As described earlier in this chapter, these processes are executed sequentially in a single iteration or multiple iterations across the project. Each of the process groups involves several different processes and requires input into the process group and produces some form of project output (see figure 27.12).

In order to better explain the process groups, a fictitious case study will be used. This case will be applied across each of the process groups to

Figure 27.12.   Process group framework

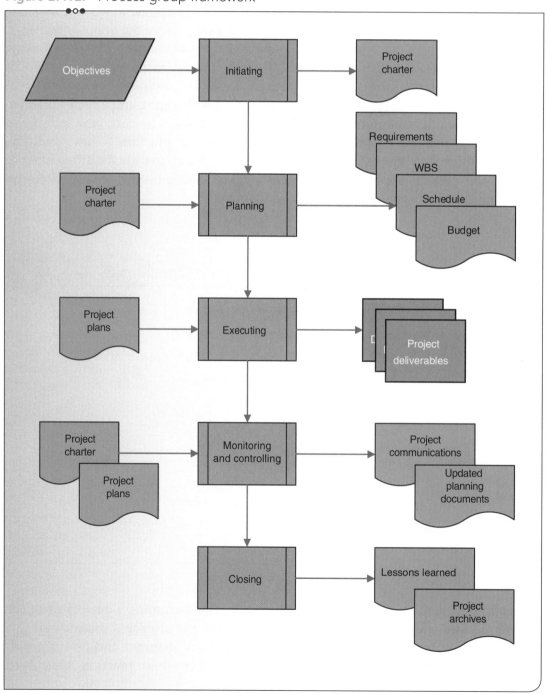

demonstrate the application of the project management process. While this case is a simplification of project management, it helps illustrate how the project management process is applied to a project without having to understand the complexities of the project.

Case Study: Continuing Education Event
Betsy is a medical records supervisor and a member of a local HIM professional organization. She has always enjoyed learning more about her field and would like to organize a continuing education event for her staff and other HIM professionals in the area. Betsy is also studying to become a project manager so she thought planning and hosting a continuing education event would be a great opportunity to practice her project management skills by treating this event like a project. She decides to begin by initiating the continuing education event and following all process groups through project closing. Betsy cannot wait to connect with her colleagues in the HIM field and hopes the project management process will make this continuing education event successful.

Initiating

Projects begin with the initiation process group where the project is first defined. This process group uses a project definition and scope, schedule, and budget estimates as inputs and results in an output of a completed project charter. The purpose of this first phase of the life cycle is to identify the project goals and gain agreement on the project constraints (scope, schedule, and budget). During the initiation phase, the project is formed. Using the definition of a project as being a temporary endeavor executed to reach specific objectives while constrained by time and resources, the initiation phase describes the effort using these attributes of a project. The objectives are determined and limited to fit within a temporary period of time, the period of time the effort will take is determined, and the type and quantity of resources (both human, financial, and other resources) are estimated. All of these factors are required to create a project and therefore identifying and agreeing upon these factors must be completed at the beginning of any project.

As part of creating the project, the project objectives are first established to justify the project. The purpose of the project is based on one of the three sources of projects (revenue, expense, compliance) and should be associated with some form of benefit to the organization to help justify the organization's financial investment (Levine 2005). Ideally, the benefits described should include some form of measurable objective that can be evaluated once the project is completed in order to evaluate the contributions to the organization.

In addition to the project objectives, the three project constraints must be defined beginning with the project scope. The scope of the project describes both what and how much. The scope identifies the project work that will be completed by the team and clearly defines the project deliverables as well as states what will not be included in the project. The project scope is defined so that the project will have a definitive end where all of the scope is delivered. The project also provides a basis for the schedule and budget constraints.

Once the scope is defined, the project schedule can be prepared. A high-level plan is developed to identify the work that must be done to complete the project and deliver all of the project scope. Using this plan, the time required to complete all of this work is estimated. These time estimates may be in the form of hours for a short project or days or weeks for a longer project. Regardless of the units used for these time estimates, the units should be consistent. For instance, if days are used to estimate some of the work and it was determined this was the best way to estimate the project, then the estimation of all the work should be calculated in days. The results of the schedule estimate should be the total amount of time (hours, days, weeks) required to complete all of the work needed to deliver the entire project scope.

The next step is to use the work previously defined to determine the resources needed to complete the project. These resources will include the money needed to purchase the raw materials for the project, money needed to pay the additional specialists required to complete the work for the project, and money needed for the tools or project logistics. These cost estimates are calculated for each of the tasks required and then added up to determine the total costs for the project. These costs form the project budget.

Once the project objectives and project constraints are determined, a project charter is created. This project charter documents the objectives, benefits, and project constraints so that the project manager and project team along with the project owner all have the same baseline expectations. In some organizations this project charter is signed and treated as a binding document while in other organizations this charter is simply used to document the initial vision for the project.

Case Study: Project Initiating

Betsy begins her education event project by first creating a project charter. She does this by simply writing in her notebook the objectives and project constraints. Betsy begins by identifying the project objective of increasing knowledge of current HIM practices and improved collaboration across local HIM professionals. In her project charter, she identifies the scope as providing a speaker, food and beverages for everyone attending the event, and inviting her colleagues and all other members of her local professional association. She estimates that she will need approximately 60 days to reserve a conference hall, purchase the food and drinks, recruit a speaker, and send out invitations. Betsy doesn't yet know the menu she will serve or supplies that are needed but she calculates that $30 per attendee should be enough to cover all expenses and she anticipates 100 people will attend the event. After summarizing the objectives, scope, schedule, and budget for the education event, she decides the effort, time, and costs are worth the benefits she and her colleagues will gain from learning more about the profession and networking with other local professionals. Based on this benefit, Betsy decides to go ahead with the educational event and moves on to complete her detailed planning for the HIM educational event project.

Planning

Once the initiation is complete the planning process group begins. The planning phase uses the completed project charter and several planning tools as input and produces a detailed project plan and updated project constraints as the output for the project planning process. The purpose of this process is to investigate the project further to gain a complete understanding of the project and the work to be completed in order to establish a detailed plan to execute it. The initial project constraints of scope, schedule, and budget from the project charter were educated guesses and must be better defined as the work is planned.

During the planning phase, the project scope specifications can be captured, the work is broken down into individual tasks, a detailed schedule of the tasks is prepared, and all expenses associated with completing the project based on the plan are identified and summarized. Common outputs from the planning phase include a requirements document, work breakdown structure (WBS), project schedule, and detailed project budget.

The project requirements may be captured in a requirements document or through other means of capturing the attributes of the expected project deliverables. Through interactions with the project owner, project users, and other project stakeholders, the project team establishes a detailed collection of expectations for the project output. In order to ensure these specifications are communicated correctly, they are expressed in a **requirements document**. There are many forms of requirements documents but one of the most basic forms of capturing these requirements is through a requirements matrix document (table 27.6).

While the requirements are collected, a detailed plan of the work to be completed is prepared. The

Table 27.6. Sample project requirements matrix

Requirement ID	Description	Priority
1	Hold event on a weekday evening to maximize the number of attendees	A
2	Meeting room should hold at least 150 people	B
3	Meeting location should be within 10 miles from office	B
4	The meeting location must allow external catering	A
5	The speaker must have experience related to the educational topic	A
6	It would be nice if the speaker has never presented at a previous event	C
7	The food should be healthy	B
8	The food must be served in individual portions	A

work is often broken down into major deliverables or phases, individual components of each deliverable or phase, activities needed to create these deliverables, and individual tasks (referred to as work packages) assigned and carried out during the activity. The **work breakdown structure (WBS)** diagram tool is developed to summarize and illustrate the project work. This form of project artifact (figure 27.13) is commonly used due to the analytical nature where the project is dissected into manageable components. In addition to the ability to dissect the project, the visual nature of this tool provides simplicity for communicating the complex work structure of the project.

Once the WBS is complete and verified, the work can be scheduled. Scheduling the project is commonly planned and managed through a Gantt chart. The **Gantt chart** captures each of the work packages identified in the WBS as tasks for the project team, assigns each task to a project team member, identifies the dates when the work begins and when it will be completed, and identifies any scheduling dependencies with other tasks. The Gantt chart can be used to display the schedule in a hierarchical form similar to the WBS. The resulting Gantt chart (figure 27.14) is used to communicate the schedule and to monitor the progress of the project during execution.

The **project budget** must also be planned. The resource expenses must be captured and calculated to determine the detailed project budget. These resource expenses may include procuring materials for the project, purchasing the tools or project shipping and transportation costs, and employing additional specialists from outside of the organization to complete the work for the project. In many projects where internal employees work on the project, the labor costs for these employees are not included in the budget. However, when projects are conducted on behalf of another organization, the employees' time may need to be captured using a billing rate for each type of team member and the number of hours expected to be used by each role in the project.

Once all material resource estimates and, if appropriate, team resource estimates are collected, a budget is prepared. The expenses are calculated for each work package and then are either reported by phase or by the work package for the project. Another method of reporting the budget is to categorize the planned expenses (table 27.7).

In addition to the requirements, WBS, Gantt chart, and project budgets, other outputs may be produced based on the size and complexity of the project. These additional project artifacts include project organizational structure, change management plan, test plans, risk management plan, stakeholder analysis and communications plan, and many other artifacts prepared to address any planning needs anticipated for the project.

Continuing Education Event Case Study: Project Planning

After deciding to go ahead with the continuing education event, Betsy begins her detailed project plans. Using a work breakdown structure Betsy outlines the work that needs to be done to reserve a location, send out invitations, order the food and drinks, and recruit the speaker. She then develops a Gantt chart to schedule the tasks to be completed and delegates the work of reserving a location to her assistant, Emily. Betsy knows that attendance ranged from 75 to 95 people for the past five continuing education events so she is planning to host a total of 100 people. She decides to serve lasagna, salad, asparagus, water and ice tea, and cupcakes. She also plans to recruit two separate speakers for the event. Betsy now recalculates the budget and finds out that the cost to host 100 attendees will be $2,700 (or $27 per person). Having a better understanding of the effort required, time needed, and costs, Betsy reevaluates her educational event idea and determines the benefits of the event still outweigh the costs and decides to begin executing her plan.

Executing

Project execution begins during the end of the planning process. The project plans are carried out and the project work products are delivered. This phase includes forming the project team, purchasing supplies and materials for the project, inspecting the project deliverables for quality issues while they are being produced, communicating with the project stakeholders, and managing the expectations of all project stakeholders.

One of the main priorities for the project manager during project execution is to maintain

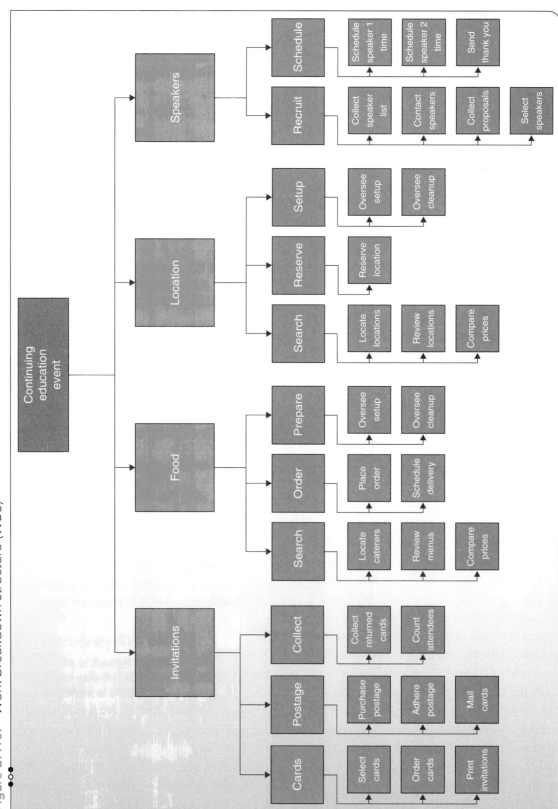

Figure 27.13.   Work breakdown structure (WBS)

Figure 27.14. Sample Gantt chart

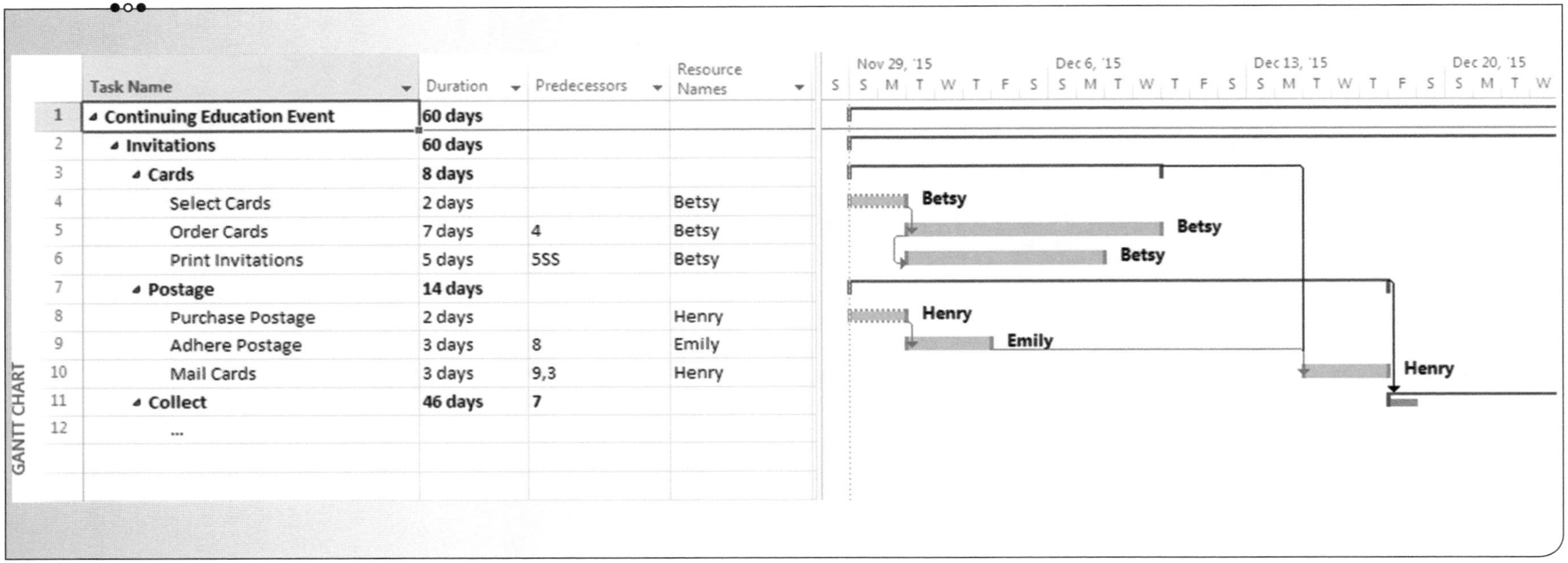

Table 27.7.   Project resource budget

Continuing education event			
Category	Planned	Actual	Variance
Room reservation	$ 400.00		
Speaker 1	$ 300.00		
Speaker 2	$ 300.00		
Catering (100 people)	$ 1,500.00		
Invitations	$ 150.00		
Postage	$ 50.00		
Total:	$ 2,700.00	$ –	$ –

communications with and among the project team members and project stakeholders. This requires publishing project planning documents and updates, frequent project meetings with the project team, maintaining an issues log to track problems and resolutions as they occur, status reporting to communicate current project progress to the project stakeholders, and frequent personal interactions with the project stakeholders to maintain interest and participation in the project.

Continuing Education Event Cast Study: Project Executing

After reevaluating the continuing education event plans and deciding to go ahead with the event, Betsy begins carrying out her plan. Betsy first sends out social media messages and email messages to all invitees to let them know she is planning the event and informs them that invitations to the event will be sent soon. She then contacts her assistant Emily to ask her to find and reserve a location for the event and gives her some general guidelines, including cost ($200), for selecting a good location. Betsy then prepares her detailed menu and purchases invitations and postage stamps. Next she recruits her colleague Henry to prepare and send out the invitations for the event. As the event day draws near, Betsy places her order with the caterer and schedules a delivery date and time. When the day of the event finally arrives, she recruits her assistant Emily and colleague Henry to help her welcome the attendees as they arrive. After the event ends, Betsy, Henry, and Emily say goodbye to their attendees and begin cleaning up.

Monitoring and Controlling

While the project team is executing the project plan, the project is also being monitored and controlled by the project manager. During this phase

of the life cycle, the project is evaluated to ensure it is on track according to the plan; alterations are made to the plans as changes occur, and variances to the baseline are reported. The scope, schedule, and budget are regulated using a change management plan (described later in the chapter), issues are identified and addressed, risks are evaluated, and appropriate contingency plans are made. This project's progress is continually evaluated and any deviations or anticipated deviations from the plan are communicated to the project stakeholders, and appropriate actions are taken to resolve the variances.

The executing and monitoring and controlling phases are very fluid. Although the project begins with detailed plans, changes occur that cause the project to deviate from the plan. The monitoring and controlling phase is where the project manager ensures the plans and the project execution are aligned so that the project adheres to the project stakeholder's scope, schedule, and budget expectations established in the project baseline.

Continuing Education Event Case Study: Project Monitoring and Controlling

While Betsy, Emily, and Henry were preparing for the educational event, Betsy ordered the food and drinks and discovered the food was more expensive than she anticipated. Rather than the $1,500 she budgeted for food and beverages, the total came to $1,650. Discovering that she was $150 over budget, Betsy wrote down this issue in her notebook and decided it was important enough to try to resolve this problem. She then contacted Emily to encourage her to find a location that was less expensive than the original budget of $250. A day later Emily informed Betsy that she was able to *reserve a location for $200 rather than the $400 budgeted. Betsy was happy to see that she was now under her budgeted costs and she made the update to her project budget and captured the result of the issue in her notebook. The rest of the preparation and the event itself went as planned.*

Closing

The final process group in the project management life cycle is the closing process group. During this phase, the project is reflected upon and evaluated by the project team and all stakeholders, all project expenditures are concluded, and the project documents and other artifacts are archived for future reference or reuse. During this closing phase, it is important for the project manager to identify the lessons learned from the project and document these lessons to help the team, stakeholders, and the organization learn from the project to improve future projects. This final phase also results in the project team disbanding and moving on to a new project or returning to their operational roles.

Continuing Education Event Case Study: Project Closing
Once Betsy, Emily, and Henry finished cleaning up after the event, they sat down and enjoyed a cold beverage and talked about the event and their preparations. Betsy told her colleagues how much she appreciated their help and commended Emily for finding a good location for less than the planned $400. The three of them shared the comments they heard from attendees about the educational event and discussed what they would do differently for the next time they planned a similar event and what they thought worked well and will do again. While they talked about their experience with the event and preparations, Betsy took out her notebook and wrote down the comments about the event so she could remember these ideas. Once Betsy returned to work the next day, she placed her notebook in her file drawer to refer to next year when she begins planning the next educational event.

Check Your Understanding 27.5

Instructions: **Answer the following questions on a separate piece of paper.**

1. What are the major deliverables in the initiating process group?
2. What are the major deliverables in the planning process group?
3. What are the major deliverables in the executing process group?
4. What are the major deliverables in the monitoring and controlling process group?
5. What are the major deliverables in the closing process group?

Managing Project Change

Change is important to project management. Earlier in this chapter, change was described as the catalyst for projects. Projects are the response to the organization's need or desire to change. In addition to becoming the origins of the project, change is also very important during the project. Change occurs frequently during the project, and the project team must respond to change to keep it on track and to ensure the project work products remain relevant and valuable to the organization. Failure to respond correctly to change is the most common source of project failures (Whitten and Bentley 2007). In this section, change will be discussed in terms of the different types of change occurring during the project and how the project manager must respond.

Types of Change

Project change occurs through several different means. Change may originate from the project team, project owner, project stakeholders, the organization, or the external environment and regulations (see table 27.8). Regardless of the source of the change, the project manager and project team must respond and shift the project plans to accommodate the change. Also, the project manager must engage the project stakeholders to reset project expectations as a result of the change.

The project manager must be aware of change and look for it throughout the project, particularly during the monitoring and controlling phase. It must be acknowledged that change will most likely occur and the project plans will have to be adjusted. However, change must also be appreciated. While change creates more work in project planning and coordinating, change and the project team's response to it provides a great deal of benefit to the organization. The project manager needs to know how to respond to change and reap the benefits of a proper response.

Benefits of Change

Although not all change is positive, responding properly to change contributes positively toward the project outcomes. For instance, if a project member resigns from the organization, the project manager can quickly respond to this negative change by acquiring another team member from the corresponding functional area and updating the project plans while informing the stakeholders of any delay resulting from this change in the team. By responding quickly and communicating the change and corresponding effect on the project,

the project manager is able to minimize the delay and also maintain the stakeholder's expectations. The stakeholders will be pleased that the change was responded to quickly and they were able to readjust their expectations early rather than learning of the delays later in the project, thus reducing their time to respond.

Change itself is also good for the project team. Changes in the business environment or changes to functional needs require the project team to change the project deliverables and will most likely lead to delays and increased costs. However, without a response to this change, the project team would have produced work products that did not adequately meet the needs of the functional department or organization resulting in a decrease in the value of the project. Properly responding to change ensures the project work products continue to provide value to the organization and meet the stakeholder's expectations.

A project manager should look favorably at change. First understanding that change will indeed occur during the project, the project manager responds to ensure project objectives are achieved and the project stakeholder's expectations are met. Lack of a proper response to change can detract from the project value and result in unmet stakeholder expectations. Project managers must be able to negotiate with the project owner and other stakeholders when responding to change in order to maintain their expectations while meeting the project goals and project constraints.

Negotiating Change and Managing Expectations

Any change encountered in the project has potential to affect the three project constraints—scope,

Table 27.8. Examples of project change

Origin of change	Examples
Project team	A project team member leaves the organization and a replacement must be requested from the functional department resulting in delays in the project products
Project owner	A new feature is requested that will benefit the organization
Project stakeholders	Disagreements occur between project stakeholders and the project owner over some of the project specifications resulting in more time to collect detailed specifications
Organization	Two business units are merged requiring a redesign of the project products
External	A new government regulation has been passed adding a new design consideration for the project

schedule, and budget. The project manager must monitor the project and the environment to recognize potential changes with the project constraints. As changes occur, the project manager recognizes the relationship between the change and the project constraints and needs to adjust the plans accordingly. Unfortunately, all stakeholders may not understand the relationship between changes to the project and the project constraints. As part of managing the stakeholder expectations, the project manager must educate the stakeholders so that they understand this relationship and will be more open to changes to the project constraints as they occur.

Using the project constraint triangle (figure 27.4), the project manager should communicate with the project owner and other stakeholders early in the relationship between the three constraints (schedule, budget, and scope). The project manager should explain that all three constraints are related and any change to one of the constraints may affect the other two. Using an example of introducing a new addition to the project scope, the project manager should be able to explain how the project team must expend additional work to deliver the new scope and this work will take time and resources and the change results in a potential increase to the project schedule and potential increase in the project budget. The stakeholders should learn to expect adjustment to the project variables as changes are introduced. Failure to understand this relationship will force the project team to respond to changes without revising the project constraints and results in the inability to meet the expectations of the project stakeholders due to missed scope, delayed delivery, or budget overage.

Project managers establish awareness of the constraint relationships early in the project and use this understanding to renegotiate the project constraints as changes occur during the project. The project stakeholders should learn to anticipate change but expect the project manager to take actions to minimize the effect the change has on the project constraints. Once the constraint relationship awareness is established, the project stakeholders will be open to working with the project team in responding to change during the project.

Change Management Process

Managing all of the change can be difficult for the project manager and the project team. One of the most significant changes during a project is a change to the project scope. Various stakeholders frequently wish to add new or enhanced project requirements after the initial requirements were gathered, and the schedule and budget were established based on these requirements. Over time, these small changes in scope create significant changes and require more resources and time than originally planned. These incremental changes are commonly referred to as scope creep. In order to best deal with the volume of changes that occur as a result to changes in the project scope, a change management process must be established and enforced.

The change management process illustrated in figure 27.15 outlines the steps that should be taken when a change to the project scope is requested. The process begins by the stakeholder formalizing a request for a new enhancement or new addition to the project scope. The requested change and its benefits to the organization should be clearly explained. Ideally these benefits are assigned a monetary value. The change request is then reviewed by the project manager and project team and a change proposal is prepared. The change proposal reiterates the change and value to the organization and describes the work required to implement the change. This includes the changes to the project scope and the effect the proposed change has on the project schedule and budget. Once the project change proposal is prepared, it is reviewed by the project owner and other stakeholders to determine if the benefits of the proposed change outweigh the changes in project schedule (typically schedule delay) and budget (typically budget increase). If the project owner and stakeholders reject the change proposal, the originator of the change request is notified by the project manager. If the project owner and stakeholder determine the change should be approved, then the project manager adjusts the scope document and updates the schedule and budget to reflect the new project baseline constraints. The updated project plans are then communicated to the stakeholders so all stakeholders are aware of the revised scope, schedule, and budget.

Figure 27.15.   Change management process

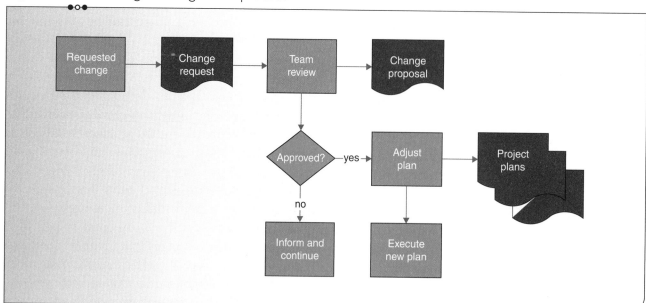

 Check Your Understanding 27.6

Instructions: **Answer the following questions on a separate sheet of paper.**

1. How does scope creep affect a project?

2. What can a project manager do to control scope creep?

3. What happens to the schedule or budget if there is a significant increase in scope?

4. What happens to the scope if there is a significant decrease in budget or schedule?

5. Why does a project manager encourage a formalized change order process?

Beyond Project Management

Every project has a purpose or an objective that is associated with some benefit to the organization. The organization will achieve a benefit that in most cases will exceed the cost of the project and will place the organization in position to either continue to operate or improve its ability to operate. These projects exist alongside other projects within the organization and in some cases have similar or related objectives. These project objectives are connected to the organization's goals so the project is helping the organization realize its long-term goals. Given the organizational value and connectedness of projects, and the contributions to the organizational goals, it is important to view projects not as isolated work but rather within the context of the entire organization.

Projects and project management have traditionally been viewed from an operational perspective. The goals of projects have been primarily focused on the three variables of scope, schedule, and budget. In the past, a project was successful if the entire scope was delivered on time and within budget. However, this operational perspective of project management is shifting to be combined with a more strategic perspective of project management. Projects are becoming viewed as contributors to the organization's goals and their association with other projects are recognized. As a result, the ways projects are selected and how they are managed are changing.

Project Selection

Organizations function within the limitations of their resources. Every organization has finite limits to the number of financial resources, employees, and time available to accomplish their goals. Since there are limits to the amount of time, money, and employees available to assign to projects, the organization cannot complete every project. The organization then must determine in which projects to invest. Given the need to select only a subset of the available projects, the organization needs to use a method to select projects to pursue and then delay or turn down other project opportunities. Regardless of the project selection method used, organizations must recognize that not all projects can be pursued and a method of selecting projects is needed. The selection method should reflect the needs, culture, and goals of the organization and should be consistently applied to all projects.

Program Management

Projects become difficult to manage as they become large and complex. The scale of the scope and the large resource investments creates a high degree of risk for the organization. These projects become increasingly prone to failure and this means the organization has a higher degree of risk of not achieving the benefits of the project while still investing resources into the project. In order to reduce this risk and increase the likelihood the project will succeed, projects can be broken down into a smaller projects where the entire set of projects is referred to as a **program**. The program is made up of several related projects and each project contributes to the overall objectives of the program.

Program management is used as another layer of management over projects where a program manager guides and coordinates the set of individual projects to ensure they produce deliverables that can be used by the other projects within the program. The result of a successful program is that the entire set of projects produce complete and integrated deliverables on time and within the overall budget. While the project manager continues to control the individual project and manages the three project constraints, the program manager focuses on connections between the projects and making sure the set of projects will be successful in meeting the organization's needs while completing them on time and within the established budget.

Project Portfolio Management

Project portfolio management (PPM) is the method that some organizations use to optimize the benefits gained from limited project resources. **Project portfolio management** is the method used to identify, select, and prioritize projects and programs in a manner to make best use of the limited resources. The purpose of this method is to leverage the suite of projects and programs to achieve the highest value to the organization. This means that the organization distributes resources to the collection of projects and that will result in the greatest benefit to the organization.

The project portfolio management method enables the organization to better connect the project objectives with the organization's goals. Similar to the project and program managers, a portfolio also has a manager. The **project portfolio manager** is responsible for ensuring all projects and programs within the portfolio produce benefits to the organization. Since each project and program begins with clearly stated objectives, the projects and programs are expected to achieve some form of benefit to the organization. The project portfolio manager's role is to monitor, guide, and direct the projects and programs to ensure each project or program within the portfolio will produce the benefits promised as part of its objectives. The project portfolio manager is not as concerned with individual budgets and schedules but rather the benefits gained from the projects and programs.

As part of managing the suite of projects and programs within the portfolio, the project portfolio manager cancels projects or programs that are no longer able to produce sufficient benefit to the organization in order to shift the resources to another project that has potential to deliver greater benefit. In addition to cancelling projects, new projects and programs are added to the portfolio as existing projects and programs are completed and new resources become available to invest in further projects and programs. As a result, projects and programs are continually added and removed from the portfolio and the portfolio changes to reflect the organization's current goals.

Project management and the related fields of program management and portfolio management are an important function in any organization. Not all organizations have formalized a project management practice, but projects and managing projects occurs in almost every organization. Projects and effective management of these projects allow the organization to respond to change and make changes in order to improve. Change is a certainty in the modern organization and project management exists to help ensure these changes occur.

Check Your Understanding 27.7

Instructions: **Answer the following questions on a separate sheet of paper.**

1. What are the three project goals from the operational project management perspective?

2. What is the perspective of strategic project management?

3. How does a program differ from a project?

4. What are the objectives of a program manager?

5. How does a portfolio differ from a program or project?

6. What are the objectives of a portfolio manager?

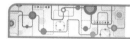

References

Besteiro, E., J. Pinto, and O. Novaski. 2015. Success factors in project management. *Business Management Dynamics* 4(9)19–34.

Brewer, J.L. and K.C. Dittman. 2013. *Methods of IT Project Management,* 2nd ed. West Lafayette, IN: Purdue University Press.

Gray, C.F., and E.W. Larson. 2014. *Project Management: The Managerial Process,* 6th ed. New York, NY: McGraw-Hill Irwin.

Kerzner, H. 2013. *Project Management: A Systems Approach to Planning, Scheduling, and Controlling,* 11th ed. Hoboken, NJ: Wiley.

Kwak, Y.H. 2003. Brief History of Project Management. In *The Story of Managing Projects.* Edited by Carayannis, E.G., Y.H. Kwak, and F.T. Anbari. West Port, CT: Praeger.

Levine, H.A. 2005. *Project Portfolio Management: A Practical Guide to Selecting Projects, Managing Portfolios,* *and Maximizing Benefits.* San Francisco, CA: Jossey-Bass.

Project Management Institute. 2015 (Nov.). PMI fact file. *PMI Today* 4.

Project Management Institute. 2013a. PMI's Pulse of the Profession: The High Cost of Low Performance. http://www.pmi.org/~/media/PDF/Business-Solutions/PMI-Pulse%20Report-2013Mar4.ashx

Project Management Institute. 2013b. *A Guide to the Project Management Body of Knowledge (PMBOK Guide),* 5th ed. Newtown Square, PA: PMI.

Project Management Institute. 2007. *Project Manager Competency Development Framework,* 2nd ed. Newtown Square, PA: PMI.

Whitten, J.L. and L.D. Bentley. 2007. *Systems Analysis and Design Methods,* 7th ed. New York, NY: McGraw-Hill Irwin.

28

Ethical Issues in Health Information Management

Morley L. Gordon, RHIT
Leslie L. Gordon, MS, RHIA, FAHIMA

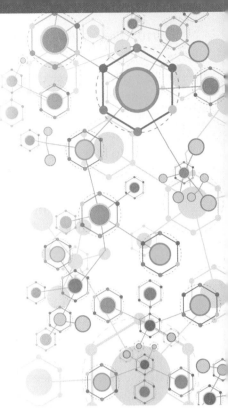

Learning Objectives

- Examine ethics and ethical dilemmas
- Interpret the concepts of morality, code of conduct, and moral judgment
- Assess the AHIMA Code of Ethics
- Differentiate how cultural issues affect health and healthcare quality, cost, and health information management
- Evaluate the consequences of a breach of healthcare ethics
- Determine the ethical issues related to research
- Apply HIM ethical standards of practice
- Evaluate the culture of a department and policies that support a culture of diversity

Key Terms

Altruism
Autonomy
Beneficence
Bias
Blanket authorization
Code of Ethics
Confidentiality
Consequentialism
Cultural audit
Cultural competence
Cultural diversity
Culture

Deontology
Double billing
Egoism
Ethical principles
Ethics
Ethics committee
Integrity
Leadership
Least harm
Medical identity theft
Moral values
Need-to-know principle

Nonmaleficence
Prejudice
Privacy
Quality
Respect
Retrospective documentation
Security
Stereotyping
Unbundling
Upcoding
Utilitarianism
Values

The phrase "first do no harm" is well known in healthcare as a long standing code of conduct for medical professionals, meaning first and foremost the goal of a healthcare professional is to not cause harm to those being treated; the legal term is **nonmaleficence**. Health information management (HIM) professionals are guided by a similar code of conduct and adhere to a professional **code of ethics**, a set of principles regarding business practices and professional behavior and described in detail in this chapter. HIM professionals do not have direct patient care contact but they do interact with patients in terms of coding, release of information, data quality, and so forth. **Ethics** is a field of study addressing moral principles, theories, and values. In healthcare, ethics involves formal decision making needed when dealing with competing perspectives and obligations of the people who have an interest in a common problem.

An individual has the right to determine what does or does not happen to him or her in terms of healthcare. **Autonomy** is a core ethical principle centered on this fact, meaning a patient has the right to choose their course of treatment. A clinical application of this concept is a cancer patient's right to refuse chemotherapy, radiation, or surgical treatment. **Beneficence** is a legal term that means promoting good for others or providing services that benefit others, such as releasing health information that will help a patient receive care or that will ensure payment of services received.

People are guided by their own sets of values and ethical principles according to their personal beliefs and cultural upbringing. It is important for HIM professionals to understand cultural competency and diversity to help guide their interactions in the workplace as well as when associating with patients. Understanding a person's background, culture, beliefs, and values makes it possible to comprehend why they act in a certain way and can help guide professional interactions.

Moral Values and Ethical Principles

A system of principles by which one guides one's life, usually with regard to right or wrong, is considered the **moral values** of the individual (AHIMA 2015a). In healthcare, employees need to be mindful of the moral values of the people they work with, including fellow employees and patients. The moral values people hold can be very strong and cause conflict with others. As an HIM professional, it is also important to understand **ethical principles** to help with decision making and to understand why others may make the decisions they do. The following principles explain the ways in which ethical decisions are made.

- *Altruism*: **Altruism** is the belief that other people are more important than an individual person, wherein a personal sacrifice must take place. An example would be donating a kidney to a stranger (Allen 2013).

- *Autonomy*: As defined earlier, autonomy is an individual's right to self-determination, a patient has the right to decide what does or does not happen to him or her (AHIMA 2015a). A patient's right to refuse treatment for cancer is one example.

- *Beneficence*: Beneficence is promoting good for others or providing services that benefit others; for example, releasing health information to help a patient receive further care (AHIMA 2015a).

- *Consequentialism*: **Consequentialism** considers the consequences before making a decision and this decision is based on the end result. For example, when documenting in a patient chart a provider understands that certain medical codes receive higher reimbursement, but the consequence of miscoding could result in legal charges against the provider.

- *Deontology*: **Deontology** is the duty or responsibility guiding the decision based on action and not the end result. For example, a release of information (ROI) specialist in a small town will not release information to a police officer who is threatening to take her to jail until consent from the patient is received (Allen 2013).

- *Egoism:* Instead of taking others into consideration, **egoism** involves only considering oneself in the decision-making process. For example, a person donating blood plasma for money during a financial emergency, not to help people in need.

- *Least harm:* **Least harm** deals with situations where two choices may both be less than ideal. One should choose the situation that will do the least amount of harm to the fewest number of people. For example, a physician choosing to treat the patient in the emergency room with the greatest chance for survival instead of the patient with greater injuries.

- *Utilitarianism:* **Utilitarianism** deals with situations that may provide the greatest benefit to the most people; for example, one person's organ donations can benefit many (Allen 2013).

Ethical decision making involves consideration of what is right and what is wrong based on a code of conduct or behavior. An ethical dilemma occurs when one is faced with a choice between two or more situations; for example, should life support be discontinued or continued, or who decides which patient will receive a single kidney. An HIM professional who has strong beliefs against assisted suicide may not be comfortable working in a facility where it is practiced. Many ethical decisions are based on one's **culture**, which includes the values, beliefs, attitudes, languages, symbols, rituals, behaviors, and customs unique to a particular group of people (Simmers et al. 2014). **Values** include the social and cultural belief system of a person or a healthcare organization. Culture is learned, shared, social in nature, dynamic, and changing—meaning people generally have similar beliefs and values based on their upbringing, what they were taught by parents, peers, and surroundings. The values of an individual can shift over time based on changing environments and social networks. For example, a student who leaves home for the first time to go away to college will be exposed to new and different experiences and, as a result, over time the values developed at home may shift and reflect those from his or her college environment.

Cultural Competence in the Healthcare Environment

Cultural competence is the ability to accept and understand the beliefs and values of other people and groups and is vital to the overall health of an organization, whereas **cultural diversity** is the perceived or actual difference among people. For example, the seemingly simple question of gender is very complex and complicated for some people: a person born male may relate to being female, may be in the final stages of transitioning to female, or may not be considering transitioning. Accepting diversity is important to cultural competence and acceptance. Culture includes the following:

- Ethnicity (classification of people based on national origin or culture)
- Socioeconomic status (classification of people based on economic or social welfare status)
- Religion
- Gender or gender identity
- Sexual orientation
- Age
- Education
- Occupation

Attitudes that affect one's cultural competence include prejudice, stereotyping, and bias. **Prejudice** judges a person based on one of the cultural elements listed previously without reviewing all of the information; for example, liking a person because she has green eyes. **Stereotyping** is an assumption that everyone within a certain group are the same; for example, believing surgeons are hard to communicate with. A **bias** prevents a person from having an impartial judgment; for example, an HIM manager who prefers to work with only women.

Healthcare professionals should be mindful of the differences in culture, beliefs, and values of other people, particularly coworkers and patients, and avoid prejudice, stereotyping, and bias. This can be done by exploring different cultures, values, and beliefs, and remaining sensitive to the ways other people conduct their lives (Simmers et al. 2014). The following topics will introduce cultural competence and how cultural issues affect healthcare, provide a background on self-awareness of one's own culture, suggest ideas for training programs related to expanding culture in the workplace, and explore regulations in regard to cultural competence. Labor and employment laws are discussed in chapter 23.

Cultural Disparities in US Healthcare

Many factors, including the influence of culture, have an effect on health and healthcare including health status, disease risk factors, and access to healthcare. The World Health Organization (WHO) defines the social determinants of health as the conditions in which persons are born, grow, live, work, and age, including differences in health status (WHO 2012). Health disparities exist disproportionately in certain populations; for example, people who live in a predominately low income neighborhood have less access to quality healthcare than people who live in a predominately high income neighborhood. Data shows that residents in mostly minority communities have lower socioeconomic status, greater barriers to healthcare access, and greater risks for disease compared with the general population (Meyer et al. 2013).

The US Department of Health and Human Services (HHS) Office of Minority Health established national standards for culturally and linguistically appropriate services (CLAS) in health and healthcare with the intention to advance health quality, improve the quality of the healthcare provided, and help eliminate healthcare disparities in the United States. The principal standard is to provide effective, equitable, understandable, and respectful quality care while being responsive to diverse cultural beliefs and practices, preferred languages, health literacy, and other communication needs (HHS 2015). By providing these basic services patients feel they are respected and understood, and they are able to understand the medical care direction their provider is asking them to take.

Healthcare Professionals and Cultural Competence

Healthcare professionals across the nation struggle to respond to the needs of people from diverse groups and to incorporate cultural competence in healthcare settings; however, doing so has many benefits for patients (Cohen and Goode 2003). Some of the reasons to incorporate cultural competence into organizational policies and procedures include the following:

- Respond to current and projected demographic changes in the United States
- Eliminate long-standing disparities in the health status of people of diverse racial, ethnic, and cultural backgrounds
- Improve the quality of services and health outcomes
- Meet legislative, regulatory, and accreditation mandates
- Gain a competitive edge in the market place
- Decrease the likelihood of liability or malpractice claims (NCCC 2015)

Assessing the cultural awareness and competence of a healthcare organization's employee involves training to help employees understand their own attitudes and practices, as well as understanding and practicing the policies of the organization. The national CLAS standards recommend healthcare organizations conduct ongoing assessments of their progress toward reaching the goals of CLAS-related actives with the purpose of assessing performance, monitoring progress, obtaining information about the organization and customers, and assessing the value of activities that fulfill governance, leadership, and workforce responsibilities (HHS 2015).

Healthcare Organizations' Cultural Competence Awareness

Addressing how one individually views language, communication style, belief systems, customs, attitudes, perceptions, and values in others is a way to assess personal cultural competence. Each employee of the healthcare organization should determine if he or she has biases and assess if those biases affect his or her actions and thinking toward fellow employees, patients, healthcare providers, vendors, and such.

When an organization requires employees to complete a self-assessment of their cultural awareness, the organization should encourage cultural acceptance in the following situations.

- Challenge colleagues when they make racial, ethnic, or sexually offensive comments or jokes; for example, if a fellow employee is overheard telling a racially-toned joke, other co-workers should let the employee know the behavior is unacceptable.

- Include diversity in social circles; for instance, many people are comfortable with the same group of co-workers and friends while having lunch. Inviting new people to the group increases cultural competence of the group, which positively affects the organization.

- Do not make assumptions about a person before the facts are verified. If a new person is hired in the HIM department and speaks broken English, an employee who is not culturally competent may assume the new person is not able to perform the job functions because of the language barrier, when in fact he or she may be able to perform the job very well.

- As an HIM professional, honestly assess individual and department strengths

and weaknesses in the area of accepting diversity. It is important for healthcare organizations to educate and train employees in the areas of diversity and competence. For example, the manager of an HIM department should provide training to employees on acceptance, understanding, and tolerance for others (NCCC 2015).

Healthcare organizations need to be sensitive to the background of patients and employees. An understanding and sensitivity to the beliefs and cultures of others can help alleviate misunderstanding and offensives that may happen because an employee has not been trained to be sensitive. For example, patients may not feel respected and listened to by healthcare providers who use medical language and do not try to explain their medical condition to them in terms they understand.

Training Programs

Cultural awareness training for all employees is an important component of an organization's overall cultural competence. By providing training to all employees of the organization in terms of cultural competence and awareness, team members will gain the knowledge, skills, and abilities to understand peoples' beliefs and culture and perhaps practice tolerance if they have prejudice, biases, and such. A **cultural audit** is a strategy to define an organization's values, symbols, and routines and identify areas for improvement. When it comes to cultural competence an organization should assess the following:

- Availability of interpreter services
- Effectiveness of cultural and linguistic competency training for staff
- Differences in services among diverse populations
- The impact of providing culturally competent services in improving the health outcomes and health status of patients

Healthcare organizations have established continuous quality improvement programs to measure the quality of a service or product through systems or process evaluation and implementation of revised processes that result in better healthcare outcomes. Organizations should incorporate CLAS measures into their ongoing quality improvement activities to determine how well they assess cultural competence as a hiring entity to abide by federal and state regulations. Information on employee training and development is discussed in greater detail in chapter 24.

Regulations for Cultural Awareness

Legal responsibilities of healthcare organizations determined by federal law prohibit discrimination based on ethnicity, religious faith, physical disability, or age. In 1961, President Kennedy used the term *affirmative action* in an Executive Order that directed government contractors to ensure that employees are treated equally without regard to their race, creed, color, or national origin. The Equal Employment Opportunity Commission (EEOC) was established to help provide equal employment opportunities for minority groups, women, people with disabilities, and veterans. Healthcare organizations must follow federal regulations and laws to remain in compliance with cultural awareness in hiring practices. (Refer to chapter 23 for more information on related regulations.)

Check Your Understanding 28.1

Instructions: **Answer the following questions on a separate piece of paper.**

1. Name at least four principles that explain the ways in which ethical decisions are made.

2. List five examples of culture.

3. List three attitudes that affect one's cultural competence.

4. What are some reasons to incorporate cultural competence into organizational policies and procedures?

5. The impact of providing culturally competent services in improving the health outcomes and health status of patients?

Ethical Foundations of Health Information Management

Ethical principles and values have been important to the HIM profession since its beginning in 1928. The first ethical pledge was presented in 1934 by Grace Whiting Myers, a visionary leader who recognized the importance of protecting information in medical records. The HIM profession was launched with recognition of the importance of privacy and the requirement of an authorization for the release of health information.

> I pledge myself to give out no information from any clinical record placed in my charge, or from any other source to any person whatsoever, except upon order from the chief executive officer of the institution which I may be serving. (Huffman 1972, 135)

Today, it is the patient who authorizes the release of their medical information and not the chief executive officer (CEO) of the healthcare organization, as was stated in the original pledge. The most important values embedded in this pledge are to protect patient privacy and confidential information and to recognize the importance of the HIM professional as a moral agent in protecting patient information. The HIM professional has a clear ethical and professional obligation not to give any information to anyone unless the release has been authorized (Harman 2012).

Professionals working in the field of HIM are guided by ethical foundations to protect privacy, maintain confidentiality, and ensure data are secure.

The guidance is detailed in a professional code of ethics that outlines the values and obligations for HIM professionals.

Protection of Privacy, Maintenance of Confidentiality, and Assurance of Data Security

HIM professionals are responsible for protecting patient privacy and confidentiality and maintaining the security and control of health records. This is accomplished by adhering to ethical principles guiding that responsibility—privacy, confidentiality, and security. **Privacy**, or freedom from unauthorized intrusion in healthcare, includes the right of a patient to control the disclosure of protected health information (PHI). **Confidentiality** is a legal and ethical concept that requires healthcare providers to protect health records and other personal and private information from unauthorized use or disclosure. **Security** is the means to control and protect access of health information and records (AHIMA 2015a). See chapter 11 for more information on privacy and security.

Professional Code of Ethics

A professional code of ethics is adopted by an organization to guide the members in determining right and wrong conduct when performing the duties of their job. The American Health Information Management Association (AHIMA) Code of Ethics applies to all AHIMA members and is based on the core values of the association. The preamble to the AHIMA Code of Ethics states:

> The ethical obligations of the HIM professional include the safeguarding of privacy and security of health information; disclosure of health information; development, use, and maintenance of health information systems and health information; and ensuring the accessibility and integrity of health information. (AHIMA 2011)

Healthcare consumers are increasingly concerned about security and the potential loss of privacy and the inability to control how their personal health information is used and disclosed. Core health information issues include what information should be collected, how the information

should be handled, who should have access to the information, under what conditions the information should be disclosed, how the information is retained and when it is no longer needed, and how is it disposed of in a confidential manner. All of the core health information issues are performed in compliance with state and federal regulations and employer policies and procedures.

Ethical obligations are central to the professional's responsibility, regardless of the employment site or the method of collection, storage, and security of health information. In addition, sensitive information (for example, genetic, adoption, drug, alcohol, sexual health, and behavioral information) requires special attention to prevent misuse. In the world of business and interactions with consumers, expertise in the protection of the information is required (AHIMA 2011). HIM professionals have access to sensitive information contained within the health record. Patients trust the information they share with their healthcare provider will be protected.

The professional working in the field of HIM is obligated to demonstrate actions that reflect values, ethical principles, and the ethical guidelines. The seven purposes listed in the AHIMA Code of Ethics are descriptions of the values and principles used to guide the conduct of HIM professionals. (See figure 28.1.)

The code includes core principles and guidelines that are aspirational and enforceable. Alleged violations of ethical principles is taken seriously by AHIMA and reviewed by a team dedicated to that purpose. AHIMA provides the Standards of Ethical Coding to assist coding professionals and managers more specifically in decision making when it comes to coding situations. It outlines expectations for making ethical decisions in the workplace and demonstrates coding professionals' commitment to integrity during the coding process (AHIMA 2015b).

Professional Values and Obligations

The HIM professional is ethically responsible for preserving, protecting, and securing health information in all mediums. This responsibility should be what the HIM professional values as part of

Figure 28.1.   The AHIMA Code of Ethics

The Code of Ethics serves seven purposes

1. Promote high standards of HIM practice
2. Identify core values on which the HIM mission is based
3. Summarize broad ethical principles that reflect the profession's core values
4. Establish a set of ethical principles to be used to guide decision making and actions
5. Establish a framework for professional behavior and responsibilities when professional obligations conflict or ethical uncertainties arise
6. Provide ethical principles by which the general public can hold the HIM professional accountable
7. Mentor practitioners new to the field to HIM's mission, values, and ethical principles

Principles and guidelines form the foundation of the Code of Ethics

Principle	Example
1. Advocate, uphold, and defend the individual's right to privacy and the doctrine of confidentiality in the use and disclosure of information.	Safeguard all confidential patient information to include, but not limited to, personal, health financial, genetic, and outcome information.
2. Put service and the health and welfare of persons before self-interest and conduct oneself in the practice of the profession so as to bring honor to oneself, peers and to the health information management profession.	Act with integrity, behave in a trustworthy manner, elevate service to others above self-interest and promote high standards of practice in every setting.
3. Preserve, protect, and secure personal health information in any form or medium and hold in the highest regards health information and other information of a confidential nature obtained in an official capacity, taking into account the applicable statutes and regulations.	Take precautions to ensure and maintain the confidentiality of information transmitted, transferred, or disposed of in the event of termination, incapacitation, or death of a healthcare provider to other parties through the use of any media.
4. Refuse to participate in or conceal unethical practices or procedures and report such practices.	Act in a professional and ethical manner at all times.
5. Advance health information management knowledge and practice through continuing education, research, publications, and presentations.	Develop and enhance continually professional expertise, knowledge, and skills (including appropriate education, research, training, consultation, and supervision). Contribute to the knowledge base of health information management and share one's knowledge related to practice, research, and ethics.
6. Recruit and mentor students, staff, peers, and colleagues to develop and strengthen professional workforce.	Provide directed practice opportunities for students.
7. Represent the profession to the public in a positive manner.	Be an advocate for the profession in all settings and participate in activities that promote and explain the mission, values, and principles of the profession to the public.
8. Perform honorably health information management association responsibilities, either appointed or elected, and preserve the confidentiality of any privileged information made known in any official capacity.	Perform responsibly all duties as assigned by the professional association operating within bylaws and policies and procedures of the association and any pertinent laws.
9. State truthfully and accurately one's credentials, professional education, and experiences.	Claim only those relevant professional credentials actually possessed and correct any inaccuracies occurring regarding credentials.
10. Facilitate interdisciplinary collaboration in situations supporting health information practice.	Foster trust among group members and adjust behavior in order to establish relationships with teams.
11. Respect the inherent dignity and worth of every person.	Treat each person in a respectful fashion, being mindful of individual differences and cultural and ethnic diversity.

Source: Adapted from AHIMA Code of Ethics 2011.

his or her duties. The professional values AHIMA identifies as important are quality, integrity, respect, and leadership and are demonstrated as follows:

- **Quality:** An abiding commitment to innovation, relevance, and continuous improvement in programs, products, and services.

- **Integrity**: Openness in decision making, honesty in communication and activity, and ethical practices that command trust and support collaboration.

- **Respect**: Appreciation of the value of differing perspectives, enjoyable experiences, courteous interaction, and celebration of achievements that advance our common cause.

- **Leadership**: Visionary thinking, decisions responsive to membership and mission, and accountability for actions and outcomes (AHIMA 2015b).

An HIM professional's ethical obligations include the duty to the patient and the healthcare team to protect health information, provide service to those who seek access to their information, preserve and secure health information, promote the quality and advancement of healthcare, function within the scope of responsibility, and refrain from passing clinical judgment. Obligations also include those to the employer such as loyalty; protection of committee deliberations (for example, a committee may involve decisions related to who will receive an organ donation from a donation list, those deliberations are protected much like patient information); compliance with all laws, regulations, and policies that govern the health information system; recognition of the authority and power of the job responsibilities; and acceptance of compensation only in relationship to work responsibilities. Ethical obligations to the public include advocating change when patterns or system problems are not in the best interest of the patients, as follows.

- Reporting violations of practice standards to the proper authorities
- Promoting interdisciplinary cooperation and collaboration
- Ethical obligations to self, peers, and professional associations include being honest about degrees, credentials, and work experiences
- Bringing honor to oneself by committing to lifelong learning

- Strengthening HIM membership in AHIMA and state associations
- Representing the HIM profession to the public
- Promoting and participating in HIM research (Harman 2012, 724)

HIM professionals are ethically obligated to give back to the HIM community by providing practice opportunities for students, such as being involved in student professional practice experience opportunities. HIM professionals also have a responsibility to pass on knowledge to new health information management professionals and students.

Ethical Issues Related to Medical Identity Theft

Identity theft is illegally obtaining another person's personal information and using it to commit theft or fraud, usually for the purpose of financial transactions. **Medical identity theft** is the fraudulent use of an individual's identifying information in a healthcare setting. This fraudulent information in a health record corrupts the record with erroneous information and can lead to incorrect diagnosis and treatment (McNabb and Rhodes 2014). The two primary ways medical identity theft happens is consensual—knowingly sharing information—and nonconsensual, someone unknown to the victim uses their information. A thief may use another person's insurance information, including social security numbers, to see a doctor, get prescription drugs, or fraudulently bill for healthcare services. Medical identity theft can be hard to detect because people do not always pay close attention to their medical bills and insurance claims. If healthcare professionals do not recognize this impact on patient records and do not fix the error, the theft can remain on the record of the patient, potentially causing misdiagnosis or treatment (McNabb and Rhodes 2014). For example, a healthcare provider sees a patient and provides treatment for diabetes. The patient seen was using the insurance card of his brother because the patient does not have healthcare coverage. The diagnosis of diabetes is now a part of his brother's health record and when the brother is seen for treatment in the future, he may receive erroneous treatment for diabetes.

The patient and the HIM professional each have a unique perspective on medical identity theft and each are responsible for identifying, reporting, and combating the crime.

HIM professionals serve patients well by educating them about what to look for in terms of medical identity theft. For example, HIM professionals should work with patients and explain the signs of identity theft. They can explain to patients that if they receive a bill for medical services that they do not recognize that they should check for fraudulent behavior in their name by requesting a complete copy of their medical bills to determine if claims are inaccurately being submitted in their name. Patients can detect medical identity theft by reviewing their credit reports annually. A credit report will indicate accounts opened in the patient's name by healthcare organizations; if the patient does not recognize the organization, he or she can begin the steps to rectify the situation and identify the fraud.

Consider a thief using a patient's insurance card to obtain prescription drugs from multiple providers and pharmacies. The patient is unaware of this use; months later the patient returns to his provider and needs medication but his record has been flagged as "drug seeking" and his provider will not prescribe the medication he needs. It can take some time for the patient to identify where and when his information was stolen and to clear his record.

With an increase in medical identity theft, it is important for HIM professionals to help find and correct fraudulent information within a health record. The California Attorney General's Office created an information sheet for consumers—First Aid for Medical Identity Theft: Tips for Consumers. The information sheet describes five signs of possible medical identity theft and provides tips on what to do in response to each.

- If a patient receives a Receipt of a Breach Notice from a healthcare organization, it indicates that the patient's protected health

information was involved in a data breach. Depending on the type of information involved in the breach, a security freeze on the patient's credit records may be required. Breach notification will be addressed in greater detail later in this chapter.

- If a patient notices an unknown item in the Explanation of Benefits from an insurance company and he or she does not recognize the service being paid for, the insurer and the provider who billed for the services must be contacted to correct the information.

- If a patient receives a notification from the insurance provider that he or she is close to or have reached the benefit limit for a service, the patient needs to request and review all claims; for example, a patient is notified that the limit of available refills for a certain medication has been reached, so the patient may need to obtain a complete list of all benefits paid on his or her behalf to determine erroneous charges.

- A call from a debt collector for medical services that the patient did not receive should prompt the patient to contact the healthcare provider who sent the bill to collections for a copy of all medical bills and related documents for that service, so the patient can dispute the collection.

- Patients should listen carefully to the questions asked of them when they are registering for a healthcare visit, meaning they should always verify their own demographic information when being seen by a provider and should always address incorrect information (OAG CA DOJ 2013).

HIM professionals are able to assist patients with the process of finding out what happened in cases of medical identity theft and help guide the patient to fixing the errors in their record.

Ethical Decision Making

When a healthcare professional is faced with ethical decisions and dilemmas, several factors are included in the decision-making process. These include but are not limited to: cost, technological feasibility, federal and state laws, medical staff bylaws, accreditation and licensing standards, and employer policies, rules, and regulations (Harman 2012, 745–746).

An example of an ethical decision-making process for a healthcare organization would be the case of an elderly patient who is not able to make their own healthcare decisions and has a limited chance of long time survival. The patient has a daughter who wants the facility to do everything possible to keep the patient alive and her brother wants to remove all care and let the patient pass. The ethics committee would consider the cost to the organization, the technological feasibility to care for the patient, the bylaws of the organization, and so forth.

HIM professionals should be guided by the AHIMA Code of Ethics in making ethical decisions. Figure 28.2 shows seven considerations that should be asked by HIM professionals faced with an ethical decision.

Decisions made due to an ethical dilemma need to go through the process identified in figure 28.2. For example, Kristi, a new graduate of an HIM program, takes the RHIA examination and fails. She does not want her employer to know she failed

so she tells all her coworkers that she passed the examination. Kristi then starts using the RHIA credential after her name in work correspondence. A coworker, Camille, discovered that Kristi is using the RHIA credential fraudulently and notifies their supervisor Darcy. It is the responsibility of both Camille and Darcy, as HIM professionals, to prevent this activity from happening. Darcy should contact AHIMA and report the abuse. Using the considerations listed in figure 28.2, Kristi's ethical dilemma is outlined as illustrated in figure 28.3.

Breach of Healthcare Ethics

Breach of healthcare ethics is the situation in which ethics are violated, whether it be intentional or accidental. Healthcare facilities establish an **ethics committee**, which is a committee of the organization tasked with reviewing ethics violations and determining the course of action required to remedy the violations. Most ethics committees involve people from varied backgrounds and have three major functions—providing clinical ethics consultation, developing policies pertaining to clinical ethics, and facilitating education on topical issues in clinical ethics (Pearlman 2013).

Figure 28.2. Ethical decision making process

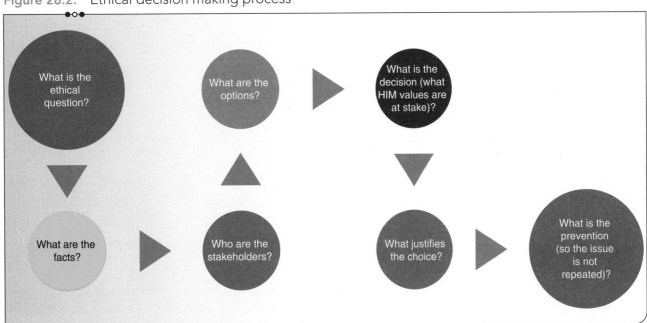

Source: Adapted from Harman 2012, 747.

Figure 28.3. Example of ethical decision making process

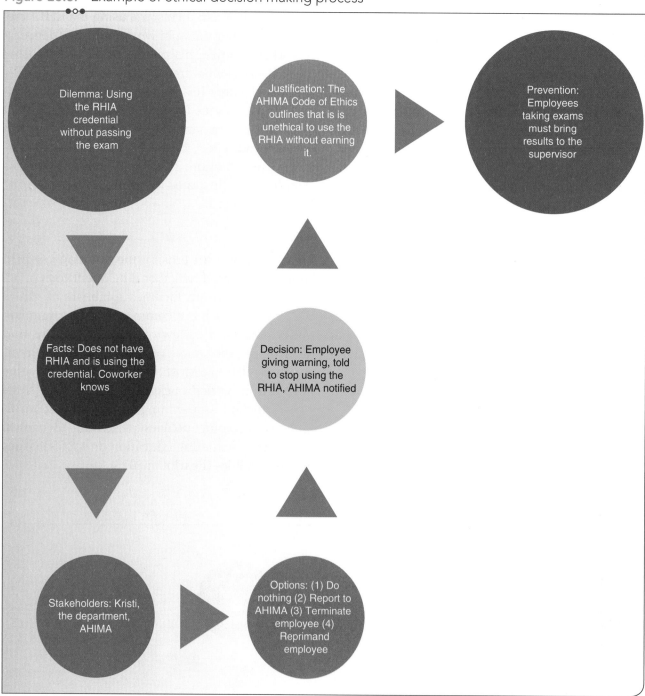

Source: Adapted from Harman 2012, 747.

The goals of the ethics committee include identifying and ensuring the rights of patients, establishing processes to ensure shared decision making between patients and clinicians, and ensuring the process does not interfere with the ethical practices of the facility (Pearlman 2013).

Important Health Information Ethical Problems

Some areas in health information management have specific ethical problems, such as documentation, privacy, coding, ROI, quality management, decision support, and public health.

Ethical Issues Related to Documentation and Privacy

It is the responsibility of an HIM professional to ensure patient documentation is accurate, timely, and created by authorized parties. This is accomplished by developing policies and procedures, in accordance with laws and regulations, to ensure the integrity of patient information is upheld by the organization. Healthcare providers are required to document their decision-making processes, this means that educational sessions are important to provide training on documentation that can help protect against unethical behaviors. By providing training on documenting how physicians came to the clinical decisions they did, the healthcare organization is helping to protect itself from malpractice claims.

An example of unethical documentation an HIM professional can help with includes retrospective documentation practice. **Retrospective documentation** is when healthcare providers add documentation after care has been given. This could be for the purpose of increasing reimbursement or avoiding a medical legal action.

Ethical Issues Related to Release of Information

Release of information (ROI) specialists should embody the value of integrity. The HIM professional must "release information only with valid authorization from a patient or a person legally authorized to consent on behalf of a patient" (AHIMA 2011). There are two primary ethical issues that arise from ROI—the need-to-know-principle and blanket authorizations. The **need-to-know principle** is based on the minimum necessary standard; for example, if there is a request to verify an admission for lap-band surgery and the ROI specialist gives out the history and physical, labs, discharge summary, and operative report to an insurance company, the documentation could reveal a lot more information than requested, which in turn results in the patient's privacy being violated because more information is being released than just the verification of the admission. An ROI specialist must only give out the need-to-know or the

least amount of information necessary, in this case just the admission information.

The other ethical concern for ROI is misuse of the **blanket authorization**, which is when the patient signs an authorization allowing the ROI specialist to release any and all information from that point forward. This is an issue because under a blanket authorization the patient is giving authorization for future diagnosis and treatment, one of which they may not want authorized. For example, if the patient signs the blanket authorization today to be able to release their annual examination to their employer and in five years the patient is diagnosed with cancer, the employer could find out about the cancer because the information was automatically released to the employer, and the patient may not remember because they signed the blanket authorization five years prior. HIM professionals need to be aware of this dilemma and help with the education of the patient to what the blanket authorization means.

Ethical Issues Related to Coding

Codes are associated with reimbursement rates and, therefore, there are inherent incentives to code so the healthcare facilities will receive the highest reimbursement dollar amount possible. Coding professionals need to be guided by ethical coding practices because they may be asked by a provider to fraudulently code to receive higher payment for services rendered. It is important for a coder to only assign codes where data is clearly stated in the health record. If more information is needed, or the information needs to be clarified, a query should be sent to the physician. This process is discussed in chapter 9.

The Standards of Ethical Coding are based on AHIMA's Code of Ethics with the guidelines outlining eleven standards for ethical coding.

- Apply accurate, complete, and consistent coding practices for the production of high-quality healthcare data
- Report all healthcare data elements required for external reporting purposes completely and accurately, in accordance with regulatory and documentation standards

and requirement and applicable official coding conventions, rules, and guidelines

- Assign and report only the codes and data that are clearly and consistently supported by health record documentation in accordance with applicable code set and abstraction conventions, rules, and guidelines

- Query provider for clarification and additional documentation prior to code assignment when there is conflicting, incomplete, or ambiguous information in the health record regarding a significant reportable condition or procedure or other reportable data element dependent on health record documentation

- Refuse to change reported codes or the narratives of codes so that meanings are misrepresented

- Refuse to participate in or support coding or documentation practices intended to inappropriately increase payment, quality for insurance policy coverage, or skew data by means that do not comply with federal and state statues, regulations, and official rules and guidelines

- Facilitate interdisciplinary collaboration in situations supporting proper coding practices

- Advance coding knowledge and practice through continuing education

- Refuse to participate in or conceal unethical coding or abstraction practices or procedures

- Protect the confidentiality of the health record at all times and refuse to access protected health information not required for coding-related activities

- Demonstrate behavior that reflects integrity, shows a commitment to ethical and legal coding practices and fosters trust in professional activities (AHIMA 2015c)

Other coding ethical dilemmas are upcoding, unbundling, and double billing. **Upcoding** is the practice of assigning diagnostic or procedural codes that represent higher payment rates than the codes that actually reflect the services provided to patients via the documentation. For example, a physician examines a patient briefly for the flu, but the bill submitted for the visit includes an hour long, complex exam that did not occur. **Unbundling** is the practice of using multiple codes to bill for the various individual steps in a single procedure rather than using a single code that includes all of the steps. For instance, a patient goes in for a new cast on a broken leg and instead of billing for one bundled visit (all of the services related to treating the fracture are billed as one service), the bill lists codes for each step as individual procedures resulting in a larger reimbursement. **Double billing** is when two providers bill for one service provided to one patient. An example of this is a surgeon who was an assistant for a procedure bills Medicare as if she were the primary surgeon, with the primary surgeon also billing Medicare for the same surgery on the same patient.

Ethical Issues Related to Quality Management, Decision Support, and Public Health

Healthcare costs are increasing and organizations are trying to find ways to keep costs down while still providing quality services, which can be a difficult task. Some examples of issues created by this challenge include:

- Healthcare organizations falsifying their performance information to the public

- Negative patient outcomes, such as inattentive patient care

- Failure to ensure a physician's license is valid

- When accreditation or licensure surveys occur, health records are hidden or not available to the surveyors.

- Repetition of unsuitable healthcare (Harman 2012, 734)

The HIM professional is put in a position where they are required to advocate so the interest of both the public and the individual patient can be served. An example of this is global infections, or bioterrorism, where it is pertinent to keep the balance between protecting the privacy of those injured or affected and delivering information to the government and healthcare professionals so the medical crisis can be resolved.

Ethical Issues Related to Managed Care

Healthcare can be expensive. Managed care helps control the cost of healthcare by providing services at a fixed cost and by minimizing variation in clinical practice; for example, all patients seen for hypertension receive the exact standard of care and service, with little variation for individual patients. Ethical issues that arise with this type of care involve physicians missing a clinical indication that a patient needs more than what the standard care provides. In some managed care settings, the goal is to increase productivity while keeping costs the same, wherein physicians have less time with patients, leaving room for the physician to miss some key information. Managed care incentives may affect provider behavior or have a negative effect on patient care.

Ethical Issues Related to Sensitive Health Information

All health information must be protected, however there is some information that requires special attention because it is considered sensitive health information such as genetic, adoption, drug, alcohol, sexual health, and behavioral information. This type of information not only often has stricter rules and regulations, but provides a more ethical "gray area" when it comes to releasing and providing records.

When developing policies and procedures for ROI that can contain substance abuse, sexually transmitted disease, and mental health information, extra caution is required on the HIM professional's part because there may be competing interests between public safety and patient privacy. Federal and state legislation provides some guidance, but often extra legal counsel may be needed.

Ethical Issues Related to Research

Research is important for the growth and advancement of the healthcare profession. The Institutional Review Boards for the Protection of Human Subjects (IRBs) is the committee that oversees the clinical research conducted for healthcare and has responsibility over the ethical application of research (Adams and Callahan 2013). More information about IRB can be found in chapter 20. Without research, common medications or cures would not exist. However, with research comes an ethical obligation to provide patient safety and protection. This obligation is cited in the Belmont Report, which provides the foundation for ethical research. The intent of the Belmont Report is to protect the autonomy, safety, privacy, and welfare of human research subjects (Adams and Callahan 2013). There are three primary ethical principles the Belmont Report provides:

- *Autonomy:* Defined earlier, autonomy includes the informed consent process for human research subjects and starts with a full disclosure of the nature of the study, the risks, benefits, and gives the participant the opportunity to back out of the study if he or she wants. The idea behind this is that the potential participant has full knowledge of what he or she is doing, and can confidently say yes or no.

- *Beneficence:* Defined earlier, beneficence is when a researcher determines what the maximum potential is for society, compared to the minimum risk of harm done to the participants in the research study. An example would be a researcher looking at a trial for finding a cure for the common cold. The risk to the research participants would be low and the maximum potential for the trial is high because the common cold effects a large number of people each year.

- *Justice:* This principle involves impartial selection of participants in a research study. The research study must stay within the law when choosing participants. It is important to avoid unfairly coercing participants, such as prisoners who have historically been coerced into taking part in medical research against their will (Adams 2013).

The HIM department is involved in the IRB process by making the medical records of patients enrolled in a research study available to external monitors and auditors. Agreements between the HIM department and researchers to ensure patient consent and policies and procedures are followed. In the case of electronic health information there are agreements outlining the exact information to be released to researchers. The HIM department offers training to researchers and HIM staff for the procedures in place for the consent process and maintenance of the records. More information can be found in chapter 20.

Ethical Issues Related to Electronic Health Record Systems

The access to electronic health record (EHR) systems is a complex challenge in regard to record integrity, information security, linkage of information for continuum of care within different e-health systems, and the development of software for HIM purposes. HIM professionals need to be part of the implementation team to provide their unique understanding of the federal rules and regulations regarding privacy and security, and can help facilitate a successful core in the implementations of these issues.

Healthcare professionals are trained in the ethical issues related to EHR systems because staff may have access to more information then what is needed to do their job. Employees accessing the record should not explore information out of curiosity, this would be unethical. When a patient's health information is shared or linked within an EHR without his or her knowledge the patient's autonomy is breached. Providers sometimes may use the copy paste option to copy information from one patient record to another and may inadvertently add incorrect information into a record.

Check Your Understanding 28.2

Instructions: **Answer the following questions on a separate piece of paper.**

1. What would you call an authorization that allows the release of information from the point it is signed and includes release of information for future care? What issues can arise?

2. Name the practice of assigning diagnostic or procedural codes that represent higher payment rates.

3. List three examples of quality outcome problems due to the trends of keeping costs down while still providing quality services?

4. Identify seven purposes served by the AHIMA Code of Ethics.

   Seven purposes served by the AHIMA Code of Ethics include:

5. The AHIMA Code of Ethics states that HIM professionals shall recruit and mentor students. What does that mean?

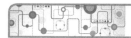

References

Adams, L. and T. Callahan. 2013. Research Ethics. Ethics in Medicine. University of Washington School of Medicine. https://depts.washington.edu/bioethx/topics/resrch.html

Allen, J. 2013. Health Law & Medical Ethics for Healthcare Professionals. Pearson Education, Inc. As Prentice Hall.

American Health Information Management Association. 2015a. Mission Vision and Values. http://www.ahima.org/about/aboutahima?tabid=mission

American Health Information Management Association. 2015b. Ethics. http://www.ahima.org/about/aboutahima?tabid=ethics

American Health Information Management Association. 2015c. American Health Information Management Association Standards of Ethical Coding. http://library.ahima.org/xpedio/groups/public/documents/ahima/bok2_001166.hcsp?dDocName=bok2_001166

American Health Information Management Association. 2011. Code of Ethics. http://library. ahima.org/xpedio/groups/public/documents/ ahima/bok1_024277.hcsp?dDocName=bok1_024277

Cohen, E. and T.D. Goode.1999, revised Goode, T.D. and C. Dunne. 2003. Policy Brief 1: Rational for Cultural Competence in Primary Care. Washington, DC: National Center for Cultural Competence, Georgetown University Center for Child and Human Development.

Harman, L.B. 2012. Ethical Issues in Health Information Management. Chapter 12 in *Health Information Management Technology: An Applied Approach,* 4th ed. Edited by N.B. Sayles. Chicago: AHIMA.

Huffman, E.K. 1972. *Manual for Medical Record Librarians,* 6th ed. Chicago: Physician's Record Company.

McNabb, J. and H.B. Rhodes. 2014. Combating the privacy crime that can kill. *Journal of AHIMA* 85(4):26–29.

Meyer, P., P. Yoon, and R. Kaufmann. 2013. Introduction: CDC Health Disparities and Inequalities Report. http://www.cdc.gov/mmwr/preview/ mmwrhtml/su6203a2.htm?s_cid=su6203a2_w

National Center for Cultural Competence. 2015. The Compelling Need for Cultural and Linguistic Competence. Georgetown University. http://nccc. georgetown.edu/foundations/need.html

Office of the Attorney General, California Department of Justice. 2013. First Aid For Medical Identity Theft Tips for Consumers. http://www.oag.ca.gov/sites/all/ files/agweb/pdfs/privacy/cis_16_med_id_theft.pdf

Pearlman, R. 2013. Ethics Committees, Programs and Consultation. Ethics in Medicine, University of Washington School of Medicine. https://depts. washington.edu/bioethx/topics/ethics.html

Simmers, L., K. Simmers-Nartker, and S. Simmers-Kobelak. 2014. Simmers DHO Health Science, 8th ed. Cengage Learning.

US Department of Health and Human Services, Office of Minority Health. n.d. National Standards for Culturally and Linguistically Appropriate Services (CLAS) in Health and Health Care. https://www.thinkculturalhealth.hhs.gov/pdfs/ EnhancedNationalCLASStandards.pdf

US Department of Health and Human Services, Office of Minority Health. 2015. What are the National CLAS Standards? https://www.thinkculturalhealth.hhs. gov/CLAS/clas_standard10.asp

World Health Organization. 2012. Social Determinants of Health. http://www.who.int/social_determinants/ sdh_definition/en/

29

Strategic Thinking and Management

Susan E. McClernon, PhD, FACHE

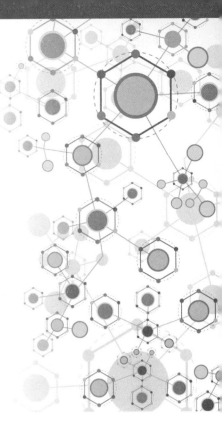

927

Setting strategy is often viewed as the work of senior managers and boards of trustees. Strategy is thought of as being handed down from on high, embodied in slogans, and generally not very relevant to the day-to-day work of most employees in the organization. Sometimes strategy is detailed in a three- to five-year plan that lays out objectives and key actions to meet the organization's goals. But strategy is no longer the sole purview of senior managers, planning departments, or consultants. The ability to develop effective strategies is a key attribute and skill of successful managers and leaders at all levels in today's organizations. Employers cite strategic thinking, which includes strategic management and change leadership, as competencies they look for in health information management (HIM) professionals (AHIMA 2015a). Managers and directors should be able to lead the development of strategic plans at their department or division level as well as contribute significantly in strategic thinking and planning at an organizational level.

Simply stated, strategy is the art and science of planning and marshaling resources for their most efficient and effective use to position your organization for the future. **Strategy** has been defined as "a plan for getting from a point in the present to some point in the future in the face of uncertainty and resistance" (Beckham 2000). Strategy means consciously choosing to be clear about your company's direction in relation to what is happening in a dynamic environment (Olsen 2006, 10).

Strategic management is the process a leader and his or her leadership team uses for assessing a changing environment to create a vision of the future; determining how the organization fits into the future environment based on its mission, vision, and knowledge of its strengths, weaknesses, opportunities, and threats; and then setting in motion a strategic plan of action to position the organization accordingly.

Strategic planning is the formalized roadmap that describes how the company executes the chosen strategy. A strategic plan spells out where an organization is going over the next three to five years and how it is going to get there. A strategic plan is a management tool that serves the purpose of helping an organization do a better job, because a plan focuses the energy, resources, and time of everyone in the organization in the same direction (Olsen 2006, 12).

Strategic planning is different than operations improvement planning. Operations improvement focuses on improving how existing programs and services are carried out. These objectives are usually evaluated and updated on an annual basis. Typically the operating objectives included in the operations plan are internally focused, yet should be related to achieving the overall strategic plan.

Management theories about the importance of strategy and how to set strategy are changing. This reconsideration is a reflection of the speed of change in every facet of contemporary life, including healthcare. One of the key components seen as missing or poorly done in current strategic planning processes is strategic thinking. **Strategic thinking** is the thought process of the CEO and the key people around him or her that helps them determine the vision for the organization at some point in the future. Strategic thinking is different from strategic planning and operational planning; it is the framework for the strategic and operational improvement plans. It combines an understanding of a strategic plan and an operational plan, which then supports comprehensive strategic thinking within an organization (Robert 2006, 51–54).

This chapter explores the importance of strategic thinking and planning to effective strategic management, describes approaches to making and communicating strategic choices, provides approaches for maximizing organizational learning, and illustrates how HIM professionals can use strategy to shape and influence change in their department and organization.

From Strategic Planning to Strategic Management and Thinking

Strategic planning was described in management literature in the 1960s and the decades that followed. It was a prominent and highly touted organizational function. Strategic planning was developed to prevent organizations from crisis planning—when they realized that their competitors outpaced them in innovation and they quickly had to develop reactive strategies to keep this from happening again. Early applications were characterized by rigorous and formal analysis of data to deduce a desired future and the steps to achieve it. In large corporations, departments of planners prepared forecasts with the aid of computer analysis. The complex reports were delivered to senior managers, who were largely uninvolved in the process.

These approaches have fallen out of favor for several key reasons. First, forecasting the future, particularly in such rapidly changing times, is difficult. Second, by the time a complex multi-year plan is finalized and delivered to its managers and employees, it is undoubtedly out of date. If customers, employees, and all levels of managers are involved in strategy development, the plan is likely to be seen as relevant and likely to be implemented. Third, for strategic planning and thinking to really be more than an operations improvement plan, the plan needs to include a clear vision for the future and innovative strategies that not only help the organization redefine its existing products and services, but creates new products and services that strategically move the organization forward toward its vision.

In order to stay strong and viable as an organization, the HIM professional must understand the organizational vision. He or she must engage the best thinking of everyone in and outside his or her area, look at where the organization is today and where it needs to be in the future, and then design the path to the new vision as a team. When departmental and organizational strategic plans are updated at least annually, the effort will result in plans that cause transformative organizational change.

No one phrase is the accepted successor for this type of comprehensive strategic planning and thinking. In fact, today managers and directors in many organizations are likely to still hear the activity referred to as strategic planning. However, it is important to get beneath the words to understand the process being followed. It may be called strategic planning, but it can embody many of the newer concepts that often are called strategic management and thinking.

- It is framed by the organization's vision, mission, and values.
- It takes into account possible future scenarios rather than trying to forecast only one future.
- It is truly the work of management and involves key stakeholders including employees, even when guided by consultants, and has broad input and participation.
- It is action oriented and measurable, with a commitment to bringing about change.
- It results in organizational innovation, change, and learning.

Strategic thinking is a way of introducing innovation into decision making and engaging others in the change process. With the rapid changes in the healthcare industry and HIM practice, this discussion of strategic thinking is not academic. The skills that distinguish a strategic thinker include the following:

- An ability to plan (consensus building) and formulate strategy (leadership)
- Flexibility and creativity

- Comfort with uncertainty and risk
- A sense of urgency and vision of how to move change forward positively
- An understanding of how to gain a powerful core of organizational supporters and customers
- An ability to communicate the vision and plans

Strategic management and thinking should be viewed as a component of each of the four functions of management discussed in chapter 22. Every aspect of management involves a strategic management component, as described here. With organizational learning as a centerpiece, the approach described in this chapter unifies change management, strategy development, and leadership. In all three, managers learn by observing and reflecting on the results of their experiences. To undertake deliberate change, individuals reflect on their experiences and become aware of new patterns and trends that they did not previously perceive. They form new ways of looking at the opportunities and the implications of their experiences. They evaluate new theories about what can and should be and then apply these theories and test their implications. They then observe and reflect on the results of their experiences (Kolb 1988, 68–88).

Skills of Strategic Managers and Strategic Thinkers

The definition of strategy is straightforward, but the skills for setting and executing strategy are far from simple. HIM professionals must take advantage of opportunities to learn and develop skills for strategic management and thinking, including:

- Monitoring industry trends in healthcare and information management
- Reflecting on how industry trends can affect existing and new products and services
- Considering how changes in one area can affect others in the organization
- Considering how a strategic course for change is set for their departments and organizations
- Helping others visualize the need for change and recruiting them as partners in moving a change agenda forward
- Implementing and measuring strategic plans effectively
- Questioning the status quo on a continuing basis and leading innovative change
- Being self-reflective and lifelong learners

Strategy is no longer a management domain reserved for only senior managers. Today, all managers must develop skills and competencies that enable them to think and act strategically. These skills include sharpening their ability to observe the world around them. Strategic managers watch for changes in the larger environment beyond the healthcare industry, including political, economic, social, and technological changes. Such changes may involve staff attitudes, public policy, ethics, or inventions and innovations within the healthcare industry or externally. Managers must consider how these changes are affecting—or might affect—healthcare and the organizations in which they work. For example, shifts in public attitudes regarding the value placed on personal privacy have implications for health information policies and practices regarding patients who are using online access to or request copies of their personal health records.

Strategic managers develop skills reflecting the implications and opportunities afforded by trends. Whether reading a journal or discussing new ideas with others, strategic managers are always testing new ideas, identifying those that have merit, and discarding those that do not. They are creating links between the trends and the value-adding actions they can take. For example, federal programs to adjust provider reimbursement on the basis of certain quality parameters suggest a need to elevate organizational health information standards for data integrity so that pay-for-performance determinations are accurate and fair.

Effective strategic managers and thinkers are creative in how they make associations among trends, ideas and new opportunities. These associations are not always direct, as in the examples about privacy and public policy or data quality and pay for performance. Making strategy choices may be the result of drawing lessons from analogous situations. When faced with an unfamiliar problem or opportunity, experienced managers often learn from connecting with colleagues who may have faced similar situations and apply what they have learned elsewhere to their current situation (Gavetti and Rivkin 2005, 54–63). For example, faced with a shortage of trained coders, the HIM director institutes a coder training program in partnership with a local community college, modeled after a similar program used to address the shortage of nurses in the community.

Strategic managers also continually look for opportunities to improve on the status quo. They do not accept the old adage, "If it's not broken, don't fix it." They always look for ways to make things better and are willing to take some risks and evaluate new approaches through trial and error. They understand that taking no action may be less tolerable than trying something even if it does not fully succeed. For example, the quality of coded data for inpatient services is at 94 percent and the data quality manager thinks that adjusting staff assignments may make better use of staff skills and improve performance.

New managers may lack the confidence to initiate change and may have few analogous experiences to draw on. Still, they should guard against accepting or perpetuating artificial barriers to creativity characterized by common squelchers, such as "We've never done that before," "We have always done it that way," or "That's not my job." Confidence comes from experience, and experience requires asking focused questions, action, and thoughtful reflection on what did and did not work.

Finally, strategic managers learn to help their organization contribute to new thinking and new ideas. They know that the best solutions represent the best thinking of all key stakeholders. Thus, strategic managers learn techniques to bring out the greatest thinking of their staff, superiors, colleagues, and customers for their change agenda. For example, in pursuit of a goal to decrease the amount of printing of electronic records by physicians, the health information manager knew that support from nursing and other staff in the patient care units was essential for success. He oversaw implementation of a multifaceted plan to reduce the rate of printing on the units and shared credit with nursing when the print rate began to decline.

The science and art of leadership skills needed to become a strategic manager can be learned. Learning begins by recognizing the importance of the strategy to today's successful managers. For HIM professionals, that learning begins with their professional coursework and directed learning experiences. Skills are learned and subsequently sharpened through work experience, particularly in opportunities to be part of—and to lead—change management projects.

Elements of Strategic Thinking and Strategic Management

As shown in figure 29.1, strategic thinking and strategic management are logical processes that comprise a number of steps in strategic planning that may be explicit or implicit. It begins with a current description and internal assessment of the organization, and an assessment of the external environment. Most commonly a **SWOT analysis** tool is used in this step. A SWOT outlines the organization's strengths (S) and weaknesses (W),

Figure 29.1.   Elements of strategic planning

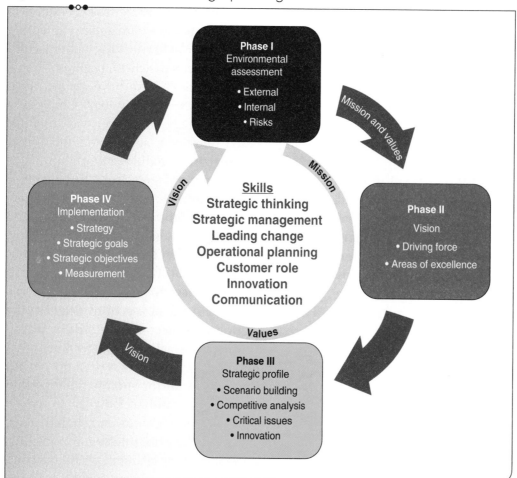

which are internal to the organization, and the opportunities (O) and threats (T) that are external to the organization.

The strategic planning process is depicted as circular because overall strategic management is a never-ending process and often requires revisiting steps as more information is discovered. The best strategies may emerge from trial and error, but an effective strategy will not emerge without a clear idea of where the leader wants to move the organization and a realistic assessment of the issues to overcome. Moreover, strategic management cannot happen in isolation. Stakeholders—whether staff, customers, caregivers, patients, or managers—must be engaged in each phase of the strategic planning process.

Each step involves learning, which in turn enables plans to be improved upon, therefore making subsequent efforts more effective. Thus, experience sharpens and clarifies understanding of the issues, allowing managers to be more precise in setting goals. Strategies and tactics are continually modified with experience. Strategic management is a process that leads to organizational learning and improvement over time.

In contrast to traditional strategic planning, where all steps are neatly outlined before implementation is begun, strategic management requires a willingness to learn and change as the leader guides an organization through the process. In a fast-paced, changing environment, constant review of strategy, goals, and objectives is required, as well as new skills focused on strategic thinking, planning, and management.

Check Your Understanding 29.1

Instructions: **Answer the following questions on a separate sheet of paper.**

1. What is a formalized road map that describes how a company executes a chosen strategy?

2. True or False: Strategic thinking is the same as a strategic planning and operational planning.

3. True or False: Today, with fast-paced change, the healthcare industry is finding it important to involve key stakeholders including employees in successful strategic planning.

4. List three key skills a strategic thinker needs to possess.

5. True or False: The four phases or elements of planning are: Phase 1: Environmental assessment; Phase 2: Vision; Phase 3: Strategy profile; Phase 4: Implementation.

Phase 1: Environmental Assessment: Internal and External

The beginning stage in developing a new or updated strategic plan is to develop a solid understanding of the organization's current profile through the internal and external assessment of the organization. This approach assesses the current mission, vision, and values of the organization or department; completes an internal analysis of the trends within the organization or department; and conducts an external assessment of trends. The final step in completing the current profile is to assess the potential impact of the uncertainties and risks in the internal and external environment on the organization's strategic thinking and plan. Based on all the information and intelligence gathered throughout this profiling process, the strategic thinking tools and techniques described here are then utilized to develop a strategic future profile.

Understand Environmental Assessment Trends

Knowledge of the current internal and external environment is essential to vision and strategy formulation. An environmental assessment is conducted, which is defined as a thorough review of the internal and external conditions in which an organization operates (Jennings 2000, 39). This data-intensive process is the continuous process of gathering and analyzing intelligence about trends that are—or may be—affecting HIM and the healthcare organization and industry. It is both internally focused on the healthcare organization and HIM and externally focused on industry, market, and environmental trends.

Internal Assessment

It is important to fully evaluate and understand the current internal environment of both the department and the organization. This is a critical step to understand the organization's current strategic direction. It is also an opportunity to gain multiple perspectives from key stakeholders on the current state. During this step in the process, differing perspectives that are held by various key stakeholders will emerge. Key themes of consensus will also begin to show.

Assess the Current Mission, Vision, and Values

It is important to review the current mission, vision, and values of the organization and department. A **mission statement** is defined as an enduring statement of purpose for an organization that identifies the scope of its operations in services and products, customer or users, and market segments and geography; and reflects its values and priorities (Abrahams 1999, 14). As described previously, the mission differs from the vision. It is also important to understand the organizational values that are used to describe the basic philosophy, principles, or ideals of the organizational culture and behavioral expectations. Any strategic plan needs to be developed in accordance with the mission, vision, and values of the organization in order to drive change that will be supported by staff and senior leaders.

Develop a Current Strategic Profile

The organizational description needs to include a current strategic profile that identifies the existing key services or products of the department or organization, nature of its customers and users, nature of its industry and market segments, and nature of its geographic markets (Robert 2006, 53–54).

Another critical step in the assessment process is to conduct a SWOT (strengths, weaknesses, opportunities, and threats) analysis of the department and organization. A SWOT analysis

> evaluates the internal organization based on its strengths compared to competitors and regional and societal demands, weaknesses compared to competitors or related to just the internal functions, opportunities for advancing ahead of competitors or serving a patient population not served well currently, and threats from external or internal agents that could stymie the organization's success. (Dunn 2010, 135)

This process should involve multiple key stakeholders and will be an opportunity to begin consensus building. At this point in the process, planning assumptions, data analysis, and identification of potential risks and uncertainties should occur.

The internal environmental assessment includes analysis of:

- *Role statements and organizational framework:* Organization-wide strategy and priorities; evaluating whether the organization is meeting its mission, vision, and value statements; and whether its structure and processes are designed to achieve business aims; includes an assessment of program development, governance, and management.

- *Performance indicators:* Budgeted staff, key statistics, educational resources, competencies, and organizational culture; information management strategy, information systems plans and priorities, compliance programs, products and services, and business processes

- *Primary market research:* Information on organization and its market place, staff and customer engagement feedback

- *Financial performance:* Budget targets and results, financials, performance, and productivity measures (Zuckerman 2012, 38–39)

When the internal assessment is complete, there should be a comprehensive view of the organization's past and current performance and strategy. Developing a comprehensive strategic profile should clearly identify the organization's advantages and disadvantages in the current environment and key planning issues. The information will be useful in the next steps of the strategic thinking and planning process. Involving employees and leaders in this step of the process is critical.

External Assessment

The external environmental assessment is conducted to understand the organization's performance as it relates to its marketplace and includes the following:

- *Review forces of the healthcare industry:* Demographic, economic, political, health status, social, technological, and educational factors that may be impacting the organization

- *Conduct primary market research:* Comparative information on the organization and its competitors and other likely key external factors including the community

- *Assess market forecasts and implications:* Healthcare reimbursement systems, patient and customer engagement trends and regulatory trends

- *Analyze competitors:* Collect competitor data rigorously using multiple sources

- *Identify potential collaborators:* Current and potential collaborators and partners
- *Assess market trends:* A review of the state of the healthcare industry and other related industries and organizations (Zuckerman 2012, 40–43)

Other key pieces of information needed for the external assessment phase of the strategic plan include the following:

- Demographics
- Innovative trends in the industry
- Technology
- Market structure
- Market share
- Market forecasts and implications
- Customers
- Competitors
- Centers of excellence

An HIM manager who focuses exclusively on his or her own area of responsibility, whether managing a department, a service, or a project, will have a difficult time succeeding as a strategic manager. Understanding the environment provides the context for the tough decisions involved in setting direction, designing strategy, and leading change. Some ways to develop access to be better able to gather internal and external assessment information in your environment include:

- Taking inventory of sources of internal and external information to identify and fill information gaps
- Building performance measures to gain perspective on trends over time
- Becoming involved in projects and task forces within the organization to interact with a wide range of coworkers
- Developing a personal reading list to follow the thinking of experts in the field
- Reading what futurists are saying about how things will change
- Becoming active in AHIMA and other professional associations and groups

- Building a network of professional colleagues
- Making full use of the information resources that AHIMA and other local, state, and national organizations make available
- Contributing to the professional body of knowledge when developing new HIM practice solutions by presenting at seminars or submitting journal articles

The process of assessing the internal and external environment should be done together and summarized with succinct graphs and tables. After reviewing all of the information gathered during this phase, the organization's strengths, weaknesses, opportunities, and threats should be evident. The assumption about the future environment should now be identified. The product of this phase in the process should be a list of critical issues that will need to be addressed and resolved in the next phase of the strategic planning process (Zuckerman 2012, 46–54).

How to Assess and Manage Risk and Uncertainty

Analyzing the changing environment and envisioning the future is an analytic and a highly creative activity. Understanding internal and external trends and forces of risks and uncertainties requires analysis of

- Relationships between trends
- Sequence of events
- Causes and effects
- Priority among items

As a strategic thinker, this ability to consider the internal and external environment is a critical skill that requires an understanding that there is risk and uncertainty as an organization begins to predict possible future trends and design strategies to manage them. It also gives the manager an opportunity to find ways for developing strategies to avoid possible pitfalls or counteract external or internal forces. Examples of key risks and uncertainties to review include:

- Demand structure—market and industry trends that affect the demand for the service or the organization

- Supply structure—access to trained employees, physicians, or supplies needed by the service or organization

- Competitors—information technology (IT), outsourcing, mergers, and acquisitions

- External forces—payers, employers, and customer trends

- Regulation—federal or state government regulatory or legal changes

- Time (immediately, six months, one year, or several years)—when the forces of risk and uncertainty described earlier are predicted to potentially change or not change (Jennings 2000, 7–14).

Another aspect that is helpful in reviewing the key forces that may bring risk and uncertainty is to understand there are three possible levels of uncertainty to consider. A clear trend is one that is known to be happening with certainty. An "unknown that is knowable" is a force or trend where current facts or information may not be known, but can be researched and become known. A residual uncertainty would be defined as a level of uncertainty that will not be able to be determined as the information will not be knowable during the current time frame, thus assumptions about its level of risk must be made. Part of the strategic process must evaluate each of the identified risks

and uncertainties by these three levels (Jennings 2000, 10–13). Examples within HIM of these levels are:

- Clear trends—moving from a paper medical record to the electronic personal health record (PHR)

- Unknowns that are knowable—consumer preferences of the electronic PHR

- Residual uncertainty—fate of information technology (IT) companies that make electronic PHRs

When assessing the levels of risk and uncertainty, it is important to understand that there may be elements the leaders will not be able to understand or they may become clearer over time. Organizations must decide whether it is important to continue tracking each of the risks or uncertainties or if they continue to have a high level of importance. The levels of risk and uncertainty that seem important will be helpful to include in the next phase, which focuses on tools for strategic thinking, especially the scenario-building exercise.

The last step in the environmental assessment process is to determine the strategic critical issues facing the organization. This list should serve as an important step in understanding what operational and strategic matters may need to be addressed by strategy development. The review of critical issues can assist in prioritizing key issues that are truly important to the organization's future, not just current operations.

Check Your Understanding 29.2

Instructions: **Answer the following questions on a separate sheet of paper.**

1. List four key types of information that should be collected during the external environmental assessment phase.

2. True or False: It is important to stay focused on healthcare and ignore trends in other industries when developing the internal and external assessment phase.

3. Identify the three categories that are used to assess the possible levels of sources of uncertainty.

4. The current strategic profile requires description of four key aspects of the organization (or department). List these four key elements.

5. True or False: A SWOT analysis is used to assess only internal strength, weaknesses, opportunities, and threats of the organization.

Phase 2: From Vision to Strategy

As defined earlier, a strategy is an action or the set of actions that moves the organization toward its vision. Strategic management is about pursuing a new set of activities or prioritizing ways of carrying out current activities that move the organization toward its vision. It may take the form of new or redesigned programs or services. It may involve implementing new systems, outsourcing certain operations, or merging functions with another organizational entity. It also may entail phasing out an outdated program or adopting new technologies. Finally, it may be aimed at bringing an organization into compliance with new regulations or finding new ways to reduce operating costs.

It is important to remember that strategic management is not the same as operations management improvement. Operations improvement is ongoing and internally focused and if aligned with the strategic plan, will assist in bringing the organization toward its goals. Strategic management seeks to improve the position of the organization for the future and in the broader marketplace in which it operates. The vision statement may require review and alignment of the organization's mission and values.

Create a Commitment to Change with Vision

The organization's vision sets the broad directional strategy, leaving the details to be worked out. A **vision** is a picture of the desired future state of the organization (Kemp et al. 1993). An effective organizational vision statement has the following characteristics:

- Conveys a picture of what the future will look like
- Appeals to the long-term interests of the stakeholders
- Sets forth realistic and achievable goals
- Is clear enough to provide guidance in decision making
- Is flexible so that alternative strategies are possible as conditions change

- Is easy to describe and communicate (Kotter 2012b, 72)

An organization may never realize a vision in its entirety. Today's technology may not yet support lifetime electronic PHRs or autocoding of 100 percent of cases, but that does not mean these bold visions should be ignored. Digitalizing all health information may be difficult, but that does not mean this vision should be abandoned. Visions must be worth pursuing; otherwise, why would others become engaged?

Visions should evoke a sense of excitement and urgency from those closest to the process. If the designers are not getting excited about the possibilities the vision presents, others are not likely to generate excitement. A sense of urgency is essential to overcome the forces that protect the status quo.

A "vision describes a bold and ideal image of the future" (Kouzes and Posner 1995, 94). It is the catalyst for change. It has been said that "if leaders are going to take us to places we've never been before, constituents of all types demand that they have a sense of direction" (Kouzes and Posner 1995, 95).

As described, a vision states the direction for organizational change and helps motivate people to take action. In 2012 and revised again in 2014, the American Health Information Management Association (AHIMA) convened an interdisciplinary panel of experts to craft a vision and strategy for the HIM profession in regard to electronic health information management (e-HIM):

> AHIMA proactively promotes the technological advancement of health information systems that enhance the delivery of quality healthcare (AHIMA 2015a).

This vision statement describes features of e-HIM that work in real time to support critical decision making across healthcare and reflects a more diverse field with a critical change focused on health and wellness worldwide. It has been used to help catalyze the field to embrace e-HIM as a change strategy. The 2014 AHIMA vision articulates even newer insights about the organization that would secure a strong future for the profession with an even more compelling update.

> AHIMA…leading the advancement and ethical use of quality health information to promote health and wellness worldwide (AHIMA 2015a).

Designing a compelling vision requires a solid understanding of the internal and external environmental assessment. It also requires the ability to break free of the current paradigms and to think creatively about a new reality for the future. Paradigm is broadly defined as a philosophical or theoretical framework within which a discipline formulates its theories and is often used to create shifts or new perspectives in thinking and direction, in this case AHIMA has had a paradigm shift (Merriam-Webster 2015).

The following are examples of effective and ineffective vision statements within HIM organizations. A director of HIM services for a health system envisions services that make the fullest use of staff and technology to provide high-quality, cost-effective information to authorized users. He expresses this idealized vision as follows:

> Utilizing state-of-the-art information technology and evidence-based practices, we will deliver accurate electronic information to support patient care and healthcare operations.

This is an example of an effective vision that lays out a substantial challenge, yet it provides focus. First, the overarching vision is to be able to deliver all information electronically to all users of HIM services. It acknowledges that technology is only as effective as the enabling processes; therefore, it promises use of evidence-based or research-proven practices, which are practices substantiated by applied research that demonstrate their validity. The vision statement acknowledges that achieving this vision will require new ways of working. First, success will require gaining a deeper understanding of the needs of those in patient care and healthcare operations, who rely on the information and whose collaboration is needed to achieve the vision. Second, it will require effective teamwork among HIM staff, who must become more comfortable with both change and risk taking.

In another example, an HIM consultant for a long-term care system was having difficulty gaining support for her vision of what an electronic health record (EHR) could contribute to the residents,

staff, and overall organization. She developed the following description of her vision:

> All members of the care team have immediate access to complete and accurate information for each resident. This information recaps care delivered and presents the status of all health, social, activity of daily living (ADL) and other resident-specific issues being managed. Information needs to be entered just once and is available for a variety of patient care, quality improvement, and administrative uses. Summary reports are used as the basis for shift change briefings and for periodic care conferences. The information system prompts caregivers to actions that need to be taken and alerts them to changes in status that require special vigilance. Data entered into the system summarizing observations, care given, orders, and activities produce a record of care that meets licensing and other external requirements. The system also automatically accumulates the information needed for care and operations management and for external reporting.

This vision is ineffective because it highlights the difficulty many have in creating a brief, compelling vision that does not include specific objectives. The vision could be simplified and revised as follows: *All members of the care team will have immediate access to complete and accurate information for each resident to improve patient care, quality, and timeliness.* The vision statement serves as a starting point for creating a more detailed set of specifications and evaluating potential system vendors.

Visions also can be created to more narrowly focus on a particular project. For example, a data quality manager for a multispecialty group practice clinic prepared the following vision statement to help the physicians and coding staff rally around a proposed project to improve the timeliness and accuracy of billing processes through the use of computer-assisted coding tools:

> During each patient visit, the physician will document using a handheld personal digital assistant (PDA). This will assist the practice in achieving 90 percent of visits billed within one business day, 95 percent within three business days, and the balance within five business days.

This vision statement has three major elements. It sets an aggressive goal of billing 90 percent of visits on the day of service, 95 percent within three business days, and the balance within five business days. To do so, physicians must initiate the process using electronic tools (PDA) to eliminate time-consuming handling of handwritten information. It also requires physician coding specialists with advanced data quality and compliance management skills to do concurrent coding.

These vision statements relate to HIM challenges. However, it is important that the HIM vision complements the organization's overall vision and mission. For example, the organization's vision is to be known for its advanced clinical services in cardiac and oncology care. To achieve this vision, the organization is pursuing a strategy of attracting clinical talent with national reputations and expanding clinical research programs. This overall vision and these strategies should be accounted for when crafting the HIM vision and strategies.

Strategic managers must understand the overall organizational goals and take them into account when crafting their own plans. First, they seek ways to support and further the overall goals of the organization through the priorities they set for their areas of responsibility. For example, will the cancer registry program need to be upgraded to support the more sophisticated information needs of a world-class oncology service? As a practical matter, it is hard to sell a plan that is out of step with priorities. Advancing the organization's goals through synergistic efforts is the mark of a successful strategic manager.

Understanding the Driving Force

The most important strategic thinking skill to understand prior to determining strategy is to understand the driving force of the department or organization. Driving force is the concept of what a department or an organization uses to determine which products or services to offer, which markets to seek, and which customers to attract (Robert 2006, 56–57). With intentional analysis, it is critical to understand the driving force or strategic drive that propels a department or an organization forward toward its vision.

When using the driving force model, every organization is assessed using 10 important strategic areas, or driving forces that exist within all business. The 10 basic components of a business are as follows.

1. Every company offers product(s) or service(s) for sale.
2. Every company sells its product(s) or service(s) to a certain class of customer or end user.
3. These customers or end users always reside in certain categories of markets.
4. Every company employs technology in its product or service.
5. Every company has a production facility located somewhere that has a certain amount of capacity or certain in-built capabilities in the making of a product or service.
6. Every company uses certain sales or marketing methods to acquire customers for its product or service.
7. Every company employs certain distribution methods to get a product or service from its location to a customer's location.
8. Every company makes use of natural resources to one degree or another.
9. Every company monitors its size and growth performance.
10. Every company monitors its return or profit performance (Robert 2006, 56–57).

Only one of the above 10 forces is strategically most important to the company and is the engine that propels or drives the company forward to success (Robert 2006, 56–57). While all forces are part of a company, there is only one key driving strategy. After the internal and external assessments, it is important to decide if the current driving force identified within the organization should continue or if there is a strategic need to change to a different future driving force to achieve the organization's vision.

For example, AHIMA's driving force is defined as a user or customer class organization that is strategically focusing its business around a describable and specific category of customers—HIM professionals. AHIMA responds by providing a wide variety of services and products that are aimed at this user class. Therefore, it is helpful to keep the key driving force in mind when it determines its future strategies. It becomes the major filter of determining what new strategies or initiatives will continue moving the organization toward its vision.

Defining Areas of Excellence

Once an organization identifies its driving force, understanding and developing clear areas of excellence is another key concept of strategic thinking. This concept refers to a describable skill, competence, or capability that a department or company cultivates to a level of proficiency greater than anything else it does (Robert 2006, 62–63). To determine a strategic direction, the leader must develop a clear understanding of current key areas of excellence in the organization and what areas of excellence will be needed to achieve the new vision. Over time, the strategy of an organization, like a person, can become stronger and healthier or it can get weaker and sicker. What determines the future success of the strategy are the areas of excellence that a department or an organization deliberately cultivates to keep the strategy strong and healthy (Robert 2006, 62). For an HIM director, understanding special capabilities—such as managing the collection of patient and clinical quality data to improve quality of patient care—can be an important area of excellence. It becomes much easier to make difficult choices involving resources and time allocation if it is clear which strategies and areas of excellence are being pursued.

Defining Key Strategies

The next step in strategic planning is to develop and refine key strategies that are aligned with the driving force and areas of excellence needed to achieve the identified vision. The strategies need to address the critical issues identified earlier. For example, implementing the strategy "Acquire and implement electronic signature software" requires research about areas of excellence within technology vendors that offer software compatible with the clinical data repository.

Building a strategy grounded in a vision provides a context in which one can continually assess whether the organization is on track and if it is making progress. The AHIMA Board of Directors identified five key strategies in its future visioning sessions that were supported by the e-HIM vision and a deep understanding of the external environment. They were cast as transformative "from-to" statements, reflecting the key changes that AHIMA must lead over the next decade:

- Informatics: Transform data into health intelligence
- Leadership: Develop HIM leaders across all healthcare sectors
- Information governance: Be recognized as the healthcare industry experts in information governance
- Innovation: Increase thought leadership and evidence-based HIM research
- Public good: Empower consumers to optimize their health through management of their personal health information (AHIMA 2015a)

It is important to look at the range of strategies being pursued to be clear about priorities, recognize opportunities for synergy and integration, and identify strategies to delete that no longer add value. When formulating strategies, question whether the leaders are getting too deeply into how something will be done. Remember that strategy is *what* direction in which the organization is going; goals and objectives are *how* the organization plans to do it.

 ## Check Your Understanding 29.3

Instructions: **Answer the following questions on a separate piece of paper.**

1. List three characteristics of an effective vision statement.

2. True or False: A vision statement for a department does not need to be aligned with the organization's vision.

3. True or False: An organization's driving force can be more than one of the 10 important strategic areas.

4. A(n) _____ refers to a describable skill, competence and capabilities to which an organization cultivates to be excellent.

5. True or False: AHIMA has built a strategy that is grounded in its vision.

Phase 3: Creating Innovative Strategy and a Future Strategic Profile

The third phase in the strategic planning process requires using the information and strategy development from phases 1 and 2 to build the future strategic profile, innovate, and assess the competition. If all these aspects are done correctly, strategic thinking will be ensured. The final strategies and strategic profile can then be confirmed before moving into the implementation phase (phase 4).

Identifying a Future Strategic Profile

Based on the findings and conclusions from the internal and external assessment, a new or updated vision statement and strategies are identified. It is important to review the current strategic profile to determine if a new or updated future strategic profile of the organization needs to be developed. The future strategic profile serves as a filter to determine what products or services the organization will offer in the future, what markets it should geographically be located in, what customers and users will be served, and the industry market segments that will be more emphasized and less emphasized in the future (Robert 2006, 54). This is the time for the organization to re-evaluate what it is focused on and where it will be located. This future strategic profile serves as a way to better allocate resources of staff, time, and money. For example, an updated vision for a managed care health plan might be to fully engage members with chronic diseases who are focused on maintaining their health as partners with the health plan. The health plan's new future strategic profile may now emphasize electronic PHR and chronic

disease managers as its key products, rather than traditional types of insurance plans. It may choose to partner with specific market segments within healthcare that provide better outcomes for patients with chronic diseases (a change in its future customers and market segments). This new future strategic profile will be helpful in allocation of resources, determining if new market opportunities should be pursued, and ensuring that strategic thinking is included in the plan.

Tools for Strategic Thinking—Scenario Building

To bring out the best strategic thinking of a team or workgroup, it is often helpful to use techniques that help participants consider factors from different perspectives. A number of group process techniques such as brainstorming, storytelling, scenario building, nominal group technique, and other techniques help unleash each individual's strategic thinking.

Storytelling is a powerful group process technique. Stories are defined as one way to transmit an organization's truths, insights, and commitments. Using compelling stories is a powerful way to persuade people by uniting an idea with an emotion. Essentially, a story expresses how and why life changes (McKee 2003). Telling stories about possible futures suggested by the external and internal assessment of trends has a number of advantages including findings that can be presented in an understandable and real-world context. Stories are memorable and easier to remember essential points, and generate excitement.

One storytelling technique that is used in more sophisticated strategic planning is that of scenario planning. The word *scenario* means a script of a play or story, or a projected sequence of events. **Scenarios** are "focused descriptions of fundamentally different futures presented in a coherent script-like or narrative fashion" (Schoemaker 1995, 25–41). They are plausible stories about how the future might unfold. They are not meant to predict but, rather, simply to interpret and clarify how internal and external environmental trends may influence the organization's strategy and how it might play out.

Scenario planning is based on analysis and interaction of environmental variables. Environmental assessment, along with assessing risks and uncertainties, are important preparatory steps in scenario development. Based on the study of the environment, two to four scenario themes are developed, reflecting alternate possible futures using differing potentials around the key forces or risks and uncertainties described earlier. Scenarios are constructed that describe possible ways in which each of these themes might be played out. These scenarios or stories are refined through input and further study until they reflect the decision maker's best thinking about what futures might be in store for the organization under various circumstances. Productive scenarios meet four tests: they are relevant, are internally consistent, describe clearly different futures, and are long term in perspective (Shoemaker 1995, 25–41). Other approaches that promote strategic thinking include contingency planning, sensitivity analysis, simulation, decision analysis and game theory, and blue ocean strategy (Zuckerman 2012, 212).

To understand how the role of HIM professionals needs to change in the future, an AHIMA strategic planning task force studied environmental trends and developed scenarios, each highlighting a slightly different, but plausible, future. Strategic managers can then develop plans focused on the key strategic variables that may shape the future vision. Using multiple possible scenarios, an AHIMA strategic plan was developed and continues to be updated (AHIMA 2015a).

The HIM professional should build a portfolio of techniques that a leader can use to bring out the best strategic thinking of others; peruse the business shelves of major bookstores for guidebooks containing exercises and techniques to improve group process; observe techniques used by facilitators to improve how groups work and think together; and keep a notebook or computer file of such techniques and practice them whenever the opportunity arises. Effective strategic managers know how to facilitate groups to help them think and work well together.

Determine Impact of Competition

Developing ways to understand the department's and organization's competitors is also valuable during the strategic planning process. Innovations or changes are also being planned by the competition. During the strategic planning process, it is important to take time to understand the current and potential strengths and weaknesses of the organization's key competitors. The organization's strategies should be developed in order to have the most influence on increasing its market share. Once the organization has selected a strategic direction, it should take time to evaluate and anticipate any impact that competitors, current or future, might have on the strategy. As the industry has matured, more and more secondary industry providers such as biomedical, pharmaceutical, and retail organizations are revising their strategies for healthcare. This is an example of how stealthy competitors need to be considered and may have a significant impact on an organization's plan.

Create a Platform for Strategic Innovation

Techniques such as scenario development and environmental assessment are useful in formulating strategy because they include a focus on both the internal and external environments. However, one should not expect to identify exciting new strategies by only looking at the past, looking inward, or looking within the healthcare industry. As a critical part of this process, time should be taken to seek information by looking outside the organization and outside the healthcare industry; as well as looking to the future in formulating innovative strategy. New or innovative services or products come from identifying potential new needs based on determining the possible future scenarios that might occur.

Organizations should seek to find or develop innovations that will actually differentiate its services or products from competitors. Strategic product or service innovations are often overlooked when finalizing key organizational strategies.

> Product or **service innovations** create new market opportunities, and in many industries are the driving force behind growth and profitability. **Process innovations** enable firms to produce existing products or services more efficiently. As such, process and service innovations are one of the main determinants of productivity growth. (Robert 2006, 118–119)

It takes understanding the department's and organization's strategic capabilities and anticipating what future needs will come from reviewing and predicting future trends. It takes a willingness to be able to take risks and think strategically. For example, having access to personal health information on the Internet 24 hours a day is an innovation in healthcare. Many of the innovations in healthcare have come from unexpected industry stress, research and development, and a willingness to test new services or products with the ultimate goal of improving the health of a population. The strategic plan needs to include time for thoughtful development of product, service, and process innovations.

An important part of strategic planning that is often overlooked, yet vital to developing effective strategy, is the role of the customer. Traditional ways of collecting customer information include consumer focus groups, patient advisory boards, and patient surveys. If designed correctly, these tools can be effective in gathering information within the proper context of strategic planning. Unfortunately, the strategic planning process often ignores customers, users, and suppliers or involves them too late to provide effective feedback. In the case of the PHR, it would mean involving patients and their families in the design of the strategies, strategic goals and objectives, and implementation plan for the PHR. During this process, the organization would begin to understand needs and expectations from the customers' perspective. It becomes easier to develop ways to provide a truly innovative product and service. These customers are often readily available, whether it involves using volunteers, staff members, or their family members who are customers of the PHR. Also, physicians and office staff who get calls from patients on a regular basis are well versed in understanding what their customers want and need.

Develop Final Strategic Profile Findings and Conclusions

After reviewing all the information from both internal and external assessments, a shared list of findings is developed with the strategic planning team. Based on these findings, the leader should determine if there are further informational needs or data points that will be important for developing a set of strategic findings and conclusions. Strategic findings and conclusions help solidify the new vision, driving force, and areas of excellence and lead to identifying key strategies for achieving the vision. After completing all aspects of strategic planning, the leaders will now need to put a strategic "stake in the ground" to move forward.

Check Your Understanding 29.4

Instructions: Answer the following questions on a separate piece of paper.

1. Name two important tools often used for strategic thinking.

2. True or False: Strategies and vision describe where an organization wants to go in the future.

3. True or False: A future strategic profile, when developed, is always identical to the current strategic profile.

4. List the four tests that scenarios need to meet.

5. True or False: The future strategic profile includes identifying the key products or services, customers and users, industry and market segments, and geographic markets that the organization wants to emphasize to achieve its future vision.

Phase 4: Strategic Management and Implementation

The essence of strategy is deciding what not to do. Managers are urged to view strategy as a series of trade-offs (Porter 1996, 61–78). Major strategic change will impact current activities and may well require their modification or even elimination. No organization has the resources to take on major new programs without considering their impact on current programs. Making trade-offs is difficult for most managers. Letting go of even a marginal program may produce a backlash. Determining implementation plans is the final critical phase in effective strategic plan. Unless strategy is implemented, it is of no value. In addition, resources must be reallocated to those programs that will enable the organization to operate at a new level of strategy. The final phase in strategic planning will outline the strategic goals and objectives in accomplishing strategy.

Defining Strategic Goals and Strategic Objectives

The next step in iterative strategic planning is to develop strategic goals and objectives to carry out each identified key strategy. A few key strategies, based on resolving the critical issues, are needed for this vision to be realized, and these must be identified and understood. Strategies are the most important high-level, directional goals to pursue to achieve the vision. Once the core strategies are identified, a set of strategic goals for each strategy needs to be developed that define a series of longer-term action steps of how to achieve each strategy. For example, a strategy for the health plan may be to develop a marketing campaign to promote the use of the PHR to focus on members who are needing increased self-management, especially those with chronic diseases. Some of the strategic goals might involve a way to develop incentives for patients to engage in wellness activities and use their PHRs and to provide easy access to computer and health literacy education. The next step would be to take each strategic goal and identify the strategic objectives or short-term action plans that are needed to accomplish each strategic goal. Major strategic goals and objectives that are needed to move toward the vision need to be described. These become more precise than the overall vision and strategy. Providing all citizens with access to lifetime electronic PHRs might be a strategy to achieve the vision of empowered and self-managing consumers. The vision describes where the organization wants to go and the strategies are how the organization intends to pursue its vision. The strategic goals and objectives describe specific action plans to be implemented and how to get there. For instance, implementing the strategy "acquire and implement electronic signature software" requires research about technology vendors that offer software compatible with the clinical data repository. It requires budgeting for this technology, securing support for the action plan, issuing a request for proposal (RFP), checking references, connectivity, and so on.

The Role of Strategic Goals

Strategic goals and objectives should not be confused with operational tactics or annual tactical planning. Often strategic plans are written as operational goals or objectives rather than at a strategic level. Strategic goals are needed to describe how to carry out each of the selected key strategies. A **strategic goal** is defined as a long-term, continuous strategic area that identifies strategic objectives (key activities) needing to be performed to achieve the new organizational vision (Olsen 2006, 37). For example, if the strategy is to have 95 percentile performance on timely billing to payers, the strategic goal might be to reduce the accounts receivable days attributable to coding backlogs, and strategic objectives may include authorizing overtime, hiring contract coders, and redesigning the record completion processes.

The Role of Strategic Objectives

Strategic objectives are more detailed ways to meet a strategic goal and include timelines, resource allocation needs, and assignment of responsibility to the person(s) accountable for implementation. From the timely billing example, the strategic objectives would state (in more detail) the person responsible and the action steps of how to authorize more overtime, who and how to hire the contract coders, and who and how the record completion process will be redesigned. For example, for the strategic objective of hiring contract coders, the objective would state with whom the organization will be contracting, how many contract coders are needed, the timelines for implementation, and who is responsible for making it happen.

Importance of Implementation and Action Plans

In order for any strategic plan to become effective and to ensure a successful implementation plan, detailed strategic goals and objectives must be written and supported by those responsible for the implementation. This requires having involvement in the design and an understanding of the rationale for and the outline of detailed responsibilities and expectations required of all leaders and staff in the department or organization. The strategic goals and objectives need to be clearly outlined, with assignments for who will be accountable, timelines, allocation of resources, and measurements that will be used to ensure success of implementation. When a detailed implementation includes the elements laid out clearly—with time frames and regular updates provided within the organization—the likelihood of strategic success increases significantly (see table 29.1). The measurement of these detailed implementation plans must be done on a regular basis, more often than annually or periodically, because what is measured becomes a priority of employees and leaders in the organization.

Check Your Understanding 29.5

Instructions: **Answer the following questions on a separate piece of paper.**

1. True or False: Implementation of strategic plans is well done in most healthcare organizations.

2. Identify two differences between a strategic goal and a strategic objective.

3. True or False: Measurement is required only once annually to determine progress on the implementation plan.

4. True or False: Vision and strategy are the drivers to moving an organization forward strategically, but implementation is critical to realizing that vision.

5. One of the most common issues that healthcare organizations fail to do well in the strategic process is:
    A. Develop a vision
    B. Develop strategies
    C. Execute the implementation plan
    D. Communicate the plan

Support for the Change Program

Sound change strategies and tactics alone do not ensure success. Success depends on great execution, including securing support for the needed organizational change efforts. Healthcare organizations are highly complex with many competing priorities. Gaining approval, even for the best-designed efforts, may be difficult. Refer to chapter 22 for more detail on change management theories.

Table 29.1.   Detailed implementation plan

Strategy #1: Transcribed reports will be dictated using voice recognition software and become part of the EHR in digital form.			
Strategic goal	**Strategic objectives**	**Implementation plan**	**Measurements**
A. Physicians are able to review and modify dictated reports online in a digital form by the third quarter of the fiscal year.	1. Implement electronic signature software 2. Design and pilot test a process where physicians can authenticate, edit, and reassign a transcribed report online 3. Design a phased plan for implementation of online physician review that is coordinated with the availability of online access to electronic reports	Timeline: RFP—First quarter Purchased by second quarter Installed by third quarter Who's Responsible: HIM supervisor and IT supervisor Resource needs: Capital and operating budget support $210,000 0.5 FTE medical staff HIM committee	Physicians' digital dictation achieved: By Q3 = 100% By Q4 = 75% Physician quality survey of dictation system: Score 4.0–5 = 100% Score 3.5–3.99 = 80% Score 3.0–3.49 = 60%
B. Voice recognition converts dictated reports to digital information for storage in the EHR	1. Implement voice recognition in the emergency, cardiac cath, and imaging departments 2. Upgrade the EHR to accept input from voice recognition in structured reports 3. Design and pilot test a plan for storing output in the EHR	Timeline: First quarter Who's responsible: HIM transcription manager; departmental reps from ER, CC, and imaging Resource needs: Capital ($35,000) and operating budget	Voice recognition conversion in place: Q1 = 100% Q2 = 75%

Source: Kloss 2006.

For example, an experienced HIM director, with support from the IT director, tried for three consecutive budget cycles to get funding for a document imaging program. The request was accompanied by a solid return on investment (ROI) picture in terms of reductions in full-time equivalents, cost of storage, and increased productivity. In year four, the director tied the request not merely to how change would affect the HIM service but also to how it would support improved access to health information, reduce errors caused by illegibility, and improve communication among caregivers. In light of the Joint Commission's patient safety goals, the HIM director enlisted the help of nursing leadership to make the budget case. Nursing spoke to how this solution would improve access to information at the patient care bedside and would help link various electronic documentation systems already in place. The caregivers stressed the need to link the systems to help them do their jobs better. By taking this approach, the document imaging system was presented to the board of directors by the organization's Patient Safety Council chairperson and was approved by the board without hesitation.

Take a Systems Approach

According to change management theory, there are five effective activities including: motivating change, creating a vision, developing political support, managing the transition, and sustaining momentum (Cummings and Worley 2015). As a part of creating a vision and strategic plans, it is important to include those in the organization by asking them to be involved in the visioning process. This assists in motivating change within the organization, as people tend to support what they help create. Understanding the influence political systems have on the distribution of power and influence within the organization may give insight during the process (for example, the authority of the medical staff, the approval and decision-making processes of the board of directors within an organization).

Major change may throw the organization into chaos as existing systems are deliberately unglued. This is a time of great vulnerability, leaders must be vigilant—watching for and thoughtfully managing the transition and attending to unintended effects that could make it difficult to achieve realignment. Leaders must be sensitive to the emotional relationships among individuals in a group and how change will affect relationships between individuals and between the manager and others. Times of change are times of high stress and anxiety. This may play out in a number of ways. For example, in times of great change, employees may be more inclined to look for other employment opportunities as it is threatening and unsettling to go through change. Some turnover in staff may be an acceptable and unavoidable result, but the leader should be attentive and sensitive so that turnover does not derail the ability to carry out the project.

The organization's systems are highly interdependent, and any change will have intended and unintended impact on all three systems. For example, when implementing new technology such as EHRs or other major systems, the focus is often on features and functions of the system. Securing the right champions for the system and understanding how it affects the workflow, procedures, and formal and informal interactions of staff are more challenging and important to successful implementation than the features and functions. The successful strategic manager leading wide-scale technology change will be the one who excels at helping people get behind and involved in the change. The manager who focuses only or primarily on installing the hardware and software will not succeed. Managers should not let these challenges keep them from pursuing the strategies their organization needs. However, success will depend on how well change is managed from a systems perspective. The manager must attend to all three identified system aspects throughout the implementation process. He or she also should be aware that implementation is not complete until all three systems are back in a new alignment after the changes are in place.

Create the Structure for Change

Organizational structure is an important element to ensure success of the change process. Once a new vision and strategies are determined, the current structure should be reviewed and focus placed on how to best restructure (if needed) to achieve the new vision. Structure is an organizational function often overlooked and yet important to successful implementation. As strategic goals and objectives are identified, the goals and objectives are assigned to a leader. Another important aspect of consideration regarding structure is where the department is positioned within the structure of the organization. This placement in the structure and strategy is important to understanding how allocation of resources and capital will be made. The importance of structure for accomplishing an organization's strategic goals and objectives should not be underestimated.

Manage the Politics of Change

Organizational change can be a political process. Change leadership requires the courage to persevere even in the face of criticism; however, plowing ahead without considering the political implications may be folly. While strategic planning has traditionally been a top-down process, many organizations are realizing the power of senior leaders creating a framework and having strategic planning from the bottom up. This change in focusing the planning process within the business units allows strategic planning to be with the "real" action and to be closer to the customer (Zuckerman 2012, 229). Political savvy entails skill in mediating and shaping conflicts that are inevitable when people are being offered multiple choices with significant consequences. Deliberately enlist the support of thought and opinion leaders. Reach out to those who may be most threatened by the proposed change; do not wait for them to come to you. Early engagement may turn potential resisters into supporters. At the very least, it will help change leaders build their arguments and communication plan to address the concerns of those who oppose the change.

Collaboration is one technique for managing the political dimensions of change. Change may threaten to shift the balance of power, and employees or coworkers who feel threatened may react by joining together to increase their own power so as to influence the course of events. AHIMA's strategic plan states "it is only through collaboration that the goals in this plan can be achieved" (AHIMA 2015a). The use of collaborations can be a force for positive change and leaders can use collaboration as a way to build support for change. The example of the HIM manager who gained the support of nursing to move ahead on the document management system project illustrates the power of collaboration and multidisciplinary team efforts in healthcare.

The first step in building a collaboration is to honestly assess subgroups in terms of how they will view the proposed change. Before embarking on a major change, the following questions should be considered carefully:

- Who will be most affected by the change?

- What benefits (for example, power) might these individuals perceive they will lose?

- Are their fears real? If so, what options are available to help overcome their fears?

- Does the change have the potential to create new benefits for these individuals?

- Can a negative reaction be avoided by engaging individuals or groups in the process?

- If the leader is not successful in getting them on board, is their influence likely to be strong enough to derail the change plan?

Even when a leader is not successful in getting resisters on board, he or she will have better information about the strength of their feelings and their resolve to oppose change. At the same time, leaders are always working to diffuse potential resistance and to focus on building support for the change.

Create a Sense of Urgency

When trying to change organizations and move forward strategically in tumultuous times, developing a sense of urgency to change is important (Kotter 2012a, 37). Leaders may overestimate the extent to which they can force or drive change in the organization. To increase the sense of urgency, leaders must remove or minimize the sources of complacency. With this rapid change in the healthcare industry, dynamic strategic planning has replaced static planning. Some examples of how this might be done include the following:

- Engage employees, customers, and coworkers in a dialogue about change through a series of input meetings (namely, having them participate in the SWOT analysis)

- Convene a guiding coalition (GC) committee with opinion leaders and representatives from major stakeholder groups

- Develop inspiring and stretching vision statements and strategies

- Present believable stories and scenarios that illustrate the potential futures using both head and heart that may occur if action is not taken

- Identify revolutionary goals, encourage strategic thinking, and drive decision making down to all levels

- Create new effective vehicles for communication, such as a project website or newsletter

The need for strategic planning has changed with the fast-paced environment. After the initial longer-term strategies are developed, strategic planning must be a continuous process. Strategic planning is everyone's daily job, not just an annual or periodic task for executive leaders (Zuckerman 2012, 230). "Sufficient urgency around a strategically rational and emotionally exciting opportunity is the bedrock upon which all else is built" (Kotter 2012a, 54). The need to build a sense of urgency among the employees in the organization is required for successful implementation. Creating a culture that emotionally engages employees and leaders will ensure strategic change is a priority.

Engaging with Communication

Communication is key to engaging others in the vision and change process. It has been said that "if you're a leader and you are not sick and tired of communicating you probably aren't doing a good enough job" (DePree 1992, 100). A benchmarking study of how companies have successfully communicated change showed that communication is critical at three stages of the change process: as it is being planned, throughout implementation, and after it is complete. Effective communication was shown to be critical at each stage, even to the point of releasing partial information when details are incomplete (Powers 1997, 30–33).

At the planning stage, leaders should communicate the need for change and the vision. Remember, if followers do not accept the vision, the rest of the change process is likely to be very rocky. Communicating results, even when they are incomplete, is an important reinforcement. It makes the change real and maintains the necessary momentum.

Communication is most effective if the message is tailored to the recipient. The leader identifies needs and opportunities to customize the organization's message to subgroups that have a particular set of issues. For example, the message to the medical staff will be different from the message to staff in health information services. Before implementing the use of report templates to expedite dictation, the manager may design a tactical plan that details all the elements of the communication plan for each of the constituent groups affected by, or with an interest in, the project.

The communication plan must offer groups the opportunity to talk back to leadership and share their opinions. This may mean that feedback could indicate that the proposed vision and new course is not moving the organization in the right direction. However, it is worth reconsidering and reworking the vision and strategic plans to ensure that they are moving the organization in a direction that the employees believe in and will follow (Kotter 2012b, 128). The importance of open communication and developing a culture of transparency within an organization cannot be underestimated.

Communication comes in two forms—words and actions—and the most effective communication is characterized by deeds. Behavior from important people that is inconsistent with the vision overwhelms other forms of communication (Kotter 2012a, 90). Leaders become the symbols for the change. Their motivations may be questioned and their actions scrutinized. Others will watch the leaders' actions for signals of commitment to the course of action and rightly insist on their integrity.

Ethics and integrity must be front and center all the time, but particularly during times of important change. At these times, the political, cultural, and technical systems are out of alignment. There is opportunity for events to take unexpected turns. Leaders' actions are closely scrutinized and their motives may be suspect.

Implementing Strategic Change

Once a vision and strategies are designed, the change management team is in place, and the guiding coalitions are organized, the hard work of implementation begins. Implementation requires all the managerial skills including planning, budgeting, monitoring, and producing results as described in chapter 22.

Create and Communicate Short-Term Wins

Major change takes time. The organization's vision may be compelling and its strategies right on target, but if short-term results cannot be demonstrated, the leaders may lose support and the momentum for change may begin to erode. The best way to sustain change efforts is to sequence the implementation plan through strategic objectives and goals in such a way that short-term successes are clearly demonstrated and celebrated. For example, in implementing a new compliance plan, the data quality manager for a group practice reported statistics to the chiefs of service showing the monthly claims rejection rate. As this rate began to decline, the manager organized special events such as a recognition event for office managers and staff at each improvement milestone. These touches garnered attention and maintained momentum for the project.

The implementation plan can be deliberately seeded with a number of short-term objectives and goals that have a high likelihood of success. This tactic enables the implementation team to work together to assess how much effort and how many resources will be required for later phases. It demonstrates that the program of planned change is real and not just talk. Moreover, it strengthens the courage and commitment of the leaders and the guiding coalitions.

New programs can be launched quickly by using techniques such as rapid prototyping, demonstration projects, or pilot tests. The details do not always need to be fully worked out to create visible demonstrations. The leader may not need to secure approval for full implementation, as testing an approach to see its value is often accepted as a pilot. In test mode, all operational details do not need to be worked out before go-live. The leader need not anticipate all the intricacies up front but should just begin the journey and adjust as he or she is implementing the pilot stage. Prototyping and pilot tests also offer a way to show others how redesigned processes or new technology might work when fully implemented.

Pace and Refine Change Plans

Implementation requires managing interdependent projects at various stages of design, development, and deployment. A difficult implementation challenge is deciding what phases should be advanced first and how fast or slow to move through them. Sequencing and pacing change requires thorough knowledge of the organization and its capacity for change, again considering all organizational components—cultural, political, and technical—and the available financial and managerial resources.

The higher the stakes, the more likely it is that a proposed change will be controversial. If the only viable approach is likely to meet with resistance, more time and effort are needed up front to gain acceptance before the approach is implemented. The importance of two-way communication throughout the process cannot be overemphasized.

The timing of change is critical. Change leaders can cite examples of projects that moved too quickly and projects that moved too slowly. With rapid changing environments, there is a need

for increasing the speed of business cycles and bringing innovation to market in order to respond quickly to unanticipated changes in the market.

Implementation is critical to the success of the plan actually being realized. If the strategic plan is not implemented, all may be lost in moving an organization toward its best future. Implementation, as a process, will guide, show when adjustments are necessary, and find ways to improve as the plan moves forward. Implementing change is a highly iterative process. Leaders should expect that their plans and tactics will need to be modified as they gain experience. They should create strategies, strategic goals and objectives, budgets, and timetables that permit frequent course corrections. The organizations that are able to act quickly will see immediate and long-term success; those who lag will suffer, if they survive at all (Kotter 2012a, 58).

Maintain Momentum and Stay the Course

Because leading change is a process of learning and adjusting, change leaders must learn to tolerate—and even enjoy—uncertainty. Change sponsors are eager to see their well-crafted strategies take hold and inevitably feel discouraged by a lengthy process. In addition to celebrating short-term wins, other ways to maintain momentum and keep moving include the following:

- Work quickly to resolve the difficult issues.
- Reiterate what will happen if change either does not occur or is watered down by compromise. If possible, focus on the consequences due to external trends.
- Stay focused on the prize. Put every action in context. Regularly revisit the vision, strategies, goals, and objectives to regenerate a sense of purpose. Help others by making the goals as tangible as possible.
- Remember that resistance to change is natural. Do not take it personally.

- Rethink the tactics, sequence, and pace regularly to keep from getting bogged down. If momentum slows, institute actions that will produce short-term gains. Keep moving forward.
- Maintain the sense of urgency. Although it is important to celebrate short-term wins, do not let these celebrations mitigate the sense of urgency the organization has created. Also, do not let intermediate gains be mistaken for the bigger goals.

For maximum and sustained impact, the change being introduced must become part of the fabric of the organization. It must become the way the organization operates, thinks, and behaves. At some point, it must become part of the culture. Even after change is implemented, there often continues to be a tug backward toward the old reality. So strong is the effect of culture, leaders should be on the lookout for signs of slippage and for opportunities to reinforce the value of the new reality. To ensure that change is lasting and to prepare the organization for more change, leaders should quantify the impact, benefits, and value of the changes and use data to identify the direction for future change. As noted previously, continue intensive communication on issues facing HIM and the organization. The leaders will need to integrate change competencies and behaviors into performance appraisal and management development programs. Finally, due to the rapid changing times, approach strategy, change, and organizational development as an ongoing process.

Measure Your Results

Environmental assessment was shown to be an important prerequisite to launching major change. It is also the way to measure the impact of change and to determine what further change is needed. Any time strategic change is undertaken, the measures by which its success will be judged should be made part of the performance measures data set. Environmental assessment, both internal

and external, must become a core competency of the organization and part of its routine work. It need not be an elaborate system, but it should be systematic and ongoing, and it must include information on performance, trends, attitudes, and satisfaction.

Once the key strategies are identified, a strategy map is designed that begins with a brief description of the current state and the desired future state. A **strategy map** is a tool that provides a visual representation of an organization's critical strategies and the relationships among them that drive organizational performance toward its vision (Norton et al. 2000, 2, 55). Depicting strategies as a road map is a useful way to help others understand the next steps of implementation, which focuses on developing strategic goals and objectives to lead to the needed strategy change.

The **balanced scorecard methodology** is a technique for measuring organizational performance across the following four perspectives (Kaplan and Norton 2004, 31):

- *Customer perspective:* To achieve the vision, how should the organization appear to internal and external customers?
- *Financial perspective:* How must the organization be held financially accountable?
- *Internal process perspective:* To satisfy customers, in which operational processes must the organization excel?
- *Learning and growth perspective:* How will the organization enhance its ability to change and improve?

A strategy map enables examination of the cause-and-effect relationships among the preceding perspectives. Figure 29.2 shows a sample balanced scorecard using these four perspectives which becomes the basis of a strategy map for improving the real and perceived value of HIM services. The purpose of using the balanced scorecard methodology is to demonstrate how a strategy is more clearly defined using a strategic goal, strategic objectives, detailed implementation plans, and measurements.

Figure 29.2.   Balanced scorecard with strategy map

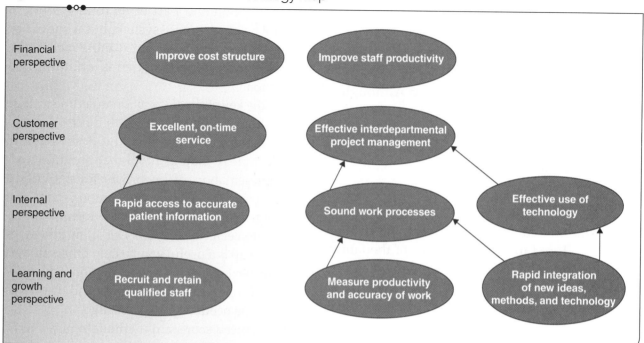

 ## Check Your Understanding 29.6

Instructions: **Answer the following questions on a separate piece of paper.**

1. True or False: Change management and collaboration can improve strategic planning outcomes because they engage other important stakeholders in the process.

2. What is one of the most important skills required of a leader that is engaging the other employees and key stakeholders in conducting strategic planning?

3. True or False: Implementation planning is not a major tactic needed to execute the business plan.

4. What is the tool that enables examination of the cause-and-effect relationships among the balanced scorecard perspectives?

5. True or False: Strategic planning becomes solely the responsibility of an organization's leaders on an annual or periodic basis.

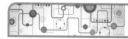 # References

Abrahams, J. 1999. *The Mission Statement Book.* Berkeley, CA: Ten Speed Press.

American Health Information Management Association. 2015a. *AHIMA Strategic Plan 2014–2017.* Chicago: AHIMA. http://bok.ahima.org/PdfView?oid=107449

American Health Information Management Association. 2015b. AHIMA Mission Vision and Values. http://www.ahima.org/about/aboutahima

Beckham, J.D. 2000. Strategy: What it is, how it works, why it fails. *Health Forum Journal* 43(6):55–59.

Cummings, T. and C. Worley. 2015. *Organization Development and Change,* 10th ed. Connecticut: Cengage Learning.

Dunn, R.T. 2010. *Haimann's Healthcare Management,* 9th ed. Chicago: Health Administration Press.

Gavetti, G. and J.W. Rivkin. 2005. How strategists really think: Tapping the power of analogy. *Harvard Business Review* 83(4):54–63.

Jennings, M.C. 2000. *Health Care Strategy for Uncertain Times.* San Francisco: Jossey-Bass.

LaTour, K., Eichenwald, S., and Oachs, P., 2013. *Health Information Management Concepts, Principles, and Practice.* 4th ed. Chicago: AHIMA Press.

Kaplan, R.S. and D.P. Norton. 2004. *Strategy Maps: Converting Intangible Assets into Tangible Outcomes.* Boston: Harvard Business School Press.

Kemp, E., R. Funk, and D. Eadie. 1993. Change in chewable bites: Applying strategic management at EEOC. *Public Administration Review* 130.

Kloss, L.L. 2006. Strategic Management. Chapter 28 in Eichenwald, S., LaTour, K., Oachs, P. *Health Information Management: Concepts, Principles, and Practices.* Chicago: AHIMA.

Kolb, D.A. 1988. Integrity, Advanced Professional Development, and Learning. In *Executive Integrity.* Edited by Srivastra, S. San Francisco: Jossey-Bass.

Kotter, J.P. 2012a. *Leading Change: Why Transformation Efforts Fail.* Boston: Harvard Business Review Press.

Kotter, J.P. 2012b. The big idea: Accelerate! *Harvard Business Review* 90(11):44–58.

Kouzes, J.M. and B.Z. Posner. 1995. *The Leadership Challenge: How to Keep Getting Extraordinary Things Done in Organizations.* San Francisco: Jossey-Bass.

McKee, R. 2003 (June). Storytelling that moves people: A conversation with screenwriting coach Robert McKee. *Harvard Business Review* 81(6).

Merriam-Webster. 2015. Paradigm. http://www.merriam-webster.com/

Norton, R., S. Kaplan, and P. David. 2000 (Sep.–Oct.). Having trouble with your strategy? Then map it. *Harvard Business Review* 78. http://hbr.org/2000/09/having-trouble-with-your-strategy-then-map-it/ar/6

Olsen, E. 2006. *Strategic Planning for Dummies.* Indianapolis: John Wiley & Sons.

Porter, M.E. 1996. What is strategy? *Harvard Business Review* 74(6):61–78.

Powers, V.J. 1997. Benchmarking study illustrates how best-in-class achieve alignment, communicate change. *Communication World* 14(2):30–33.

Robert, M. 2006. *The New Strategic Thinking: Pure and Simple.* New York, NY: McGraw-Hill.

Schoemaker, P.J.H. 1995. Senario planning: A tool for strategic thinking. *Sloan Management Review* 36(2):25–41.

Zuckerman, A. 2012. *Healthcare Strategic Planning.* Chicago: Health Administration Press.

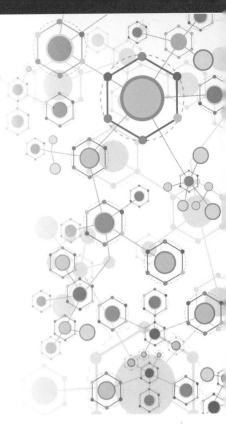

APPENDIX A
Answers to Odd-numbered Check Your Understanding Exercises

Chapter 1

Check Your Understanding **1.1**

1. B
3. D
5. C
7. D

Check Your Understanding **1.2**

1. B
3. A
5. I
7. F
9. G

Check Your Understanding **1.3**

1. C
3. D

5. B
7. B

Check Your Understanding **1.4**

1. True
3. True
5. False. Retail clinics treat routine illnesses and perform preventative care.
7. True
9. False. Patients in post-acute care often require ongoing medical management or therapeutic, rehabilitative, or nursing services.

Check Your Understanding **1.5**

1. True
3. True
5. True

7. True

9. True

Check Your Understanding 1.6

1. D

3. C

5. B

7. B

Check Your Understanding 1.7

1. True

3. False. Medicaid was created to allow lower-income Americans access to healthcare.

5. True

7. True

Chapter 2

Check Your Understanding 2.1

1. The three related subsystems of government are the executive, legislative, and judicial branches.

3. The two types of jurisdiction that determine whether a case will be brought in federal court are subject matter jurisdiction and diversity jurisdiction.

5. The court of last resort in the United States legal system is the US Supreme Court.

7. Civil law involves relations between individuals, corporations, government entities, and other organizations. The typical remedy for a civil wrong is monetary. Criminal law involves matters between individuals or groups of people and the government. Criminal law addresses crimes, which are wrongful acts against public health, safety, and welfare. It also addresses punishment for offenders.

9. The parties are the government, which brings charges, and the defendant, who is believed to have committed a crime. The accused defendant may plead guilty and be sentenced to probation or imprisonment and/or pay a fine. He or she may instead plead not guilty, which results in a trial. Upon conclusion of the trial, a verdict of either guilty or not guilty is rendered. When a defendant is found not guilty (acquitted), the charges are dismissed. A defendant found to be guilty is sentenced to probation or imprisonment and/or to pay a fine.

Check Your Understanding 2.2

1. The two most common types of civil healthcare causes of action are torts and contracts.

3. The three categories of negligence are malfeasance, misfeasance, and nonfeasance. The four elements of negligence are duty of care, breach of duty of care, causation, and injury or harm.

5. A healthcare organization might commit defamation of character if false information (either written or verbal) is shared or published with a third party, and there is no defense of privilege protecting the disclosure (for example, privilege exists if the disclosure was made in good faith or to one who had a legal or otherwise legitimate reason to receive the information).

7. A contract is a written or oral agreement that is legally enforceable. The required elements of a contract are agreement, offer, acceptance, and consideration.

9. A contract action arises when one party alleges that another party has failed to meet an obligation that was established in the valid contract (namely, the contract was breached). A party to a contract may also claim a contract is valid based on fraud, mistake of fact, duress, impossibility, or illegality.

Check Your Understanding 2.3

1. The two types of information collected in the health record are demographic (name, address, birth date, sex, age, insurance information) and clinical (diagnosis, complaint, medical history, family history, social history, documentation of ongoing medical care, diagnostic tests, procedure reports, consultant reports).

3. Licensure requirements (often determined by state law); certification requirements (for example, Medicare Conditions of Participation); accreditation requirements (for example, Joint Commission and the American Osteopathic Association); and other applicable statutes and regulations must be taken into consideration when a healthcare organization makes decisions about the form and content of its health records.

5. The Privacy Act of 1974 and the Freedom of Information Act of 1967 also address privacy.

7. The legal health record should be defined by taking into consideration the documents and data that will be released upon a legal request; the format of the data; the purpose of the record; state and federal statutes, regulations and standards defining health record content; internal documents; and whether the information meets the rules of evidence requirements.

The electronic record becomes more complicated because of the existence of metadata, along with the ability to readily bring together inpatient and outpatient records; personal health records; records from other providers; and intermingled administrative, financial, and clinical data. Information that in the past was separate from the medical record can now be considered part of it (for example, electronic scheduling records or communications between the patient and provider). These factors should all be taken into consideration.

9. External (legal) factors that must be taken into consideration include federal and state statutes and regulations (for example, Medicare Conditions of Participation and state laws that define minimum retention periods) and the applicable statutes of limitations for bringing legal actions such as medical malpractice and breach of contract. Internal (operational) factors that should be taken into consideration include patient treatment, communication among providers, continuity of care, proof of services provided to justify reimbursement; evaluation of quality and efficiency of care, statistical needs, research, education, and facilitation of an organization's operations management.

Check Your Understanding 2.4

1. The health record custodian may testify that the record was documented in the normal course of business and at the time the events occurred. The custodian may also testify about the creation of the record, including the system or process used, and maintenance of the record in ways that prevent it from being altered.

3.

Durable power of attorney for healthcare decisions	Executed by a competent adult on his or her own behalf.
	Designates another person (proxy) to make healthcare decisions consistent with the individual's wishes on the individual's behalf.
Living will	Executed by a competent adult on his or her own behalf.
	Expresses one's wishes to limit treatment if a medical condition renders the individual unable to communicate on his or her own behalf.
	May be limited to certain medical conditions (for example, vegetative state), depending on state law.
	Most often used elderly or in chronically ill health.
Do-not-resuscitate order	Directs healthcare providers to refrain from CPR if the individual experiences cardiac or respiratory arrest.

5. It serves as documentation of care provided in civil cases such as medical malpractice (for example, a patient alleges wrongdoing against healthcare providers) or other personal injury (for example, vehicle accidents) and in criminal cases (for example, rape, homicide, and healthcare fraud).

7. The physician–patient privilege provides that the physician is not permitted to testify as a witness about certain information gained as a result of his or her relationship with the patient. This protection may be removed if the patient has given consent; through waiver (for example, the patient places his or her medical condition at issue in a lawsuit); or there is overriding law or public policy (for example, disclosing a communicable disease in the interest of public safety).

9. Yes. One may be authorized to gain access to a health record, but that does not give the individual ownership—custodial rights and responsibilities associated with that record. Ownership includes the responsibilities of ensuring record integrity and security.

Check Your Understanding 2.5

1. Five types of highly sensitive information that require special disclosure protections are behavioral health, substance abuse, HIV/AIDS, genetics, and adoption.

3. Medical identity theft is the inappropriate or unauthorized misrepresentation of another's identity to do one of two things: obtain medical services or goods or falsify claims for medical services in an attempt to obtain money. It can cause both financial harm and medical harm to its victims. If incorrect information is entered into a victim's health record, improper and harmful medical treatment could result.

5. Concurrent quality review activities are carried out as care is being given.

Retrospective quality review activities are carried out after a patient–provider encounter has ended.

7. An incident is an occurrence that is inconsistent with the standard of care (for example, a medication error that results in harm to the patient). Incident reports may be protected from discovery under the following theories: (1) state statutes that protect QI studies and activities; or (2) attorney–client privilege.

Chapter 3

Check Your Understanding 3.1

1. A
3. B
5. C

Check Your Understanding 3.2

1. D
3. C
5. C

Chapter 4

Check Your Understanding 4.1

1. The primary purpose of patient health information is patient care and treatment.

3. Factors influencing the content of the health record include provider preference; process of care; data sets; external standards and regulations from accrediting and certifying bodies and state licensure standards; and internal standards like medical staff bylaws.

5. A longitudinal health record is a birth-to-death record that acts as an ongoing reference for and about the patient. The problem with achieving a longitudinal health record with a hybrid system is that the patient has paper records in multiple settings that cannot be linked.

Check Your Understanding 4.2

1. D
3. J
5. B
7. I
9. H

Check Your Understanding 4.3

1. Source-oriented health record

3. Integrated health record

5. The P stands for plan, which states the methods to be followed in addressing the problems identified

Check Your Understanding 4.4

1. Voice recognition technology will turn medical transcriptionists into editors and proofreaders.

3. Quantitative analysis is a review of the record for completeness and accuracy. For example, a quantitative analysis checks that the proper reports for each patient exist, that signatures are in place, and that the organization of the record is correct. Qualitative analysis is a more thorough review of the quality and accuracy of the documentation, ensuring that it meets standards and regulations.

5. Incomplete records can hold up a facility's billing process and affect the timely reimbursement for patient care.

7. The HIM professional educates providers in proper documentation and sets up procedures within the HIM department to provide lists of what is needed to complete the record, to conduct concurrent analysis, to flag or mark what needs to be signed, and to complete other tasks to make it easier for providers to complete records quickly.

9. Providers wanting a new form should go through the approval process to ensure control of forms, especially as the transition to imaging or computerized systems continues. The person developing the form may be unaware of the impact the form may have on the patient care process.

Check Your Understanding 4.5

1. The master patient index (MPI) is the key locator for records in a numerical filing system because it contains the patient numbers by which the records are filed.

3. Some of the reasons why incorrect patient information is obtained are that someone other than the patient provides the information; incorrect spelling; different names and/or initials are used for the same patient; clerical mistakes; and language differences.

5. Common attributes used to help identify patients includes patient full name, date of birth, address, gender, race, health record number, physician name, or billing account number.

7. Terminal-digit filing allows for a more even distribution of files within the filing area and thus a more even distribution of work. In straight numerical filing, newer records are at the end of the file and most of the file work will be concentrated in the area with the new files.

9. The four primary steps in an effective record retention program are conducting inventory, determining storage format and location, assigning retention periods, and destroying unnecessary records.

Chapter 5

Check Your Understanding 5.1

1. A clinical classification is "a clinical vocabulary, terminology, or nomenclature that lists words or phrases with their meanings; provides for the proper use of clinical words as names or symbols; and facilitates mapping of standardized terms to broader classifications for administrative, regulatory, oversight, and fiscal requirements" (AHIMA 2011). A classification system provides easy storage, retrieval, and analysis of data for the purposes of transmitting and comparing data.

   A clinical vocabulary is "a formally recognized list of preferred medical terms" (AHIMA 2014). The definition for the vocabulary is similar to that of terminology except that it includes the meanings or definitions of words.

   A terminology is "a set of terms representing a system of concepts" (Giannangelo 2015, 4). A clinical terminology is "a set of standardized terms and their synonyms that record patient findings, circumstances, events, and interventions with sufficient detail to support clinical care, decision support, outcomes research, and quality improvement" (AMIA and AHIMA Terminology and Classification Policy Task Force 2007, 41).

   Each plays a specific yet interdependent role in data standardization.

3. Example of classification systems: ICD-10-CM and ICD-10-PCS

   Example of a terminology: LOINC

5. Standardization is important for the purposes of recording patient findings, circumstances, and interventions in a consistent way. Consistency supports clinical care, decision support, outcomes research, and allows for quality improvement.

Check Your Understanding 5.2

1. ICD-10-CM is a US clinical modification of WHO's ICD-10 and is maintained by the National Center for Health Statistics (NCHS). It is a morbidity classification system that classifies diagnoses and other reasons for healthcare encounters. The code structure is alphanumeric, with codes comprised of three to seven characters.

   ICD-10-PCS is a procedure coding system developed under contract by the Centers for Medicare and Medicaid Services (CMS) as a replacement of the ICD-9-CM procedure coding system for hospital reporting of inpatient procedures. It has a seven-character alphanumeric code structure (CMS 2015a).

3. HCPCS is used to report services and supplies primarily for reimbursement purposes in the outpatient or ambulatory setting. The system is divided into two sections referred to as levels. Level I of HCPCS is composed of the CPT codes as published by the AMA and represents medical services and procedures performed by physicians and other healthcare providers. Level II of HCPCS contains codes that represent products, supplies, and services not included in the CPT codes.

5. It serves as a universal product identifier for human drugs and identifies the labeler/vendor, product, and trade package size. It is an approved HIPAA billing/financial transaction code set for reporting drugs and biologicals. In 2004, the NDCs were adopted as a federal healthcare information interoperability standard to enable the federal healthcare sector to share information regarding drug products (USHIK 2008).

Check Your Understanding 5.3

1. Interoperability is "the ability to communicate and exchange data accurately, effectively, securely, and consistently with different information technology systems, software applications, and networks in various settings, and exchange data such that clinical or operational purpose and meaning of the data are preserved and unaltered" (Bush 2006).

   Healthcare terminologies facilitate health information exchange by standardizing the data collected. Through this standard representation of data, terminologies provide shared meaning and a sense of context for the information being used. In simple terms, this ability to exchange information between computer systems is referred to as interoperability.

3. (a) laboratory data, LOINC; (b) nursing documentation, Clinical Care Classification; and (c) problem list documentation, SNOMED CT

5. RxNorm is a standardized nomenclature for clinical drugs that provides information on a drug's ingredients, strengths, and form in which it is to be administered or used. It is produced by the National Library of Medicine (NLM) and allows various systems using different drug nomenclatures to share data efficiently at the appropriate level of detail.

   MEDCIN is a proprietary clinical terminology owned and maintained by Medicomp Systems. The system was initially developed by Peter Goltra in 1978 and has been updated regularly (NLM 2015g). MEDCIN'S approximately 270,000 clinical elements created with a strong focus on facilitating documentation by providing clinically relevant choices in a format that is consistent with the provider's clinical thought processes. Because of this feature, the system is considered to be an interface terminology (Bowman 2005; Fraser 2005). MEDCIN is licensed by EHR developers that incorporate the terminology into their EHR systems. For example, MEDCIN is the clinical terminology used by the DoD in its Armed Forces Health Longitudinal Technology Application (AHLTA) system. MEDCIN also identifies relationships through multiple hierarchies for each of its clinical elements. These linkages support other functionalities of the system such as clinical alerts, automated note generation, and computer-assisted coding for CPT evaluation and management codes (Goltra 1997; Medicomp Systems 2012).

Check Your Understanding 5.4

1. No single terminology, vocabulary, or classification has the depth and breadth to represent the broad spectrum of medical knowledge; thus, a core group of well-integrated, nonredundant methods will be needed to serve as the backbone of clinical information (Open Clinical 2012).

3. Both private organizations and government agencies such as ONC, CSM, FDA, the Agency for Health Care Policy and Research, the Office of the Assistant Secretary for Planning and Evaluation, and the CDC work collaboratively in the development and maintenance of these standards.

5. HIM professionals can assist in the development, policy, and governance of receiving data in an understandable and usable manner through data standardization for describing, classifying, and exchanging medical terms and concepts. Use of standardization facilitates electronic data collection at the point of care; retrieval of relevant data, information, and knowledge; and reuse of data for multiple purposes (Aspen et al. 2003).

Chapter 6

Check Your Understanding 6.1

1. A primary data source is created by the healthcare professionals providing the care. The medical record is considered a primary data source. A secondary data source is made up of data taken from a primary data source and put in a different format, such as a registry.

3. Secondary data sources are created to put the information from the primary record into a format that is easier to query and manipulate. For example, it is difficult and time-consuming for a cancer registrar to determine the number of patients with each type of cancer by looking at individual records. A database, which is a secondary record, can be queried to provide this information in a report from the secondary data that have been entered, thus accelerating the process.

5. Within a healthcare facility, internal users include medical, administrative, and management staff.

Check Your Understanding 6.2

1. HIM departments use facility-specific indexes to locate data as requested by internal and external users. The operation index, for example, could be used to locate medical records for patients with a specific operation for a quality assessment study. It could also be used to provide information to external users. For example, residents often must provide data on the types of operations they have performed during their residency to the appropriate board for certification in their specialty.

3. An index is a report from a database that enables locating records by diagnosis, procedure, or physician.

5. The purpose of the physician index is to locate medical records of patients who have been treated by a particular physician. It must, at a minimum, include the physician's name or a code number assigned and the patient's name or health record number.

Check Your Understanding 6.3

1. Registries are collections of secondary data related to a patient's specific diagnosis, condition, or procedure. They are created and maintained to provide specific information from the medical record in an easily retrievable form.

3. Case definition refers to the process used by each registry to define the cases to be included in it. Case finding is a method used to identify patients who have been seen or treated in the facility for the particular disease or condition of interest to the registry.

5. Cancer Registry

   - For a facility-based registry, patient records are reviewed to collect demographic information, type and site of the cancer, diagnostic methodologies, and treatment methodologies.

   - For a population-based registry, information is submitted by facilities within the population covered.

   Trauma Registry

   - Abstracting data from the medical record including demographic information, hospital care provided, status of patient at the time of admission, diagnosis and procedure codes, abbreviated injury scale, and injury severity score.

   Birth Defects Registry

   - Abstracting information from the sources used in case finding. Abstracted information includes demographic information, diagnosis codes, birth weight, status at birth, autopsy, cytogenetic reports, mother's and father's use of alcohol and drugs, and family history of birth defects.

   Diabetes Registry

   - Abstracting information from physician office or clinic record including demographic information and laboratory values.

Implant Registry

- Abstracting information from the health record including demographic data and data required by the FDA.

Transplant Registry

- Recipient information: Demographic data, patient diagnosis, medical urgency, functional status, life support status, and previous transplants
- Donor information/living donor: Relationship to recipient, clinical information, organ recovery information, and histocompatibility
- Donor information/deceased donor: Cause and circumstances of death, organ procurement and consent process, medications taken, and other donor history

7. Cancer Registry

- Reviewing medical records for treatment in the last year; contacting the patient's physician; contacting the patient, newspaper obituaries, or websites

Trauma Registry

- Follow-up is done by some, but not all, registries; emphasis is on patient's quality of life

Birth Defects Registry

- Not routinely done

Diabetes Registry

- Done to ensure appropriate continued care

Implant Registry

- Follow-up is done to assess performance of the implant over time

Transplant Registry

- At intervals throughout the first year and then annually
- Living donor: Complications of the procedure, length of hospital stay
- Recipient: Status at time of follow-up, functional status, graft status, treatment

Immunization Registry

- Follow-up reminders that immunizations are due, by postcard, telephone call, or autodialed call

9. Cancer Registry

- On-the-job training, seminars, and/or cancer registry program in a college; AHIMA's online Cancer Registry program

Trauma Registry

- Varies; may use RHITs, RHIAs, RNs, LPNs, EMTs, or other health professionals or workshops and on-the-job training

Birth Defects Registry

- None specified (not specified)

Diabetes Registry

- None specified (not specified)

Implant Registry

- None specified (not specified)

Transplant Registry

- None specified (not specified)

Immunization Registry

- None specified (not specified)

Check Your Understanding 6.4

1. The three phases of database design are conceptual, logical, and physical phases.

3. NoSQL database scale out instead of up, so it is easy to add storage space when needed. When relational databases reach capacity the entire system needs to be migrated, which is a cumbersome and expensive task. NoSQL databases also have quicker response times for large datasets.

5. Structured Query Language

Check Your Understanding 6.5

1. The MEDPAR file provides data on Medicare patients including demographic patient data, provider data, Medicare coverage, total charges, charges by service, diagnosis and procedure codes, and DRGs.

3. The National Practitioner Data Bank was developed to make information on malpractice claims, sanctions by boards of medical examiners, and professional review actions available among all states. Before, physicians who had incurred such actions could move to another state and practice without anyone in the new state knowing his or her background. The Health Care Quality Improvement Act of 1986 mandated the creation of the NPDB. The Healthcare Integrity and Protection Data Bank was developed because there was no central repository for information on healthcare fraud and abuse. The data bank was mandated by the Health Insurance Portability and Accountability Act of 1996.

5. Healthcare organizations use the National Practitioner Data Bank in the credentialing process. They must query the data bank when a physician initially applies for medical staff privileges and every two years thereafter. Federal and state government agencies and health plans may access the Healthcare Integrity and Protection Data Bank. Practitioners, providers, and suppliers may only query about themselves.

7. The source of data for the Healthcare Cost and Utilization Project is data collected at the state level on claims data from the UB-04 or discharge abstracted data including the UHDDS reported by individual hospitals and, in some cases, ambulatory care centers.

9. The Healthcare Integrity and Protection Data Bank was developed because there was no central repository for information on healthcare fraud and abuse. The data bank was mandated by the Health Insurance Portability and Accountability Act of 1996.

Check Your Understanding 6.6

1. Increased use of automated data entry is a current trend in the collection of secondary data. The development of the electronic patient record will ensure that less data will have to be abstracted from the medical record into secondary records. Emphasis by stakeholders on issues such as ownership of secondary data has increased. The HIM stewardship role is becoming increasingly important in the area of secondary data.

3. Data stewardship is the responsible management of data during managing, viewing, storing, sharing, and disclosing tasks.

5. The patient health record is shifting into database.

Check Your Understanding 6.7

1. Timeliness and accuracy are listed in both AHIMA's data quality model and the MRI essential principles of documentation.

3. The 10 dimensions of data quality are accuracy, accessibility, comprehensiveness, consistency, currency, definition, granularity, precision, relevancy, and timeliness.

5. An enterprise-wide data dictionary contains descriptions of common data and their formats.

Chapter 7

Check Your Understanding 7.1

1. Medicare Part B (Supplemental Medical Insurance) covers the following services and supplies:

   - Physicians' and surgeons' services, including some covered services furnished by chiropractors, podiatrists, dentists, and optometrists; and services provided by the following Medicare-approved practitioners who are not physicians—certified registered nurse anesthetists, clinical psychologists, clinical social workers (other than those employed by a hospital or an SNF), physician assistants, nurse practitioners, and clinical nurse specialists working in collaboration with a physician

   - Services in an emergency department or outpatient clinic, including same-day surgery and ambulance services

   - Home healthcare not covered under Medicare Part A

   - Laboratory tests, x-rays, and other diagnostic radiology services, as well as certain preventive care screening tests

   - Ambulatory surgery center (ASC) services in Medicare-approved facilities

   - Most physical and occupational therapy and speech pathology services

   - Comprehensive outpatient rehabilitation facility services and mental healthcare provided as part of a partial hospitalization psychiatric program when a physician certifies that inpatient treatment would be required without the partial hospitalization services

   - Radiation therapy, renal dialysis and kidney transplants, and heart and liver transplants under certain limited conditions

   - DME approved for home use, such as oxygen equipment; wheelchairs; prosthetic devices; surgical dressings, splints, and casts; walkers; and hospital beds needed for use in the home

   - Drugs and biologicals that cannot be self-administered, such as hepatitis B vaccines and transplant and immunosuppressive drugs (plus certain self-administered anticancer drugs)

   - Preventive services such as bone mass measurements, cardiovascular screening blood tests, colorectal cancer screening, diabetes services, glaucoma testing, Pap test and pelvic exam, prostate cancer screening, screening mammograms, and vaccinations (flu, pneumococcal, hepatitis B)

3. The Consolidated Omnibus Budget Reconciliation Act of 1985 (COBRA) established an employee's right to continue healthcare coverage beyond the scheduled benefit termination date (including HMO coverage).

5. Private commercial insurance plans are financed through the payment of premiums. When a claim for medical care is submitted to the insurance company, the claim is paid out of the fund's reserves.

   Before payment is made, the insurance company reviews every claim to determine whether the services described on the claim are covered by the patient's policy. The company also reviews the claim to ensure that the services provided were medically necessary. Payment then is made to either the provider or the policyholder.

   Most insurance policies include the following information:

   - What medical services the company will cover
   - When the company will pay for medical services
   - How much and for how long the company will pay for covered services
   - What process is to be followed to ensure that covered medical expenses are paid

   The cost of employer-based self-insurance funding is lower than the cost of paying premiums to private insurers because the premiums reflect more than the actual cost of the services provided to beneficiaries. Private insurers build additional fees into premiums to compensate them for assuming the risk of providing insurance coverage. In self-insured plans, the employer assumes the risk. By budgeting a certain amount to pay its employees' medical claims, the employer retains control over the funds until the time when group medical claims need to be paid.

Employer-based self-insurance has become a common form of group health insurance coverage. Many employers enter into administrative services only (ASO) contracts with private insurers and fund the plans themselves. The private insurers administer self-insurance plans on behalf of the employers.

Check Your Understanding 7.2

1. Fee-for-service reimbursement methodologies issue payments to healthcare providers on the basis of the charges assigned to each of the separate services that were performed for the patient. The total bill for an episode of care represents the sum of all the itemized charges for every element of care provided. Independent clinical professionals such as physicians and psychologists who are not employees of the facility issue separate itemized bills to cover their services after the services are completed or on a monthly basis when the services are ongoing.

3. Global payments are lump-sum payments distributed among the physicians who performed the procedure or interpreted its results and the healthcare facility that provided the equipment, supplies, and technical support required. The procedure's professional component is supplied by physicians (for example, radiologists), and its technical component (for example, radiological supplies, equipment, and support services) is supplied by a hospital or freestanding diagnostic or surgical center

5. The capitated managed care plan negotiates a contract with an employer or a government agency representing a specific group of individuals. According to the contract, the managed care organization agrees to provide all the contracted healthcare services that the covered individuals need over a specified period of time (usually one year). In exchange, the individual enrollee or third-party payer agrees to pay a fixed premium for the covered group. Like other insurance plans, a capitated insurance contract stipulates as part of the contract exactly which healthcare services are covered and which ones are not.

Check Your Understanding 7.3

1. A hospital's case-mix index (types or categories of patients treated by the hospital) is based on the relative weights of the MS-DRG. The case-mix index can be figured by multiplying the relative weight of each MS-DRG by the number of discharges within that MS-DRG.

This provides the total weight for each MS-DRG. The sum of all total weights divided by the sum of total patient discharges equals the case-mix index. A hospital may relate its case-mix index to the costs incurred for inpatient care.

3. Discounting applies to multiple surgical procedures furnished during the same operative session. For discounted procedures, the full APC rate is paid for the surgical procedure with the highest rate, and other surgical procedures performed at the same time are reimbursed at 50 percent of the APC rate.

5. The long-term care community falls under the MS-LTC-DRGs, which are based on the MS-DRGs.

Check Your Understanding 7.4

1. In many instances, patients have more than one insurance policy, and the determination of which policy is primary and which is secondary is necessary so that there is no duplication of benefits paid. This process is called the coordination of benefits (COB) or the coordination of benefits transaction. The monies collected from third-party payers cannot be greater than the amount of the provider's charges.

3. Medicare sends a Medicare summary notice (MSN) to a beneficiary to show how much the provider billed, how much Medicare reimbursed the provider, and what the patient must pay the provider by way of deductible and copayments.

5. A Medicare Administrative Contractor (MAC) is a private healthcare insurer that has been awarded a geographic jurisdiction to process Medicare Part A and Part B (A/B) medical claims or Durable Medical Equipment (DME) claims for Medicare Fee-For-Service (FFS) beneficiaries. CMS relies on a network of MACs to serve as the primary operational contact between the Medicare FFS program and the healthcare providers enrolled in the program. MACs are multistate, regional contractors responsible for administering both Medicare Part A and Medicare Part B claims. MACs perform many activities including:

- Process Medicare FFS claims
- Make and account for Medicare FFS payments
- Enroll providers in the Medicare FFS program
- Handle provider reimbursement services and audit institutional provider cost reports
- Handle redetermination requests (1st stage appeals process)
- Respond to provider inquiries
- Educate providers about Medicare FFS billing requirements
- Establish local coverage determinations (LCDs)
- Review medical records for selected claims
- Coordinate with CMS and other FFS contractors (CMS 2015j)

Chapter 8

Check Your Understanding 8.1

1. National Coverage Determinations and Local Coverage Determination policies list diagnoses supporting medical necessity

3. Answer could include any of the following:

   - Incorrect insurance plan listed
   - Policy number or group number missing or invalid
   - Patient not eligible on date of service
   - Patient with insurance listed as private pay
   - Medicare listed when plan is Medicare HMO
   - Medicare listed as primary when should be secondary
   - Minors listed as guarantors
   - More than one health record number per patient
   - Accident claims without occurrence codes
   - Patient relationship to insurance subscriber code errors
   - Failure to list medical necessity
   - Missing guarantor or employer information
   - Physician orders incomplete or missing
   - Internal coding mismatches (for example, financial class to patient type to stay type to service code to admit code)
   - Missing prior authorization or pre-certification required for service provided
   - Transposed digits: Social Security number, date of birth, policy number, group number
   - Invalid punctuation in specified text fields
   - Misspelled name
   - Insurance eligibility verification failure
   - Address verification failure (returned mail cost)
   - Observation patient with inpatient stay type
   - Point-of-service collection failure
   - Incomplete or inaccurate Medicare secondary payer questionnaire

5. Answer could include any of the following:

   - Determinations of medical necessity must adhere to the standard of care that applies to the actual direct care and treatment of the patient.
   - Medical necessity is the standard terminology that all healthcare professionals and entities will use in the review process when determining if medical care is appropriate and essential.
   - Determinations of medical necessity must reflect the efficient and cost-effective application of patient care including, but not limited to, diagnostic testing, therapies (including activity restriction, aftercare instructions, and prescriptions), disability ratings, rehabilitating an illness, injury, disease or its associated symptoms, impairments or functional limitations, procedures, psychiatric care, levels of hospital care, extended care, long-term care, hospice care, and home healthcare.

   - Determinations of medical necessity made in a concurrent review should include discussions with the attending provider regarding the current medical condition of the patient whenever possible. A physician advisor or reviewer can make a positive determination regarding medical necessity without necessarily speaking with the treating provider if the advisor has enough available information to make an appropriate medical decision. A physician advisor cannot decide to deny care as not medically necessary without speaking to the treating provider and these discussions must be clearly documented.
   - Determinations of medical necessity must be unrelated to payers' monetary benefit.
   - Determinations of medical necessity must always be made on a case-by-case basis consistent with the applicable standard of care and must be available for peer review.
   - Recommendations approving medical necessity may be made by a nonphysician reviewer. Negative determinations for the initial review regarding medical necessity must be made by a physician advisor who has the clinical training to review the particular clinical problem (clinically matched) under review. A physician reviewer or advisor must not delegate his or her review decisions to a nonphysician reviewer.
   - The process to be used in evaluating medical necessity should be made known to the patient.
   - All medical review organizations involved in determining medical necessity shall have uniform, written procedures for appeals of negative determinations that services or supplies are not medically necessary.

Check Your Understanding 8.2

1. Complete and accurate charges must be posted to the claim because reimbursement rates are often related to the individual charges, the charges posted to the claim claims can drive specific prices and reimbursement rates, and payers also use historical claim information to set current and future reimbursement rates, The charges reflect the resources that were used to provide the services and they help organizations measure labor costs and staff productivity.

3. The case-mix index is calculated by adding the Medicare DRG weight for every inpatient discharge and dividing by the number of discharges.

5. Charges set up in the source systems, whether electronic or on paper, must identically match the charge found in the CDM.

Check Your Understanding 8.3

1. The greater the bill hold days and the lower the percentage of clean claims, the higher the accounts receivable days. Conversely, the shorter the bills hold days and the higher the clean claims submission, the lower the accounts receivable days.

3. Answer could include any of the following:

   - Beneficiary not covered
   - Lack of medical necessity—not reasonable or necessary
   - Lack of precertification
   - Inappropriate utilization, noncovered services
   - Incorrect charging—unbundled code, late charges/timely filing
   - Incorrect coding such as procedure code does not match patient sex, diagnosis procedure code does not match service provided
   - Procedure code inconsistent with modifier used
   - Procedure code inconsistent with place of service
   - Diagnosis is inconsistent with age, sex, and procedure
   - Modifier not provided

5. Account receivable days are the average number of days between the provision of services discharge date and the receipt of payment for those services rendered.

Check Your Understanding 8.4

1. Key strategies of success for the revenue cycle include: organization-wide focus on revenue cycle improvement and a dedicated team; metrics to conduct root cause analysis to facilitate changes throughout the healthcare system; a shared sense of accountability for revenue cycle performance; collaboration with other departments to enhance the revenue cycle performance; a comprehensive approach needs to be developed to address uncompensated care; innovative ways to enhance customer service; and the organization must focus on improving the total patient experience.

3. The purpose of MAP keys is to develop the standard for consistent measurement and revenue cycle excellence.

5. Numerator: Total number of verified encounters

   Denominator: Total number of registered encounters

Chapter 9

Check Your Understanding 9.1

1. Clinical documentation improvement is a process to facilitate the accurate representation of a patient's clinical status in the patient health record, which is then transformed into coded data.

3. Clinical documentation is the foundation for communication between providers as well as multiple reimbursement, quality, and public health measures.

5. Composition of the CDI staff, alignment of the CDI program, identification of the types of records to review, frequency of health record reviews, budget, training needs, reporting and performance monitoring need to be considered when planning to implement a CDI process.

Check Your Understanding 9.2

1. Compliance means adhering to rules, laws, standards, or regulations.

3. Optimization seeks the most accurate documentation, coded data, and resulting payment in the amount the provider is rightly and legally entitled to receive as opposed to maximization, which focuses on collecting the highest rate of payment.

5. Exclusion is significant because the government is the largest purchaser and provider of services in the United States.

Chapter 10

Check Your Understanding 10.1

1. The four compliance goals as identified by the Office of Inspector General are (1) fight fraud, waste, and abuse; (2) promote quality and safety; (3) secure the future; and (4) advance innovation.

3. EMTALA was enacted to ensure public access to emergency services regardless of ability to pay. The components of this obligation include providing medical screening examinations (MSE), providing stabilization treatment, and transferring patients (transferring in terms of to another organization or released from the ED).

5. The Red Flags Rule requires many businesses and organizations to implement a written identity theft prevention program designed to detect the "red flags"

of identity theft in day-to-day operations, take steps to prevent the crime, and mitigate its damage. The intent is to deter identity theft and have a plan in place for quick detection if suspicious activity is suspected.

Check Your Understanding 10.2

1. OIG workplans are issued at the beginning of each fiscal year and provide for new and ongoing reviews or audits in programs administered by the Department of Health and Human Services (HHS). The goals of the reviews are to protect the integrity of both state and federal programs by detecting and preventing fraud, waste, and abuse; identifying opportunities for improvement in economy, efficiency, and effectiveness; and holding accountable those who do not meet program requirements or violate federal laws. The intent of a compliance program is to help mitigate the likelihood of fraud, waste, and abuse.

3. Three examples of fraud surveillance approaches from the external audit perspective are whistleblower incentives, complaint audits, and RAC audits.

5. CIAs are negotiations as part of the settlement of federal healthcare program investigations, providers or entities agree to the obligations in exchange for the OIG to not seek their exclusion from participation in federal healthcare programs. CIAs may last for many years and are imposed when serious misconduct (fraud and abuse) is discovered through an audit or self-disclosure.

Check Your Understanding 10.3

1. Risk management is the process of planning, organizing, directing, and controlling resources to achieve given objectives when events are possible. The purpose of a risk management program is to protect an organization and its assets against negative risks (loss), including accidental losses.

3. An incident report is a form used to record unplanned or unusual occurrences in detail. Any employee or patient can file the form. It is important to capture any dates, times, and locations of incident occurrences. Each incident report can be reviewed individually or used to create report data that is tabulated and analyzed to help identify trends and establish probable cause.

5. Each incident report can be reviewed individually or to create report data that is tabulated and analyzed to help identify trends and help to establish probable cause. Tabulated incident report data can include types of occurrences, severity of the injuries, frequencies and patterns, demographics, and effectiveness of corrective measures.

7. Three major categories of types of threats are:

- Natural threats (floods or earthquakes)
- Technical/manmade (that is, mechanical, biological)
- Intentional acts (namely, terrorism, computer security, and such)

9. The seven components defined by NIST to a viable contingency planning program are:

- Identify specific regulatory requirements related to contingency planning
- Conduct a business impact analysis to prioritize critical systems, business processes, and components
- Identify and implement preventive controls and measures
- Develop recovery strategies
- Develop contingency plans with guidance and procedures
- Plan and implement testing and training to both validate and identify gaps, as well as prepare staff
- Maintain contingency plans, updating regularly

Chapter 11

Check Your Understanding 11.1

1. B

3. Privacy is the right of an individual to be let alone; refers to who should have access, what constitutes the patient's rights to confidentiality, and what constitutes inappropriate access to health records.

   Confidentiality is when data or information is not made available or disclosed to unauthorized persons or processes, and establishes how the records (or the systems that hold those records) should be protected from inappropriate access.

   Security is the means by which the privacy and confidentiality of information is maintained.

5. D

Check Your Understanding 11.2

1. D

3. True

5. Answer should include:

- Documentation to release records:
  ○ Authorization for Disclosure of PHI signed by the patient (or representative)
- Verification:
  ○ Identification of attorney
  ○ Link to the law firm by attorney (request on letter head, business card, and such)

Check Your Understanding 11.3

1. A

3. B

5. A

7. Answer should include:

   - Data are in plain text—data available to anyone who can get access to it and is considered unsecure.
   - Cryptographic key is applied to the data—the key is the process that changes the data from plain text to cipher text allowing encryption to occur.
   - Data are in cipher text—the data are considered unusable, indecipherable, and unreadable. The information is secure.

Check Your Understanding 11.4

1. False. A healthcare organization needs to be aware of all devices that are accessing patient information to evaluate if any information is being stored or transmitted over the device. If a data breach occurred due to a personal device with an organization's data, the organization would still be held responsible. Proper safeguards should be established for the management of mobile technology, compliance with HIPAA, and protection of the security and privacy of patient information

3. True

5. The areas that should be covered when educating the workforce about HIE include

   - Process for consent and authorization
   - Process for education to patients and families
   - Process for adequate patient searching and patient matching
   - Process for assurance of selection of the correct patient
   - Process for patient information to be utilized to support care
   - Process for processing patient information if used to support care
   - Process for reporting any issues or concerns with the HIE and data being used
   - Information regarding organization's evaluation of audit trails and supporting of patient care for accessing PHI in the HIE

Check Your Understanding 11.5

1. False. HIPAA defines workforce as Employees, volunteers, trainees, and other persons whose conduct, in the performance of work for a covered entity or business associate, is under the direct control of such covered entity or business associate, whether or not they are paid by the covered entity or business associate.

3. D

5. True

Chapter 12

Check Your Understanding 12.1

1. Informatics applies information management in the context of computer-based systems that are designed to support specific types of users in performing their work (for example, decision-making support). Information management, however, is a more generalized discipline with similar aims that are applied in both paper-based and computer-based environments.

3. Due to the ease and availability of web-based commerce, online banking, ATMs, and other technologies, healthcare appears to lag behind. The healthcare industry is just beginning to adopt web-based services for patients such as appointment scheduling, demographic and insurance updates, and e-mail contact with physicians or clinicians. This perception may be changed by informing healthcare consumers of the advances in healthcare technology, the importance of privacy and standards when sharing patient information, and the subjectivity of clinical practice, which makes healthcare different from other industries.

5. False, the ONC updated its strategic plan through 2020.

Check Your Understanding 12.2

1. Both diagnostic images and document images are bitmapped data. All document images and some diagnostic images are based on analog documents (paper or photographic film) that must be scanned to digitize the data for electronic storage. However, some diagnostic images are based on digital modalities, such as images resulting from computed radiography (CR), magnetic resonance (MR), and computed tomography (CT).

3. The difference is

   (a) Speech recognition technology employs basic natural language processing capabilities as it translates spoken words (natural language voice bytes) into text. However, speech recognition technology does not yet employ the advanced capabilities of natural language processing; for instance, speech recognition technology is not yet capable of taking two sound-alike terms (such as ileum and ilium) with different meanings and then selecting the correct term based on an analysis of the context.

(b) Natural language processing technology and Boolean searching differ from each other in that the former considers sentence structure (syntax), meaning (semantics), and context to accurately extract data from free text. For example, "no shortness of breath, chest pain aggravated by exercise" and "no chest pain, shortness of breath aggravated by exercise" look the same to a Boolean word search engine when it identifies occurrences of chest and pain in the same sentence. Natural language processing technology, however, would discern the syntactical and semantic differences between these two phrases.

5. Document imaging technology electronically captures, stores, identifies, retrieves, and distributes documents that are not generated digitally or are generated digitally but are stored on paper.

   Workflow/business process management (BPM) technology allows computers to add and extract value from document content as the documents move throughout an organization. The documents can be automatically assigned, routed, activated, and managed through system-controlled rules that mirror business operations.

   Computer output laser disk (COLD)/enterprise report management (ERM) technology electronically stores, manages, and distributes documents that are generated in a digital format and whose output data are report-formatted. These documents can be distributed through fax, e-mail, web, and hard copy.

   Automated forms processing technology allows users to electronically enter data into online forms and electronically extract the data from the online forms for data manipulation. The form document is stored in a form format, as the user sees it on the screen, for ease of interpretation.

   Digital signature management technology offers both signer and document authentication for analog or digital documents. Signer authentication is the ability to identify the person who digitally signed the document. Document authentication ensures that the document and the signature cannot be altered.

Check Your Understanding 12.3

1. Electronic data interchange (EDI) was the healthcare industry's first venture into direct electronic transmission of data between the computer system of one organization and the computer system of another organization (often called a business partner). By 2000, EDI as a term (not as a concept) had become dated and was replaced by e-commerce and e-health. E-health now refers to the practice of e-commerce within the healthcare industry.

3. Barcoding is commonly used in healthcare; examples include labels, patient wristbands, specimen containers, and medication packets. Optical character recognition (OCR) technology is used on a limited basis; examples include the indexing of scanned documents and the

digitizing of text documents. Intelligent character recognition (ICR) technology is being adopted slowly; examples include pen-based and handheld input devices. Radio frequency identification (RFID) is rapidly evolving; examples include the tracking of moveable patients, clinicians, medications, and equipment. Intelligent document recognition (IDR) has recently been developed; examples include document and form type identification.

5. Secure clinical messaging is not dependent upon time zones, it can be done in each clinical user's own timeframe, it gives clinical recipients time to think over and respond to issues appropriately, and it does not require all participants to be available at the same time.

7. Benefits of open source technology are its availability, extensibility to be customized, and the collaborative nature of this technology allowing users and developers to interact and improve upon the product. Drawbacks include the need for skilled developers within the organization and the lack of technical support.

Check Your Understanding 12.4

1. Distinct examples of diagnostic tests that involve physiological signal processing include electrocardiograms (EKGs), electroencephalograms (EEGs), electromyograms (EMGs), fetal tracings, digital blood pressure (BP) monitors, and digital thermometers.

3. Second- and third-generation telehealth applications rely on patient interaction and consultation, whereas first-generation applications relied on the transfer of patient information only. The use of guided robotics is evident in third-generation telehealth applications. For example, telesurgeons in New York City performed a gallbladder surgery on a patient in France via robots fed by high-speed signals sent across the Atlantic Ocean through fiber-optic cables.

5. Based upon the definitions provided by NAHIT, the major difference between an EHR and EMR is whether the system conforms to nationally recognized interoperability standards.

Check Your Understanding 12.5

1. Cryptography is an applied science in which mathematics transforms intelligible data and information into unintelligible strings of characters and back again. Encryption technology uses cryptography to code digital data and information. The use of cryptography and encryption allows data to be securely exchanged.

3. Delegating responsibility to users for examining their audit histories is one way to establish user trust. Another way to instill user trust is to frequently sample system usage by organizational managers and publish results of audit trails.

5. Public key infrastructure (PKI) is a type of encryption technology. It involves a private key (known to one

computer) and a public key that is given to a second computer. The second computer receives an incoming message from the first computer and decodes it with the public key and its own private key. PKI is becoming the standard encryption technology for securing data transfers and online authentication. Public key infra-structure is receiving much attention within the health-care industry because secure data transfers and online authentication are vital in meeting the HIPAA security regulations.

Check Your Understanding 12.6

1. D
3. D
5. F
7. A
9. C
11. C

Chapter 13

Check Your Understanding 13.1

1. False. The focus is health information technology and human factors.
3. False. Senior management and information technology leadership should be involved in governance.
5. B
7. A
9. C

Check Your Understanding 13.2

1. G
3. H
5. A
7. C
9. E

Check Your Understanding 13.3

1. False. Data quality management is the business process that ensures the integrity of an organization's data.
3. False. There are several discovery processes to identify issues.
5. True

Chapter 14

Check Your Understanding 14.1

1. A
3. A
5. C

Check Your Understanding 14.2

1. D
3. False. Social determinants of health include the condi-tions in which people are born, grow, work, live, and age, and the wider set of forces and systems shaping the conditions of daily life.
5. False. There are currently numerous valid and reliable measures of health literacy, including the SAHL–S&E.

Check Your Understanding 14.3

1. B
3. B
5. True

Check Your Understanding 14.4

1. D
3. D
5. False. It is the use of telecommunications to connect individuals across geographic distance.

Check Your Understanding 14.5

1. C
3. False. Personalized medicine uses very specific attributes to tailor treatment to meet individual needs.
5. True

Chapter 15

Check Your Understanding 15.1

1. Health information exchange is intended to facilitate access to and retrieval of clinical data to provide safer, timelier, efficient, effective, equitable, patient-centered care.

3. CEHRT standards were implemented to inform technology vendors and providers about the functionality required to receive incentive payments for the implementation of EHR technology in the CMS EHR incentive program.

5. Care quality is intended to be improved by making critical patient information available at the point of care delivery and through the aggregation and mining of data to determine best practices in diagnosis and treatment.

Check Your Understanding 15.2

1. Interoperability is the ability of different information technology systems and software applications to communicate, exchange data, and use the information that has been exchanged.

3. The purpose of the NHIN is to provide a nationwide information technology architecture, consisting of rules and standards to use the Internet for exchanging health information in a secure and timely fashion.

5. Examples of information complexity include: The multiple descriptors assigned to pharmaceuticals, the different formats used for clinical document transmission, or the different protocols used for information transmission within and between systems.

Check Your Understanding 15.3

1. The five categories of value are Improved communications; improved patient safety; increased use of evidence-based medical practice; improved metrics reporting; and greater support of preventative medicine initiatives.

3. The ONC has led the way in the implementation of interoperable health information exchange by providing the vision, initiating pilot programs through funding and guidance initiatives, and ensuring that the efforts of public and private stakeholders are coordinated to fulfill the goals of interoperable health information exchange.

5. Once organizations have agreed to agree to exchange patient data the establishment of policies, procedures and the metrics against which to monitor their progress toward their stated goals must be established.

Check Your Understanding 15.4

1. Meaningful Use was implemented to incentivize the adoption of electronic health records in the healthcare industry.

3. The ONC published the interoperability roadmap as a high-level guidance document for healthcare industry stakeholders to provide focus, milestones, and expectations for the path toward interoperability within the next 10 years.

5. As the consumer is nudged toward more involvement in their wellness care they will make greater demands for more efficient and better care using all of the technical capabilities that are available.

Chapter 16

Check Your Understanding 16.1

1. 5:1

3. 30.86

5. 32

Check Your Understanding 16.2

1. Match the term to the correct definition:

C = A patient who is provided with room, board, and continuous general nursing service in an area of an acute-care facility where patients generally stay at least overnight

E = A hospital patient who receives services in one or more of the hospital's facilities when he or she is not currently an inpatient or home care patient.

B = A patient born in the hospital at the beginning of the current patient hospitalization

F = An acute-care facility's formal acceptance of a patient who is to be provided with room, board, and continuous nursing service in an area of the facility where patients generally stay overnight

G = The termination of hospitalization through the formal release of an inpatient by the hospital

A = The unit of measure denoting the services received by one inpatient in one 24-hour period; it is often referred to in the shortened version of patient day

D = Indicates the number of patients present in the healthcare facility at a particular point in time

3. 247

5.

Date	Number of patients discharged	Discharge days	Average length of stay
June 2	16	89	5.56
June 3	22	119	5.41
June 4	12	54	4.5
June 5	19	105	5.53
June 6	15	45	3
June 7	24	118	4.92
June 8	18	68	3.78

Check Your Understanding 16.3

1.

	Gross death rate	Net death rate
City Hospital reported 49 deaths in June. There were 489 discharges. Eight of those deaths occurred within 48 hours of admission.	10.02%	8.52%
County Hospital reported 62 deaths in May. There were 524 discharges. Seventeen of those deaths occurred within 48 hours of admission.	11.83%	8.88%

Check Your Understanding 16.4

1. C

3. D

5. D

7. A

9. D

Chapter 17

Check Your Understanding 17.1

1. B

3. B

5. A

Check Your Understanding 17.2

1. A

3. B

5. C

Check Your Understanding 17.3

1. B

3. C

5. B

Check Your Understanding 17.4

1. C

3. D

5. A

Chapter 18

Check Your Understanding 18.1

1. A pie chart uses area to present data. The area of each group presented in a pie chart must be compared to understand which group represents a higher and lower proportion of the whole.

3. False. Graphical techniques can be ranked based on the most accurate presentation methods. The most accurate method to graph an object is position along a common scale.

Check Your Understanding 18.2

1. A table presenting the cholesterol levels would be preferred since the task requires the patient to identify a discrete value.

3. A

5. True

Check Your Understanding 18.3

1. B

3. C

5. D

Chapter 19

Check Your Understanding 19.1

1. False. This statement defines research methodology.

3. False. This statement defines a theory.

5. True

Check Your Understanding 19.2

1. False. The first component is defining the research question. This statement represents the third component.

3. False. This statement defines the problem statement.

5. False. Using a research model is a good practice because research models show all the factors and relationships of a theory.

Check Your Understanding 19.3

1. True

3. False. While information sources can be printed publications, they can also be audiovisual and electronic media.

5. True

7. True

9. False. Synthesis makes sense of all the details to create information by comparing and contrasting results of previous studies, critically evaluating previous studies' methods and analytical tools, interpreting the findings, and drawing conclusions about the information presented by previous articles.

Check Your Understanding 19.4

1. True

3. False. Positive relationships move in the same direction. In this case, if the relationship were positive the supervisor's feelings of personal efficacy would increase, not decrease.

5. False. Variables that reflect the outcome of the research's interventions are the dependent variables. Dependent variables reflect the results that the researcher theorizes. Independent variables, on the other hand, are the antecedent or prior factors upon which the outcomes depend.

Check Your Understanding 19.5

1. False. Sample surveys collect data from representative members of a population. Census surveys collect data from all members of a population.

3. True

5. True

Check Your Understanding 19.6

1. False. Being able to apply results to other types of healthcare organizations is external validity.

3. False. Developing an instrument takes time and selecting an instrument with established validity and reliability is easier.

5. True

7. True

9. False. A pilot study assists both experienced and unexperienced researchers in working out logistical details and, thereby, enhances the likelihood of their research's successful completion.

Check Your Understanding 19.7

1. True

3. False. Qualitative analytical softwares assist researchers in their data analysis. The researchers are deriving the keywords, categories, and the logical relationships from their data.

5. False. For an audience of practitioners, researchers should focus on their actual findings or implications for practice—in this case, the "take home message."

Check Your Understanding 19.8

1. False. Researchers who conduct secondary analyses must comply with HIPAA, other applicable rules and regulations, and the policies of the source of the data.

3. True

5. False. All paper records have not been digitized.

Chapter 20

Check Your Understanding 20.1

1. The Nuremberg Code outlines research ethics to guide the conduct of research involving human subjects. It was developed during the trials of Nazi war criminals following World War II. Its basic tenets are that informed consent is essential, research should be based on prior animal work, and the risks should be justified by the anticipated benefits.

3. Respect for persons

5. A summary of the changes include: broadening protections for research subjects, such as more focused informed consent documents that are shorter and clearer; and a focus on more oversight for those studies that hold more risk for the research subject and less oversight on those that pose less risk.

Check Your Understanding 20.2

1. Research that is exempt does not mean that the researchers have no ethical obligations to the participants, but that the regulatory requirements such as informed consent and yearly renewal from the IRB do not apply to this type of research. The IRB still reviews research protocols to determine their exempt status. Examples include:

   - Educational settings (45 CFR 46.101(b)(1))
   - Use of educational tests, surveys, interviews, or observation (45 CFR 46.101 (b)(2))
   - Use of educational tests, surveys, interviews, or observation (45 CFR 46.101 (b)(3))
   - Research involving the collection or study of existing data, documents, records, pathological specimens, or diagnostic specimens (45 CFR 46.101 (b)(4))
   - Research and demonstration projects that are conducted by or subject to the approval of department or agency heads, and are designed to study, evaluate, or otherwise examine (45 CFR 46.101 (b)(5))
   - Taste and food quality evaluation and consumer acceptance studies (45 CFR 46.101 (b)(6))

3. False. The researcher, the research sponsor, and/or the organization in which the research is conducted are not exculpable for any harm caused to the human subject.

5. True

Check Your Understanding 20.3

1. The HIPAA Privacy Rule protects medical records and other individually identifiable information from disclosure. It informs human subjects about how information about them will be used or disclosed. It also outlines their rights to access the information.

3. Common types of research designs include epidemiological studies, case-control studies, cohort studies, cross-sectional study, and clinical trials.

5. In case-control studies, groups are defined on the basis of an outcome and then assessed on the basis of past exposure to possible risk factors. Case-control studies are quick and easy to conduct and inexpensive. However, because a case-control study is a retrospective study, recall bias may be a limitation or disadvantage of this type of study design.

7. Relative risk is a ratio that compares the risk of disease or the incidence rate between two groups; it is also referred to as risk ratio.

Check Your Understanding 20.4

1. The purpose of the measures developed by the NCQA is to provide purchasers of healthcare, primarily employers, with information about the cost and effectiveness of organizations with which they contract for services. The Joint Commission measures also are designed primarily to encourage organizations to improve their own performance and to provide a comprehensive picture of the care provided within the organization.

3. A priority of the National Quality Strategy in Person and Family-Centered Care is to increase the use of EHRs by integrating patient-generated data in EHRs and routinely measuring patient engagement, self-management, shared decision making, and patient-reported outcomes. One of its indicators for doing this is to collect the percentage of patients asked for feedback. This is an example of how the EHR will be used to demonstrate at what rate the patient is involved in his or her care, and patient-centered outcomes research will be a major component in this data analysis.

5. Patient-centered outcomes research will include research that is most important to the patient and will include data elements related to survival, functional status, and health-related quality of life, and such, instead of just clinical data elements collected by investigators. It will also ask questions most important to patients such as: What are the benefits and harms related to different treatment options provided?

Chapter 21

Check Your Understanding 21.1

1. D
3. D
5. D

Check Your Understanding 21.2

1. D
3. A
5. D

Check Your Understanding 21.3

1. Patient function, quality of life, patient satisfaction, and mortality

3. AHRQ is the sponsor of HCUP. HCUP is a robust online query system that provides instant access to the largest set of all payer healthcare databases that are publicly available. It can be used to identify, track, analyze, and compare trends in hospital care at the national, regional and state levels.

5. Four types of AHRQ quality indicators are
   - Prevention indicators identify hospital admissions that could have been avoided through high quality outpatient care.
   - Inpatient indicators reflect the quality of care inside hospitals, including inpatient mortality for medical conditions and surgical procedures.
   - Patient safety indicators reflect quality of care inside hospitals focusing on potentially avoidable complications and iatrogenic events.
   - Pediatric indicators use one or more of the previous three indicators and adapt them for use with children and neonates.

Check Your Understanding 21.4

1. A
3. D
5. C

Chapter 22

Check Your Understanding 22.1

1. The acceptance and popularity of management ideas is related to how easily they are understood, evidence present to support them, continuity with previous ideas, and ability to more effectively solve problems. In other cases, a promise of a quick fix has led to premature adoption and higher expectations.

3. In many cases, the companies became too impressed with their successes and stayed with the strategy that initially provided success. They did not attend to the changing market and need to continually revise their approaches.

5. Use grid paper to break the project down into discrete steps. On the upper line of the chart, designate the days over time to complete the project. Then draw a bar from the beginning to the end of each task as the tasks progress across the time grid.

Check Your Understanding 22.2

1. As you review the job description, categorize each task description as conceptual, interpersonal, and technical. Given the level of the job (front-line, supervisor, middle management, and so forth) estimate the percentage of each type of skills.

3. Quality can mean fewer errors, meeting or exceeding customer expectations, sophistication of the product, satisfaction with the service, and such. If, for example, you were interested in the quality of your data entry, a metric might be the number of errors per hour, or time taken to enter information.

5. Ask a manager to list the job description or tasks done throughout the week. Then go back and code each one according to their match with Mintzberg's roles. Notice any differences in which tasks and roles are more prominent.

Check Your Understanding 22.3

1. Indications of cohesion include: team members may be unwilling to listen to outside or divergent opinions or sanction those who express them; they are highly unified in a strategy without considering possible risks; they have excessive certainty that they will succeed; individuals feel pressure to conform to the group's decision.

3. A diverse team is more likely to approach a problem from different perspectives; wider representation on a team makes acceptance and trust more likely by other stakeholders; they are less susceptible to groupthink; different cohort experiences and different values add perspectives to problem solving and often better choices; low levels of conflict can help identify real issues as well as highlight important value differences.

5. Suggestions may include: Bring in external experts, evaluate team interactions and decision making effectiveness, assign members to other teams so their team identity is more diffused, have the leader attend late so the team can discuss its own decisions without undue leader influence, and such.

Check Your Understanding **22.4**

1. Identify two different situations such as your work team and sports team. Under each, list your personal traits and skills, placing a plus or minus next to each depending whether it is an advantage or disadvantage on that particular team.

3. Make two columns—one for effective and one for ineffective. Identify the situation in which you are evaluating the leader and then list their characteristics.

5. Start with a decision and the circumstances driving it. Draw and connect the subsequent events or ripple effects that are impacted by the decision. When possible, identify feedback loops that go back to a previous stage and have implications for the decision.

7. Adding people to a late project is a good intention, but adding them requires training and orientation time, may not merge with group interpersonal processes, will probably have an initial error rate, will require time to master the task, and may create a further unintended delay in completion.

9. You might find examples of what appeared to be simple problems but were, in fact, more complex and produced unexpected and adverse consequences. You might also explain that what may be a solution in one limited context, may create problems further down the chain of actions in the organization, or later in time.

Check Your Understanding **22.5**

1. Each of the roles involves a special skill at a key time period in innovation. The inventor role occurs when the idea is created, but the inventor may not have the skill or authority to move further with it. The champion role is important and next in sequence since it involves recognition of the value of the idea and provides resources for development. The sponsor provides authority and legitimacy, while the final role of critic ensures that it is thought through clearly.

3. Each adopter group is motivated by different values and outcomes. By identifying each one and their unique needs, the innovation can be presented in ways that is meaningful to them and engenders less resistance to the innovation.

5. People need time to think about a change and consider how it affects their lifestyle, habits, and work. Some people are not as current regarding emerging ideas and information and take longer to hear about it. Still others may be aware of it but resist change or don't feel sufficient support for the adoption.

Check Your Understanding **22.6**

1. People may resist change due to not knowing what will happen to their jobs, whether they will lose prestige or turf, they feel they have lost control, don't have time to get used to the change, the change is suddenly presented without warning, concerns about competence, feel overwhelmed with the prospect of more work, and such. For all of these reasons, managers and leaders need to prepare them early for change, let them know what will be the same and what will be different, reassure them that they will get through the change, provide training for new skills, and such.

3. People may react with anxiety regarding whether they are qualified for the new position; they may wonder whether they are targeted to be forced out; they may take it as a message to look elsewhere for a job. Management can reduce the stress by explaining why the position is being restructured, identify the skills that are required, and holding information sessions on the pending change.

Chapter 23

Check Your Understanding **23.1**

1. True

3. False. This reporting requirement is part of the Occupational Safety and Health Act.

5. They provide key guidelines for managing compensation and benefits.

Check Your Understanding **23.2**

1. True

3. False. Individuals applying for professional level positions must submit a resume and a cover letter.

5. True

7. One can delegate authority but not responsibility.

Check Your Understanding 23.3

1. True

3. False. Federal regulations specify exemptions from some or all of the FLSA provisions for several groups of employees; they are called exempt employees and are paid a salary per pay period.

5. True

7. True

9. Grievance taken to the highest levels for resolution will likely be resolved through mediation and arbitration.

Chapter 24

Check Your Understanding 24.1

1. Training refers to content that develops entry-level skills; development is associated with continuing employee development and upgrading competencies to prepare for increased career opportunities.

3. Among the items to consider when designing a training program are the curriculum, budget, who will teach the program, materials to be developed, location, and method of delivery.

5. Outcomes of the needs analysis include:

   - An understanding of where training is needed in the organization
   - A list of the tasks to be learned at each level (entry-level, remedial, and management development)
   - An analysis of the deficiencies in employee knowledge and skills (accomplished by a comparison of desired and current levels of competence)

7. Feedback provides important communication with those involved in the training program in order to maintain interest and support.

Check Your Understanding 24.2

1. The purposes of the employee orientation program are to introduce employees to the:

   - Organization's mission, policies, rules, and culture
   - Department or workgroup
   - Specific job he or she will be performing

   The orientation program also provides a period of socialization in which the employee learns the values, behavior patterns, and expectations of the organization.

3. Orientation of overseas workers should include English proficiency, American etiquette, and cultural understanding, as well as quality standards such as turnaround time and performance expectations. In addition, training on HIPAA requirements and confidentiality are important.

5. The top two skills include electronic health record (EHR) management and skills in managing privacy and security.

Check Your Understanding 24.3

1. The five models are:

   - Sensory: Does the learner prefer to listen, read or practice in order to learn best?
   - Personality: One's personality traits affect how a person views the world
   - Information processing: People differ in how they receive and process information
   - Social interaction: Learning style differs by gender and social context
   - Instructional and environmental preference: The environment and its structure determine learning style

3. Motivation plays a role in developing a training program because individual employee needs vary and even a single employee may have needs that differ at different points in his or her life or career. By calling attention to the relevance of training to specific needs and connecting the knowledge learned with a work goal, training can be facilitated for each employee.

5. The best combination of learning methods is a combination of verbal instruction, demonstration, and hands-on experience.

Check Your Understanding 24.4

1. Factors that influence selection of a training method include:

   - Purpose of the training
   - Level of education and experience of the trainees
   - Amount of space, equipment, and media available for training
   - Number of trainees and their location
   - Cost of the method
   - Need for special accommodation due to disability or cultural differences

3. Mobile learning (m-learning) is effective for delivering multimedia information to a large number of people quickly and delivering key points and short updates. Participants can respond using social media or discussion. It is not effective for long courses with a large amount of material.

5. Distance learning removes training barriers associated with location and timing, both for individuals and groups. Learners can attend at a time and place of their choosing.

7. There are many ways that a healthcare organization can use an intranet to deliver training. Intranets are useful for distributing policies and procedures as well as for uploading educational courses for employee self-study. Electronic material can be installed and delivered to the employee's desktop or customized for specific needs.

9. Social networking sites can be used to share files or website bookmarks. Training materials can be distributed via blogs. A collaborative website can be built using wikis. MUVEs can simulate work environments and scenarios and can be used to practice role-play of leadership or anti-harassment situations.

Check Your Understanding 24.5

1. Managers can empower employees by:

   - Getting others involved in selecting their work assignments and methods for accomplishing tasks
   - Creating an environment of cooperation, information sharing, discussion, and shared ownership of goals
   - Encouraging others to take initiative and make decisions
   - When problems arise, finding out what others think and letting them help design solutions
   - Giving others the freedom to put their ideas and solutions into practice
   - Recognizing successes and encouraging high performance

3. Mentors are senior employees who work with employees early in their careers. Mentoring is a form of coaching in that it helps employees become self-sufficient but is usually done on a one-on-one basis. Mentors share their knowledge of management styles and teach interpersonal skills, primarily for future job advancement. A coach, on the other hand, may work with several employees at the same time and is concerned more with helping them do the best job they can in their current job by removing obstacles and offering suggestions.

5. Hospitals are required to train employees in fire safety and other job-related safety measures to reduce unsafe practices.

Chapter 25

Check Your Understanding 25.1

1. Space may need to be redesigned if new technology requiring a new workflow is implemented; if employees begin to work remotely freeing up individual workspace yet requiring temporary space; and if the work area needs to move per the master facility plan. Also space may need to be redesigned if there is a change in number of staff, a shift in staff functions, or there are new functions or methods of doing work.

3. The fundamental elements that must be addressed in good work environment planning are workflow, space, equipment, aesthetics, and ergonomics.

5. Lighting should be sufficiently bright; exposure to natural light is easiest on the eyes, desk or task lighting is more physically supportive than overhead fluorescent lighting. Glare from light or PC screens should be avoided. Color influences how people feel; for instance, neutral colors have a calming effect. Certain kinds of music can reduce tension and sound proofing can keep an office less noisy; carpeting, drapes, and partitioning all affect the noise level because they absorb sound. Air that is too warm or cold can be distracting, so temperature is also important for an effective work space.

Check Your Understanding 25.2

1. A service level agreement (SLA) includes the detail of what services are needed and the performance expectations, price and payment terms, reporting chain of command, terms for termination of the agreement, and confidentiality expectations of the vendor and vendor staff.

3. Work distribution analysis can reveal the following potential problem areas:

   - There is too much or too little job function specialization
   - There is duplication of efforts of functions
   - Some employees are overloaded while others do not have enough work to keep them busy
   - Large amounts of time are spent on functions of minor importance
   - Small amounts of time are spent on functions of key importance

5. Serial work division is the consecutive handling of tasks and products by individuals who perform a specific function in sequence, similar to an assembly line. Parallel work division is the concurrent handling of tasks; for example, each employee completes the function from start to finish and there may be several employees doing that function. Unit work division is when all staff perform a different specialized task at the same time; the tasks are not dependent on each other.

Check Your Understanding 25.3

1. True

3. False. Turnaround times and error rates are examples of qualitative standards.

5. True

Check Your Understanding 25.4

1. Preventive controls are put in place at the front end of a process to ensure an error isn't made, such as edits in a computer system or employee training. Feedback controls occur after a task is done offering information regarding the performance, such as an employee review or a customer satisfaction survey.

3. Performance measurement is the process of comparing the outcomes of an organization, work unit, or employee to pre-established performance standards. Performance measurement is a fundamental management activity that supports two basic functions of management—controlling and planning. The manager must ensure the work unit or organization is doing what it should be doing in the right way, and the manager must define the expectations of performance, the processes required to achieve those expectations, and the desired outcomes of performance.

5. Examples of changes to address performance issues could be additional staff training, modifications in

procedures, adjustments in workflow, revision of policies, or purchase of updated equipment.

Check Your Understanding 25.5

1. False. The components of an open, cybernetic system are input, process, output, controls and standards, feedback, and external environment.

3. True

5. False. The three goals of performance efforts are effectiveness, efficiency, and adaptability.

Check Your Understanding 25.6

1. False. An organization has many customers and sometimes the expectations of one group of customers conflict with those of another group. Nevertheless, the goal of CQI is an admirable one and should be pursued because it can only serve to improve an organization's performance.

3. True

5. False. Soft tools include tools as ground rules, a team agenda, a parking lot to track ideas, and progress reports.

Chapter 26

Check Your Understanding 26.1

1. The HIM department is responsible for the coding of the records. While this is important in the billing process, the actual claims are filed by the patient accounts department. Therefore, the insurance company should be referred to the patient accounts department for resolution. If there is an individual who is specifically responsible for handling billing audits, that individual is an appropriate referral. Part of the claims audit may involve a review of the medical records. In that case, the HIM department will provide access to the records in the department, if necessary.

3. This is not a good strategy as it violates the matching principle (figure 26.2). While the hospital should certainly make every effort to capture all of the associated expenses for this fiscal year, next year's expenses must be booked next year. If some of next year's expenses are actually paid this year, they would not be booked as expenses but rather as assets under the heading prepaid expenses.

5. Purely on the basis of the information in this chapter, yes, the hospital can sell these services. The hospital would book nonoperating revenue. However, a not-for-profit hospital may potentially incur income tax

liability—a problem if the revenue is substantial, since the income is unrelated to its main business.

Check Your Understanding 26.2

1. 50/600 = 0.083 or 8.3%

3. The three key reports are the income statement, statement of retained earnings, and balance sheet.

   The income statement includes revenues and expenses. The statement of retained earnings expresses the change in retained earnings from the beginning of the balance sheet period to the end. The balance sheet lists the major account categories grouped under their equation headings—assets, liabilities, and equity and fund balance—and employs the equation: assets = liabilities + fund balance.

5. The best ratio to use for this analysis is the current ratio—an organization's ability to pay current liabilities with current assets is important to lenders. Current assets implicitly will be (or could be) converted to cash at some point within a year, either through collections, sales, or other business activity. The current ratio compares total current assets with total current liabilities.

Check Your Understanding 26.3

1. Direct costs are directly traceable to a specific product or service. Examples in healthcare include medications and nursing care that is directly traceable to a patient. Indirect costs are incurred in the process of providing goods and services and are difficult or impossible to trace to a patient. Examples of indirect costs include human resource department expenses, marketing expenses and janitorial services. Fixed costs remain the same despite changes in volume and examples include mortgage payments and copy machine depreciation expense. Variable expenses are sensitive to volume and examples include medication and nursing staff time. Direct costs can be classified as either fixed or variable while indirect costs are often fixed.

3. Three types of internal controls are preventive, detective, and corrective controls. Preventive controls are designed to stop an error before it happens. Detective controls are designed to find errors that have already been made. Corrective controls are designed to correct problems after they have been detected.

5. The four methods of allocation of overhead are

   - Direct method of cost allocation distributes the cost of overhead departments solely to the revenue-producing areas. Allocation is based on each revenue-producing area's relative square footage, number of employees, or actual usage of supplies and services.

   - Step-down allocation distributes overhead costs once beginning with the area that provides the least amount of nonrevenue-producing services.

   - Double distribution allocates overhead costs twice, which takes into consideration the fact that some overhead departments provide services to each other.

   - Simultaneous equations method distributes overhead costs through multiple iterations allowing maximum distribution of interdepartmental costs among overhead departments.

Check Your Understanding 26.4

1. Both branches of accounting deal with the recording, reporting, and analysis of transactions. However, financial accounting focuses on the financial statements and the needs of the users of those statements; and managerial accounting focuses on internal measurements of financial performance, such as budgets.

3. Preventive, corrective, and detective controls.

5. This is a favorable variance, since the payroll amount is actually less than budgeted. However, for a complete analysis, other line items, such as temporary employees and consulting expenses, must be analyzed. For example, a $2,000 favorable payroll variance due to the resignation of a coder may be offset by a $3,000 consulting fee for temporary coding services.

Chapter 27

Check Your Understanding 27.1

1. Organizations create projects as a temporary structure to initiate a change to processes, services, or products.

3. Projects are unique and temporary with a specific goal while operations are ongoing actions designed around consistency.

5. Expense projects have a goal of decreasing the cost of operating the organization.

7. No. While some compliance projects may yield a cost savings or increase revenue, the true purpose of a compliance project is to deliver the change needed to satisfy the internal or external expectations.

Check Your Understanding 27.2

1. The scope is the collection of work to be completed as part of the project effort and may include new or revised processes, products, or services.

3. The project champion is a senior executive who aligns the project with the organization's goals, ensures

continued organizational support for the project, and works with the project manager to secure resources needed to meet the project goals.

5. The stakeholders are the individuals who have an interest in the project. The individuals consist of the project team, project champion, end users of the project deliverables, and anyone else who will be affected by the project outcomes.

Check Your Understanding 27.3

1. In a purely functional organization the manager controls the resources and operates independently of other departments. Projects may exist within the department but this structure is challenged by projects requiring coordination across departments. In cross-departmental projects, the project coordination takes place across all managers contributing to the project. Each manager directly controls and directs the resources within the department.

3. Strong matrix organizations include a functional area dedicated to project management. This group is responsible for managing projects across other departments. In the

weak matrix organization, a member of an operational department is tasked with leading a project. Strong matrix organizations include project management as an area of specialty while weak matrix organizations view project management as a part-time need.

5. A distributed team consists of team members who work in different locations. These different locations may be on different floors within the same building, different buildings within the same city, or in different cities across the country or across the world. Distributed teams rely on several forms of communication outside of in-person meetings to collaborate on the project.

Check Your Understanding 27.4

1. An administrative supervisor is responsible for hiring, promoting, and firing an employee and, as a result, has direct authority over the employee. On the other hand, a functional supervisor has no direct authority over the employee and only provides direction and supervision over the work performed. In the project setting, a team member continues to report to the administrative supervisor while working under the direction of the functional supervisor.

3. Organizations are separated by layers of management and functional silos. These boundaries form islands of groups with a specific operational focus. These islands allow the groups to specialize a specific function but make it challenging to communicate and coordinate work with other areas. Project management is used to cross these boundaries and coordinate work and communications across the layers of management and functional silos.

5. The organization experience provides the project manager with the context for the project. The project is executed within the organization and is affected by the politics, sources of power, established formalized and informal processes, and the culture of the organization. Experience working within the organization provides the environmental awareness needed to support the project manager's actions and decisions.

Check Your Understanding 27.5

1. The major deliverables in the initiating process group are the project charter and the scope, budget, and schedule baseline estimates.

3. The major deliverables for the executing process group are the project product deliverables that are a part of the project's scope.

5. The major deliverables for the closing process group are the outcomes from the lessons learned reflection and the archived project artifacts.

Check Your Understanding 27.6

1. Scope creep slowly increases the project scope and does not allow for supporting resources and time to deliver the increased scope. This may result in a project exceeding the planned budget and schedule.

3. An increased scope requires more work to be performed to complete the additional scope. This additional work increases the resources and time needed to complete the new work and results in increased resources and schedule.

5. A formalized changer order process allows the project team to recognize and react to changes to the project scope. The project team is then able to renegotiate the project budget and project schedule based on the new scope items included in the change request.

Check Your Understanding 27.7

1. The project goals from the operational perspective of executing the project are complete delivery of the scope, resource spending within the planned budget, and project completion on or before the targeted completion date. In other words, delivering the entire scope, on time and within budget.

3. A program consists of a set of related projects where each project contributes the changes needed for a larger program change.

5. A portfolio is a collection of projects and programs. Unlink a program, the subparts are not always related. The portfolio's projects and programs may fall within a specific area of the organization or may include all of the organization's projects and programs.

Chapter 28

Check Your Understanding 28.1

1. Principles that explain the ways in which ethical decisions are made are altruism, autonomy, beneficence, consequentialism, deontology, egoism, least harm, and utilitarianism.

3. Prejudice, stereotyping, and bias affect one's cultural competence.

5. An organization should assess the availability of interpreter services, effectiveness of cultural and linguistic competency training for staff, and differences in services among diverse populations.

Check Your Understanding 28.2

1. Blanket authorization. Issues include the potential of someone finding out about a diagnosis that they did not have before signing the release.

3. Examples of quality outcome problems due to the trends of keeping costs down while still providing quality services include: healthcare organizations falsifying their performance information to the public; negative patient outcomes, such as inattentive patient care; failure to ensure a physician's license is valid; when accreditation or licensure surveys occur, health records are hidden or not available to the surveyors; or repetition of unsuitable healthcare.

5. HIM professionals should provide directed practice opportunities for students.

Chapter 29

Check Your Understanding 29.1

1. A strategic plan spells out where an organization is going over the next 3 to 5 years and how it is going to get there.

3. True

5. True

Check Your Understanding 29.2

1. Four types of information that should be collected during the external environmental assessment phase include: forces of the healthcare industry, primary market research, market forecasts and implications, competitor analysis, collaborator identification, or assessment of market trends.

3. Three categories that are used to assess the possible levels of sources of uncertainty are clear trends, unknowns that are knowable, and residual uncertainty.

5. False. A SWOT analysis is both an internal analysis (strengths and weaknesses) and an external analysis (opportunities and threats) facing the organization.

Check Your Understanding 29.3

1. Characteristics of an effective vision statement are it: appeals to the long-term interests of the stakeholders; conveys a picture of what the future will look like; sets forth realistic and achievable goals; is clear enough to provide guidance in decision making; is flexible so that alternative strategies are possible as conditions change; and is easy to describe and communicate.

3. False. An organization's driving force can only be one of the 10 strategic areas, as this force is the most evident reason for the current and future success and focus of the organization.

5. True

Check Your Understanding 29.4

1. Important tools often used for strategic thinking include: scenario building and storytelling, contingency planning, brainstorming, nominal group technique, sensitivity analysis, simulation, decision analysis and game theory, and blue ocean strategy.

3. False. Often when reassessing products and services offered, what customers to serve, what industry markets to focus on and what geography to work in, one or all of these key areas may have changed as the future strategy of the organization has been identified.

5. True

Check Your Understanding 29.5

1. False. The implementation phase of strategic planning has been the weakest link in the process as often organizations either fail to provide adequate resources, capital, structure, or measurement to complete the strategic plan.

3. False. Measurement should be an ongoing process and key implementation plans should be measured either monthly or quarterly at a minimum.

5. C

Check Your Understanding 29.6

1. True

3. False. Implementation planning is an important part of the execution of the business plan.

5. False. For it to be successful, the implementation and planning process must engage all of the employees and leadership working together.

Glossary

A

A&C: Adults and children (in a daily census)

A&D: Patients who are admitted and discharged on the same day

Abbreviated Injury Scale (AIS): An anatomically-based, consensus-derived global severity scoring system that classifies each injury by region according to its relative importance on a 6-point ordinal scale (1 = minor and 6 = maximal). AIS is the basis for the Injury Severity Score (ISS) calculation of the multiply injured patient

Abstracting: 1. The process of extracting information from a document to create a brief summary of a patient's illness, treatment, and outcome 2. The process of extracting elements of data from a source document or database and entering them into an automated system

Abuse: Describes practices that, either directly or indirectly, result in unnecessary costs to the Medicare Program. Abuse includes any practice that is not consistent with the goals of providing patients with services that are medically necessary, meet professionally recognized standards, and are fairly priced

Accept the risk: Understanding that residual risk would exist as no additional controls would be implemented leaving some risk to the organization

Acceptance: In contract law, requires a meeting of the minds between the parties about terms that are sufficiently definite and complete

Accession number: A number assigned to each case as it is entered in a cancer registry

Accession registry: A list of cases in a cancer registry in the order in which they were entered

Accountability: 1. The state of being liable for a specific activity 2. All information is attributable to its source (person or device)

Accountable care organization (ACO): A legal entity that is recognized and authorized under applicable state, federal, or tribal law, is identified by a Taxpayer Identification Number (TIN), and is formed by one or more ACO participant(s) that is (are) defined at 425.102(a) and may also include any other ACO participants described at 425.102(b) (42 CFR 425.20 2011)

Accounting: 1. The process of collecting, recording, and reporting an organization's financial data 2. A list of all disclosures made of a patient's health information

Accounting of disclosure: 1. Under HIPAA, a standard that states (1) An individual has a right to receive an accounting of disclosures of protected health information made by a covered entity in the six years prior to the date on which the accounting is requested, except for disclosures: (i) To carry out treatment, payment, and health care operations as provided in 164.506; (ii) To individuals of protected health information about them as provided in 164.502; (iii) Incident to a use or disclosure otherwise permitted or required by this subpart, as provided in 164.502; (iv) Pursuant to an authorization as provided in 164.508; (v) For the facility's directory or to persons involved in the individual's care or other notification purposes as provided in 164.510; (vi) For national security or intelligence purposes as provided in 164.512(k)(2); (vii) To correctional institutions or law enforcement officials as provided in 164.512(k)(5); (viii) As part of a limited data set in accordance with 164.514(e); or (ix) That occurred prior to the compliance date for the covered entity (45 CFR 164.528 2002) 2. On May 31, 2011 a notice of proposed rule-making (NPRM) was issued that would modify the AOD standard. The purpose of these modifications is, in part, to implement the statutory requirement under the Health Information Technology for Economic and Clinical Health Act ("the HITECH Act" or "the Act") to require covered entities and business associates to account for disclosures of protected health information to carry out treatment, payment, and health care operations if such disclosures are through an electronic health record. Pursuant to both the HITECH Act and its more general authority under HIPAA, the department proposes to expand the accounting provision to provide individuals with the right to receive an access report indicating who has accessed electronic protected health information in a designated record set. Under its more general authority under HIPAA, the department also proposes changes to the existing accounting requirements to improve their workability and effectiveness

Accounting rate of return (ARR): The projected annual cash inflows, minus any applicable depreciation, divided by the initial investment

Accounts payable: Records of the payments owed by an organization to other entities

Accounts receivable (A/R) days: 1. Records of the payments owed to the organization by outside entities such as third-party payers and patients 2. Department in a healthcare facility that manages the accounts owed to the facility by customers who have received services but whose payment is made at a later date

Accreditation: 1. A voluntary process of institutional or organizational review in which a quasi-independent body created for this purpose periodically evaluates the quality of the entity's work against preestablished written criteria 2. A determination by an accrediting body that an eligible organization, network, program, group, or individual complies with applicable standards 3. The act of granting approval to a healthcare organization based on whether the organization has met a set of voluntary standards developed by an accreditation agency

Accreditation Association for Ambulatory Health Care: A professional organization that offers accreditation programs for ambulatory and outpatient organizations such as single-specialty and multispecialty group practices, ambulatory surgery centers, college/university health services, and community health centers

Accrue: The process of recording known transactions in the appropriate time period before cash payments/receipts are expected or due

Acquittal: Lack of proven guilt

Activity-based budget: A budget based on activities or projects rather than on functions or departments

Acute care: Medical care of a limited duration that is provided in an inpatient hospital setting to diagnose and treat an injury or a short-term illness

Acute-care prospective payment system: The Medicare reimbursement methodology system referred to as the inpatient prospective payment system (IPPS). Hospital providers subject to the IPPS utilize the Medicare severity diagnosis-related groups (MS-DRGs) classification system, which determines payment rates

ADDIE model: Training and development method that is defined as Analyze, Design, Develop, Implement, Evaluate

Addressable standards: As amended by HITECH, the implementation specifications of the HIPAA Security Rule that are designated "addressable" rather than "required"; to be in compliance with the rule, the covered entity must implement the specification as written, implement an alternative, or document that the risk for which the addressable implementation specification was provided either does not exist in the organization, or exists with a negligible probability of occurrence (45 CFR 164.306 2013)

Adhesion contract: A contract provision that places a healthcare provider in a significant position of power over a patient who relies on the provider's services may be against public policy

Administrative applications: Application that must also connect to EHR systems include admission, discharge, transfer (R-ADT); enterprise master patient index or master patient index (EMPI or MPI); encoders, chart tracking, chart deficiency management, release of information; order communication/results reporting (OC/RR); quality assurance (QA), including core measures abstracting (which pulls specified, quality-related data from health records for reporting to the Joint Commission and Centers for Medicare and Medicaid Services); and many others

Administrative data: Coded information contained in secondary records, such as billing records, describing patient identification, diagnoses, procedures, and insurance

Administrative law: A body of rules and regulations developed by various administrative entities empowered by Congress; falls under the umbrella of public law

Administrative management theory: A subdivision of classical management theory that emphasizes the total organization rather than the individual worker and delineates the major management functions

Administrative metadata: This type of metadata is programmed to be generated by the information technology and provides information about how and when data were created and used; it also is a record of the instructions given to users about actions to be taken with the information technology and what the user response was

Administrative safeguards: Under HIPAA, are administrative actions and policies and procedures, to manage the selection, development, implementation, and maintenance of security measures to protect electronic protected health information and to manage the conduct of the covered entity's or business associate's workforce in relation to the protection of that information (45 CFR 164.304 2013)

Administrative services only (ASO) contract: An agreement between an employer and an insurance organization to administer the employer's self-insured health plan

Administrative supervisor: The supervisor from the functional area to where the employee reports

Administrative system: System that controls governmental administrative operations and operates through federal and state administrative agencies that enact regulations

Admit-discharge-transfer (ADT): The name given to software systems used in healthcare facilities that register and track patients from admission through discharge including transfers; usually interfaced with other systems used throughout a facility such as an electronic health record or lab information system

Adoption: Refers to the stage where every intended user is fully using the basic functionality of the system

Advance directive: A legal, written document that describes the patient's preferences regarding future healthcare or stipulates the person who is authorized to make medical decisions in the event the patient is incapable of communicating his or her preferences

Adverse determination: Occurs when a health care insurer denies payment for proposed or already rendered healthcare service

Affinity grouping: A technique for organizing similar ideas together in natural groupings

Age Discrimination in Employment Act (1967): The federal act that states, it is unlawful for an employer to discriminate against an individual in any aspect of employment because that individual is 40 years old or older, unless one of the statutory exceptions applies. Favoring an older individual over a younger individual because of age is not unlawful discrimination under the ADEA, even if the younger individual is at least 40 years old. However, the ADEA does not require employers to prefer older individuals and does not affect applicable state, municipal, or local laws that prohibit such preferences

Agency for Healthcare Research and Quality (AHRQ): The branch of the US Public Health Service that supports general health research and distributes research findings and treatment guidelines with the goal of improving the quality, appropriateness, and effectiveness of healthcare services

Agile approach: The project life cycle is repeated in many iterations

Aggregate data: Data extracted from individual health records and combined to form de-identified information about groups of patients that can be compared and analyzed

All patient diagnosis-related group (AP-DRG): A case-mix system developed by 3M and used in a number of state reimbursement systems to classify non-Medicare discharges for reimbursement purposes

All-patient refined diagnosis-related group (APR-DRG): An expansion of the inpatient classification system that includes four distinct subclasses (minor, moderate, major, and extreme) based on the severity of the patient's illness

Allied health professional: A credentialed healthcare worker who is not a physician, nurse, psychologist, or pharmacist (for example, a physical therapist, dietitian, social worker, or occupational therapist)

Allied Health Reinvestment Act (2005): Legislation that encourages individuals to seek and complete high-quality allied health education and training programs by providing funding for their schooling

Alternative hypothesis: A hypothesis that states that there is an association between independent and dependent variables

Altruism: The belief that other people are more important than an individual person, wherein a personal sacrifice must take place

Ambulatory care: Preventive or corrective healthcare services provided on a nonresident basis in a provider's office, clinic setting, or hospital outpatient setting

Ambulatory surgery center (ASC): Under Medicare, an outpatient surgical facility that has its own national identifier; is a separate entity with respect to its licensure, accreditation, governance, professional supervision, administrative functions, clinical services, recordkeeping, and financial and accounting systems; has as its sole purpose the provision of services in connection with surgical procedures that do not require inpatient hospitalization; and meets the conditions and requirements set forth in the Medicare Conditions of Participation

American College of Radiology: Accredits radiology facilities and offers accreditation programs in CT, MRI, breast MRI, nuclear medicine and PET as mandated under the Medicare Improvements for Patients and Providers Act as well as for modalities mandated under the Mammography Quality Standards Act

Americans with Disabilities Act of 1990 (ADA): Federal legislation which ensures equal opportunity for and elimination of discrimination against persons with disabilities (Public Law 110-325 2008)

Analog: Data or information that is *not* represented in an encoded, computer-readable format

Analysis: Review of health record for proper documentation and adherence to regulatory and accreditation standards

Ancillary systems: Clinical department applications that include laboratory information systems (LISs), radiology information systems (RISs), pharmacy information systems, and others

Anti-Kickback Statute (AKS): Statute that makes knowingly offering, paying, soliciting, or receiving any remuneration that rewards referrals for services reimbursable by a Federal program a criminal offense

Answer: Response prepared by the defendant or attorney on the defendant's behalf

Apology statute: Also known as "I'm Sorry" laws, these statutes protect a healthcare provider's apology from being admitted into evidence during a court proceeding as an admission of liability

Appellate court: Courts that hear appeals on final judgments of the state trial courts or federal trial courts

Application service provider (ASP): A third-party service company that delivers, manages, and remotely hosts standardized applications software via a network through an outsourcing contract based on fixed, monthly usage, or transaction-based pricing

Applied research: A type of research that focuses on the use of scientific theories to improve actual practice, as in medical research applied to the treatment of patients

Arbitration: A proceeding in which disputes are submitted to a third party or a panel of experts outside the judicial trial system

Arithmetic mean: The sum of all of the numbers in a group of data is divided by the number of items in that group of data

Arm's length transaction: A transaction in which parties are dealing from equal bargaining positions, neither party is subject to the other's control or dominant influence, and the transaction is treated with fairness, integrity, and legality

Arraign: To call before the court

Artifacts: Developed through architecture data management such as data models, use cases, data flow diagrams, and data dictionaries, these

abstractions and models are used describe data and the relationships among data and the processes they support

Assault: A deliberate threat, along with apparent ability, to cause contact with another person that either can either be offensive or cause physical harm

Assessment: The systematic collection and review of information pertaining to an individual who wants to receive healthcare services or enter a healthcare setting

Assets: The human, financial, and physical resources of an organization

Assumption of risk: The plaintiff who voluntarily places himself or herself at risk to a known or appreciated danger may not recover damages for injury resulting from the risk

Asynchronous: Not at the same time; web-based courses where learners and instructors interact through e-mail or discussion forums

Attributable risk (AR): A measure of the impact of a disease on a population (for example, measuring additional risk of illness as a result of exposure to a risk factor)

Attributes: 1. Data elements within an entity that become the column or field names when the entity relationship diagram is implemented as a relational database 2. Properties or characteristics of concepts; used in SNOMED CT to characterize and define concepts

Audioconferencing: A learning technique in which participants in different locations can learn together via telephone lines while listening to a presenter and looking at handouts or books

Audit: 1. A function that allows retrospective reconstruction of events, including who executed the events in question, why, and what changes were made as a result 2. To conduct an independent review of electronic system records and activities in order to test the adequacy and effectiveness of data security and data integrity procedures and to ensure compliance with established policies and procedures

Audit log: A chronological record of electronic system(s) activities that enables the reconstruction, review, and examination of the sequence of events surrounding or leading to each event or transaction from its beginning to end. Includes who performed what event and when it occurred

Audit trail: 1. A chronological set of computerized records that provides evidence of information system activity (log-ins and log-outs, file accesses)

used to determine security violations 2. A record that shows who has accessed a computer system, when it was accessed, and what operations were performed

Authentication: 1. The process of identifying the source of health record entries by attaching a handwritten signature, the author's initials, or an electronic signature 2. Proof of authorship that ensures, as much as possible, that log-ins and messages from a user originate from an authorized source 3. As amended by HITECH, means the corroboration that a person is the one claimed (45 CFR 164.304 2013)

Authenticity: The genuineness of a record, that it is what it purports to be; information is authentic if proven to be immune from tampering and corruption

Authority: The right to make decisions and take actions necessary to carry out assigned tasks

Authorization: 1. As amended by HITECH, except as otherwise specified, a covered entity may not use or disclose protected health information without an authorization that is valid under section 164.508 2. When a covered entity obtains or receives a valid authorization for its use or disclosure of protected health information, such use or disclosure must be consistent with the authorization (45 CFR 164.508 2013)

Autocratic leadership: Leadership where the manager makes decisions without others' input and gives very specific direction

Automated drug dispensing machines: System that makes drugs available for patient care

Automated forms-processing (e-forms) technology: Technology that allows users to electronically enter data into online digital forms and electronically extract data from online digital forms for data collection or manipulation

Autonomy: A core ethical principle centered on the individual's right to self-determination that includes respect for the individual; in clinical applications, the patient's right to determine what does or does not happen to him or her in terms of healthcare

Autopsy: The postmortem examinations of the organs and tissues of a body to determine the cause of death or pathological conditions

Avatar: Created representation of a user in a multiuser virtual environment

Average daily census: The mean number of hospital inpatients present in the hospital each day for a given period of time

B

Balance sheet: A report that shows the total dollar amounts in accounts, expressed in accounting equation format, at a specific point in time

Balanced Budget Refinement Act (BBRA) of 1999: Mandated the establishment of a per-discharge, DRG-based PPS for longer-term care hospitals beginning October 1, 2002

Balanced matrix organization: In this organizational structure, a project organization exists within the existing functional hierarchy and a project manager is recruited from one of the functional departments to serve as the leader of the project

Balanced scorecard (BSC) methodology: A strategic planning tool that identifies performance measures related to strategic goals

Bar plot: Used for presenting data as a position along a common scale

Barcoding technology: A method of encoding data that consists of parallel arrangements of dark elements, referred to as bars, and light elements, referred to as spaces, and interpreting the data for automatic identification and data collection purposes

Basic interoperability: Relates to the ability to successfully transmit and receive data from one computer to another

Basic research: A type of research that focuses on the development and refinement of theories

Battery: The intentional and nonconsensual touching of another person's body

Bed turnover rate: The average number of times a bed changes occupants during a given period of time

Behavioral description interview: An interview format that requires applicants to give specific examples of how they have performed a specific procedure or handled a specific problem in the past

Benchmarking: The systematic comparison of the products, services, and outcomes of one organization with those of a similar organization; or the systematic comparison of one organization's outcomes with regional or national standards

Benchmarks: A comparison of one's own results of measure and performance statistics with the results of other individuals, departments, or organizations

Beneficence: A legal term that means promoting good for others or providing services that benefit others, such as releasing health information that will help a patient receive care or will ensure payment for services received

Benefits realization: The point in time when the organization believes all end users are trained, the system has gone live, and there has been some period of time to get acclimated and adopt as much of the process changes and functionality as possible

Best of breed: A vendor strategy used when purchasing an EHR that refers to system applications that are considered the best in their class

Best of fit: A vendor strategy used when purchasing an EHR in which all the systems required by the healthcare facility are available from one vendor

Bias: Idea or notion that prevents a person from having an impartial judgment

Bibliographic database: Databases of published literature such as journals, magazines, newspaper articles, books, book chapters, and other information sources

Big data: Data sets so large and complex that new tools for analysis are required

Bill hold period: The span of time during which a bill is suspended in the billing system awaiting late charges, diagnosis or procedure codes, insurance verification, or other required information

Biomedical research: The process of systematically investigating subjects related to the functioning of the human body

Biometric authentication: Allows a user to be uniquely identified and access the system based on one or more biometric traits such as fingerprints, hand geometry, retinal pattern, or voice waves

Biotechnology: The field devoted to applying the techniques of biochemistry, cellular biology, biophysics, and molecular biology to addressing practical issues related to human beings, agriculture, and the environment

Blanket authorization: The patient signs an authorization allowing the ROI specialist to release any and all information from that point forward

Blended learning: A training strategy that uses a combination of techniques—such as lecture, web-based training, or programmed text—to appeal to a variety of learning styles and maximize the advantages of each training method

Blogs: Web logs that provide a web page where users can post text, images, and links to other websites

Boxplot: Displays the descriptive statistics of a continuous variable including the minimum, first quartile, medium, third quartile, maximum, and potential outlier values

Brainstorming: A group problem-solving technique that involves the spontaneous contribution of ideas from all members of the group

Breach: Under HITECH, the acquisition, access, use, or disclosure of protected health information in a manner not permitted under subpart E of this part that compromises the security or privacy of the protected health information (45 CFR 164.402 2013)

Breach notification: As amended by HITECH, a covered entity shall, following the discovery of a breach of unsecured protected health information, notify each individual whose unsecured protected health information has been, or is reasonably believed by the covered entity to have been, accessed, acquired, used, or disclosed as a result of such breach (45 CFR 164.404 2013)

Breach Notification Rule: Requires covered entities and business associates to establish policies and procedures to investigate an unauthorized use or disclosure of protected health information to determine if a breach occurred, conclude the investigation, and to notify affected individuals and the secretary of the Department of Health and Human Services within 60 days of date of discovery of the breach

Breach of warranty: A broken promise where the plaintiff must show there was an express or implied warranty

Bring your own device: Refers to personal devices that are allowed to be used within a healthcare organization and interact with electronic protected health information (ePHI)

Brooks' Law: States adding people actually slows down team productivity due to different work styles, low team cohesion, and learning curve or orientation to the task time

Burden of proof: 1. A legal term that obligates an individual to prove or disprove a fact 2. Under HITECH, a covered entity or business associate, as applicable, shall have the burden of demonstrating that all notifications were made as required by this subpart or that the use or disclosure did not constitute a breach, as defined at 164.402 (45 CFR 164.414 2009)

Bureaucracy: A formal organizational structure based on a rigid hierarchy of decision making and inflexible rules and procedures

Business associate: 1. A person or organization other than a member of a covered entity's workforce that performs functions or activities on behalf of or affecting a covered entity that involve the use or disclosure of individually identifiable health information 2. As amended by HITECH, with respect to a covered entity, a person who creates, receives, maintains, or transmits PHI for a function or activity regulated by HIPAA, including claims processing or administration, data analysis, processing or administration, utilization review, quality assurance, patient safety activities, billing, benefit management, practice management, and repricing or provides legal, actuarial, accounting, consulting, data aggregation, management, administrative, accreditation, or financial services (45 CFR 160.103 2013)

Business associate agreement: As amended by HITECH, a contract between the covered entity and a business associate must establish the permitted and required uses and disclosures of protected health information by the business associate and provides specific content requirements of the agreement. The contract may not authorize the business associate to use or further disclose the information in a manner that would violate the requirements of HIPAA, and requires termination of the contract if the covered entity or business associate are aware of noncompliant activities of the other (45 CFR 164.504 2013)

Business case: An economic argument, or justification, usually for a capital expenditure

Business intelligence (BI): The end product or goal of knowledge management

Business process reengineering (BPR): The analysis and design of the workflow within and between organizations

Bylaws: Operating documents that describe the rules and regulations under which a healthcare organization operates

C

Cancer staging: The process of determining the size and extent of spread of the tumor throughout the body

Capital budget: Budget that focuses on long-term investments

Capitation: A specified amount of money paid to a health plan or doctor. This is used to cover the cost of a health plan member's healthcare services for a certain length of time

Cardinality: The maximum number of occurrences of each entity that occurrences of other entities can link to

Care coordination: The act of organizing patient care activities and sharing information among all of the participants concerned with a patient's care to achieve safer and more effective care

Care path: A care-planning tool similar to a clinical practice guideline that has a multidisciplinary focus emphasizing the coordination of clinical services

Career plan: A strategic plan for an individual, providing direction, goals, and an action plan to reach those goals

Case-control (retrospective) study: A study that investigates the development of disease by amassing volumes of data about factors in the lives of persons with the disease (cases) and persons without the disease

Case definition: A method of determining criteria for cases that should be included in a registry

Case finding: A method of identifying patients who have been seen or treated in a healthcare facility for the particular disease or condition of interest to the registry

Case management: 1. A process used by a doctor, nurse, or other health professional to manage a patient's healthcare 2. The ongoing, concurrent review performed by clinical professionals to ensure the necessity and effectiveness of the clinical services being provided to a patient

Case manager: A nurse, doctor, or social worker who arranges all services that are needed to give proper healthcare to a patient or group of patients

Case mix: 1. A description of a patient population based on any number of specific characteristics, including age, gender, type of insurance, diagnosis, risk factors, treatment received, and resources used 2. The distribution of patient into categories reflecting differences in severity of illness or resource consumption

Case-mix groups (CMGs): The 97 function-related groups into which inpatient rehabilitation facility discharges are classified on the basis of the patient's level of impairment, age, comorbidities, functional ability, and other factors

Case-mix group (CMG) relative weight: Factors that account for the variance in cost per discharge and resource utilization among case-mix groups

Case-mix index: The average relative weight of all cases treated at a given facility or by a given physician, which reflects the resource intensity or clinical severity of a specific group in relation to the other groups in the classification system; calculated by dividing the sum of the weights of diagnosis-related groups for patients discharged during a given period by the total number of patients discharged

Case study: A type of nonparticipant observation in which researchers investigate one person, one group, or one institution in depth

Categorically needy eligibility group: Categories of individuals to whom states must provide coverage under the federal Medicaid program

Causal relationship: A type of relationship in which one factor results in a change in another factor (cause and effect)

Causal-comparative research: A research design that resembles experimental research but lacks random assignment to a group and manipulation of treatment

Centralized model: In this model of health information exchange architecture, data are stored in a shared data repository

Centers for Medicare and Medicaid Services (CMS): The Department of Health and Human Services agency responsible for Medicare and parts of Medicaid. Historically, CMS has maintained the UB-92 institutional EMC format specifications, the professional EMC NSF specifications, and specifications for various certifications and authorizations used by the Medicare and Medicaid programs. CMS is responsible for the oversight of HIPAA administrative simplification transaction and code sets, health identifiers, and security standards. CMS also maintains the HCPCS medical code set and the Medicare Remittance Advice Remark Codes administrative code set

Certification: 1. The process by which a duly authorized body evaluates and recognizes an individual, institution, or educational program as meeting predetermined requirements 2. An evaluation performed to establish the extent to which a particular computer system, network design, or application implementation meets a prespecified set of requirements

Certified electronic health records technology (CEHRT): Standards used to inform technology vendors and providers about the functionality required to receive incentive payments for the implementation of EHR technology in the CMS EHR incentive program

Champion: An individual within an organization who believes in an innovation or change and promotes the idea by building financial and political support

Change agent: A specialist in organization development who facilitates the change brought about by the innovation

Change control: A formal process of documenting what change in an information system is needed, the rationale for the change, necessary approvals, when the change was made, who made the change, that related documentation has been updated to reflect the change, and that monitoring for a period of time was performed

Change driver: Large-scale forces such as demographic, social, political, economic, technical, and more recently, global and informational factors that require organizations to revise how they operate

Change management: The formal process of introducing change, getting it adopted, and diffusing it throughout the organization

Charge capture: The process of collecting all services, procedures, and supplies provided during patient care

Charge description master (CDM): A financial management form that contains information about the organization's charges for the healthcare services it provides to patients

Charitable immunity: A doctrine that shielded hospitals (as well as other institutions) from liability for negligence because of the belief that donors would not make contributions to hospitals if they thought their donation would be used to litigate claims combined with concern that a few lawsuits could bankrupt a hospital

Charity care: Services for which healthcare organizations did not expect payment because they had previously determined the patients' or clients' inability to pay

Chart conversion: An EHR implementation activity in which data from the paper chart are converted into electronic form

Charting by exception: A system of health record documentation in which progress notes focus on abnormal events and describe any interventions that were ordered and the patient's response

Check sheet: A data collection tool permitting the recording and compiling of observations or occurrences; it consists of a simple listing of categories, issues, or observations on the left side of the chart and a place on the right for individuals to record checkmarks next to the item when it is observed or counted

Chief executive officer (CEO): The senior manager appointed by a governing board to direct an organization's overall long-term strategic management

Chief information officer (CIO): The senior manager responsible for the overall management of information resources in an organization

Chief medical informatics officer (CMIO): Physicians who have special interest in health information systems and technology; they typically are practicing physicians who can put policy into practice

Chief nursing officer (CNO): The senior manager (usually a registered nurse with advanced education and extensive experience) responsible for administering patient care services

Chief technology officer (CTO): Individual responsible for overseeing current technology and creating relevant policy for its use

Children's Health Insurance Program (CHIP): (Title XXI of the Social Security Act) A program initiated by the BBA that allows states to expand existing insurance programs to cover children up to age 19; it provides additional federal funds to states so that Medicaid eligibility can be expanded to include a greater number of children

Cipher text: A text message that has been encrypted, or converted into code, to make it unreadable in order to conceal its meaning

Circuit: Geographic area covered by the US Court of Appeals

Circuit court: One of 13 federal appellate courts

Civil law: The branch of law involving court actions among private parties, corporations, government bodies, or other organizations, typically for the recovery of private rights with compensation usually being monetary

Civil Monetary Penalties Law: Authorizes the imposition of substantial civil money penalties against an entity that engages in activities including, but not limited to 1. knowingly presenting or causing to be presented a claim for services not provided as claimed or which is otherwise false or fraudulent in any way; 2. knowingly giving or causing to be given false or misleading information reasonably expected to influence the decision to discharge a patient; 3. offering or giving remuneration to any beneficiary of a federal healthcare program likely to influence the receipt of reimbursable items or services; 4. arranging for reimbursable services with an entity which is excluded from participation from a federal health care programs; 5. knowingly or willfully soliciting or receiving remuneration for a referral of a federal health care program beneficiary; or 6. using a payment intended for a federal health care program beneficiary for another use (42 USC §1320a–7a 2015)

Civil Rights Act, Title VII (1964): The federal legislation that prohibits discrimination in employment on the basis of race, religion, color, sex, or national origin (Public Law 88-352 1964)

Civil Rights Act (1991): The federal legislation that focuses on establishing an employer's responsibility for justifying hiring practices that seem to adversely affect people because of race, color, religion, sex, or national origin (Public Law 102-166 1991)

Civilian Health and Medical Program—Uniformed Services (CHAMPUS): Run by the Department of Defense, provided medical care to active duty members of the military, military retirees, and their eligible dependents. This program is now called TRICARE

Civilian Health and Medical Program—Veterans Administration (CHAMPVA): The federal healthcare benefits program for dependents (spouse or widow[er] and children) of veterans rated by the Veterans Administration (VA) as having a total and permanent disability, for survivors of veterans who died from VA-rated service-connected conditions or who were rated permanently and totally disabled at the time of death from a VA-rated service-connected condition, and for survivors of persons who died in the line of duty

Claim: A request for payment for services, benefits, or costs by a hospital, physician or other provider that is submitted for reimbursement to the healthcare insurance plan by either the insured party or by the provider

Claims scrubber software: A type of computer program at a healthcare facility that checks the claim elements for accuracy and agreement before the claims are submitted

Clean claim: A completed insurance claim form that contains all the required information (without any missing information) so that it can be processed and paid promptly

Clinical: refers to work done with real patients, about or relating to the medical treatment that is given to patients in facilities such as hospitals and clinics

Clinical Care Classification (CCC): Two interrelated taxonomies, the CCC of Nursing Diagnoses and Outcomes and the CCC of Nursing Interventions and Actions, that provide a standardized framework for documenting patient care in hospitals, home health agencies, ambulatory care clinics, and other healthcare settings

Clinical classification: a clinical vocabulary, terminology, or nomenclature that lists words or phrases with their meanings; provides for the proper use of clinical words as names or symbols; and facilitates mapping of standardized terms to broader classifications for administrative, regulatory, oversight, and fiscal requirements

Clinical data: Data produced by healthcare providers in the process of diagnosing and treating patients

Clinical data analyst: Individuals who contribute to configuring information systems specific to organizational needs, conduct training on use of technology and specific healthcare applications, and may be engaged in creating reports and monitoring data usage for specific clinical applications—especially those related to clinical research

Clinical decision support (CDS) systems: interactive programs designed to assist clinicians in making patient care decision

Clinical Document Architecture (CDA): An HL7 XML-based document markup standard for the electronic exchange model for clinical documents (such as discharge summaries and progress notes). The implementation guide contains a library of CDA templates, incorporating and harmonizing previous efforts from HL7, Integrating the Healthcare Enterprise (IHE), and Health Information Technology Standards Panel (HITSP). It includes all required CDA templates for Stage I Meaningful Use, and HITECH final rule.

Clinical documentation improvement (CDI): The process an organization undertakes that will improve clinical specificity and documentation that will allow coders to assign more concise disease classification codes

Clinical information model (CIM): An outcome of the transitions of care (ToC) initiative consisting of unambiguous, clinically-relevant definitions of the core data elements that should be included in care transitions

Clinical Laboratory Improvement Amendments: Established quality standards for all laboratory testing to ensure the accuracy, reliability, and timeliness of patient test results regardless of where the test is (Public Law 90-174 1967)

Clinical pathways: A tool designed to coordinate multidisciplinary care planning for specific diagnoses and treatments

Clinical privileges: The authorization granted by a healthcare organization's governing board to a member of the medical staff that enables the physician to provide patient services in the organization within specific practice limits

Clinical terminology: A set of standardized terms and their synonyms that record patient findings, circumstances, events, and interventions with sufficient detail to support clinical care, decision

support, outcomes research, and quality improvement

Clinical transformation: Profound changes including optimization focusing on using a health information system to improve the clinical practice of medicine

Clinical trial: 1. The final stages of a long and careful research process that tests new types of medical care to see if they are safe 2. Experimental study in which an intervention or treatment is given to one group in a clinical setting and the outcomes compared with a control group that did not have the intervention or treatment or that had a different intervention or treatment

Clinical vocabulary: A formally recognized list of preferred medical terms

Clinical workstation: The presentation of healthcare data and the launching of applications in the most effective way for healthcare providers

Clinician/physician web portal: The media for providing physician/clinician access to the provider organization's multiple sources of data from any network-connected device

Closed record: 1. A health record that has been closed following analysis to ensure all documentation components are met, for example, signatures and dictated reports 2. Documentation or a note that has been closed due to system requirements or after a defined period of time

Closed-record review: A review of records after a patient has been discharged from the organization or treatment has been terminated

Closed systems: Systems that operate in a self-contained environment

Cloud computing: 1. The application of virtualization to a variety of computing resources to enable rapid access to computing services via the Internet; 2. Refers to servers that may be located anywhere in the world and that supply data and functionality via the Internet, rather than a local place that provides data and functionality via virtual private network (VPN) or even direct cabling to a healthcare organization

Cluster sampling: The process of selecting subjects for a sample from each cluster within a population (for example, a family, school, or community)

Coaching: 1. A training method in which an experienced person gives advice to a less-experienced worker on a formal or informal basis 2. A disciplinary method used as the first step for employees who are not meeting performance expectations

Code of ethics: A statement of ethical principles regarding business practices and professional behavior

Coefficient of determination (r^2): r^2 measures how much of the variation in one variable is explained by the second variable

Cognitive complexity: The ability to see the many parts of a problem, process conflicting information, and integrate that diversity into a coherent picture

Cohort study: A study, followed over time, in which a group of subjects is identified as having one or more characteristics in common

Collaborative Stage Data Set: A new standardized neoplasm-staging system developed by the American Joint Commission on Cancer

Commission on Accreditation of Rehabilitation Facilities: An international, independent, nonprofit accreditor of health and human services that develops customer-focused standards for areas such as behavioral healthcare, aging services, child and youth services, and medical rehabilitation programs and accredits such programs on the basis of its standards

Common cause variation: The source of variation in a process that is inherent within the process

Common law: Unwritten law originating from court decisions where no applicable statute exists

Comorbidity: 1. A medical condition that coexists with the primary cause for hospitalization and affects the patient's treatment and length of stay 2. Pre-existing condition that, because of its presence with a specific diagnosis, causes an increase in length of stay by at least one day in approximately 75 percent of the cases

Comparative effectiveness research (CER): Research that generates and synthesizes evidence that compares the benefits and harms of alternative methods to prevent, diagnose, treat, and monitor a clinical condition, or to improve the delivery of care

Comparative negligence: The plaintiff's conduct contributed in part to the injury the plaintiff suffered, but the plaintiff's recovery is reduced by some amount based on his or her percentage of negligence

Compensable factor: A characteristic used to compare the worth of jobs (for example, skill, effort, responsibility, and working conditions)

Competencies: Demonstrated skills that a worker should perform at a high level

Complex adaptive system: Refer to the complexity of structures and processes involved in healthcare, and the ongoing changes and rearrangements of these structures and processes

Compliance: 1. The process of establishing an organizational culture that promotes the prevention, detection, and resolution of instances of conduct that do not conform to federal, state, or private payer healthcare program requirements or the healthcare organization's ethical and business policies 2. The act of adhering to official requirements 3. Managing a coding or billing department according to the laws, regulations, and guidelines that govern it

Complaint: In litigation, a written legal statement from a plaintiff that initiates a civil lawsuit

Compliance projects: Projects that include self-imposed initiatives organizations place on themselves, industry imposed compliance where organizations must meet a minimum level of stakeholder expectations, and government or regulatory compliance that organizations must meet in order to remain in business

Complication: 1. A medical condition that arises during an inpatient hospitalization (for example, a postoperative wound infection) 2. Condition that arises during the hospital stay that prolongs the length of stay at least one day in approximately 75 percent of the cases

Compound authorization: Under HIPAA, an authorization for use or disclosure of protected health information may not be combined with any other document to create a compound authorization, except as follows: (i) an authorization for the use of disclosure of protected health information for a research study may be combined with any other type of written permission for the same or another research study; (ii) an authorization for a use or disclosure of psychotherapy notes may only be combined with another authorization for a use or disclosure of psychotherapy notes; (iii) when a covered entity has conditioned the provision of treatment, payment, enrollment in the health plan, or eligibility for benefits under this section on the provision of one of the authorizations (45 CFR 164.508 2013)

Compressed workweek: A work schedule that permits a full-time job to be completed in less than the standard five days of eight-hour

Compromise: Method of conflict management where both parties must be willing to lose or give up a piece of their position

Computer-assisted coding: The process of extracting and translating dictated and then transcribed free-text data (or dictated and then computer-generated discrete data) into ICD-10-CM and CPT evaluation and management codes for billing and coding purposes

Computer-based training (CBT): A type of training that is delivered partially or completely using a computer

Computer output laser disk/enterprise report management (COLD/ERM) technology: Technology that electronically stores documents and distributes them with fax, e-mail, web, and traditional hard-copy print processes

Computerized provider order entry (CPOE) system: Electronic prescribing systems that allow physicians to write prescriptions and transmit them electronically. These systems usually contain error prevention software that provides the user with prompts that warn against the possibility of drug interaction, allergy, or overdose and other relevant information

Concept: A unique unit of knowledge or thought created by a unique combination of characteristics

Conceptual skills: One of the three managerial skill categories that includes intellectual tasks and abilities such as planning, deciding, and problem solving

Concurrent analysis: A review of the health record while the patient is still hospitalized or under treatment

Concurrent review: Review that occurs while the patient care is ongoing, often the reviewers are alongside the healthcare providers on the patient care units to facilitate communication

Conditions for Coverage: Standards applied to facilities that choose to participate in federal government reimbursement programs such as Medicare and Medicaid

Conditions of Participation: The administrative and operational guidelines and regulations under which facilities are allowed to take part in the Medicare and Medicaid programs; published by the Centers for Medicare and Medicaid Services, a federal agency under the Department of Health and Human Services

Confidence interval: A healthcare statistic that is calculated from the standard error of the mean, it is an estimate of the true limits within which the true population mean lies; the range of values that may reasonably contain the true population mean

Confidentiality: 1. A legal and ethical concept that establishes the healthcare provider's responsibility for protecting health records and other personal and private information from unauthorized use or disclosure 2. As amended by HITECH, the practice that data or information is not made available or disclosed to unauthorized persons or processes (45 CFR 164.304 2013)

Conflict management: A problem-solving technique that focuses on working with individuals to find a mutually acceptable solution

Confounding variable: In research an event or a factor that is outside a study but occurs concurrently with the study

Consent: 1. A patient's acknowledgement that he or she understands a proposed intervention, including that intervention's risks, benefits, and alternatives 2. The document signed by the patient that indicates agreement that protected health information (PHI) can be disclosed

Consequentialism: Ethical principle where one considers the consequences before making a decision and this decision is based on the end result

Conservatism: Compliance of financial data in that they fairly represent the financial results of the period and do not overstate or understate information in a significant (material) way

Consideration: 1. Refers to attention to the interpersonal aspects of work, including respecting subordinates' ideas and feelings, maintaining harmonious work relationships, collaborating in teamwork, and showing concern for the subordinates' welfare 2. A contract must be supported by legal and bargained-for consideration, which is what the parties will receive from each other in exchange for performing the obligations of the contract

Consistency: Principle that requires that the accounting method not change over the life of the asset

Constructive confrontation: A method of approaching conflict in which both parties meet with an objective third party to explore perceptions and feelings

Consultant: Individual who provides specialized expertise to the project that may not exist within the current employees

Consultation: Opinions of physicians with specialty training beyond general board certification such as oncologists, cardiologists, or dermatologists

Consumer health informatics: Field devoted to informatics from multiple consumer or patient views; includes patient-focused informatics, health literacy, and consumer education, with a focus on information structures and processes that empower consumers to manage their own health

Consumer mediated exchange: Provides patients with access to their health information allowing them to manage their healthcare online in a similar fashion to how they might manage their finances through online banking

Content analysis: A method of research that provides a systematic and objective analysis of communication effectiveness, such as the analysis performed on tests

Content management: The management of digital and analog records using computer equipment and software. It encompasses two related organization-wide roles: content management and records management

Contingency plan: 1. Documentation of the process for responding to a system emergency, including the performance of backups, the line-up of critical alternative facilities to facilitate continuity of operations, and the process of recovering from a disaster 2. A recovery plan in the event of a power failure, disaster, or other emergency that limits or eliminates access to facilities and electronic protected personal health information (ePHI)

Contingency planning: A comprehensive plan that highlights potential vulnerabilities and threats as well as to identify the approaches to either prevent them or at least minimize the impact; there are three major categories or types of threats: natural threats (floods, earthquakes); technical or man-made (mechanical, biological); intentional acts (terrorism, computer security)

Contingency theory of leadership: Contends that the greater the favorability toward the leader, the more the subordinates can be relied on to carry out the task and the fewer challenges to leadership

Continuing education (CE): Training that enables employees to remain current with advancing knowledge in their profession

Continuity of care document (CCD): The result of ASTM's Continuity of Care Record standard content being represented and mapped into the HL7's Clinical Document Architecture specifications to enable transmission of referral information between providers; also frequently adopted for personal health records

Continuity of care record (CCR): Is a core data set of the most relevant administrative, demographic, and clinical information about a patient's healthcare, covering one or more healthcare encounters. It provides a means for one healthcare practitioner, system, or setting to aggregate all of the pertinent data about a patient and forward it to another practitioner, system, or setting to support the continuity of care

Continuous data: In healthcare statistics, data that represent measurable quantities but are not restricted to certain specified values

Continuous quality improvement (CQI): 1. A management philosophy that emphasizes the importance of knowing and meeting customer expectations, reducing variation within processes, and relying on data to build knowledge for process improvement 2. A component of total quality management (TQM) that emphasizes ongoing performance assessment and improvement planning

Continuous speech input: Speech recognition software that does not require the user to pause between words to let the computer distinguish between the beginning and ending of words

Continuous variables: Discrete variables measured with sufficient precision

Continuum of care: Patients are provided care by different caregivers at several different levels of the healthcare system

Contract: (1) A legally enforceable agreement (2) an agreement between a union and an employer that spells out details of the relationship of management and the employees

Contract law: A branch of law based on common law that deals with written or oral agreements that are enforceable through the legal system

Contract negotiation: The process of going back and forth with the vendor on the issues identified until all are resolved to the satisfaction of both parties

Contractor: Individual added to the team for his or her specialized skills and detailed knowledge not available within the existing employees; or who may be added to increase the work capacity of the existing project team

Contrary: State law cannot be complied with when (1) a covered entity determines that it is impossible to comply with both the federal and state privacy regulations; or (2) compliance with the state law would create a barrier to compliance with the federal regulations under HIPAA

Contributory negligence: The plaintiff's conduct contributed in part to the injury the plaintiff suffered and, if found to be sufficient, can preclude the plaintiff's recovery for the injury

Control: (1) One of the four management functions in which performance is monitored in accordance with organizational policies and procedures (2) Under ICD-10-PCS, a root operation that involves stopping, or attempting to stop, postprocedural bleeding

Control group: A comparison study group whose members do not undergo the treatment under study

Controlling: Refers to the monitoring of performance and use of feedback to ensure that efforts are on target toward prescribed goals, making course corrections as necessary

Controls: Measures and functionality established for the purpose of preventing and mitigating risks

Coordination of benefits (COB) transaction: Process for determining the respective responsibilities of two or more health plan that have some financial responsibility for a medical claim

Corporate integrity agreement (CIA): A compliance program imposed by the government, which involves substantial government oversight and outside expert involvement in the organization's compliance activities and is generally required as a condition of settling a fraud and abuse investigation

Corporation: An organization that may have one or many owners in which profits may be held or distributed as dividends (income paid to the owners)

Correlation: The existence and degree of relationships among factors

Correlational research: A design of research that determines the existence and degree of relationships among factors

Cost accounting: The specialty branch of accounting that deals with quantifying the resources expended to provide the goods and services offered by the organization to its customers, clients, or patients

Cost outlier: Exceptionally high costs associated with inpatient care when compared with other cases in the same diagnosis-related group

Cost outlier adjustment: Additional reimbursement for certain high-cost home care cases based on the loss-sharing ratio of costs in excess of a threshold amount for each home health resource group

Counterclaims: In a court of law, a countersuit

Covered entity: As amended by HITECH, (1) a health plan, (2) a healthcare clearinghouse, (3) a healthcare provider who transmits any health information in electronic form in connection with a transaction covered by this subchapter (45 CFR 160.103 2013)

Credentialing: The process of reviewing and validating the qualifications (degrees, licenses, and other credentials) of physicians and other licensed independent practitioners, for granting medical staff membership to provide patient care services

Criminal law: A branch of law that addresses crimes that are wrongful acts against public health, safety, and welfare, usually punishable by imprisonment or fine

Criminal negligence: An individual may be found liable if his or her behavior is categorized as reckless disregard or deliberate indifference

Critic: A role in organizational innovation in which an idea is challenged, compared to stringent criteria, and tested against reality

Criticality analysis: Consists of evaluating each of the different systems in the organization to determine how crucial the information in the system is to day-to-day healthcare operations and patient care

Cross-claim: 1. In law, a complaint filed against a codefendant 2. A claim by one party against another party who is on the same side of the main litigation

Cross-functional: A term used to describe an entity or activity that involves more than one healthcare department, service area, or discipline

Cross-sectional study: A biomedical research study in which both the exposure and the disease outcome are determined at the same time in each subject

Cross-training: The training to learn a job other than the employee's primary responsibility

Cryptographic key: Tool applied to the data in order to turn the information into cipher text as well as converting the data from cipher text back to plain text

Cryptography: 1. The art of keeping data secret through the use of mathematical or logical functions that transform intelligible data into seemingly unintelligible data and back again 2. In information security, the study of encryption and decryption techniques

Culture: The values, beliefs, attitudes, languages, symbols, rituals, behaviors and customs unique to a particular group of people

Cultural competence: Skilled in awareness, understanding, and acceptance of beliefs and values of the people of groups other than one's own

Cultural diversity: Any perceived difference among people, such as age, functional specialty, profession, sexual orientation, geographic origin, lifestyle, or tenure with the organization or position

Current Dental Terminology (CDT): A reference manual maintained and updated annually by the American Dental Association (ADA); included in the manual is the Code on Dental Procedures and Nomenclature (the Code), which is a classification system for dental treatment procedures and services

Current Procedural Terminology (CPT): A comprehensive, descriptive list of terms and associated numeric and alphanumeric codes used for reporting diagnostic and therapeutic procedures and other medical services performed by physicians; published and updated annually by the American Medical Association

Current ratio: The total current assets divided by total current liabilities

Curriculum: A prescribed course of study in an educational program

Cybernetic systems: Systems that have standards, controls, and feedback mechanisms built in to them

Cyclical staffing: A transitional staffing solution wherein workers are brought in for specific projects or to cover in busy times

D

Dashboard: Reports of process measures to help leaders follow progress to assist with strategic planning; method that has been developed for presenting a variety of data on a single display in an easy-to-read format

Data administrator: Persons who apply domain expertise to the logical design of a database, establish policies and standards governing creation and use of data, maintain data dictionaries, and manage the quality of data

Data analytics: The science of examining raw data with the purpose of drawing conclusions about that information. It includes data mining, machine language, development of models, and statistical measurements. Analytics can be descriptive, predictive, or prescriptive

Data architecture: an integrated set of specification artifacts (models and diagrams) used to define data requirements, guide integration and control of data assets, and align data investments with business strategy

Data at rest: Data is in storage within a database or on a server where it is no longer being used or access

Data backup plan: A plan that ensures the recovery of information that has been lost or becomes inaccessible

Data conversion: The task of moving data from one data structure to another, usually at the time of a new system installation

Data dictionary: A descriptive list of the names, definitions, and attributes of data elements to be collected in an information system or database whose purpose is to standardize definitions and ensure consistent use

Data governance: The overall management of the availability, usability, integrity, and security of the data employed in an organization or enterprise

Data governance steering committee: Composed of representatives from various business or functional organizational units, this group serves as the coordinating body for the data governance (DG) program; it develops the goals of the DG program, identifies and sequences project and task priorities, coordinates the data steward committees, monitors DG program outcomes, recommends policy and standards, and reports the status of the DG program to the executive data governance council

Data governance office (DGO): Led by an individual with the title of chief data officer (CDO) or data governance program director, among the responsibilities of the DGO are: providing centralized communication and archive for data governance (DG) initiatives; working with stakeholders, coordinating DG initiatives; facilitating and coordinating data steward committees, task forces, and meetings; supporting the data governance council; and collecting and analyzing DG metrics

Data in motion: Data that are in the process of being transmitted from one location to another location such as an e-mail

Data, information, knowledge and wisdom (DIKW) hierarchy: An essential of computer information and library sciences, in this hierarchy data are facts and when a fact is related to some other fact (data), the relationship produces a piece of information; each level in the hierarchy is dependent on the previous levels

Data life cycle: Made up of a series of successive stages and has beginning and end points, a typical cycle includes the following stages: data planning, data inventory and evaluation, data capture, data transformation and processing, data access and distribution, data maintenance, data archival, and data destruction

Data mining: The process of extracting and analyzing large volumes of data from a database for the purpose of identifying hidden and sometimes subtle relationships or patterns and using those relationships to predict behaviors

Data model: 1. A picture or abstraction of real conditions used to describe the definitions of fields and records and their relationships in a database 2. A conceptual model of the information needed to support a business function or process

Data modeling: The process of determining the users' information needs and identifying relationships among the data

Data provenance: Type of administrative data that refers to where data originated and where data may have moved between databases

Data quality management: The business processes that ensure the integrity of an organization's data during collection, application (including aggregation), warehousing, and analysis; a continuous process for defining the parameters for specifying acceptable levels of data quality to meet business needs, and for ensuring that data quality meets these levels

Data quality measurement: Measurement in which a data quality measure is a mechanism to assign a quantity to quality of care by comparison to a criterion

Data security: The process of keeping data, both in transit and at rest, safe from unauthorized access, alteration, or destruction

Data security management: Policies and procedures that address confidentiality and security concerns of organizational stakeholders (for example, patients, providers, and employees), protecting organizational proprietary interests, and compliance with government and regulatory requirements while accommodating legitimate access needs

Data stakeholders: Those who have an interest or stake in organizational data and can include customers, front line workers, business units, managers, executives, and even external groups such as state and federal agencies, accreditation bodies, and others

Data steward: An individual appointed with responsibility and accountability for data, usually in a specific domain

Data use and reciprocal service agreement (DURSA): A legally binding contract that draws from federal and local laws and defines the requirements for participation in the eHealth Exchange national network

Data warehouse: A database that makes it possible to access data from multiple databases and combine the results into a single query and reporting interface

Database administrator: The individual responsible for the technical aspects of designing and managing databases

Database management system: Software tools used to store, analyze, modify and access data

Days in accounts receivable: The ending accounts receivable balance divided by an average day's revenues

Debt ratio: The total liabilities divided by the total assets

Debt service: The current obligations of an organization to repay loans

Decision rights: Appointing authority to specific individuals or categories of individuals to make data-related decisions and designating when and how those decisions are made

Decision support: A computer-based system that gathers data from a variety of sources and assists in providing structure to the data by using various analytical models and visual tools in order to facilitate and improve the ultimate outcome in decision-making tasks associated with nonroutine and nonrepetitive problems

Decryption: The process of transforming the information from cipher text to plain text

Deductive reasoning: The process of developing conclusions based on generalizations

Deemed status: An official designation indicating that a healthcare facility is in compliance with the Medicare Conditions of Participation

Defamation of character: A false communication about someone to a person other than the subject that tends to injure that person's reputation

Default judgment: A court ruling against a defendant in a lawsuit who fails to answer a summons for a court appearance

Defendant: In civil cases, an individual or entity against whom a civil complaint has been filed; in criminal cases, an individual who has been accused of a crime

Deficiency assignment: Each facility must develop its own procedures for quantitative analysis and responsibility for completion of the record must be assigned to each responsible provider; the deficiencies, or parts of the record needing completion or signature, are entered into the HIS or on paper worksheets attached to the incomplete, or deficient, health record

Deidentification: (1) The act of removing from a health record or data set any information that could be used to identify the individual to whom the data apply in order to protect his or her confidentiality (2) to remove the names of the principal investigator (PI), coinvestigators, and affiliated organizations to allow reviewers to maintain objectivity

Delegation: The process by which managers distribute work to others along with the authority to make decisions and take action

Delinquent health record: An incomplete record not finished or made complete within the time frame determined by the medical staff of the facility

Democratic leadership: Involves members in decision making

Denial: When a bill has been returned unpaid for any of several reasons (for example, sending the bill to the wrong insurance company, patient not having current coverage, inaccurate coding, lack of medical necessity, and so on)

Deontology: The duty or responsibility guiding the decision based on action and not the end result

Dependency: The relationship between two tasks in a project plan; also exists when one component cannot operate without another component

Dependent variable: A measurable variable in a research study that depends on an independent variable

Deposition: A method of gathering information to be used in a litigation process

Depreciation: The allocation of the dollar cost of a capital asset over its expected life

Descriptive metadata: Describes each data element to be captured and processed by information technology

Descriptive statistics: A set of statistical techniques used to describe data such as means, frequency distributions, and standard deviations; statistical information that describes the characteristics of a specific group or a population

Descriptive research: A type of research that determines and reports the current status of topics and subjects

Designated record set (DRS): As amended by HITECH: 1. A group of records maintained by or for a covered entity that is: (i) The medical records and billing records about individuals maintained by or for a covered health care provider; (ii) The enrollment, payment, claims adjudication, and case or medical management record systems maintained by or for a health plan; or (iii) Used, in whole or in part, by or for the covered entity to make decisions about individuals 2. For purposes of this paragraph, the term means any item, collection, or grouping of information that includes protected health information and is maintained, collected, used, or disseminated by or for a covered entity (45 CFR 164.501 2013)

Development: Maintaining or upgrading competencies

Diagnosis-related group (DRG): 1. A unit of case-mix classification adopted by the federal government and some other payers as a prospective payment mechanism for hospital inpatients in which diseases are placed into groups because related diseases and treatments tend to consume similar amounts of healthcare resources and incur similar amounts of cost; in the Medicare and Medicaid programs, one of more than 500 diagnostic classifications in which cases demonstrate similar resource consumption and length-of-stay patterns. Under the prospective payment system (PPS), hospitals are paid a set fee for treating patients in a single DRG category, regardless of the actual cost of care for the individual. 2. A classification system that groups patients according to diagnosis, type of treatment, age, and other relevant criteria. Under the prospective payment system, hospitals are paid a set fee for treating patients in a single DRG category, regardless of the actual cost of care for the individual

Diagnostic image data: Data such as a digital chest x-ray or a computed tomography (CT) scan

Diagnostic Statistical Manual of Mental Disorders, 5th edition (DSM-5): A nomenclature developed by the American Psychiatric Association to standardize the diagnostic process for patients with psychiatric disorders

Digital dictation: The process by which voice sounds are recorded and converted into a digital format

Digital signature management technology: Offers both signer and document authentication for analog or digital documents

Direct costs: Resources expended that can be identified as pertaining to specific goods and services (for example, medications pertain to specific patients)

DIRECT exchange: Launched in March 2010 as a part of the Nationwide Health Information Network, the Direct Project was created to specify a simple, secure, scalable, standards-based way for participants to send (push) authenticated, encrypted health information directly to known, trusted recipients over the Internet

Disaster recovery plan: The document that defines the resources, actions, tasks, and data required to manage the businesses recovery process in the event of a business interruption

Discharge summary: A summary of the resident's stay at a healthcare facility that is used along with the postdischarge plan of care to provide continuity of care upon discharge from the facility

Discharged, no final bill (DNFB): A report that includes all patients who have been discharged from the facility but for whom, for one reason or another, the billing process is not complete

Discipline: A field of study characterized by a knowledge base and perspective that is different from other fields of study

Disclosure: As amended by HITECH, the release, transfer, provision of access to, or divulging in any manner of information outside the entity holding the information (45 CFR 160.103 2013)

Discounting: A reduction from the full rate of payment. This can be the result of a fee for service contract, multiple procedures, or due to third party payer guidelines

Discrete data: Data that represent separate and distinct values or observations; that is, data that contain only finite numbers and have only specified values

Discrimination: The act of treating one entity differently from another

Disease index: A listing in diagnosis code number order for patients discharged from the facility during a particular time period

Disease registry: A centralized collection of data used to improve the quality of care and measure the effectiveness of a particular aspect of healthcare delivery

Disposition: A description of the patient's status at discharge

District court: The lowest tier in the federal court system, which hears cases involving felonies and misdemeanors that fall under federal statute and suits in which a citizen of one state sues a citizen of another state

Diversity jurisdiction: Legal matters belonging only to federal courts where the parties do not live in the same state

Diversity training: Training that facilitates an environment that fosters tolerance and appreciation of individual differences within the organization's workforce

DMAIC: A scientific methodology that involves the following steps: define, measure, analyze, improve, and control

Do-Not-Resuscitate Order (DNR): An order written by the treating physician stating that in the event the patient suffers cardiac or pulmonary arrest, cardiopulmonary resuscitation should not be attempted

Document imaging technology: The practice of electronically scanning written or printed paper documents into an optical or electronic system for later retrieval of the document or parts of the document if parts have been indexed

Document management technology: Automatically organizes, assembles, secures, and shares documents

Dot plot: Presents the frequency or means to compare many groups using dots

Double billing: Two providers bill for one service provided to one patient

Double-blind study: A type of clinical trial conducted with strict procedures for randomization in which neither researcher nor subject knows whether the subject is in the control group or the experimental group

Driving force: The concept of what a department or an organization uses to determine which products or services to offer, which markets to seek, and which customers to attract

Due diligence: The actions associated with making a good decision, including investigation of legal, technical, human, and financial predictions and ramifications of proposed endeavors with another party

Durable power of attorney: A power of attorney that remains in effect even after the principal is incapacitated; some are drafted so that they only take effect when the principal becomes incapacitated

E

Early adopter: Accounts for about 13.5 percent of the organization. The individuals in this group have a high degree of opinion leadership, and they are more localized than cosmopolitan and often look to the innovators for advice and information; these are the leaders and respected role models in the organization, and their adoption of an idea or practice does much to initiate change

Early majority: Compromises about 34 percent of the organization; although usually not leaders, the individuals in this group represent the backbone of the organization, are deliberate in thinking and acceptance of an idea, and serve as a natural bridge between early and late adopters

e-commerce: The integration of all aspects of business-to-business (B2B) and business-to-consumer (B2C) activities, processes, and communications, including electronic data interchange (EDI)

e-discovery: Refers to Amendments to Federal Rules of Civil Procedure and Uniform Rules Relating to Discovery of Electronically Stored Information;

wherein audit trails, the source code of the program, metadata, and any other electronic information that is not typically considered the legal health record is subject to motion for compulsory discovery

Egoism: Ethical principle that involves only considering oneself in the decision-making process

e-health: The application of e-commerce in the healthcare industry

eHealth Exchange: A group of federal agencies and non-federal organizations that came together under a common mission and purpose to improve patient care, streamline disability benefit claims, and improve public health reporting through secure, trusted, and interoperable health information exchange. Participating organizations mutually agree to support a common set of standards and specifications that enable the establishment of a secure, trusted, and interoperable connection among all participating Exchange organizations for the standardized flow of information

Eighty-five/fifteen (85/15) rule: The total quality management assumption that 85 percent of the problems that occur are related to faults in the system rather than to worker performance

e-learning: Refers to training courses delivered electronically

Electronic data interchange (EDI): A standard transmission format using strings of data for business information communicated among the computer systems of independent organizations

Electronic document/content management (ED/CM) system: Any electronic system that manages an organization's analog and digital documents and content (that is, not just the data) to realize significant improvements in business work processes

Electronic health record (EHR): An electronic record of health-related information on an individual that conforms to nationally recognized interoperability standards and that can be created, managed, and consulted by authorized clinicians and staff across more than one healthcare organization

Electronic medical record: An electronic record of health-related information on an individual that can be created, gathered, managed, and consulted by authorized clinicians and staff within one healthcare organization

Electronic performance support system (EPSS): Sets of computerized tools and displays that automate training, as well as documentation, and integrate this automation with the computer application

Electronic records management technology: Systems that capture data from print files and other report-formatted digital documents, such as e-mail, e-fax, instant messages, web pages, digital dictation, and speech recognition and stores them for subsequent viewing

Electronic signature: A generic, technology-neutral term for the various ways that an electronic record can be signed, such as a digitized image of a signature, a name typed at the end of an e-mail message by the sender, a biometric identifier, a secret code or PIN, or a digital signature

Emergency Medical Treatment and Active Labor Act (EMTALA): A 1986 law enacted as part of the Consolidated Omnibus Reconciliation Act largely to combat "patient dumping"—the transferring, discharging, or refusal to treat indigent emergency department patients because of their inability to pay (Public Law 99-272 1986)

Emergency mode operation plan: A plan that defines the processes and controls that will be followed until the operations are fully restored

Emotional intelligence (EI): The sensitivity and ability to monitor and revise one's behavior based on the needs and responses of others

Employee handbook: Presentation of policies and requirements that all employees must know, such as insurance programs, payroll requirements, and personnel policies, in a guide given to new employees during orientation

Employee self-logging: A form of self-reporting in which the employees simply track their tasks, volume of work units, and hours worked

Employer-based self-insurance: An umbrella term used to describe health plans that are funded directly by employers to provide coverage for their employees exclusively in which employers establish accounts to cover their employees' medical expenses and retain control over the funds but bear the risk of paying claims greater than their estimates

Employment-at-will: Concept that employees can be fired at any time and for almost any reason based on the idea that employees can quit at any time and for any reason

Empowerment: The condition of having the environment and resources to perform a job independently

Encryption: The process of transforming text into an unintelligible string of characters that can be transmitted via communications media with a high degree of security and then decrypted when it reaches a secure destination

End user: Individual using the system for everyday tasks

Enterprise health information management: 1. Ensuring the value of information assets, requiring an organization-wide perspective of information management functions; it calls for explicit structures, policies, processes, technology, and controls 2. The infrastructure and processes to ensure the information is trustworthy and actionable

Enterprise master patient index (EMPI): An index that provides access to multiple repositories of information from overlapping patient populations that are maintained in separate systems and databases

Entity: A class of objects that exist in the real world and have related properties

Entity relationship diagram (ERD): A specific type of data modeling used in conceptual data modeling and the logical-level modeling of relational databases

Environmental scan: A systematic and continuous effort to search for important cues about how the world is changing outside and inside the organization

Epidemiological study: Study concerned with finding the causes and effects of diseases and conditions

Epidemiology: Is the study of the distribution and determinants of health problems in specified populations and the application of this study to control health problems

Episode-of-care (EOC) reimbursement: Method that issues lump-sum payments to providers to compensate them for all the healthcare services delivered to a patient for a specific illness or over a specific period of time

Equal Employment Opportunity Act: The 1972 amendment to the Civil Rights Act of 1964 prohibiting discrimination in the workplace on the basis of age, gender, race, color, religion, sex, or national origin (Public Law 92-261 1972)

Equal Employment Opportunity Commission: Created by Title VII of the Civil Rights Act of 1964 as the agency responsible for investigating discrimination claims emanating from the Civil Rights Act of 1991, finally giving legal voice to a process that formally had none

Equal Pay Act of 1963: The federal legislation that requires equal pay for men and women who perform substantially the same work (Public Law 88-38 1963)

Equity: Securities that are shared in the ownership of the organization

Ergonomics: A discipline of functional design associated with the employee in relationship to his or her work environment, including equipment, workstation, and office furniture adaptation to accommodate the employee's unique physical requirements so as to facilitate efficacy of work functions

E-Rx (e-prescribing): When a prescription is written from the personal digital assistant and an electronic fax or an actual electronic data interchange transaction is generated that transmits the prescription directly to the retail pharmacy's information system

Esprit de corps: One of Henry Fayol's principles of management that emphasized the work climate in which harmony, cohesion, and high morale promoted good work

Ethical principles: Principles taken into consideration when making ethical decisions or to understand how and why others make the decisions they do

Ethics: A field of study that deals with moral principles, theories, and values; in healthcare, a formal decision-making process for dealing with the competing perspectives and obligations of the people who have an interest in a common problem

Ethics committee: A committee of an organization tasked with reviewing ethics violations and determining the course of action required to remedy the violations

Ethics training: Training that includes how to recognize ethical dilemmas and draw upon codes of conduct to resolve problems

Ethnography: A method of observational research that investigates culture in naturalistic settings using both qualitative and quantitative approaches

Evaluation research: A design of research that examines the effectiveness of policies, programs, or organizations

Evidence: The means by which the facts of a case are proved or disproved

Evidence-based management: Management that is information based

Evidence-based practice: the application of the best available research results (evidence) when making decisions about health care

Exchange relationship: Relationship in which a leader offers greater opportunities and privileges to a subordinate in exchange for loyalty, commitment, and assistance

Exclusions Provisions: A component of the Social Security Act that indicates that the Office of

Inspector General has the authority to exclude individuals from participating in federal healthcare programs and will not pay for items or services furnished by an excluded individual or entity

Exclusive provider organization (EPO): Hybrid managed care organization that provides benefits to subscribers only when healthcare services are performed by network providers; sponsored by self-insured (self-funded) employers or associations and exhibits characteristics of both health maintenance organizations and preferred provider organizations

Executive dashboard: An information management system providing decision makers with regularly updated information on an organization's key strategic measures

Executive data governance council: Committee or board that leads the data governance (DG) program and is responsible for making the business case for the DG program, providing the authorization for the DG program, establishing the program's mission and scope, setting the program's strategic direction, securing funding and resources for the program, and evaluating and measuring the overall program success

Exempt employees: Specific groups of employees who are identified as not being covered by some or all of the provisions of the Fair Labor Standards Act

Exit interview: The final meeting an employee has with his or her employer before leaving the organization

Expectancy theory of motivation: Proposes that one's efforts will result in the attainment of desired performance goals

Expense projects: Projects where new and improved information is created

Expenses: Amounts that are charged as costs by an organization to the current year's activities of operation

Experimental (study) group: A group of participants in which the exposure status of each participant is determined and the individuals are followed forward to determine the effects of the exposure

Experimental method: Researchers randomly assign participants into an experimental group or into a control group and actively intervene to test a hypothesis; they manipulate an independent variable (treatment or intervention) in order to assess its effect on the dependent variable (the outcome)

Experimental research: 1. A research design used to establish cause and effect 2. a controlled investigation in which subjects are assigned randomly to groups that experience carefully controlled interventions that are manipulated by the experimenter according to a strict protocol

Experimental study: The exposure status for each individual in the study is determined and the individuals are then followed to determine the effects of the exposure

Expert determination method: Data elements that could identify an individual are removed from the data and then an expert, such as a statistician, applies scientific methodology to determine the likelihood of identification of the individual; the expert that the organization hires to statistically analyze the information provides documentation of the probability that the information would be identified

Explanation of benefits (EOB): A statement issued to the insured and the healthcare provider by an insurer to explain the services provided, amounts billed, and payments made by a health plan

Explicit knowledge: Documents, databases, and other types of recorded and documented information

Express warranty: The seller makes specific promises to the buyer

External benchmarking: Comparison that occurs when an organization uses comparative data between organizations to judge performance and identify improvements that have proven to be successful in other organizations

External customers: Individuals from outside the organization who receive products or services from within the organization

External validity: An attribute of a study's design that allows its findings to be applied to other groups

Extranet: A system of connections of private Internet networks outside an organization's firewall that uses Internet technology to enable collaborative applications among enterprises

Extrapolation method: This method of auditing claims looks at a small sample of records and applies the correction in payment/reimbursement across a large number of claims in a time period or service area

F

Facility-based registry: A registry that includes only cases from a particular type of healthcare facility, such as a hospital or clinic

Facility charge: Allows the capture of an E/M charge that represents those resources not included with the CPT code for the clinic environment

Factor comparison method: A complex quantitative method of job evaluation that combines elements of both the ranking and point methods

Fair Labor Standards Act of 1938: The federal legislation that sets the minimum wage and overtime payment regulations

False Claims Act: Legislation passed during the Civil War, amended in 1986, that prohibits contractors from making a false claim to a governmental program; used to reinforce the prevention of healthcare fraud and abuse (Public Law 99-562 1986)

False imprisonment: Intentional tort in healthcare where excessive force is used to restrain a patient

Family and Medical Leave Act (FMLA) of 1993: The federal legislation that allows full-time employees time off from work (up to 12 weeks) to care for themselves or their family members with the assurance of an equivalent position upon return to work (Public Law 103-3 1993)

Favorable variance: The positive difference between the budgeted amount and the actual amount of a line item, that is, when actual revenue exceeds budget or actual expenses are less than budget

Federal Register: The daily publication of the US Government Printing Office that reports all changes in regulations and federally mandated standards, including HCPCS and ICD-10-CM codes

Federated model: Model of health information exchange where there is not a centralized database of patient information; also known as decentralized model

Fee-for-service reimbursement: A method of reimbursement through which providers retrospectively receive payment based on either billed charges for services provided or on annually updated fee schedules

Feedback control: Back-end processes that monitor and measure output and then compare it to expectations and identify variations that then must be analyzed so corrective action plans can be developed and implemented

Felony: A serious crime such as murder, larceny, rape, or assault for which punishment is usually severe

Fetal death: The death of a product of human conception before its complete expulsion or extraction from the mother regardless of the duration of the pregnancy

Fetal death rate: A proportion that compares the number of intermediate or late fetal deaths to the total number of live births and intermediate or late fetal deaths during the same period of time

Financial Accounting Standards Board (FASB): An independent organization that sets accounting standards for businesses in the private sector

Financial counselor: Staff dedicated to helping patients and physicians determine sources of reimbursement for healthcare services; counselors are responsible for identifying and verifying the method of payment and debt resolution for services rendered to patients

Financial data: The data collected for the purpose of managing the assets and expenses of a business (for example, a healthcare organization, a product line); in healthcare, data derived from the charge generation documentation associated with the activities of care and then aggregated by specific customer grouping for financial analysis

Firewall: A computer system or a combination of systems that provides a security barrier or supports an access control policy between two networks or between a network and any other traffic outside the network

Fiscal year: Any consecutive 12-month period an organization uses as its accounting period

Fishbone diagram: A performance improvement tool used to identify or classify the root causes of a problem or condition and to display the root causes graphically

Fixed budget: A type of budget based on expected capacity with no consideration of potential variations

Fixed costs: Resources expended that do not vary with the activity of the organization (for example, mortgage expense does not vary with patient volume)

Flexible budget: A type of budget that is based on multiple levels of projected productivity (actual productivity triggers the levels to be used as the year progresses)

Flextime: A work schedule that gives employees some choice in the pattern of their work hours, usually around a core of midday hours

Float employee: An employee who is not assigned to a particular shift, function, or unit and who may fill in as needed in cases of standard employee absence or vacation

Flowchart: A graphic tool that uses standard symbols to visually display detailed information, including time and distance, of the sequential flow of work of an individual or a product as it progresses through a process

Focus group: A group of approximately 6 to 12 subjects, usually experts in the particular area of study, brought together to discuss a specific topic using the focused interview method, usually with a moderator who is not on the research team

Focused study: A study in which a researcher orally questions and conducts discussions with members of a group

Force-field analysis: A performance improvement tool used to identify specific drivers of, and barriers to, an organizational change so that positive factors can be reinforced and negative factors reduced

For-profit organization: The tax status assigned to business entities that are owned by one or more individuals or organizations and that earn revenues in excess of expenditures that are subsequently paid out to the owners or stockholders

Framework: A conceptual structure for classifying, organizing, and showing interrelationships among activities used as a guide for taking action to achieve a goal

Fraud: The intentional deception or misrepresentation that an individual knows, or should know, to be false, or does not believe to be true, and makes, knowing the deception could result in some unauthorized benefit to himself or some other person(s)

Freedom of Information Act (FOIA): The federal law established in 1967, amended in 1986, that is applicable only to federal agencies, through which individuals can seek access to information without the authorization of the person to whom the information applies (Public Law 99-570 1986)

Functional organization: Organization where each employee has a single supervisor and employees are grouped in departments by specialty or subspecialty

Functional interoperability: Refers to sending messages between computers with a shared understanding of the structure and format of the message

G

Gantt chart: A graphic tool used to plot tasks in project management that shows the duration of project tasks and overlapping tasks

General consent: Permits healthcare providers to perform overall medical care, from a patient for routine treatment

General Equivalence Mapping (GEM): A program created to facilitate the translation between ICD-9-CM and ICD-10-CM/PCS

General jurisdiction: Courts that hear more serious criminal cases or civil cases that involve large amounts of money; may hear all matters of state law except for those cases that must be heard in courts of special jurisdiction

General ledger: A master list of individual revenue and expense accounts maintained by an organization

Generalizability: The ability to apply research results, data, or observations to groups not originally under study

Generally accepted accounting principles (GAAP): An accepted set of accounting principles or standards, and recognized procedures central to financial accounting and reporting

Genetic Information Nondiscrimination Act (2008): Legislation which prohibits genetic information discrimination against employees or applicants

Geographic practice cost index (GPCI): An index developed by the Centers for Medicare and Medicaid Services to measure the differences in resource costs among fee schedule areas compared to the national average in the three components of the relative value unit (RVU): physician work, practice expenses, and malpractice coverage; separate GPCIs exist for each element of the RVU and are used to adjust the RVUs, which are national averages, to reflect local costs

Gesture recognition technology: Collectively, the recognition of constrained or unconstrained, handwritten, English language free text like intelligent character recognition technology or recognition of hand-marked characters like mark sense technology

Global payment: A form of reimbursement used for radiological and other procedures that combines the professional and technical components of the procedures and disperses payments as lump sums to be distributed between the physician and the healthcare facility

Global surgery payment: Covers all the healthcare services entailed in planning and completing a specific surgical procedure; every element of the procedure from the treatment decision through normal postoperative patient care is covered by a single bundled payment

Goal: A specific description of the services or deliverable goods to be provided as the result of a business process

Going concern: Organization's ability to operate for the foreseeable future after an analysis of an entity's financial data

Go-live: The first day users use the system in actual practice

Good Samaritan statutes: State law or statute that protects healthcare providers from liability for not obtaining informed consent before rendering care to adults or minors at the scene of an emergency or accident

Governance: Refers to the establishment of policies and the continual monitoring of their implementation for effectively and efficiently managing an organization's assets

Governmental immunity: Precludes anyone from bringing a lawsuit against a governmental entity unless that entity consents to the lawsuit

Grand jury: Has the authority to issue subpoenas for its investigative process, and all evidence considered by the grand jury remains confidential unless an indictment is returned

Graphical perception: The visual interpretation process and was originally described as the ability to unconsciously extract information from graphics

Great person theory: The belief that some people have natural (innate) leadership skills

Grievance: A formal, written description of a complaint or disagreement

Grievance procedures: The steps employees may follow to seek resolution of disagreements with management on job-related issues

Gross autopsy rate: The number of inpatient autopsies conducted during a given time period divided by the total number of inpatient deaths for the same time period

Gross death rate: The number of inpatient deaths that occurred during a given time period divided by the total number of inpatient discharges, including deaths, for the same time period

Gross negligence: An extreme departure from the ordinary standard of care; it represents reckless disregard

Grounded theory: A theory about what is actually going on instead of what should go on

Group discussion: Learners form smaller groups to generate ideas through interactive sharing of ideas; effective following a lecture

Group model HMO: A type of health plan in which an HMO contracts with an independent multispecialty physician group to provide medical services to members of the plan

Group practice without walls (GPWW): A type of managed care contract that allows physicians to maintain their own offices and share administrative services

Groupthink: Refers to the tendency of a highly cohesive team to seek consensus, often at the detriment of sound decision making

H

Harassment: The act of bothering or annoying someone repeatedly

Hawthorne effect: A research study that found that novelty, attention, and interpersonal relations have a motivating effect on performance

Hay method of job evaluation: A modification of the point method of job evaluation that numerically measures the levels of three major compensable factors: know-how, problem-solving ability, and accountability

Health data: Raw facts or figures that are processed into useful health information

Health data stewardship: Pertains to responsibilities that best ensure appropriate use of health data

Health informatics: Scientific discipline that is concerned with the cognitive, information-processing, and communication tasks of healthcare practice, education, and research, including the information science and technology to support these tasks

Health information: As amended by HITECH, any information, including genetic information, whether oral or recorded in any form or medium, that: 1. Is created or received by a health care provider, health plan, public health authority, employer, life insurer, school or university, or health care clearinghouse; and 2. Relates to the past, present, or future physical or mental health or condition of an individual; the provision of health care to an individual; or the past, present, or future payment for the provision of health care to an individual (45 CFR 160.103 2013)

Health information exchange: The exchange of health information electronically between providers and others with the same level of interoperability, such as labs and pharmacies

Health information system: Refers to all the components—human and computer—that ensure health data are processed into useful health information

Health information technology: Under HITECH, hardware, software, integrated technologies or related licenses, intellectual property, upgrades, or packaged solutions sold as services that are designed for or support the use by health care entities or patients for the electronic creation, maintenance, access, or exchange of health information (Public Law 111-5 2009)

Health Information Technology for Economic and Clinical Health (HITECH) Act: Legislation created to promote the adoption and meaningful use of health information technology in the United States. Subtitle D of the Act provides for additional privacy and security requirements that will develop and support electronic health information, facilitate information exchange, and strengthen monetary penalties. Signed into law on February 17, 2009, as part of ARRA (Public Law 111-5 2009)

Health Information Technology Standards Committee (HITSC): An HHS advisory committee that recommends standards, implementation specifications, and certification criteria for the electronic exchange and use of health information

Health Insurance Portability and Accountability Act (HIPAA) of 1996: The federal legislation enacted to provide continuity of health coverage, control fraud and abuse in healthcare, reduce healthcare costs, and guarantee the security and privacy of health information; limits exclusion for pre-existing medical conditions, prohibits discrimination against employees and dependents based on health status, guarantees availability of health insurance to small employers, and guarantees renewability of insurance to all employees regardless of size; requires covered entities (most healthcare providers and organizations) to transmit healthcare claims in a specific format and to develop, implement, and comply with the standards of the Privacy Rule and the Security Rule; and mandates that covered entities apply for and utilize national identifiers in HIPAA transactions (Public Law 104-191 1996)

Health literacy: The ability to understand instructions on prescription drug bottles, appointment cards, medical education brochures, doctor's directions, and consent forms; it also includes the ability to navigate complex health care systems; it requires a complex group of reading, listening, analytical, and decision-making skills and the ability to apply these skills to health situations

Health maintenance organization (HMO): Entity that combines the provision of healthcare insurance and the delivery of healthcare services, characterized by: 1. an organized healthcare delivery system to a geographic area, 2. a set of basic and supplemental health maintenance and treatment services, 3. voluntarily enrolled members, and 4. predetermined fixed, periodic prepayments for members' coverage

Health record banking model: This PHR model would allow patients and healthcare providers to share information by making deposits of health information into a bank. The health record bank would have to protect the privacy and security of the health information

Health reform: Major policy changes to improve the quality and manage the cost of healthcare

Health Research Extension Act: Federal legislation that established guidelines for the proper care of animals used in biomedical and behavioral research (Public Law 99-158 1985)

Health savings account (HSA): Savings accounts designed to help people save for future medical and retiree health costs on a tax-fee basis; part of the 2003 Medicare bill; Also called medical savings accounts

Health services research: Research conducted on the subject of healthcare delivery that examines organizational structures and systems as well as the effectiveness and efficiency of healthcare services

Health statistics: Providing information for understanding, monitoring, improving, and planning the use of resources to improve the lives of people, provide services, and promote their well-being

Health technology assessment (HTA): The evaluation of the usefulness (utility) of a health technology in relation to cost, efficacy, utilization, and other factors in terms of its impact on social, ethical, and legal systems

Healthcare Common Procedure Coding System (HCPCS): A medical code set that identifies healthcare procedures, equipment, and supplies for claim submission purposes. It has been selected for use in the HIPAA transactions. HCPCS Level I contains numeric CPT codes which are maintained by the AMA. HCPCS Level II contains alphanumeric codes used to identify various items and services that are not included in the CPT medical code set. These are maintained by HCFA, the BCBSA, and the HIAA. HCPCS Level III contains alphanumeric codes that are assigned by Medicaid state agencies to identify additional items and services not included in levels I or II. These are usually called "local codes," and must have W, X, Y, or Z in the first position. HCPCS Procedure Modifier Codes can be used with all three levels, with the WA–ZY range used for locally assigned procedure modifiers.

Healthcare Cost and Utilization Project (HCUP): A family of databases and related software tools and products developed through a Federal-State-Industry partnership and sponsored by AHRQ. HCUP databases are derived from administrative data and contain encounter-level, clinical and nonclinical information including all-listed diagnoses and procedures, discharge status, patient demographics, and charges for all patients, regardless of payer (such as, Medicare, Medicaid, private insurance, uninsured), beginning in 1988

Healthcare data analytics: The practice of using data to make business decisions in healthcare

Healthcare Fraud Statute: Identifies that it is illegal to defraud any healthcare benefit program or to obtain fraudulent funds or property by any of the healthcare benefit programs

Healthcare informatics: The field of information science concerned with the management of all aspects of health data and information through the application of computers and computer technologies

Healthcare Integrity and Protection Data Bank (HIPDB): Developed in response to HIPAA mandate of the collection of information on healthcare fraud and abuse because there was no central place to obtain this information

Healthcare Quality Improvement Act of 1986: A federal law that established standards and requirements related to peer review among physicians

Heterogeneity: The state or fact of containing various components

Histogram: A graphic technique used to display the frequency distribution of continuous data (interval or ratio data) as either numbers or percentages in a series of bars

Historical research: A research design used to investigate past events

History: A summary of the patient's illness from his or her point of view

HITECH-HIPAA Omnibus Privacy Act: Includes some of the most significant changes to patient privacy since HIPAA was first enacted in 2003; it went into effect on March 26, 2013, and covered entities were to ensure compliance by September 23, 2013; also known as the Omnibus Rule, this Act strengthens the privacy and security of patient health information, modifies the breach notification rule, strengthens privacy protections for genetic information by prohibiting health plans from using or disclosing such information for underwriting, makes business associates of HIPAA-covered entities liable for compliance, strengthens limitations on the use and disclosure of PHI for marketing, research and fundraising, and allows patients increased restriction rights

Home Assessment Validation and Entry (HAVEN): A type of data-entry software used to collect Outcome and Assessment Information Set (OASIS) data and then transmit them to state databases; imports and exports data in standard OASIS record format, maintains agency/patient/employee information, enforces data integrity through rigorous edit checks, and provides comprehensive online help. HAVEN is used in the home health prospective payment system (HHPPS)

Home health agency (HHA): A program or organization that provides a blend of home-based medical and social services to homebound patients and their families for the purpose of promoting, maintaining, or restoring health or of minimizing the effects of illness, injury, or disability; these services include skilled nursing care, physical therapy, occupational therapy, speech therapy, and personal care by home health aides

Home health resource group (HHRG): A classification system for the home health prospective payment system (HHPPS) derived from the data elements in the Outcome and Assessment Information Set (OASIS) with 80 home health episode rates established to support the prospective reimbursement of covered home care and rehabilitation services provided to Medicare beneficiaries during 60-day episodes of care; a six-character alphanumeric code is used to represent a severity level in three domains

Home healthcare: A wide-range of healthcare services that can be delivered in the home and it is the fastest-growing sector to offer services for Medicare recipients

Hospice care: An interdisciplinary program of palliative care and supportive services that addresses the physical, spiritual, social, and economic needs of terminally ill patients and their families

Hospital: A healthcare entity that has an organized medical staff and permanent facilities that include inpatient beds and continuous medical or nursing services and that provides diagnostic and therapeutic services for patients as well as overnight accommodations and nutritional services

Hospital-acquired conditions (HAC): CMS identified eight hospital-acquired conditions (not present on admission) as "reasonably preventable," and hospitals will not receive additional payment for cases in which one of the eight selected conditions was not present on admission; the eight originally selected conditions include: foreign object retained after surgery, air embolism, blood incompatibility, stage III and IV pressure ulcers, falls and trauma, catheter-associated urinary tract infection, vascular catheter-associated infection, and surgical site infection—mediastinitis after coronary artery bypass graft; additional conditions were added in 2010 and remain in effect: surgical site infections following certain orthopedic procedures and bariatric surgery, manifestations of poor glycemic control, and deep vein thrombosis (DVT)/pulmonary embolism (PE) following certain orthopedic procedures

Hospital autopsy rate: The total number of autopsies performed by a hospital pathologist for a given time period divided by the number of deaths of hospital patients (inpatients and outpatients) whose bodies were available for autopsy for the same time period

Hospital death rate: The number of inpatient deaths for a given period of time divided by the total number of live discharges and deaths for the same time period

Hospital inpatient: A patient who is provided with room, board, and continuous general nursing services in an area of an acute care facility where patients generally stay at least overnight

Hospital-issued notice of noncoverage (HINN): If the hospital determines that the care the beneficiary is receiving, or is about to receive, is not covered because it: is not medically necessary, is not delivered in the most appropriate setting, or is custodial in nature, hospitals have the responsibility to issue notification to Medicare beneficiaries prior to admission, at admission, or at any point during an inpatient stay

Hospital newborn inpatient: A patient born in the hospital at the beginning of the current inpatient hospitalization

Hospital outpatient: A hospital patient who receives services in one or more of a hospital's facilities when he or she is not currently an inpatient or a home care patient

Human subjects: Individuals whose physiologic or behavioral characteristics and responses are the object of study in a research program

Hung jury: Occurs when members of a jury cannot agree on the defendant's guilt or lack of proven guilt

Hybrid model: A cross between the centralized and the decentralized models of health information exchange, which combines the functionality of a record locator service and a centralized data repository

Hybrid record: A combination of paper and electronic records; a health record that includes both paper and electronic elements

Hypothesis: A statement that describes a research question in measurable terms

Hypothesis test: Allows the analyst to determine the likelihood that a hypothesis is true given the data present in the sample with a predetermined acceptable level of making an error

I

Identity theft: A fraud attempted or committed using identifying information of another person without authority

Implementation: The process in which the system is configured to meet a specific organization's needs

Implementation plan: Plan used to manage the thousands of tasks in selecting, acquiring, and implementing the various hardware, software, and operational components of the health information system

Implied warranty: Exists when the law implies such a warranty exists "as a matter of public policy" to protect the public from harm

Incentive pay: A system of bonuses and rewards based on employee productivity; often used in transcription areas of healthcare facilities

Incidence: Refers to the number of new cases of a disease

Incidence rate: A computation that compares the number of new cases of a specific disease for a given time period to the population at risk for the disease during the same time period

Incident: An occurrence in a medical facility that is inconsistent with accepted standards of care

Incident report: A quality or performance management tool used to collect data and information about potentially compensable events (events that may result in death or serious injury)

Income statement: A statement that summarizes an organization's revenue and expense accounts using totals accumulated during the fiscal year

Independent practice association (IPA): An open-panel health maintenance organization that provides contract healthcare services to subscribers through independent physicians who treat patients in their own offices; the HMO reimburses the IPA on a capitated basis; the IPA may reimburse the physicians on a fee-for-service or a capitated basis

Independent variable: The factors in experimental research that researchers manipulate directly

Index: An organized (usually alphabetical) list of specific data that serves to guide, indicate, or otherwise facilitate reference to the data

Indian Health Service (IHS): The federal agency within the Department of Health and Human

Services that is responsible for providing federal healthcare services to American Indians and Alaska natives

Indictment: Formal charge; needed for a felony crime to be prosecuted

Indirect costs: Resources expended that cannot be identified as pertaining to specific goods or services (for example, electricity is not allocable to a specific patient)

Indirect standardization: Appropriate to use for risk adjustment when the risk variables are categorical and the rate or proportion for the variable of interest is available for the standard or reference group at the level of the risk categories, the expected outcome rate for each risk category is calculated based on the reference group and then weighted by the volume in each risk group at population to be compared to the standard

Individually identifiable health information: As amended by HITECH, information that is a subset of health information, including demographic information collected from an individual, and: 1. is created or received by a health care provider, health plan, employer, or health care clearinghouse; and 2. relates to the past, present, or future physical or mental health or condition of an individual; the provision of health care to an individual; or the past, present, or future payment for the provision of health care to an individual; and (i) that identifies the individual; or (ii) with respect to which there is a reasonable basis to believe the information can be used to identify the individual (45 CFR 160.103 2013)

Inductive reasoning: A process of creating conclusions based on a limited number of observations

Industry knowledge: Awareness of regulatory and legal requirements, past and future trends within the industry, and experience with projects in the industry

Infection rate: The ratio of all infections to the number of discharges, including deaths

Inferential statistics: 1. Statistics that are used to make inferences from a smaller group of data to a large one 2. A set of statistical techniques that allows researchers to make generalizations about a population's characteristics (parameters) on the basis of a sample's characteristics

Infliction of emotional distress: A person can be held liable for the intentional or reckless mental suffering resulting from such things as despair, shame, grief, and public humiliation

Information governance: The accountability framework and decision rights to achieve enterprise information management (EIM). IG is the responsibility of executive leadership for developing and driving the IG strategy throughout the organization. IG encompasses both data governance (DG) and information technology governance (ITG)

Information management: The generation, collection, organization, validation, analysis, storage, and integration of data as well as the dissemination, communication, presentation, utilization, transmission, and safeguarding of the information

Information overload: A difficulty in making decisions due to the presence of excessive amounts of information

Informed consent: 1. A legal term referring to a patient's right to make his or her own treatment decisions based on the knowledge of the treatment to be administered or the procedure to be performed 2. An individual's voluntary agreement to participate in research or to undergo a diagnostic, therapeutic, or preventive medical procedure

In-group: Subordinates who form a group around the leader

Initiating structure: Leaders in this group were more task-focused and centered on giving direction, setting goals and limits, and planning and scheduling activities

Injury Severity Score (ISS): An overall severity measurement maintained in the trauma registry and calculated from the abbreviated injury scores for the three most severe injuries of each patient

Innovator: An early adopter of change who is eager to experiment with new ways of doing things

Inpatient: A patient who is provided with room, board, and continuous general nursing services in an area of an acute care facility where patients generally stay at least overnight

Inpatient admission: An acute-care facility's formal acceptance of a patient who is to be provided with room, board, and continuous nursing service in an area of the facility where patients generally stay at least overnight

Inpatient bed occupancy rate: The total number of inpatient service days for a given time period divided by the total number of inpatient bed count days for the same time period

Inpatient census: Indicates the number of patients present in the healthcare facility at a particular point in time

Inpatient discharge: The termination of hospitalization through the formal release of an inpatient from a hospital

Inpatient Rehabilitation Validation and Entry (IRVEN) system: A computerized data-entry system used by inpatient rehabilitation facilities (IRFs). Captures data for the IRF Patient Assessment Instrument (IRF PAI) and supports electronic submission of the IRF PAI. Also allows data import and export in the standard record format of the Centers for Medicare and Medicaid Services (CMS)

Inpatient service day: The unit of measure denoting the services received by one inpatient in one 24-hour period

In-service education: Training that teaches employees specific skills required to maintain or improve performance, usually internal to an organization

Installation: The process a vendor uses to load software onto the hardware being acquired

Institutional Review Board (IRB): An administrative body that provides review, oversight, guidance, and approval for research projects carried out by employees serving as researchers, regardless of the location of the research (such as a university or private research agency); responsible for protecting the rights and welfare of the human subjects involved in the research. IRB oversight is mandatory for federally funded research projects

Instrument: A standardized and uniform way to measure and collect data

Insurance verification: A vital component of the prearrival process for scheduled patients, substantiation of the patient's insurance for unscheduled patients occurs at the time of their registration for clinical services or shortly thereafter; yhe verification process entails validating that the patient is a member of the insurance plan given and is covered for the scheduled service date, as well as whether the patient's insurance plan is in-network versus out-of-network, whether the scheduled service expenses will be covered, whether a referral or an authorization is required prior to the service being rendered, and whether the patient will incur an out-of-pocket expense

Integrated delivery system (IDS): A system that combines the financial and clinical aspects of healthcare and uses a group of healthcare providers, selected on the basis of quality and cost management criteria, to furnish comprehensive health services across the continuum of care

Integrated health record: A system of health record organization in which all the paper forms are arranged in strict chronological order and mixed with forms created by different departments

Integrated provider organization (IPO): An organization that manages the delivery of healthcare services provided by hospitals, physicians (employees of the IPO), and other healthcare organizations (for example, nursing facilities)

Integrity: 1. The state of being whole or unimpaired 2. The ability of data to maintain its structure and attributes, including protection against modification or corruption during transmission, storage, or at rest. Maintenance of data integrity is a key aspect of data quality management and security

Intelligent document recognition (IDR) technology: A form of technology that automatically recognizes analog items, such as tangible materials or documents, or recognizes characters or symbols from analog items, enabling the identified data to be quickly, accurately, and automatically entered into digital systems

Intent: An individual committed an act purposely or knowing that harm would likely occur

Interface: The zone between different computer systems across which users want to pass information (for example, a computer program written to exchange information between systems or the graphic display of an application program designed to make the program easier to use)

Interface terminology: Terminology concerned with facilitating clinician documentation within the standardized structure needed for an electronic health record

Internal benchmarking: Comparison used to identify best practices within an organization, to compare best practices within an organization, and to compare current practice over time

Internal customer: Customers located within the organization

Internal rate of return (IRR): An interest rate that makes the net present value calculation equal zero

Internal Revenue Service: Entity that regulates and collects federal taxes

Internal validity: An attribute of a study's design that contributes to the accuracy of its findings

International Classification of Diseases (ICD): Facilitates the storage and retrieval of diagnostic information and serves as the basis for compiling mortality and morbidity statistics reported by World Health Organization members

International Classification of Diseases, 9th Revision, Clinical Modification (ICD-9-CM): A coding and classification system previously used in the United States to report diagnoses in all healthcare settings and inpatient procedures and services as well as morbidity and mortality information

International Classification of Diseases, 10th Revision, Clinical Modification (ICD-10-CM): The coding classification system that replaced ICD-9-CM, Volumes 1 and 2, on October 1, 2015. ICD-10-CM is the United States' clinical modification of the WHO's ICD-10. ICD-10-CM has a total of 21 chapters and contains significantly more codes than ICD-9-CM, providing the ability to code with a greater level of specificity.

International Classification of Diseases, 10th Revision, Procedure Coding System (ICD-10-PCS): The coding classification system that replaced ICD-9-CM, Volume 3, on October 1, 2015. ICD-10-PCS has 16 sections and contains significantly more procedure codes than ICD-9-CM, providing the ability to code procedures with a greater level of specificity.

International Classification of Diseases, 11th Revision (ICD-11): The coding classification system developed to integrate medical data discovered since ICD-10 was published; it still needs to be clinically modified for use in the United States

International Classification of Diseases for Oncology, 3rd edition (ICD-O-3): A system used for classifying incidences of malignant disease

International Classification of Primary Care (ICPC-2): Classification used for coding the reasons of encounter, diagnoses, and interventions in an episode-of-care structure

International Classification on Functioning, Disability, and Health (ICF): Classification of health and health-related domains that describe body functions and structures, activities, and participation

International Health Terminology Standards Development Organization (IHTSDO): An international nonprofit organization based in Denmark that maintains and distributes the Systemized Nomenclature of Medicine–Clinical Terminology

Internet forum: Web application for holding discussions and posting user generated content, also commonly referred to as web forums, newsgroups, message boards, discussion boards, bulletin boards or simply a forum

Interoperability: The capability of different information systems and software applications to communicate and exchange data

Interpersonal skills: An early adopter of change who is eager to experiment with new ways of doing things

Interprofessional education: Occurs when two or more professions learn about, from, and with each other to enable effective collaboration to improve health outcomes

Interrater reliability: A measure of a research instrument's consistency in data collection when used by different abstractors

Interrogatories: Discovery devices consisting of a set of written questions given to a party, witness, or other person who has information needed in a legal case

Interval data: A type of data that represents observations that can be measured on an evenly distributed scale beginning at a point other than true zero

Interview survey: A formal meeting, often between a job applicant and a potential employer

Intranet: A private information network that is similar to the Internet and whose servers are located inside a firewall or security barrier so that the general public cannot gain access to information housed within the network

Intrarater reliability: A measure of a research instrument's reliability in which the same person repeating the test will get reasonably similar findings

Invasion of privacy: The intrusion upon one's solitude

Inventor: A role in organizational innovation that requires idea generation

Investor-owned hospital chain: Group of for-profit healthcare facilities owned by stockholders

Iterative approach: Executing projects in releases

Iterative process: Process that initially prioritizes initiatives and focuses on small select business imperatives that quickly deliver value and expands as the program matures

J

Job classification method: 1. A method of job evaluation that compares a written position description with the written descriptions of various classification grades 2. A method used by the federal government to grade jobs

Job evaluation: The process of applying predefined compensable factors to jobs to determine their relative worth

Job procedure: A structured, action-oriented list of sequential steps involved in carrying out a specific task or solving a problem

Job ranking: A method of job evaluation that arranges jobs in a hierarchy on the basis of each job's importance to the organization, with the most important jobs listed at the top of the hierarchy and the least important jobs listed at the bottom

Job rotation: A work design in which workers are shifted periodically among different tasks

Job sharing: A work schedule in which two or more individuals share the tasks of one full-time or one full-time-equivalent position

Job specifications: A list of a job's required education, skills, knowledge, abilities, personal qualifications, and physical requirements

Joinder: Codefendant where the defendant brings a claim against an outsider

Joint Commission: An independent, not-for-profit organization, the Joint Commission accredits and certifies more than 20,000 healthcare organizations and programs in the United States. Joint Commission accreditation and certification is recognized nationwide as a symbol of quality that reflects an organization's commitment to meeting certain performance standards

Judicial system: The count system where a person or entity has the opportunity to bring a civil action against another person or entity believed to have caused harm

Jurisdiction: The power and authority of a court to hear, interpret, and apply the law to and decide specific types of cases

Justice: Requires that people be treated fairly and that benefits and risks be shared equitably among the population

Just-in-time training: Training provided anytime, anyplace, and just when it is needed

K

Key performance indicators: A quantifiable measure used over time to determine whether some structure, process, or outcome in the provision of care to a patient supports high-quality performance measured against best practice criteria

L

Labor-Management Relations Act (Taft-Hartley Act): Federal legislation passed in 1947 that imposed certain restrictions on unions while upholding their right to organize and bargain collectively

Labor-Management Reporting and Disclosure Act of 1959 (Landrum-Griffin Act): Federal legislation passed in 1959 to ensure that union members' interests were properly represented by union leadership; created, among other things, a bill of rights for union members (Public Law 86-257 1959)

Labor relations: Human resources management activities associated with unions and collective bargaining

Laggards: A category of adopters of change who are very reluctant to accept proposed changes and may resist transition

Late majority: Skeptical group that comprises another 34 percent of the organization: individuals in this group usually adopt innovations only after social or financial pressure to do so

Latency: The amount of time it takes to answer a question, compactness of the display, and user preference

Layoffs: Unpaid leaves of absence initiated by the employer as a strategy for downsizing staff in response to a change in the organization's status

Leader–member exchange (LMX): Micro theory that focuses on dyadic relationships, or those between two people or between a leader and a small group; explains how in-group and out-group relationships form with a leader or mentor, and how delegation may occur

Leader–member relations: Group atmosphere much like social orientation; includes the subordinates' acceptance of, and confidence in, the leader as well as the loyalty and commitment they show toward the leader

Leadership: Roles or functions that advance an organization toward meetings its goals; visionary thinking, decisions responsive to membership and mission, and accountability for actions and outcomes

Leading: One of the four management functions in which people are directed and motivated to achieve goals

Lean: A management strategy in which the core idea is to maximize value while minimizing waste; basically creating more value with fewer resources

Learning: What occurs in the individual to achieve the changes in behavior, knowledge, attitudes, abilities, and skills that are desired

Learning content management system (LCMS): Management system that provides a technical framework to develop the content and permit sharing and reusing content

Learning curve: The time required to acquire and apply certain skills so that new levels of productivity and performance exceed prelearning levels (productivity often is inversely related to the learning curve)

Learning health system: An ecosystem where all stakeholders can securely, effectively, and efficiently contribute, share, and analyze data and create new knowledge that can be consumed by a wide variety of electronic health information systems to support effective decision making leading to improved health outcomes

Learning management system (LMS): A software application that assists with managing and tracking learners and learning events and collating data on learner progress

Least harm: Ethical principle that deals with situations where two choices may both be less than ideal; one should choose the situation that will do the least amount of harm to the fewest number of people

Least preferred co-worker (LPC) scale: Fred Fiedler's brief test that assessed the degree to which a manager was task or relationship oriented

Lecture: Method in which the instructor delivers content and the student listens and observes primarily one-way communication

Legacy system: A type of computer system that uses older technology but may still perform optimally

Legal health record (LHR): Documents and data elements that a healthcare provider may include in response to legally permissible requests for patient information

Legal hold: A communication issued because of current or anticipated litigation, audit, government investigation, or other such matters that suspend the normal disposition or processing of records. Legal holds can encompass business procedures affecting active data, including, but not limited to, backup tape recycling. The specific communication to business or IT organizations may also be called a "hold," "preservation order," "suspension order," "freeze notice," "hold order," or "hold notice"

Legal system: A process through which members of society settle dispute

Legislative system: System that enacts laws and controls many activities related to industry, including the healthcare industry

Length of stay: The total number of patient days for an inpatient episode, calculated by subtracting the date of admission from the date of discharge

Lexicon: 1. The vocabulary used in a language or a subject area or by a particular speaker or group of speakers 2. A collection of words or terms and their meanings for a particular domain, used in healthcare for drug terms

Liability: 1. A legal obligation or responsibility that may have financial repercussions if not fulfilled

2. An amount owed by an individual or organization to another individual or organization

Libel: Written form of defamation

Licensure: The legal authority or formal permission from authorities to carry on certain activities that by law or regulation require such permission (applicable to institutions as well as individuals)

Likert scale: An ordinal scaling and summated rating technique for measuring the attitudes of respondents; a measure that records level of agreement or disagreement along a progression of categories, usually five (five-point scale), often administered in the form of a questionnaire

Limited jurisdiction: Lower-level trial courts may only hear certain types of cases and include courts such as probate, family, juvenile, surrogate, and criminal

Line authority: The authority to manage subordinates and to have them report back, based on relationships illustrated in an organizational chart

Line plot: Presents trends or patterns in the number of occurrences between groups; presents trends or patterns in the mean of a variable between groups

Liquidity: The degree to which assets can be quickly and efficiently turned into cash, for example, marketable securities are generally liquid, the assumption being that they can be sold for their full value in a matter of days, whereas buildings are not liquid, because they cannot usually be sold quickly

Litigation: A civil lawsuit or contest in court

Living will: A legal document, also known as a medical directive, that states a patient's wishes regarding life support in certain circumstances, usually when death is imminent

Local coverage determination (LCD): Established by Section 522 of the Benefits Improvement and Protection Act, a decision by a fiscal intermediary or carrier whether to cover a particular service on an intermediary-wide or carrier-wide basis in accordance with Section 1862(a)(1)(A) of the Social Security Act, which is a determination regarding whether the service is reasonable and necessary. LCDs consist only of reasonable and necessary information. Effective December 7, 2003, CMS's contractors will begin issuing LCDs instead of LMRPs

Logic bombs: Malware that will execute a program, or a string of code, when a certain event happens

Logical Observation Identifiers Names and Codes (LOINC): A database protocol developed by the Regenstrief Institute for Health Care aimed at standardizing laboratory and clinical codes for use in clinical care, outcomes management, and research that enable exchange and aggregation of electronic health data from many independent systems

Longitudinal: A type of time frame for research studies during which data are collected from the same participants at multiple points in time

Longitudinal health record: A permanent, coordinated patient record of significant information listed in chronological order and maintained across time, ideally from birth to death

Long-term care: A variety of services that help people with health or personal needs and activities of daily living over a period of time. Long-term care can be provided in the home, in the community, or in various types of facilities, including nursing homes and assisted living facilities

Long-term care hospital (LTCH): According to the Centers for Medicare and Medicaid Services (CMS), a hospital with an average length of stay for Medicare patients that is 25 days or longer, or a hospital excluded from the inpatient prospective payment system and that has an average length of stay for all patients that is 20 days or longer

Low-utilization payment adjustment (LUPA): An alternative (reduced) payment made to home health agencies instead of the home health resource group reimbursement rate when a patient receives fewer than four home care visits during a 60-day episode

M

Major diagnostic category (MDC): Under diagnosis-related groups (DRGs), one of 25 categories based on single or multiple organ systems into which all diseases and disorders relating to that system are classified

Malfeasance: A wrong or improper act

Malware: Any program that causes harm to systems by unauthorized access, unauthorized disclosure, destruction, or loss of integrity of any information

Managed care: 1. Payment method in which the third-party payer has implemented some provisions to control the costs of healthcare while maintaining quality care 2. Systematic merger of clinical, financial, and administrative processes to manage access, cost, and quality of healthcare

Managed care organization (MCO): A type of healthcare organization that delivers medical care and manages all aspects of the care or the payment for care by limiting providers of care, discounting payment to providers of care, or limiting access to care; *Also called* coordinated care organization

Management by objectives (MBO): A management approach that defines target objectives for organizing work and compares performance against those objectives

Management service organization (MSO): Under diagnosis-related groups (DRGs), one of 25 categories based on single or multiple organ systems into which all diseases and disorders relating to that system are classified

Managerial accounting: The development, implementation, and analysis of systems that track financial transactions for management control purposes, including both budget systems and cost analysis systems

MAP key: Measures a specific revenue cycle function and provides the purpose for the measurement, the value of the measure, and the specific equation (numerator and denominator) to consistently calculate the measure

Mapping: The process of associating concepts from one coding system with concepts from another coding system and defining their equivalence in accordance with a documented rationale and a given purpose

Maslow's Hierarchy of Needs: A theory developed by Abraham Maslow suggesting that a hierarchy of needs might help explain behavior and guide managers on how to motivate employees

Massed training: Training in a highly concentrated session

Massive open online course (MOOC): An online course with unlimited participation and open access offered via the Internet

Master data management: Master data that an enterprise maintains about key business entities such as customers, employees, or patients, and reference data that is used to classify other data or identify allowable values for data such as codes for state abbreviations or products

Master patient index (MPI): A patient-identifying directory referencing all patients related to an organization and which also serves as a link to the patient record or information, facilitates patient identification, and assists in maintaining a longitudinal patient record from birth to death

Matching: A concept that enables decision makers to look at expenses and revenues in the same period to measure the organization's income performance

Materiality: The significance of a dollar amount based on predetermined criteria

Maternal death: The death of any woman from any cause related to, or aggravated by, pregnancy or its management, regardless of the duration of the pregnancy or the site of the death

Matrix organization: Organization where employees report to an administrative supervisor from the original functional area to carry out their operational work but may also report to a functional supervisor to manage their work on the project

Maximization: Using unbundling or upcoding to make the most of reimbursement to the highest possible amount through coded data

Mean: A measure of central tendency that is determined by calculating the arithmetic average of the observations in a frequency distribution

MEDCIN: A proprietary clinical terminology developed as a point-of-care tool for electronic medical record documentation at the time and place of patient care

Median: A measure of central tendency that shows the midpoint of a frequency distribution when the observations have been arranged in order from lowest to highest

Mediation: When an objective third party unrelated to the dispute is invited to bring the parties to mutual agreement

Medical identity theft: The fraudulent use of an individual's identifying information in a healthcare setting

Mediation: Occurs when cases are heard by a mediator and the parties involved reach a mutual agreement

Medicaid: A joint federal and state program that helps with medical costs for some people with low incomes and limited resources. Medicaid programs vary from state to state, but most healthcare costs are covered if a patient qualifies for both Medicare and Medicaid

Medical device: An instrument, machine, implement or apparatus intended for use in the diagnosis of disease or for monitoring or treatment of a condition

Medical foundation: Multipurpose, nonprofit service organization for physicians and other healthcare providers at the local and county level; as managed care organizations, medical foundations have established preferred provider organizations, exclusive provider organizations, and management service organizations, with emphases on freedom of choice and preservation of the physician–patient relationship

Medical home: A program to provide comprehensive primary care that partners physicians with the patient and their family to allow better access to healthcare and improved outcomes

Medical identity theft: The inappropriate or unauthorized misrepresentation of another's identity to do one of two things: obtain medical services or goods, or falsify claims for medical services in an attempt to obtain money

Medical Literature, Analysis, and Retrieval System Online (MEDLINE): MEDLINE is the US National Library of Medicine's (NLM) premier bibliographic database that contains over 19 million references to journal articles in life sciences with a concentration on biomedicine

Medical malpractice liability: Refers to instances where a civil claim for damages against a healthcare provider successfully proves that the provider was negligent in their care of the patient leading to injury or death

Medical necessity: 1. The likelihood that a proposed healthcare service will have a reasonable beneficial effect on the patient's physical condition and quality of life at a specific point in his or her illness or lifetime 2. As amended by HITECH, a covered entity or business associate may not use or disclose protected health information, except as permitted or required (45 CFR 164.502 2013) 3. The concept that procedures are only eligible for reimbursement as a covered benefit when they are performed for a specific diagnosis or specified frequency (42 CFR 405.500 1995)

Medical peer review: The process by which a professional review body considers whether a practitioner's clinical privileges or membership in a professional society will be adversely affected by a physician's competence or professional conduct

Medical staff: The staff members of a healthcare organization who are governed by medical staff bylaws; may or may not be employed by the healthcare organization

Medical staff bylaws: Standards governing the practice of medical staff members; typically voted upon by the organized medical staff and the medical staff executive committee and approved by the facility's board; governs the business conduct, rights, and responsibilities of the medical staff; medical staff members must abide by these bylaws in order to continue practice in the healthcare facility

Medical staff classification: The organization of physicians according to clinical assignment

Medical Subject Headings database (MeSH): The National Library of Medicine's controlled vocabulary thesaurus. It consists of terms naming descriptors in a hierarchical structure that permits searching at various levels of specificity

Medically needy option: An option in the Medicaid program that allows states to extend eligibility to persons who would be eligible for Medicaid under one of the mandatory or optional groups but whose income and resources fall above the eligibility level set by their state

Medicare: A federally funded health program established in 1965 to assist with the medical care costs of Americans 65 years of age and older as well as other individuals entitled to Social Security benefits owing to their disabilities

Medicare administrative contractor (MAC): Required by section 911 of the Medicare Prescription Drug, Improvement and Modernization Act of 2003, CMS is completing the process of awarding Medicare claims processing contracts through competitive procedures resulting in replacing its current claims payment contractors, fiscal intermediaries and carriers, with new contract entities called MACs. Initially 19 MACs were expected through three procurement cycles. Currently there are 15 A/B MAC jurisdictions that have served as the foundation for CMS's initial series of A/B MAC procurements. CMS will continue to consolidate to 10 A/B MAC jurisdictions

Medicare Advantage plan: A type of Medicare health plan offered by a private company that contracts with Medicare to provide the beneficiary with all Part A and Part B benefits. These plans include Health Maintenance Organizations, Preferred Provider Organizations, Private Fee-for-Service Plans, Special Needs Plans, and Medicare Medical Savings Account Plans. Enrollees in Medicare Advantage Plans have their services are covered through the plan are not paid for under original Medicare

Medicare fee schedule (MFS): A feature of the resource-based relative value system that includes a complete list of the payments Medicare makes to physicians and other providers

Medicare Prescription Drug, Improvement, and Modernization Act: Enacted to amend title XVIII of the Social Security Act to provide for a voluntary program for prescription drug coverage under the Medicare Program, to modernize the Medicare Program, to amend the Internal Revenue Code

of 1986 to allow a deduction to individuals for amounts contributed to health savings security accounts and health savings accounts, to provide for the disposition of unused health benefits in cafeteria plans and flexible spending arrangements, and for other purposes

Medicare Provider Analysis and Review (MEDPAR): File made up of acute-care hospital and skilled nursing facility (SNF) claims data for all Medicare claims

Medicare severity diagnosis-related groups (MS-DRGs): The US government's 2007 revision of the DRG system, the MS-DRG system better accounts for severity of illness and resource consumption

Medicare summary notice (MSN): A summary sent to the patient from Medicare that summarizes all services provided over a period of time with an explanation of benefits provided

Medication administration record (MAR): The records used to document the date and time each dose and type of medication is administered to a patient

Medigap: Private, supplemental health insurance that pays, within limits, most of the healthcare service charges not covered by Medicare Parts A or B

Mental ability (cognitive) tests: Examinations that assess the reasoning capabilities of individuals

Mentor: A trusted advisor or counselor; an experienced individual who educates and trains another individual within an occupational setting

Meta-analysis: A specialized form of systematic literature review that involves the statistical analysis of a large collection of results from individual studies for the purpose of integrating the studies' findings

Metadata: Descriptive data that characterize other data to create a clearer understanding of their meaning and to achieve greater reliability and quality of information. Metadata consist of both indexing terms and attributes. Data about data: for example, creation date, date sent, date received, last access date, last modification date

mHealth: The use of mobile cellular devices and other wireless personal devices focused on health and fitness monitoring

Migration path: A series of coordinated and planned steps required to move a plan from one situation level to another

Minimum Data Set 3.0 (MDS): Document created when OBRA required CMS to develop an assessment instrument to standardize the collection of SNF patient data; the MDS is the minimum core of defined and categorized patient assessment data that serves as the basis for documentation and reimbursement in an SNF

Minimum necessary: Privacy Rule standard that requires that a covered entity or business associate make reasonable efforts to limit protected health information to the minimum necessary to accomplish the intended purpose of the use, disclosure, or request; it is meant to limit unnecessary or inappropriate access to and disclosure of PHI so that it is only used or disclosed to carry out necessary functions for treatment, payment, and healthcare operations

Misdemeanor: A crime that is less serious than a felony

Misfeasance: Relating to negligence or improper performance during an otherwise correct act

Mission: A written statement that sets forth the core purpose and philosophies of an organization or group; defines the organization or group's general purpose for existing; also known as a *mission statement*

Mitigate the risk: The process of reducing or eliminating a risk by implementing a control

Mixed methods research: Research method approach that combines quantitative and qualitative techniques within a single study or across multiple, complementary studies

M-learning: Mobile learning; the application of e-learning to mobile computing devices and wireless networks

Mode: A measure of central tendency that consists of the most frequent observation in a frequency distribution

Model: The representation of a theory in a visual format, on a smaller scale, or with objects

Moral values: A system of principles by which one guides one's life, usually with regard to right or wrong

Morality: A composite of the personal values concerning what is considered right or wrong in a specific cultural group

Morphology: The science of structure and form of organisms without regard to function

Motion for summary judgment: A request made by the defendant in a civil case to have the case ruled in his or her favor based on the assertion that the plaintiff has no genuine issue to be tried

Motivation: The inner drive to accomplish a task

Movement diagram: A chart depicting the location of furniture and equipment in a work area and showing the usual flow of individuals or materials as they progress through the work area

Multiaxial: The ability of a nomenclature to express the meaning of a concept across several axes

Multihospital system: A system that includes two or more hospitals owned, leased, sponsored, or contract managed by a central organization

Multimedia: The combination of free-text, raster or vector graphics, sound, or motion video or frame data

Multiuser virtual environment (MUVE): Sometimes called virtual worlds, MUVEs are accessed over the Internet and can be used to simulate a work environment and bring a new dimension to learning

Multivoting technique: A decision-making method for determining group consensus on the prioritization of issues or solutions

N

Narrative: The author details the processes of the procedure in a step-by-step descriptive method; most common format for procedure writing

National Center for Health Statistics (NCHS): The federal agency responsible for collecting and disseminating information on health services utilization and the health status of the population in the United States; developed the clinical modification to the International Classification of Diseases, Tenth Revision (ICD-10) and is responsible for updating the diagnosis portion of the ICD-10-CM

National Committee for Quality Assurance (NCQA): A private not-for-profit organization dedicated to improving healthcare quality. Since its founding in 1990, NCQA has been a central figure in driving improvement throughout the healthcare system, helping to elevate the issue of healthcare quality to the top of the national agenda

National conversion factor (CF): A mathematical factor used to convert relative value units into monetary payments for services provided to Medicare beneficiaries

National coverage determination (NCD): An NCD sets forth the extent to which Medicare will cover specific services, procedures, or technologies on a national basis. Medicare contractors are required to follow NCDs

National Drug Codes (NDC) directory: A list of all drugs manufactured, prepared, propagated, compounded, or processed by a drug establishment registered under the Federal Food, Drug, and Cosmetic Act

National Health Care Survey: A national public health survey that contains data abstracted manually from a sample of acute care hospitals and discharged inpatient records, or obtained from state or other discharge databases

National Labor Relations Act (Wagner Act): Federal pro-union legislation that provides, among other things, procedures for union representation and prohibits unfair labor practices by unions, such as coercing nonstriking employees, and by employers, such as interference with the union selection process and discrimination against employees who support a union

National Library of Medicine (NLM): The world's largest medical library and a branch of the National Institutes of Health

National Practitioner Data Bank (NPDB): A confidential information clearinghouse created by Congress with the primary goals of improving healthcare quality, protecting the public, and reducing healthcare fraud and abuse in the United States. The NPDB is primarily an alert or flagging system intended to facilitate comprehensive review of the professional credentials of healthcare practitioners, healthcare entities, providers, and supplies

National Vital Statistics System (NVSS): The oldest and most successful example of intergovernmental data sharing in public health, and the shared relationships, standards, and procedures that form the mechanism by which NCHS collects and disseminates the nation's official vital statistics. These data are provided through contracts between NCHS and vital registration systems operated in the various jurisdictions and legally responsible for the registration of vital events—births, deaths, marriages, divorces, and fetal deaths

Nationwide Health Information Network (NHIN): Established by the ONC in 2004, it was initiated to create a governance, standards, and policy structure that could be easily adopted and scaled to enable health information exchange across organizational, regional and state boundaries; it is a set of guidelines, recommended technology standards, and data use and service level agreements that can facilitate data exchange

Natural language processing (NLP): A technology that converts human language (structured or unstructured) into data that can be translated then manipulated by computer systems; branch of artificial intelligence

Naturalistic observation: A type of nonparticipant observation in which researchers observe certain behaviors and events as they occur naturally

Needs assessment: A procedure performed by collecting and analyzing data to determine what is required, lacking, or desired by an employee, a group, or an organization

Need-to-know principle: The release-of-information principle based on the minimum necessary standard

Negligence: A legal term that refers to the result of an action by an individual who does not act the way a reasonably prudent person would act under the same circumstances

Net assets: The organization's resources remaining after subtracting its liabilities

Net autopsy rate: The ratio of inpatient autopsies compared to inpatient deaths calculated by dividing the total number of inpatient autopsies performed by the hospital pathologist for a given time period by the total number of inpatient deaths minus unautopsied coroners' or medical examiners' cases for the same time period

Net death rate: The total number of inpatient deaths minus the number of deaths that occurred less than 48 hours after admission for a given time period divided by the total number of inpatient discharges minus the number of deaths that occurred less than 48 hours after admission for the same time period

Net income: The difference between total revenues and total expenses

Net loss: The condition when total expenses exceed total revenue

Net present value (NPV): A formula used to assess the current value of a project when the monies used were invested in the organization's investment vehicles rather than expended for the project; this value is then compared to the allocation of the monies and the cash inflows of the project, both of which are adjusted to current time

Network: 1. A type of information technology that connects different computers and computer systems so they can share information 2. Physicians, hospitals, and other providers who provide healthcare services to members of a managed care organization; providers may be associated through formal or informal contracts and agreements

Network model HMO: Program in which participating HMOs contract for services with one or more multispecialty group practices

Network provider: A physician or another healthcare professional who is a member of a managed care network

Neural network: Nonlinear predictive models that, using a set of data that describe what a person wants to find, detect a pattern to match a particular profile through a training process involving interactive learning

Newborn death rate: The number of newborns who died divided by the total number of newborns, both alive and dead

Nomenclature: A recognized system of terms that follows preestablished naming conventions; a disease nomenclature is a listing of the proper name for each disease entity with its specific code number

Nominal data: A type of data that represents values or observations that can be labeled or named and where the values fall into unordered categories

Nominal group technique (NGT): A group process technique that involves the steps of silent listing, recording each participant's list, discussing, and rank ordering the priority or importance of items; allows groups to narrow the focus of discussion or to make decisions without becoming involved in extended, circular discussions

Nonexempt employees: All groups of employees covered by the provisions of the Fair Labor Standards Act

Nonfeasance: A type of negligence meaning failure to act

Nonmaleficence: A legal principle that means "first do no harm"

Nonparticipant observation: A method of research in which researchers act as neutral observers who do not intentionally interact or affect the actions of the population being observed

Nonrandom (nonprobability) sampling: A type of convenience or purposive sampling in which all members of the target population do not have an equal or independent chance of being selected for a research study

Nonprogrammed decision: A decision that involves careful and deliberate thought and discussion because of a unique, complex, or changing situation

Normal distribution: A theoretical family of continuous frequency distributions characterized by a symmetric bell-shaped curve, with an equal mean, median, and mode; any standard deviation; and with half of the observations above the mean and half below it

Normalization: 1. A formal process applied to relational database design to determine which variables should be grouped in a table in order to reduce data redundancy 2. Conversion of various representational forms to standard expressions so those with the same meaning will be recognized as synonymous by computer software in a data search

Normative decision model: A decision tree developed by Vroom-Yetton to determine when to make decisions independently or collaboratively or by delegation

Nosocomial infection rate: The number of hospital-acquired infections for a given time period divided by the total number of inpatient discharges for the same time period

No-SQL: Not only SQL (structured query language) model used in database management systems; it differs from the relational model in that it does not provide a table-based representation but uses either a document or graph-oriented model

Not-for-profit organization: An organization that is not owned by individuals whose profits are retained by the organization and reinvested back into the organization for the benefit of the community it serves

Notice of privacy practices: As amended by HITECH, a statement (mandated by the HIPAA Privacy Rule) issued by a healthcare organization that informs individuals of the uses and disclosures of patient-identifiable health information that may be made by the organization, as well as the individual's rights and the organization's legal duties with respect to that information (45 CFR 164.520 2013)

Notifiable diseases: A disease that must be reported to a government agency so that regular, frequent, and timely information on individual cases can be used to prevent and control future cases of the disease

Null hypothesis: A hypothesis that states there is no association between the independent and dependent variables in a research study

O

Objective: A statement of the end result expected, stated in measurable terms, usually with a time limitation (deadline date) and often with a cost estimate or limitation

Observational research: A method of research in which researchers obtain data by watching research participants rather than by asking questions

Observational study: Study where the exposure and outcome for each individual in the study is studied (observed)

Occupational Safety and Health Act (OSHA) of 1970: The federal legislation that established comprehensive safety and health guidelines for employers (Public Law 91-596 1970)

Odds ratio: A relative measure of occurrence of an illness; the odds of exposure in a diseased group divided by the odds of exposure in a nondiseased group

Offer: One party promises to either do something or not do something if the other party agrees to either do something or not do something

Office of the Inspector General (OIG): Mandated by Public Law 95-452 (as amended) to protect the integrity of HHS programs, as well as the health and welfare of the beneficiaries of those programs. The OIG has a responsibility to report both to the Secretary and to the Congress program and management problems and recommendations to correct them. The OIG's duties are carried out through a nationwide network of audits, investigations, inspections, and other mission-related functions performed by OIG components

Office for Human Research Protections (OHRP): Provides leadership in the protection of the rights, welfare, and well-being of subjects involved in research conducted or supported by the US Department of Health and Human Services (HHS). OHRP helps ensure this by providing clarification and guidance, developing educational programs and materials, maintaining regulatory oversight, and providing advice on ethical and regulatory issues in biomedical and social-behavioral research

Office of Research Integrity (ORI): Promotes integrity in biomedical and behavioral research supported by the US Public Health Service (PHS) at about 4,000 institutions worldwide. ORI monitors institutional investigations of research misconduct and facilitates the responsible conduct of research (RCR) through educational, preventive, and regulatory activities

Offshoring: Outsourcing jobs to countries overseas, wherein local employees abroad perform jobs that domestic employees previously performed

OIG workplan: Yearly plan released by the OIG that outlines the focus for reviews and investigations in various healthcare settings

Omnibus Budget Reconciliation Act (OBRA): Federal legislation passed in 1987 that required the Health Care Financing Administration (renamed the Centers for Medicare and Medicaid Services) to develop an assessment instrument (resident assessment instrument) to standardize the collection of patient data from skilled nursing facilities (Public Law 100-203 1987)

Onboarding: Formal new employee orientation process

One-on-one training: In this type of training, the employee learns by first observing a demonstration and then performing the task

One sample t-test: Used to compare a population to a standard value

On-the-job training: A method of training in which an employee learns necessary skills and processes by performing the functions of his or her position

Open-record review: A review of the health records of patients currently in the hospital or under active treatment; part of the Joint Commission survey process

Open source technology: Software products with applications whose source (human-readable) code is freely available to anyone who is interested in downloading the code

Open system: A system which permits other parties to produce products that interoperate with it; a computer is an open system

Operation index: A list of the operations and surgical procedures performed in a healthcare facility, which is sequenced according to the code numbers of the classification system in use

Operational budget: A type of budget that allocates and controls resources to meet an organization's goals and objectives for the fiscal year

Operational plans: Tactical plans that that are ultimately implemented as daily activities at the lower departmental levels

Operations: Organization plans that do not have a specified end date and the work is repeated routinely

Operations management: An application of statistical, mathematical, and quantitative methods to decision making in the business setting in order to better understand how products and services could be manufactured and delivered

Optical character recognition (OCR) technology: A method of encoding text from analog paper into bitmapped images and translating the images into a form that is computer readable

Optical imaging technology: The process by which information is scanned onto optical disks

Optimization: Seeking the most accurate documentation, coded data, and resulting payment in the amount the provider is rightly and legally entitled to receive; includes activities that extend use of information systems beyond the basic functionality

Ordinal data: A type of data that represents values or observations that can be ranked or ordered

Ordinary negligence: Failure to do what a reasonably prudent person would do, or doing something that a reasonably prudent person would not do, in the same or a similar situation

Organization development (OD): The application of behavioral science research and practices to planned organizational change

Organizational chart: A graphic representation of an organization's formal reporting structure

Organizational culture: Refers to an organization's norms, beliefs and values, or generally "how we do things here"; what is felt by staff on any given day that is intangible but greatly influences how an employee feels about their job and the environment in which they perform it

Organizational experience: Provides the project manager with an understanding of how projects are executed within the context of the organization

Organizational safeguards: Measures like business associate agreements so arrangements are made to protect electronic protected health information (ePHI) between organizations

Organized healthcare delivery: Care providers have established relationships and mechanisms for communicating and working to coordinate patient care across health conditions, services, and care settings over time

Organizing: The way in which the managed system is designed and operated to attain the desired goals; it involves the way that tasks are grouped into departments and resources are distributed to them

Orientation: A set of activities designed to familiarize new employees with their jobs, the organization, and its work culture

Original jurisdiction: State civil and criminal cases are initiated in the lower-level trial courts, which have the authority to first hear a case on a given matter

Out-group: Subordinates not included in the group that forms around a leader

Outcome and Assessment Information Set (OASIS): A standard core assessment data tool developed to measure the outcomes of adult patients receiving home health services under the Medicare and Medicaid programs

Outcome evaluation: Collecting and analyzing data at the end of an implementation or operating cycle to determine whether the program, project, or other activity or object has achieved its expected or intended impact, product, or other outcome

Outcomes research: Research aimed at assessing the quality and effectiveness of healthcare as measured by the attainment of a specified end result or outcome, improved health, lowered morbidity or mortality, and improvement of abnormal states

Outpatient code editor (OCE): A software program linked to the Correct Coding Initiative that applies a set of logical rules to determine whether various combinations of codes are correct and appropriately represent the services provided

Outpatient prospective payment system (OPPS): The Medicare prospective payment system used for hospital-based outpatient services and procedures that is predicated on the assignment of ambulatory payment classifications

Outsourcing: The hiring of an individual or a company external to an organization to perform a function either on site or off site

Outsourcing agency: A company that enters into a contract with a healthcare organization to perform services such as clinical coding or transcription

Overhead costs: The expenses associated with supporting but not providing patient care services

Overlap: Situation in which a patient is issued more than one medical record number from an organization with multiple facilities

Overlay: Situation in which a patient is issued a medical record number that has been previously issued to a different patient

P

Packaging: A payment under the Medicare outpatient prospective payment system that includes items such as anesthesia, supplies, certain drugs, and the use of recovery and observation rooms

Panel interview: An interview format in which the applicant is interviewed by several interviewers at once

Parallel work division: A type of concurrent work design in which one employee does several tasks and takes the job from beginning to end

Pareto chart: A bar graph that includes bars arranged in order of descending size to show decisions on the prioritization of issues, problems, or solutions

Partial hospitalization: A structured program of active treatment for psychiatric care that is more intense than the care a patient receives in a doctor or therapist's office

Participant observation: A research method in which researchers also participate in the observed actions

Partnership: Business relationship where two people share in the responsibility for the business, and income still flows through the individuals' tax returns

Path–goal theory: A situational leadership theory that emphasizes the role of the leader in removing barriers to goal achievement

Patient activation measure (PAM): Developed as a way to be able to predict the patient's level of engagement in healthcare, including the knowledge, beliefs, skills, and behaviors that are necessary to manage one's health, the PAM is a 13-item Likert survey instrument that scores patients on a scale of 1-100 and classifies patients as falling into one of four categories based upon their total score; the levels describe four progressive domains of activation—from passive health consumer to active health advocate

Patient-centered care: Relationship-based primary care that meets the individual patient and family's needs, preferences, and priorities

Patient-centered medical home (PCMH): A program to provide comprehensive primary care that partners physicians with the patient and their family to allow better access to healthcare and improved outcomes

Patient engagement: Actions individuals must take to obtain the greatest benefit from the health care services available to them

Patient-focused care: A concept developed to contain hospital inpatient costs and improve quality by restructuring services so that more of them take place in the nursing units (patient floors) and not in specialized units in dispersed hospital locations

Patient-generated health data: Health-related data created, recorded, or gathered by or from patients (or family members or other caregivers) to help address a health concern

Patient-identifiable data: Personal information that can be linked to a specific patient, such as age, gender, date of birth, and address

Patient medical record information (PMRI): Information in which SNOMED CT is part of a core set of terminology

Patient/member web portals: Portal that allows patients to pay their bills online and to securely view all or portions of their provider-based, electronic health record, such as current medical conditions, medications, allergies, and test results

Patient Protection and Affordable Care Act (ACA): The product of the healthcare reform agenda of the Democratic 111th Congress and the Obama administration. The act is designed at increasing the rate of health insurance coverage for Americans and reducing the overall costs of healthcare (Public Law 111-148 2010)

Patient portal: Information system that allows patient to log in to obtain information, register, and perform other functions

Patient safety: Preventing harm to patients, learning from errors, and building a culture of safety

Patient Self-Determination Act: The federal legislation, passed through an Amendment to the Omnibus Budget Reconciliation Act of 1990, that requires healthcare facilities to provide written information on the patient's right to issue advance directives and to accept or refuse medical treatment

Payback period: A financial method used to evaluate the value of a capital expenditure by calculating the time frame that must pass before inflow of cash from a project equals or exceeds outflow of cash

Pay for performance: 1. A type of incentive to improve clinical performance using the electronic health record that could result in additional reimbursement or eligibility for grants or other subsidies to support further HIT efforts 2. The Integrated Healthcare Association initiative in California based on the concept that physician groups would be paid for documented performance

Payment status indicator (PSI): An alphabetic code assigned to CPT/HCPCS codes to indicate whether a service or procedure is to be reimbursed under the Medicare outpatient prospective payment system

Peer review: 1. Review by like professionals, or peers, established according to an organization's medical staff bylaws, organizational policy and procedure, or the requirements of state law; the peer review system allows medical professionals to candidly critique and criticize the work of their colleagues without fear of reprisal 2. The process by which experts in the field evaluate the quality of a manuscript for publication in a scientific or professional journal

Performance: The action or process of carrying out or accomplishing an action, task, or function

Performance improvement: The continuous study and adaptation of a healthcare organization's functions and processes to increase the likelihood of achieving desired outcomes

Performance measurement: The process of comparing the outcomes of an organization, work unit, or employee to pre-established performance standards

Performance review: An evaluation of an employee's job performance

Performance standards: The stated expectations for acceptable quality and productivity associated with a job function

Personal health data: data maintained by an individual, often in a personal health record

Personal health record (PHR): An electronic or paper health record maintained and updated by an individual for himself or herself; a tool that individuals can use to collect, track, and share past and current information about their health or the health of someone in their care

Personalized medicine: the tailoring of medical treatment to the individual characteristics, needs, and preferences of a patient during all stages of care, including prevention, diagnosis, treatment, and follow-up

Persuasive authority: Though a precedent in one state does not bind courts in other states, states may use each other's precedents as guidance in analyzing a specific legal problem

Petition for writ of certiorari: A request for the US Supreme Court to consider a case

Physical safeguards: As amended by HITECH, security rule measures such as locking doors to safeguard data and various media from unauthorized access and exposures;, including facility access controls, workstation use, workstation security, and device and media controls (45 CFR 164.310 2013)

Physician champion: An individual who assists in communicating and educating medical staff in areas such as documentation procedures for accurate billing and appropriate EHR processes; also known as physician advisor

Physician–hospital organization (PHO): An integrated delivery system formed by hospitals and physicians (usually through managed care contracts) that allows for cooperative activity but permits participants to retain some level of independence

Physician index: A list of patients and their physicians usually arranged according to the physician code numbers assigned by the healthcare facility

Physician-patient privilege: The legal protection from confidential communications between physicians and patients related to diagnosis and treatment being disclosed during civil and some misdemeanor litigation

Physiological signal processing system: Systems that store data based on the body's signals and create output based on the lines plotted between the signals' points

Picture archiving and communication systems (PACS): An integrated computer system that obtains, stores, retrieves, and displays digital images (in healthcare, radiological images)

Pie chart: A graphic technique in which the proportions of a category are displayed as portions of a circle (like pieces of a pie); used to show the relationship of individual parts to the whole

Piece-rate incentive: An adjustment of the compensation paid to a worker based on exceeding a certain level of output

Pilot study: A trial run on a smaller scale

Plain text: A message that is not encrypted; a form of text that does not support text formatting such as bold, italic, or underline; most efficient way to store text

Plaintiff: The group or person who initiates a civil lawsuit

Plan-do-check-act (PDCA): A performance improvement model developed by Walter Shewhart, but popularized in Japan by W. Edwards Deming

Planning: An examination of the future and preparation of action plans to attain goals; one of the four traditional management functions

Planning horizon: For the strategic planning of a health information system, this refers to both the scope of the system to be addressed and the number of years estimated for planning, acquiring, and implementing the components identified

Playscript: This procedural documentation format describes each player in the procedure, the action of the player, and the player's responsibility regarding the process from the start to completion of a specific task within the procedure

Point-of-care information system: System that allows healthcare providers to capture and retrieve data and information at the location where the healthcare service is performed

Point-of-service (POS) collection: The collection of the portion of the bill that is likely the responsibility of the patient prior to the provision of service

Point of service (POS) plan: A type of managed care plan in which enrollees are encouraged to select healthcare providers from a network of providers under contract with the plan but are also allowed to select providers outside the network and pay a larger share of the cost

Point method: A method of job evaluation that places weight (points) on each of the compensable factors in a job whereby the total points associated with a job establish its relative worth and jobs that fall within a specific range of points fall into a pay grade with an associated wage

Policies: 1. Governing principles that describe how a department or an organization is supposed to handle a specific situation or execute a specific process 2. Binding contracts issued by a healthcare insurance company to an individual or group in which the company promises to pay for healthcare to treat illness or injury; such contracts may also be referred to as health plan agreements and evidence of coverage

Policy analysis: Identifying options to meet goals and estimating the costs and consequences of each option prior to the implementation of any option

Population-based registry: A type of registry that includes information from more than one facility in a specific geopolitical area, such as a state or region

Population-based statistics: Statistics based on a defined population rather than on a sample drawn from the same population

Population health data: Data on the quality, cost, and risk associated with the health of a specific set of individuals

Position (job) description: A detailed list of a job's duties, reporting relationships, working conditions, and responsibilities

Position power: Refers to the authority the leader has to direct others and to use reward and coercive power

Post-acute care: Care that supports patients who require ongoing medical management or therapeutic, rehabilitative, or skilled nursing care

Potentially compensable event: An event (for example, an injury, accident, or medical error) that may result in financial liability for a healthcare organization, for example, an injury, accident, or medical error

Preauthorization: 1. the requirement that a healthcare provider obtain permission from the health insurer prior to predefined services being provided to the patients 2.Control number issued when a healthcare service is approved

Precedent: Binding force for future cases addressing the same issues in that state

Predictive modeling: A process used to identify patterns that can be used to predict the odds of a particular outcome based on the observed data

Preemption: In law, the principle that a statute at one level supersedes or is applied over the same or similar statute at a lower level (for example, the federal HIPAA privacy provisions trump the same or similar state law except when state law is more stringent)

Preferred provider organization (PPO): A managed care contract coordinated care plan that: (a) has a network of providers that have agreed to a contractually specified reimbursement for covered benefits with the organization offering the plan; (b) provides for reimbursement for all covered benefits regardless of whether the benefits are provided with the network of providers; and (c) is offered by an organization that is not licenses or organized under state law as an HMO

Pregnancy Discrimination Act (1978): The federal legislation that prohibits discrimination against women affected by pregnancy, childbirth, or related medical conditions by requiring that affected women be treated the same as all other employees for employment-related purposes, including benefits (Public Law 95-555 1978)

Prejudice: Pre-judging a person based on culture, gender, sexual orientation, age, and such

Premium: Amount of money that a policyholder or certificate holder must periodically pay an insurer in return for healthcare coverage

Present on admission (POA): A condition present at the time of inpatient admission

Prevalence: The proportion of people in a population who have a particular disease at a specific point in time or over a specified period of time; also known as *prevalence rate*

Preventive control: Internal controls implemented prior to an activity and designed to stop an error from happening

Primary analysis: Refers to analysis of original research data by the researchers who collected them

Primary care physician (PCP): 1. Physician who provides, supervises, and coordinates the healthcare of a member and who manages referrals to other healthcare providers and utilization of healthcare services both inside and outside a managed care plan. Family and general practitioners, internists, pediatricians, and obstetricians and gynecologists are primary care physicians 2. The physician who makes the initial diagnosis of a patient's medical condition

Primary data source: Source that contains information about a patient documented by the professionals who provided care or services to that patient (namely, the health record)

Primary source: An original work of a researcher who conducted an investigation

Principal diagnosis: e disease or condition that was present on admission, was the principal reason for admission, and received treatment or evaluation during the hospital stay or visit *or* the reason established after study to be chiefly responsible for occasioning the admission of the patient to the hospital for care

Principal investigator (PI): The individual with primary responsibility for the design and conduct of a research project

Privacy: The quality or state of being hidden from, or undisturbed by, the observation or activities of other persons, or freedom from unauthorized intrusion; in healthcare-related contexts, the right of a patient to control disclosure of protected health information

Privacy Act of 1974: A law that requires federal agencies to safeguard personally identifiable records and provides individuals with certain privacy rights (Public Law 93-579 1974)

Private law: The collective rules and principles that define the rights and duties of people and private businesses

Privacy Rule: The federal regulations created to implement the privacy requirements of the simplification subtitle of the Health Insurance Portability and Accountability Act of 1996; effective in 2002; afforded patients certain rights to and about their protected health information

Privilege: The professional relationship between patients and specific groups of caregivers that affects the patient's health record and its contents as evidence; the services or procedures, based on training and experience, that an individual physician is qualified to perform; a right granted to a user, program, or process that allows access to certain files or data in a system

Problem-oriented medical record: A patient record in which clinical problems are defined and documented individually

Problem statement: A single sentence with an action verb, such as explore or compare, that specifically and succinctly states what the researcher will be doing to investigate the problem or question

Procedure: 1. A document that describes the steps involved in performing a specific function 2. An action of a medical professional for treatment or diagnosis of a medical condition 3. The steps taken to implement a policy

Procedure manual: A compilation of all of the procedures used in a specific unit, department, or organization

Process: A systematic series of actions taken to create a product or service

Process evaluation: Monitoring programs, projects and other activities or objects to check whether their development or implementation is proceeding as planned

Process innovation: Innovation that enables firms to produce existing products or services more efficiently

Process knowledge: Competency developed by identifying and understanding all of the processes used across one or more project management methodologies

Process redesign: The steps in which focused data are collected and analyzed, the process is changed to incorporate the knowledge gained from the data collected, the new process is implemented, and the staff is educated about the new process

Productivity: A unit of performance defined by management in quantitative standards

Professional behavior: Consists of the ability to manage project resources, guide a team through motivation and goal setting, communicate effectively with all project stakeholders, understand the project complexities as well as the external environments affecting the project, applying good judgment in evaluation of the project environment leading to good decisions, and demonstrating ethical and professional behaviors to achieve the desired project results

Profitability: Refers to an organization's ability to increase in value

Program: Made up of several related projects and each project contributes to the overall objectives of the program

Program evaluation and review technique (PERT): A project management tool that diagrams a project's time lines and tasks as well as their interdependencies

Program management: Another layer of management over projects where a program manager guides and coordinates the set of individual projects to ensure they produce deliverables that can be used by the other projects within the program

Programmed decision: An automated decision made by people or computers based on a situation being so stable and recurrent that decision rules can be applied to it

Programmed learning: Learning that allows students to progress at their own pace; it presents material, questions the learner, and provides immediate responses with either positive or negative reinforcement

Programmed learning modules: Lead learners through subject material that is presented in short sections, followed immediately by a series of questions that require a written response based on the section just presented; answers are provided in the module for immediate feedback

Programs of All-Inclusive Care for the Elderly (PACE): Provides an alternative to institutional care for individuals 55 years old or older who require a level of care usually provided at nursing facilities; it offers and manages all of the health, medical, and social services needed by a beneficiary and mobilizes other services, as needed, to provide preventive, rehabilitative, curative, and supportive care

Progress notes: The documentation of a patient's care, treatment, and therapeutic response, which is entered into the health record by each of the clinical professionals involved in a patient's care, including nurses, physicians, therapists, and social workers

Progressive discipline: A four-step process for shaping employee behavior to conform to the requirements of the employee's job position that begins with a verbal caution and progresses to written reprimand, suspension, and dismissal upon subsequent offenses

Project: A temporary and single instance of work involving specialized individuals working together to achieve a specific goal within resource and time limitations

Project budget: Resource expenses are calculated to determine how much money can be spent

Project champion: An executive in the organization who believes in the benefits of the project and advocates for the project

Project coordinator: Typically a HIM professional with experience working with different departments within the HIM area, who works with the functional manager of each department to get work completed

Project expeditor: Tasked with materials management and logistics for the project, this individual works as a staff assistant and communications coordinator

Project failure: Occurs when the entire scope identified is not delivered, all work is not completed before the targeted date, or all work cannot be completed while remaining within the defined resource budget

Project management: A formal set of principles and procedures that help control the activities associated with implementing a usually large undertaking to achieve a specific goal, such as an information system project

Project management constraints: Schedule, budget, and scope of a project

Project management life cycle: The period in which the processes involved in carrying out a project are completed, including project definition, project planning and organization, project tracking and analysis, project revisions, change control, and communication

Project manager: Individual responsible to ensure the work is planned, organized, assigned, directed, and monitored and that the project is completed within the constraints of scope, schedule, and budget

Project performance: Represents the project manager's ability to apply the project process knowledge and technical skills to the project environment

Project plan: This plan for a health information system will very likely have hundreds, if not close to a thousand or more tasks; details of each task's timeline, dependencies, and resources required are included

Project portfolio management: Method used to identify, select, and prioritize projects and programs in a manner to make best use of the limited resources

Project portfolio manager: Individual responsible for ensuring all projects and programs within the portfolio produce benefits to the organization

Project scope: 1. The intention of a project 2. The range of a project's activities or influence

Project sponsor: Project owner; often either the functional leader expressing the need for change or a leader over the functional area most likely to be affected or benefited by the project

Project stakeholder: Anyone with an interest in the project deliverables

Project team: Individuals with knowledge or skills specific to the project needs

Projectized organization: Organization where the operational department structures focused on a specialty or subspecialty are replaced by multidisciplinary project teams lead by a project manager

Promotion: The act of being raised in position or rank

Prosecutor: An attorney who prosecutes a defendant accused of a crime on behalf of a local, state, or federal government

Prospective payment system (PPS): A type of reimbursement system that is based on preset payment levels rather than actual charges billed after the service has been provided; specifically, one of several Medicare reimbursement systems based on predetermined payment rates or periods and linked to the anticipated intensity of services delivered as well as the beneficiary's condition

Prospective study: A study designed to observe outcomes or events that occur after the identification of a group of subjects to be studied

Protected health information (PHI): As amended by HITECH, individually identifiable health information: 1. Except as provided in paragraph two of this definition, that is: (i) transmitted by electronic media; (ii) maintained in electronic media; or (iii) transmitted or maintained in any other form or medium. 2. Protected health information excludes individually identifiable health information: (i) in education records covered by the Family Educational Rights and Privacy Act, as amended, 20 U.S.C. 1232g; (ii) in records described at 20 U.S.C. 1232g(a)(4)(B)(iv); (iii) in employment records held by a covered entity in its role as employer; and (iv) regarding a person who has been deceased for more than 50 years (45 CFR 160.103 2013)

Protocol: In healthcare, a detailed plan of care for a specific medical condition based on investigative studies; in medical research, a rule or procedure to be followed in a clinical trial; in a computer network, a rule or procedure used to address and ensure delivery of data

Public Company Accounting Oversight Board (PCAOB): Created by the Sarbanes-Oxley Act, this board oversees the audits of companies that are publicly traded. Sarbanes-Oxley had a significant impact on the degree of scrutiny and testing of internal controls, financial reporting, and governance of organizations

Public health: An area of healthcare that deals with the health of populations in geopolitical areas, such as states and counties

Public key infrastructure (PKI): A system of digital certificates and other registration authorities that verify and authenticate the validity of each party involved in a secure transaction

Public health data: Data used to prevent the spread of disease

Public law: A type of legislation that involves the government and its relations with individuals and business organizations

Punitive damages: Damages awarded to punish or deter wrongful conduct over and above compensation for injury

P-value: The probability of making a Type I error based on a particular set of data

Q

Qualitative analysis: A review of the health record to ensure that standards are met and to determine the adequacy of entries documenting the quality of care

Qualitative approach: A philosophy of research that assumes that multiple contextual truths exist and bias is always present

Qualitative standards: Service standards in the context of setting expectations for how well or how soon work or a service will be performed

Quality: The degree or grade of excellence of goods or services, including, in healthcare, meeting expectations for outcomes of care

Quality indicators: A standard against which actual care may be measured to identify a level of performance for that standard

Quality management: Evaluation of the quality of healthcare services and delivery using standards and guidelines developed by various entities, including the government and independent accreditation organizations

Quality professional: One who possesses a variety of knowledge and skills including those related to data analytics and information management, quality and performance improvement, leadership, and patient safety and risk management

QualityNet: A Centers for Medicare and Medicaid Services (CMS) website that provides information about quality measurement and serves as the basis for communication between CMS, their contractors, and healthcare providers regarding quality data and metric

Quantified Self: A global movement that promotes and supports the collection and use of large amounts of information regarding personal activity—diet, physical activity, psychological states and traits, mental and cognitive traits, environmental variables, and social variables

Quantitative analysis: A review of the health record to determine its completeness and accuracy

Quantitative approach: A philosophy of research that assumes that there is a single truth across time and place and that researchers are able to adopt a neutral, unbiased stance and establish causation

Quantitative standard: Criteria that specify the level of measurable work, or productivity, expected for a specific function

Quasi-experimental method: In this method, researchers cannot randomly assign participants into two groups but, rather, observe the effect of an intervention that has already occurred; these interventions could be diagnostic or therapeutic procedures, risk factors, exposures, or other events

Query: A routine communication and education tool used to advocate for complete and compliant documentation

Query-based exchange: Used by providers to search and discover accessible clinical sources on a patient; a query on a database asks a question of the database and pulls information based on the keywords that are used in the query; this type of exchange is often used when delivering unplanned care such as ED visits

Questionnaire survey: A type of survey in which the members of the population are questioned through the use of electronic or paper forms

Qui tam relators: The "whistleblower" provisions of the False Claims Act which provides that private persons, known as relators, may enforce the Act by filing a complaint, under seal, alleging fraud committed against the government

R

Radio frequency identification (RFID): An automatic recognition technology that uses a device attached to an object to transmit data to a receiver and does not require direct contact

Random ovals: Similar to systematic ovals—A graphical technique that displays stacked ovals with the height of the stack corresponding to the maximum of the scale—but not as uniform; the ovals are randomly filled in.

Range: A measure of variability between the smallest and largest observations in a frequency distribution

Random sampling: An unbiased selection of subjects that includes methods such as simple random sampling, stratified random sampling, systematic sampling, and cluster sampling

Randomization: The assignment of subjects to experimental or control groups based on chance

Randomized clinical trial (RCT): A special type of clinical trial in which the researchers follow strict rules to randomly assign patients to groups

Randomized controlled trial (RCT): A special type of clinical trial in which the researchers follow strict rules to randomly assign patients to groups

Rate: A measure used to compare an event over time; a comparison of the number of times an event did happen (numerator) with the number of times an event could have happened (denominator)

Ratio: 1. A calculation found by dividing one quantity by another 2. A general term that can include a number of specific measures such as proportion, percentage, and rate

Ratio data: Data that may be displayed by units of equal size and placed on a scale starting with zero and thus can be manipulated mathematically (for example, 0, 5, 10, 15, 20)

RAT-STATS: OIG offers this statistical package that is free to download and use for both sample size determination and the generation of the random numbers required for sampling

Reasonable cause: As amended by HITECH, an act or omission in which a covered entity or business associate knew, or by exercising reasonable diligence would have known, that the act or omission violated an administrative simplification provision, but in which the covered entity or business associated did not act with willful neglect (45 CFR 160.401 2013)

Record locator service (RLS): Provides the ability to identify where records are located based upon criteria such as a person ID and/or record data type as well as provides functionality for the ongoing maintenance of this location information

Recruitment: The process of finding, soliciting, and attracting employees

Red Flags Rule: Requires many businesses and organizations to implement a written identity theft prevention program designed to detect the "red flags" of identity theft in day-to-day operations, take steps to prevent the crime, and mitigate its damage

Redundancy: As data is entered and processed by one server, data is simultaneously being entered and processed by a second server. The concept of building a backup computer system that is an exact version of the primary system and that can replace it in the event of a primary system failure

Reference check: Contact made with an individual that a prospective employee has listed to provide a favorable account of his or her work performance or personal attributes

Reference terminology: A set of concepts and relationships that provide a common consultation point for the comparison and aggregation of data about the entire healthcare process, recorded by multiple individuals, systems, or institutions

Refreezing: Lewin's last stage of change in which the new behaviors are reinforced to become as stable and institutionalized as the previous status quo behaviors

Registry: A collection of care information related to a specific disease, condition, or procedure that makes health record information available for analysis and comparison

Regulations: A rule established by an administrative agency of government. The difference between a statute and a regulation is regulations must be followed by any healthcare organization participating in the related program. Administrative agencies are responsible for implementing and managing the programs instituted by state and federal statutes

Reidentification: An organization can apply a specific code, or other means, to the data for future identification purposes; however, the specific code cannot be derived from any type of data elements that come from the patient's health information

Reinforcement: The process of increasing the probability of a desired response through reward

Relational database: A type of database that stores data in predefined tables made up of rows and columns

Relationship: A type of connection between two terms

Relative risk (RR): A ratio that compares the risk of disease between two groups

Relative value unit (RVU): A number assigned to a procedure that describes its difficulty and expense in relationship to other procedures by assigning weights to such factors as personnel, time, and level of skill

Reliability: A measure of consistency of data items based on their reproducibility and an estimation of their error of measurement

Remittance advice (RA): An explanation of payments (for example, claim denials) made by third-party payers

Request for production: A discovery device used to compel another party to produce documents and other items or evidence important to a lawsuit

Request for proposal (RFP): A collection of care information related to a specific disease, condition, or procedure that makes health record information available for analysis and comparison

Required standards: As amended by HITECH, under the Security Rule are implementation specifications which are detailed instructions for implementing a particular standard. Each set of safeguards comprise a number of standards, which in turn are generally composed of specifications that are required. If a specification is required, the covered entity must implement policies and procedures that meet what

the implementation specification requires (45 CFR 164.306 2013)

Requirements analysis: The step that identifies, in detail, the precise requirements needed for both health information technology (that is, hardware and software) and operational components (people, policy, and process) of the health information system to meet the goals specified in the strategic plan

Requirements document: A detailed collection of expectations for the project output

Requirements specification: A formal document conveyed to vendors identifying all the requirements that need to be acquired from the vendor

Research: 1. An inquiry process aimed at discovering new information about a subject or revising old information. Investigation or experimentation aimed at the discovery and interpretation of facts, revision of accepted theories or laws in the light of new facts, or practical application of such new or revised theories or laws; the collecting of information about a particular subject 2. As amended by HITECH, a systematic investigation, including research development, testing, and evaluation, designed to develop or contribute to generalized knowledge

Research data: Data used for the purpose of answering a proposed question or testing a hypothesis

Research design: Structure of a study ensuring that the evidence collected will be relevant and that the evidence will unambiguously and convincingly answer the research question; the design includes a detailed plan that, in a quantitative study includes controlling variance

Research frame: Comprises the theory underpinning the study and the model illustrating the factors and relationships that the study is investigating; it also includes the assumptions of the researcher's field and the field's typical methods and analytical tools; and provides an overarching structure for a research project

Research method: A set of specific procedures used to gather and analyze data

Research methodology: A set of procedures or strategies used by researchers to collect, analyze, and present data

Research question: A clear statement in the form of a question of the specific issue within a topic that a researcher wishes to study

Resident Assessment Validation and Entry (RAVEN): Data-entry software that imports and exports data in standard MDS record format; maintains facility, resident, and employee information; enforces data integrity via rigorous edit checks; and provides comprehensive online help

Residual risk: Risk that remains after no additional controls are implemented

Resource-based relative value scale (RBRVS): A scale of national uniform relative values for all physicians' services. The relative value of each service must be the sum of relative value units representing the physicians' work, practice expenses net of malpractice insurance expenses, and the cost of professional liability insurance

Resource Utilization Groups, Version IV (RUG-IV): A case mix–adjusted resident classification system based on the MDS used in skilled nursing facilities for resident assessments; the RUG-IV classification system uses resident assessment data from the MDS collected by SNFs to assign residents to one of 66 groups

Respect: Appreciation of the value of differing perspectives, enjoyable experiences, courteous interaction, and celebration of achievements that advance our common cause

Respect for persons: The principle that all people are presumed to be free and responsible and should be treated accordingly

Respite care: Temporary or periodic care provided in a nursing home, assisted living residence, or other type of long-term care program so that the usual caregiver can rest or take some time off

Respondent superior: "Let the master answer"; liability of employers for any job-related acts of their employees or agents

Responsibility: The accountability required as part of a job, such as supervising work performed by others or managing assets or funds

Restitution: The act of returning something to its rightful owner, of making good or giving something equivalent for any loss, damage, or injury

Retail clinics: Clinics that treat non–life-threatening acute illnesses and offer routine wellness services such as flu shots, sports physicals, and prescription refills

Retention: 1. Mechanisms for storing records, providing for timely retrieval, and establishing the length of times that various types of records will be retained by the healthcare organization 2. The ability to keep valuable employees from seeking employment elsewhere

Retrospective documentation: Occurs when healthcare providers add documentation after care has been given

Retrospective review: The part of the utilization review process that concentrates on a review of clinical information following patient discharge

Retrospective payment system: Type of fee-for-service reimbursement in which providers receive recompense after health services have been rendered

Retrospective study: A type of research conducted by reviewing records from the past (for example, birth and death certificates or health records) or by obtaining information about past events through surveys or interviews

Return on investment (ROI): The financial analysis of the extent of value a major purchase will provide

Revenue: The recognition of income earned and the use of appropriated capital from the rendering of services during the current period

Revenue cycle: 1. The process of how patient financial and health information moves into, through, and out of the healthcare facility, culminating with the facility receiving reimbursement for services provided 2. The regularly repeating set of events that produces revenue

Reverse mentoring: The new employee mentors a senior person on subjects in which he or she may have more expertise, such as use of social media or digital technologies

Revenue Principle: States that earnings as a result of activities and investments may only be recognized when they have been earned, can be measured, and have a reasonable expectation of being collected

Revenue projects: Projects that result in new or expanded products or services

Right to privacy: The right "to be let alone"; this includes the rights of individuals to be free from surveillance and interference, as well as the right to keep one's information from being disclosed

Risk analysis: The process of identifying possible security threats to the organization's data and identifying which risks should be proactively addressed and which risks are lower in priority

Risk management: A comprehensive program of activities intended to minimize the potential for injuries to occur in a facility and to anticipate and respond to ensuring liabilities for those injuries that do occur. The processes in place to identify, evaluate, and control risk, defined as the organization's risk of accidental financial liability

Role playing: A training method in which participants are required to respond to specific problems they may actually encounter in their jobs

Role theory: Thinking that attempts to explain how people adopt specific roles, including leadership roles

Rootkit: Type of malicious software that will remotely access or control a computer without being detected by users or security programs

Rules of engagement: Principles and regulations that specify the way that policy makers, data owners, data stewards and other stakeholders interact with each other

Run chart: A type of graph that shows data points collected over time and identifies emerging trends or patterns

RxNorm: A clinical drug nomenclature developed by the Food and Drug Administration, the Department of Veterans Affairs, and HL7 to provide standard names for clinical drugs and administered dose forms

S

Safe harbor method: Deidentification method that requires the covered entity or business associate to remove 18 data elements from the health information; the data elements are defined as the following: names; all Geographic subdivision smaller than state (street address, city, county, precinct, zip code, and any other equivalent geocodes); all elements of dates excluding year (birth date, admission date, discharge date, death date). If over 89 years of age, all elements of dates including year; telephone number(s); fax number(s); Social Security Number; medical record number; health plan beneficiary numbers (insurance information); account numbers; certificate/license numbers; vehicle identification numbers and series numbers (example: license plate numbers); device numbers or identifiers; Web universal resource locator (URL); Internet protocol (IP) address; biometric identifiers (finger tips, voice recognition, palm reading); full face photographs; any other unique identifiable number, characteristic, or code

Sample: A set of units selected for study that represents a population

Scalar chain: A theory in the chain of command in which everyone is included and authority and responsibility flow downward from the top of the organization

Scale: Measure with progressive categories, such as size, amount, importance, rank, or agreement

Scanning: The process by which a document is read into an optical imaging system

Scatter diagram: A graph that visually displays the linear relationships among factors

Scatterplot: A visual representation of data points on an interval or ratio level used to depict relationships between two variables

Scenarios: Stories describing the current and feasible future states of the business environment

Schema mapping: Converting entity relationship diagrams into tables using rules such as determining table structuring based on the cardinality of the relationship

Scientific management: An effort to apply scientific principles and practices to business processes

Scope creep: A process in which the scope of a project grows while the project is in process, virtually guaranteeing that it will be over budget and behind schedule

Scribe: An individual who perform data entry functions at the point of care

Secondary analysis: A method of research involving analysis of the original work of another person or organization

Secondary data source: Data derived from the primary patient record, such as an index or a database

Secondary source: A summary of an original work, such as an encyclopedia

Secure information: Unreadable, unusable, and indecipherable encrypted information

Secure messaging: A system that eliminates the security concerns that surround e-mail, but retains the benefits of proactive, traceable, and personalized messaging

Securities and Exchange Commission (SEC): The federal agency that regulates all public and some private transactions involving the ownership and debt of organizations

Security: 1. The means to control access and protect information from accidental or intentional disclosure to unauthorized persons and from unauthorized alteration, destruction, or loss 2. The physical protection of facilities and equipment from theft, damage, or unauthorized access; collectively, the policies, procedures, and safeguards designed to protect the confidentiality of information, maintain the integrity and availability of information systems, and control access to the content of these systems

Security Rule: The federal regulations created to implement the security requirements of HIPAA

Self-monitoring: The act of observing the reactions of others to one's behavior and making the necessary behavioral adjustments to improve the reactions of others in the future

Semantic interoperability: Mutual understanding of the meaning of data exchanged between information systems

Serial-unit numbering system: In this system, the patient is issued a different number for each admission or encounter for care and the records of past episodes of care are brought forward to be filed under the last number issued

Serial work division: The consecutive handling of tasks or products by individuals who perform a specific function in sequence

Servant leadership: The leader's role is viewed as serving others

Service innovation: Product innovation that creates new market opportunities and, in many industries, is the driving force behind growth and profitability

Service level agreement (SLA): A contract between a customer and a service provider that records the common understanding about service priorities, responsibilities, guarantees, and other terms, especially related to availability, serviceability, performance, operation, or other attributes of the service like billing and penalties in the case of violation of the SLA

Settlement: Official agreements made out of court before going to trial or any time during trial

Shift differential: An increased wage paid to employees who work less desirable shifts, such as evenings, nights, or weekends

Shift rotation: The assignment of employees to different periods of service to provide coverage, as needed

Simple linear regression: A type of statistical inference that not only measures the strength of the relationship between two variables, but also estimates a functional relationship between them

Simple random sample: The process of selecting units from a population so that each one has exactly the same chance of being included in the sample

Simulation: A training technique for experimenting with real-world situations by means of a computerized model that represents the actual situation

Simulation observation: A type of nonparticipant observation in which researchers stage events rather than allowing them to happen naturally

Single-blind study: A study design in which (typically) the investigator but not the subject knows the identity of the treatment and control groups

Situational theory of leadership: Refers to the idea that the leader's style should be adjusted to different situations and employees encountered

Six Sigma: Disciplined and data-driven methodology for getting rid of defects in any process

Skilled nursing facility (SNF): A facility which primarily provides inpatient skilled nursing care and related services to patients who require medical, nursing, rehabilitative services but does not provide the level of care or treatment available in a hospital

Skilled nursing facility prospective payment system (SNF PPS): A per-diem reimbursement system implemented in July 1998 for costs (routine, ancillary, and capital) associated with covered skilled nursing facility services furnished to Medicare Part A beneficiaries

Slander: Spoken form of defamation

Slicing and dicing: The process of taking what is known at the highest level of understanding and working downward to identify the underlying causes for the high-level observation

SMART goals: statements that identify results that are: Specific, Measurable, Attainable, Relevant, and Time-based

Social determinants of health: The conditions in which people are born, grow, work, live, and age, and the wider set of forces and systems shaping the conditions of daily life; these forces and systems include economic policies and systems, development agendas, social norms, social policies and political systems

Socialization: The process of influencing the behavior and attitudes of a new employee to adapt positively to the work environment

Software as a Service (SaaS): A subscription service to EHRs delivered over the cloud; it houses the servers and delivers data and functionality to the users via secure connection, but also provides the software

Sole proprietorship: A venture with one owner in which all profits are considered the owner's personal income

Source-oriented health record: A system of health record organization in which information is arranged according to the patient care department that provided the care

Source systems: 1. A system in which data was originally created 2. Independent information system application that contributes data to an EHR, including departmental clinical applications (for example, laboratory information system, clinical pharmacy information system) and specialty clinical applications (for example, intensive care, cardiology, labor and delivery)

Spaced training: The process of learning a task in sections separated by time

Span of control: Concept of classical organization theory that suggests managers are capable of supervising only a limited number of employees

Spatial representation: Allows information to be viewed at a glance utilizing perceptual processes without needing to address the individual elements of the information separately or analytically

Special cause variation: An unusual source of variation that occurs outside a process but affects it

Speech recognition technology: Technology that translates speech to text

Spoliation: Intentional destruction, mutilation, alteration, or concealment of evidence

Sponsor: Usually a high-level manager who approves and protects the idea, expedites testing and approval, and removes barriers within the organization

Staff authority: The lines of reporting in the organizational chart in which the position advises or makes recommendations

Staff model HMO: A type of health maintenance that employs physicians to provide healthcare services to subscriber

Stages of grief: Elizabeth Kubler-Ross examined the stress of change in her classic study of grief experienced by terminally ill patients and their families; a five stage model resulted, outlining the sequence of grief reactions as shock and denial; anger; despair; bargaining; acceptance

Staging system: A method used in cancer registers to identify specific and separate different stages or aspects of the disease

Stakeholder analysis: A process that identifies and analyzes the attitudes or opinions of stakeholders

Standard: 1. A scientifically based statement of expected behavior against which structures, processes, and outcomes can be measured 2. A model or example established by authority, custom, or general consent or a rule established by an authority as a measure of quantity, weight, extent, value, or quality 3. Under HITECH, a technical, functional, or performance-based rule, condition, requirement, or specification that stipulates instructions, fields, codes, data, material, characteristics or actions (45 CFR 170.102 2012) 4. As amended by HITECH at section 160.103, a rule, condition, or requirement: (1) describing the following information for products, systems, services, or practices: (i) classification of components; (ii) specification of materials, performance, or operations; or (iii) delineation of procedures; or (2) with respect to the privacy of protected health information (45 CFR 160.103 2013)

Standard deviation: A measure of variability that describes the deviation from the mean of a frequency distribution in the original units of measurement; the square root of the variance

Standard of care: An established set of clinical decisions and actions taken by clinicians and other representatives of healthcare organizations in accordance with state and federal laws, regulations, and guidelines; codes of ethics published by professional associations or societies; regulations for accreditation published by accreditation agencies; usual and common practice of equivalent clinicians or organizations in a geographical region

Stare decisis: "Let the decision stand"— principle that states that in cases in a lower court involving a fact pattern similar to that in a higher court within the court system, the lower court is bound to apply the decision of the higher court

Stark Law: Law that prohibits a physician from referring certain health service to an entity in which the physician (or member of immediate family) has an ownership or investment or with which the physician has a compensation arrangement, unless an exception applies

Statement of cash flow: A statement that details the reasons that cash changed from one balance sheet period to another

Statement of retained earnings: A statement expressing the change in retained earnings from the beginning of the balance sheet period to the end

Statement of stockholder's equity: A statement detailing the reasons for changes in each stockholder's equity accounts

Statistics: A branch of mathematics concerned with collecting, organizing, summarizing, and analyzing data

Statistical process control (SPC) chart: A type of run chart that includes both upper and lower control limits and indicates whether a process is stable or unstable

Statutes: A piece of legislation written and approved by a state or federal legislature and then signed into law by the state's governor or the president

Statute of limitations: A specific time frame allowed by a statute or law for bringing litigation

Statutory (legislative) law: Written law established by federal and state legislatures

Steering committee: A representative group of key stakeholders who provide advice and guidance in the acquisition of the health information system components under consideration

Stereotyping: An assumption that everyone within a certain group are the same

Stewardship: Taking care of something you own or have been entrusted with

Straight numeric filing system: In this system, records are filed in numerical order according to the number assigned

Strategic goals: Long-term objectives set by an organization to improve its operations

Strategic IM plan: The document in which the leadership of a healthcare organization identifies the organization's overall mission, vision, and goals to help set the long-term direction of the organization as a business entity

Strategic management: The process a leader and their leadership team uses for assessing a changing environment to create a vision of the future; determining how the organization fits into the future environment based on its mission, vision, and knowledge of its strengths, weaknesses, opportunities, and threats; and then setting in motion a strategic plan of action to position the organization accordingly

Strategic objectives: More detailed ways to meet a strategic goal and include timelines, resource allocation needs, and assignment of responsibility to who will be accountable for implementation

Strategic plan: The document in which the leadership of a healthcare organization identifies the organization's overall mission, vision, and goals to help set the long-term direction of the organization as a business entity

Strategic planning: The formalized roadmap that describes how the company executes the chosen strategy

Strategic profile: Identification of the existing key services or products of the department or organization, the nature of its customers and users, the nature of its industry and market segments, and the nature of its geographic markets

Strategic thinking: The process of thinking that goes on in the head of the CEO and the key people around him or her that helps them determine the look for the organization at some point in to the future

Strategy: A course of action designed to produce a desired (business) outcome

Strategy map: A visual representation of the cause-and-effect relationships among the components of an organization's strategy

Stratified sample: The process of selecting the same percentages of subjects for a study sample as they exist in the subgroups (strata) of the population

Strict liability: Occurs when a person or entity is held for acts or omissions regardless of whether there was fault

Stringent: State law is considered stringent if the law prohibits or restricts use or disclosure in circumstances under which such use or disclosure would be permitted under federal law. State law is considered to be more stringent if it: gives an individual greater rights to acquire, copy, or amend their PHI; further prohibits the use and disclosure of protected health information; provides the individual greater rights of access to the information; requires greater authorization requirements for compliance; requires more privacy protections; requires greater protection with sensitive notes such as mental health or HIV/AIDS

Strong matrix organization: In these organizations, project managers are not functional staff members assuming the role of project manager but rather project manager specialists reporting to a manager of project management; it is very similar to the balanced matrix but includes a department of project managers

Structural metadata: Describes how the data for each data element are captured, processed, stored, and displayed

Structured data: Data that are organized and easily retrievable and interpreted by traditional databases and data models; data that can be captured in a fixed field; data that are comprised of values that can be stored as either numbers or a finite number of categories

Structured interview: An interview format that uses a set of standardized questions that are asked of all applicants

Structured Query Language (SQL): A fourth-generation computer language that includes both DDL and DML components and is used to create and manipulate relational databases

Subject matter jurisdiction: Legal matters that include federal crimes, such as racketeering and bank robbery

Subpoena: A command to appear at a certain time and place to give testimony on a certain matter

Succession planning: A specific type of promotional plan in which senior-level position openings are anticipated and candidates are identified from within the organization; the candidates are given training through formal education, job rotation, and mentoring so that they can eventually assume these positions

Summons: An instrument used to begin a civil action or special proceeding and is a means of acquiring jurisdiction over a party

Sunsetting: Refers to the action taken by a vendor to no longer support ongoing maintenance or upgrades for a legacy system

Super users: Typically staff members who will ultimately be end users (those using the system for everyday tasks), but who have agreed to help with the implementation, testing, training, and post go-live trouble shooting

Supreme Court: The highest court in the US legal system; hears cases from the US Courts of Appeals and the highest state courts when federal statutes, treaties, or the US Constitution is involved

Surgeon general: Appointed by the president of the United States, this individual provides leadership and authoritative, science-based recommendations about the public's health; the surgeon general has responsibility for the public health service workforce

Survey: A method of self-report research in which the individuals themselves are the source of the data

Swimlane diagram: Diagram that shows an entire business process from beginning to end and is especially popular because it highlights relevant variables (who, what, and when) while requiring little or no training to use and understand

SWOT analysis: Analysis tool used to outline the organization's strengths (S) and weaknesses (W), which are internal to the organization, and the opportunities (O) and threats (T) external to the organization

Symbolic representation: Requires analytical processes where information is extracted from specific data values

Synchronous: Occurring at the same time

Systematic ovals: A graphical technique that displays stacked ovals with the height of the stack corresponding to the maximum of the scale

Systematic review: A comprehensive review of the evidence on a clearly formulated question that uses systematic and explicit methods to identify, select, and critically appraise relevant published and unpublished research studies; to extract and analyze data from the studies that are included in the review; and to present integrated and synthesized information

Systemized Nomenclature of Medicine–Clinical Terminology (SNOMED CT): The most comprehensive, multilingual clinical healthcare terminology in the world. SNOMED CT contributes to the improvement of patient care by underpinning the development of electronic health records that record clinical information in ways that enable meaning-based retrieval

System: A set of components that work together to achieve a common purpose

System configuration: Also known as system build, this includes loading data tables and master files, adjusting decision support rules for transitioning, writing interfaces, customizing screens, and numerous other tasks that make the system work for the specific organization

System development life cycle: Refers to the steps taken from an initial point of recognizing the need for a desired result, through the steps taken to ensure that all components needed for the system to achieve the desired result are addressed, to repeating this cycle whenever the result of the system fails to continue to produce the desired result

System integrator: A company that acquires products and develops permanent interfaces between them, selling them then as a single technology offering

Systematic random sampling: The process of selecting a sample of subjects for a study by drawing every *n*th unit on a list

Systematized Nomenclature of Medicine–Reference Terminology (SNOMED RT): In 1997, the College of American Pathologists (CAP) worked with a team of physicians and nurses from Kaiser Permanente to begin development of SNOMED RT, which came to be recognized as a reference terminology by the inclusion of an elementary mapping to ICD-9-CM

Systems: The foundations of caregiving, which include buildings (environmental services), equipment (technical services), professional staff (human resources), and appropriate policies (administrative)

Systems thinking: An objective way of looking at work-related ideas and processes with the goal of allowing people to uncover ineffective patterns of behavior and thinking and then finding ways to make lasting improvements

T

Tacit knowledge: The actions, experiences, ideals, values, and emotions of an individual that tend to be highly personal and difficult to communicate (for example, corporate culture, organizational politics, and professional experience)

Tactical plan: A type of decision making that usually affects departments or business units (and sometimes policies and procedures) and includes short- and medium-range plans, schedules, and budgets

Task analysis: A procedure for determining the specific duties and skills required of a job

Task and bonus plan: Management plan of Henry Gantt that provided bonus payment for workers who exceeded their production standards for the day

Task structure: Refers to how clearly and how well defined the task goals, procedures, and possible solutions are

Tax Equity and Fiscal Responsibility Act of 1982 (TEFRA): The federal legislation that modified Medicare's retrospective reimbursement system for inpatient hospital stays by requiring implementation of diagnosis-related groups and the acute care prospective payment system (Public Law 97-248 1982)

Team building: The process of organizing and acquainting a team and building skills for dealing with later team processes

Technical safeguards: As amended by HITECH, the Security Rule means the technology and the policy and procedures for its use that protect electronic protected health information and control access to it (45 CFR 164.304 2013)

Technical skills: One of the three managerial skill categories, related to knowledge of the technical aspects of the business

Telecommuting: A work arrangement in which at least a portion of the employee's work hours is spent outside the office (usually in the home) and the work is transmitted back to the employer via electronic means

Telehealth: A telecommunications system that links healthcare organizations and patients from diverse geographic locations and transmits text and images for (medical) consultation and treatment

Telemedicine/telehealth: Professional services given to a patient through an interactive telecommunications system by a practitioner at a distant site

Terminal-digit filing system: Records are filed according to a three-part number made up of two-digit pairs; the basic terminal-digit filing system contains 10,000 divisions, made up of 100 sections ranging from 00 to 99 with 100 divisions within each section ranging from 00 to 99

Termination: The act of ending something (for example, a job)

Terminology: A set of terms representing the system of concepts of a particular subject field; a clinical terminology provides the proper use of clinical words as names or symbols

Terminology and classification management: Processes for managing the breadth of healthcare terminologies, vocabularies, classification systems, and data sets that an organization may use; serves as a terminology authority for the enterprise

Text mining: The process of extracting and then quantifying and filtering free-text data

Theory: A systematic organization of knowledge that predicts or explains the behavior or events

Theory X: Douglas McGregor management theory that presumed that workers inherently disliked work and would avoid it, had little ambition, and mostly wanted security; therefore, managerial direction and control were necessary

Theory X and Y: A management theory developed by McGregor that describes pessimistic and optimistic assumptions about people and their work potential

Theory Y: Douglas McGregor management theory that assumed that work was as natural as play, that motivation could be both internally and externally driven, and that under the right conditions people would seek responsibility and be creative

Thoughtflow: Refers to a process and its sequence when the process is largely conducted mentally

360-degree evaluation: A method of performance evaluation in which the supervisors, peers, and other staff who interact with the employee contribute information

Time and motion studies: Studies in which complex tasks are broken down into their component motions to determine inefficiencies and to develop improvements

Time ladder: A document used by the employee to record the amount of time worked on various tasks

Topography: Code that describes the site of origin of the neoplasm and uses the same three- and four-character categories as in the neoplasm section of the second chapter of ICD-10; description of a part of the body

Tort: An action brought when one party believes that another party caused harm through wrongful conduct and seeks compensation for that harm

Total margin ratio: Measurement of overall profitability of an organization that compares excess of revenue over expense by total revenue

Total quality management: A management philosophy that includes all activities in which the needs of the customer and the organization are satisfied in the most efficient manner by using employee potentials and continuous improvement

Tracer methodology: A process the Joint Commission surveyors use during the on-site survey to analyze an organization's systems, with particular attention to identified priority focus areas, by following individual patients through the organization's healthcare process in the sequence experienced by the patients; an evaluation that follows (traces) the hospital experiences of specific patients to assess the quality of patient care; part of the new Joint Commission survey processes

Training: A set of activities and materials that provide the opportunity to acquire job-related skills, knowledge, and abilities

Train the trainer: A method of training certain individuals who, in turn, will be responsible for training others on a task or skill

Trait approach: Proposes that leaders possess a collection of traits or qualities that distinguish them from nonleaders

Transfer the risk: Outsourcing or insuring the risk against any potential loss to the organization

Transitions of care (ToC) initiative: One of the projects of the Standards and Interoperability (S&I) Framework, this initiative's charter states that the exchange of clinical summaries is hampered by ambiguous common definitions of what data elements must at a minimum be exchanged, how they must be encoded, and how those common semantic elements map to Meaningful Use specified formats (C32/CCD and CCR)

Traumatic injury: A wound or another injury caused by an external physical force such as an automobile accident, a shooting, a stabbing, or a fall

Treatment: As amended by HITECH, the provision, coordination, or management of health care and related services by one or more health care providers, including the coordination or management of health care by a health care provider with a third party; consultation between health care providers relating to a patient; or the

referral of a patient for health care from one health care provider to another

Trial court: The lowest tier of state court, usually divided into two courts: the court of limited jurisdiction, which hears cases pertaining to a particular subject matter or involving crimes of lesser severity or civil matters of lower dollar amounts; and the court of general jurisdiction, which hears more serious criminal cases or civil cases that involve large amounts of money

Triangulation: The use of multiple sources or perspectives to investigate the same phenomenon

TRICARE: The federal healthcare program that provides coverage for the dependents of armed forces personnel and for retirees receiving care outside military treatment facilities in which the federal government pays a percentage of the cost; formerly known as Civilian Health and Medical Program of the Uniformed Services

Trier of fact: Judge or jury

Triple constraint: Schedule, budget, and scope as project management constraints

Triple Aim: Created by the Institute for Healthcare Improvement, the Triple Aim identifies that vast and systematic improvements are needed in order to improve experiences for patients in their pursuit of healthcare, enhance health among the population, and lower per capita costs

Trojan horses: A destructive piece of programming code hidden in another piece of programming code (such as a macro or e-mail message) that looks harmless

Trust community: A group of organizations that have identified a set of mutual goals and dependencies that through collaborative effort lead to mutual benefit

Two-factor authentication: Security control for e-prescribing, namely a password and token

Type I error: The probability of incorrectly rejecting the null hypothesis given the values present in the sample

Type II error: Occurs when the null hypothesis is not rejected when it is actually false

U

Unbundling: The practice of using multiple codes to bill for the various individual steps in a single procedure rather than using a single code that includes all of the steps of the comprehensive procedure

Unfreezing: The first stage of Lewin's change process in which people are presented with disconcerting information to motivate them to change

Unified Medical Language System (UMLS): A program initiated by the National Library of Medicine to build an intelligent, automated system that can understand biomedical concepts, words, and expressions and their interrelationships; includes concepts and terms from many different source vocabularies

Uniformed Services Employment and Reemployment Rights Act (1994): Federal legislation that prohibits discrimination against individuals because of their service in the uniformed services (Public Law 103-353 1994)

Union: Labor organizations that enter into negotiations with employers on behalf of groups of employees who have elected to join

Unique identifier: A combination of numbers or alphanumeric characters assigned to a particular patient

Unit numbering system: A health record identification system in which the patient receives a unique medical record number at the time of the first encounter that is used for all subsequent encounters

Unit work division: Simultaneous assembly in which everyone performs a different specialized task at the same time

Unity of command: A human resources principle that assumes that each employee reports to only one specific management position

Unstructured data: Nonbinary, human-readable data

Upcoding: The practice of assigning diagnostic or procedural codes that represent higher payment rates than the codes that actually reflect the services provided to patients

Usability: The overall ability of a user to capture and retrieve data efficiently and effectively; the efficiency, effectiveness, and satisfaction with which users achieve results from health information systems

Use: As amended by HITECH, with respect to individually identifiable health information, the sharing, employment, application, utilization, examination, or analysis of such information within an entity that maintains such information (45 CFR 160.103 2013)

Use case analysis: A technique to determine how users will interact with a system. Uses the designed future (to-be) process and describes how a user will interact with the system to complete process steps and how the system will behave from the user perspective

User authentication: The process where an end user logs into an electronic system using specific credentials defined by the organization

Users: All internal and external stakeholders who are directly affected by the project deliverables

Utilitarianism: Ethical principle that deals situations that may provide the greatest benefit to the most people

Utilization management: 1. A collection of systems and processes to ensure that facilities and resources, both human and nonhuman, are used maximally and are consistent with patient care needs 2. A program that evaluates the healthcare facility's efficiency in providing necessary care to patients in the most effective manner

V

Validity: 1. The extent to which data correspond to the actual state of affairs or that an instrument measures what it purports to measure 2. A term referring to a test's ability to accurately and consistently measure what it purports to measure

Value: A combination of quality, cost, and patient experience of care

Values: 1. The social and cultural belief system of a person or a healthcare organization 2. A descriptive list of the organization's fundamental principles or beliefs

Values-based leadership: An approach that emphasizes values, ethics, and stewardship as central to effective leadership

Value-based purchasing: CMS incentive plan that links payments more directly to the quality of care provided and rewards providers for delivering high-quality and efficient clinical care. It incorporates clinical process-of-care measures as well as measures from the Hospital Consumer Assessment of Healthcare Providers and Systems (HCAHPS) survey on how patients view their care experiences; also known as *value-based payments*

Values statement: A short description that communicates an organization's social and cultural belief system

Variable: A characteristic or property that may take on different values

Variable costs: Resources expended that vary with the activity of the organization, for example, medication expenses vary with patient volume

Variance: A disagreement between two parts; the square of the standard deviation; a measure of variability that gives the average of the squared deviations from the mean; in financial management, the difference between the budgeted amount and the actual amount of a line item; in project management, the difference between the original project plan and current estimates

Vector graphic data: Digital data that have been captured as points and are connected by lines (a series of point coordinates) or areas (shapes bounded by lines)

Vertical dyad linkage: Micro theory that focuses on dyadic relationships, or those between two people or between a leader and a small group; explains how in-group and out-group relationships form with a leader or mentor, and how delegation may occur

Videoconferencing: A learning technique that offers one- or two-way video together with two-way audio

Virtual reality: Computer-based training approach that utilizes devices or programs replicating tasks away from the job site

Virtualization: The emulation of one or more computers within a software platform that enables one physical computer to share resources across other computers

Viruses: A computer program, typically hidden, that attaches itself to other programs and has the ability to replicate and cause various forms of harm to the data

Vision: A picture of the desired future that sets a direction and rationale for change

Vision statement: A short description of an organization's ideal future state

Vital statistics: Data related to births, deaths, marriages, and fetal deaths

Voice recognition technology: A method of encoding speech signals that do not require speaker pauses (but uses pauses when they are present) and of interpreting at least some of the signals' content as words or the intent of the speaker

Volume log: Sometimes used in conjunction with a time ladder to obtain information about the volume of work units received and processed in a day by simply keeping track of the number of products produced or activities done

Vulnerable subjects: A subject who has limited mental capacity or is unable to freely volunteer

W

Waste: To encompass overutilization, underutilization, or misuse of resources; anything that does not add value to a product or service from the standpoint of the customer

Waterfall method: Sequential method of completing the project phases

Weak matrix organization: In this organization, the project manager role does not exist but a project expediter role is used to work directly with the functional staff rather than through the functional managers

Web content management system: Systems in which information placed on a website can be labeled and tracked so that it can be easily located, modified, and reused

Web portal: A website entryway serving as a starting point to access, find, and deliver information and including a broad array of resources and services, such as e-mail, forums, and search engines

Web service: An open, standardized way of integrating disparate, web browser-based and other applications

Webinar: Seminar delivered via a web browser, either real-time or as a recorded broadcast

Whistleblowers: Individuals, including employees, patients, and competitors who bring lawsuits based on their knowledge of fraud

Wikis: A collection of webpages that together form a collaborative website

Willful neglect: As amended by HITECH, conscious, intentional failure or reckless indifference to the obligation to comply with the administrative simplification provision violated (45 CFR 160.401 2013)

Wireless systems: Systems that use wireless networks and wireless devices to access and transmit data in real time

Work: The effort, usually described in hours, needed to complete a task

Work breakdown structure (WBS): A hierarchical structure that decomposes project activities into levels of detail

Work distribution analysis: An analysis used to determine whether a department's current work assignments and job content are appropriate

Work distribution chart: A matrix that depicts the work being done in a particular workgroup in terms of specific tasks and activities, time spent on tasks, and the employees performing the tasks

Work measurement: The process of studying the amount of work accomplished and the amount of time it takes to accomplish it

Work sampling: A technique of work measurement that involves using statistical probability (determined through random sample observations) to characterize the performance of the department and its functional work units

Worker immaturity–maturity: Concept borrowed from Chris Argyris, who suggested that job and psychological maturity also influences leadership style; job maturity refers to how much work-related ability, knowledge, experience, and skill a person has; psychological maturity refers to willingness, confidence, commitment, and motivation related to work

Workers' Adjustment Retraining and Notification (WARN) Act: Federal legislation that requires employers to give employees a 60-day notice in advance of covered plant closings and covered mass layoffs (Public Law 100-379 1988)

Workers' compensation: Insurance that employers are required to have to cover employees who get sick or injured on the job

Workflow: Any work process that must be handled by more than one person

Workflow technology: Technology that automatically routes electronic documents into electronic in-baskets of its department staff for disposition decisions

Worms: A special type of computer virus, usually transferred from computer to computer via e-mail, that can replicate itself and use memory but cannot attach itself to other programs

Writs: Legal written commands

Z

Zero-based budgets: Types of budgets in which each budget cycle poses the opportunity to continue or discontinue services based on available resources so that every department or activity must be justified and prioritized annually to effectively allocate resources

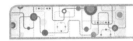

References

42 USC § 1320a–7a. 2015. Civil Monetary Penalties and Affirmative Exclusions. http://oig.hhs.gov/fraud/enforcement/cmp/

45 CFR 160.103. 65 FR 82798, Dec. 28, 2000, as amended at 78 FR 5687, Jan. 25, 2013. www.ecfr.gov.

45 CFR 160.401. 74 FR 56130, Oct. 30, 2009, as amended at 78 CFR 5691, Jan. 25, 2013. www.ecfr.gov.

45 CFR 164.304. 68 FR 8376, Feb. 20, 2003, as amended at 78 FR 5693, Jan. 25, 2013. www.ecfr.gov.

45 CFR 164.306. 68 FR 8376, Feb. 20, 2003 as amended at 78 FR 5693, Jan. 25, 2013. www.ecfr.gov.

45 CFR 164.404. 74 FR 42767, Aug. 24, 2009, as amended at 78 FR 5695, Jan. 25, 2013. www.ecfr.gov.

45 CFR 164.414. 74 FR 42767, Aug. 24, 2009. www.ecfr.gov.

45 CFR 164.501. 65 FR 82802, Dec. 28, 2000, as amended at 78 FR 5695, Jan. 25, 2013. www.ecfr.gov.

45 CFR 164.502. 65 FR 82802, Dec. 28, 2000, as amended at 78 FR 5696, Jan. 25, 2013. www.ecfr.gov.

45 CFR 164.504. 65 FR 82802, Dec. 28, 2000, as amended at 78 FR 5697, Jan. 25, 2013. www.ecfr.gov.

45 CFR 164.508. 67 FR 53268, Aug. 14, 2002, as amended at 78 FR 5699, Jan. 25, 2013. www.ecfr.gov.

45 CFR 164.520. 65 FR 82802, Dec. 28, 2000, as amended at 78 FR 5701, Jan. 25, 2013. www.ecfr.gov.

45 CFR 164.528. 65 FR 82802, Dec. 28, 2000, as amended at 67 FR 53271, Aug. 14, 2002. www.ecfr.gov.

42 CFR 405.500. 60 FR 63175, Dec. 9, 1995. www.ecfr.gov.

42 CFR 425.20. 76 FR 67973, Nov. 2, 2011. www.ecfr.gov.

Public Law 86-257. 1959. 73 Stat. 519 (29 U.S.C. 401 et seq.) Short title, see 29 U.S.C. 401 note. http://uscode.house.gov/.

Public Law 88-38. 1963. 77 Stat. 56. Short title 29 U.S.C. 201. www.uscode.house.gov/.

Public Law 90-174. 1967. 81 Stat. 536 (42 U.S.C. 263a), short title 42 U.S.C. 201 note. http://uscode.house.gov/.

Public Law 91-596. 1970. 84 Stat. 1590 Short Title, see 29 U.S.C. 651 note.

Public Law 92-261. 1972. 86 Stat. 103, short title 42 U.S.C. 2000a note. www.uscode.house.gov/.

Public Law 93-579. 1974. 88 Stat. 1896, Short Title see, 5 U.S.C. 552a note. www.uscode.house.gov/.

Public Law 95-555. 1978. 92 Stat. 2076 (42 U.S.C. 2000e(k)). www.uscode.house.gov/.

Public Law 97-248. 1982. 96 Stat. 324, Short Title, see 26 U.S.C. 1 note.

Public Law 99-158. 1985. 99. Stat. 401. Short title, see 42 U.S.C. 201 note. www.uscode.house.gov/.

Public Law 99-272, title IX, 9121(b). 1986. 100 Stat. 164, short title, see 42 U.S.C. 1395dd note. http://uscode.house.gov/.

Public Law 99-562. 1986. 100 Stat. 3153. www.uscode.house.gov/.

Index